Guidelines for adult intensive care patients

(in general order of priority)

1. **Airway**
   - If blocked, intubation or tracheotomy
2. **Maintain arterial oxygen** >70 mm Hg (9.3 kPa) (ideally, 90–100 mm Hg [12–13.3 kPa]).
   - Intranasal oxygen (15 L/min for adults, 9 L/min for foals) if needed
3. **Treat hypovolaemia.**
   - Indicators of hypovolaemia (none are pathognomic)
     - Tachycardia
     - Venous oxygen <32 mm Hg (4.27 kPa)
     - Lactate >1.4 mmol/L
     - Increasing PCV
     - Poor jugular fill
   - Shock dose for crystalloids is 60–80 ml/kg as fast as possible
   - Shock dose for 10% Pentastarch is 10–15 ml/kg; for 10% Hetastarch is 10 ml/kg
   - Hypertonic saline dose is 2–4 ml/kg **(do NOT give to foals)**—must be followed by at least half shock dose crystalloids
   - Usually give half shock dose and reassess before giving second half.
4. **Treat cardiac dysrhythmias.**
   - Ventricular tachycardias (>100 bpm—if less than 100 bpm, address underlying causes, page 437)
     - Procainamide (1 mg/kg/min IV not to exceed 20 mg/kg)
     - Magnesium sulphate (2–5 mg/kg/min not to exceed 50 mg/kg total dose)
   - Sinus bradycardia, third-degree AV block
     - Check for hyperkalaemia
     - Atropine or glycopyrrolate (0.005–0.1 mg/kg)
   - Supraventricular tachycardia (>150 bpm—if less than 150 bpm, seek advice)
     - Digoxin 0.0022 mg/kg IV
     - Propanolol 0.03–2 mg/kg IV
5. **Treat dehydration, provide maintenance fluid requirements and cover ongoing losses.**
   - Maintenance for adult horse with no other fluid intake (food or water) is 2.5 ml/kg/hr.
   - Dehydration should be estimated (5–12%) and replaced in first 24 hours.
     - Treatment given for hypovolaemia should not be included in calculations for first 24 hours.
   - Ongoing losses (reflux, diarrhoea, heavy sweating) should be estimated and added to fluid requirements.
   - First 24 hours = dehydration + maintenance + ongoing losses. Subsequent 24 hours = maintenance + ongoing losses
6. **Maintain potassium** between 3.5 and 5.0 mmol/L.

- **Hyperkalaemia**
  - If symptomatic (bradycardia, muscle weakness) or >7.0 mmol/L
    - Calcium gluconate 40%; 0.5 ml/kg IV over 10 minutes
    - 50% dextrose or glucose solution; 2 ml/kg IV over 5 minutes ± followed by regular insulin 0.1 unit/kg bolus
    - (if these unsuccessful) Sodium bicarbonate 1–2 mEq/kg IV over 15 minutes
  - If not symptomatic and <7.0 mmol/L
    - Diurese with at least 5 ml/kg/hr lactated Ringer's
    - Possibly 1 mg/kg frusemide if horse well perfused
- **Hypokalaemia**
  - Always treat low normal potassium or mild hypokalaemia if animal acidotic.
    - Never infuse potassium at greater than 0.5 mmol/kg/hr.
    - Rule of thumb—if fluids no faster than 5 L/hr, horse >400 kg (continuous infusion, periodically check K^+ and adjust)
    - If K^+ <2.5 mmol/L add 40 mmol/L (= 77 ml of 20% [13 mEq/5 ml] KCl per 5-L bag) and 0.1–0.2 g/kg per os (if appropriate)
    - If K^+ <2.9 mmol/L add 30 mmol/L (= 58 ml of 20% [13 mEq/5 ml] KCl per 5-L bag) and 0.1–0.2 g/kg per os (if appropriate)
    - If K^+ <3.2 mmol/L add 20 mmol/L (= 39 ml of 20% [13 mEq/5 ml] KCl per 5-L bag)
    - If K^+ <3.5 mmol/L add 10 mmol/L (= 19 ml of 20% [13 mEq/5 ml] KCl per 5-L bag)
  - If horse remains hypokalaemia despite aggressive K^+ supplementation, supplement Mg^{2+} unless hypermagnesaemic.

7. **Maintain ionized magnesium** between 0.35 and 0.7 mmol/L (0.85–1.7 mg/dl) (or total magnesium between 0.4 and 0.9 mmol/L [0.97–2.2 mg/dl]).
   - Treat hypomagnesaemia with 4–32 mg/kg magnesium sulphate per 5-L bag of crystalloid fluids and remeasure magnesium within 12 hours.
   - Investigate renal function with hypermagnesaemia.
     - If hypermagnesaemia symptomatic (weakness, recumbency)
       - Treat with 125–250 ml of 40% calcium gluconate IV over 15 minutes.
8. **Maintain ionized calcium** between 0.9 and 1.8 mmol/L (3.6 –7.2 mg/dl).
   - Treat hypocalcaemia with 0.1–0.5 ml/kg 40% calcium gluconate solution over 2–3 hours—consider vitamin D_3, especially in foals.
   - Treat hypercalcaemia (rare) with magnesium sulphate IV 4–16 mg/kg.
   - Evaluate magnesium as may require concurrent treatment.
9. **Maintain blood glucose** between 4.4 and 9.0 mmol/L (80–163 mg/dl) **and triglycerides** below 2.5 mmol/L (220 mg/dl).
   - Treat hyperglycaemia with insulin (starting dose 0.01 unit/kg/hr). Monitor blood glucose hourly until stable.
     - Do not change insulin rate by more than 0.02 unit/kg/hr in any 1 hour.
     - Monitor potassium concentration carefully during insulin infusion.
   - Treat iatrogenic hypoglycaemia by decreasing insulin and/or increasing glucose infusion.
     - If hypoglycaemic on insulin, decrease insulin rate.
     - If given insulin overdose, give 1 ml/kg of 50% dextrose or glucose solution and remeasure glucose hourly. Repeat as necessary.
   - Treat hypertriglyceridaemia and persistent hypoglycaemia with parenteral nutrition.
     - If triglycerides increased, start partial parenteral nutrition (dextrose 50%, amino acids 15%) with a minimum final target rate of 10 kcal/kg/day.
     - Start PPN at half final target rate. Monitor blood glucose hourly. Increase PPN rate to 75% after 4 hours and 100% after 8 hours.
10. **Maintain creatinine** below 200 µmol/L (2.26 mg/dl)
    - Evaluate aminoglycoside, NSAID and ceftiofur treatment, if relevant.
    - If horse urinating, get urine sample (submit for dipstik, cytology. gGT/creatinine ratio).
    - If horse urinating, treat with at least 4 ml/kg/hr lactated Ringer's solution—consider aminophylline (4–8 mg/kg IM q12h).
    - If animal not urinating
      - Double-check no signs of hypovolaemia—low-dose fluid challenge: 2 ml/kg of crystalloids
      - Consider dobutamine (1–2 µg/kg/min) and/or aminophylline (4–8 mg/kg IM q12h) or theophylline (5 mg/kg PO q12h).
      - Frusemide (furosemide) 1 mg/kg IV up to q3h

The Equine Hospital Manual

The Equine Hospital Manual

Edited by:

Kevin Corley
BVM&S PhD DECEIM DACVIM DACVECC MRCVS

and

Jennifer Stephen
BVMS MRCVS DipECVS

Anglesey Lodge Equine Hospital
The Curragh, Co. Kildare, Ireland

with illustrations by **Stephen Cahalan,** MVB

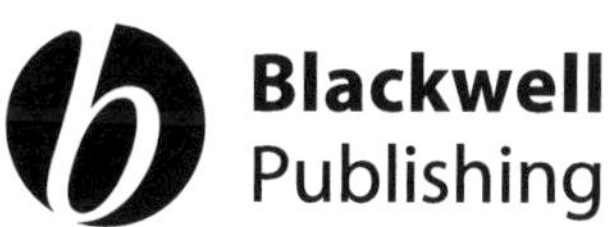

Blackwell
Publishing

This edition first published 2008

Blackwell Publishing was acquired by John Wiley & Sons in February 2007. Blackwell's publishing programme has been merged with Wiley's global Scientific, Technical, and Medical business to form Wiley-Blackwell.

Registered office
John Wiley & Sons Ltd, The Atrium, Southern Gate, Chichester, West Sussex, PO19 8SQ, United Kingdom

Editorial office
9600 Garsington Road, Oxford, OX4 2DQ, United Kingdom

For details of our global editorial offices, for customer services and for information about how to apply for permission to reuse the copyright material in this book please see our website at www.wiley.com/wiley-blackwell.

Library of Congress Cataloging-in-Publication Data

The equine hospital manual / edited by Kevin Corley and Jennifer Stephen ; with illustrations by Stephen Cahalan.
p. ; cm.
Includes bibliographical references and index.
ISBN 978-1-4051-3016-5 (alk. paper)
1. Horses–Diseases. 2. Veterinary hospitals. I. Corley, Kevin. II. Stephen, Jennifer.
[DNLM: 1. Horse Diseases–therapy. 2. Hospital Administration. 3. Hospitals, Animal. SF 951 E6376 2008]
SF951.E554 2008
636.1′089–dc22
2007050953

A catalogue record for this book is available from the British Library.

Set in 10 pt Minion Regular by SNP Best-set Typesetter Ltd., Hong Kong

2 2009

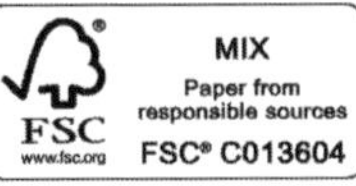

To our wonderful family, especially our parents, David, Ros, Roger, and Brigitte, for their unfailing love and support.

Contents

Preface xii
Contributors xiii
Abbreviations xvi

Chapter 1 Procedures in the adult horse **3**

1.1 Endotracheal intubation 3
Kevin Corley
1.2 Cardiopulmonary resuscitation 5
Kevin Corley
1.3 Physical examination 7
Anna Hammond
1.4 Examination per rectum 8
Emma Rowe
1.5 Collection of blood samples and intravenous injection 10
Kevin Corley
1.6 Intramuscular injections 13
Jennifer O. Stephen
1.7 Passage of a nasogastric tube and indwelling nasogastric tube 15
Bettina Dunkel
1.8 Abdominocentesis 16
Jennifer O. Stephen
1.9 Peritoneal lavage 18
Emma Rowe
1.10 Gastroscopy 21
Tim Brazil
1.11 Percutaneous trocharisation 24
Emma Rowe
1.12 Rectal mucosal biopsy 25
Anna Hammond
1.13 Liver biopsy 26
Kevin Corley
1.14 Jugular catheterisation 28
Kevin Corley
1.15 Catheterisation of the cephalic and lateral thoracic veins 30
Kevin Corley
1.16 Fluid administration sets 36
Kevin Corley
1.17 Electronic infusion pumps and syringe drivers 37
Kevin Corley
1.18 Blood and plasma transfusion 40
Anna Hammond
1.19 Collection of arterial blood gas samples 42
Harold McKenzie

1.20 Arterial catheterisation 43
Harold McKenzie
1.21 Indirect arterial blood pressure measurement 44
Kevin Corley
1.22 Direct arterial blood pressure measurement 45
Kevin Corley
1.23 Central venous pressure measurement 47
Mary Durando
1.24 Electrocardiography 49
Mary Durando
1.25 Echocardiography 52
Mary Durando
1.26 Cardiac output measurement 55
Mary Durando
1.27 Pericardiocentesis 58
Mary Durando
1.28 Emergency tracheotomy 60
Jennifer O. Stephen
1.29 Intranasal oxygen administration 62
Harold McKenzie
1.30 Nebulisation 63
Harold McKenzie
1.31 Endoscopy of the respiratory tract 65
Jennifer O. Stephen
1.32 Endoscopy of the guttural pouch 66
Harold McKenzie
1.33 Tracheal aspiration 68
Harold McKenzie
1.34 Bronchoalveolar lavage 70
Harold McKenzie
1.35 Pleurocentesis 71
Harold McKenzie
1.36 Evacuation of pneumothorax 72
Harold McKenzie
1.37 Lung biopsy 74
Harold McKenzie
1.38 Sinocentesis 77
Jennifer O. Stephen
1.39 Lumbosacral spinal fluid collection 79
Martin Furr
1.40 Atlanto-occipital cerebrospinal fluid collection 80
Martin Furr
1.41 Epidural injection and catheterisation 81
Lydia Donaldson
1.42 Urinary catheterisation 84
Anna Hollis
1.43 Endoscopy of the bladder and ureters 86
Anna Hollis
1.44 Endometrial biopsy 86
Anna Hollis
1.45 Uterine lavage 87
Anna Hollis
1.46 Renal biopsy 88
Anna Hollis
1.47 Bone marrow biopsy 89
Roger Smith

1.48 Regional anaesthesia of the eye 91
Mary Utter
1.49 Placement of a subpalpebral lavage catheter 93
Mary Utter
1.50 Regional analgesia of the limb 96
Jennifer O. Stephen
1.51 Bandaging of the limb 100
Louise L. Southwood
1.52 Application of splints 106
Jennifer O. Stephen
1.53 Application of a tourniquet and regional limb perfusion 108
Jennifer O. Stephen
1.54 Bandaging of the head 110
Louise L. Southwood
1.55 Muscle biopsy 112
Nicola Menzies-Gow
1.56 Suture materials and suture patterns for skin closure 114
Jennifer O. Stephen

Chapter 2 Procedures in the neonatal foal 120

2.1 Nasotracheal and orotracheal intubation 120
Kevin Corley
2.2 Cardiopulmonary resuscitation 122
Kevin Corley
2.3 Mechanical ventilation 125
Kevin Corley
2.4 Restraint of the neonatal foal 129
Kevin Corley
2.5 Placing an indwelling nasogastric tube 130
Kevin Corley
2.6 Jugular vein catheterisation 133
Kevin Corley
2.7 Indirect blood pressure measurement 137
Kevin Corley
2.8 Collection of arterial blood gas/arterial catheterisation 139
Kevin Corley
2.9 Placement of a urinary catheter 142
Kevin Corley
2.10 Ultrasonography of the umbilicus 144
Kevin Corley

Chapter 3 Hospital design and organisation 147

3.1 Designing and building an equine hospital 147
Tim Greet
3.2 Diagnostic imaging 164
Renate Weller, Fiona M. Ripley, Nick Bolas and Jennifer O. Stephen
3.3 Biosecurity for equine hospitals: Protecting the patient and the hospital 180
Helen Wheeler Aceto and Barbara Dallap Schaer
3.4 Hospital forms 200
Veronica Roberts and Shaun McKane

Chapter 4 Anaesthesia 226

4.1 General anaesthesia 226
Lydia Donaldson
4.2 Anaesthesia for some specific situations 246
Lydia Donaldson

4.3 Total intravenous anaesthesia 252
Lydia Donaldson
4.4 Standing surgery sedation and anaesthesia 253
Lydia Donaldson
4.5 Postanaesthetic morbidity 254
Lydia Donaldson

Chapter 5 Nutritional management of the hospitalised horse 261
5.1 The adult horse 261
Meri Stratton-Phelps
5.2 Nutritional management of the hospitalised foal 297
Meri Stratton-Phelps

Chapter 6 Common treatments 312
6.1 Standing sedation 312
Lydia Donaldson
6.2 Pain management in the hospitalised horse 324
Lydia Donaldson
6.3 Antimicrobial therapy 337
Steeve Giguère
6.4 Aerosolised antimicrobials 361
Harold C. McKenzie III
6.5 Fluid therapy 364
Kevin Corley

Chapter 7 Common problems encountered in the hospitalised horse 393
7.1 Unexplained fever 393
Veronica Roberts and Shaun McKane
7.2 Thrombophlebitis 395
Harold C. McKenzie III
7.3 Inappetence 397
Bettina Dunkel
7.4 Unwillingness to drink 398
Harold C. McKenzie III
7.5 Hyperlipaemia 399
Bettina Dunkel

Chapter 8 Monitoring and treating the coagulation system 401
8.1 Monitoring the coagulation system 401
Luis Monreal
8.2 Management of horses with coagulopathies 409
Luis Monreal and Escolástico Aguilera

Chapter 9 Monitoring and treating the cardiovascular system 417
9.1 Monitoring the cardiovascular system 417
Mary Durando and Kevin Corley
9.2 Treating the cardiovascular system 436
Mary Durando and Kevin Corley

Chapter 10 Monitoring and treating the respiratory system 457
10.1 Monitoring the respiratory system 457
Harold C. McKenzie III
10.2 Management of horses with respiratory disorders 466
Harold C. McKenzie III

Chapter 11 Monitoring and treating the gastrointestinal system **484**
11.1 Monitoring the gastrointestinal system 484
Emma Rowe, Jennifer O. Stephen, Kevin Corley and Tim Brazil
11.2 Management of horses with gastrointestinal disorders 499
Emma Rowe

Chapter 12 Monitoring and treating the liver **520**
12.1 Monitoring the hepatic system 520
Andy Durham
12.2 Management of horses with hepatic disorders 524
Andy Durham

Chapter 13 Monitoring and treating the urogenital system **533**
13.1 Monitoring the urogenital system 533
Anna Hollis and Kevin Corley
13.2 Treating the urogenital system 543
Anna Hollis and Kevin Corley

Chapter 14 Monitoring and treating the neurological system **557**
14.1 Monitoring the neurological system 557
Martin Furr
14.2 Management of horses with neurological disorders 561
Martin Furr

Chapter 15 Monitoring and treating common musculoskeletal problems in hospitalised horses **572**
15.1 Monitoring the musculoskeletal system 572
Louise L. Southwood
15.2 Laminitis 581
Louise L. Southwood and Nicola Menzies-Gow
15.3 Biochemical monitoring of the muscles 585
Nicola Menzies-Gow
15.4 Management of rhabdomyolysis and myopathy 587
Nicola Menzies-Gow
15.5 Monitoring horses with implants 591
Louise L. Southwood
15.6 Monitoring surgical incisions 596
Ehud Eliashar
15.7 Ultrasonography of surgical incisions 597
Ehud Eliashar
15.8 Management of surgical site infections 598
Louise L. Southwood and Eric Parente
15.9 External coaptation (splinting) 605
Jennifer O. Stephen
15.10 Application of casts 607
Ehud Eliashar

Chapter 16 Management of horses with problems of the integument **609**
16.1 Wound management in hospitalised horses 609
Louise L. Southwood
16.2 Simple skin grafting techniques 623
Jennifer O. Stephen

Chapter 17 Monitoring and treatment of eyes **628**

17.1 Ophthalmic examination 628
Mary E. Utter

17.2 Management of horses with specific ophthalmic conditions 628
Mary E. Utter

17.3 Management of ocular problems in the neonatal foal 636
Mary E. Utter

Chapter 18 Physiotherapy: indications and treatment techniques **638**
Bairbre Sharkey and Patrick Herbots

Chapter 19 Appendix **654**

19.1 Drug doses 654
19.2 Normal physiological values 654
19.3 Anticoagulants needed for various blood tests 654
19.4 Haematology 654
19.5 Biochemistry and electrolytes 654
19.6 Blood gas analysis 654
19.7 Peritoneal fluid analysis 654
19.8 Transtracheal and bronchoalveolar fluid analysis 681
Harold McKenzie
19.9 Normal values for pleural fluid 681
19.10 Normal values for cerebrospinal fluid 681
Martin Furr
19.11 Normal values for urine and urine production 681
19.12 Normal and abnormal values for joint fluid 684
19.13 Normal haemodynamics of adults and foals 684
19.14 Diagnosis of pituitary pars intermedia dysfunction (Cushing's disease) 686
Jocelyn Habershon-Butcher
19.15 The oral glucose tolerance test 688
Jocelyn Habershon-Butcher
19.16 Ageing horses by dentition 688

Index 689

Inside Front Cover

Guidelines for adult intensive care patients

Inside Back Cover

Flowchart for CPR in the newborn foal

Preface

The idea of a text covering all aspects of equine hospital management stems from our experiences as students, interns, residents and clinicians. We have had the benefit of working and visiting many excellent institutions around the world, and we wanted a book that would bring together all the practical tips and information that clinicians gain from years of personal experience that are often not to be found in texts. We wanted this book to be easy to use and extremely practical and yet still have a sound basis in evidence-based medicine.

We hope that this book will be useful to all who work in specialist equine practice from students in clinics to experienced clinicians. We were frustrated that no one text covered all the routine procedures necessary in the workup and management of both medicine and surgery cases. How often have we all struggled to find that excellent description of a technique that we think we remembered among a huge stack of textbooks? Or been stuck for a dose rate because the key book is back at the practice?

This book is not a complete guide to equine medicine, nor is it intended to be a complete equine surgical manual. Instead, it covers all the vital practical areas where information is so often difficult to find in one place—from the very basics such as bandaging, to more difficult procedures such as arterial blood sampling, to the very advanced such as mechanical ventilation of the neonatal foal. This book includes quick reference sections for all major procedures, reference ranges and drug doses combined with in-depth chapters. It also aims to address some of the practical concerns in designing and setting up an equine facility suitable for the care of inpatients.

We are very grateful to all our contributors who have been generous enough to share their hard-earned experience and knowledge to create this book. We give special thanks to Stephen Cahalan for creating such beautiful and clear illustrations for us. Editing a book for the first time proved to be a very challenging experience, and we must thank all the staff at Wiley-Blackwell for their support, advice and patience, especially Sophie Gillanders, Adam Burbage, Justinia Seaman, Samantha Jackson and Allison Frank Esposito.

Many other people deserve our thanks, not least our fantastic family and friends, who deserve the highest praise for their constant support. Of course, we both owe a huge debt of gratitude to all the students, interns, residents, colleagues, clients and patients we have worked with who have made life so interesting. Jen would particularly like to thank Angus Callegari, Keith Baptiste, Dean Richardson, Anna Hammond, Renate Weller, Angus Adkins and Marie Harty. Kevin would like to thank all those who inspired and challenged him, particularly Robert Livie, Celia Marr, Lydia Donaldson, Martin Furr, Harold McKenzie and Jane Axon. We would both like to thank all the staff at Anglesey Lodge Equine Hospital for providing such a happy workplace where we have learnt so much.

Jennifer O. Stephen
Kevin T.T. Corley

Contributors

Helen Wheeler Aceto PhD VMD
Director of Biosecurity
Assistant Professor, Dept. of Clinical Studies
New Bolton Center
382 W. Street Rd.
Kennett Square, PA 19348, USA
helenwa@vet.upenn.edu

Escolástico Aguilera DVM PhD DECEIM
Facultad de Veterinaria
Universidad de Córdoba
Córdoba, Spain

Nicholas M Bolas MA DPhil MBA
Hallmarq Veterinary Imaging Ltd
Unit 1K
Merrow Business Centre
Guildford, Surrey GU4 7WA, UK

Tim Brazil BVSc PhD Cert EM (Internal Medicine) DECEIM MRCVS
Equine Medicine on the Move Ltd
Moreton-in-Marsh
GLOUCS, GL56 0DU, UK
TimBrazil@emotm.com

Stephen Cahalan MVB
25 Ardlui Park
Blackrock
Co. Dublin, Ireland
stiofain1982@gmail.com

Kevin Corley BVM&S PhD DECEIM DACVIM DACVECC MRCVS
Specialist (Internal Medicine and Critical Care)
Anglesey Lodge Equine Hospital
The Curragh
Co. Kildare, Ireland
kttcorley@gmail.com

Barbara L. Dallap Schaer VMD DACVS DACVECC
Service Chief, Emergency Services
Assistant Professor, Dept. of Clinical Studies
New Bolton Center
382 W. Street Rd.
Kennett Square, PA 19348, USA
bldallap@vet.upenn.edu

Lydia Donaldson VMD PhD DACVA
P.O. Box 1100
Middleburg, VA 20118, USA
ldonldsn@earthlink.net

Bettina Dunkel DVM DACVIM DACVECC
Department of Veterinary Basic Sciences
The Royal Veterinary College
Hawkshead Campus
Hertfordshire, UK
bdunkel@rvc.ac.uk

Mary M. Durando DVM PhD DipACVIM
University of Minnesota
College of Veterinary Medicine
Veterinary Population Medicine Department
225 Veterinary Teaching Hospitals
1365 Gortner Avenue
St. Paul, MN 55108, USA

Andy Durham BSc BVSc CertEP DEIM DECEIM MRCVS
The Liphook Equine Hospital
Hampshire, GU30 7JG, UK
andy@TheLEH.co.uk

Ehud Eliashar BSc DVM DECVS MRCVS
Lecturer in Equine Surgery
Equine Referral Hospital
Royal Veterinary College
Hawkshead Lane
N. Mymms, Herts AL9 7TA, UK
EEliashar@RVC.AC.UK

Martin O. Furr DVM PhD DACVIM
Adelaide C. Riggs Chair in Equine Medicine
Marion duPont Scott Equine Medical Center
Virginia-Maryland Regional College of Veterinary Medicine
17690 Old Waterford Road at Morven Park
P.O. Box 1938
Leesburg, VA 20177, USA
mfurr@vt.edu

Steeve Giguère DVM PhD DACVIM
Associate Professor of Large Animal Internal Medicine
Director, Hofmann Equine Neonatal Intensive Care Unit
Department of Large Animal Clinical Sciences
College of Veterinary Medicine
University of Florida
P.O. Box 100136
Gainesville, FL 32610, USA
gigueres@mail.vetmed.ufl.edu

Timothy R.C. Greet BVMS MVM CertEO DESTS DECVS FRCVS
Rossdales Equine Hospital
Cotton End Road
Exning, Newmarket CB8 7NN, UK
tim.greet@rossdales.com

Jocelyn Habershon-Butcher BVetMed MRCVS
Equine Referral Hospital
Royal Veterinary College
Hawkshead Lane
N. Mymms, Herts AL9 7TA, UK
jbutcher@rvc.ac.uk

Anna N. Hammond BVM&S CertEM MRCVS
Mayes and Scrine
Equine Veterinary Practice
Dawes Farm
Warnham, Horsham, West Sussex, UK

P. Herbots DVM
Veterinary Physiotherapist
Dierenarts-dierfysiotherapeut
B-9050 Ledeberg (Gent), Belgium
patrick.herbots@village.uunet.be

Anna R. Hollis BVetMed MRCVS
New Bolton Center
School of Veterinary Medicine
University of Pennsylvania
382 W. Street Rd.
Kennett Square, PA 19348, USA
ahollis@vet.upenn.edu

Shaun McKane BVSc BSc(vet) PhD DACVIM MRCVS
Lecturer in Equine Medicine
Equine Hospital
Leahurst, Neston
South Wirral, CH64 7TE, UK
samckane@liv.ac.uk

Harold C. McKenzie III DVM MS DACVIM
Assistant Professor of Equine Medicine
Marion duPont Scott Equine Medical Center
Virginia-Maryland Regional College of Veterinary Medicine
17690 Old Waterford Road at Morven Park
P.O. Box 1938
Leesburg, VA 20177, USA
hmckenzi@vt.edu

Nicola Menzies-Gow MA VetMB PhD DECEIM MRCVS
Lecturer in Equine Medicine
Equine Referral Hospital
Royal Veterinary College
Hawkshead Lane
N. Mymms, Herts AL9 7TA, UK
nmenziesgow@rvc.ac.uk

Luis Monreal DVM PhD DECEIM
Associate Professor of Equine Medicine
Servei de Medicina Interna Equina
Facultat de Veterinària
Universitat Autònoma de Barcelona
Barcelona, Spain
lluis.monreal@uab.es

Eric Parente DVM DACVS
Associate Professor of Surgery
University of Pennsylvania School of Veterinary Medicine
382 West Street Rd.
Kennett Square, PA 19348-1692, USA

Fiona M. Ripley
Equine Diagnostic Imaging Technician
Royal Veterinary College
Hawkshead Lane
N. Mymms
Herts AL9 7TA, UK

Veronica Roberts MA VetMB MA (Oxon) MRCVS
Equine Hospital
Leahurst, Neston
South Wirral, CH64 7TE, UK
v.roberts@liverpool.ac.uk

Emma L. Rowe BSc BVMS(Hons) MS DACVS
Senior Lecturer in Equine Surgery
Murdoch University Equine Hospital
South Street
Murdoch, Western Australia 6150

Bairbre Sharkey BSc (Hons) Physiotherapy MSc Veterinary Physiotherapy MISCP Cat A ACPAT
H2 Calenders Mill
Simmonstown Manor, Celbridge
Co. Kildare. Ireland
bairbresharkey@hotmail.com

Roger K.W. Smith MA VetMB PhD DEO DECVS MRCVS
Professor of Equine Orthopaedics
Equine Referral Hospital
Royal Veterinary College
Hawkshead Lane
N. Mymms
Herts AL9 7TA, UK
rksmith@rvc.ac.uk

Louise Southwood BVSc PhD DACVS DACVECC
Assistant Professor Emergency Medicine and Critical Care (CE)
University of Pennsylvania School of Veterinary Medicine
382 West Street Rd.
Kennett Square, PA 19348-1692, USA
southwoo@vet.upenn.edu

Jennifer Stephen BVMS MRCVS DECVS
Anglesey Lodge Equine Hospital
The Curragh
Co. Kildare, Ireland
corley.jennifer@gmail.com

Meri Stratton-Phelps DVM MPVM DACVIM DACVN
Adjunct Assistant Clinical Professor
Department of Large Animal Medicine
College of Veterinary Medicine
The University of Georgia
Athens, GA 30602, USA
Owner, All Creatures Veterinary Nutrition Consulting
West Sacramento, CA, USA
msp@allcreaturesnutrition.com

Mary E. Utter DVM PhD DACVO
Assistant Professor of Ophthalmology
New Bolton Center
School of Veterinary Medicine
University of Pennsylvania
382 W. Street Rd.
Kennett Square, PA 19348, USA
utter@vet.upenn.edu

Renate Weller Dr Med Vet PhD MRCVS
Lecturer in Diagnostic Imaging
Equine Referral Hospital
Royal Veterinary College
Hawkshead Lane
N. Mymms
Herts AL9 7TA, UK
rweller@rvc.ac.uk

Abbreviations

Drug doses and frequency of administration used in this book

Abbreviation	Meaning	Comments
IV	intravenously	Administer into a vein or a venous catheter
IM	intramuscularly	Administer into an appropriate muscle (see Chapter 1.6)
PO	*per os* (by mouth)	Administer into the mouth
pNGT	per nasogastric tube	Administer via a previously placed nasogastric tube (see Chapter 1.7)
SQ	subcutaneously	Administer by injection into the subcutaneous tissue
MDI	metered-dose inhaler	Administer via metered-dose inhaler and appropriate mask (see Chapter 10.2 and Figures 10.18 and 10.19)
mg/kg	milligrams per kilogram	Dose per kilogram body weight
mg/450 kg	milligrams per 450 kg	Dose for a 450-kg (1000-lb) horse
µg/kg	micrograms per kilogram	Dose per kilogram body weight
mcg/kg	micrograms per kilogram	Dose per kilogram body weight
U/kg	units per kilogram	Dose per kilogram body weight
IU/kg	international units per kilogram	Dose per kilogram body weight
µg/kg/min	micrograms per kilogram per minute	Dose per kilogram body weight per minute
IU/kg/hr	international units per kilogram per hour	Dose per kilogram body weight per hour
PRN	*pro re nata* (as necessary)	Give drug when clinical signs dictate
q	*quaque* (every)	Frequency of drug administration (e.g., q12h = every 12 hours)
SID	*semel in die* (once daily)	Give the drug once daily (at 24-hour intervals)
BID	*bis in die* (twice daily)	Give the drug twice daily (at 12-hour intervals)
TID	*ter in die* (three times daily)	Give the drug three times daily (at 8-hour intervals)
QID	*quater in die* (four times daily)	Give the drug four times daily (at 6-hour intervals)

The Equine Hospital Manual

1

Procedures in the adult horse

1.1 Endotracheal intubation
1.2 Cardiopulmonary resuscitation
1.3 Physical examination
1.4 Examination per rectum
1.5 Collection of blood samples and intravenous injection
1.6 Intramuscular injections
1.7 Passage of a nasogastric tube and indwelling nasogastric tube
1.8 Abdominocentesis
1.9 Peritoneal lavage
1.10 Gastroscopy
1.11 Percutaneous trocharisation
1.12 Rectal mucosal biopsy
1.13 Liver biopsy
1.14 Jugular catheterisation
1.15 Catheterisation of the cephalic and lateral thoracic veins
1.16 Fluid administration sets
1.17 Electronic infusion pumps and syringe drivers
1.18 Blood and plasma transfusion
1.19 Collection of arterial blood gas samples
1.20 Arterial catheterisation
1.21 Indirect arterial blood pressure measurement
1.22 Direct arterial blood pressure measurement
1.23 Central venous pressure measurement
1.24 Electrocardiography
1.25 Echocardiography
1.26 Cardiac output measurement
1.27 Pericardiocentesis
1.28 Emergency tracheotomy
1.29 Intranasal oxygen administration
1.30 Nebulisation
1.31 Endoscopy of the respiratory tract
1.32 Endoscopy of the guttural pouch
1.33 Tracheal aspiration
1.34 Bronchoalveolar lavage
1.35 Pleurocentesis
1.36 Evacuation of pneumothorax
1.37 Lung biopsy
1.38 Sinocentesis
1.39 Lumbosacral spinal fluid collection
1.40 Atlanto-occipital cerebrospinal fluid collection
1.41 Epidural injection and catheterisation
1.42 Urinary catheterisation
1.43 Endoscopy of the bladder and ureters
1.44 Endometrial biopsy
1.45 Uterine lavage
1.46 Renal biopsy
1.47 Bone marrow biopsy
1.48 Regional anaesthesia of the eye
1.49 Placement of a subpalpebral lavage catheter
1.50 Regional analgesia of the limb
1.51 Bandaging of the limb
1.52 Application of splints
1.53 Application of a tourniquet and regional limb perfusion
1.54 Bandaging of the head
1.55 Muscle biopsy
1.56 Suture materials and suture patterns for skin closure

1.1 Endotracheal intubation

Kevin Corley

Intubation of the adult horse is a routine procedure for maintenance of anaesthesia for surgery. It is also required for cardiopulmonary resuscitation. Compared to other species, it is relatively easy and unlikely to result in complications. The animal should be anaesthetised (see Chapter 4) or unconscious prior to endotracheal intubation, which is not possible in the conscious animal. Nasotracheal intubation can be performed in the conscious adult horse in a similar manner to that described for the foal (see Chapter 2.1) but is rarely used in the adult. One indication for nasotracheal intubation is protection of the airway during vigorous lavage to relieve oesophageal obstruction (choke).

Equipment required

The equipment required is listed in Box 1.1. The internal diameter of the tube should be matched to the size of the horse (Table 1.1).

Table 1.1. Matching the size (internal diameter) of the endotracheal tube to the weight of the horse

Weight of foal	Typical breeds	Typical sizes for orotracheal intubation
150–350 kg	Pony Yearling Thoroughbred	18 mm 20 mm 22 mm
350–500 kg	Arabian Larger pony breeds	22 mm 24 mm 26 mm
450–600 kg	Thoroughbred Warmblood	26 mm 30 mm
600–800 kg	Draft breeds	30 mm

Smaller tubes are easier to pass but provide more resistance to airflow.

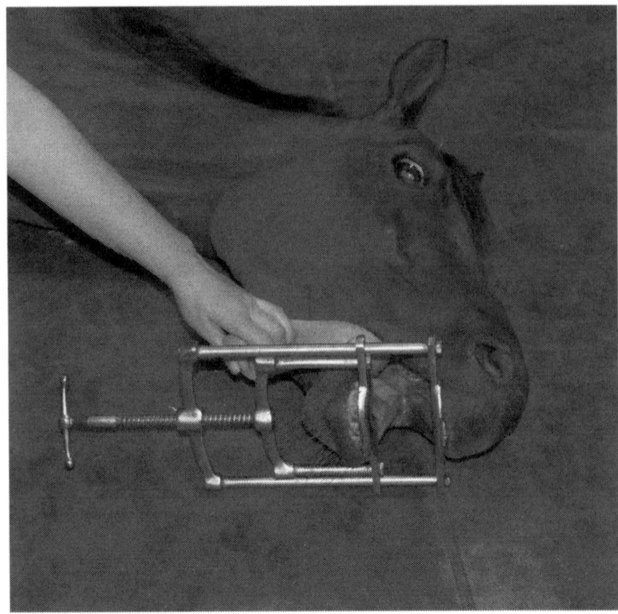

Figure 1.1 Opening the mouth of a horse with a gag, prior to intubation. The tongue is grasped to steady and control the larynx, and to stop the tongue interfering with the passage of the endotracheal tube. ©Kevin Corley 2007.

Box 1.1. Equipment for endotracheal intubation of the adult horse

Required
Endotracheal tube* (see Table 1.1)
50–60-ml syringe to inflate endotracheal tube cuff
Gag or bite block to open mouth

Optional
End-tidal carbon dioxide monitor

*Bivona Inc., Gary, IN, USA.

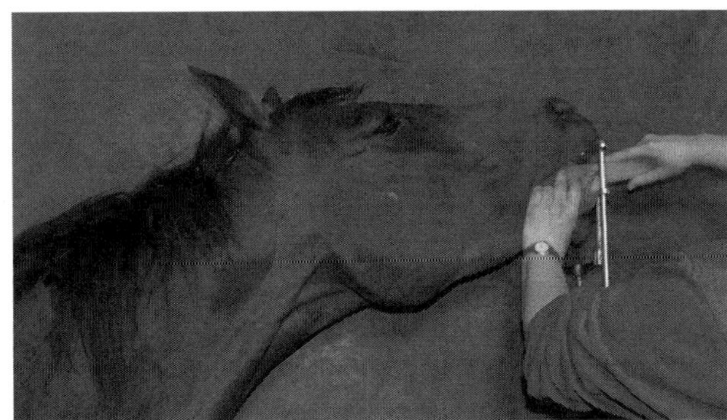

Figure 1.2 The head should be stretched out, so that it is almost at a straight line with the neck. ©Kevin Corley 2007.

Procedure

With the horse on the ground, the mouth should be opened with a gag or bite block (Figure 1.1). The head should be stretched out so that it is almost in line with the neck (Figure 1.2). It may be helpful to have a second person kneel or push against the poll of the animal, to help straighten the head relative to the neck. The tongue is grasped and gently pulled out to one side of the mouth (Figures 1.2 and 1.3). The endotracheal tube is held so that any curve points towards the bottom of the mouth. The tube is pushed over the middle of the tongue towards the back of the mouth (Figure 1.2). As the tube approaches the larynx, it may be necessary to gently twist it, so that the bevel passes between the arytenoid cartilages of the larynx. If resistance to being passed is felt, the tube should be withdrawn slightly, twisted and readvanced.

Once the tube is believed to be in the trachea, it should be checked. The usual method for checking the tube is by one person pressing on the thorax, whilst another feels for expiration of air from the end of the tube. It is also possible to connect the tube to an end-tidal carbon dioxide monitor. If the tube is in the trachea, carbon dioxide should be detected on expiration. If the tube is in the oesophagus, no carbon dioxide will be detected.

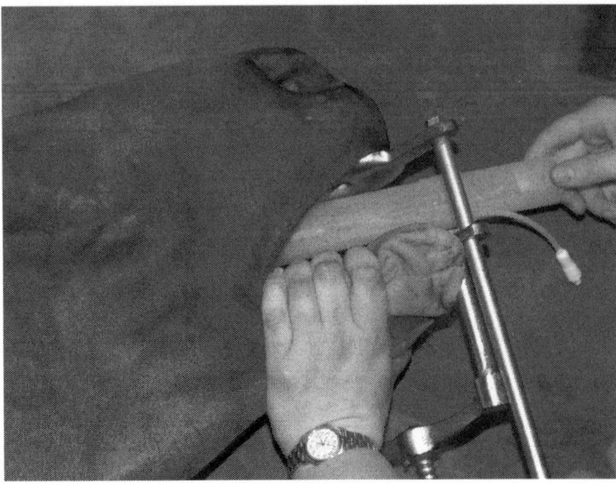

Figure 1.3 The tube may have to be twisted to pass past the larynx. ©Kevin Corley 2007.

Difficult intubations

Difficult intubations are extremely rare in the adult. If the tube cannot be passed, and the situation is not emergent, an endoscope should be passed down the nasal passage to inspect the pharynx and larynx (see Chapter 1.31). For example, if this occurs in a horse undergoing routine surgery, anaesthesia can be maintained with injectable anaesthetic agents (see Chapter 4) until the larynx can be inspected. If the larynx appears normal, the endotracheal tube should be advanced whilst observing the nasopharynx and larynx with the endoscope. If the larynx is grossly abnormal, or it is vital to intubate the horse immediately, an emergency tracheotomy should be performed (see Chapter 1.28).

1.2 Cardiopulmonary resuscitation

Kevin Corley

Cardiopulmonary resuscitation (CPR) in the adult horse, as opposed to in the neonatal foal (see Chapter 2.2), is technically challenging and rarely clinically worthwhile. The few horses that are successfully resuscitated usually rearrest very shortly afterwards, as a result of the primary pathology that caused the initial arrest. The one exception to this is horses that arrest during anaesthesia, which can often be saved. These horses are intensively monitored and already intubated and connected to a circuit with a rebreathing bag, meaning that the arrest is immediately identified and precious time is saved. Furthermore, horses may arrest during anaesthesia as an effect of the anaesthetic protocol (drugs, positioning etc.) with no underlying life-threatening pathology.

Equipment required

The equipment needed is given in Box 1.2. Self-inflating resuscitation bags (Ambu bags) of sufficient size for adult horses are not available commercially. For this reason, most clinicians use the anaesthetic circuit to ventilate horses, using the rebreathing bag (see Figure 4.5) to manually inflate the lungs.

CPR for the anaesthetised horse

Recognising the need for CPR

If the horse is being monitored with an electrocardiogram (ECG), the ECG trace may show abnormalities, such as asystole (Figure 1.4), ventricular rhythm (Figure 1.5) or ventricular fibrillation (Figure 1.5). Markedly irregular or slow ECG activity may possibly be the sign of a possible impending arrest (Figure 1.4). The significance of irregular rhythms during anaesthesia is discussed in Chapter 4, and treatments for dysrhythmias are discussed in Chapter 9.2. If an unusual ECG rhythm is noted, the pulse rhythm and quality should be immediately checked.

Box 1.2. Equipment for cardiopulmonary resuscitation of the adult horse

Required
Nasotracheal tube (see Table 1.1)
50-ml syringe to inflate nasotracheal tube cuff
Anaesthetic machine with 5-L or larger rebreathing bag
Small pen torch (flashlight)
Epinephrine (adrenaline) bottle*
Five 10-ml sterile syringes
18-Gauge $1\frac{1}{2}$-inch needles

Equipment that should be available if possible
Oxygen supply
Direct arterial pressure monitor
End-tidal carbon dioxide monitor

*Epinephrine injection 1:1000, Butler, Dublin, OH, USA.

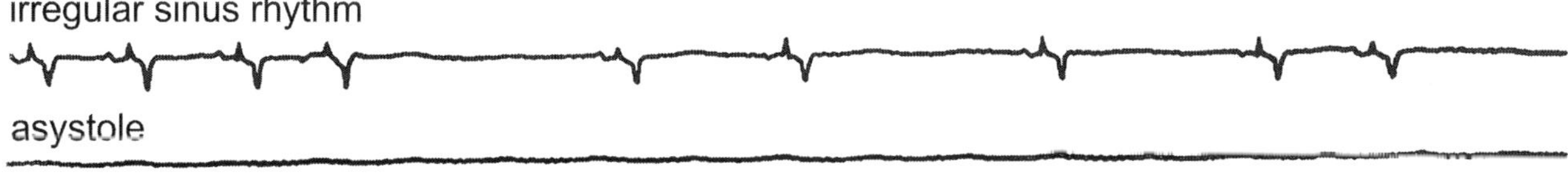

Figure 1.4 Irregular sinus rhythm progressing to asystole in a horse. Asystole is recognised by the complete absence of discernable QRS complexes. ©Kevin Corley 2001.

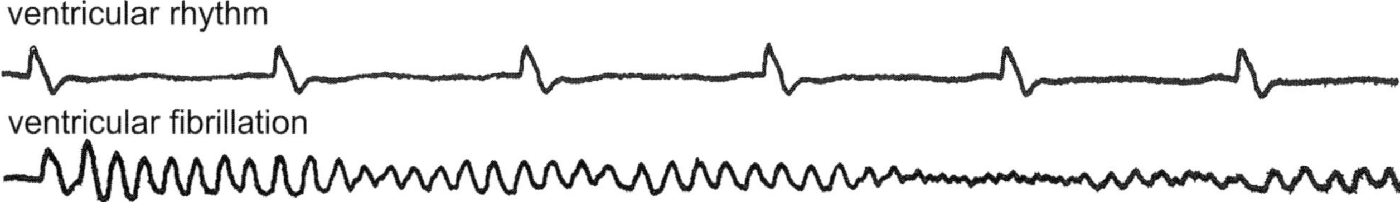

Figure 1.5 Ventricular rhythm progressing to ventricular fibrillation in a horse. The ventricular rhythm is recognised by the slow rate (typically 18 to 22 bpm) and wide QRS complexes, showing that they originate from the ventricle. The ventricular fibrillation is characterised by jagged undulating electrical activity with no discernable QRS complexes. ©Kevin Corley 2001.

Box 1.3. Triggers for initiating CPR during anaesthesia

Two or more of the following occurring simultaneously should trigger immediate CPR

- No palpable pulse or weak, intermittent pulse
- No arterial waveform on arterial pressure monitor
- Asystole or ventricular fibrillation on the ECG
- End-tidal carbon dioxide less than 10 mm Hg (1.33 kPa)
- No palpebral or corneal reflex despite light plane of anaesthesia

The horse may also stop spontaneously breathing. This should be viewed in the context of the stage of anaesthesia, as this is common on induction.

If only one of the above occurs, the result should be double-checked (e.g., by feeling for the pulse at a separate point, checking the piece of machinery is functioning correctly, checking depth of anaesthesia, etc) whilst intensively monitoring the horse and deciding on the need for CPR.

The triggers for immediate CPR are given in Box 1.3. A low venous oxygen concentration may indicate that an imminent arrest is likely.[1]

Procedure

Firstly, it should be decided whether resuscitation is appropriate for this patient. This depends on the reason for the surgery. Horses that arrest during elective surgery appear to have a good chance of survival based on the two horses I have seen in this circumstance and two further ones I have had reported to me. I was also involved with one horse that arrested during stitching at the end of colic surgery, in which successful CPR was performed. An outline for CPR of the anaesthetised horse is given in Box 1.4. Placing the horse in lateral recumbency can obviously be problematic when the horse is in dorsal recumbency with an open abdomen. Depending on the circumstances, packing the abdomen quickly and securing with two or three sutures through all layers of the abdominal wall, or simply trying to keep the abdominal contents sterile and on the table, is an option. It is not possible to successfully resuscitate a horse in dorsal recumbency.

There is no effective way to perform thoracic compressions in the adult horse. Most people try to use their body weight to squeeze the heart and lungs. The most effective way to do this is to jump from the ventral side of the thorax onto the midpoint of the thorax just behind the triceps muscle mass, landing on the knee and shin.[2] This can result in injury to the person doing the thoracic compressions either by damaging the leg they land on or possibly from the legs of the horse if it moves. The technique also may cause rib fractures in the horse, especially if done by a heavier person. An alternative is to thump the middle of the thorax, just behind the triceps muscle mass, which might be effective in small horses and ponies. Thumping the thorax risks bruising and possible breakage of the hand of the person doing the thumping.

Box 1.4. CPR during anaesthesia

1. Turn the vapouriser for inhaled anaesthetic agent to zero. If on any gases other than oxygen, turn these off to give 100% oxygen.
2. Open the pressure-relief valve and press the emergency oxygen flush to try and flush out as much anaesthetic agent as possible. Squeeze the rebreathing bag.
3. If using an inflatable mattress or support, let all the air out.
4. Position the horse in lateral recumbancy on the hardest surface available quickly.
5. Intubate the horse, if not already intubated (see Chapter 1.1).
6. Connect the horse to anaesthetic machine, if not already done so.
7. Turn the oxygen flowmeter to high flow (10–15 L/min).
8. Half close the pressure-relief valve on the anaesthetic machine.
9. Squeeze the rebreathing bag to give the horse a breath.
10. Check the pulse and ECG.
11. If there is no pulse, start thoracic compressions.
12. Jump onto horse, landing with knee and shin on the high point of the thorax just behind the triceps muscle mass*.
13. Aim for 80 compressions per minute.
14. Continue squeezing the rebreathing bag to give 10–20 breaths per minute.
15. Adjust oxygen flowmeter and valve to refill the rebreathing bag between breaths.
16. Check for pulse and ECG waveform after 30 seconds of thoracic compressions.
17. If no return of circulation, give 1–2 ml/100 kg body weight of 1 mg/ml epinephrine (adrenaline) intravenously (NOT direct cardiac injection).
18. Continue thoracic compressions and squeezing the rebreathing bag.
19. Check for pulse every 60 seconds.
20. Repeat epinephrine (adrenaline) at 3-minute intervals.
21. Stop if no return of spontaneous circulation after 15 minutes.
22. If there is a return of spontaneous circulation, maintain the horse on mechanical ventilation or continued manual squeezing of the rebreathing bag for the rest of the procedure.
23. Make a plan to finish the surgery as rapidly as possible, under the minimum anaesthetic agent possible. Consider regional or systemic analgesia to reduce anaesthetic agent requirements.

*This risks injury to the person doing the thoracic compressions.

The ideal rate for thoracic compressions in the adult horse is 80 compressions per minute.[2] This is obviously hard to maintain for any length of time and will require several people to take turns to try and maintain this rate.

CPR for the nonanaesthetised adult horse

A nonanaesthetised horse that undergoes a cardiopulmonary arrest is likely to rapidly lose consciousness, fall to the ground and have no palpable pulse or auscultable heartbeat. It is most important to decide whether CPR is appropriate in this circumstance. Most of the horses I have seen arrest are horses with severe colic lesions shortly after arrival at the hospital. I have attempted CPR on a couple of these horses, mostly to satisfy owner demand. None have been successful.

If CPR is attempted on a nonanaesthetised horse, the same general scheme applies as for the anaesthetised horse. The plan in Box 1.4 can be followed, starting at point 4.

References

1. McGoldrick TM, Bowen IM, Clarke KW: Sudden cardiac arrest in an anaesthetised horse associated with low venous oxygen tensions. Vet Rec 142:610-611, 1998
2. Hubbell JA, Muir WW, Gaynor JS: Cardiovascular effects of thoracic compression in horses subjected to euthanasia. Equine Vet J 25:282-284, 1993

1.3 Physical examination

Anna Hammond

The clinical examination is a vital, and often partially neglected, component of the diagnostic puzzle presented by patients. This is especially true in the hospitalised patient where there is a danger of overreliance on the use of sophisticated diagnostic technology. The following description should serve only as a basic guide to the process of clinical examination and may not apply to every case. In the emergent case, such as the collapsed foal or violently colicking horse, the principles of triage must apply and a shortened version should be used to gather vital information quickly. A full examination can then follow resuscitation or instigation of pain relief. The ability to recognise an abnormality is built upon a sound knowledge of what is normal; thorough clinical examination of normal horses is never time wasted.

Equipment needed

Little equipment is required for the physical examination (Box 1.5). Generally, money invested in a stethoscope is well spent. More subtle abnormalities, particularly of the heart, are hard to appreciate with inferior stethoscopes.

Box 1.5. Equipment for physical examination of the horse

Required
Stethoscope, with a large (adult, not paediatric) bell
Thermometer
Small flashlight or pen-torch
Physical examination form or notebook
Pen

Physical examination

Knowledge of the patient's history, including previous and concurrent disease, management, other animal contact and transportation, provides a useful background to the examination. It is important to try and avoid leading questions, as some owners may bias their answers in an attempt to help.

There is a great deal of information that can be obtained from standing back and observing the animal's behaviour: Is it aware of its surroundings? Is it interested in what's going on? Does it appear painful? Subtle changes in the animal's behaviour may only be apparent to the owner, so it is worth asking (and listening) whether there has been any recent change. From a distance, one can also observe any nasal/ocular discharge or asymmetry, the respiratory pattern and rate (normal: 8 to 12 breaths per minute), any asymmetry in the musculature, unwillingness to bear weight on a particular limb, reluctance to move and the stance of the animal. Palpation of the animal follows observation. Many clinicians adopt a "head-to-toe" approach; others work through each body system in turn. It matters less which approach is adopted than it does to have a routine so that no parts are overlooked.

Using a head-to-toe approach: Starting at the head, movement of air though each of the external nares is observed and any nostril flaring or discharge is noted and characterised. Parting the lips then allows assessment of the gingival mucous membranes for colour and, by pressing on the gum, the capillary refill time (this is, however, very subjective). Mucous membrane colour can also be assessed in the conjunctiva and vulva. Moving to the eyes, presence of symmetry, discharge and ptosis are again noted. Ptosis is most easily observed by assessing the angle of the eyelashes. Ears should display symmetry in position and movement in response to the presence of the observer. Assessing the inside of the ear often requres sedation. Percussion of the frontal and maxillary sinuses should then be performed. The areas medial, dorsal and ventral to eye level are tapped with one knuckle. A "dullness" or reduced resonance may indicate the presence of fluid or soft tissue within the sinus cavity. Palpation of the submandibular lymph nodes is achieved within the V-shaped groove between the mandibular rami. The pharynx should also be pinched in an attempt to elicit a cough reaction, which may suggest airway inflammation. Such a response is, however, highly variable. The muscles of the head and neck should be palpated for symmetry, presence of masses, wasting and a painful response to touch. Running the hands down the fore limbs will enable localisation of any areas of heat, pain or swelling. Particular attention should be paid to each joint. This process should end at the feet, where the pulsation in the palmar digital vessels is palpated as they course over the lateral, proximal sesamoid bone. The feet are also palpated for general warmth.

Moving to the thorax, the left and right lung fields are carefully auscultated for any abnormal noises (e.g., crackles and wheezes) superimposed on the normal quiet bronchovesicular sounds. The normal sounds should be audible in all areas of the lungs. These sounds can be very difficult to hear in an overweight individual. To exaggerate any abnormalities, an airtight bag is placed over the nostrils, which is kept in place until the respiratory rate and effort is increased. The thorax is auscultated during the period of increased rate, and on recovery. This procedure is known as a rebreathing examination and is not performed in horses that have obvious respiratory symptoms. If pleuritis is suspected, it can be helpful to place both hands on the sternum and give a sudden push upwards, often eliciting a marked pain response in such cases. Auscultation of the heart should cover the entire cardiac area, underneath the triceps muscles on the left and right sides, in the third to fifth intercostal spaces. The heart rate should be counted (normal: 28 to 36 beats per minute), allowing for increases if the horse is nervous or excited. In a nervous animal, it is often a good idea to auscultate the heart over a more prolonged period. The heart rate will gradually decrease more towards its true resting rate as the horse gets used to the auscultation procedure. If there is any abnormal rhythm, the heart rate should be counted over several minutes. Any murmurs should be auscultated whilst simultaneously palpating the pulse (usually using the facial artery) to confirm their presence in systole or diastole. Accurate description of any murmur heard requires its localisation physically and within the cardiac cycle.

The abdomen is normally auscultated in separate quadrants: upper and lower, left and right. Each quadrant is auscultated for a minute to assess borborygmi and any "tinkling" associated with gas accumulation. The rectal temperature should be taken (normal: 37.5° to 38.5° C or 99.5° to 101.5° F) and at the same time the rectal and tail tone can be appreciated. Palpation and observation then continues over the hindquarters and hind limbs noting any swelling or muscle wastage, often best done by careful observation from behind the animal. Once this examination is completed, abnormal findings are recorded and, in association with the history, form the basis of a diagnostic plan.

1.4 Examination per rectum

Emma Rowe

It is only possible to palpate the caudal 30% to 40% of the horse's abdomen, as the peritoneal cavity is so large.[1] Because of this, not all structures and areas within the abdomen can be palpated, and therefore it may not always be possible to arrive at a definitive diagnosis following rectal examination. However, it is rare that useful information is not gained. Usually, the findings of the rectal examination are evaluated in conjunction with the results of other diagnostic procedures. For example, a horse hospitalised for colic with worsening pain may have a rectal examination performed in addition to a physical examination, nasogastric intubation, abdominocentesis and blood work in order to decide the appropriate course of action. The severity of the problem and necessity of surgery are often made judged mainly on the findings of the rectal examination, even if the specific lesion cannot be identified. In certain cases, the rectal examination will allow diagnosis of certain conditions such as nephrosplenic entrapment, ileal impaction, uterine torsion or inguinal ring herniation of the small intestine.[1,2]

Equipment needed

Little equipment is required for examination per rectum (Box 1.6). It is extremely important to have very good control of the horse when performing the technique and a competent handler is required to hold the horse.

Preparation for the examination

To perform a rectal examination, it is vitally important that the horse is properly restrained. Ideally, the horse should be restrained in stocks to increase the safety of the veterinarian. In most purpose-built equine hospitals, stocks are available for restraint. Sedation, an experienced handler and application of a nose twitch can also be very effective. In some cases the horse will be in the stall, connected to intravenous fluids and possibly continuous rate drug infusion. For these horses, it will be easier to perform the rectal examination in the stall rather than disconnecting all the infusions and moving the horse to the stocks.

The handler should stand the same side as the veterinarian performing the rectal. The horse should have a nose

Box 1.6. Equipment for examination per rectum

Required
Rectal sleeve
Obstetrical lubricant
Competent horse holder

Optional
Sedation
Twitch
Stocks to restrain the horse
Mepivacaine* or lidocaine to instil in the rectum
75-cm (30-inch) fluid extension set†
50–60-ml syringe

*Intra-epicaine, Arnolds Veterinary Products, Shrewsbury, UK; Carbocaine-V, Pfizer Animal Health, New York, NY, USA.

†2C5645; Baxter Healthcare, Deerfield, IL, USA.

twitch applied and should be sedated, if necessary. A nose twitch helps restrain the horse and promotes relaxation of the rectum.[1] The horse can be sedated with an α_2-agonist such as xylazine or detomidine, which improves control of the patient and also relaxes the rectum. If the horse is very young or fractious or has a suspected rectal tear, it may be necessary to perform epidural anaesthesia with 2% lidocaine (lignocaine) (0.22 mg/kg) or xylazine (0.17 mg/kg expanded to the appropriate volume with sterile saline)[3] (see Chapter 1.41).

Long rectal sleeves should be worn for the examination. It is preferable to turn the sleeve inside out if there are prominent seams in the sleeve. Some examiners prefer to use a surgical glove over the rectal sleeve, which can increase the sensitivity of palpation. This is often preferable if palpating a rectal tear, or the examiner may choose to wear no protection so the tear can be felt with the gentlest palpation. It is extremely important for the examiner to use a large amount of lubrication over the sleeve on the hand and arm to ensure there is minimal irritation to the rectal mucosa, minimal discomfort to the horse and minimal chance of a rectal tear. The most common lubricant is hydrated methylcellulose.[3] When the veterinarian initially places the hand into the rectum, if the horse is not standing in stocks, he or she should stand to one side of the hind end, adjacent to the hind limb, facing caudally. There is a certain amount of force required to manipulate the hand through the anus into the rectum, which should be done in a slow, controlled manner. The thumb and fingers should be together in the extended position, and once the hand has moved passed the anus, the examiner can move directly behind the horse and remove the faeces from the rectum.

Examination per rectum

After the faeces have been removed, the examiner can replace the hand in the rectum very slowly, after applying more lubricating gel to the sleeve, using the same technique. Once inside the rectum, the examiner should relax and leave the arm in place for 20 to 30 seconds (allows the rectum to relax around the arm), and then the arm can be advanced cranially. Initial examination of the caudal abdomen with the arm only inserted halfway into the rectum is not recommended as the horse may start straining, which can result in excessive peristaltic contractions of the rectum.[1] It is extremely important that advancement of the examiner's arm is slow, and if any resistance is felt, the examiner should cease cranial movement immediately. If a peristaltic contraction is felt, the arm should be retracted and the contraction allowed to pass. The most serious complication of the rectal examination is iatrogenic perforation of the rectum: Withdrawing the hand at the appropriate times will avoid rectal injury in most cases. If the horse is straining or tense, intrarectal administration of local anaesthetic (lidocaine [lignocaine] or mepivacaine) can be useful to provide analgesia and relax the rectum. It is rare that a broodmare would require this, but a tense Arabian horse or young gelding unaccustomed to the rectal examination may require this in addition to sedation. Local anaesthetic can be administered into the rectum with a fluid extension set attached to a 50- to 60-ml syringe filled with 2% lidocaine (lignocaine) or mepivacaine.

Once the arm is in as far comfortably as possible, the examiner should relax again for 15 to 30 seconds and allow the anal sphincter, rectum and small colon to relax. If the bladder is very full, it may prevent palpation of the rest of the abdomen, and in that case the horse should be encouraged to urinate by terminating the examination and placing the horse in a stall. If voluntary urination does not occur, then a urinary catheter should be placed (Chapter 1.42). The rectal examination should be performed in a systematic manner to ensure that problems are not missed. The particular order of the structures that are palpated may vary between examiners, but a common approach is to start in the left dorsal quadrant of the abdomen and systematically move around in a clockwise direction (Figure 1.6). Staring in the left dorsal quadrant, the spleen is located with the caudal edge against the left body wall. The examiner can follow the caudal edge of the spleen up to the nephrosplenic ligament and caudal pole of the left kidney and into the nephrosplenic space. No intestine or other material is present in the nephrosplenic space in the normal horse, and three or four fingers can be placed into it.[3] However, in larger breeds of horses, the nephrosplenic space may not be able to be reached. From this location, the examiner moves the hand to the right side across midline and the aorta can be palpated. The root of the mesentery may also be palpated, but in large horses the mesentery may be out of reach or may just be reached with the tips of the fingers.[4] The aortic pulse is easily palpable, whereas the pulse within the mesenteric stalk is only occasionally palpable.[3] The right upper quadrant of the abdomen is then palpated. The duodenum is located dorsal to the base of the caecum and can sometimes be palpated if it is distended or distends during a peristaltic wave[4] but is not often felt during rectal examination. The examiner's hand can then move down to the base of the caecum and palpate the ventral and medial caecal bands (taenia). These bands run in a dorsocaudal-to-ventrocranial direction and are usually relaxed and can be moved with gentle manipulation by the examiner's fingers. The examiner then moves caudally and to the left ventral quadrant, where pelvic flexure and the dorsal colon may be felt, if there are enough ingesta and that part of the large colon is sitting caudally. The pelvic flexure may occasionally be out of reach, even in the normal horse. The left dorsal colon is identified by the fact that there are no palpable haustra or taenia, compared to the left ventral colon, which has two palpable taenia and haustrations.[3] The small colon can also often be palpated in the left ventral quadrant but may be palpable in various regions. The small colon usually contains formed faecal balls, which make it easily identified. In the normal

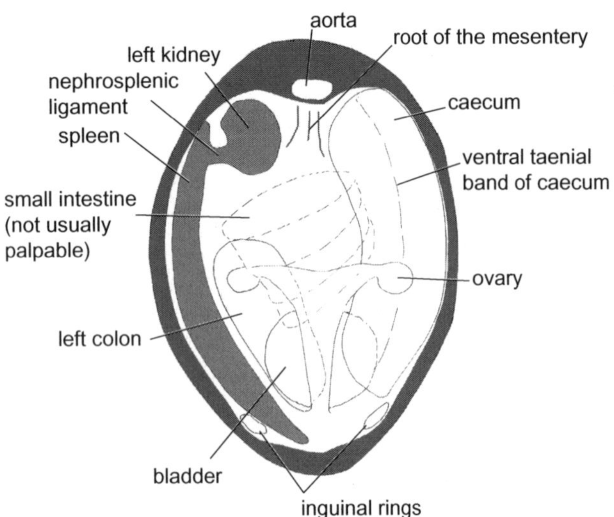

Figure 1.6 Schematic diagram illustrating structures palpable on examination per rectum.

horse, it is rare to palpate the small intestine, which is usually only felt when it is distended. The examiner should then move caudally at the end of the examination to palpate the reproductive structures including uterus, ovaries and cervix for the mare and internal inguinal rings for the stallion or gelding. The inguinal rings can be located by moving the hand across the pelvic rim and then feeling cranial and just ventral and lateral to the cranial edge of the pelvis.[4] In some stallions, a finger can be inserted into the inguinal ring and the ductus deferens is then palpable in the caudomedial aspect of the vaginal ring. However, the inguinal ring is much smaller in geldings and decreases in size with age, making the vas deferens nonpalpable.[5] The bladder should also be palpated for thickening or the presence of uroliths.

Abnormal findings on examination per rectum are described in Chapter 11.1.

References

1. Kopf N: Rectal examination in the colic patient, in Robinson NE (ed): Current Therapy in Equine Medicine. Philadelphia, WB Saunders, 1997, pp 170-174
2. Mueller P, Moore J: Colic in the late-term pregnant mare, in Orsini J, Divers T (eds): Manual of Equine Emergencies. Philadelphia, WB Saunders, 1998, pp 211-215
3. Mueller POE, Moore JN: Rectal examination of horses with acute abdominal pain. Comp Cont Educ Pract Vet 22:606-615, 2000
4. White NA: Examination and diagnosis of the acute abdomen, in White NA (ed): The Equine Acute Abdomen. Philadelphia, Lea & Febiger, 1990, pp 102-142
5. O'Connor J: Rectal examination of the cryptorchid horse. Irish Vet J 25:129-131, 1971

Box 1.7. Equipment for collection of blood samples and intravenous injection

Vacutainer blood collection
18–20-gauge vacutainer needle
Vacutainer sleeve
Appropriate vacutainer* (see Box 19.3)

Syringe and needle blood collection
Appropriate sized syringe (usually 10–30 ml)
18–20-gauge 2.5–3.75-cm (1–1½-inch) needle
Appropriate vacutainer or blood sample bottle (see Box 19.3)

Blood collection for packed cell volume measurement only
23–25-gauge 1.6-cm (⅝-inch) needle
Microhaematocrit tube containing EDTA
Microhaematocrit tube sealant

Intravenous injection
Appropriate-sized syringe filled with drug
18–20-gauge 2.5–3.75-cm (1–1½-inch) needle

Required for all techniques
Competent horse handler

Optional for all techniques
Alcohol- or antiseptic-soaked cotton wool or gauze swab (4 × 4)
Twitch

*Becton Dickinson (http://catalog.bd.com).

1.5 Collection of blood samples and intravenous injection

Kevin Corley

Blood sampling and intravenous injections are fairly straightforward in the horse. The main vein used is the jugular vein, which is usually the safest and most practical from which to collect. Venipucture can result in sudden, sometimes violent, movements by the horse. Appropriate restraint techniques by a competent handler are required to reduce the risk to the person attempting venipuncture.

Equipment needed

The equipment needed is listed in Box 1.7.

Procedure

Disinfection prior to venipuncture

It is debated whether disinfection prior to venipuncture is necessary or effective. Proponents argue that not disinfecting the skin prior to venipuncture increases the chance of thrombophlebitis or local cellulitis. Opponents suggest that a single wipe with disinfectant is ineffective. Alcohol-based disinfection works primarily by drying and desiccation. Most people who use disinfection do not allow any time for the alcohol to dry. It is argued that a quick wipe simply puts resident bacteria into suspension, making it easier to introduce them into the subcutaneous tissues and vein. If the area over the vein is grossly contaminated, it should certainly be cleaned and disinfected prior to venipuncture.

Collection of blood and injection from the jugular vein

It is easiest to collect blood from and inject into the jugular vein in the upper half of the neck. The carotid artery lies in closer proximity to the jugular vein in the lower half of the neck, making inadvertent carotid puncture less likely in the upper neck.

The vein should be raised below the site of venipuncture (Figure 1.7), using the nondominant hand. The needle is held with the bevel facing outwards (with the tip closest to the skin), and at a narrow angle to the vein (Figure 1.7). The aim should be to push the needle through the skin over the middle of the vein. It is important to observe how the vein runs above the venipuncture site, and to make sure that the needle is on the same line as it. Otherwise, it is easy to push the needle through the vein and into the tissue on the other side. If using a vacutainer system, it is important not to push the vacutainer completely onto the piercing needle until the needle is securely into the vein (Figure 1.7).

The needle should be pushed firmly through the skin and into the vein, whilst keeping the vein raised. Donkeys and ponies have tougher skin than do Thoroughbred horses, necessitating more force to get the needle through the skin. Once through the skin, the angle should be flattened, and the needle advanced to the hub (Figure 1.8). With a vacutainer system, the vacutainer should be pushed firmly onto the piercing needle, taking care not to move the needle in the vein. It may be easiest to place one or two fingers of the hand holding the vacutainer sleeve onto the skin of the horse to make sure that the sleeve, and therefore the needle in the vein, does not move relative to the horse and the vein (Figure 1.8). The vacutainer can be pushed onto the piercing needle with the heel of the hand raising the vein (Figure 1.8), or the little finger of the hand holding the vacutainer sleeve. The vein should be raised until the vacutainer is full. If no blood flows into the vacutainer, it should be pulled off the piercing needle. The sleeve and needle are then redirected, and the vacutainer is again pushed onto the piercing needle. If the vacutainer is fully on the piercing needle, and the needle inadvertently comes out of the skin of the horse, the vacuum in the vacutainer will be lost. The vacutainer should be replaced before reattempting venipuncture.

When using a syringe and needle for collection of blood or injection, it is generally easier to take the needle off the syringe and introduce it fully into the vein before connecting the syringe. This is particularly the case in fractious horses. If the horse moves suddenly in response to the needle placement, there is a good chance that a needle will stay in place, allowing connection of syringe once the reaction is over. A second advantage of disconnecting the needle is that, if it is inadvertently placed in the carotid, pulsatile flow of bright red blood can be seen, avoiding accidental intra-arterial injection of potentially very harmful drugs. The disadvantage of disconnecting the needle is that it increases the chance of dropping the needle, which may become hidden in the horse's bedding material and could potentially penetrate part of the horse or the person cleaning out the stable. Once

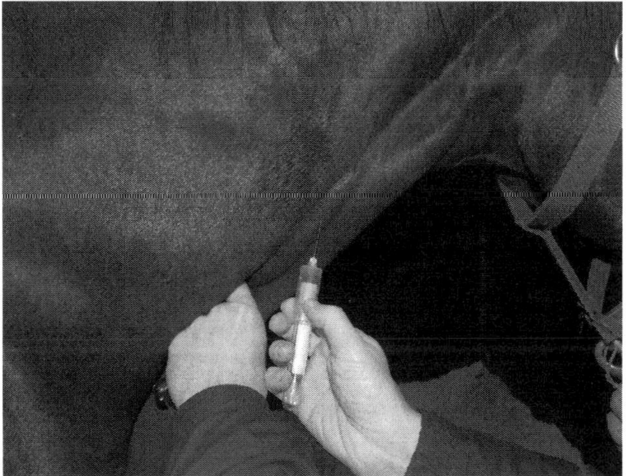

Figure 1.7 The vein is raised with one hand, whilst the needle is pushed into the centre of the vein at a narrow angle. The bevel of the needle should be pointing out (i.e., the tip is closest to the skin of the horse. The vacutainer is held in light contact with the piercing part of the needle, without puncturing the top of the vacutainer. ©Kevin Corley 2007.

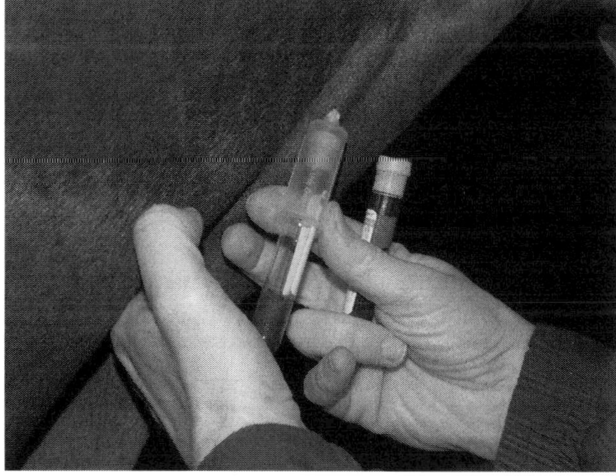

Figure 1.8 After the needle has been slid into the vein, the vacutainer is pushed onto the piercing needle, which allows the blood to flow. It is important not to accidentally push the needle out of the vein when pushing up the vacutainer. ©Kevin Corley 2007.

the needle is through the skin, it should be redirected into the middle of the raised vein. The syringe should be connected whilst holding the hub of the needle, taking care not to inadvertently push the needle through the vein. If collecting blood, once the syringe is connected, the plunger should be slowly drawn back, whilst keeping the vein raised. If the blood stops flowing, the needle should be carefully redirected to allow blood to flow again. Often, just slightly pulling the needle back is sufficient to restore blood flow.

When injecting a drug, once the syringe has been reconnected, the plunger should be slightly withdrawn to allow a small amount of blood into the syringe. This confirms that the needle is still in the vein and should be repeated two or three times during injection of the drug. Once it is confirmed that the needle is still in the vein, the plunger should be slowly depressed. Some drugs, such as potassium penicillin and oxytetracycline, require very slow injection over several minutes (see Chapter 6.3). The vein should not be continuously raised during injection of a drug, unless it is the intention to give the drug as a bolus.

The jugular veins are the most accessible and easy veins from which to collect blood and in which to inject drugs. However, bilateral jugular thrombophlebitis can have serious consequences for the horse, including profound swelling of the head due to impaired venous drainage, potentially causing respiratory distress and necessitating placement of a tracheotomy (see Chapter 7.2). Therefore, in high-risk patients (such as those with fulminant colitis, see Chapter 8.1) and those with a preexisting jugular thrombophlebitis (see Chapter 7.2), jugular venipuncture should be limited as much as possible, and alternative sites such as the facial sinus should be used.

Collection of blood from the facial sinus

The facial sinus is a good site for collection of blood for a number of reasons. Firstly, noninfectious thrombophlebitis in this area seems to be of little consequence. Secondly, placing a needle in the facial sinus is surprisingly well tolerated by a majority of horses. It is possible to collect quite large volumes of blood (20 to 30 ml) easily from this site. Blood may be collected either by needle and syringe or vacutainer from this site. People unfamiliar with blood collection from this site are advised to use a needle and syringe for the first few horses on which they attempt this technique. The author usually leaves the syringe attached to the needle for this collection site, although it is also possible to place the needle and then connect the syringe.

The facial sinus is just below the facial crest on the side of the face. It is directly below the centre of the eye (Figure 1.9). The needle should be placed at 90° to the skin, approximately 1 to 1.5 cm ($\frac{2}{5}$ to $\frac{3}{5}$ inch) below the facial crest. The needle should be pushed until it just touches the bone, and then very slightly withdrawn. The plunger of the syringe is gently withdrawn, and the syringe is filled with blood. If no blood is obtained, the needle should be slightly redirected. Initial redirection should be to angle the needle slightly towards the muzzle of the horse.

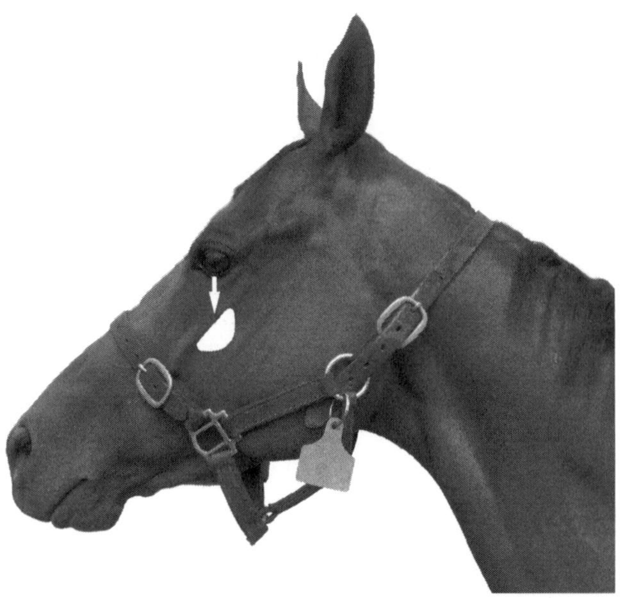

Figure 1.9 The facial sinus (*white semicircle*) is located just below the facial crest, at the level of the middle of the eye (*arrow*). ©Kevin Corley 2007.

Collection of blood and injection into other veins

Blood can be collected, and drugs injected into other veins in the horse. The cephalic vein can be used but is potentially dangerous for the operator, as it involves crouching next to the front leg of the horse. The cephalic vein is described in Chapter 1.15 and Figure 1.38. Collection is similar to that from the jugular vein, except that it should be raised above the site of venipuncture. The lateral thoracic vein (see Chapter 1.15 and Figure 1.45) is very difficult to collect blood from or inject, without first placing a catheter.

Collection of blood for packed cell volume and total solids only

If collecting blood for packed cell volume (PCV) and total solids only, a needle hub technique may be used. A small-gauge (23- to 25-gauge) needle is placed in the jugular vein, facial sinus or other site. When the hub of the needle has filled with blood, the end of a microhaematocrit tube is placed directly into the hub of the needle to collect the blood. The blood should flow along the microhaematocrit tube via capillary action, although it may be necessary to slightly point it downwards to allow the blood to fill it. The microhaematocrit tube is immediately pushed into tube sealant clay or putty at the side of the horse and then carried to the laboratory for centrifugation.

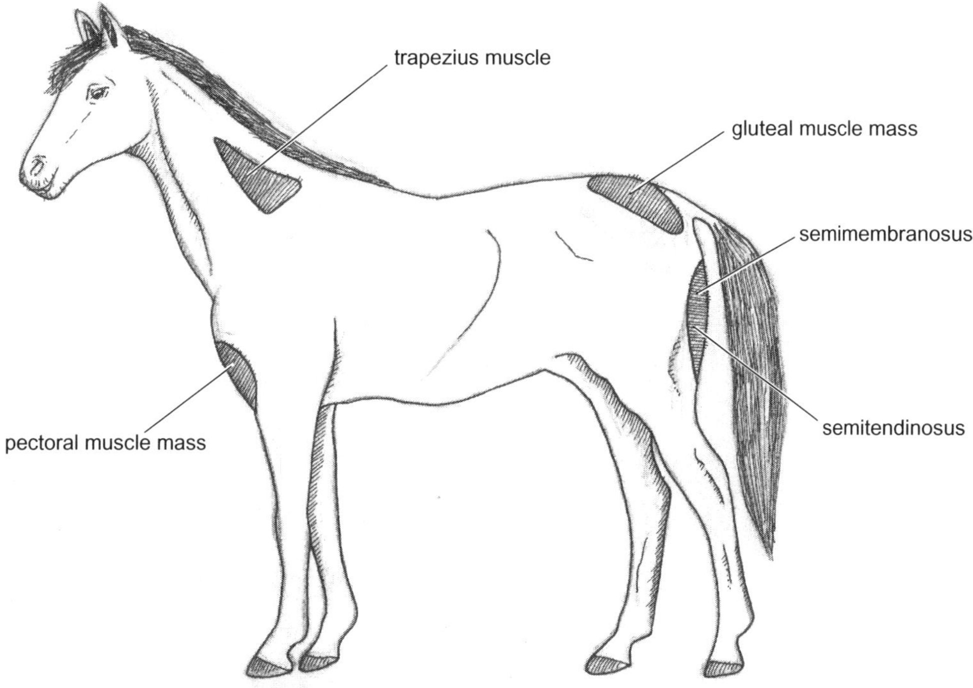

Figure 1.10 Sites for intramuscular injection in the horse.

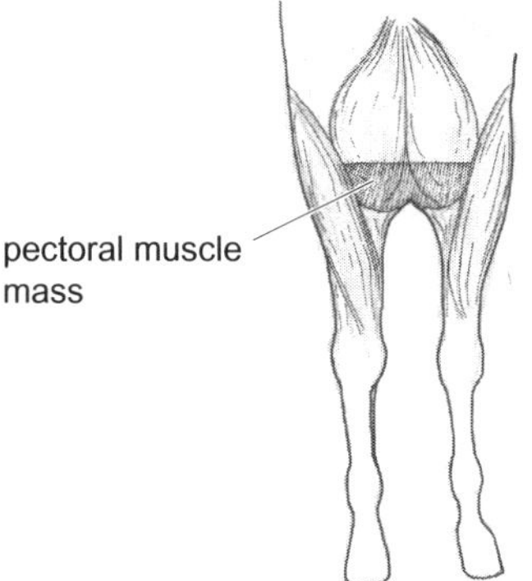

Figure 1.11 Schematic of the cranial aspect of the front legs, showing the site of intramuscular injection into the pectoral muscles.

Box 1.8. Equipment for intramuscular injection

Required

Syringe

$1\frac{1}{2}$-inch, 22–18-gauge needle (depends on viscosity of medicine to be delivered)

Optional

Alcohol- or antiseptic-soaked cotton wool or gauze swab (4 × 4)

1.6 Intramuscular injections

Jennifer O. Stephen

Potential sites for intramuscular injection in the horse

1. Neck: above the cervical vertebrae, below the nuchal ligament and in front of the scapula (Figure 1.10)
2. Lower half of semitendinosus and semimembranosus muscles (Figure 1.10)
3. Pectoral muscles (Figure 1.11)
4. Gluteal muscles (Figure 1.10)

Equipment needed

The equipment needed is listed in Box 1.8. Some authors recommend cleaning the skin with alcohol prior to injection.[1] However, it is important to check the manufacturer's data sheet, as this is contraindicated with some products, particularly vaccinations. If alcohol is used, sufficient time must be left for the alcohol to dry for it to be effective.

Technique

The horse must be properly restrained by an assistant. The needle should be inserted through the skin as quickly as possible. The initial insertion is likely to cause a reaction;

most horses will settle once the needle is in. The needle should be pushed in to the hub. The syringe should then be securely attached and drawn back. If there is any sign of blood when the plunger is drawn back, the needle must be redirected and the procedure repeated. The needle may be redirected to a different site without the needle leaving the skin. Ideally, no more than 5 to 10 ml should be delivered per site.

Complications

Abscess formation is an occasional complication. A disadvantage of using the neck or gluteal muscles for injection is that, should abscessation occur, these are difficult sites to drain. Some veterinarians will avoid giving intramuscular injections, including vaccinations, in these areas to competition horses. Muscle soreness is a common complication related to the volume injected and site of administration. Rotating the sites used can help to avoid this, especially when the horse is on twice-daily medication. If muscle soreness develops, no further injections should be administered at that site. Topical heat packs may provide some analgesia for this problem. Severe reactions including seizure may be seen with certain drugs (classically the injection of procaine penicillin G) if the drug is inadvertently injected into a blood vessel. This can generally be prevented by drawing back on the syringe to ensure there is no blood, prior to injection.

"Needle-shy" horses

Horses that resent intramuscular injections are a common problem. Where possible, these horses should be put on to intravenous or oral medications. If intramuscular injections are absolutely necessary, they should only be administered by experienced personnel, with good horse handling and injection skills. Injecting the horse in stocks can help. However, in some cases, getting the horse into the stocks can become very difficult and dangerous, especially once the horse associates this with being injected. Using a twitch is obviously helpful in horses that respond well to this. Horses may become difficult to catch in the box. These horses should be kept in leather head collars with a 1.5-foot length of lead rope attached. Every effort to make the injection as painless and quick as possible should be taken. Use as small a needle as possible. Make the drug up in as small a volume as possible. Chilling the skin prior to injection with an ice pack may help desensitise these patients, but some horses will not tolerate this. When dealing with difficult horses with limited sites for injection, it is even more important to rotate sites to prevent muscle soreness.

When dealing with these horses, choose a site for injection that will allow you to be in as safe a position as possible. This will depend on the behaviour of the horse—whether it bites, rears, attempts to crush people against walls, strikes with front limbs or with hind limbs or all of the above. It obviously also depends on the height/reach of the veterinarian and his or her injection technique. Generally, the pectoral muscle or neck can offer a relatively safe site to inject. If using the neck, a skin twitch should be taken with the left hand whilst the right hand slides the needle in behind this. Both the person holding the horse and the person performing the injection should stand on the same side of the horse. The person injecting should stand as close to the horse's shoulder as possible.

When using the pectoral muscle site in a horse that rears and strikes, it may be safest for one person to hold the horse and administer the injection, providing that person is experienced both in horse handling and injecting. You should stand as close to the horse as possible at the level of the shoulder (Figure 1.12), holding the horse with your nondominant hand and the needle in your dominant hand. If the horse barges forward, you should pull it in a tight circle towards you, using your body against the horse as a pivot. Do not let the horse turn its head away from you, or you may suddenly be faced by a kick from the back legs. Keep your body against the horses at all times, whilst being aware that the horse may strike at your feet. Hold the needle between your thumb and forefingers with the needle pointing into the palm of your hand as shown in Figure 1.13. Use the side of this hand to gently pat the horse on the left and right pectoral muscles several times until the horse has accepted your presence; then, continuing this motion, suddenly thrust the needle through the skin into the middle of a pectoral muscle. Have an assistant pass you the syringe and if possible hold the horse whilst you connect it and draw back and inject. This is not always possible, so it is useful to practice doing this procedure with one hand.

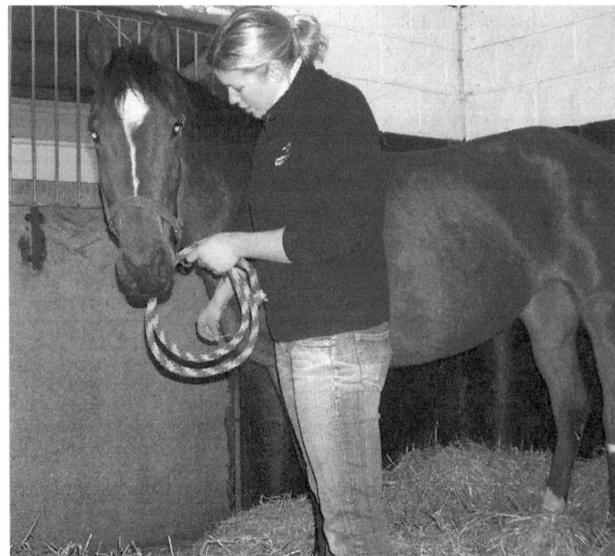

Figure 1.12 Intramuscular injection in the pectoral muscle. The handler stands next to the shoulder of the horse, and holds the needle so that it points backwards along the palm of the hand. ©Kevin Corley 2007.

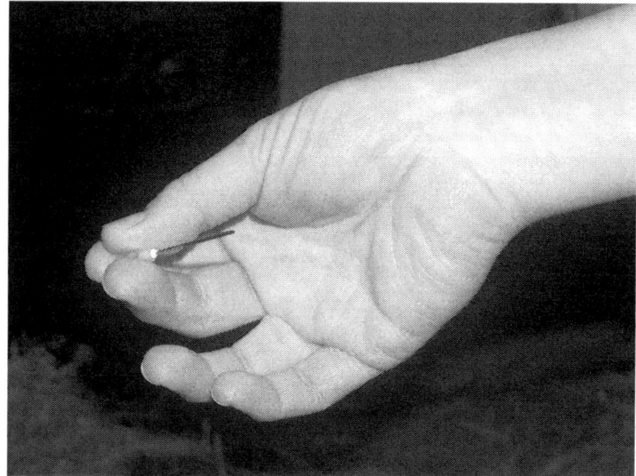

Figure 1.13 Close up of the hand holding the needle in Figure 1.12, demonstrating the position that the needle is held. ©Kevin Corley 2007.

Reference

1. Orsini JA: Medication administration, in Orsini JA, Divers TJ (eds): Manual of Equine Emergencies. Philadelphia, WB Saunders, 1998, pp 7-9

1.7 Passage of a nasogastric tube and indwelling nasogastric tube

Bettina Dunkel

Nasogastric tubes are frequently used in the equine hospital. They are used to evacuate the stomach if reflux is building up, for direct hydration of the gastrointestinal contents and for delivery of certain drugs (e.g., quinidine sulfate). Indwelling nasogastric feeding tubes can be used to provide constant enteral fluids (see Chapter 6.5), and occasionally for providing nutrition (see Chapter 5).

Equipment needed

The equipment for nasogastric intubation is listed in Box 1.9. Nasogastric tubes can be purchased in several sizes from many different suppliers. A medium (outer diameter: 15.9 mm) or large tube is suitable for most adult horses. Ponies and yearlings may require a smaller tube (outer diameter: 12.7 mm). Special tubes designed for foals (outer diameter: 9.5 mm) tube are also available.[1]

Nasogastric intubation

The person passing the tube should be positioned on one side of the horse, with the person holding the horse on the opposite side. The end of the tube should be moistened or lubricated with K-Y Jelly. The tube should be held approximately 20 to 30 cm from its end in one hand. The other hand is placed lightly on the nostrils of the horse, without occluding them. This hand is used to ensure that the tube is passed into the ventral meatus, by applying pressure with one finger ventrally and medially (Figure 1.14). It is very important to keep the tube ventral to avoid the ethmoid turbinate bone. Once the pharynx is reached, resistance to further passage is noted. Swallowing can be induced by careful rotation or gentle pressure on the pharynx. As the horse swallows, a gentle swift forward movement allows the tube to pass into the oesophagus. There is just noticeable resistance of the collapsed oesophagus against the tube as it is passed. There may be moderately increased resistance as the tube passes through the cardia, into the stomach. If the horse does not swallow or the tube repeatedly glides into the trachea, bending of the horse's neck to bring the horse's chin towards the chest can help. It is important to keep the horse's head on a straight line with

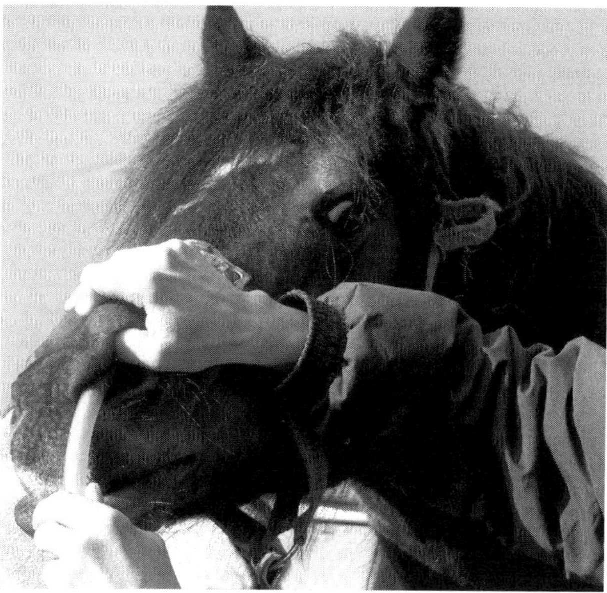

Figure 1.14 Passing a nasogastric tube in a horse. The thumb is used to guide the tube ventrally and medially, into the ventral meatus. ©Bettina Dunkel 2006.

Box 1.9. Equipment for nasogastric intubation

Nasogastric intubation
Translucent equine nasogastric tube*†

Indwelling stomach tube
Enteral feeding tube (18Fr, 250 cm suitable for most adults)‡

Optional
K-Y Jelly§
Sedation
Twitch

*Arnolds Veterinary Products, Shropshire, UK.
†Portex Ltd., Kent, UK.
‡MILA International, Florence, KY, USA.
§Johnson and Johnson, New Brunswick, NJ, USA.

the body. Other options include passage of the tube through the other nostril, using a larger or smaller diameter tube and blowing air or water through the tube into the pharynx.

Correct placement is ensured by observation of the left jugular grove. The tube can be seen and felt as it proceeds down the neck and can be palpated dorsal to the larynx or, at the left base of the neck, lateral to the trachea deep to the jugular vein. Placement in the stomach can be confirmed by flushing the tube with water, and retrieving gastric material by siphoning. No resistance against passage, air movement in and out of the tube, vigorous coughing and the inability to see or palpate the tube suggest that the tube has passed into the trachea. If there is any doubt about the correct placement, the tube should be removed and placed again.

Passage of an indwelling nasogastric feeding tube

Indwelling nasogastric feeding tubes are passed in a similar manner. However, the small diameter of the tube and its pliable nature make the procedure and verification of correct placement more difficult. Before the tube is placed, one should ensure that the guide wire can be removed easily. If necessary, the wire can be lubricated (with K-Y Jelly) to enable easy removal once the tube has been placed. An upper airway endoscope, operated by a third person, can greatly simplify the procedure. The endoscope is passed up the opposite nostril to the tube, until the pharynx can be visualised. The person handling the scope can now direct the person passing the tube, and ensure correct placement in the oesophagus. The tube can also be placed without endoscopic guidance, but the procedure requires more patience and some experience for palpatory confirmation of correct placement.

Once the tube is passed into the stomach or distal oesophagus, the guide wire is removed. The proximal end should be closed and the tube secured with tape on the head collar. Correct placement must be confirmed by palpation and flushing of the tube with water before each use.

Reference

1. Lopes M, Hepburn RJ, McKenzie HC, et al: Enteral fluid therapy for horses. Comp Contin Educ Pract Vet 25:390-397, 2003

1.8 Abdominocentesis

Jennifer O. Stephen

Abdominocentesis may be indicated in the workup of cases with abdominal pain (colic), weight loss or pyrexia. Abdominocentesis of the acute colic case should be performed only after the physical examination and rectal examination have been completed, and then only if it is not clear whether the animal should be treated medically or surgically. The procedure is not always necessary and should be avoided in cases with an increased risk of bowel penetration, such as horses with large colon impaction or severe distension of viscera.

Box 1.10. Equipment for abdominocentesis

Both techniques

Clippers with a fine (No. 40) blade
Small gauze swabs (4 × 4) soaked in chlorhexidine (4%) scrub solution*
Small gauze swabs (4 × 4) soaked in surgical spirit (alcohol)
Sterile surgery gloves
Collection tube containing EDTA for cytological analysis
Sterile collection tube for protein analysis and bacteriological culture

Teat cannula technique

Mepivacaine 2%†: 2 ml drawn up in a 2–3-ml syringe with a 23–25-gauge needle
No. 15 scalpel blade
Bovine teat cannula

Needle technique

18-Gauge, 3.75-cm ($1\frac{1}{2}$-inch) needle

Optional

Sedation
Twitch

*Hibiscrub; Mölnlycke Health Care, Dunstable, UK.
†Intra-epicaine, Arnolds Veterinary Products, Shrewsbury, UK; Carbocaine-V; Pfizer Animal Health, New York, NY, USA.

Equipment needed

The equipment needed for abdominocentesis is given in Box 1.10. Abdominocentesis can be performed with either a needle or a bovine teat cannula. The needle technique is faster, and there is less risk of bleeding from a skin vessel contaminating the sample. There may be less chance of inadvertent enterocentesis (entry into the intestinal lumen) with a teat cannula.

Preparation

The clinician should be aware of the risk of injury from being kicked at all times during the procedure. Good restraint of the patient is essential. Sedation or twitching might be necessary. If the horse has violent colic signs, decompression of the stomach with a nasogastric tube or administration of analgesics may help to achieve restraint. The clinician should stand on the right side of the horse, at the horse's shoulder facing the tail. The clinician should then crouch down and look up at the abdomen. Never place your head under the horse's abdomen. If the horse is in lateral recumbency, the technique should be performed with the clinician standing behind the horses back and reaching over towards the abdomen.

The site for abdominocentesis is usually at the most dependent part of the abdomen, slightly (2 to 3 cm) to the right of midline. The site should be clipped and aseptically prepared. The clinician performing the technique should wear sterile gloves.

Technique

If using a hypodermic needle, thrust the needle through the body wall at the site described. To avoid blood contamination, try to avoid sites with obvious superficial veins. Twist and withdraw slightly and/or turn the hub to encourage the flow of peritoneal fluid.

If using a teat cannula, a small bleb of local anaesthetic should first be infused under the skin using a 25-gauge, 15-mm ($\frac{5}{8}$-inch) needle. Insert the cannula through a sterile swab prior to use (Figure 1.15). A guarded number 15 scalpel blade is then used to make small stab incision through the skin, to a depth of about 1 cm into the body wall. The teat cannula should then be slid through this incision and then pushed through the body wall with a short sharp thrust.

Fluid samples should be collected into sterile plain tubes and into EDTA tubes. Protein measurements on refractometers should only be carried out on samples from plain tubes as the specific gravity of EDTA in solution may influence the value, especially if only a small sample is obtained.

If no fluid is obtained, either the needle/cannula should be rotated or repositioned. Injection of air with sterile syringe may assist drainage of fluid. Attempts to aspirate peritoneal fluid using a syringe are usually unsuccessful and will often cause occlusion of the needle by peritoneum or omentum. If fluid is not obtained whilst using a needle, a second needle should be placed a few centimetres from the first. It is advisable to leave the first needle in place as the release of pressure by the second needle may cause a flow of fluid from the first needle. Several needles may be placed this way. It is not usually necessary to use this technique with a cannula. If after prolonged manipulation of the cannula abdominocentesis is nonproductive, or blood contaminated, a second attempt should be made 8 to 10 cm distant to the first site. If using a needle and no sample is obtained in a fat patient, consider using a teat cannula.

Ultrasonography can be very useful in determining a good site for abdominocentesis. A 2.5- to 6-MHz probe can be used to give an estimate of the thickness of the body wall and the position of underlying abdominal viscera. Peritoneal fluid is simply seen as a hypoechoic (black) area above the body wall (Figure 1.16). The spleen is the most homogeneous and echogenic of the abdominal organs (Figure 1.17) and can extend across midline in some patients. Large bowel is usually recognised by its hyperechoic sacculated appearance (Figure 1.17). The hyperechogenicity is due to the gas within the lumen of the bowel, which also obscures the content of the bowel.

Blood in the abdominocentesis specimen may be the result of superficial haemorrhage, perforation of a blood vessel on the serosal surface, perforation of an abdominal organ, especially the spleen, haemorrhagic diapedesis or haemoperitoneum. Taking the PCV of the sample can help to determine the source of bleeding. Samples from splenic puncture will have a higher PCV than the venous blood of the patient. Bleeding from accidental splenic puncture will generally stop with no further treatment. Accidental enterocentesis has been reported to occur in 2% to 5% of cases without any significant clinical sequelae.[1–3] However, one study identified that whilst no clinical symptoms are observed, a local peritonitis may develop.[4] Therefore, if

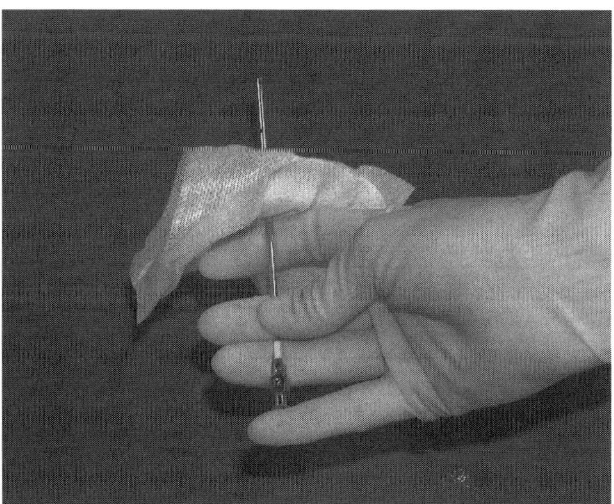

Figure 1.15 Teat cannula pushed through a sterile gauze swab for abdominocentesis. The swab prevents blood from the skin or superficial vessels running down the outside of the cannula and into the sample collection tube. ©Jennifer Stephen 2006.

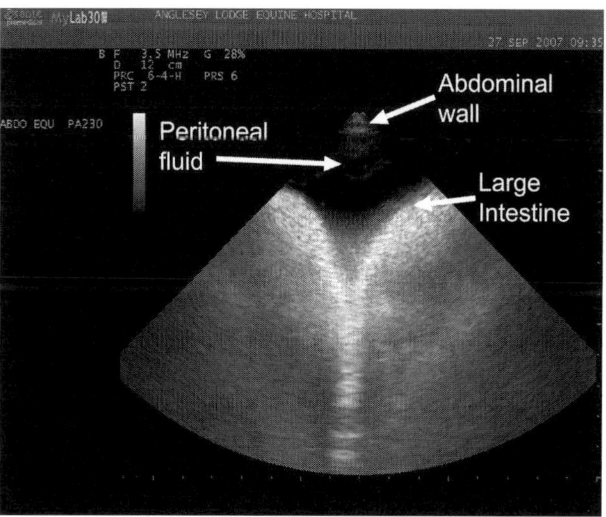

Figure 1.16 Ultrasound of peritoneal fluid. Increased amount of peritoneal fluid between two sections of large intestine, in a 6-month-old foal. ©Kevin Corley 2007.

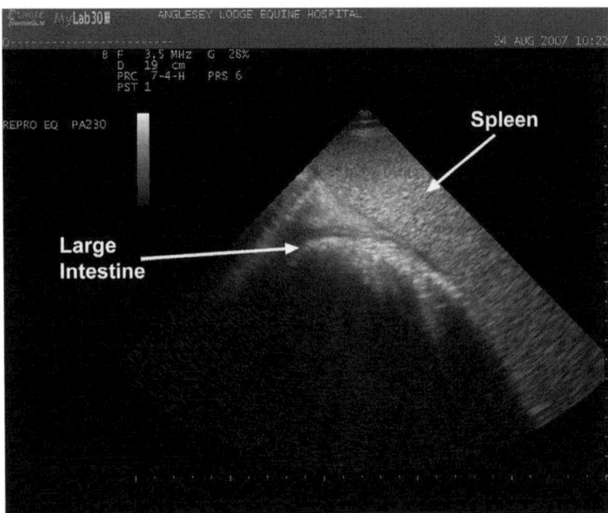

Figure 1.17 Ventral abdominal ultrasound of a mare, showing the spleen and ventral large colon. ©Kevin Corley 2007.

enterocentesis is suspected, 3 to 5 days of broad-spectrum systemic antibiotics should be administered.

Normal values for peritoneal fluid are given in the Appendix (see Table 19.11). Interpretation of peritoneal fluid results is described in Chapter 11.2 and Box 19.24.

References

1. Bach LG, Ricketts SW. Paracentesis as an aid to the diagnosis of abdominal disease in the horse. Equine Vet J 6:116-121, 1974
2. Swanwick RA, Wilkinson JS. A clinical evaluation of abdominal paracentesis in the horse. Aust Vet J 52:109-117, 1976
3. Schneider RK, Meyer DJ, Embertson RM, et al. Response of pony peritoneum to four peritoneal lavage solutions. Am J Vet Res 49:889-894, 1988
4. Schumacher J, Spano JS, Moll HD. Effects of enterocentesis on peritoneal fluid constituents in the horse. JAVMA 186:1301-1303, 1985

Box 1.11. Equipment for peritoneal lavage

Required

Abdominal drain

- 32Fr thoracic drain*
- 16Fr–30Fr thoracic drain, made from polyvinylchloride and Silastic
- 19Fr polyvinylchloride fenestrated drain†
- Argyle catheter‡

2-0 Nonabsorbable suture on a straight needle§
Sterile surgery gloves
No. 15 scalpel blade
Heimlich valve, condom, syringe or other one-way valve
Clamp
Two-lead arthroscopic irrigation set** or uterine flushing tube
Warmed sterile fluids for flushing (usually 3–5-L balanced electrolyte solution)

Required for the standing horse

Clippers with a No. 40 blade
Small gauze swabs (4 × 4) soaked in chlorhexidine (4%) scrub solution††
Small gauze swabs (4 × 4) soaked in surgical spirit (alcohol)
Mepivacaine‡‡ as a local anaesthetic
2-ml syringe and 25-gauge needle
Competent horse holder

Optional

Sedation
Twitch

*Trochar Catheter; Deknatel Inc, Fall River, MA, USA.
†Fenestrated drain $\frac{1}{4}$-inch (19Fr); Wound Drainage Devices, Zimmer, Warsaw, IN, USA.
‡Trochar-catheters, Argyle; Sherwood Medical Industries Inc., St. Louis, MO, USA.
§628H; Ethilon Nylon; Ethicon, Somerville, NJ, USA.
**Baxter Healthcare Corp., Deerfield, IL, USA.
††Hibiscrub; Mölnlycke Health Care, Dunstable, UK.
‡‡Intra-epicaine; Arnolds Veterinary Products, Shrewsbury, UK; Carbocaine-V; Pfizer Animal Health, New York, NY, USA.

1.9 Peritoneal lavage

Emma Rowe

The placement of abdominal drains and peritoneal lavage facilitates the removal and dilution of blood, bacteria, proteolytic enzymes, cellular debris and fibrin,[1,2] whilst also enhancing the mechanical separation of bowel loops, which may reduce adhesion formation.[3,4] Thus, peritoneal lavage is used in the treatment of peritonitis or as a prophylactic treatment for those horses at risk of developing septic peritonitis and abdominal adhesions.[4]

Equipment needed

The equipment for peritoneal lavage is given in Box 1.11. Tube drains used for abdominal lavage are readily available, the most common ones being made from silicone or polyvinylchloride (PVC). Silicone may be the best as minimal reaction has been noted with silicone drains when placed in the abdomen compared with a moderate reaction observed with PVC drains.[2] The use of silicone abdominal drains has also been reported to have a lower incidence of obstruction.[7] Plastic and rubber are more likely to be irritating than silicone or PVC; however, plastic causes less reaction than rubber.[2] Argyle catheters have a mushroom-tipped catheter that is very useful as an abdominal drain. Thoracic drains are very popular but may be stiffer compared with other drains and may cause patient discomfort or bowel damage.[4] The abdominal drain can be placed standing or before closure of the ventral midline incision following an exploratory laparotomy.

Passive (function by overflow, gravity or capillary action) or active (external vacuum source applied) drains can be placed.[2,5,6]

Inserting abdominal drain under general anaesthesia

The drain can be inserted into the abdomen just prior to closure of the ventral midline incision following exploratory laparotomy. A full-thickness stab incision can be made to the right side of the cranial to middle third of the incision (4 to 10 cm lateral to the incision). The drain can then be inserted through the stab incision. Placement through the stab incision is usually smooth, as most drains have a trochar allowing easy placement. If a Foley catheter is being placed, then the catheter can be stretched over a sterile female canine urinary catheter to allow placement through the body wall.[9] Once the drain is in place, it is secured to the body wall externally. The drain should be occluded with a sterile syringe for recovery. The drain can also exit the abdomen at two sites with fenestrations in between by placing a sharp trochar on the end of a PVC fenestrated drain*, and the trochar can be passed from the peritoneal surface to the skin 8 to 10 cm lateral to the caudal end of the incision.[4] The trochar can then be detached and attached to the other end of the tubing and the procedure repeated at the cranial end of the incision on the same side with the both ends of the drain being secured to the skin externally with suture.[4] The drain ends are both capped immediately for recovery.[4]

Inserting a drain in the standing horse

The drain should be inserted in the most ventral part of the abdomen. A transabdominal ultrasound examination is very useful to confirm the best location and to identify any bowel adhered to body wall that may be inadvertently punctured with placement of the drain. This would be very important in the case of long-standing peritonitis.[6] In most cases, the insertion site will be to the right of midline (5 to 10 cm), or on midline, in the most dependent part of the abdomen.

Once the location is chosen, the region is clipped and aseptically prepared. The horse must be restrained adequately (in most cases, sedation is necessary), and then approximately 2 ml of local anaesthetic is infiltrated in the region where the stab incision for drain placement is to be performed. Using a number 15 scalpel blade, a stab incision (approximately 1 cm) is made into the skin and through into the external sheath of the rectus abdominis muscle. If the drain chosen includes a trochar, it can then be inserted through the stab incision. The drain is inserted through the rectus abdominis muscle, internal rectus sheath and peritoneum very carefully, and once the abdominal cavity is punctured, the trochar is removed to reduce the risk of puncture to the viscera.[6] A blunt hollow trochar can be placed through the stab incision and the drain tube inserted into the trochar and the trochar removed after the drain is in place. A custom-design blunt hollow trochar has been used (inside diameter of 6.4 mm; custom designed from a mare urinary catheter).[4] The thoracic trochars are generally the more popular choice for percutaneous puncture. Many people choose to add fenestrations to these catheters before placement.[6] This is done by cutting extra holes (approximately 1 cm long × 0.5 cm wide) towards the end of the catheter. Ideally, this should be done before the catheter is sterilised, to allow careful cutting of the holes and prevention of sharp edges. It may also be done immediately prior to placement, if sterility is not broken.

Securing the drain

The drain needs to be secured externally, and there are several different effective suture patterns to achieve this. Two suture patterns commonly used are the "Chinese finger trap" suture or the "double clove-hitch" pattern.[6,10] The "Chinese finger trap" suture is placed by placing a purse-string suture around the drain, as it exits from the animal (Figure 1.18). The suture is crossed several times behind and in front of the drain. Each time the suture is passed in front of the drain, a surgeon's knot is thrown. These crosses are placed progressively along the drain, under reasonable tension (Figure 1.19). This suture firmly

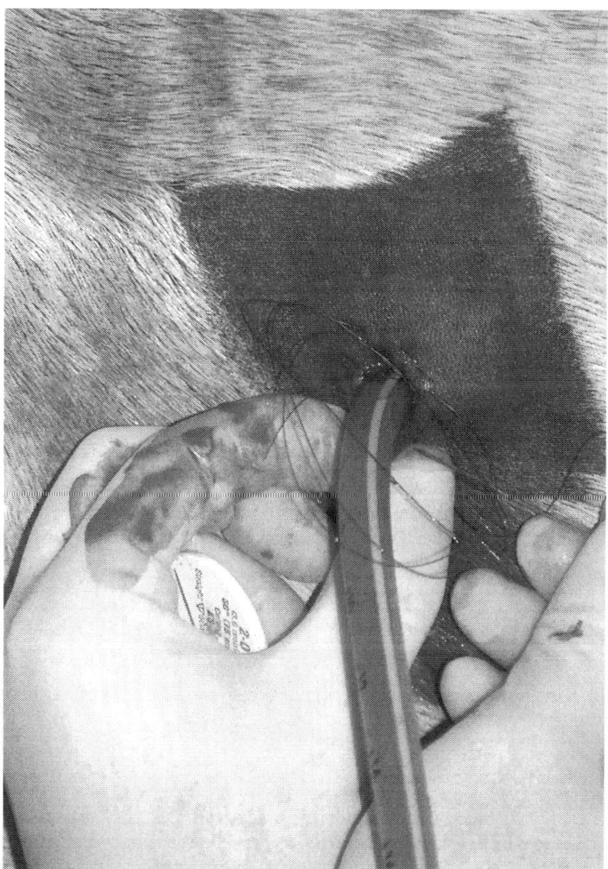

Figure 1.18 Placing a purse-string suture, around the base of a drain, before continuing to a "Chinese finger trap" suture. ©Kevin Corley 2004.

*Fenestrated drain $\frac{1}{4}$-inch (19Fr) Wound Drainage Devices; Zimmer, Warsaw, IN, USA.

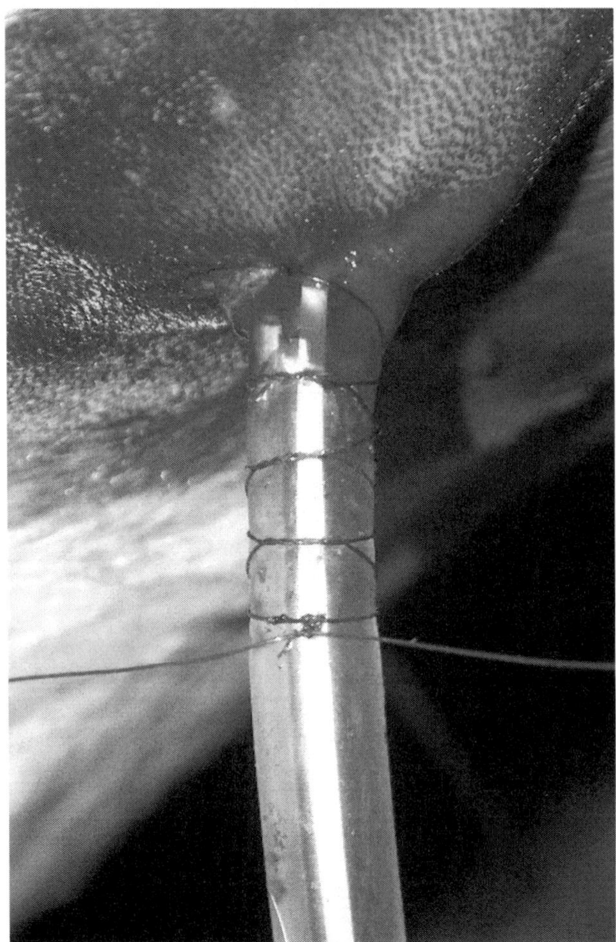

Figure 1.19 The "Chinese finger trap" suture around a drain. ©Kevin Corley 2004.

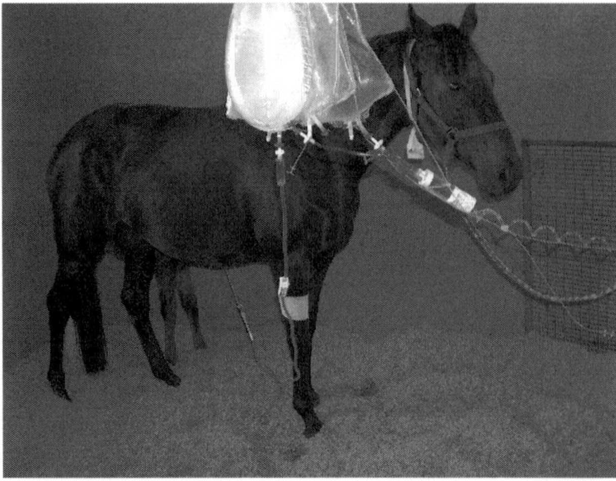

Figure 1.20 Gravity-flow of fluids into the abdomen via a peritoneal drain in a broodmare. ©Kevin Corley 2004.

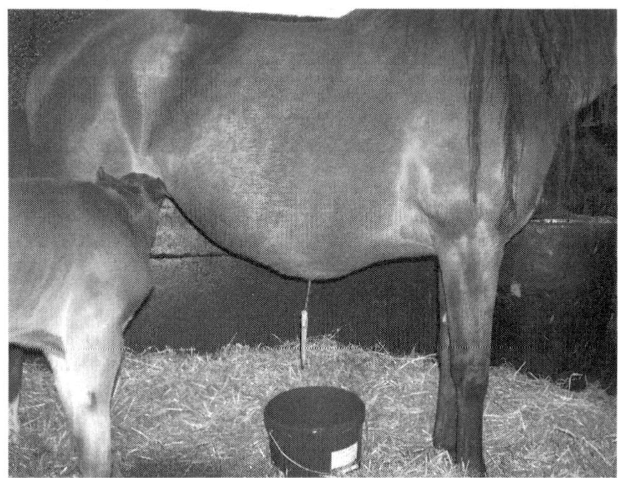

Figure 1.21 Draining the abdomen in a broodmare. A latex condom with the end cut off has been placed on the end of the drain to act as a one-way valve. ©Kevin Corley 2007.

holds the drain in place, and prevents it moving out of the animal. The drain end needs to be protected to prevent ascending infection by attaching a syringe, a latex condom with the end cut off (acts as a one-way valve) or a Heimlich valve. The Heimlich valve has been designed for thoracic drainage and has a latex liner that allows air and fluid to exit during expiration and collapses during inspiration.[4] A closed-suction system can also be used, by attaching the drain end or ends to a suction reservoir with a Y connector.[4]

Performing the lavage

To perform the lavage, lactated Ringer's solution or saline are usually the fluids of choice. The best solution and volume for peritoneal lavage has not been determined in horses.[3] Peritoneal lavage with saline has been shown to cause a mild inflammatory response in the abdomen and povidone-iodine solutions in saline (as dilute as 3%) are irritating to peritoneal surfaces.[8] The volume used will depend on clinician preference, the size of the horse and the condition being treated and may range from 1 to 15 L[4]; however, commonly 10 L is administered. Fluid bags are connected with large-bore tubing to the abdominal drain and the fluids are infused by gravity (Figure 1.20). The author's preference is to administer fluids through a two-lead arthroscopic irrigation set, as also described by others.[4]

Some horses may become painful as the fluid is being infused. If this occurs, the fluid administration is discontinued. Some clinicians will sedate the horse to infuse as close to 10 L of fluid as possible; however, it is the author's preference to discontinue fluids when the horse becomes uncomfortable. After fluid administration, the abdominal drain can be clamped, and the horse may be walked for 10 minutes to redistribute the fluid within the abdomen. The fluid is then allowed to drain from the abdomen, and the volume is measured and colour is noted (Figure 1.21).

Possible complications

In a recent study, the most common complications with the use of an active intra-abdominal drain and lavage included obstruction or slow passage of fluid through the drain, leakage of fluid around the drain and subcutaneous fluid accumulation around the drain.[4] Other complications may include pneumoperitoneum, perforation of viscera within the abdomen, ascending infection and electrolyte and protein disturbances.

References

1. Chase J, et al.: Open peritoneal drainage in horses with experimentally induced peritonitis. Vet Surg 25:189-194, 1996
2. Lee AH, Swaim SF: Surgical drainage. Comp Continu Educ Pract Vet 8:94-105, 1986
3. Hague B, et al.: Evaluation of postoperative peritoneal lavage in standing horses for prevention of experimentally induced abdominal adhesions. Vet Surg 27:122-126, 1998
4. Nieto J, et al.: Use of an active intra-abdominal drain in 67 horses. Vet Surg 32:1-7, 2003
5. Arighi M: Drains, dressings and external coaptation devices, in Auer JA (ed): Drains, Dressings and External Coaptation Devices. Philadelphia, WB Saunders, 1992, pp 159-176
6. Stone WC: Drains, dressings and external coaptation devices, in Auer JA (ed): Drains, Dressings and External Coaptation Devices. Philadelphia, WB Saunders, 1992, pp 104-113
7. Rout RW: Drainage of abdmoinal wounds, in Zuidema GD (ed): Drainage of abdominal Wounds. Philadelphia, WB Saunders, 1996, pp 328-329
8. Schneider JR, et al.: Response of pony peritoneum to four peritoneal lavage solutions. Am J Vet Res 49:889-894, 1988
9. Valdez H, Scrutchfield WL, Taylor TS: Peritoneal lavage in the horse. J Am Vet Med Assoc 175:388-391, 1979
10. Wigle R: A simple technique for securing tubes and drains. Surg Gynecol Obstet 174:233, 1992

1.10 Gastroscopy

Tim Brazil

Gastroduodenoscopy is well tolerated by horses. A competent examination requires detailed knowledge of the relevant anatomy and recommended techniques, patience and practice! An assistant experienced in passing the gastroscope greatly facilitates both passage into and down the oesophagus and navigation within the stomach.

Equipment needed

The equipment for gastroscopy is listed in Box 1.12. A 3-metre endoscope is required for adult horses of greater than 400 kg body weight. It may be possible to perform a complete examination in smaller horses with a shorter endoscope. In foals, a narrower external diameter endoscope may be required to pass through the nasal passages. An air pump is essential for insufflation of the stomach. Often, the air pumps incorporated into the endoscope control towers are insufficient for rapid insufflation of the stomach, and many clinicians prefer to use adapted garden spray pumps (Figure 1.22). Often, feed material is stuck to the stomach wall, obscuring the view of any ulcers. This can be washed off via the biopsy channel with a pressurised water pump, an adapted garden spray pump (as for air) or 60-ml syringes filled with water. Long biopsy forceps are used for lesion probing, facilitating entry into the pylorus, and for harvest of transendoscopic mucosal biopsy specimens. Instruments for harvest of larger glandular mucosal samples have been described.[1]

Box 1.12. Equipment for gastroscopy

Required

3 m × 12 mm external diameter videoendoscope*
High-intensity light source
Air pump
Pressurised water pump or 60-ml syringes
325–350-cm biopsy forceps
Sedation
Twitch

Equipment that should be available if possible

Suction pump
325–350-cm aspiration catheter

Optional

Short length of stomach tube
Hausmann's gag

*Endoscopes with wider external diameters can be used but are not suitable for smaller patients and may be less flexible and manoeuvrable.

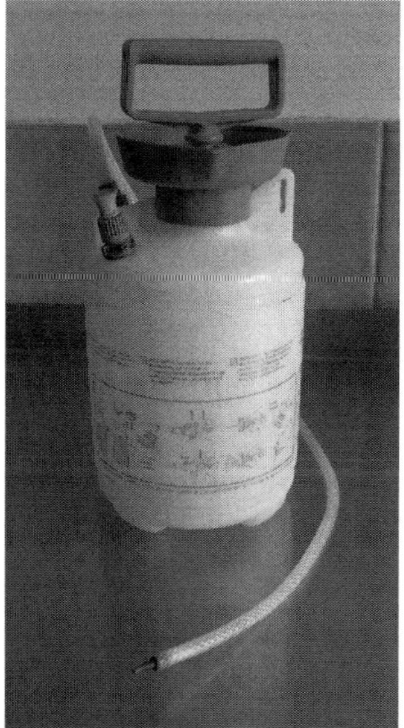

Figure 1.22 Adapted garden spray pump for insufflation of the stomach. The spray unit has been cut off from the end of the hose and replaced with a Christmas tree adapter. ©Kevin Corley 2007.

It is useful to have a suction pump to evacuate gastric fluid if necessary and insufflated air after the procedure. Some clinicians use a stomach tube after the procedure to evacuate insufflated air. An aspiration catheter is useful for local lavage, probing lesions and aspiration of gastric and/or duodenal fluid under sterile conditions if necessary (the end of the catheter can be plugged with sterile agar transport medium from a bacteriological swab).

Patient preparation

Food should be withheld for at least 12 hours and water for at least 4 hours prior to the procedure. The fluid-phase gastric emptying time is short (30 minutes), but a longer period facilitates the examination. The horse should be stabled on rubber matting or inedible bedding during the period of starvation.

The procedure can be performed in a stable or with horse restrained in stocks. Light to moderate sedation is required (α_2-agonist, with butorphanol if necessary; see Chapter 6.1) depending on the animal's temperament.

A twitch may be required in some animals to aid passage of the endoscope into the ventral nasal meatus.

To eliminate the risk of inadvertent retroflexion into the oropharynx, some practitioners pass a short length of nasogastric tube in to the proximal oesophagus, through which the gastroscope is then passed. It is necessary to lubricate the outside of the gastroscope so that it passes freely through the stomach tube without damage to its outer skin. Other clinicians attempt to minimise the risk of damage to the gastroscope by the horse's teeth if it should become retroflexed by placing a Hausmann's gag on the horse prior to gastroscopy.

Gastroscopy

The assistant should pass the endoscope in the manner of nasogastric tube (see Chapter 1.7) whilst the endoscopist directs the tip of the gastroscope dorsal to the arytenoid cartilages of the larynx. When the tip is in place, pressing the air/water piston to pass water through the flushing channel helps to stimulate swallowing; gently touching the mucosa above the arytenoids with the end of the endoscope will also stimulate swallowing.

Once the tip of the gastroscope has been swallowed, the assistant should stop passing the endoscope momentarily to ensure correct positioning in oesophagus (Figure 1.23). Insufflation of air allows dilation of the oesophagus and the characteristic mucosa to be imaged. The gastroscope should then be advanced down the oesophagus. Continuous insufflation assists passage of the gastroscope.

If undue resistance is encountered or the image is unclear, the gastroscope should be retracted slightly. Air should be insufflated, then passage of the gastroscope can be resumed. Some horses "grab" the gastroscope in the pharynx by displacing the palate, causing great resistance to forward passage. If the gastroscope is forced against this resistance, there is a great danger of retroflexion into the mouth and damage to the gastroscope. Stimulating the horse to swallow by placing a hand on the tongue through the bars of the mouth, or by injecting a small amount of water into the mouth, can relieve this "grabbing".

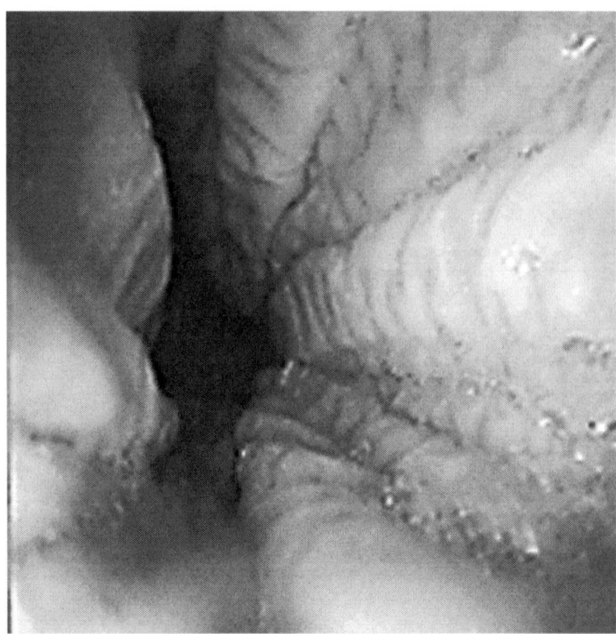

Figure 1.23 Endoscopic view of the oesophagus. ©Kevin Corley 2007.

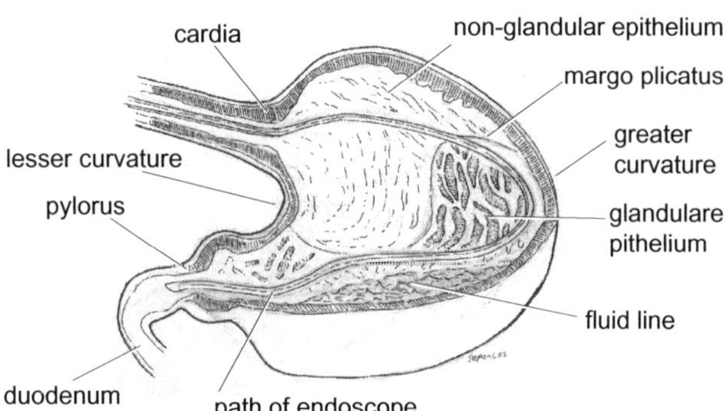

Figure 1.24 Anatomy of the stomach, and path along which a gastroscope should be passed to image the pyloric antrum, pylorus and duodenum.

In most average-sized (400 to 600 kg; 900 to 1300 lb) horses, the cardia is approximately 2 metres from the nares. After entering the stomach, the endoscope should be orientated such that gastric fluid line is horizontal and below the endoscope. The stomach should be insufflated with air to flatten out the mucosal folds and allow complete mucosal examination. Insufflation and "rounding" of the stomach greatly ease passage of the endoscope around greater curvature toward the pylorus. Once the stomach has been inflated, the margo plicatus should be visible on the left of the cardia (Figure 1.24).

The endoscope should be turned to the left to be in contact with the wall of the stomach. It should remain in contact with the wall of the stomach as it is advanced and directed on a line just dorsal to the margo plicatus, around the greater curvature of the stomach. Once the gastroscope has passed around the greater curvature, the lesser curvature can be viewed. The endoscope can be seen leaving the cardia, just above the lesser curvature (Figure 1.25). Further insufflation may be required to view the entrance to the pyloric antrum.

On occasion, a route ventral to the margo plicatus must be used. This may be hindered by retained gastric fluid and solid contents, leading to a loss of orientation. A glandular mucosal fold running obliquely from left dorsal to right ventral at the entrance to the antrum can be difficult to negotiate.

The endoscope should be passed into antrum to view the pylorus.[2] Waiting may allow antral motility to move the endoscope toward the pylorus. If it is not possible to enter the antrum, the endoscope should be retracted to the cardia and reorientated. It may be necessary to reinflate the stomach. If the antrum or pylorus is visible but cannot be approached, the biopsy instrument should be passed down the endoscope and anchored on the mucosa of the antrum, pylorus or lesser curvature, as appropriate. The biopsy instrument should be withdrawn as the endoscope is passed, to direct the tip towards this point. This can be repeated as necessary. Rarely, gastric fluid must be suctioned to visualise the entrance to the antrum. Suctioning through the endoscope commonly leads to blockage of the suction channel by food material.

The pylorus can be inspected (Figure 1.26) and lesions graded. The remainder of the squamous and glandular mucosae of the stomach can be examined and lesions graded during this procedure (Box 1.13).

Duodenoscopy

Usually, as the endoscope is passed into the antrum, it ends up lined up with the pylorus on the lefthand side. Turning the gastroscope to the left allows it to pass through the pylorus into the bulb-like duodenal ampulla. Occasionally, antral and pyloric motility will push the endoscope into the duodenum without any operator effort. From the pylorus, the endoscope is directed hard to the left and up to bring the lumen of the duodenum into view. The duodenal

Box 1.13. Equipment for percutaneous trocharisation

Required

14-Gauge catheter*
75 cm (30 inch) fluid extension set†
Small specimen jar filled with sterile water
Sterile surgery gloves
Mepivacaine‡ as a local anaesthetic
2-ml syringe with a 25-gauge needle
No. 15 scalpel blade
Clippers with a No. 40 blade
Small gauze swabs (4 × 4) soaked in chlorhexidine (4%) scrub solution§
Small gauze swabs (4 × 4) soaked in surgical spirit (alcohol)

Optional

Sedation
Twitch
Stocks to restrain the horse

*Abocath, 14-gauge, 13 cm; Abbott Laboratories, Abbott Park, IL, USA.
†2C5645; Baxter Healthcare, Deerfield, IL, USA.
‡Intra-epicaine; Arnolds Veterinary Products, Shrewsbury, UK; Carbocaine-V; Pfizer Animal Health, New York, NY, USA.
§Hibiscrub; Mölnlycke Health Care, Dunstable, UK.

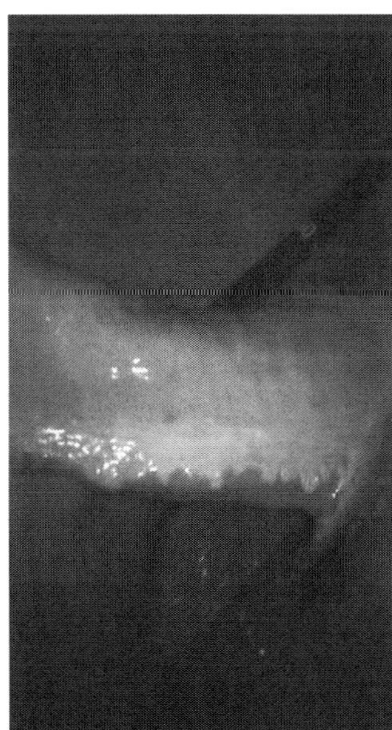

Figure 1.25 Endoscopic view of the lesser curvature, cardia and pyloric antrum of the stomach. ©Kevin Corley 2005.

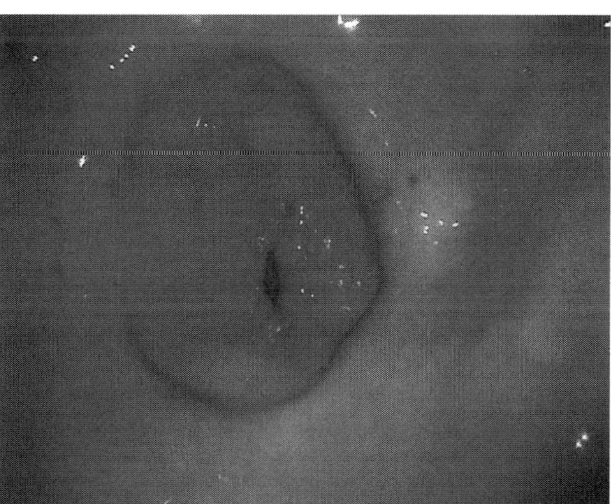

Figure 1.26 Endoscopic view of the pylorus. There are several small erythematous lesions around the pylorus. ©Kevin Corley 2005.

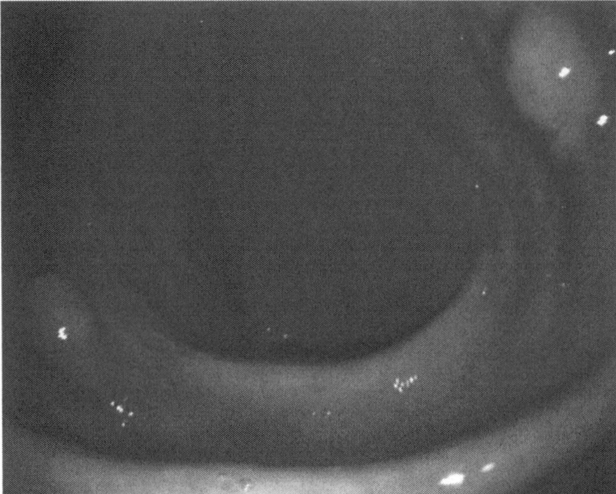

Figure 1.27 Endoscopic view of the major (*right* of image) and minor (*left* of image) papillae in the duodenum. ©Kevin Corley 2005.

mucosa is recognised by its pale pink/brown (bile)-tinged colour and obvious villous mucosa. Insufflation and redirection of the tip may be required to maintain this view. Patience to allow peristalsis to assist aboral movement of the endoscope is often rewarded. From this point, with the endoscope "hooked" in the duodenum, gradual retraction of the endoscope will move the tip in an aboral direction (i.e., farther into the duodenum). Following the initial sharp bend, the lumen narrows and turns to the left (cranial duodenal flexure) into the duodenum proper, where the major (right of image, common outlet of hepatic and pancreatic ducts) and minor (slightly further aboral and left of image, accessory pancreatic duct) duodenal papillae are seen approximately 10 cm beyond the pylorus (Figure 1.27). The typical circular duodenal mucosal folds are seen during peristalsis.

References

1. Murray MJ, Hepburn RJ, Sullins KE: Preliminary study of use of a polypectomy snare to obtain large samples of the equine gastric antrum by endoscopy. Equine Vet J 36:76-78, 2004
2. Murray MJ, Nout YS, Ward DL: Endoscopic findings of the gastric antrum and pylorus in horses: 162 cases (1996-2000). J Vet Intern Med 15:401-406, 2001
3. Bain FT, Petrizzi L, Valbonetti L, Muttini A: Gastroscopy and duodenoscopy. In Slovis NM (ed): Atlas of Equine Endoscopy. St. Louis, Mosby, 2004, pp. 147-168

1.11 Percutaneous trocharisation

Emma Rowe

Percutaneous trocharisation is a technique that involves placing a catheter into a gas-distended large colon or caecum to allow decompression in a standing horse.

Equipment needed

The equipment needed for percutaneous trocharisation is given in Box 1.13.

Indications

The main indication for trocharisation is a horse with severe abdominal distension and pain that is not responsive to analgesia and fluid therapy, when surgery is not an option. It should only be attempted in horses where distension of the large intestine, such as the large colon or caecum, has been identified on examination per rectum (see Chapters 1.4 and 11.1.1). It is not to be performed to relieve distension of the small intestine or small colon. Severe large colon distension can result in compromise of the cardiovascular system due to compression of veins draining the abdomen (so-called "abdominal compartment syndrome"). Furthermore, the pain associated with the distension may become unrelenting, necessitating euthanasia of the horse for humane reasons. Percutaneous trocharisation can be performed to relieve some of the gas distension, which may decrease the abdominal pain. In some cases, in combination with the intravenous fluid therapy and analgesia, this decompression may be sufficient to allow intestinal motility to return and the abdominal pain to resolve. This procedure should ideally only be reserved for horses in which surgery is not an option. As the procedure is not without complications and may contaminate the abdomen, it should not be performed before an exploratory laparotomy whenever possible.

Caecal trocharisation has been advocated for horses with primary gas distension of the caecum and colon secondary to physical obstruction or ileus. In these cases of tympany, trocharisation has been recommended when the clinical signs appear to be resolving, the pain is manageable and medical treatment is preferable to surgery.[1] Careful consideration should always be made before performing the procedure, as there are potential complications. However, if done correctly, complications such as laceration of the viscera and peritonitis can be reduced.

Performing the procedure

Great care must be taken when performing this procedure. If ultrasound is not available, trocharisation should only be performed on the right upper flank region. This is the most common site and is a safe location, if there has been accurate identification of gas-distended intestine close to the body wall. Careful percussion with identification of gas "pings" and examination per rectum will allow accurate identification of the gas-distended intestine and the correct location for catheter placement. In smaller horses or foals, radiographs and/or ultrasound will be necessary to identify the distended intestine and location for catheter placement. It is very important that the catheter used for trocharisation only penetrates the intended distended large colon or caecum. It is possible with incorrect placement to

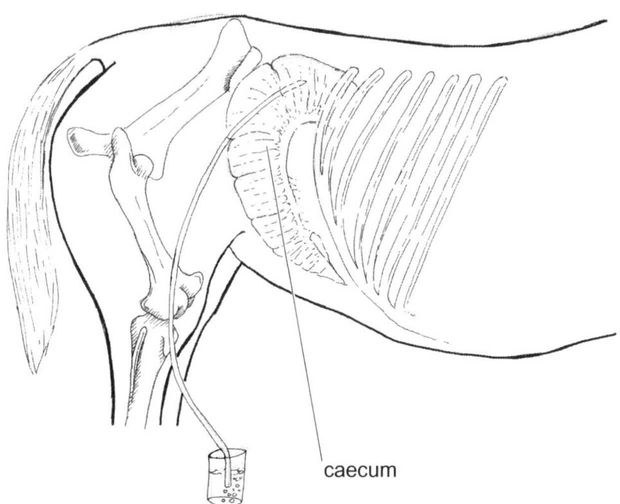

Figure 1.28 Anatomy of the caecum and site for percutaneous trocharisation.

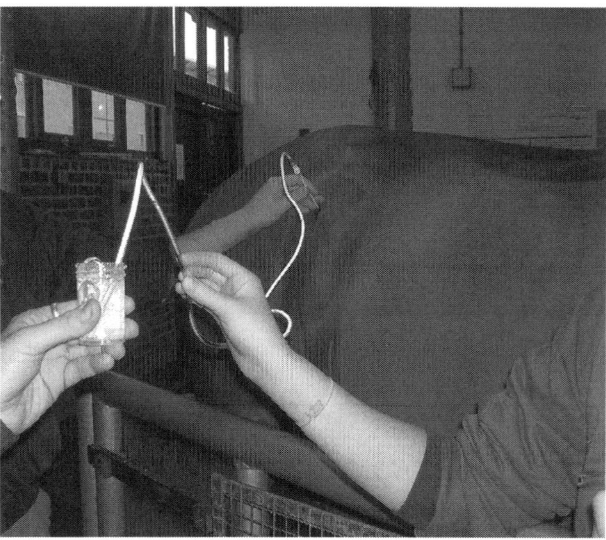

Figure 1.29 Percutaneous trocharisation of the caecum. The gas released is bubbled through sterile water. ©Kevin Corley 2004.

puncture the diaphragm or other structures such as the kidney or spleen. Transabdominal ultrasound is very useful for identifying a safe location and reduces the risk of inadvertent puncture of a vital structure. There is a high chance of complication on the left side of the abdomen, without ultrasound-derived knowledge of the location of vital structures.

If the trocharisation is to be performed on the right side without ultrasound localisation, it should be done just cranial to the greater trochanter where the caecal base is located. A definite ping should be auscultated in this region to confirm accurate placement.

Once the correct location has been identified, the region is clipped and aseptically prepared and 2 to 5 ml of local anaesthetic is infiltrated under the skin and into the subcutaneous tissue over the small area where the catheter is to be placed. Sterile gloves should be worn for the procedure. A 14-gauge catheter is placed through and perpendicular to the skin, through the area infiltrated with local anaesthetic, towards the distended viscus (Figure 1.28). A sterile 75-cm (30-inch) extension tube is attached to the catheter and placed into a small specimen jar filled with water, held by an assistant. The end of the extension tube is placed below the surface of the water to allow bubbles to form when the gas starts to escape after the intestine has been entered (Figure 1.29). The catheter tip is gently advanced and positioned until the gas starts escaping, indicating penetration of the intestine. Once gas is obtained, the clinician should withdraw the trochar part of the catheter, to avoid inadvertent laceration of the bowel as the distension decreases and the bowel wall changes location. The catheter may need to be repositioned several times during the procedure. When no more gas can be obtained, the catheter is withdrawn. Many clinicians will inject an antibiotic, usually gentamicin, into the tissue as the catheter is withdrawn, to reduce the risk of local abscessation. Parenteral antibiotics should not be required unless the clinician is concerned that there may be a high risk of peritonitis developing, such as secondary to laceration of the viscus following a traumatic trocharisation. The two most common complications of trocharisation are peritonitis and local abscessation.

Reference

1. Dart A, Dowling B, Hodgson DR: Large intestine, in Auer J, Stick J (eds): Equine Surgery, ed 2. Philadelphia, WB Saunders, 1999, pp 257-285

1.12 Rectal mucosal biopsy

Anna Hammond

Samples of rectal mucosa can be collected with relative ease. This is a valuable technique as histopathological examination may reveal cellular infiltration, reflecting changes at more proximal, and inaccessible, locations. Analysis is not straightforward and it cannot be assumed that the inflammation, if observed, is consistent throughout the intestinal tract. Although rectal biopsy can be useful in a proportion of cases,[1–4] a lack of standardisation in histopathological interpretation limits this usefulness. A system of standardisation has been proposed.[1]

Equipment needed

The equipment required is listed in Box 1.14.

Technique

This procedure is easiest to perform with the horse in a set of stocks. Sedation is optional and dependent on the patient's temperament. The tail is held to one side and the

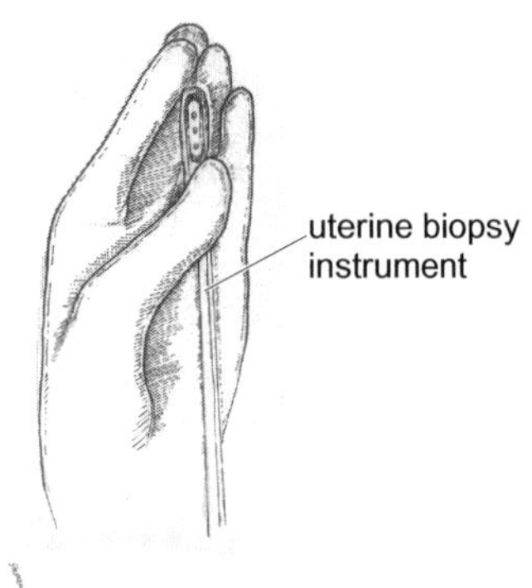

Figure 1.30 Holding the uterine biopsy instrument for introduction into the rectum.

Box 1.14. Equipment for rectal mucosal biopsy

Required
Sharp, long-handled biopsy forceps*
Rectal sleeve
Obstetrical lubricant
Competent horse holder
Sample pot containing 10% neutral buffered formalin
23-Gauge or 25-gauge needle

Optional
Sedation
Twitch
Stocks to restrain the horse
Mepivacaine† or lidocaine to instil in the rectum
75-cm (30-inch) fluid extension set‡
50–60-ml syringe

*141700, uterine biopsy instrument 60 cm; Kruuse, Marslev, Denmark.
†Intra-epicaine; Arnolds Veterinary Products, Shrewsbury, UK; Carbocaine-V; Pfizer Animal Health, New York, NY, USA.
‡2C5645; Baxter Healthcare, Deerfield, IL, USA.

rectum emptied of faeces. Instillation of a local anaesthetic agent appears unnecessary, unless the horse strains excessively during initial evacuation of faeces. Areas of the rectum that feel abnormal should be sampled, although usually a random site is selected. The forceps are introduced with the hand guarding the cutting blades (Figure 1.30). The sample is normally taken approximately 30 cm proximal to the anus at the 10 or 2 o'clock positions (away from the aorta). The mucosa is immobilised between finger and thumb and pulled away from the muscular layers. The sample is collected just behind the operator's hand on the aboral side (Figure 1.31). Before withdrawing the forceps, ensure that the sample of mucosa is totally separated from the rectum, by passing the fingers around the forceps blade. The forceps are withdrawn completely from the rectum and the sample is placed in a sample container containing 10% neutral buffered formalin. It may be necessary to tease

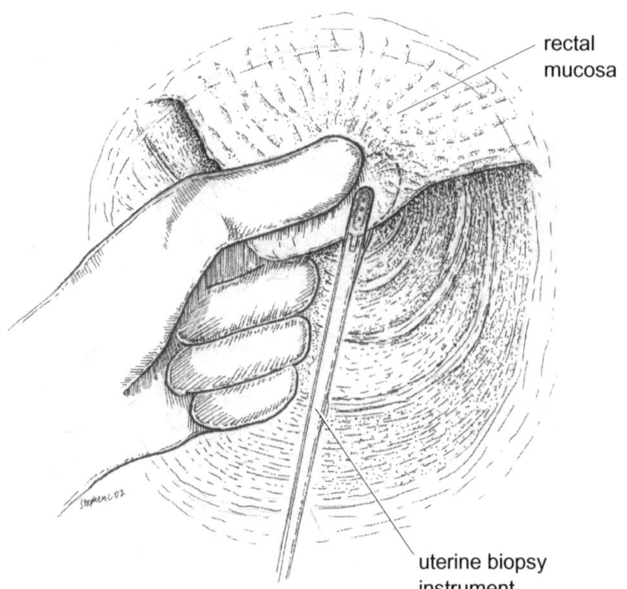

Figure 1.31 The rectal mucosa is pinched and placed in the jaws of the biopsy instrument.

the sample from the instrument blades with a small gauge needle, taking care not to damage it. Antibiotics may be administered although many clinicians do not routinely prescribe them following this procedure and do not report any associated complications.

References

1. Lindberg R, Nygren A, Persson SG: Rectal biopsy diagnosis in horses with clinical signs of intestinal disorders: a retrospective study of 116 cases. Equine Vet J 28:275-284, 1996
2. Gibson KT, Alders RG: Eosinophilic enterocolitis and dermatitis in two horses. Equine Vet J 19:247-252, 1987
3. Kemper DL, Perkins GA, Schumacher J, et al: Equine lymphocytic-plasmacytic enterocolitis: a retrospective study of 14 cases. Equine Vet J Suppl:108-112, 2000
4. Ricketts SW: Rectal biopsy—a piece of the diagnostic jigsaw puzzle. Equine Vet J 28:254-255, 1996

1.13 Liver biopsy

Kevin Corley

Liver biopsy is indicated when liver enzymes or function tests are increased (see Chapter 12.1) and further diagnostic or prognostic information is needed. The main potential problems associated with liver biopsy in the horse are collection of an unrepresentative biopsy and adverse effects of the procedure itself including haemorrhage, colic, peritonitis, pleuritis and pneumothorax.[1] In the author's experience, all of these problems are rare, especially when the technique is performed under ultrasonographic guidance, and the requirement for prebiopsy coagulation assessment is questionable.[2] A quarter of human patients report some degree of abdominal pain following liver biopsy,[3] and

Box 1.15. Equipment for liver biopsy

Required

14-Gauge 16-cm biopsy needle*
Sample pot containing 10% neutral buffered formalin
23-Gauge or 25-gauge needle
Sedation
Sterile surgery gloves
Mepivacaine† as a local anaesthetic
2-ml syringe with a 25-gauge needle
No. 15 scalpel blade
Clippers with a No. 40 blade
Small gauze swabs (4 × 4) soaked in chlorhexidine (4%) scrub solution‡
Small gauze swabs (4 × 4) soaked in surgical spirit (alcohol)

For ultrasound guided technique

Ultrasound machine with a 3.5–7.5 MHz sector or linear array probe
Biopsy guide to fit the ultrasound probe
Sterile coupling gel§ or alcohol

Optional

Sterile sample pot, if culture of a biopsy specimen is required
Skin stapler**
Sterile staple remover
Topical antiseptic spray
Twitch
Stocks to restrain the horse

*Ranfac Cut Biopsy Needle; Ranfac Corporation, Avon, MA, USA.
†Intra-epicaine; Arnolds Veterinary Products, Shrewsbury, UK; Carbocaine-V; Pfizer Animal Health, New York, NY, USA.
‡Hibiscrub; Mölnlycke Health Care, Dunstable, UK.
§K-Y Jelly (Johnson and Johnson, New Brunswick, NJ, USA) is suitable for this purpose.
**Auto Suture Appose ULC 35W; United States Surgical, Tyco Healthcare Group, Norwalk, CT, USA.

therefore routine systemic analgesia should also be administered in horses. Interpretation of liver biopsies is discussed in Chapter 12.1.

Equipment needed

The equipment needed is listed in Box 1.15.

Technique

The horse should be sedated for this technique (see Chapter 6.1). Ideally, the technique should be performed with ultrasonographic guidance. In this case, an ultrasound examination of the right cranial abdomen is performed. The site for biopsy is selected either as one where a lesion is evident, or where the liver is apposed to the peritoneum and reasonably thick. If it is not possible to perform an ultrasound exam during the biopsy collection, the selected site should be marked by placing a skin staple. If ultrasound is not available, the preferred site is the right 13th intercostal space midway between two lines drawn between the point of the shoulder and the *tuber coxae* and the point of the elbow and the *tuber coxae* (Figure 1.32). A 6- to 8-cm square around the biopsy site is clipped and aseptically prepared. Local anaesthetic should be infiltrated at the biopsy site subcutaneously and through the intercostal muscles to the parietal peritoneum.

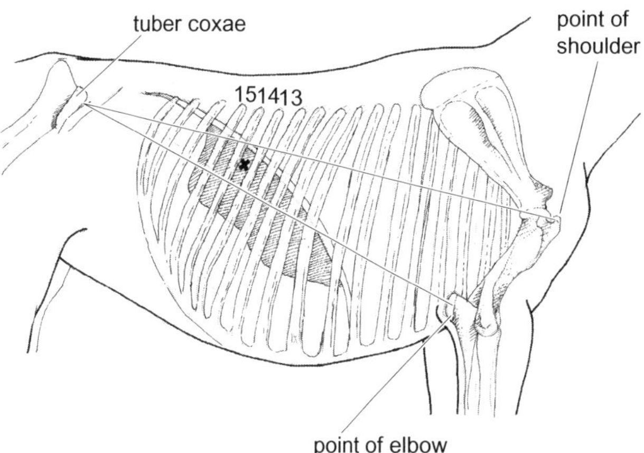

Figure 1.32 Preferred site for liver biopsy (when ultrasound guidance is not available). The site is over the right 13th intercostal space midway between two lines drawn between the point of the shoulder and the *tuber coxae* and the point of the elbow and the *tuber coxae*.

For the ultrasound-guided technique, a sterile sleeve should be placed over the probe. With most probes, it is possible to put them into the thumb of a large pair of sterile surgical gloves. Ultrasound coupling gel should be put in the sterile sleeve or surgical glove. Biopsy guides are available for many ultrasound probes, which fix the biopsy needle in the plane of the ultrasonographic image and may facilitate the procedure. A small amount of sterile coupling gel or alcohol is applied to the skin or probe.

A small stab incision should be made through the skin. If a staple was used to mark the site, the stab incision should be made alongside the staple, which should then be removed with sterile staple removers. The biopsy needle is advanced perpendicularly to the skin until rhythmic movement of diaphragm is felt (typically between 5 and 10 cm from skin surface). The needle is further advanced by about 2 to 3 cm and the biopsy sample is collected. There is often a "crunchy" feel as the needle is advanced into the liver. With ultrasonographic guidance, the biopsy needle can be seen advancing into the liver. The biopsy specimen is collected. For ultrasonographic guidance, two or three attempts at collection may be required. For the "blind" technique, several attempts may be necessary, but they should be limited to five or six. The specimen may have to be teased off the needle into the sample container using a small-gauge needle. Care should be taken not to damage the sample. Samples for histopathology should be collected into 10% neutral buffered formalin. Samples for culture should be collected into a sterile sample container.

After collection of the biopsies, some clinicians choose to spray the skin over the site with an antiseptic spray. Other clinicians may choose to close the stab incision with a staple, especially if a larger stab was made. The animal should be given an analgesic, such as phenylbutazone, flunixin or an opioid (see Chapter 6.2).

References

1. Modransky PD: Ultrasound-guided renal and hepatic biopsy techniques. Vet Clin North Am (Equine Pract) 2:115-125, 1986
2. Divers TJ, Bernard WV, Reef VB: Equine liver disease and liver failure—causes, diagnosis and treatment. Proc Bain-Fallon Mem Lect 10:35-46, 1988
3. Vautier G, Scott B, Jenkins D: Liver biopsy: blind or guided? Br Med J 309:1455-1456, 1994

1.14 Jugular catheterisation

Kevin Corley

Intravenous catheters are essential for fluid therapy in the hospital. They are also useful for horses that are scheduled to have repeated intravenous injections, as they improve patient compliance and decrease the chance of thrombophlebitis compared to repeated needlesticks. In the horse, the easiest vein to catheterise is the external jugular vein.

Equipment needed

The equipment for jugular catheterisation is listed in Box 1.16. The choice of catheter depends on the clinical status of the horse. Large-gauge catheters are essential for rapid reversal of moderate to severe hypovolaemia but have the disadvantage of being more thrombogenic. A 10- or 12-gauge catheter is recommended for severely hypovolaemic adult horses, and a 12- or 14-gauge catheter for moderately hypovolaemic horses. Large-bore short extension sets should be used for 10- and 12-gauge catheters. Sixteen-gauge catheters are sufficient for moderately hypovolaemic weanlings and miniature horses. Smaller-bore (14- or 16-gauge) catheters should be used in adult horses requiring medication and not fluids. For administration of parenteral nutrition (PN), double-lumen catheters can provide a dedicated line for the PN and avoid the need to interrupt the PN when administering incompatible drugs. The technique for placing a double-lumen catheter is described in Chapter 2.6.

Placement of an over-the-needle catheter

The vein should be raised and checked to see that it fills easily, with no obvious bulges, heat, hardness or defects. If there is a minor lesion over (but not involving) the vein, the contralateral jugular vein should be catheterised. If there is evidence of thrombophlebitis, the lateral thoracic or cephalic vein should be catheterised (see Chapter 1.15). A rectangle of hair approximately 10 cm long and 6 to 8 cm

Box 1.16. Equipment for placing a jugular catheter in the adult horse

Suitable catheters

For prolonged use

- 14-Gauge 13-cm (5.25-inch) over-the-needle polyurethane catheter*
- 14-Gauge single-lumen 20-cm (8-inch) over-the-wire catheter†‡
- 16-Gauge, 13-cm (5.25-inch) over-the-needle polyurethane catheter§
- 16-Gauge single-lumen 20-cm (8-inch) over-the-wire catheter**††

For short-term (1–2 day) use

- 10-Gauge 15-cm (6-inch) over-the-needle catheter‡‡
- 12-Gauge 13-cm (5.25-inch) over-the-needle catheter§§

Other required equipment

Clippers with a fine (No. 40) blade
Small gauze swabs (4 × 4) soaked in chlorhexidine (4%) scrub solution***
Small gauze swabs (4 × 4) soaked in surgical spirit (alcohol)
2–0 Nonabsorbable monofilament suture on a straight needle†††
10–20-ml syringe of 0.9% sterile saline (±5 units/ml heparin)
High-flow extension set‡‡‡ (for 14-gauge and smaller catheters), if not supplied with catheter
Wide-bore extension set§§§ (for 12-gauge and larger catheters), if not supplied with catheter
Injection cap (if not supplied in catheter kit)
Surgical gloves
Zinc oxide tape
Bandage scissors

Optional

Mepivacaine 2%****: 2 ml drawn up in a 2–3 ml syringe with a 23–25-gauge needle
No. 15 scalpel blade
Twitch
Sedation

*1411; MILA International, Florence, KY, USA.
†1410; MILA International, Florence, KY, USA.
‡CS-04701; Arrow International Inc., Reading, PA, USA.
§1611; MILA International, Florence, KY, USA.
**CV-04301; Arrow International Inc., Reading, PA, USA.
††1610; MILA International, Florence, KY, USA.
‡‡1006; MILA International, Florence, KY, USA.
§§1212; MILA International, Florence, KY, USA.
***Hibiscrub; Mölnlycke Health Care, Dunstable, UK.
†††628H, Ethilon Nylon, Ethicon, Somerville, NJ, USA.
‡‡‡8590; MILA International, Florence, KY, USA.
§§§ET3002 large animal 7 inch extension set; International WIN Ltd., Kennett Square, PA, USA.
****Intra-epicaine; Arnolds Veterinary Products, Shrewsbury, UK; Carbocaine-V; Pfizer Animal Health, New York, NY, USA.

wide should be clipped over the vein and the area should be aseptically prepared, ideally with a chlorhexidine scrub solution. In young and fractious horses, a bleb of local anaesthetic placed subcutaneously at the catheter site may make catheterisation easier. The aseptic scrub should be repeated after the local anaesthetic is deposited. The extension set should be preflushed with sterile saline (with heparin, if required). The catheter should be handled and placed wearing sterile gloves. A small stab incision through the skin can be helpful when using a local anaesthetic or if 10-gauge or Seldinger ("over the wire") catheters are used. For fluid therapy, the catheter should be directed towards the heart. For collection of blood for transfusion into another animal, the catheter should be pointed up the vein, away from the heart.

The vein is raised with the knuckle of the nondominant hand at the bottom edge of the prepared site. The catheter and stylet are held at the hubs between the thumb and second and third fingers of the dominant hand (Figure 1.33). The point of the stylet should be closest to the skin of the horse (bevel pointing outwards). The stylet is pushed through the skin (or stab incision, if made) at approximately 30 to 40° to the skin (Figure 1.33). The catheter and stylet are advanced until it feels like they have pushed through into the vein. At this point, there should be a momentary pause in advancing the catheter, and the hub of the stylet should be observed for blood to confirm correct placement into the vein. If blood is not seen, the catheter and stylet should be withdrawn slightly and redirected. Once blood is seen, the angle is flattened so that the catheter is approximately 10° to the skin (Figure 1.34). The catheter and stylet are advanced about 5 to 10 mm within the lumen of the vessel. The hub is again observed for blood.

The nondominant hand is then used to hold the stylet. It is important to keep the stylet absolutely still at this point. The dominant hand is used to advance the catheter down off the stylet and into the vein (Figure 1.35). A common error is to advance the stylet too far, through the other side of the vein. The catheter hub is seated against the skin, and the stylet is completely withdrawn and discarded. The vein should again be raised at this point to both check the correct placement of the catheter and prevent air aspiration. The extension set or, if preferred, an injection cap should be connected to the catheter.

The author prefers to fix the catheter in place with a cruciate suture. Other clinicians may prefer two simple interrupted sutures. Whichever suture pattern is used, it is important to place the sutures a couple of millimetres below (in the case of downward pointing catheters) or above (for upward catheters) the hub. This acts to pull the catheter towards the entry site and prevents movement of

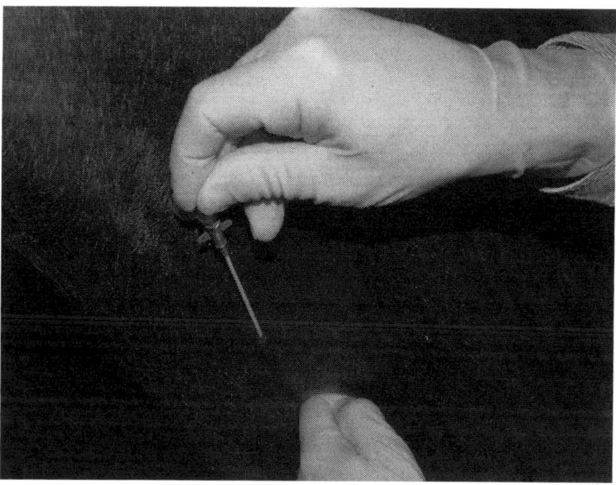

Figure 1.34 Once into the vein lumen, the catheter is flattened towards the neck, and advanced 5 to 10 mm. ©Kevin Corley 2007.

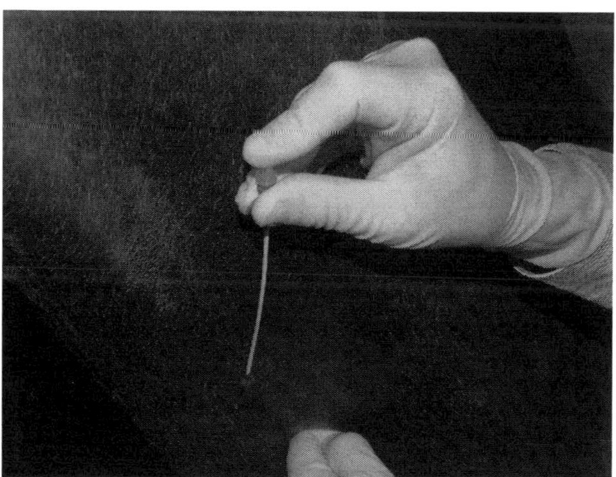

Figure 1.33 Pushing an over-the-needle catheter through the skin over the jugular vein. Unless a stab incision has been made, reasonable force needs to be used to push through the skin. ©Kevin Corley 2007.

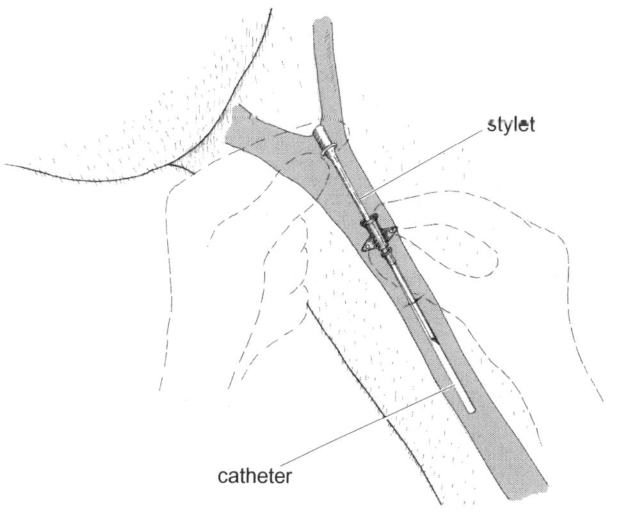

Figure 1.35 Sliding the catheter off the stylet, and into the vein.

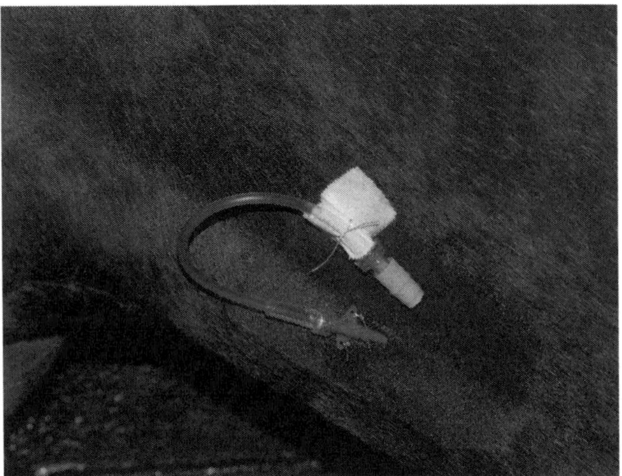

Figure 1.36 Jugular catheter with extension set. ©Kevin Corley 2007.

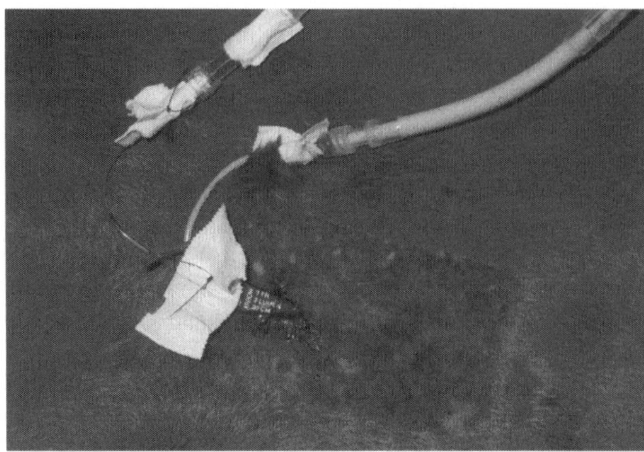

Figure 1.37 Double-lumen catheter in the jugular vein of an adult horse. ©Kevin Corley 2000.

the catheter in and out of the skin, which can promote entry of bacteria to the subcutaneous tissues or the vein. Catheters for very short-term use can be fixed with instant bonding glue.

If an injection cap was used whilst the catheter was being secured, it should now be replaced by an extension set. An extension set reduces movement of the catheter in the vein during administration of injections. If the extension set does not include a one-way valve, it should be clamped during placement to prevent air aspiration into the vein. The extension set should be set in a curve and sutured dorsal to the entry site (Figure 1.36). Placing zinc oxide tape on the extension set, close to its hub, is an easy way to affix it to the horse and prevent it from slipping. The suture is through the zinc oxide "butterfly" from outside to inside on one side of the extension set, through the skin beneath the extension set and back out through the zinc oxide tape on the other side of the extension set. This is then tied with a surgeon's knot.

After placement, the catheter should be flushed with sterile saline or heparinised saline.

Placement of an over-the-wire catheter

Placing an over-the-wire catheter is very similar to placement in the foal. A brief description is given here, but readers are referred to Chapter 2.6 for a more detailed explanation and to Figure 2.16 for identification of the parts of an over-the-wire catheter kit.

Following sterile preparation of the catheter site and placement of local anaesthetic under the skin, the vein is raised with the knuckles of the nondominant hand. Prior to raising the vein, for catheter kits without a dilator, and in ponies and donkeys with thick skin, a small stab incision should be made through the skin over the centre of vein. The needle is placed through the skin at an angle of 30° to 40°. When blood is seen, the needle is changed to an angle of 5° to 10° and advanced to the hub. The wire, having previously been slightly withdrawn into the assembly so that it is flush with the tip, is advanced through the needle, leaving 5 to 10 cm of wire exposed. It is crucial in the adult standing horse not to let go of the wire, as gravity may take the wire completely into the vein. The needle is withdrawn out of the skin and completely off the wire. The dilator is threaded onto the wire and pushed through the skin (may need to be twisted slightly) and to the hub. The dilator is then withdrawn, leaving the wire in place. The catheter is carefully threaded onto the wire, making sure that it makes no contact with the skin or hair of the animal. It is threaded down the wire, until it is seated to the hub. The wire is withdrawn and discarded. An injection cap should be placed on the catheter or extension sets, or the extension sets clamped to prevent aspiration. The catheter hub and extension sets are then sutured to the skin of the animal. If a double-lumen catheter is being used, both extension tubes should be sutured to the animal, one above the other (Figure 1.37). After placement, the catheter (both lumens, if relevant) should be flushed with sterile saline or heparinised saline.

1.15 Catheterisation of the cephalic and lateral thoracic veins

Kevin Corley

If one jugular vein is thrombosed or occluded, it is inadvisable to catheterise the contralateral jugular vein and risk bilateral jugular thrombosis, which can result in life-threatening swelling of the head. The cephalic and lateral thoracic veins carry less serious consequences if they become occluded through thrombophlebitis. However, the maximum fluid rate attainable in these smaller veins (approximately 5 L/hr in adult horses) is less than that attainable in the jugular vein. Furthermore, infectious thrombophlebitis may be serious at any site.

Box 1.17. Equipment for placing a lateral thoracic or cephalic catheter

Suitable catheters

- 14-Gauge single-lumen 20-cm (8-inch) over-the-wire catheter*
- 16-Gauge single-lumen 20-cm (8-inch) over-the-wire catheter†
- 14-Gauge 13-cm (5.25-inch) over-the-needle polyurethane catheter‡
- 16-Gauge, 13-cm (5.25-inch) over-the-needle polyurethane catheter§

Other required equipment

Clippers with a fine (No. 40) blade
Small gauze swabs (4 × 4) soaked in chlorhexidine (4%) scrub solution**
Small gauze swabs (4 × 4) soaked in surgical spirit (alcohol)
2-0 Nonabsorbable monofilament suture on a straight needle††
20–30-ml syringe of 0.9% sterile saline (±5 units/ml heparin)
No. 15 scalpel blade
Mepivacaine 2%‡‡: 2 ml drawn up in a 2–3 ml syringe with a 23–25-gauge needle
High-flow extension set§§, if not supplied with catheter
Injection cap (if not supplied in catheter kit)
7.5-cm (3-inch) wide stretchy adhesive dressing (Elastoplast***/Elastikon†††)
1 Sterile small gauze swab (4 × 4)
Surgical gloves
Zinc oxide tape
Bandage scissors

Optional

75-cm (30-inch) fluid extension set§§§
Ultrasound machine with a 6–12-MHz linear array or linear probe
Twitch
Sedation

*CS-04701, Arrow International Inc., Reading, PA, USA;1410; MILA International, Florence, KY, USA.
†CV-04301, Arrow International Inc., Reading, PA, USA; 1610, MILA International, Florence, KY, USA.
‡1411, MILA International, Florence, KY, USA.
§1611, MILA International, Florence, KY, USA.
**Hibiscrub; Mölnlycke Health Care, Dunstable, UK.
††628H, Ethilon Nylon; Ethicon, Somerville, NJ, USA.
‡‡Intra-epicaine; Arnolds Veterinary Products, Shrewsbury, UK; Carbocaine-V; Pfizer Animal Health, New York, NY, USA.
§§8590, MILA International, Florence, KY, USA.
***Johnson and Johnson, New Brunswick, NJ, USA.
†††Beiersdorf AG, Hamburg, Germany.
§§§2C5645, Baxter Healthcare, Deerfield, IL, USA.

Equipment needed

The equipment needed is given in Box 1.17. It is much easier to catheterise these veins with an over-the-wire catheter than with the over-the-needle technique. For cephalic catheters, the flexible over-the-wire catheters are much less likely to kink with leg movement than the relatively stiff over-the needle catheters. In the cephalic and lateral thoracic veins, valves can impede the passing of a catheter stylet or wire. Ultrasonography can help identify the lateral thoracic vein, which can be otherwise hard to find in fatter horses.

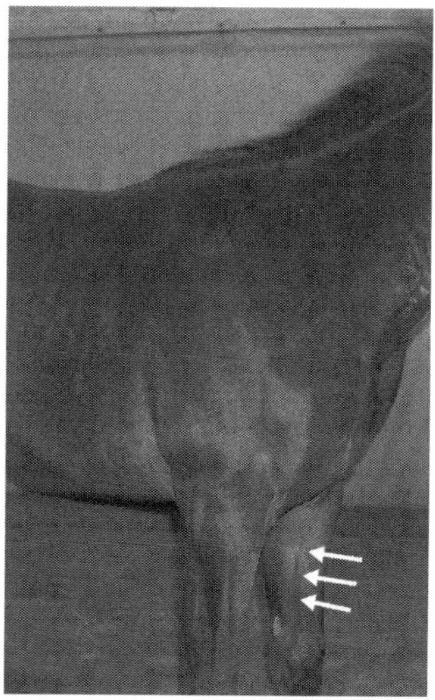

Figure 1.38 Site of the cephalic vein (*arrows*). ©Kevin Corley 2007.

Cephalic vein

The cephalic vein runs along the medial side of the upper foreleg (Figure 1.38). Not all patients are tractable for placement of a cephalic catheter. Good sedation is required (see Chapter 6.1). The author has anaesthetised 2- to 5-month-old foals with a short-acting injectable anaesthetic (ketamine after xylazine premedication) and placed these catheters with the animal in lateral recumbency.

The catheter entry site is usually best placed halfway between the midpoint of the medial upper leg and the top of the carpus. The idea is to place the catheter sufficiently far away from the carpus that it is not interfered with by movement of the leg but far enough down the leg so that the majority of the catheter is in the straight part of the vein and not overly interfered with by flexion of the shoulder joint. There is a small risk of infection associated with the catheter entry site spreading to the carpal joints, and this risk is increased if the catheter is placed too close to the carpus. There are small skin vessels in the area of the ideal entry site, and these should be avoided. Once the entry site has been chosen, the area should be clipped and aseptically prepared. A bleb of local anaesthetic should be placed over the vein (Figure 1.39), and a second bleb may be placed where it is anticipated that the extension set will be sutured to the leg.

The vein is raised above the entry site, and the needle is placed into the vein. The vein is very superficial in this area, and the needle should be placed at a flat angle to the leg (Figure 1.40). The needle does not need to be advanced all the way to the hub. The wire is fed into the needle, and the wire assembly discarded. This leaves a small amount of wire exposed out of the needle (Figure 1.40). The needle is

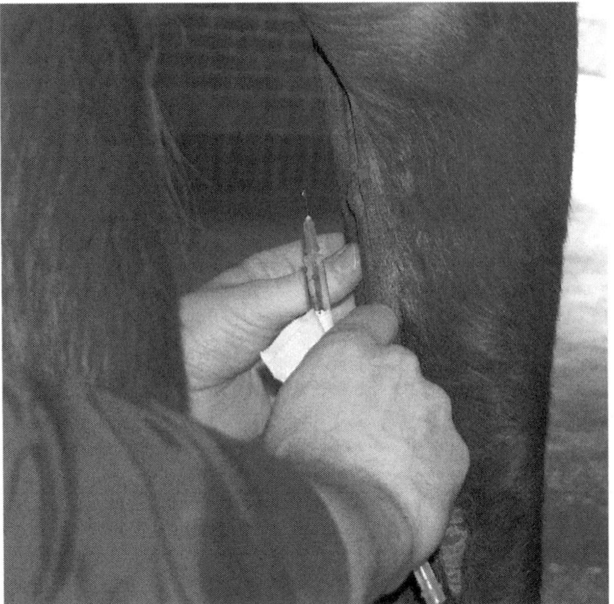

Figure 1.39 Placing local anaesthetic over the catheter entry site for a cephalic catheter. ©Kevin Corley 2003.

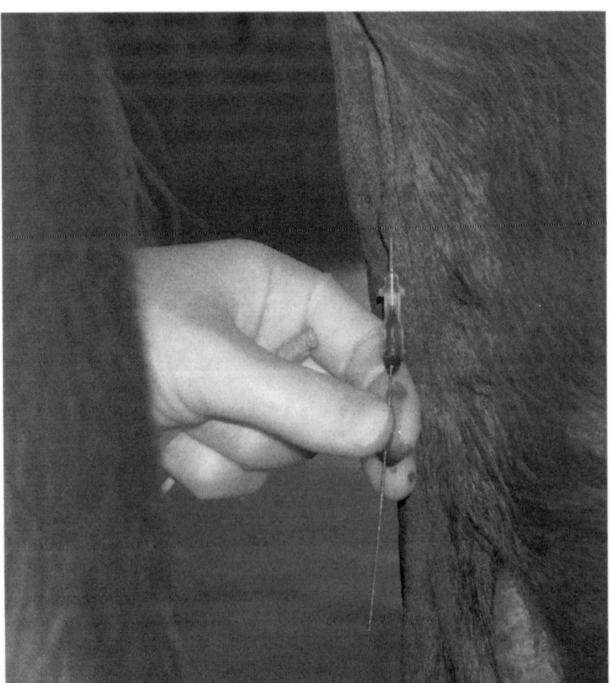

Figure 1.40 The needle is placed into the vein, and the wire is fed into the needle. ©Kevin Corley 2003.

then withdrawn with the wire, until the needle is completely out of the leg. The wire is grasped on the leg side of the needle, and the needle is pulled off the wire and discarded. In catheter designs with a dilator, this should then be fed up the wire and pushed through the skin into the vein (Figure 1.41). The dilator should be pushed up to its hub, and then withdrawn off the wire, leaving the wire in place. It is usual for the entry site to bleed reasonably profusely when the dilator is removed.

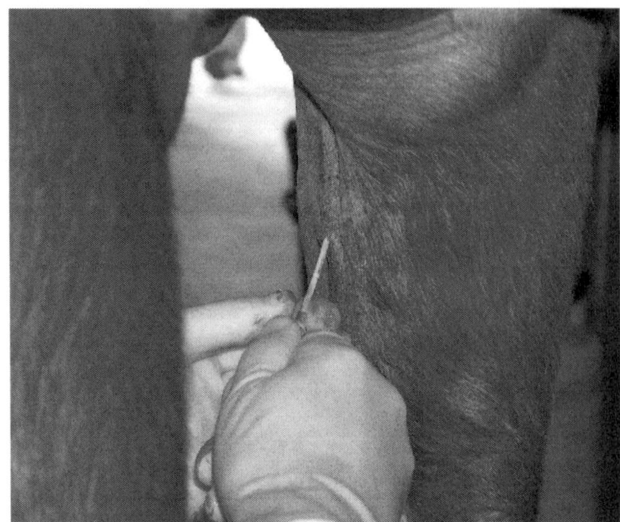

Figure 1.41 The dilator is fed up the wire, and pushed through the skin into the vein. ©Kevin Corley 2003.

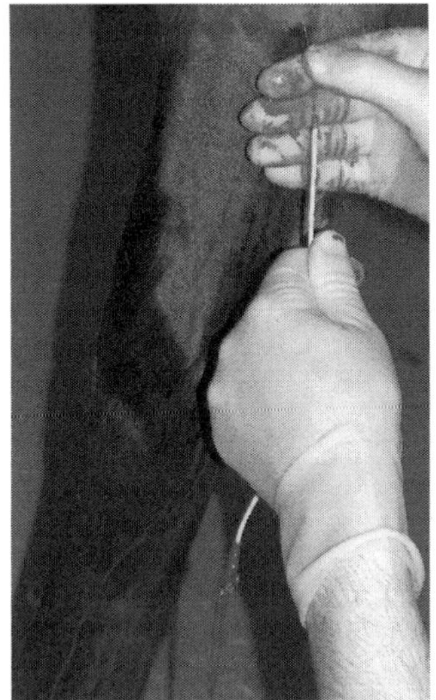

Figure 1.42 The catheter is fed up the wire, and into the vein up to the hub. ©Kevin Corley 2003.

The catheter is then carefully lifted out of the pack, taking care not to accidentally contaminate it. It is usually easiest to lift the catheter out of the box by the hub. The catheter is then threaded onto the wire (Figure 1.42), and into the vein. The catheter is seated to the hub. Some clinicians chose to suture the catheter hub to the leg at this point, before removing the wire. Other clinicians remove the wire, flush the catheter with heparinised saline and then suture the hub. Suturing the hub before removing the wire reduces the time before the catheter is secured, in case the animal moves, but may increase the chance of contamination. The author prefers to suture the catheter with a cruciate suture (Figure 1.43). If the wire was not removed before

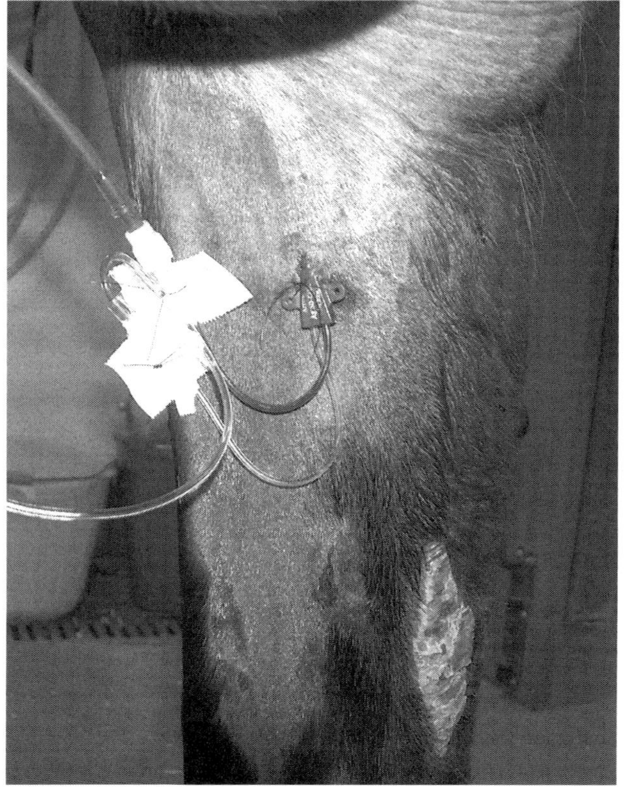

Figure 1.43 The catheter hub is sutured with a cruciate stitch. The extension sets are fixed with a zinc oxide tape "butterfly" sutured to the leg. ©Kevin Corley 2003.

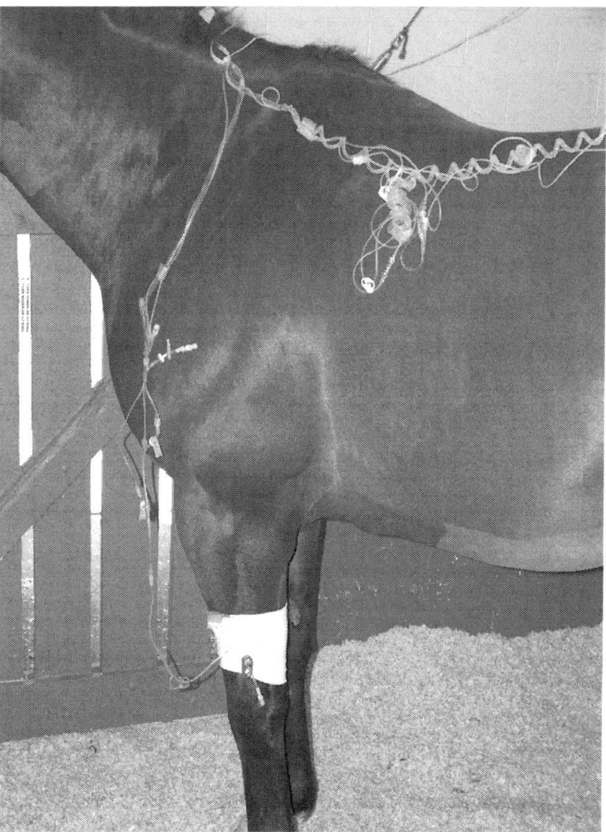

Figure 1.44 Horse connected to fluids, parenteral nutrition and insulin through a double-lumen cephalic catheter. ©Kevin Corley 2004.

suturing the hub, it should be at this point, and the catheter flushed with heparinised saline.

The extension sets should then be secured to the leg. A zinc oxide tape butterfly is placed at the extension set hub, and this is sutured to the leg (see Figure 1.43). It is usually most secure if the suture is placed through the tape on one side of the extension set hub, through the skin and out through the tape on the other side of the hub. If the catheter is to be used to give fluids, a long extension set should be attached and affixed to the mane (Figure 1.44). The catheter hub should be covered with a sterile small gauze swab, and the whole catheter should be wrapped with stretchy adhesive dressing (Elastoplast/Elastikon*).

Lateral thoracic vein

The lateral thoracic vein runs from just behind the elbow caudally along the wall of the ventral thorax (Figure 1.45). It can be hard to identify and has a flat profile, which can make it difficult to pass a catheter into the lumen. The vein is probably best catheterised using an over-the-wire catheter, although over-the-needle catheters can be successfully placed and maintained in this vein.

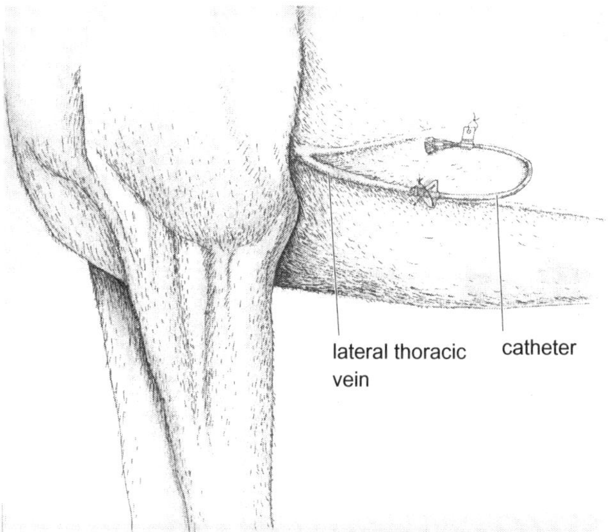

Figure 1.45 Site for catheterisation of the lateral thoracic vein.

The vein is catheterised approximately two handwidths (20 cm) behind the elbow. The vein should be held off on the cranial side of the catheterisation site (Figure 1.46). It can be identified by raising and lowering the vein, gently tapping the site and feeling a fluid-filled tubular structure or by ultrasound (Figure 1.47). The area should be clipped

---

* Johnson and Johnson, New Brunswick, NJ, USA; Beiersdorf AG, Hamburg, Germany.

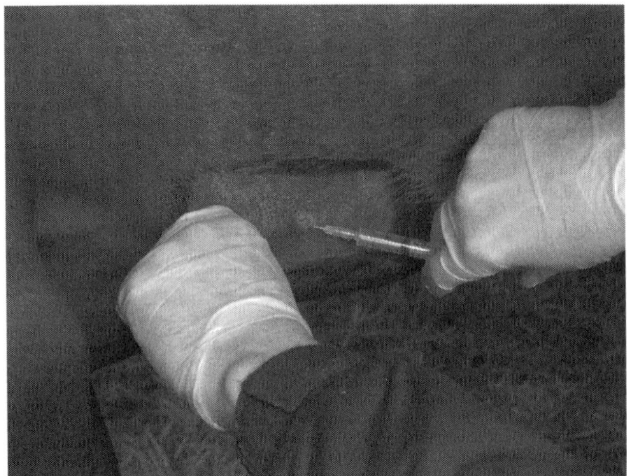

Figure 1.46 Raising the lateral thoracic vein, and placing a local anaesthetic bleb over it. ©Kevin Corley 2007.

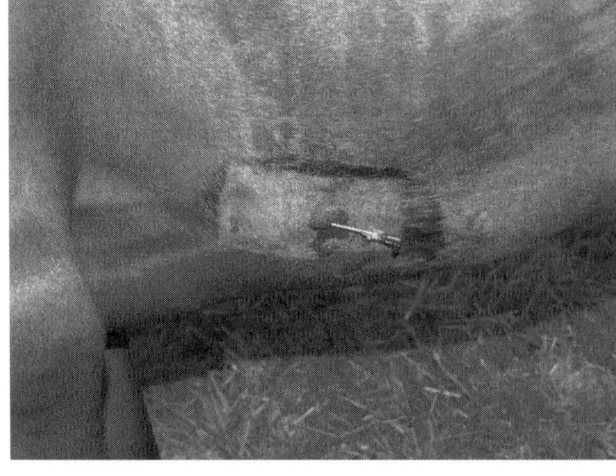

Figure 1.48 The catheter needle in the lateral thoracic vein, dripping blood. ©Kevin Corley 2007.

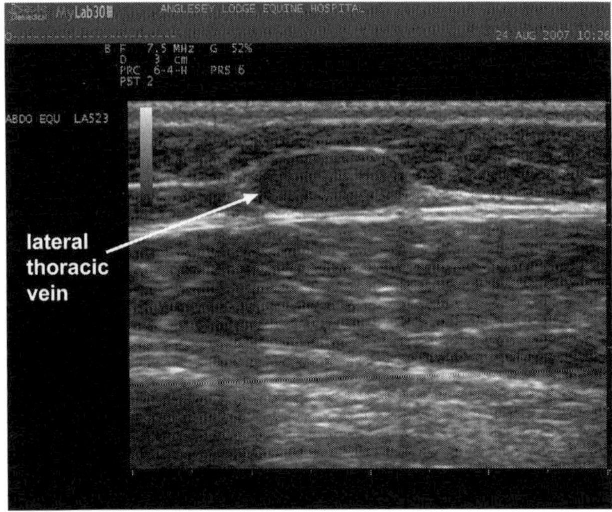

Figure 1.47 Ultrasound of the raised lateral thoracic vein in a horse, using a 7.5-MHz linear probe. ©Kevin Corley 2007.

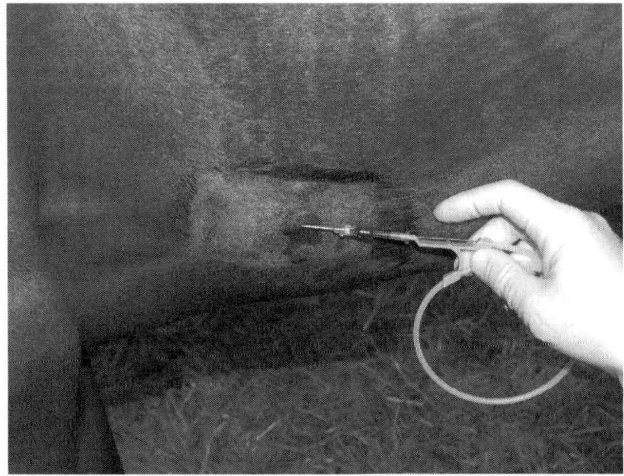

Figure 1.49 The wire is advanced into the needle, taking care not to displace the needle. ©Kevin Corley 2007.

and aseptically prepared. The catheterisation site should be chosen to avoid any obvious skin vessels, and a bleb of local anaesthetic placed over the vein there (Figure 1.46). In catheter kits without a dilator, a small stab incision should be made at this point.

The needle should be placed through the bleb (and stab incision, if present) into the vessel at a flat angle (10° to 20° to the skin), and advanced until blood is continuously dripping from the end (Figure 1.48). The needle does not need to be advanced all the way to the hub. The wire is then advanced into the vein, taking care not to displace the needle (Figure 1.49). The needle is removed, leaving the wire in place. The dilator is then threaded onto the wire, and advanced to its hub through the skin into the vein. Some force may be required to get the dilator to pass through the skin (Figure 1.50). The dilator is removed, leaving the wire in place. The catheter is then fed onto the

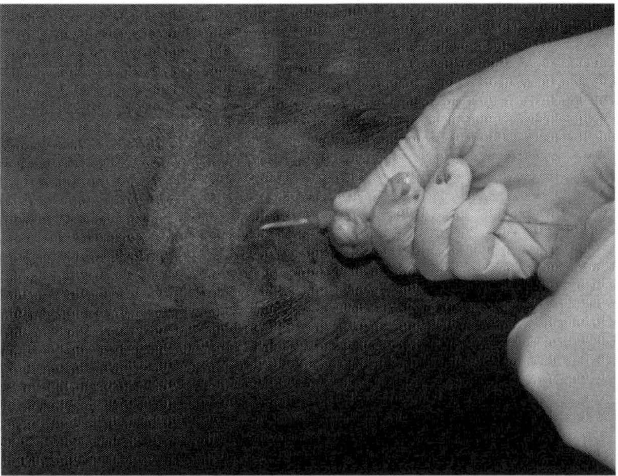

Figure 1.50 The dilator is fed onto the wire, and then pushed through the skin into the vein. It should be buried to the hub, and then removed. ©Kevin Corley 2007.

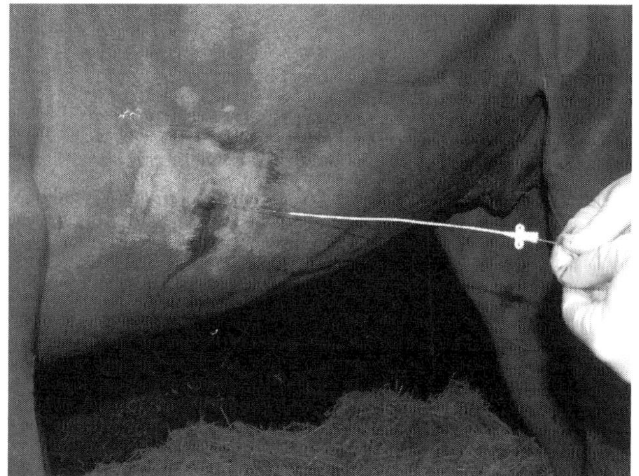

Figure 1.51 The catheter is fed onto the wire. ©Kevin Corley 2007.

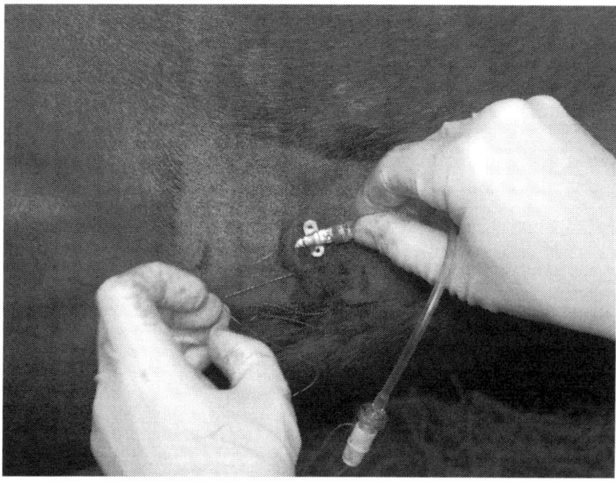

Figure 1.53 The catheter hub is secured to the skin with a cruciate suture. ©Kevin Corley 2007.

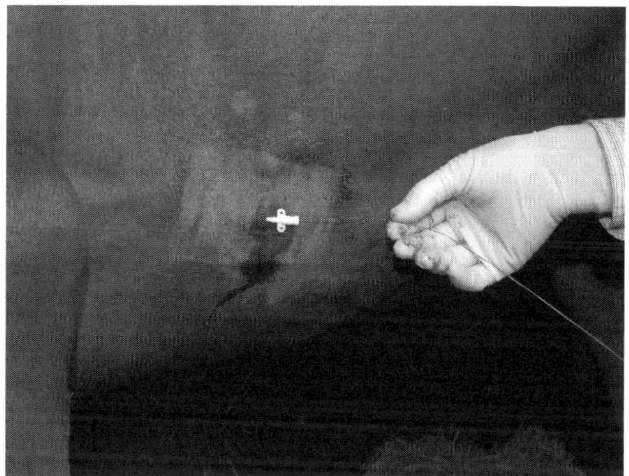

Figure 1.52 Once the catheter is seated into the vein, the wire is removed. ©Kevin Corley 2007.

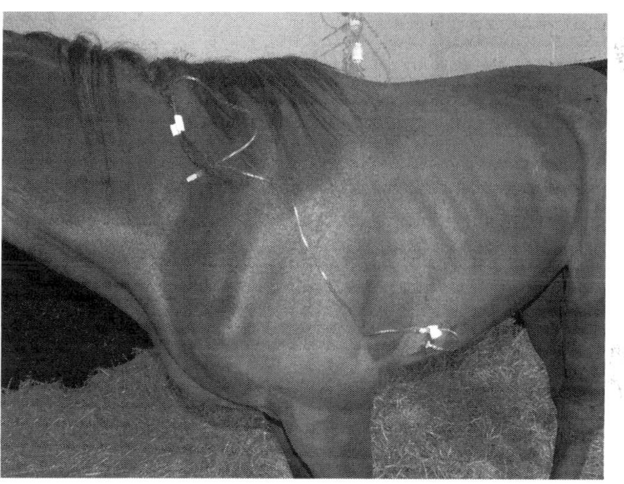

Figure 1.54 A long extension set can be attached to the mane, to allow fluid therapy. ©Kevin Corley 2007.

wire (Figure 1.51), and then advanced into the vein to its hub. Once the catheter is seated, the wire is removed (Figure 1.52). Some clinicians may chose to suture the catheter in place, prior to removing the wire. Other clinicians attach an extension set and injection cap, and flush the catheter prior to suturing, to ensure sterility. The hub is secured to the skin with a cruciate suture (Figure 1.53). A "butterfly" made from zinc oxide tape is put around the hub of the extension set, and this is sutured to the skin. A long extension set can be used to attach the catheter to the mane, for administration of fluids (Figure 1.54). Once the catheter and extension sets have been sutured in place, the catheter should be covered with a small sterile gauze swab and wrapped with stretchy adhesive dressing (Elastoplast/Elastikon) around the thorax of the horse (Figure 1.55).

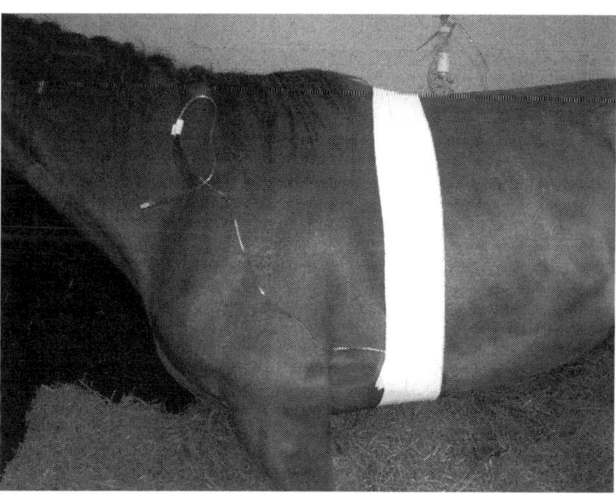

Figure 1.55 The catheter should be covered with a sterile gauze swab wrapped with stretchy adhesive dressing. ©Kevin Corley 2007.

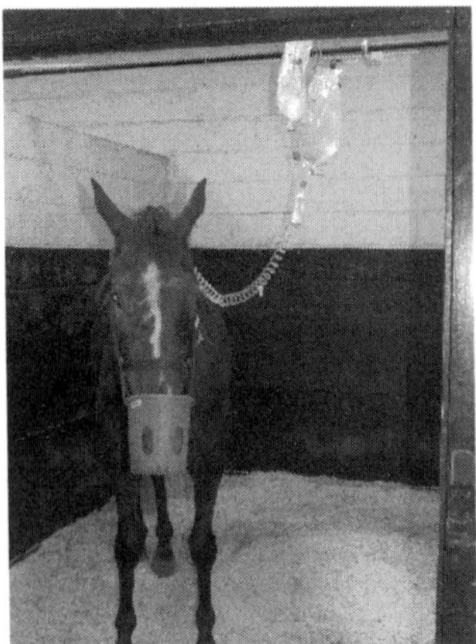

Figure 1.56 Horse on continuous intravenous fluids, using an infusion set with a coil. ©Kevin Corley 2007.

1.16 Fluid administration sets

Kevin Corley

A variety of fluid administration sets are available commercially. For adult horses, sets that include a large drip chamber, a coil so that the horse may move around the box without getting tangled in the set and wide-bore tubing* are most effective (Figure 1.56). Horses often move round the box when attached to fluids, and the fluid line will become twisted and prevent fluids flowing if the fluids are not able to swivel as the horse moves. For this reason, fluid hangers with a swivel mechanism† are highly recommended.

Four fluid bags can be hung simultaneously from one of the fluid hangers. The uppermost bags are connected to the lower bags with a transfer set‡. It is important to make sure that the bags are each hung at the appropriate heights, to ensure that all four bags flow completely into the horse (Figure 1.57).

Infusions of drugs, plasma and other fluids can be added to the drip chamber. The fluid set from these supplementary fluids is connected to a needle, which is inserted through the bung on the top of the drip chamber, and secured with zinc oxide tape (Figure 1.58). Fluid drop rates for various giving sets are given in Table 6.14.

For foals, fluid rates are usually lower and therefore are most accurately controlled with an electronic infusion pump (see Chapter 1.17). An alternative to a pump is a fluid control dial§, which is more accurate for producing lower fluid infusion rates than counting drops in the drip chamber. The giving sets from two fluid pumps can be combined into a single line, either by means of a Y-piece extension set**, or by putting a needle on the end of one giving set and taping it into the injection port on the other. If a coil†† is used between the giving set and the foal, it allows an ambulatory foal to move around the box without getting caught in the fluid line (Figure 1.59) and means

* IV8001S Coiled Primary I.V. Set; International WIN Ltd, Kennett Square, PA, USA.

† HS7003 Gyro Hanger with Supreme Swivel; International WIN Ltd, Kennett Square, PA, USA.

‡ TS2001, IV Transfer Set; International WIN Ltd, Kennett Sq., PA, USA.

§ 175480; MILA International Inc., Florence, KY, USA.

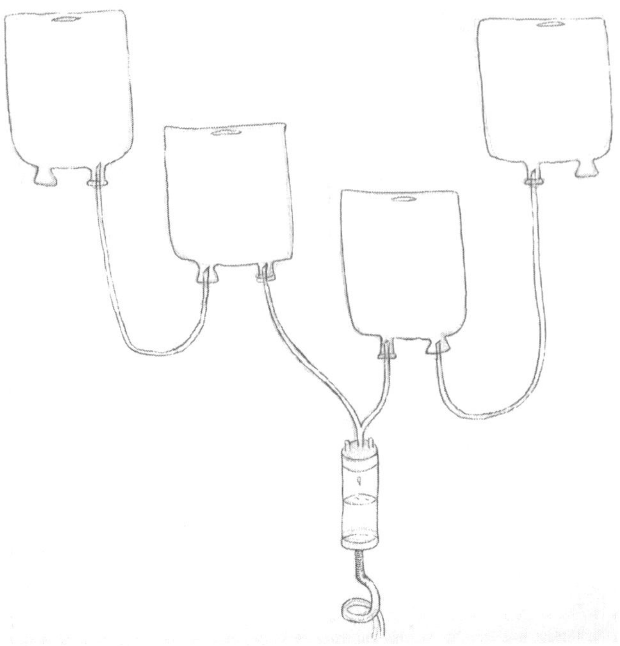

Figure 1.57 Connecting four fluid bags to a giving set with two spikes, using transfer sets.

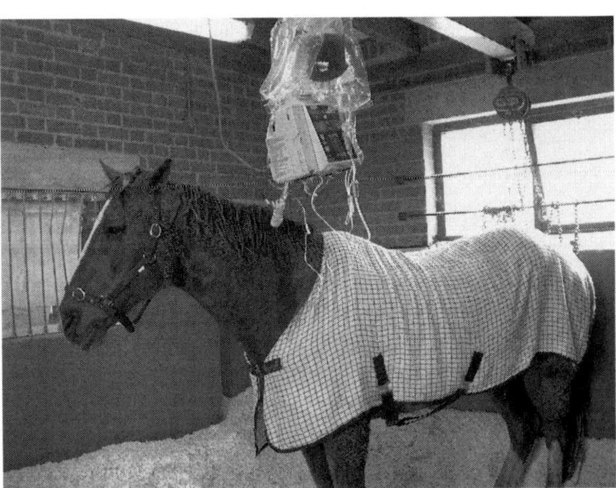

Figure 1.58 Supplementary fluids may be added to the drip chamber by connecting them to the drip chamber. A needle on the end of the drip set from the supplementary fluids can be inserted into the bung on the top of the drip chamber. ©Kevin Corley 2005.

** W21808; Arrow International Inc., Reading, PA, USA.

†† CE 8020S Coiled extension set with swivel; International WIN Ltd, Kennett Square, PA, USA.

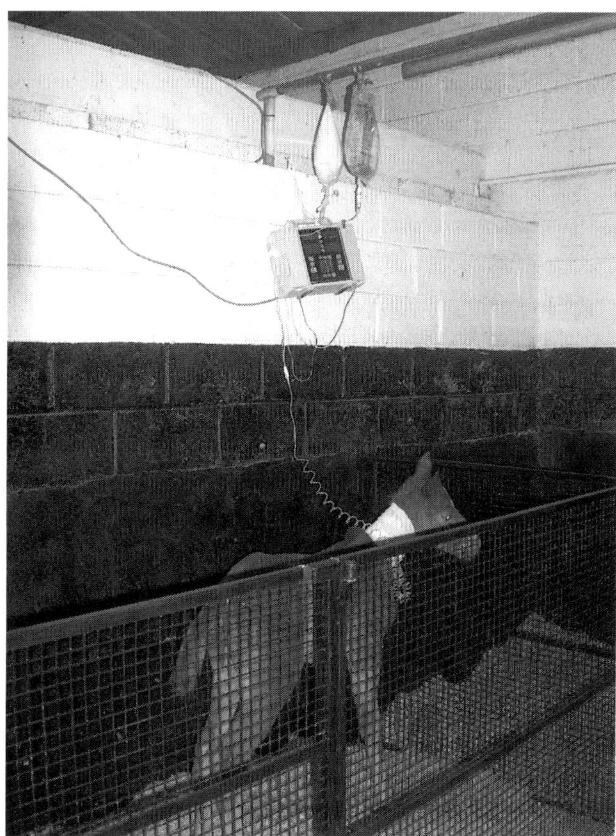

Figure 1.59 A foal connected to a fluid pump. The fluid are delivered through a coil, which allows the foal to move around the cage without getting caught in the fluid line. ©Kevin Corley 2007.

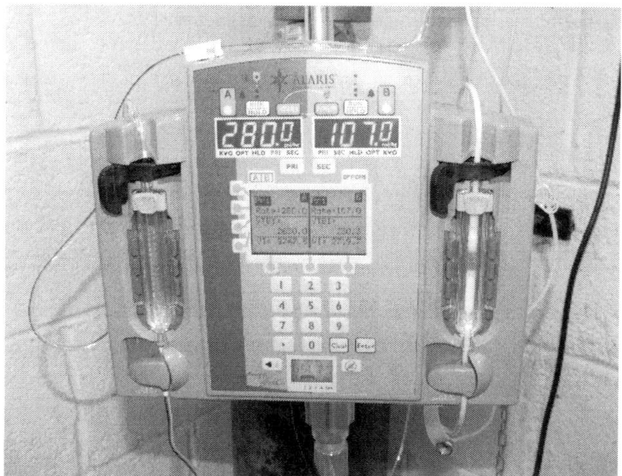

Figure 1.60 Alaris Signature Gold dual-channel pump. ©Kevin Corley 2007.

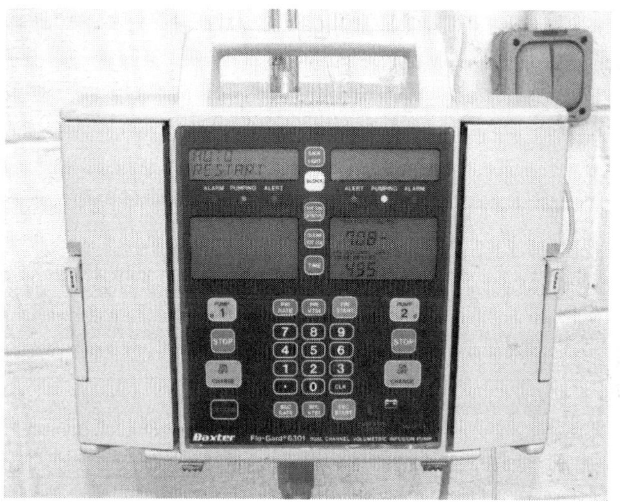

Figure 1.61 Baxter Flo-Gard 6301 dual-channel pump. ©Kevin Corley 2007.

there is less chance of accidentally disconnecting the fluids from a recumbent foal. If there is a mare in the box with the foal, she is likely to break fluid lines to the foal. Placing the foal in a cage (Figure 1.59) or behind a barrier (see Figure 3.5, A and C) can maintain the mare–foal bond but prevent damage to the fluid lines.

1.17 Electronic infusion pumps and syringe drivers

Kevin Corley

Electronic infusion pumps

Electronic infusion pumps are essential for continuous infusions of medication (e.g., lidocaine [lignocaine] infusions for postoperative colics) and very useful for controlled delivery of intravenous fluids. Many different infusion pumps are available, which vary quite considerably in design (Figures 1.60 and 1.61). However, there are some common features of their design and operation.

The part that varies most between pumps is the fluid-giving set, and how it attaches into the pump. Many pumps use proprietary giving sets. These either click into the front of the pump (Figure 1.60) or are fitted behind a door. Other pumps use regular 10 drops/ml or 20 drops/ml giving sets. These are threaded into a channel on the pump either behind a door (Figure 1.62) or on the front of the machine. Before placing the fluid set into the pump or connecting it to the patient, it should be primed with the fluid or drug to be infused, making sure that there is no air in the system. Vented fluid sets need to be used for infusing drugs or fluids in bottles. The cost of the giving sets is an important factor to consider when purchasing or renting a pump.

Basic operation of pumps

The basic operation of the pumps is broadly similar for all pumps. Before starting the pump, a rate (ml/hr) and volume to be infused (VTBI; see Box 1.18) need to be set. In some dual-channel pumps, the side of the pump ("Pump 1" or "Pump 2") needs to be selected before the rate or

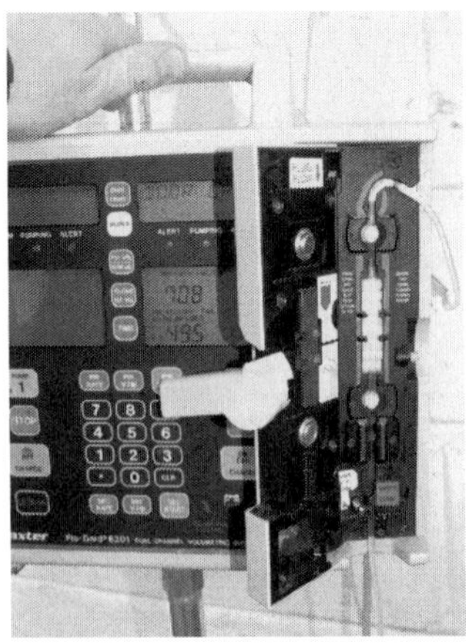

Figure 1.62 The fluid set is pressed into the fluid channel in the Baxter Flo-Gard 6301 pump. The safety clamp prevents flow of fluids when the door is open, and must be clicked open to insert or remove a giving set. ©Kevin Corley 2007.

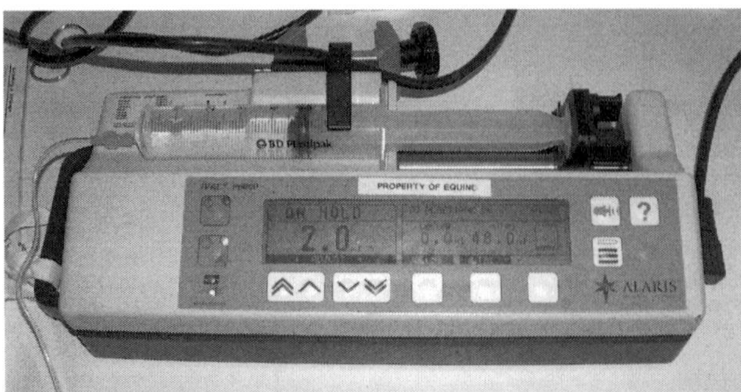

Figure 1.63 Alaris IVAC P6000 syringe driver. ©Kevin Corley 2004.

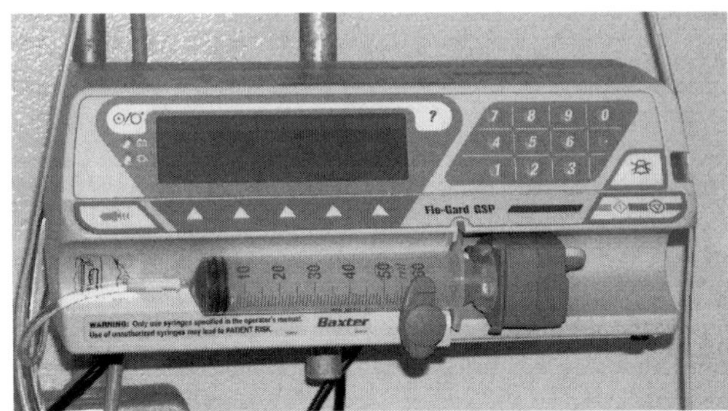

Figure 1.64 Baxter Flo-Gard GSP syringe driver. ©Kevin Corley 2006.

Box 1.18: Abbreviations used on electronic infusion pumps

VTBI = volume to be infused (i.e. what is left in the fluid bag)

VI = volume infused (can be over several fluid bags)
Called TOT VOL on some pumps

PRI = primary settings
SEC = secondary settings
PRI and SEC are used to deliver a set volume at one rate, and then automatically change the rate for the remainder of the infusion. With special infusion sets, the SEC and PRI can be of different fluids.

KVO = keep vein open
After the set volume has been infused, this continues infusion at a low rate (usually 5ml/hr) to prevent occlusion of the catheter. It is usually accompanied by an audible warning

HLD = hold (pump is paused)

VTBI button is pressed, and the number entered. For basic operation, the primary (PRI) VTBI and rate buttons are used. Other pumps require an "Enter" button to be pressed to complete numerical entry of the rate and VTBI. If the total volume to be infused is greater than the volume of the fluid bag, the VTBI should be set to a volume just less than the bag size. The machine will then alarm before the bag is empty, preventing air entering the fluid line and allowing another bag to be prepared in time to maintain an unbroken infusion. Many pumps go into KVO ("keep vein open") mode (Box 1.18) and alarm when the infusion is complete. As the pump infuses, the remaining VTBI will be displayed and counted down. The pump will also display the rate of infusion and may display the volume infused and the pressure in the line between the pump and the patient.

Syringe drivers

Syringe drivers are extremely useful for controlled continuous delivery of drugs. There are two advantages of using a syringe pump over adding the drug in question to a bag of fluids. The first is that a far lower volume of dilute drug can be used, allowing smaller amounts of drug to be opened and diluted. This is especially useful when first starting a horse on a drug, to avoid opening a large amount of drug when its effectiveness is uncertain. The second advantage is that much lower rates of infusion are possible, which avoids excessive combined fluid rates in neonatal foals when multiple continuous infusions are necessary. Examples of drugs that the author routinely uses a syringe driver for are insulin, dobutamine and norepinephrine.

Most designs of syringe driver are broadly similar in design (Figures 1.63 and 1.64). The flanges at the end of the syringe barrel are inserted into the notches or groove. The end of the plunger is inserted into the clamp. There is a release that allows the clamp to be moved up and down, so that the end of the plunger is held by the clamp. It is important to have the syringe flat in the groove, with the graduations showing (Figures 1.63 and 1.64). A side-arm clamp is then twisted across the syringe, to keep it in place. Modern syringe drivers will then read out the manufacturer and volume of the syringe. If this is not correct, the syringe should be carefully repositioned. It is advisable to connect narrow (low-volume) fluid extension sets to the syringe pump, if a low rate of infusion is to be used, to ensure accurate delivery.

The basic operation of syringe drivers is similar to that of infusion pumps. Before connecting the lines to the patient, they should be primed. Most pumps have a purge or prime button to allow brief rapid infusion for this purpose. After pressing the button, it may be necessary to confirm this action by pressing other buttons under the screen, as directed by the display. The rate of infusion and VTBI should be set, and then the pump may be started.

Alarms

Pumps and syringe drivers may alarm for a variety of reasons. Blockages to the flow of fluids will cause an alarm. Many pumps will distinguish between blockages between the fluid bag and the pump ("Upstream occlusion") and those between the fluid pump and patient ("Downstream occlusion" or "Occlusion Patient-side" or just "Occlusion"). Syringe drivers can only have downstream occlusions. Upstream occlusions are usually easily remedied by checking the line between the bag and the pump, making sure all fluid sliders and stoppers are open, and, if necessary, raising the height of the fluid bag relative to the pump.

Downstream occlusions can be much harder to solve, and more frustrating. The first response is to methodically check the fluid line between the pump and horse for any kinks or twists that could be causing a restriction. If this is unsuccessful, the catheter and extension set should be carefully checked. This will involve disconnecting the fluid line (and capping it to keep it sterile) and flushing the catheter with sterile saline or heparinised saline. If the catheter does not flush very easily, it and the extension set should be carefully checked. If the catheter has been wrapped with Elastoplast/Elastikon, this needs to be removed to completely check the catheter. If there is no twist or kink to the catheter or extension set outside the skin and flushing does not clear the blockage, the catheter will need to be replaced. It may also need to be replaced if it has become kinked or displaced. If the catheter does flush easily, then the fluid lines should be double-checked and reconnected. The most frustrating downstream occlusions are those that occur when a horse or foal with a jugular catheter is standing with its head down, but not when the head is raised (often called "positional catheters"). Sometimes increasing the acceptable pressure limit for the pump can cure this problem. In some pumps and syringe drivers, this can be done from the normal running screen. In other pumps, an "occlusion level" can be permanently changed for the pump in the configuration screen, prior to operation. More often, the problem persists or returns after the pressure level has been increased. Replacing the catheter with another jugular catheter may not cure the problem, and the author has found that placing a cephalic catheter (see Chapter 1.15) almost always eliminates this problem.

Another common alarm is for air bubbles in the fluid line ("air in line" or "air"). Often, pumps made for the human medicine market are by default very sensitive to any possible air. This is not necessary for horses, and in many pumps this sensitivity can be permanently changed in the configuration or setup screen. The first response to an air alarm is to check the fluid line and find the air. If there is a significant bubble, the fluid set should be disconnected from the patient and run through (or purged) to remove the air. It is important not to break sterility, or forget to clamp the remaining line to the patient, during this procedure. It is often possible to avoid disconnecting the patient by placing a needle through a giving port in the line, clamping the line below the giving port and running the air out of the needle. Some clinicians elect to run small air bubbles just past the pump and its air detector and then restart the pump to allow the bubble to run into the patient, with no apparent ill effects. Air embolisms can clearly cause serious pathology and death, and therefore this approach is not without risk. It is also important to remember that allowing fluids to run for a few seconds to clear the air will give the patient a small bolus of the drug being infused, and therefore is not appropriate if a high concentration of drug is being infused at a slow rate. Occasionally, pumps will continually alarm for air when there is no air in the giving set. This appears to be due to changed refraction by the wall of the giving set. Replacing the giving set is the most effective way of dealing with this problem. Occasionally, the problem can be solved by cleaning the outside of the fluid set with surgical spirit or, for pumps that use regular giving sets, changing the part of the giving set that is in the pump.

Other alarms on pumps and syringe drivers are activated when the VTBI has been reached (often, this is a different sounding alarm), when the battery is running low when disconnected from the mains, when the fluid set is incorrectly set or the door is open and when there is a malfunction.

Advanced operation

Advanced operations can differ between makes and models of pumps and syringe drivers. Many modern pumps and drivers will allow programmed dose rates. For these, the clinician enters the amount of drug in the bag or syringe and the volume it was diluted in or the concentration of the drug. The weight of the patient can be entered, if appropriate to the drug dose regime. The dose rate and units (e.g., units/kg/hr) are selected, and the pump automatically selects the infusion rate. The dose rate is displayed, and this can be adjusted up or down, rather than directly adjusting the infusion rate. Some pumps will also allow a secondary infusion (SEC; see Box 1.18), which automatically switches to a primary infusion when complete.

1.18 Blood and plasma transfusion

Anna Hammond

Whole blood or plasma transfusion is simple to perform, requires no expensive equipment and is potentially life saving. It should be considered early in the disease progression. Suitable donors are described in Box 1.19. Because of the difficulty in reliably cross matching blood in the horse,[1] it is ideal if potential donors have been blood-typed in advance. Unfortunately, with the advent of DNA typing to establish parentage in Thoroughbred horses, only a few laboratories are offering this service (e.g., Weatherbys Ireland, Irish Equine Centre, Johnstown, Naas, Co. Kildare, Ireland).

Equipment needed

The equipment needed is listed in Box 1.20. A 10-gauge catheter is useful for rapid collection of blood from the donor but carries a higher risk of damage to the vein and thrombophlebitis.

Procedure

The collection system consists of two bags—a 3-L bag for collection of the blood and a 2-L bag for separation of plasma (Figure 1.65). The connection between the 2- and 3-L bags is blocked. A 14-gauge needle is placed on the end of the collection tube, and this is inserted into the bag of anticoagulant to transfer the contents to the 3-L bag. A 10- to 12-gauge catheter is placed into the jugular vein of the donor with the tip pointing up the vein (towards the head), in a sterile manner (see Chapter 1.14). The catheter can be fixed with instant bonding glue, or a suture. Once blood is flowing from the catheter, the collection tube is attached to the catheter. Some clinicians elect to put an injection cap on the end of the catheter and use a 14-gauge needle through this injection cap to collect the blood into the collection tube. The advantage of this system is that if the donor horse moves suddenly, the needle will come out of the injection cap, rather than the catheter out of the vein.

Up to 20% of the blood volume can be safely collected from the donor. Blood volume is approximately 7% to 9% of body weight. Usually either 6 or 9 L is collected. Holding off the vein below the catheter can increase blood flow. During collection, the bag should be gently inverted on several occasions to optimise mixing with anticoagulant. It is very important to completely fill each bag of blood.

Box 1.19. Properties of an ideal donor for blood or plasma transfusion

Body weight over 400 kg
It is usually safe to take 1.5% of body weight as blood. Lighter horses may be used if only a small amount of blood is required.

Free of infectious disease
Several diseases, including equine infectious anaemia, have been inadvertently spread through blood transfusions.

Male
Female horses may have been sensitised to other blood groups via parturition. Female horses where the complete history is known, that cannot have been pregnant, are potentially suitable donors.

Never have received a transfusion
Animals that have received a blood or plasma transfusion could potentially have been sensitised to red cell antigens. However, it is rarely possible to know the complete history of a horse.

Blood-type matching the recipient
Cross matching is difficult in the horse, because of the propensity of horse blood to auto-agglutinate.
Horses that do not have the Aa and Qa antigens on their red cells are the recipients most likely to have a transfusion reaction on unmatched blood. Therefore, donors should be Aa and Qa negative, if possible. Cold-blooded (draught-type) horses are most likely to be Aa and Qa negative.

Not used as a blood donor in the past 3 weeks
Donor horses take approximately 3 weeks to recover red cell numbers and packed cell volume after donation.

Box 1.20. Equipment for blood or plasma transfusion

For collection from the donor
Blood collection kit* (see Figure 1.65)

- With acid citrate phosphate dextrose (ACD) anticoagulant
- Citrate-phosphate-dextrose with added adenine (CPDA-1) is preferable as an anticoagulant for longer-term storage

14-Gauge needle
10-Gauge† or 12-gauge‡ catheter
Clippers with a fine (No. 40) blade
Small gauze swabs (4 × 4) soaked in chlorhexidine (4%) scrub solution§
Small gauze swabs (4 × 4) soaked in surgical spirit (alcohol)
10–20-ml syringe of 0.9% sterile saline (±5 units/ml heparin)
Instant-bonding glue or suture
Injection cap
No. 15 scalpel blade

For infusion into the recipient
Venous catheter (see Chapter 1.14 or 1.15)
Blood giving set with an in-line filter**

*Arnolds Veterinary Products, Shrewsbury, UK.
†1006; MILA International, Florence, KY, USA.
‡1212; MILA International, Florence, KY, USA.
§Hibiscrub; Mölnlycke Health Care, Dunstable, UK.
**Aqufarm veterinary blood administration set; Animalcare Ltd., York, UK.

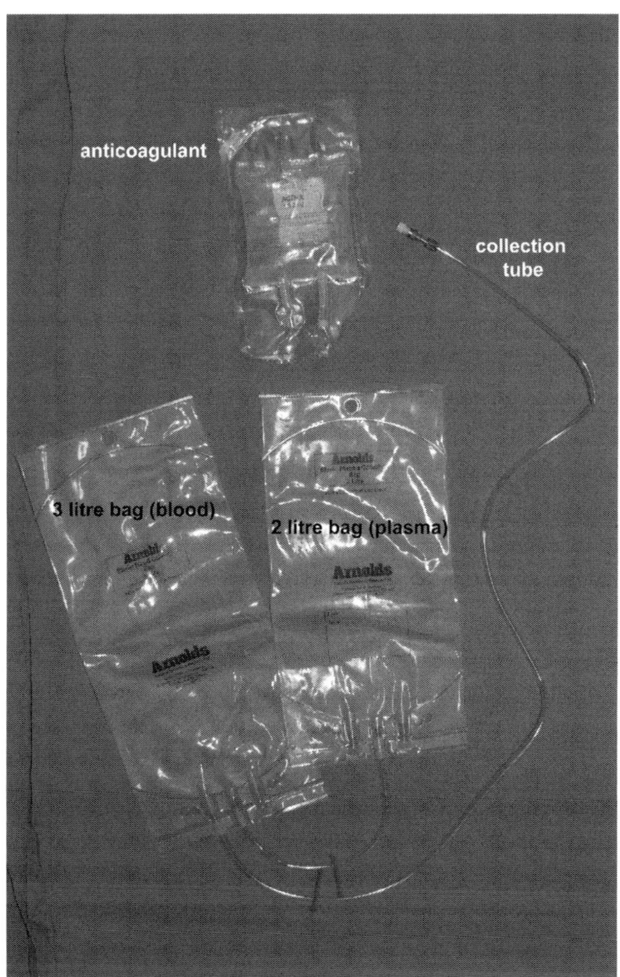

Figure 1.65 Parts of a plasma collection kit. ©Kevin Corley 2007.

Underfilling the bag can lead to an excess of anticoagulant. Excess citrate can result in toxicity in the recipient.[2] The initial clinical sign is muscle fasciculations,[3] which can progress to clinical hypocalcaemia. The clinical signs of hypocalcaemia in the horse include synchronous diaphragmatic flutter, tetany, muscle spasm and seizures (see Chapter 6.5). This should be treated with calcium gluconate or borogluconate (0.1 to 0.5 ml/kg of 40% calcium borogluconate or 0.2 to 1.0 ml/kg of 23% calcium gluconate, repeated if necessary: see also Chapter 6.5 and Table 6.16).

Separation of plasma

If plasma is to be used, the contents of the bag are left to separate (ideally in the fridge). The tube between the 2- and 3-L bags should be uppermost and clamped. The cellular components should be allowed to settle (around 4 to 6 hours; overnight if time allows). Plasma stored for longer than 6 hours may have decreased concentrations of some clotting factors (see Chapter 8.2). Once the cells have settled sufficiently, the bag can be gently squeezed from the bottom to decant the plasma into the 2-L bag. This can be done with the bag against using a large book to exert a steady pressure. Alternatively, a homemade device can be used (Figures 1.66 and 1.67). It is impossible to obtain plasma by this method without a small amount of erythrocyte contamination.

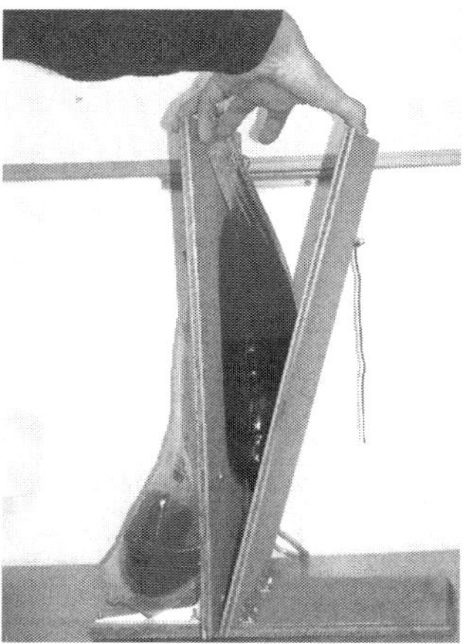

Figure 1.66 Separation of plasma using a homemade device. ©Kevin Corley 2006.

An alternative to this method of collection is to use commercially made plasma*. Plasma from reputable sources will be tested free of disease and will have the correct ratio of anticoagulant to plasma. It is also tested for antibodies against equine red blood cell antigens. It may also contain increased concentrations of antibodies to certain pathogenic organisms (hyperimmune plasma). However, it can be expensive to purchase and may still result in adverse reactions.

Administration

Collected blood or plasma is immediately transfused via a blood-giving set. The pulse, respiratory rate and rectal temperature of the recipient should be noted prior to starting the transfusion. If the clinical status of the recipient permits, the first 200 ml should be given over 30 minutes, the patient being closely monitored for signs of a transfusion reaction. Even if the recipient is in urgent need of the transfusion, only a small amount should be given in the first 5 minutes, monitoring the patient carefully during this time. The remainder may be given at a high rate, bearing in mind the risk and monitoring for adverse reactions. Transfusion reactions are usually manifested by urticaria, tachycardia, tachypnoea, dyspnoea or colic. If these signs occur, the transfusion is stopped. The patient may require analgesic drugs or corticosteroids. If an anaphylactic reaction occurs, isotonic fluids should be rapidly infused and epinephrine administered.

* Veterinary Immunogenics Ltd, Penrith, Cunbria, UK; Plasvac USA, Templeton, CA, USA; Plasvac Pty Ltd, Kalbar, Queensland, Australia.

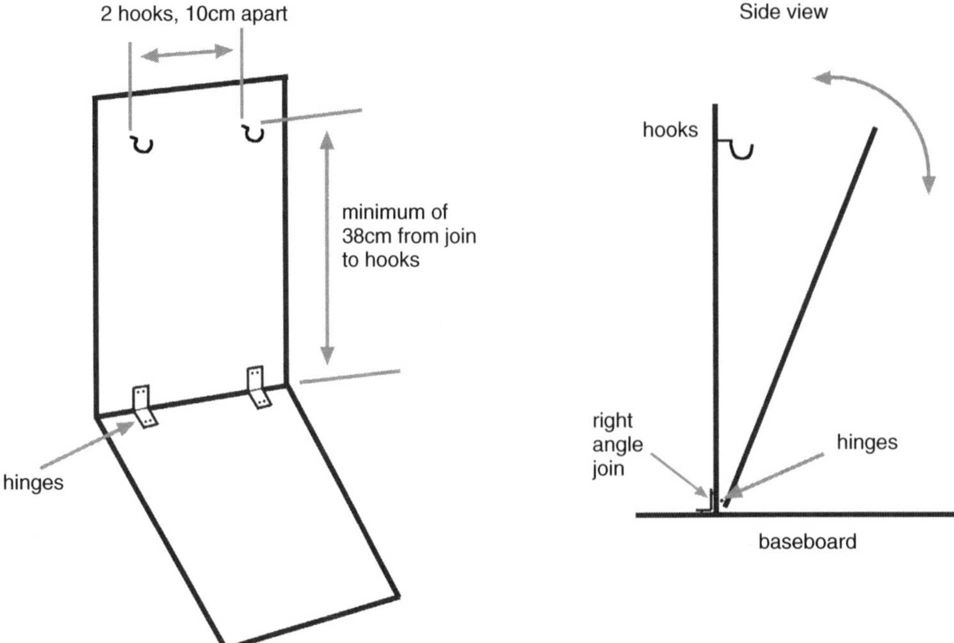

Figure 1.67 Design for homemade plasma collection device. The hooks must be capable of holding 3 kg, and the stand needs to be long enough that 3 kg of weight will not cause the device to tip over. ©Anna Hammond and Kevin Corley 2007.

References

1. Durham AE: Blood and plasma transfusion in the horse. Equine Vet Educ 8:8-12, 1996
2. MacLennan S, Barbara JA: Risks and side effects of therapy with plasma and plasma fractions. Best Pract Res Clin Haematol 19:169-189, 2006
3. Gordon BJ, Latimer KS, Murray CM, et al: Evaluation of leukapheresis and thrombocytapheresis in the horse. Am J Vet Res 47:997-1001, 1986

1.19 Collection of arterial blood gas samples

Harold McKenzie

Arterial blood gas sampling is performed primarily for evaluation of pulmonary function, although insight into the patient's acid-base status is also obtained.

Equipment needed

The equipment needed for arterial blood gas collection is given in Box 1.21.

Box 1.21. Equipment for collection of arterial blood gas samples

Required

1–3-ml blood gas syringe

- Commercial syringe with lithium heparin pellet*
- 2–3-ml syringe flushed with sodium heparin† solution

20-Gauge needle for aspiration of heparin

$1\frac{1}{2}$ cm 25 gauge needle

Optional

Mepivacaine 2%‡: 2 ml drawn up in a 2–3 ml syringe with a 23–25-gauge needle

Twitch

Sedation

*Available from many suppliers, including QS-50, Radiometer, Brønshøj, Denmark; Blood gas monovette, Sarstedt (www.sarstedt.com), Newton, NC, USA; and Nümbrecht, Germany.

†Multiparin, 5000 units/ml, CP Pharmaceuticals Ltd., Wrexham, UK.

‡Intra-epicaine; Arnolds Veterinary Products, Shrewsbury, UK; Carbocaine-V; Pfizer Animal Health, New York, NY, USA.

Procedure

Arterial blood gas sampling is most readily performed in the conscious adult horse using the transverse facial artery. Arterial samples may also be obtained from the facial, carotid or dorsal metatarsal arteries (Figure 1.68), but these sites are considerably more challenging to utilise in the conscious horse. The transverse facial artery overlies the mandible as it courses rostrally below the zygomatic process of the temporal bone from the area of the parotid gland to the bony orbit, and it is readily palpable in this location (Figure 1.69). Care must be taken when collecting the sample, as the transverse facial vein is located immediately superior to the artery.

Either commercially available blood gas syringes can be used, or a standard syringe can be preheparinised. A small volume of heparin solution (0.1 ml) is first aspirated into a 2- to 3-ml syringe, the needle is changed and the heparin

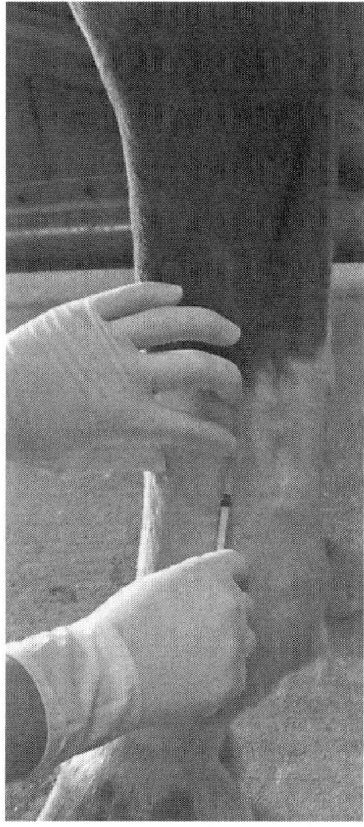

Figure 1.68 Arterial blood sampling from the dorsal metatarsal artery. ©Harold C. McKenzie III 2006.

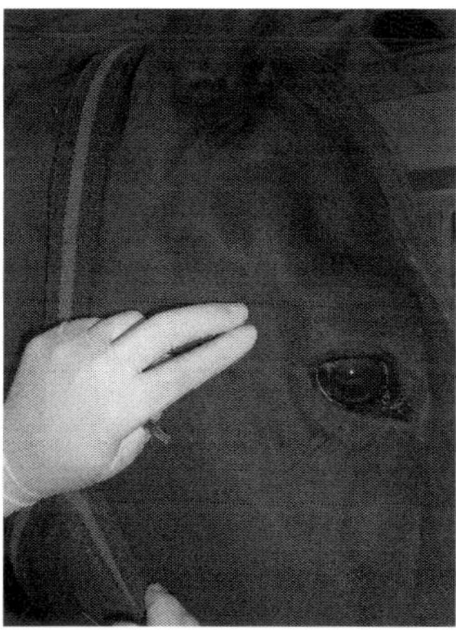

Figure 1.69 The transverse facial artery overlies the mandible as it courses rostrally below the zygomatic process of the temporal bone from the area of the parotid gland to the bony orbit, and it is readily palpable in this location. ©Harold C. McKenzie III 2006.

solution is discharged from the syringe, leaving a small but adequate amount of heparin within the syringe in order to prevent coagulation of the sample. A 1.5-cm 25-gauge needle is used for sample collection. Topical anaesthesia of the skin overlying the artery may minimise the degree of patient reaction to needle insertion.

Arterial puncture is most easily achieved using the left transverse facial artery for right-handed individuals, and the right artery for left-handed individuals. This allows the individual to rest the back of the hand holding the syringe against the side of the head, thereby minimising movement of one's hand relative to the horse's head. Leave the needle on the syringe and use the fingers of the hand not holding the syringe to palpate the pulse in the artery. Insert the needle through the skin and advance into the artery, at which point a small amount of arterial blood (the "flash") should be observed in the hub of the needle. Aspirate at least 1 ml of blood into the syringe and withdraw. Ensure that adequate pressure is placed on the arterial puncture site for at least 1 minute following sampling to avoid haematoma formation.

The tip of the needle should be immediately capped with a rubber stopper (from a small vacuum collection blood tube) to prevent gas contamination of the sample. The sample should be processed immediately or it can be placed on ice. Samples analysed for pH and $PaCO_2$ determination are fairly stable and can be held at room temperature for up to 1 hour.[1] Arterial samples for determination of PaO_2 are less stable and must be collected in glass syringes and stored on ice (for up to 2 hours) if not immediately processed.[1]

Normal values are given in the Appendix (see Table 19.10).

Reference

1. Deane JC, Dagleish MP, Benamou AE, et al. Effects of syringe material and temperature and duration of storage on the stability of equine arterial blood gas variables. Vet Anaesth Analg 31:250-257, 2004

1.20 Arterial catheterisation

Harold McKenzie

The placement of percutaneous arterial catheters is easily and safely performed in conscious horses.[1] The transverse facial artery (see Figure 1.69) is most readily utilised in adult horses, whereas the facial and dorsal metatarsal arteries are difficult to access in the conscious patient.

Equipment needed

The equipment for arterial catheterisation is given in Box 1.22. Seldinger technique catheters are generally easier to place than over-the-needle catheters but are more expensive to purchase. Over-the-wire catheters can be tricky to place in a conscious, moving horse.

Procedure

Prior to catheter placement, the skin at the insertion site should be aseptically prepared. Desensitisation of the site with a topical anaesthetic may aid in placement by minimising patient discomfort. The small catheters used in this application may be damaged during insertion through the skin, and this can be minimised by making a small incision or needle puncture at the site of insertion prior to catheter placement.

Box 1.22. Equipment for arterial catheterisation

Required

Arterial catheter

- 20-Gauge, 4.5-cm (1.75-inch) polyurethane Seldinger-technique arterial catheter*
- 3.5Fr, 5-cm (2-inch) polyurethane over-the-wire arterial catheter†
- 20-Gauge, 3.3-cm (1.3-inch) over-the needle catheter‡

Small gauze swabs (4 × 4) soaked in chlorhexidine (4%) scrub solution§
Small gauze swabs (4 × 4) soaked in surgical spirit (alcohol)
Short, narrow extension set
Injection cap
Fixing material

- Instant bonding glue (cyanoacrylate adhesive) (Superglue)**
- 2–0 Nonabsorbable monofilament suture on a straight needle††

10–20-ml syringe of 0.9% sterile saline (±5 units/ml heparin)

Optional

Clippers with a fine (No. 40) blade
Mepivacaine 2%‡‡: 1 ml drawn up in a 2–3-ml syringe with a 23–25-Gauge needle
Surgical gloves
No. 11 scalpel blade OR 18–20-gauge needle
Three-way stopcock (three-way tap)‡

*RA-04020; Arrow International Inc., Reading, PA, USA.
†ART35; MILA International, Florence, KY, USA.
‡Vygon, Ecouen, France.
§Hibiscrub; Mölnlycke Health Care, Dunstable, UK.
**Nexaband; Abbott Laboratories, North Chicago, IL, USA; Superglue; Loctite, Henkel Consumer Adhesives, Avon, OH, USA.
††628H, Ethilon Nylon; Ethicon, Somerville, NJ, USA.
‡‡Intra-epicaine; Arnolds Veterinary Products, Shrewsbury, UK; Carbocaine-V; Pfizer Animal Health, New York, NY, USA.

A Seldinger catheter (see Figure 2.27) is put in as follows: Holding the wire assembly with the dominant hand, the tip should be inserted through the area of local anaesthetic, pointing towards the rear of the horse. The whole assembly is advanced at a flat angle (10° to 20°) through the skin. As soon as blood is seen in the flash hub, the wire assembly is held very still and the nondominant hand is used to advance the wire by pushing forward the wire advancer. The wire assembly is still held still. The nondominant hand is used to smoothly advance the catheter forward off the wire assembly and into the artery, and the wire assembly is removed.

For over-the-needle catheters, the catheter and stylet should be advanced through the skin into the artery. When arterial blood is observed within the hub of the stylet, the outer catheter sheath is then advanced off the stylet into the artery. The stylet is then withdrawn.

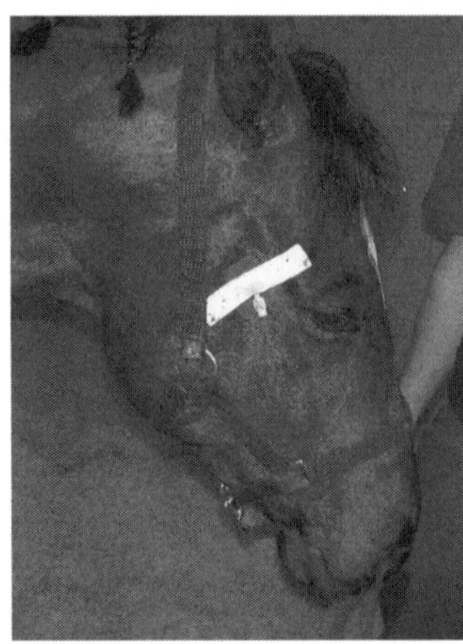

Figure 1.70 Arterial catheter in the transverse facial artery of a horse after colic surgery. ©Kevin Corley 2002.

Once the catheter is in the artery, the catheter should be temporarily capped with an injection cap and the hub sutured or glued to the skin of the patient to prevent inadvertent withdrawal (Figure 1.70). If required, an extension set primed with a heparinised saline solution is then attached to the catheter and the catheter is flushed.

Maintenance of an arterial catheter can be challenging in the conscious patient. Arterial catheters are highly susceptible to obstruction due to clot formation, and their patency must be maintained by intermittent or continuous flushing with heparinised saline. Following successful catheter placement, arterial blood samples can be drawn through the catheter, followed by flushing with heparinised saline, or blood pressure may be obtained by connecting the extension set to a pressure transducer. The use of a three-way stopcock can facilitate flushing of the catheter whilst leaving the pressure transducer connection intact. Arterial catheters represent a potential site of infection and thrombus formation, necessitating careful handling using sterile technique and close monitoring. Upon removal of an arterial catheter, firm pressure must be applied to the site for at least 1 minute to minimise the risk of local haemorrhage.

Reference

1. Riebold TW, Brunson DB, Lott RA, et al. Percutaneous arterial catheterization in the horse. Vet Med Small Anim Clin 75:1736-1742, 1980

1.21 Indirect arterial blood pressure measurement

Kevin Corley

In contrast to indirect blood pressure measurement in foals (see Chapter 2.7), it is only moderately accurate in adult horses,[1–4] and the results should always be interpreted

Box 1.23. Equipment for indirect arterial blood pressure monitoring

Required
Cuff of appropriate bladder width

- Cuffs designed for the upper arm of "medium-sized" adult humans are often close to the correct size.

Oscillometric automated sphygmomanometric monitor

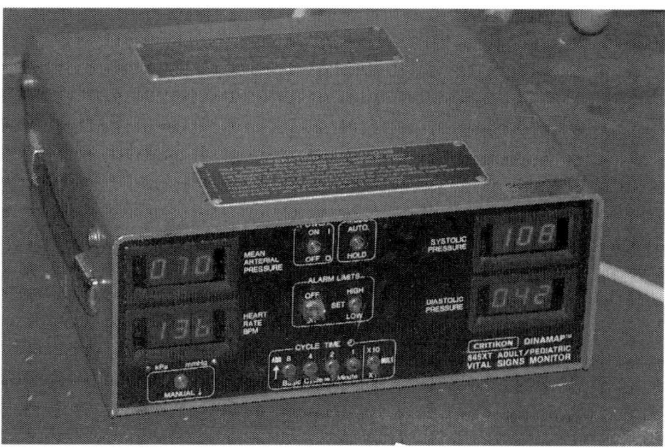

Figure 1.71 Indirect arterial pressure monitor. The monitor is connected to a critically ill foal, explaining the high heart rate (136 bpm). ©Kevin Corley 2007.

with caution. If possible, direct blood pressure should be measured.

Equipment needed

The equipment needed is listed in Box 1.23. A great many automated blood pressure machines are made for the human market. Some of these are set so that they do not measure over the prolonged periods required for the low heart rates of the horse. The majority of machines also have problems recording blood pressure when the horse is in second-degree atrioventricular block. These machines will repeatedly give error messages, rather than a reading.

Procedure

In contrast to in foals, the ratio of the width of the bladder of the cuff to the circumference of the tail base appears to be important in adult horses. For optimal accuracy of systolic blood pressure, the ratio of bladder width to tail girth circumference should be 0.34.[5] For optimal accuracy of diastolic blood pressure, the ratio of bladder width to tail girth circumference should be 0.98.[5] Where the cuff bladder width is too wide, the reading given will be falsely low.[6] If the cuff bladder width is too narrow, the reading given will be falsely high.[6]

The centre of the bladder of the cuff should be placed over the coccygeal artery. The centre is marked by an arrow on some makes of cuff or lies between the two hosepipes on models that have two hosepipes. The coccygeal artery is located on ventral midline of the tail. Measurements are most accurate when the cuff is placed as close to the base of the tail as possible. The cuff should be orientated so that the hose runs away from the body of the horse (see Figure 2.21).

Once the cuff is securely placed, a measurement can be taken. Many machines have the option of a manual measurement, or automated measurements are repeated after a set interval. The heart rate measured by the machine (Figure 1.71) should be compared to the heart rate of the horse, counted from the pulse or heart. If the heart rate measured by the machine is not accurate, the reading should be disregarded.

There are frequently problems getting measurements or repeatable measurements by the indirect technique in adult horses. The techniques discussed under "Troubleshooting" in Chapter 2.7 can also be used in the adult horse and may help obtain a reading.

References

1. Muir WW, Wade A, Grospitch B: Automatic noninvasive sphygmomanometry in horses. J Am Vet Med Assoc 182:1230-1233, 1983
2. Riebold TW, Evans AT: Blood pressure measurements in the anesthetized horse: comparison of four methods. Vet Surg 14:332-337, 1985
3. Branson KR: A clinical evaluation of an oscillometric blood pressure monitor on anesthetized horses. J Equine Vet Sci 17:537-540, 1997
4. Ellis PM: The indirect measurement of arterial blood pressure in the horse. Equine Vet J 7:22-26, 1975
5. Parry BW, McCarthy MA, Anderson GA, et al: Correct occlusive bladder width for indirect blood pressure measurement in horses. Am J Vet Res 43:50-54, 1982
6. Magdesian KG: Monitoring the critically ill equine patient. Vet Clin N Am Equine Pract 20:11-39, 2004

1.22 Direct arterial blood pressure measurement

Kevin Corley

Direct blood pressure monitoring is most frequently performed for monitoring of horses under general anaesthesia. Rarely, it is also used to monitor blood pressure in critically ill conscious horses.

Equipment needed

The equipment needed is given in Box 1.24.

Procedure

Prior to direct measurement of arterial pressure, placement of an arterial catheter is required (Figure 1.72). This is described in Chapter 1.20.

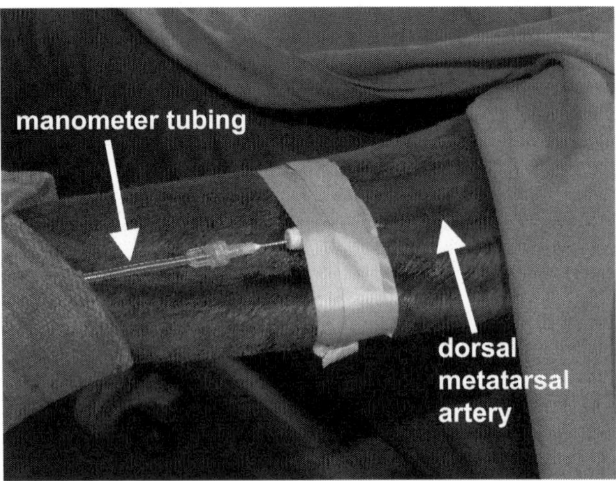

Figure 1.72 Arterial catheter in the dorsal metatarsal artery of an anaesthetised horse, for direct arterial blood pressure monitoring. The manometer tubing is connected to the arterial line via an 18-gauge needle, pushed through an injection cap. ©Kevin Corley 2007.

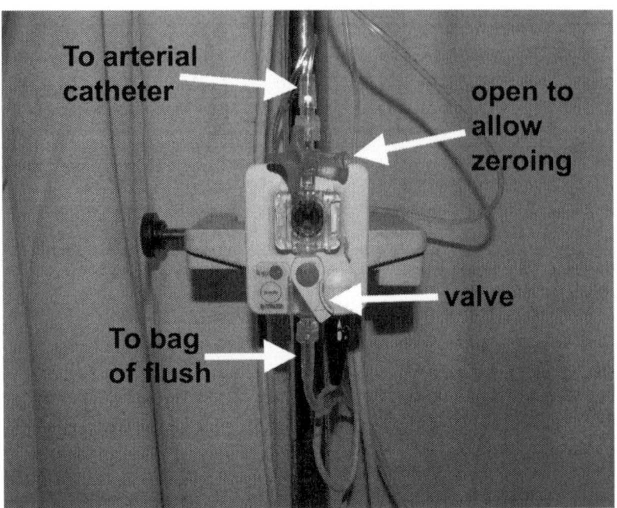

Figure 1.73 Pressure transducer for direct monitoring of arterial pressure. The valve is depressed to flush the tubing and arterial catheter. The three-way stopcock (three-way tap) may be turned 90° anti-clockwise, so that the pressure transducer is open to the atmosphere, for zeroing. ©Kevin Corley 2007.

Box 1.24. Equipment for direct arterial blood pressure monitoring

Required

Arterial catheter (see Box 1.20)
Pressure transducer*

- With appropriate lead for the electronic patient monitor

Electronic patient monitor with direct blood pressure
Manometer tubing
Three-way stopcock (three-way tap)†
Fluid stand to attach pressure transducer to
10–20-ml syringe of 0.9% sterile saline (±5 units/ml heparin)

Optional

500–100-ml bag of 0.9% sterile saline (±5 units/ml heparin)
Pressure infusion bag
Fluid-giving set

*For example: Deltran IV Disposable Blood Pressure Monitoring Systems; Utah Medical Products, Inc., Midvale, UT, USA.
†Vygon, Ecouen, France.

Setting up the pressure transducer

The patient end of the transducer is connected to a three-way stopcock (three-way tap) and then to manometer tubing. The other end of the pressure transducer is connected either to a bag of saline or heparinised saline ("flush") via a fluid-giving set or to a syringe full of heparinised saline flush. If a bag of flush is used, it can be placed in a pressure bag. Using a pressurised bag of flush connected to the transducer is the optimum method, as it allows easy flushing of the system and the arterial catheter.

The valve (Figure 1.73) should be depressed to prefill the transducer and manometer tubing. If a syringe of flush is being used, the flush from the syringe needs to be injected into the system at the same time as depressing the valve. The manometer tubing is then connected to the arterial catheter, either via a needle through an injection cap (see Figure 1.72) or via a three-way stopcock. The system is then flushed again.

Zeroing the pressure transducer

The pressure transducer should be placed at the level of the heart base (set as the level of the sternal manubrium) and fixed to a fluid stand to maintain it at a constant height. The three-way stopcock at the patient end of the transducer is turned so that the pressure transducer is open to the atmosphere (Figure 1.73). The machine is then zeroed by depressing the appropriate button. The three-way stopcock is then turned back so that it is open to the transducer and the patient, and closed to the atmosphere (Figure 1.73).

Measurement

A pressure trace should then be seen on the screen of the monitor, and the systolic, diastolic and mean pressures should be displayed (Figure 1.74). Some monitors do not display the mean pressure in their default settings, and the instruction manual should be consulted as to how to alter the display so that mean pressure is displayed.

After flushing or zeroing, the numerical readout of the pressures may take a few seconds to read accurately. The measurement should not be recorded or acted upon until the numbers are changing by less than 2 to 3 mm Hg on each beat. If a good trace (Figure 1.74) is not established or reestablished, the system should be reflushed.

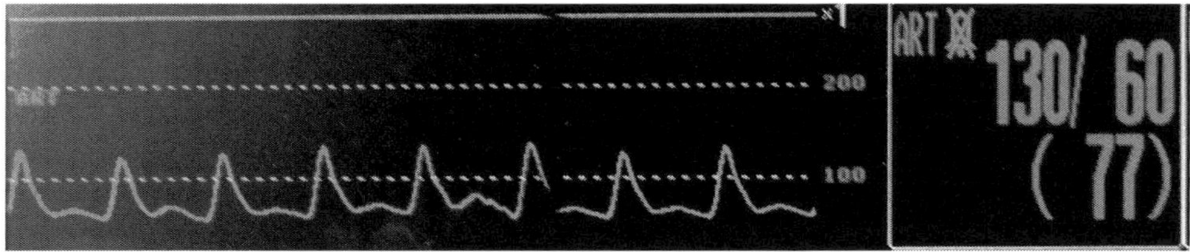

Figure 1.74 Direct arterial pressure trace from a foal. The systolic direct arterial pressure is 130 mm Hg, the diastolic pressure is 60 mm Hg and the mean pressure is 77 mm Hg. ©Kevin Corley 2007.

1.23 Central venous pressure measurement

Mary Durando

Central venous pressure (CVP) is very useful to assess venous return to the heart and to monitor fluid therapy. It is particularly useful in managing those cases at higher risk for overhydration whilst on fluid therapy, such as horses in renal failure or with significant cardiac disease. It can also be very helpful in determining if the administered fluid therapy is sufficient to meet the needs of the patient, especially those with gastrointestinal disease. CVP gives an indication of the patient's fluid requirements and the ability of the cardiovascular system to handle the administered fluid load.[1–4] It is easy to perform and minimally invasive and requires very little in the way of specialised equipment.

Equipment needed

The equipment needed is listed in Box 1.25.

> **Box 1.25. Equipment for central venous pressure monitoring**
>
> **Required**
>
> 10–14-Gauge jugular catheter (see Chapter 1.14 for placement)
> Sterile polyethylene tubing (outside diameter 1.70 mm, at least $1\frac{1}{2}$ metres long)*
> Blunt needle
> 30-ml syringe of 0.9% sterile saline (±5 units/ml heparin)
> Narrow bore extension tubing
> Three-way stopcock (three-way tap)†
> Surgical gloves
>
> **For manometer measurement**
>
> Manometer‡
> A piece of fluid extension tubing taped to a ruler may be substituted for the manometer
>
> **For electronic measurement**
>
> Pressure transducer§
> Electronic patient monitor with direct blood pressure and electrocardiogram
>
> *PE190; Strategic Applications Inc., www.sai-infusion.com; BB31695-PE/8, Scientific Commodities Inc., www.scicominc.com.
> †Vygon, Ecouen, France.
> ‡CVP35; MILA International, Florence, KY, USA.
> §For example: Deltran IV Disposable Blood Pressure Monitoring Systems; Utah Medical Products, Inc., Midvale, UT, USA.

Procedure

A catheter extending through the intrathoracic cranial vena cava to the level of the right atrium is used for measuring CVP. In adult horses, because of their size, it is easiest to use sterile polyethylene (PE) or polypropylene tubing that has been premeasured to approximately the right atrium (approximately intercostal space 4 or 5, over the heart base), passed through a 10- to 14-gauge jugular venous catheter. It is necessary to carefully insert a (blunt) needle of appropriate gauge into the end of this tubing, to create a Luer connection. The tubing (which is primed with sterile heparinised saline before placement) is connected via a three-way stopcock and narrow-bore extension tubing either to a manometer or an electronic pressure transducer. The manometer or pressure transducer should be placed at the level of the heart base[5] as a standardised way to zero the instrument and record pressures (Figure 1.75). If repeated measurements from a single patient over time are envisaged, the zero level should be marked, either on the horse (with clippers, for example) or by connecting the manometer or transducer to a fluid stand. If the end of the tubing is correctly in the right atrium (or vena cava), the pressure will vary with breathing.

A catheter of sufficient length (e.g., Intracath; 24 inch [61 cm] length, Becton Dickinson, Newark, DE, USA) may also be used, as long as it is placed distally in the jugular vein allowing it to reach the right atrium. It should be premeasured first, to determine if it is long enough.

Manometer reading

The manometer should be primed with sterile heparinised saline prior to connection. A blunt needle is used to connect the PE tubing to the three-way stopcock. The fluid column should rise and fall with respiration, reflecting intrathoracic pressure changes. The central venous pressure is read as the height of the fluid column in centimetres (Figure 1.76). An example of measurement of CVP in a horse is shown in Figure 1.77.

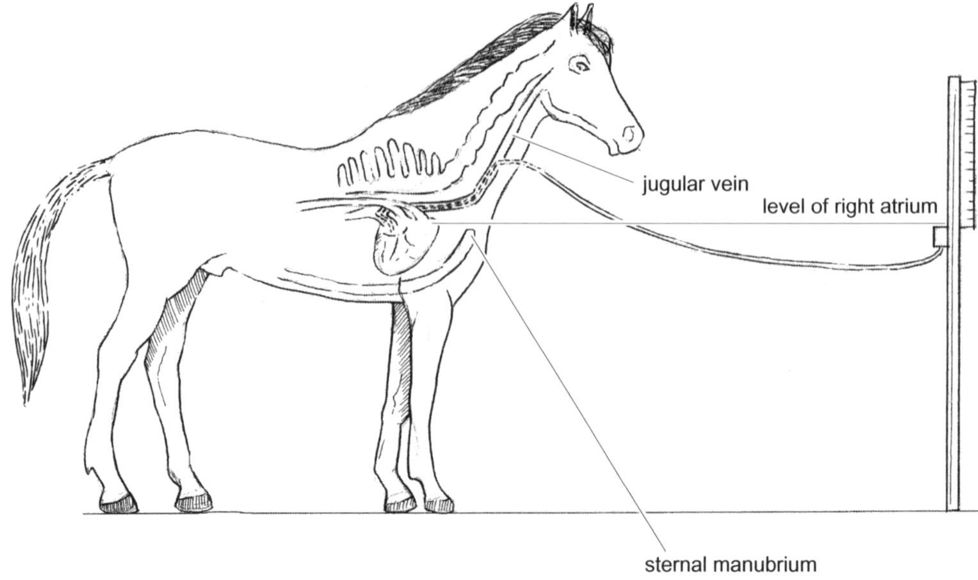

Figure 1.75 Central venous pressure measurement. The tip of the tubing or catheter is placed in the right atrium. The manometer or pressure transducer is set at the level of the sternal manubrium.

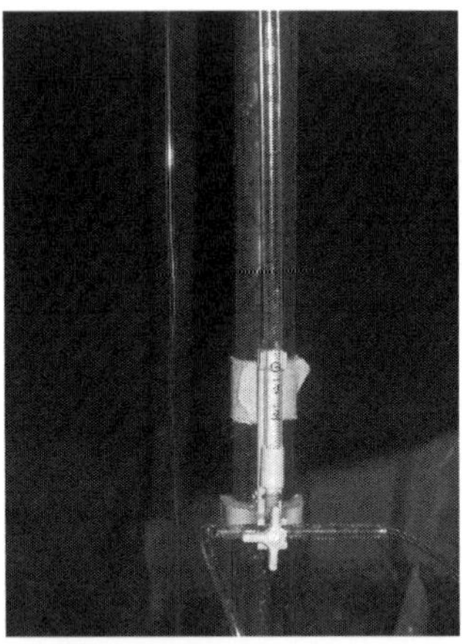

Figure 1.76 Manometer for measurement of central venous pressure Manometer and three-way stopcock attached to an IV stand to maintain a consistent position, with the zero mark at the level of the sternal manubrium (point of the shoulder). ©Mary Durando 2006.

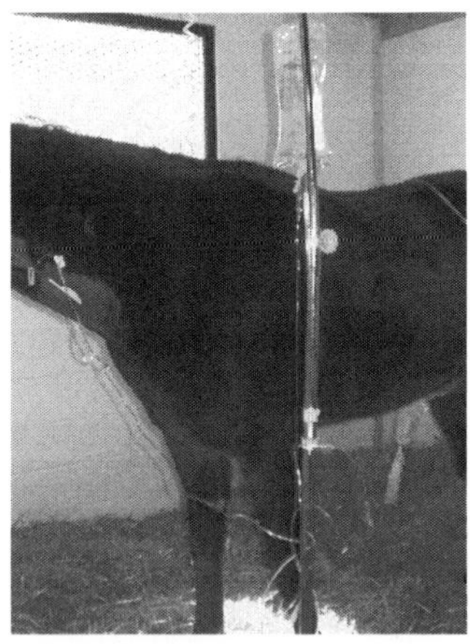

Figure 1.77 Central venous pressure measurement in a horse with gastro-intestinal disease, using the manometer method. ©Mary Durando 2006.

Electronic reading

For an electronic reading, the tubing is connected to a electronic pressure transducer. This must then be connected to a suitable monitor, which should be zeroed (see Chapter 1.22) prior to taking a measurement. The monitor is used to determine the pressure. However, because CVP varies with intrathoracic pressure, determining its absolute value requires interpretation. Simply using the electronically averaged mean displayed by the monitor may be misleading, especially during hyperpnoea or mechanical ventilation.[6]

For accurate measurement of CVP, a simultaneous electrocardiogram recording is required (Figure 1.78). This enables proper identification of the a-wave in the CVP trace, which falls in the PR interval (Figure 1.79). The central venous pressure should be measured as the mean of the a-wave at end-expiration.[6] The a-wave at end-expiration can be identified in the last waveform prior to the rapid fall in pressure indicating inspiration in spontaneously breathing animals (Figure 1.78), and in the last waveform prior to the rapid rise in pressure in mechanically ventilated animals.

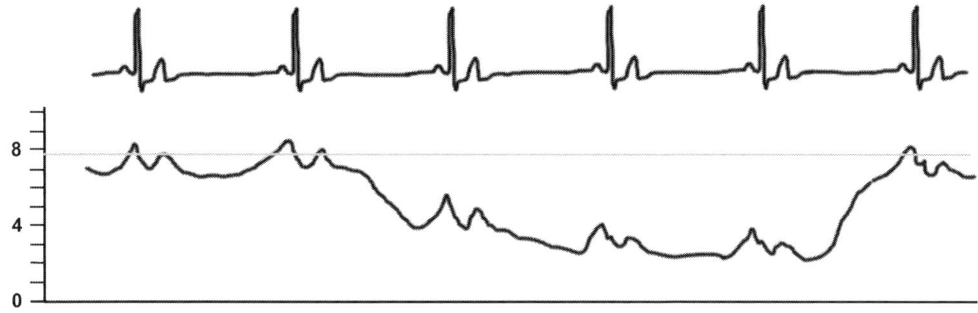

Figure 1.78 Example of a central venous pressure trace taken during spontaneous breathing. The value for central venous pressure is taken as the mean of the a-wave at end expiration. In the spontaneously breathing animal, this is the last a-wave prior to the fall in pressure (negative pressure from inspiration). ©Kevin Corley 2007.

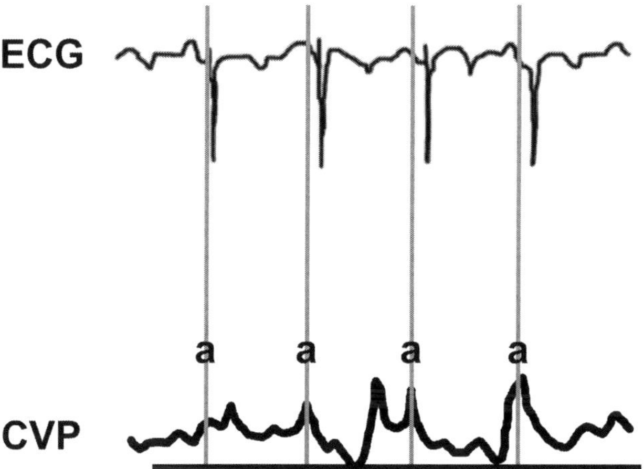

Figure 1.79 Identification of the a-wave in a complicated central venous pressure reading. The a-wave falls in the PR interval on the electrocardiogram. Trace of a central venous pressure wave and electrocardiogram from a mechanically ventilated foal. ©Kevin Corley 2007.

The normal CVP in the adult horse is approximately 7 to 12 cm H_2O.[5]

References

1. Mark JB: Central venous pressure monitoring: clinical insights beyond the numbers. J Cardiothorac Vasc Anesth 5:163-173, 1991
2. Oakley RE, Olivier B, Eyster GE, et al: Experimental evaluation of central venous pressure monitoring in the dog. J Am Anim Hosp Assoc 33:77-82, 1997
3. Pittman JA, Ping JS, Mark JB: Arterial and central venous pressure monitoring. Int Anesthesiol Clin 42:13-30, 2004
4. de Laforcade AM, Rozanski E: Central venous pressure and arterial blood pressure measurements. Vet Clin N Am: Sm Anim Pract 31:1163-1174, 2001
5. Hall LW, Nigam JM: Measurement of central venous pressure in horses. Vet Rec 97:66-69, 1975
6. Daily EK, Schroeder JS: Central venous and right atrial pressure monitoring, in Daily EK, Schroeder JS (eds): Techniques in Bedside Hemodynamic Monitoring, ed 5. St. Louis, Mosby, 1994, pp 79-98

Box 1.26. Equipment for electrocardiography

Required

Electrocardiography machine (ECG machine/EKG machine):

- Many different models are available. Can often be obtained second hand from refurbished medical equipment suppliers.

Contact

- ECG contact gel
- Surgical spirit (alcohol) in a spray bottle

1.24 Electrocardiography

Mary Durando

In horses, electrocardiograms (ECG) are most commonly used to evaluate cardiac rhythm and conduction disturbances. Although components of the ECG can be used for information about heart size and mean electrical axis in humans and small animals, this is less reliable in horses, and that information is best gained by other diagnostic means.

Equipment needed

The equipment needed is given in Box 1.26.

Procedure

Base-apex system

The base-apex lead system is the most commonly used lead system in the horse and is best suited for the purpose of evaluating rhythm.[1–4] It is well tolerated and less affected by motion artefacts than limb leads and generally gives large, easily discernible complexes, with clear P, QRS and T waves.[5,6] To apply a base-apex lead, the (+) left arm electrode (yellow or black; Table 1.2) is positioned near the

Table 1.2. Colour coding systems for electrocardiogram (ECG) leads

Name	IEC system		AHA system	
	Inscription	Colour	Inscription	Colour
Right arm	R	Red	RA	White
Left arm	L	Yellow	LA	Black
Right leg	N	Black	RL	Green
Left leg	F	Green	LL	Red
Chest	C1	White/red	V1	Brown/red
Chest	C2	White/yellow	V2	Brown/yellow
Chest	C3	White/green	V3	Brown/green
Chest	C4	White/brown	V4	Brown/blue
Chest	C5	White/black	V5	Brown/orange
Chest	C6	White/violet	V6	Brown/purple

IEC, International Electrotechnical Commission; AHA, American Heart Association.

apex of the heart, and the (−) right arm electrode (red or white; Table 1.2) is placed over the shoulder near the withers on the right side or at the right jugular furrow (Figure 1.80). A ground electrode (right leg; black or green; Table 1.2) can be placed anywhere remote from these places, and the ECG is recorded on lead I. With this configuration, the QRS complex is negative (Figures 1.81 and 1.82). In horses, the ECG is generally recorded at a paper speed of 25 mm/sec and an amplitude of 10 mm for each 1 mV, although the sensitivity may be adjusted to change the size of the complexes to make them more easily read. If sufficient tachycardia is present, recording at a paper speed of 50 mm/sec may make the complexes more easily distinguished.

Other lead systems

Although base-apex systems are usually sufficient to evaluate rhythm, occasionally more than one lead system is helpful to distinguish a supraventricular from ventricular dysrhythmia (i.e., P waves can not be discerned in a base-apex lead).[4,7] This can be done with either limb leads or a complete 12-lead ECG. For limb leads, the four leads (see Table 1.2) are placed on each of the legs. On the forelegs, the clips should be placed on the fold of skin just above or below the elbow joint. On the hind limbs, the clips should be placed on the fold of skin above or at the stifles. Some horses may object as these leads are placed, and caution is advised. Placement of limb leads allows a three-lead ECG to be recorded. The complete 12-lead ECG includes the standard bipolar limb leads, augmented unipolar limb leads and unipolar chest leads. Leads I, II, III, aVR, aVL, aVF, CV_{6LL}, CV_{6LU}, CV_{6RL}, CV_{6RU}, and V_{10} are recorded. For a more complete description of lead systems and normal values for various intervals and segments, the reader is referred to articles that explain the 12-lead system in detail.[5,8]

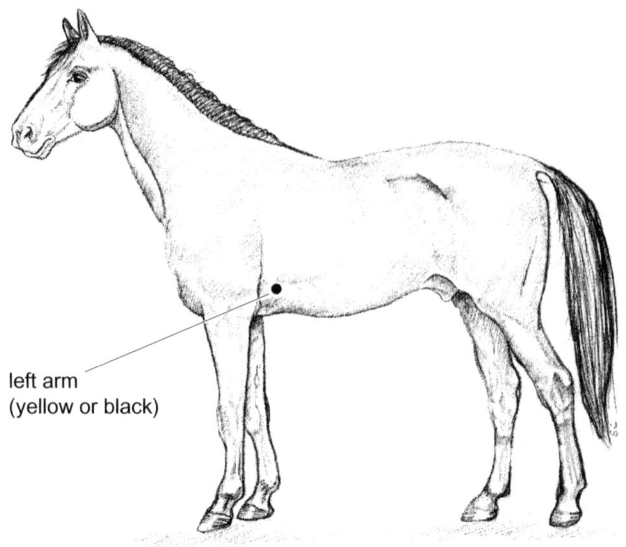

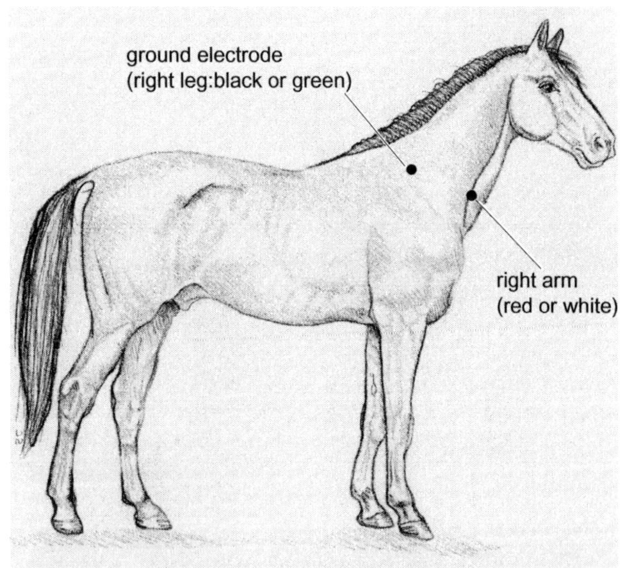

Figure 1.80 Placement of leads for recording a base-apex ECG. The *black circles* represent locations for electrode placement, and lead I is recorded. LA, left arm lead; RA, right arm lead; RL, right leg.

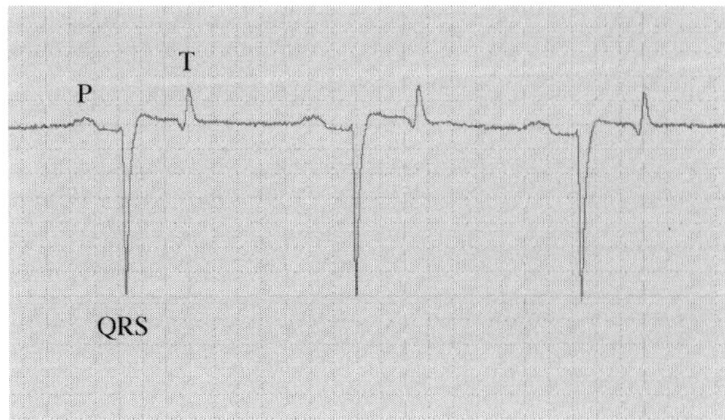

Figure 1.81 The P, QRS and T waves in a base-apex ECG. ©Mary Durando 2006.

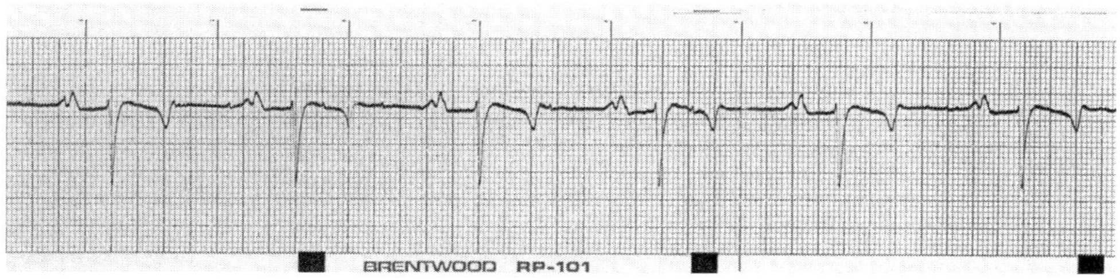

Figure 1.82 Base-apex ECG. Note the normal variations in P wave (bifid) and T wave (inverted) configurations, compared with Figure 1.81 ©Mary Durando 2006.

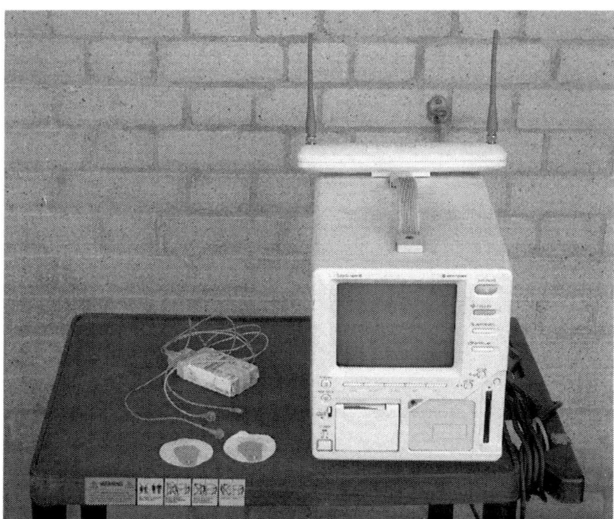

Figure 1.83 Radiotelemetry unit for recording ECGs. The transmitter box is secured to a surcingle around the horse, and the ECG may be monitored at least 80 m away. ©Kevin Corley 2003.

Continuous and remote monitoring

Two systems that record longer-term continuous ECGs, radiotelemetry and 24-hour ambulatory (Holter) monitors, are very simple to use and useful, particularly in a hospital setting.[9,10] Both systems are readily available and relatively inexpensive. They both allow monitoring of the horse's cardiac rhythm in its natural setting, without having to be confined to stocks or having a person attached. Telemetric ECG consists of the leads positioned in a modified base-apex configuration with the negative RA lead behind the dorsal portion of the shoulder on the left side, the positive LA electrode on the sternum or in the axillary region and the ECG recorded on lead I. The leads are attached to a transmitter device that converts voltage from the horse to waveforms, sends the waveforms to a receiver, which then converts them back to voltage, and displays the ECG in real-time (Figure 1.83). Holter recordings are similar; however, rather than send the ECG to a receiver, the leads are attached to a recording device, either digital or magnetic tape, for future evaluation. They typically record over a 24- to 48-hour period, allowing documentation of the horse's rhythm over time, but cannot be viewed in real-time. The leads for telemetry and Holter monitor systems are held snugly in place with a surcingle, and the device is secured to this surcingle.

Ensuring electrical contact

To obtain a diagnostic ECG by any method, alcohol or coupling gel is applied to the horse's hair to thoroughly saturate the area and provide adequate contact, although water will work in some situations. In colder climates in the winter, if contact is still poor and the horse's skin is drier, the hair may need to be clipped. Telemetry or Holter monitor systems with flat electrodes are more likely to need an area clipped in the winter than other methods that use alligator clips to attach the leads.

References

1. Durando MM, Young LE: Cardiovascular examination and diagnostic techniques, in Robinson NE (ed): Current Therapy in Equine Medicine, ed 5. St. Louis, WB Saunders, 2003, pp 572-585
2. Patteson MW: Equine Cardiology. Oxford, Blackwell, 1996, p 254
3. Reef VB: Evaluation of the equine cardiovascular system. Vet Clin N Am Equine Pract 1:275-288, 1985
4. Reef VB: Arrhythmias, in Marr CM (ed): Cardiology of the Horse. London, WB Saunders, 1999, pp 179-209
5. Buss DD, Rawlings CA, Bisgard GE: The normal electrocardiogram of the domestic pony. J Electrocardiol 8:167-172, 1975
6. Holmes JR: Equine electrocardiography: some practical hints on technique. Equine Vet J 16:477-479, 1984
7. Physick-Sheard PW: Diagnostic techniques in equine cardiology, in Robinson NE (ed): Current Therapy in Equine Medicine, ed 4. Philadelphia, WB Saunders, 1997, pp 225-233
8. Fregin GF: Electrocardiography. Vet Clin North Am Equine Pract 1:419-432, 1985
9. Reef VB: Electrocardiography and echocardiography in the exercising horse, in Robinson NE (ed): Current Therapy in Equine Medicine, ed 4. Philadelphia, WB Saunders, 1997, pp 234-239
10. Reef VB: Ambulatory and exercise electrocardiography and post-exercise echocardiography, in Marr CM (ed): Cardiology of the Horse. London, WB Saunders, 1999, pp 150-160

1.25 Echocardiography

Mary Durando

Echocardiography is the method of choice for evaluating cardiac anatomy, function and size and is safe, as well as readily available to equine practitioners.[1,2] Two-dimensional and M-mode techniques allow size, anatomy and function to be accurately evaluated, and Doppler studies help to determine normality of blood flow through the heart and great vessels. In order to use echocardiography effectively, reduce variability, avoid overlooking important findings and communicate information to others, a methodical approach using standardised views is necessary.[3]

Equipment needed

The equipment needed is given in Box 1.27. In adult horses, a low-frequency transducer (2.5 MHz or lower) with a scanning depth of 30 cm is usually needed. For neonates and older foals, a higher-frequency transducer (3.5 to 5 MHz) with a displayed depth less than that used for adults is adequate. Phased array, annular array or sector transducers are better than linear transducers for echocardiography. It is important to be able to display a simultaneous ECG for timing with the cardiac cycle, and helpful to be able to display a two-dimensional image along with M-mode or Doppler studies, for correct orientation. Most new equipment allows this.

Procedure

There are six standard two-dimensional views that are obtained from the right parasternal window, although less standard views or permutations of these views may be obtained, depending on the particular abnormality present.[1,2] From the right parasternal approach, three long-axis and three short-axis views are obtained. For the long-axis views, the reference marker on the probe is directed between 12 and 1 o'clock. The right outflow tract view is obtained by placing the probe in the fourth intercostal space (ICS), between the point of the elbow and the point of the shoulder, and angling cranially towards the opposite point of the shoulder. The structures evaluated are the right atrium and ventricle, tricuspid valve, pulmonic valve, pulmonary artery and aorta (Figure 1.84, A). For the left outflow tract view, the probe is placed in a similar position and directed straight across the chest. It is sometimes necessary to rotate the probe slightly clockwise to 1 o'clock. This allows visualisation of the aorta, aortic valve, left ventricle, right atrium and ventricle, tricuspid valve, and pulmonary artery (Figure 1.84, B). The most caudally oriented of the long axis views, the four-chamber view, is obtained by directing the probe caudally. The four chambers, right and left atria and right and left ventricles, along with the mitral and tricuspid valves, are visualised (Figure 1.84, C). The right parasternal short-axis views are obtained by rotating the probe 90°, with the reference marker at approximately 4 o'clock. The right parasternal short-axis view of the left ventricle is obtained by directing the probe caudally and looking ventrally, until just below the mitral valve, and chordae tendinae are imaged. The left ventricle is the primary structure evaluated with this view (Figure 1.85). The probe is angled dorsally to the mitral valve, and dorsally and slightly cranially to the aortic valve (Figure 1.86), to obtain the remaining images. The mitral valve, and the aortic valve, left atrial appendage and pulmonary artery, respectively, are evaluated with these views.

M-mode images are one-dimensional views of the heart displayed over time across the *x*-axis. Timing of cardiac events using a simultaneous ECG is very accurate with M-mode. They are used for measurements of chamber size, great vessels and wall thickness in systole and diastole, evaluation of valve motion and calculation of indices such as percent fractional shortening (FS).[3] M-modes are obtained by placing the cursor perpendicularly in each two-dimensional short-axis view, bisecting the desired structures, to give images of the left ventricle, mitral valve and aortic valve. It is very important to place the cursor perpendicularly in standard views that are obtained correctly, as views that are skewed may yield inaccurate or unreliable measurements.

FS is calculated from the dimensions obtained with the M-mode of the left ventricle (Figure 1.87), using the following formula:

$$\frac{(\text{LVIDd} - \text{LVIDs}) \times 100}{\text{LVIDd}}$$

where LVIDd is the internal diameter of the left ventricle at end diastole, with the beginning of the QRS as the refer-

Box 1.27. Equipment for echocardiography

Required

Ultrasound machine

- Capable of
  - B-mode and M-mode images
  - Doppler ultrasonography
  - Simultaneous display of ECG

Ultrasound coupling gel

For adult horses

2.5-MHz sector, phased array or annular array transducer with a scanning depth of 30 cm (preferable)

For foals

3.5–5 MHz sector, phased array or annular array transducer

Very helpful

Colour-flow Doppler

Optional

Clippers with a fine (No. 40) blade

Surgical spirit (alcohol)

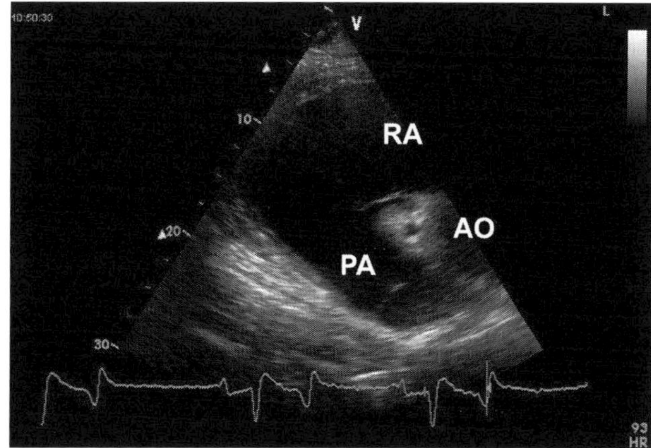

A

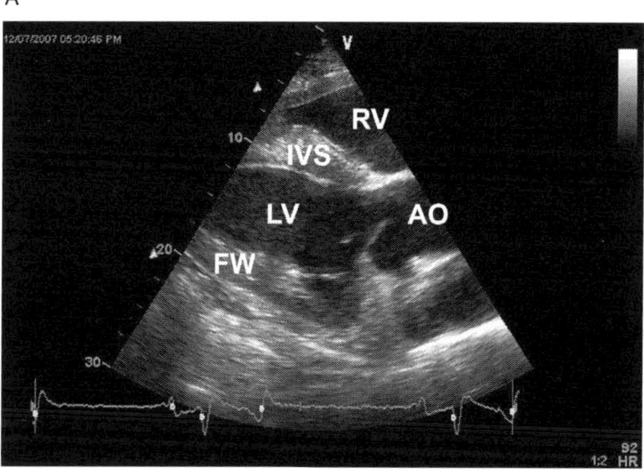

B

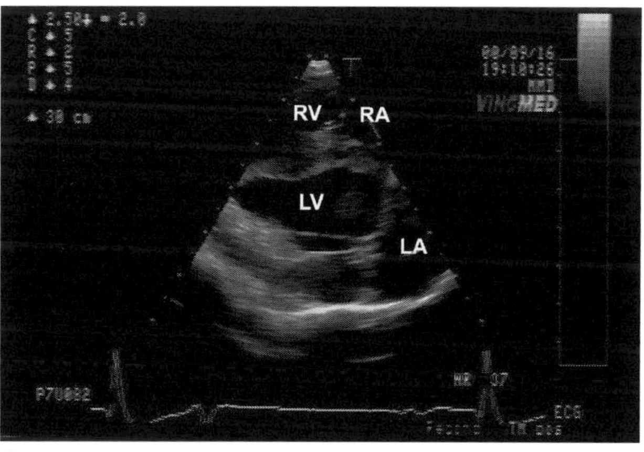

C

Figure 1.84 A-C Two-dimensional, right parasternal long-axis echocardiograms of the heart. **A,** Right outflow tract view. The right atrium and ventricle, tricuspid valve, pulmonary artery, pulmonic valve and aorta can be seen in this view. **B,** Left outflow tract view. The aortic root, aortic valve left ventricle, left ventricular free wall, interventricular septum, right ventricle, right atrium, tricuspid valve and pulmonary artery can be seen in this view. **C,** Four chamber view. The right atrium and ventricle, left atrium and ventricle, mitral valve, tricuspid valve, interventricular septum and left ventricular free wall can be seen in this view. Abbreviations are as follows: RA, right atrium; RV, right ventricle; PA, pulmonary artery; LA, left atrium; LV, left ventricle; AO, aorta; FW, free wall; IVS, interventricular septum. ©Mary Durando 2006.

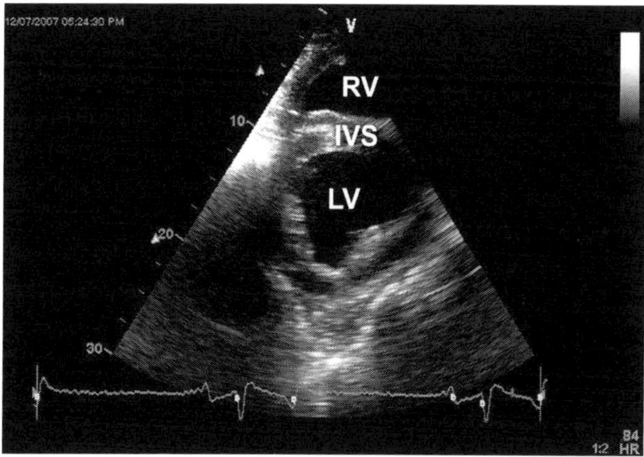

Figure 1.85 Two-dimensional, right parasternal short-axis echocardiogram of the left ventricle. The left ventricle, interventricular septum, left ventricular free wall and right ventricle are seen in this view. Abbreviations are as for Figure 1.84, A–C. ©Mary Durando 2006.

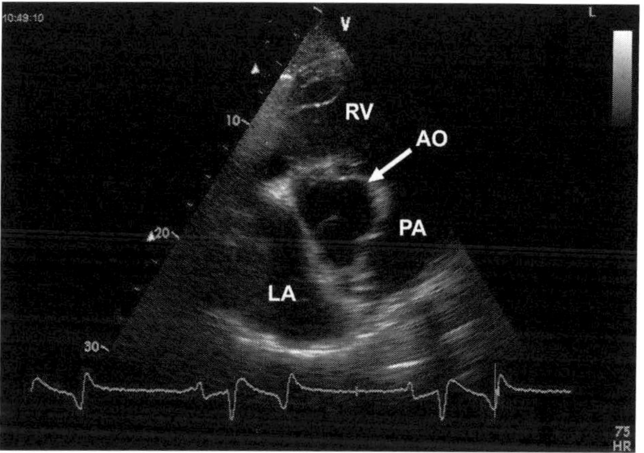

Figure 1.86 Two-dimensional, right parasternal short-axis echocardiogram of the aorta. The aorta, left atrium, pulmonary artery and right ventricle are seen in this view. Abbreviations are as for Figure 1.84, A–C. ©Mary Durando 2006.

ence point, and LVIDs is the internal diameter of the left ventricle in peak systole, at the maximum upswing of the left ventricular free wall (Figure 1.87). FS gives an estimation of contractility (thus systolic function) of the left ventricle. Normal is 30% to 40% if the horse has a normal heart rate and is in a resting state. It should be higher with sympathetic input, elevated heart rates and left ventricular volume overload.

Left parasternal images are obtained from the left third, fourth and fifth ICS. These allow better visualisation of the left atrium and mitral valve and the aortic and pulmonic valves and are useful if the entire heart does not fit on the screen from the right parasternal position. They also may allow better alignment with blood flow for Doppler studies across the mitral and aortic valves. The reference marker for the long axis views is directed at approximately 12 o'clock. The left two-chamber view is obtained from the

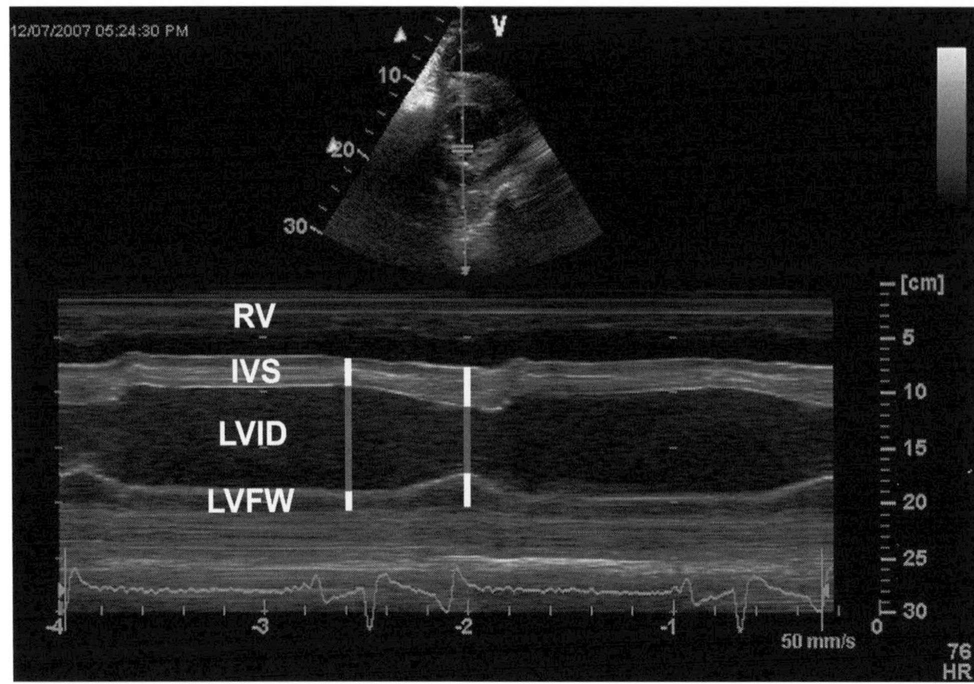

Figure 1.87 M-mode of the left ventricle. LVID, Left ventricular internal diameter. Other abbreviations are as for Figure 1.84, A–C. ©Mary Durando 2006.

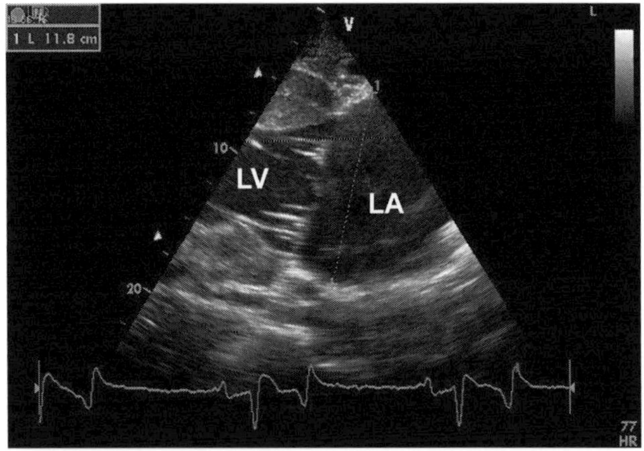

Figure 1.88 Two-dimensional left parasternal echocardiogram of the left atrium. The left atrium, mitral valve and left ventricle are seen with this view. The vertical line is placed at measurement of the left atrial diameter. A measurement of 11.8 cm is within normal limits. Abbreviations are as for Figure 1.84, A–C. ©Mary Durando 2006.

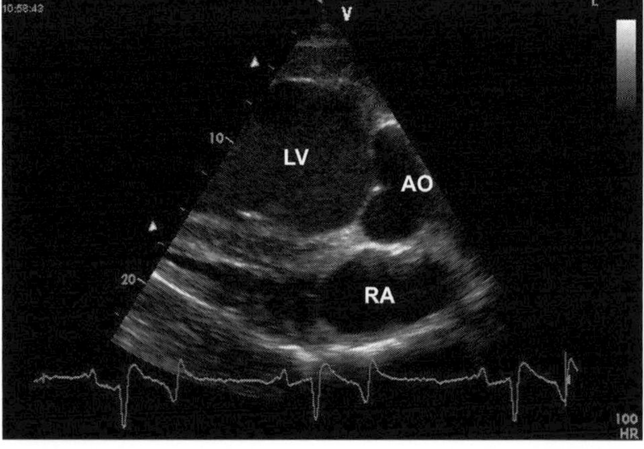

Figure 1.89 Two-dimensional left parasternal echocardiogram of the aorta. The aorta, left ventricle and right atrium are seen in this view. Abbreviations are as for Figure 1.84, A–C. ©Mary Durando 2006.

fifth ICS at a level midway between the point of the shoulder and elbow. This view allows a more representative measurement of left atrial size than right parasternal images and, in general, a more detailed look at the mitral valve and better Doppler studies (Figure 1.88). The left outflow tract view is obtained from the fourth ICS at a similar level and is used for examination of the aortic valve (Figure 1.89). The right outflow tract view, often the most difficult to obtain because it is so far cranial, is obtained from the third ICS angling slightly caudally (Figure 1.90). From this view, the pulmonic valve and pulmonary artery are evaluated. Typically, the pulmonary artery and aorta measure larger from the left side. Short-axis views are obtained by rotating the probe 90°, as for the right side.

All views are greatly facilitated by placing the horse's foreleg on the side of the examiner forward. For a more detailed description of echocardiographic technique and Doppler evaluation, the reader is referred to more comprehensive articles on the topic.[4–10]

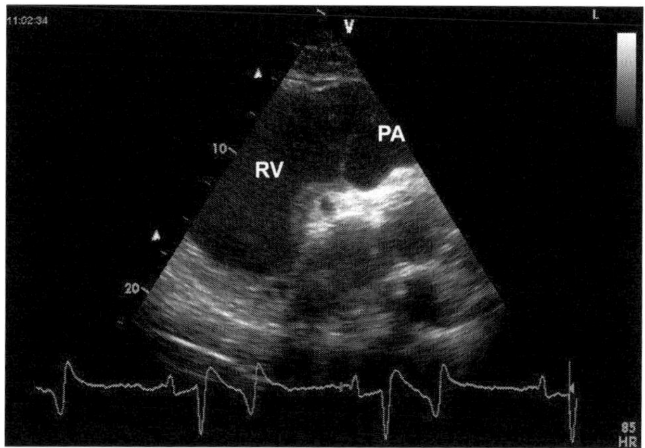

Figure 1.90 Two-dimensional left parasternal echocardiogram of the pulmonary artery. The pulmonary artery and right ventricle are seen in this view. Abbreviations are as for Figure 1.84, A–C. ©Mary Durando 2006.

References

1. Reef VB: Echocardiographic examination in the horse: the basics. Compend Contin Educ Pract Vet 12:1312-1320, 1990
2. Long KJ, Bonagura JD, Darke PG: Standardised imaging technique for guided M-mode and Doppler echocardiography in the horse. Equine Vet J 24:226-235, 1992
3. Bonagura JD, Blissitt KJ: Echocardiography. Equine Vet J Suppl:5-17, 1995
4. Blissitt KJ, Bonagura JD: Pulsed wave Doppler echocardiography in normal horses. Equine Vet J Suppl 19:38-46, 1995
5. Blissitt KJ, Bonagura JD: Colour flow Doppler echocardiography in horses with cardiac murmurs. Equine Vet J Suppl:82-85, 1995
6. Blissitt KJ, Young LE, Jones RS, et al: Measurement of cardiac output in standing horses by Doppler echocardiography and thermodilution. Equine Vet J 29:18-25, 1997
7. Reef VB: Heart murmurs in horses: determining their significance with echocardiography. Equine Vet J Suppl 19:71-80, 1995
8. Reef VB: Evaluation of ventricular septal defects in horses using two-dimensional and Doppler echocardiography. Equine Vet J Suppl:86-95, 1995
9. Reef VB, Bain FT, Spencer PA: Severe mitral regurgitation in horses: clinical, echocardiographic and pathological findings. Equine Vet J 30:18-27, 1998
10. Reef VB, Spencer P: Echocardiographic evaluation of equine aortic insufficiency. Am J Vet Res 48:904-909, 1987

1.26 Cardiac output measurement

Mary Durando

Monitoring cardiac output (CO) is useful to assess the haemodynamic status and cardiovascular function of the patient. The most common, well-validated methods of measuring CO in horses are the Fick method[1] and indicator dilution methods.[2,3] Because the Fick method requires the use of a facemask and equipment to measure oxygen consumption/CO_2 production, as well as an arterial and pulmonary artery catheter, it is too technically demanding for uses other than research and is not suitable for most clinic cases. The earlier dilution methods using indocyanine green dye[4,5] and thermodilution[6–9] also require placement of a pulmonary artery catheter; however, the development of the lithium dilution (LIDCO) method has allowed a relatively noninvasive, simpler means of measuring CO, requiring only a venous and peripheral artery catheter.[6,10,11]

Principle

Dilution methods rely on the principle that concentration A × volume A = concentration B × volume B. Therefore, if a known mass (concentration and volume) of a substance is injected into an unknown volume, and the final concentration of the substance is determined, the volume it is diluted in (CO) can be calculated. Using LIDCO, a known mass is injected rapidly into the venous side (e.g., jugular vein), and a catheter placed in a peripheral artery (e.g., transverse facial artery) withdraws the blood at a constant rate across a lithium specific electrode. The sensor calculates the concentration of lithium over time, and from this a curve is drawn. The computer program calculates the area under the curve, to give a volume of blood per unit time.[10,12,13] CO is given in litres/min, although it is more appropriate to convert this value to cardiac index, or mass specific CO, as ml/kg/min because of large variability in the size of many horses. All dilution methods rely on the substance measured not being metabolised or excreted, and the methods are not accurate in the presence of an intracardiac shunt. Because it is less invasive and cumbersome than other methods and has been validated in the horse, only the LIDCO method will be described here. References are available that contain detailed descriptions of other methods.[1,9,12]

Equipment needed

The equipment needed for measuring CO by the lithium dilution method is given in Box 1.28.

This method requires the purchase of a specialised computer (Figure 1.91) that connects to a disposable lithium sensor (Figure 1.92), to convert the readings in the sensor to the concentration of lithium (Figure 1.93), and to be able to draw and calculate the area under the curve (Figure 1.94). Other requirements are disposable lithium sensors, lithium and a pump to withdraw blood at a constant rate (Figure 1.95). The instrumentation needed is a catheter in a major vein (i.e., jugular vein works well) for rapid injection of lithium and a catheter in a peripheral artery such as the transverse facial artery, or in foals, the metatarsal artery.

Procedure

Before making a measurement, the arterial sodium and haemoglobin concentrations need to be obtained. These

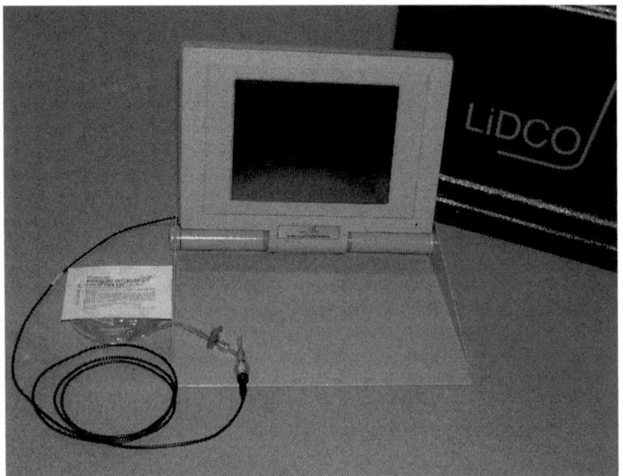

Figure 1.91 The original LiDCO computer and sensor for calculation of cardiac output. This model allows calculation of cardiac output but not continuous monitoring of cardiac output by pulse wave analysis. The microbore extension set leads from the arterial catheter to the input of the sensor via a three-way stopcock. A stopcock and tubing lead from the sensor output to a peristaltic pump. ©EK Birks 2007.

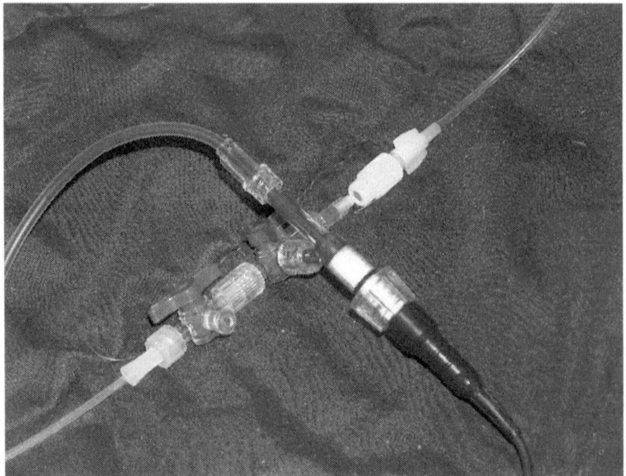

Figure 1.92 Lithium specific sensor for lithium dilution method of cardiac output monitoring. ©Kevin Corley 2005.

Box 1.28. Equipment for lithium dilution method of measuring cardiac output

Required

LiDCOplus or LiDCO computer*
Peristaltic pump
Blood collection bag
Lithium sensor
Lithium chloride solution
Venous catheter (usually jugular) (see Chapters 1.14 and 1.15)
Arterial catheter (see Chapter 1.20)
Narrow bore extension tubing
Three-way stopcock (three-way tap)†
T-port or short extension set
500-ml bag of 0.9% sterile saline (5–10 units/ml heparin)
20–30-ml syringes
Blood sodium concentration analyser
Blood haemoglobin concentration analyser

Optional (for pulse contour analysis)

Direct arterial pressure monitor
Lead to connect LiDCOplus to direct arterial pressure monitor

*LiDCO Ltd., Sawston, Cambridge, UK.
†Vygon, Ecouen, France.

values, along with the exact amount of lithium injected (in mmol), are entered into the computer before each measurement. The computer algorithm uses this information to calculate the CO from the lithium concentration determined by the sensor. The computer assumes a lithium concentration of 150 mmol/L to read out the volume of lithium injected. For each new patient, the computer also

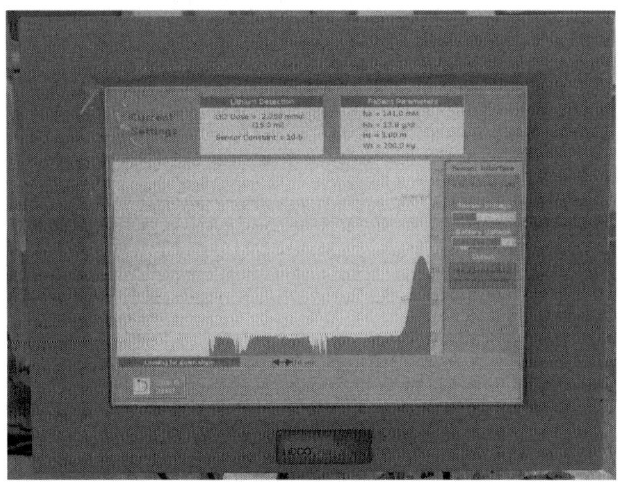

Figure 1.93 The lithium dilution is converted to a voltage, which is displayed on the screen. ©Kevin Corley 2003.

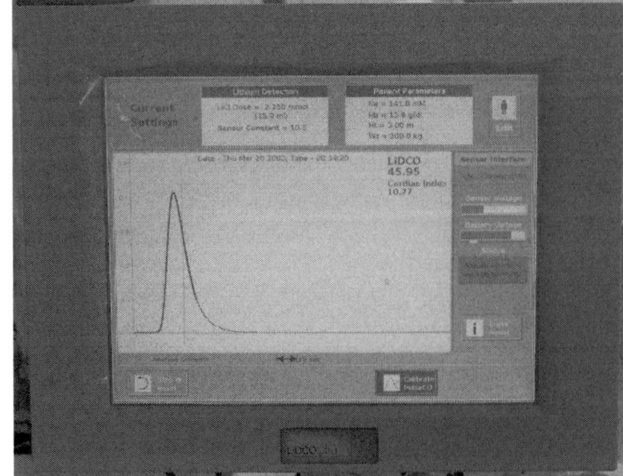

Figure 1.94 The computer program calculates the area under the curve, to give a volume of blood per unit time, i.e., the cardiac output. ©Kevin Corley 2003.

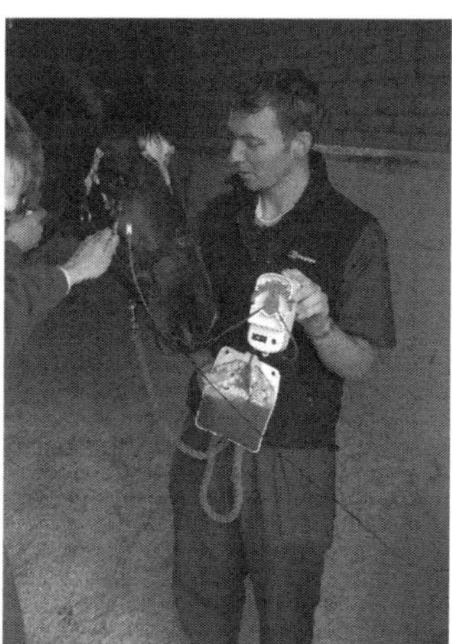

Figure 1.95 LiDCO measurement of cardiac output in a horse after colic surgery. The horse was instrumented with a transverse facial arterial catheter connected via a three-way stopcock to the lithium sensor. The arterial catheter is secured in place with super glue and zinc oxide tape. The peristaltic pump withdraws blood from the artery through the sensor at a constant rate of 4 ml/min. There is also a catheter in the right jugular vein for injection of lithium. ©Kevin Corley 2002.

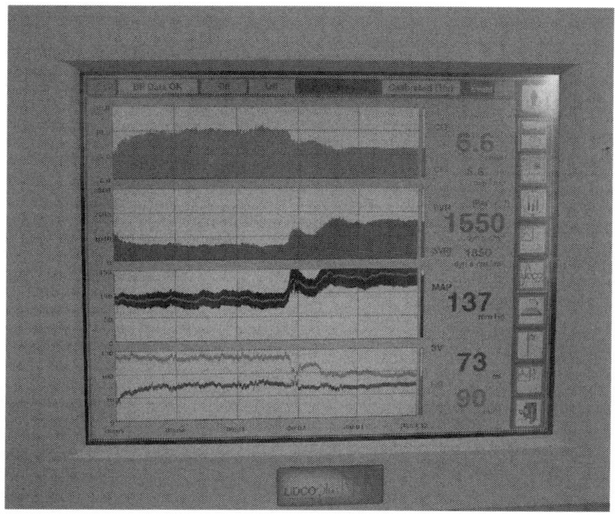

Figure 1.96 Readout from pulse contour analysis cardiac output determination in a foal. ©Kevin Corley 2006.

requires a height and weight for the patient. This information is used to calculate cardiac index based on body surface area calculations based on a human algorithm. This is not used for measurement in the horse, and any number can be entered.

The peristaltic pump must be turned on prior to making a measurement, and blood must be flowing through the sensor, in order to let it equilibrate and obtain a stable baseline. This is critical for correct operation. To quickly stabilise the baseline, the release can be pressed on the pump to allow more rapid flow of blood through the sensor. Once the baseline has stabilised, a known concentration and volume of lithium (i.e., 20 ml of 150 mmol/L lithium chloride for a standing horse; 3 to 5 ml of 150 mmol/L lithium chloride for a neonatal foal) are rapidly injected into a vein as the pump continues to withdraw blood from the artery. An "inject" button on the screen or foot-pedal must be depressed before the injection is given. The lead-time depends on the expected CO of the horse. The lithium sensor detects the concentration of lithium in blood withdrawn from the artery over time, allowing calculation of the volume of blood (CO) by the computer software, by drawing a curve and calculating the area under the curve (Figure 1.94). The COt in litres/min should be read out, and can be divided by body weight to obtain ml/kg/min. The value given for cardiac index is not accurate in the horse and should be ignored.

The rapidity of injection will influence the curve; therefore, it is easier to use a short extension set or T-port connected to the venous catheter, rather than a long extension set, and these should be primed with the lithium solution. The arterial catheter should be connected to a small-bore extension set and a three-way stopcock, which attaches to the input of the lithium sensor, as per instructions. The sensor output is attached to a three-way stopcock, tubing and the pump, to withdraw blood at a constant rate across the sensor. The catheter and sensor should be flushed with heparinised saline between readings to prevent blood clots and should not be allowed to dry out. The sensor probably cannot be used on successive days or on multiple patients, as its life span is limited. Background lithium concentrations can build up with repeated injections of lithium interfering with accurate calculation of CO, although by using a standard dose of lithium, in the typical clinical scenario, this is not likely to happen.[14,15]

Pulse contour analysis

Continuous CO measurement from the arterial pulse waveform allows beat-to-beat assessment of cardiovascular status. Pulse contour analysis calculates stroke volume (SV) from the arterial waveform. The area under the pulse waveform during systole allows calculation of CO.[12] The form of pulse waveform is, in part, due to elastic recoil of the artery, and is unique to each individual.[16,17] Therefore, the technique requires calibration in the subject prior to use.[16,17] Commercial calibration methods available for human patients are transpulmonary thermodilution and lithium dilution.[12] Pulse contour analysis, using lithium dilution for calibration, has been shown to be accurate in anaesthetised horses.[18]

This method requires direct monitoring of arterial pressure (see Chapter 1.22) and a monitor that is compatible with the LiDCOplus computer. After obtaining a lithium dilution curve, the arterial catheter is reconnected to the arterial pressure monitor (usually by turning a three-way stopcock). Once a stable arterial waveform has been reestablished, the PulseCO can be calibrated to the LiDCO. The PulseCO then gives a continuous reading of CO, systemic vascular resistance (SVR), mean arterial pressure (MAP), stroke volume (SV) and heart rate (HR) (Figure 1.96). The pulse contour reading should be recalibrated periodically (at least every 8 hours) and if there is a major or unusual change in CO.

Normal values for the horse and foal are given in the Appendix (see Tables 19.17 and 19.18).

References

1. Fedak MA, Rome L, Seeherman HJ: One-step N2-dilution technique for calibrating open-circuit VO2 measuring systems. J Appl Physiol 51:772-776, 1981
2. Kinsman JM, Moore JW, Hamilton WF: Studies on the circulation. 1. Injection method: physical and mathematical considerations. Am J Physiol 89:332, 1932
3. Stewart GN: Researches on circulation time and on the influences which affect it. IV. The output of the heart. J Physiol (Lond) 22:159-183, 1897
4. Lund-Johansen P: The dye dilution method for measurement of cardiac output. Eur Heart J 11(Suppl I):6-12, 1990
5. Mizuno Y, Aida H, Hara H, et al: Comparison of methods of cardiac output measurements determined by dye dilution, pulsed Doppler echocardiography and thermodilution in horses. J Vet Med Sci 56:1-5, 1994
6. Corley KTT, Donaldson LL, Furr MO: Comparison of lithium dilution and thermodilution cardiac output measurements in anaesthetised neonatal foals. Equine Vet J 34:598-601, 2002
7. Ganz W, Donoso R, Marcus HS, et al: A new technique for measurement of cardiac output by thermodilution in man. Am J Cardiol 27:392-396, 1971
8. Hinchcliff KW, McKeever KH, Muir WW: Hemodynamic effects of atropine, dobutamine, nitroprusside, phenylephrine, and propranolol in conscious horses. J Vet Int Med 5:80-86, 1991
9. Muir WW, Skarda RT, Milne DW: Estimation of cardiac output in the horse by thermodilution techniques. Am J Vet Res 37:697-700, 1976
10. Linton RA, Band DM, Haire KM: A new method of measuring cardiac output in man using lithium dilution. Br J Anaesth 71:262-266, 1993
11. Linton RA, Young LE, Marlin DJ, et al: Cardiac output measured by lithium dilution, thermodilution and transesophageal Doppler echocardiography in anesthetized horses. Am J Vet Res 61:731-737, 2000
12. Corley KTT, Donaldson LL, Durando MM, et al: Cardiac output technologies with special reference to the horse. J Vet Int Med 17:262-272, 2003
13. Linton RA, Linton NW, Band DM: A new method of analysing indicator dilution curves. Cardiovasc Res 30:930-938, 1995
14. Mason DJ, O'Grady M, Woods JP, et al: Effect of background serum lithium concentrations on the accuracy of lithium dilution cardiac output determination in dogs. Am J Vet Res 63:1048-1052, 2002
15. Hatfield CL, McDonnell WN, Lemke KA, et al: Pharmacokinetics and toxic effects of lithium chloride after intravenous administration in conscious horses. Am J Vet Res 62:1387-1392, 2001
16. Winer N, Sowers JR, Weber MA: Gender differences in vascular compliance in young, healthy subjects assessed by pulse contour analysis. J Clin Hypertens (Greenwich) 3:145-152, 2001
17. McVeigh GE, Bratteli CW, Morgan DJ, et al: Age-related abnormalities in arterial compliance identified by pressure pulse contour analysis: aging and arterial compliance. Hypertension 33:1392-1398, 1999
18. Hallowell GD, Corley KT: Use of lithium dilution and pulse contour analysis cardiac output determination in anaesthetized horses: a clinical evaluation. Vet Anaesth Analg 32:201-211, 2005

1.27 Pericardiocentesis

Mary Durando

Pericardiocentesis is indicated for the management of cases with rapid or large accumulations of fluid within the pericardial sac (Figure 1.97), as well as a diagnostic aid in determining the aetiology of the pericardial disease.[1–3]

Equipment needed

The equipment needed is given in Box 1.29.

Procedure

Echocardiography should be used to select the optimal site. The left cardiac window is most often selected, as there is usually no overlying lung, less chance of piercing the right ventricular free wall or lacerating a coronary artery, and less chance of entering the pleural space than on the right. The fifth ICS, between the point of the shoulder and the lateral thoracic vein, is usually the best location (Figure 1.98). Because of the risk for induction of dysrhythmias, cardiac rhythm should always be monitored during the procedure. This is most easily done with telemetry[2] (Figure 1.99). If multiple dysrhythmias are encountered during placement of the catheter, it should not be advanced

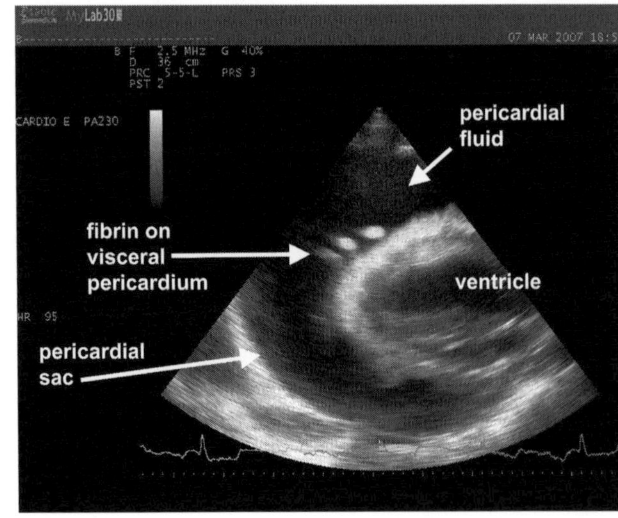

Figure 1.97 Echocardiogram showing a large pericardial effusion and fibrin deposition on the visceral pericardium (epicardium) in a 2-year-old sport horse. ©Kevin Corley 2007.

Box 1.29. Equipment for pericardiocentesis

Required

Catheter for centesis

- 10–14-Gauge 13-cm (5.25 inch) over-the-needle catheter and three-way stopcock (three-way tap)*
- Large-bore (16Fr–32Fr) Argyle chest tube and adapter to connect catheter to syringe

Clamp (haemostats)
50–60-ml syringe
Ultrasound machine for echocardiography (see Box 1.25)
Method to monitor ECG
  Ideally telemetric ECG monitor
Clippers with a fine (No. 40) blade
Small gauze swabs (4 × 4) soaked in chlorhexidine (4%) scrub solution†
Small gauze swabs (4 × 4) soaked in surgical spirit (alcohol)
Sterile small gauze swabs (4 × 4)
Mepivacaine 2%‡: 2–5-ml drawn up in a syringe with a 23–25-gauge needle
2–0 Nonabsorbable monofilament suture on a straight needle§
No. 11 scalpel blade
Surgical gloves
Intravenous catheter (Chapter 1.14 or 1.15)
Emergency anti-dysrhythmic drugs with dosages calculated

Optional

Sterile ultrasound probe cover
Sterile coupling gel**
Heimlich valve or syringe case
Serum and EDTA blood collection tubes
Material for aerobic and anaerobic cultures
Twitch
Sedation

*Vygon, Ecouen, France.
†Hibiscrub; Mölnlycke Health Care, Dunstable, UK.
‡Intra-epicaine; Arnolds Veterinary Products, Shrewsbury, UK; Carbocaine-V; Pfizer Animal Health, New York, NY, USA.
§628H, Ethilon Nylon; Ethicon, Somerville, NJ, USA.
**K-Y Jelly (Johnson and Johnson, New Brunswick, NJ, USA) is suitable for this purpose.

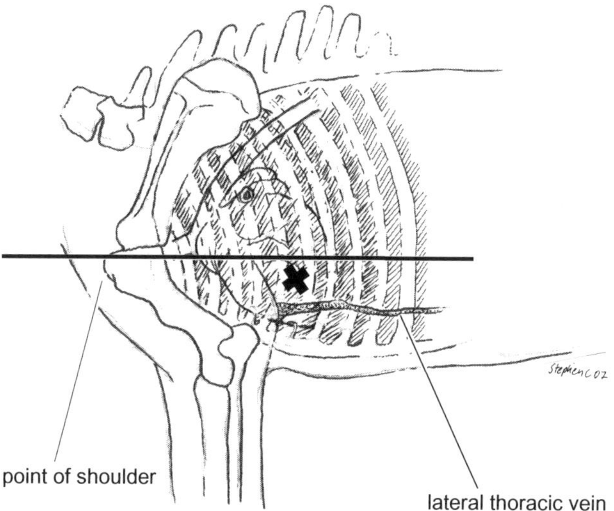

Figure 1.98 The usual site for pericardiocentesis. In the left fifth intercostal space, midway between a horizontal line from the point of the shoulder and the lateral thoracic vein.

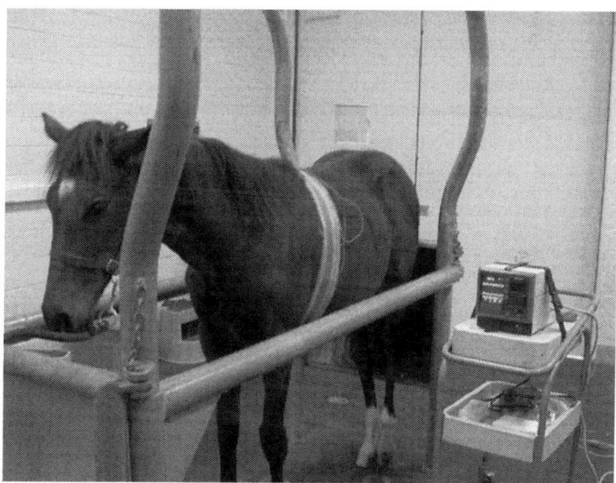

Figure 1.99 Weanling foal with telemetric ECG set up for monitoring cardiac rhythm during pericardiocentesis. Courtesy of Dr. Whitcomb, University of California, Davis, CA. ©Dr. Whitcomb 2006.

further, and/or withdrawn and repositioned. Although repositioning is usually enough to end dysrhythmias, an IV catheter should always be placed prior to centesis in the event rapid venous access and emergency therapy is needed, and appropriate antidysrhythmic drugs should be available.

The chosen site is clipped and surgically prepared and then infiltrated with local anaesthetic through the skin and subcutaneous tissues. A stab incision with a number 11 scalpel blade is made through the skin and subcutaneous tissues over the cranial portion of the rib. A large-bore French Argyle chest tube can be used (16Fr to 32Fr) for better drainage (Figures 1.100 and 1.101). The trocar of the larger tubes is more blunted and can be difficult to pass through the tissue layers; therefore, care must be taken when advancing to maintain control, as the tissue resistance can decrease suddenly when passing through the body wall. At the pericardial surface, the tube will move rhythmically with the heartbeat and should be advanced very carefully. The tube should be clamped as the trocar is removed to prevent pneumopericardium if fluid does not drain out immediately. The tube can be sutured in place with a purse-string suture and Chinese finger tie or butterfly tape, and left clamped, or closed with a sterile syringe, syringe case or a one-way Heimlich valve. If an over-the-needle type catheter system is chosen, it should be con-

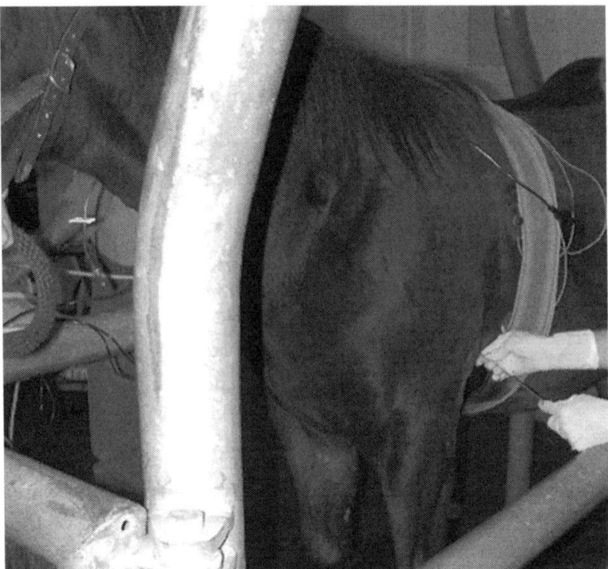

Figure 1.100 A 20Fr Argyle chest tube is being inserted in the fifth ICS between the point of the shoulder and the elbow to drain pericardial effusion. The foal has an IV catheter in place and cardiac rhythm is monitored with telemetric ECG. Courtesy of Dr. Whitcomb, University of California, Davis, CA. ©Dr. Whitcomb 2006.

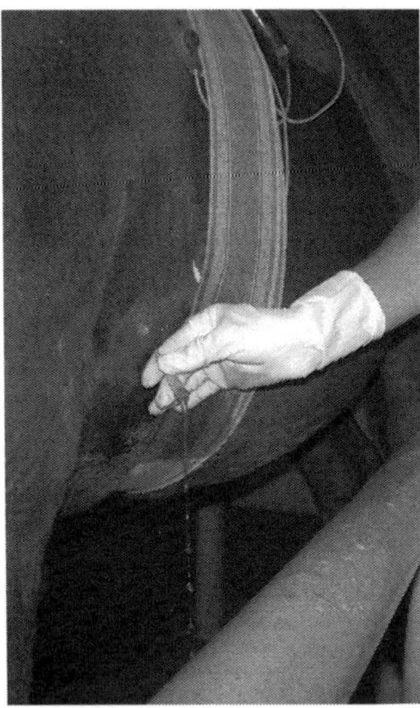

Figure 1.101 Fluid draining from the chest tube, placed in the pericardial sac. Courtesy of Dr. Whitcomb, University of California, Davis, CA. ©Dr. Whitcomb 2006.

nected to an extension set with a three-way stopcock turned to off, to prevent air from entering the thorax or pericardial space. Final tube or catheter position can be verified with echocardiography (Figure 1.102), using a sterile probe cover and surgical spirit (alcohol), and the amount of fluid remaining and cardiac function after drainage can be assessed.

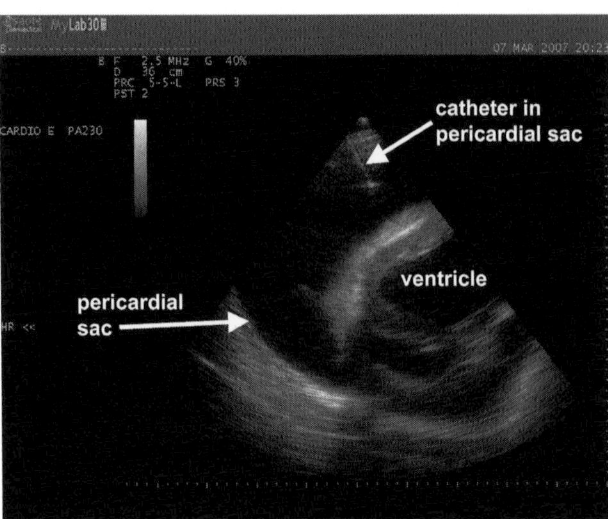

Figure 1.102 Catheter in the pericardial sac, draining pericardial fluid. ©Kevin Corley 2007.

References

1. Sleeper MM: Acquired pericardial disease, in Robinson NE (ed): Current Therapy in Equine Medicine, ed 5. St. Louis, WB Saunders, 2003, pp 622-624
2. Bernard W, Reef VB, Clark ES, et al: Pericarditis in horses: six cases (1982-1986). J Am Vet Med Assoc 196:468-471, 1990
3. Worth LT, Reef VB: Pericarditis in horses: 18 cases (1986-1995). J Am Vet Med Assoc 212:248-253, 1998

1.28 Emergency tracheotomy

Jennifer O. Stephen

Tracheotomy is performed for upper-airway obstructions. Conditions associated with acute upper airway obstructions include recovery from inhalational anaesthesia, enlargement of the retropharyngeal lymph nodes (usually due to *Streptococcus equi equi* infection), bilateral laryngeal paralysis secondary to hepatic encephalopathy and physical obstruction of the airway.

Equipment needed

The equipment needed is given in Box 1.30.

Procedure

The trachea is easily identified on palpation of the midline of the neck. The site for tracheotomy is at the junction of the cranial and middle third of the ventral neck. Ideally, the area should be clipped and aseptically prepared (Figure 1.103, A). Five to 10 ml of local anaesthetic should then be infused into the skin and subcutaneous tissue overlying the trachea, along the line where the skin incision is to be made. With sterile gloves, a 10-cm skin incision should be made over the middle of the trachea in a proximal to distal direction through the skin and subcutaneous tissue (Figure

Box 1.30. Equipment for emergency tracheotomy

Required

Tracheal tube

- Self-retaining tracheal tube
- Short silicone tube*
- Metal J tube

Clippers with a fine (No. 40) blade
Small gauze swabs (4 × 4) soaked in chlorhexidine (4%) scrub solution†
Small gauze swabs (4 × 4) soaked in surgical spirit (alcohol)
Mepivacaine 2%‡: 5–10 ml drawn up in a syringe with a 23–25-gauge needle
Surgical gloves
No. 11 scalpel blade

Optional

Twitch
Sedation

*Bivona; Smiths Medical International (UK), Watford, UK.: www.smiths-medical.com.
†Hibiscrub; Mölnlycke Health Care, Dunstable, UK.
‡Intra-epicaine; Arnolds Veterinary Products, Shrewsbury, UK; Carbocaine-V; Pfizer Animal Health, New York, NY, USA.

1.103, B). The paired muscles overlying the trachea (sternothyrohyoideus muscles) should then be bluntly dissected and retracted to expose the tracheal cartilages. An incision is made into the tracheal annular ligament between two tracheal cartilages, parallel to the cartilages (Figure 1.103, C). The incision should be large enough to insert a suitable tube, but no more than one third to one half of the circumference of the trachea.[1] A variety of tracheal tubes may be used: self-retaining tracheal tubes, short silicone tubes or metal J tubes.

In a life-threatening emergency, the surgical procedure should be performed as fast as possible—without aseptic preparation or local anaesthetic. Where no proper endotracheal tube is available, any hollow tube may be used to keep the airway open, such as a section of stomach tube or garden hose.

After placement

Once placed, the tracheal tube must be checked for patency and cleaned regularly. Potential complications of tracheotomy include infection, subcutaneous emphysema, blockage of the tracheal tube,[2] ischaemic necrosis of the tracheal mucosa from overinflation of cuffed tube[3] and tracheal stricture. Removal of the tracheal tube as soon as possible reduces long-term complications. After removal of the tube, the site should be left to heal by second intention and cleaned twice daily with dilute antiseptic solution.

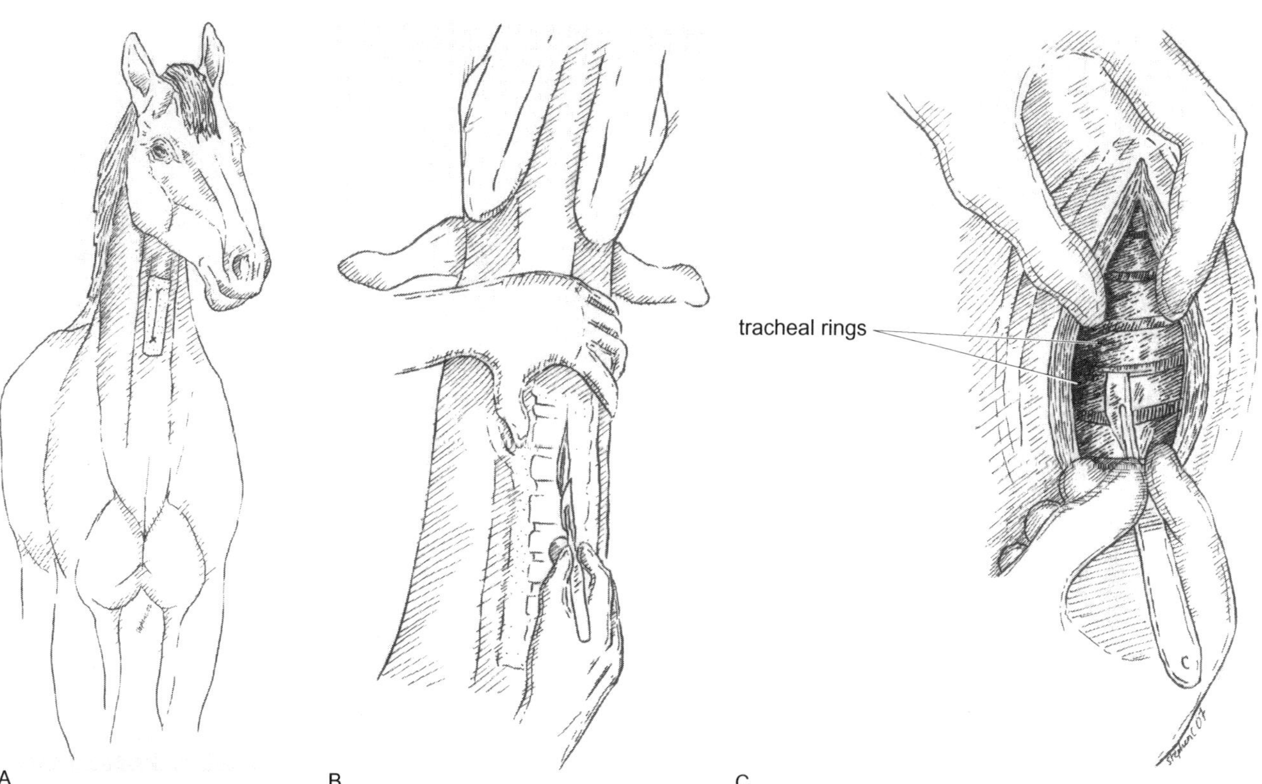

Figure 1.103 Tracheotomy. **A,** The site for tracheotomy, at the junction of the cranial and middle third of the ventral neck. **B,** A 10-cm skin incision should be made over the middle of the trachea in a proximal-to-distal direction. **C,** An incision is made into the tracheal annular ligament between two tracheal cartilages, parallel to the cartilages.

References

1. Shappell KK, Tulleners EP: Trachea, in Auer JA (ed): Equine Surgery. Philadelphia, WB Saunders, 1992, p 489
2. Krpan MK: Tracheotomy in the horse: a photo essay. Mod Vet Pract 65:9, 1984
3. Holland MH: Larnyngotracheal injury associated with naso-tracheal intubation in the horse. J Am Vet Med Assoc 189:1447, 1986.

1.29 Intranasal oxygen administration

Harold McKenzie

The provision of supplemental oxygen is easily accomplished in adults and foals by means of nasal oxygen insufflation.

Equipment needed

The placement of a nasal catheter is required for nasal oxygen insufflation, and these are available commercially (Box 1.31). The oxygen tanks should be outside the stall, and in a place where they cannot be accidentally knocked over by animals or people. A safer system is to install a piped oxygen system in the intensive care unit (Figure 1.104). The oxygen should be humidified by bubbling through sterile water prior to insufflation (Figures 1.104 and 1.105).

Procedure

It is important that the nasal catheter be positioned deep within the nasal passages but rostral to the pharynx, and this can be estimated by setting the length of the catheter to reach from the external nares to the level of the medial canthus of the eye. In foals, the catheter can be maintained in position by taping it to a 4- to 5-cm segment of tongue depressor and then taping the catheter around the rounded portion of the tongue depressor such that the catheter is directed up the nasal passages (Figure 1.106). The external portion of the catheter and the tongue depressor are fixed to the foal's face by means of a circumferential band of stretchy adhesive dressing (Figure 1.107). In some cases, it is helpful to secure the catheter to the external nares using a "butterfly" of tape placed around the catheter, which is

Box 1.31. Equipment for nasal insufflation of oxygen

Nasal oxygen cannula
For adults
14Fr–18Fr red rubber feeding tube*
For foals
14Fr × 41-cm oxygen catheter†

Required
Oxygen cylinder or piped oxygen outlet
Oxygen flowmeter
Inline oxygen humidifier‡
Sterile water
Oxygen tubing§
Zinc oxide tape
7.5-cm (3-inch) wide stretchy adhesive dressing (Elastoplast**/Elastikon††)
For foals
Tongue depressor
For adults
2-0 Nonabsorbable monofilament suture on a straight needle‡‡

Optional:
Coiled fluid administration set§§

*Kendall Sovereign; Tyco Healthcare Group, LP, Mansfield, MA, USA.
†Allegiance Healthcare Corp., McGaw Park, IL, USA.
‡Examples include Airlife prefilled humidifier; Allegiance Healthcare Corp., McGaw Park, IL, USA.
§Examples include: 6.4-metre length Airlife oxygen tubing; Allegiance Healthcare Corp., McGaw Park, IL, USA.
**Beiersdorf AG, Hamburg, Germany
††Johnson and Johnson, New Brunswick, NJ, USA.
‡‡628H, Ethilon Nylon; Ethicon, Somerville, NJ, USA.
§§Coiled extension set; International Win, Ltd., Kennett Square, PA, USA.

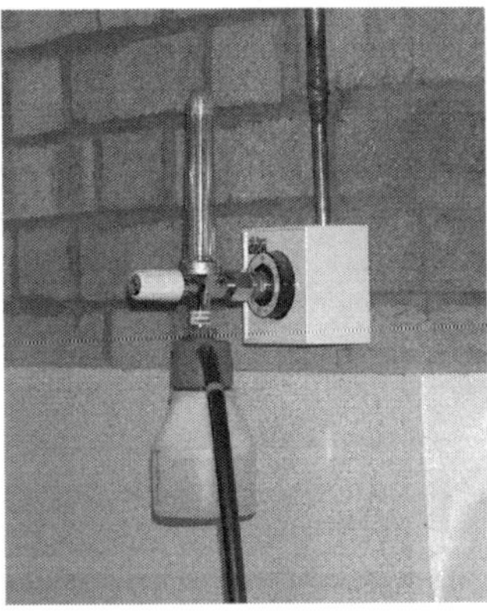

Figure 1.104 Piped oxygen outlet, flowmeter and humidifier. ©Kevin Corley 2005.

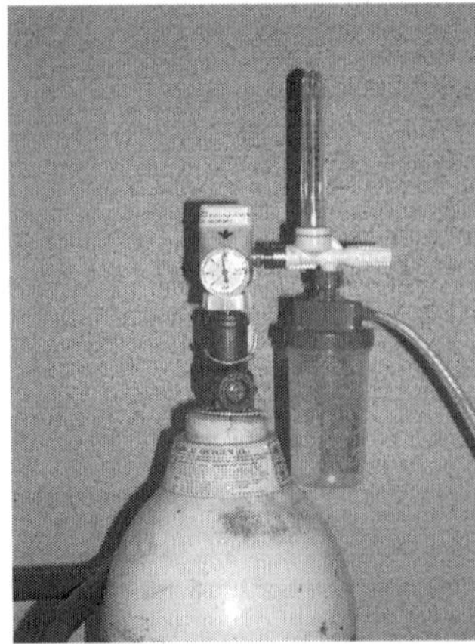

Figure 1.105 Oxygen tank, flowmeter and humidifier. ©Kevin Corley 2007.

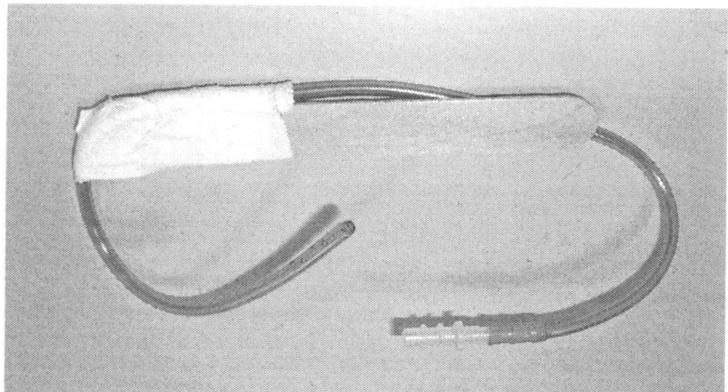

Figure 1.106 Nasal oxygen catheter taped to tongue depressor. ©Harold C. McKenzie III 2006.

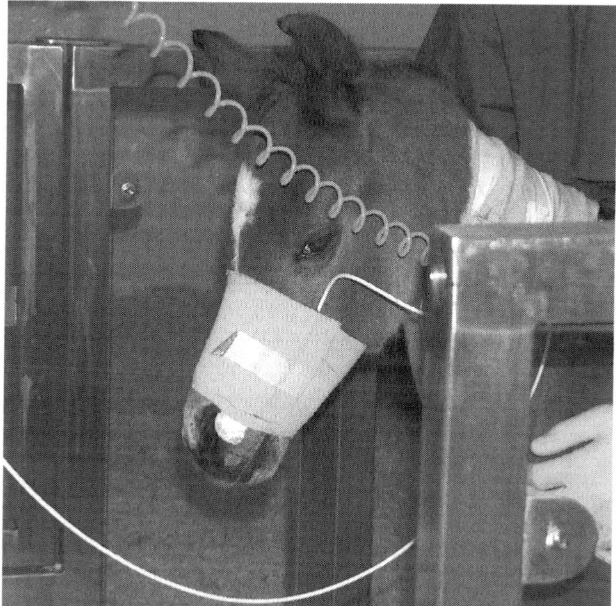

Figure 1.107 The external portion of the catheter and the tongue depressor are affixed to the foal's face by means of a circumferential band of stretchy adhesive dressing. ©Kevin Corley 2005.

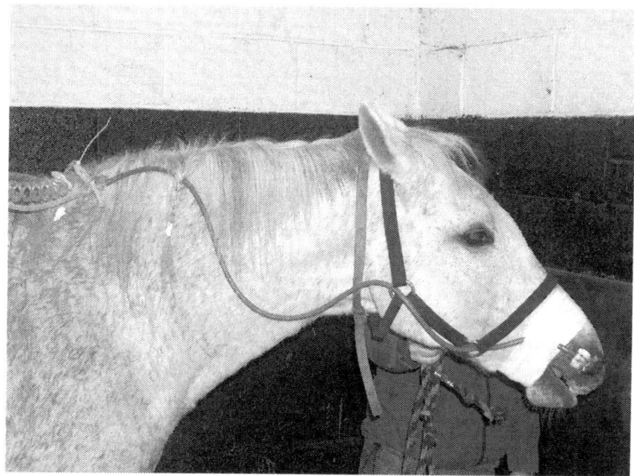

Figure 1.108 In adults, the catheter is typically sutured to the external nares and taped to the halter for stabilisation. ©Kevin Corley 2007.

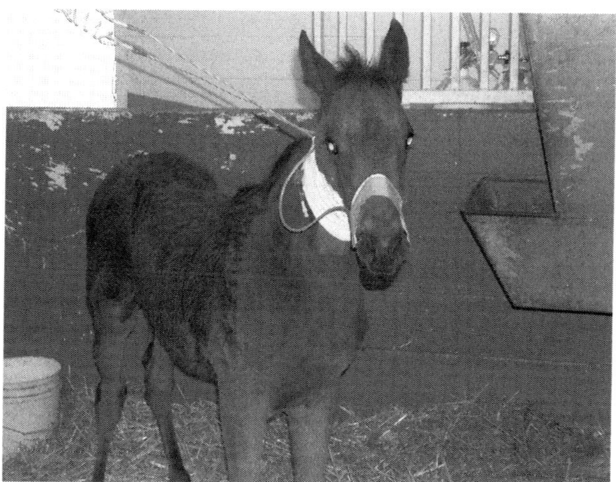

Figure 1.109 Bilateral nasal oxygen administration in a foal with severely compromised oxygenation, due to *Rhodococcus equi* infection. ©Kevin Corley 2004.

then secured with a single simple interrupted suture using nonabsorbable suture material. In adults, the catheter is typically sutured to the external nares and taped to the halter for stabilisation (Figure 1.108).

Prior to administering oxygen to the patient, the oxygen must pass through a humidification device in order to prevent the inhalation of dry gas that would result in respiratory tract injury. Delivery of the humidified oxygen to the patient is readily achieved using flexible oxygen tubing to connect the output port of the humidifier to the nasal catheter of the patient. Ambulatory patients can present a challenge, as this tubing will become tangled, but this can be minimised by delivering the oxygen through a coiled fluid administration set. Administration rates are generally limited by the delivery system to approximately 10 to 15 L/min, which is adequate for most foals but may not be adequate in adults. In cases where higher flow rates are desired, two separate systems can be utilised to deliver oxygen into both nostrils (Figure 1.109), thereby further increasing the FIO_2.

1.30 Nebulisation

Harold McKenzie

Nebulisation is the delivery of medication to the respiratory tract in the form of an aerosol derived from a liquid, typically using either a pneumatic (jet) nebuliser or an ultrasonic nebuliser. These devices generate a cloud of aerosol particles from the liquid medication, and this aerosol is then delivered to the patient for inhalation.

Equipment needed

The equipment needed for nebulisation is given in Box 1.32. In the conscious horse, nebulisation requires the use

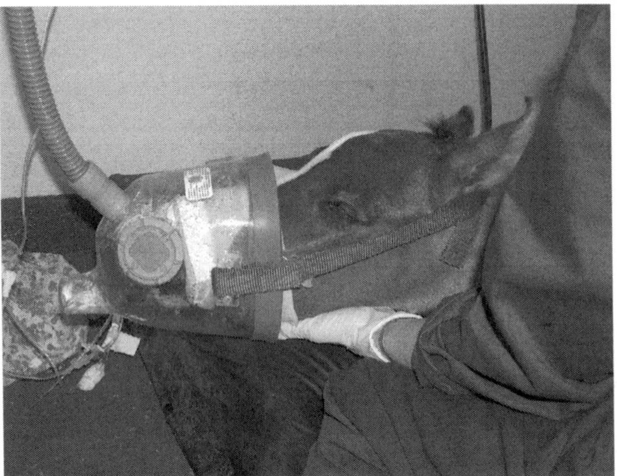

Figure 1.110 Nebulisation of a foal with a fitted, valved facemask. ©Kevin Corley 2005.

> **Box 1.32. Equipment for nebulisation**
>
> **Nebuliser**
> - Pneumatic (jet) nebuliser*
> - Ultrasonic nebuliser†
>
> **Required**
> Fitted, valved facemask‡
> Spacer device or plastic aerosol tubing
> Drug to be nebulised
>
> **Optional**
> Sedation
> Systemic or inhaled β_2-agonist bronchodilators 30–60 minutes prior to treatment
>
> *Nebul; Agritronics, Meux,. Belgium (www.vtrade.be).
> †Ultraneb; Sunrise Medical, Longmont, CO, USA. (www.sunrisemedical.com).
> ‡Aeromask ES; Trudell Medical International, London, Ont., Canada; Eramask, Biomedtech
> §Australia Pty Ltd Melbourne, Australia.

of a fitted, valved facemask connected to the nebuliser by means of a spacer device or plastic aerosol tubing (Figure 1.110). The valved facemask allows for aerosol delivery without concern for coordination with the patients respirations, as it allows the aerosol to be delivered with each inhaled breath by way of the centrally located inhalation valve, whilst the exhaled air exits the mask by way of the two exhalation valves located over the nostrils.

Procedure

The medication to be aerosolised is placed into the reservoir of the nebulisation device and the aerosol delivery system is connected to the facemask on the patient. The reservoir of pneumatic nebulisers is generally fairly small (3 to 6 ml), often necessitating that the reservoir be refilled during the procedure to allow for aerosolisation of the full volume of medication (see Figure 10.21), whilst the reservoir of ultrasonic nebulisers is larger (20 to 30 ml), allowing for placement of the entire volume of medication to be delivered without refilling the reservoir (see Figure 10.20).

When first introducing a patient to nebulisation therapy, place the facemask onto the patient for several minutes prior to initiating nebulisation to allow them to become familiarised with wearing the mask itself. Some fractious young horses may require sedation for the first few treatments, after which most individuals become adequately familiarised with the procedure. Ensure that the rubber gasket encircling the edge of the facemask is forming a good seal around the muzzle prior to initiating treatment. Connect the nebulisation device to the facemask using disposable corrugated nebuliser tubing, and turn on the nebuliser.

Pneumatic nebulisers should be run until the reservoir is empty, with as many refills as required to deliver the total dose. Ultrasonic nebulisers will not effectively aerosolise all of the solution placed within the sample cup, and treatment is complete when the device is no longer producing a visible cloud of aerosol and the solution in the cup begins to "sputter". The fact that some of the aerosolisation solution remains is normal and does not impair the ability of the device to deliver an effective dosage to the patient. While the patient is receiving the aerosol treatment, monitor the facemask to ensure that there is no leakage of aerosol around the muzzle.

After the treatment is completed, remove the facemask and clean it thoroughly using warm water and a mild detergent; then rinse well and dry the facemask prior to the next treatment. The aerosolisation tubing should be rinsed with warm water and air dried between uses, and this tubing should be replaced at least every other day. Pneumatic nebulisers can be reused but must be cleaned and dried as described for the facemask or following the manufacturer's recommendations. The sample cup and lid used in ultrasonic nebulisers are disposable and should be replaced for each treatment administration. Cleanliness is extremely important, as contamination of the aerosolisation solution or aerosol delivery equipment may result in nosocomial infections.[1]

The solution used for aerosolisation should ideally be a commercially available product intended for aerosol delivery (examples include Albuterol Sulfate Solution for Inhalation 0.5%; Astra USA, Inc., Westborough, MA, USA). Antimicrobial solutions for aerosol administration to horses must be formulated, however, and should have a concentration of 25 to 50 mg/ml in either 0.45% saline solution or sterile water (ceftiofur)[2] (see Chapter 6.4). Pretreatment with systemic or inhaled β_2-agonist bronchodilators (salbutamol [albuterol], clenbuterol) 5 to 10 minutes prior to treatment is recommended in patients receiving aerosolised medications, as some aerosolised medications may induce reflex bronchosconstriction.[2]

References

1. Pegues CF, Pegues DA, Ford DS, et al.: *Burkholderia cepacia* respiratory tract acquisition: epidemiology and molecular characterization of a large nosocomial outbreak. Epidemiol Infect 116:309-317, 1996
2. McKenzie HC: Characterization of antimicrobial aerosols for administration to horses. Vet Ther 4:110-119, 2003

1.31 Endoscopy of the respiratory tract

Jennifer O. Stephen

Equipment needed

The equipment needed is given in Box 1.33. For endoscopy of the upper airways alone, scopes of up to 12-mm outer diameter may be used in the adult. A 9-mm outer diameter scope is the largest that should be used in foals. This diameter is also adequate for adults and will allow bronchial structures to be examined.[1]

General procedure

Three people are required. One person should restrain the horse, one should pass the scope and one should "drive" the endoscope. Sedation should be avoided until the function of the larynx or pharynx has been assessed. In patients that resent examination, the use of a twitch may help. Once the larynx has been examined, sedation can aid in examination of the lower airway by preventing coughing. All of the equipment required for procedure should be prepared and ready to hand before passing the scope. If the horse cannot be restrained in stocks, it is important to position the equipment so it can be rapidly moved away from the patient.

If samples of exudates for culture are required, transtracheal aspiration should be carried out prior to endoscopy (see Chapter 1.33). Transendoscopic tracheal wash samples are suitable only for cytology as contaminants from the pharynx are introduced into the trachea during this procedure.

1. Lightly lubricate the endoscope distally with a sterile water-soluble gel. The person passing the scope should lift the horse's nostril with his or her nondominant hand. Lightly resting this hand on the muzzle, use the thumb to push the endoscope ventrally and medially as it is passed into the nose with the other hand. It is important that the scope is passed via the ventral nasal meatus to avoid trauma to the ethmoturbinates.
2. The person driving the scope should be familiar with the normal anatomy of the respiratory tract. It is important to keep the scope in the correct orientation and maintain a clear view at all times whilst the scope is passed to avoid damage to the scope or to the patient.
3. As the scope is passed to the pharynx, examine the nasal turbinates. The nasomaxillary opening is located in the caudal middle meatus and can be reached with a 9-mm scope. Look "up" (dorsally) with the scope when it has reached the middle of the head. Drainage from the paranasal sinus may be seen here. Advance the scope to examine the ethmoturbinates and then direct the scope down and forwards to the pharynx. In horses that resent endoscopic examination, it may be easier to perform the detailed examination of this area as the scope is withdrawn at the end of the examination.
4. Once the scope is in the pharynx check, both guttural pouch openings for discharge or swellings, observe the pharynx, epiglottis and arytenoid cartilages. Squirt a little water through the scope or lightly touch the pharynx with the scope so that swallowing may be observed.
5. To assess the function of the larynx, briefly occlude both nostrils by pinching the muzzle, causing the horse to breath in deeply. As this occurs, the arytenoids should be pulled back with maximum abduction.
6. To enter the trachea, the scope should be positioned centrally between the arytenoid cartilages. As the horse takes a breath in, the scope should be passed quickly through into the trachea. It is important to be able to identify a clear picture at all times. Occaisionally, the scope may retroflex over the soft palate and enter the oral cavity. Any sight of teeth should signal rapid retraction of the scope. If the picture is lost at this point, it is possible that the scope is in the oesophagus; by using the air supply, you should be able to identify this through dilation of the oesophagus or simply pull back the scope 3 to 4 inches and look for the larynx again.
7. The trachea is easily identified by the tracheal rings. The length of the trachea should be examined for mucosal inflammation, discharge, collapse or foreign material. A scoring system for mucopus is given in Box 1.34. At the end of the trachea, the two major bronchi should be readily identified as they diverge at the carina.

Box 1.33. Equipment for respiratory endoscopy

Required
Endoscope
- 60-cm long is adequate for upper airway examination.
- 100 cm allows upper airway examination plus proximal tracheal examination.
- 150–200-cm long is required for a full respiratory examination.

Endoscopic light source

Optional
K-Y Jelly*
Sedation
Twitch

*Johnson and Johnson, New Brunswick, NJ, USA.

Box 1.34. Scoring system for tracheal mucus[2]

Grade	Description
0	No visible mucus
1	Singular small blobs of mucus
2	Multiple blobs of mucus, only partly confluent
3	Mucus ventrally confluent
4	Large ventral pool
5	Profuse amounts of mucus occupying more than 25% of the tracheal lumen

Box 1.35. Laryngeal function grading system[3]

Grade	Description
I	Both left and right arytenoid cartilages abduct completely and synchronously during respiration
II	Left arytenoid cartilage abducts asynchronously during respiration. Full abduction of the left arytenoid cartilage can be induced by occluding the nares.
III	Left arytenoid cartilage abducts asynchronously during respiration. Full abduction of the left arytenoid cartilage cannot be induced by occluding the nares.
IV	Left arytenoid cartilage does not abduct during respiration and stays at or near the midline of the larynx when the right arytenoid cartilage abducts.

Box 1.36. Laryngeal function grading system (Lane)[4]

Grade	Description
1	All movements, both adductory and abductory, are synchronized at rest and after exercise. Any appearance of asymmetry arises as an artifact of the position of the endoscope; the perspective distortion is cancelled when the left and right nostrils are used in turn.
2	All major movements are symmetric with a full range of adduction and abduction. Transient asynchrony, flutter, or delayed or biphasic abduction may be seen, especially of the left arytenoids.
3	Although the left arytenoids is still capable of full adduction, activity is generally reduced on the left when compared with the right, with periods of prolonged asymmetry, particularly during quiet movements. Full bilateral abduction can be stimulated transiently by partial asphyxiation during nostril occlusion, but is not sustained.
4	The left arytenoids is no longer capable of full abduction and during adduction, compensation by the right arytenoids crossing the midline may be evident. Asymmetry is marked, but residual movements are present.
5	True hemiplegia—active movement is completely absent on the affected side and the "slap" test does not provoke any response.

8. The cranial lobar bronchus can be seen on the lateral aspect of the right principal bronchus. The right accessory lobar bronchus can be seen on its ventromedial aspect. Opposite the accessory lobar bronchus is the first segmental caudal lobar bronchus, which continues as the caudal lobar bronchus. Advancement down the right caudal lobar bronchus allows visualisation of the bifurcating segmental bronchi. Advancement of the endoscope down these segmental bronchi allows visualisation of the small segmental bronchi within the right caudal lung lobe.
9. The left principal bronchus has no accessory lobar bronchus but is otherwise similar to the right side in that the left cranial lobar bronchus branches from the lateral aspect. The first ventral caudal lobar segemental bronchus exits ventrally, and the caudal lobar bronchus continues. Advancement of the endoscope into the left caudal segmental bronchus allows visualisation of the small segmental bronchi within the left caudal lung lobe.

Laryngeal functional grading systems

Two systems are in use for grading of left laryngeal hemiplegia. These are given in Boxes 1.35 and 1.36.

References

1. Burns J: Endoscopic instrumentation, in Slovis NM (ed): Atlas of Veterinary Endosurgery. St Louis, Mosby, 2003, pp 3-27
2. Holcombe SJ, Jackson C, Gerber V, et al.: Stabling is associated with airway inflammation in young Arabian horses. Equine Vet J 33:244-249, 2001
3. Rakestraw PC, Hackett RP, Ducharme NG, et al.: Arytenoid cartilage movement in resting and exercising horses. Vet Surg 20:122-127, 1991
4. Lane JG: Equine recurrent laryngeal neuropathy (RLN): current attitudes to aetiology, diagnosis and treatment. Presented at the 15th Bain-Fallon Memorial Lectures, Canberra, Australia, 1993

1.32 Endoscopy of the guttural pouch

Harold McKenzie

Examination of the guttural pouch using endoscopy allows for the identification of accumulated exudates, retropharyngeal abscessation, mycotic plaques, temperohyoid osteopathy or other abnormalities, as well as allowing for the collection of samples for cytology and culture and facilitating drainage of accumulated exudate.

Box 1.37. Equipment for guttural pouch endoscopy

Required

Endoscope

- Fibreoptic or video endoscope of at least 1 metre length
- Maximum outer diameter of 10–12 mm

Endoscopic light source

Endoscopic biopsy forceps (at least 10–20 cm longer than endoscope)

Optional

K-Y Jelly*

Sedation

Twitch

*Johnson and Johnson, New Brunswick, NJ, USA.

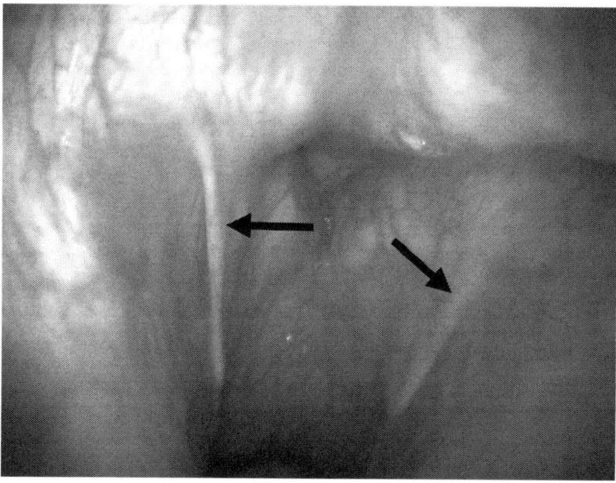

Figure 1.111 The guttural pouch openings (*black arrows*) of a 6-month-old foal, viewed from an endoscope passed up the right nasal passages. ©Kevin Corley 2007.

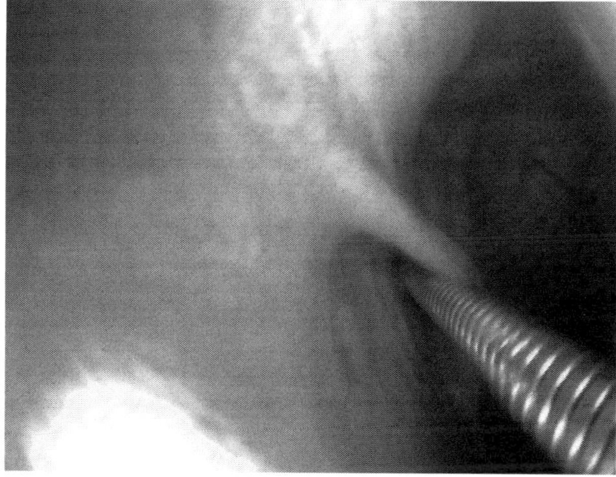

Figure 1.112 The biopsy forceps are used to open the salpingopharyngeal fold and allow entry of the endoscope into the guttural pouch. ©Kevin Corley 2007.

Equipment needed

The equipment needed is given in Box 1.37. The guttural pouch is readily examined using either a fibreoptic endoscope or a video endoscope. The outer diameter of the endoscope should be no more than 10 to 12 mm in order to easily pass through the pharyngeal opening of the guttural pouch (salpingopharyngeal orifice) and the auditory canal. The simplest way to introduce the endoscope into the guttural pouch is to utilise the endoscopic biopsy forceps. The biopsy forceps will act as a stylet to allow the endoscope to be passed into the auditory canal and the guttural pouch.

Procedure

Insert the biopsy forceps into the biopsy channel of the endoscope prior to inserting the endoscope into the nasal passages of the patient. Ensure that the forceps are not extending from the tip of the endoscope, and then insert the endoscope into the nasal passage ipsilateral to the pouch to be examined and pass the endoscope through the ventral meatus to the level of the nasopharynx. Upon visualisation of the salpingopharyngeal fold (Figure 1.111), extend the biopsy forceps (ensuring that they remain closed) and pass them lateral to the top corner of the fold and 2 to 3 cm into the auditory canal. After placing the biopsy forceps, rotate the endoscope body to the left (right guttural pouch) or the right (left guttural pouch), which will cause the biopsy forceps to raise the fold (Figure 1.112), allowing the endoscope to be advanced into the auditory canal. As the endoscope enters into the guttural pouch, the biopsy forceps should be withdrawn into the endoscope. The entire guttural pouch may then be examined (Figures 1.113 and 1.114).

To examine the contralateral guttural pouch, it is typically easiest to completely withdraw the endoscope and place it in the nasal passages on the same side of the horse as the guttural pouch to be examined, although with practice both guttural pouches can sometimes be entered without repositioning the endoscope. Following repositioning of the endoscope, the procedure is then repeated, remembering to rotate the endoscope in the opposite direction from that used on the first side. An alternative approach involves the use of a Chambers catheter or a plastic uterine infusion pipette bent approximately 20° at a point 15 cm from the distal end of the catheter. The catheter is passed through the nasal passages contralateral to the guttural pouch of interest, with the endoscope in place in the ipsilateral nares. Under endoscopic visualisation, the catheter is introduced into the pharyngeal opening of the guttural pouch, which will allow the endoscope to be passed lateral to the catheter into the guttural pouch.

Guttural pouch endoscopy should always be performed with caution, especially in the patient with a history of

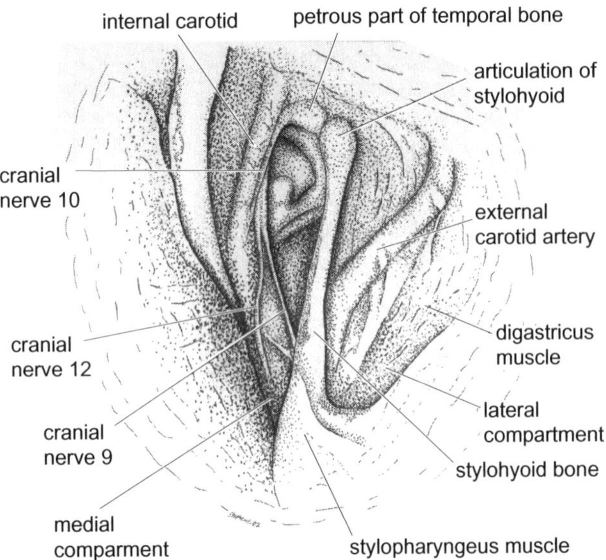

Figure 1.113 Anatomy of the left guttural pouch.

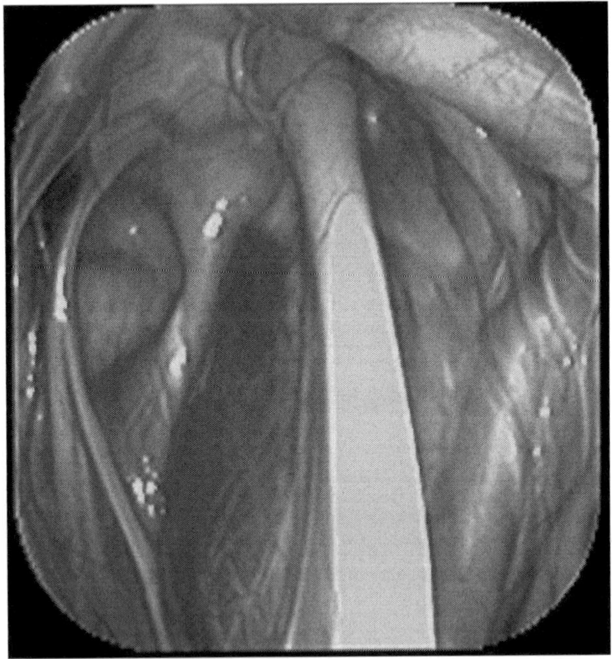

Figure 1.114 Endoscopic view of a normal left guttural pouch. ©Kevin Corley 2007.

epistaxis, as this procedure may result in the destabilisation of an existing clot within the guttural pouch, resulting in resumption of haemorrhage. In this subset of patients, one should be prepared for immediate surgical intervention prior to performing endoscopy.[1]

Reference

1. Hardy J, Leveile R: Diseases of the guttural pouches. Vet Clin North Am Equine Pract 19:123-158, 2003

1.33 Tracheal aspiration

Harold McKenzie

Two methods are commonly utilised for the collection of samples of airway fluid from the trachea for the purposes of cytological analysis and bacterial culture. The first method involves the use of guarded aspiration catheters introduced through the biopsy channel of a fiberoptic or video endoscope,[1] whilst the second uses a percutaneous approach. The endoscopic technique has the distinct advantage of being minimally invasive but may be associated with an increased likelihood of sample contamination due to passage of the endoscope through the nares.[2] The percutaneous technique may be less prone to sample contamination, as it is performed in a sterile manner, but can be associated with subcutaneous emphysema due to air leaking from the tracheal puncture site, cellulitis at the tracheal puncture site due to airway fluid contaminating the subcutaneous tissues, injury to the tracheal cartilages or the development of pneumomediastinum.[3] Despite this list of potential complications, percutaneous aspiration remains the preferred method of sample collection, especially when samples for bacterial culture are required.

Equipment needed

The equipment needed for either technique is given in Box 1.38.

Transendoscopic technique

The transendoscopic technique utilises a double- or triple-stage guarded system of tubing, which is introduced into the tracheal lumen by way of the endoscopic biopsy channel. This technique requires an endoscope of at least 1-metre length to be able to adequately enter the cervical trachea. The endoscope should be thoroughly cleansed and disinfected prior to performing the procedure to decrease the risk of sample contamination. To reach the trachea, the endoscope is passed to the level of the pharynx and then directed into the trachea and advanced to the midcervical level of the trachea, or until the small pool of fluid present within the cranial thoracic trachea is visible.

A double- or triple-stage guarded aspiration catheter is then advanced into the trachea until it is within several centimetres of the pool of tracheal fluid. The inner, guarded, segments of the catheter are then advanced sequentially and directed into the tracheal fluid, and a sample of this fluid is then aspirated using a sterile Luer-tip syringe attached to the external end of the endoscopic catheter. If no fluid is present within the tracheal lumen, a small amount of sterile saline (10 to 20 ml) can be infused via the catheter to lavage the tracheal surface, and this fluid is then aspirated. The sample should be kept in a sterile capped syringe if it is to be immediately submitted for cytology and culture. If there is to be a delay in submission, aliquots of the samples should be placed in an EDTA tube (cytology) and a plain tube (culture) for transport to the

> **Box 1.38. Equipment for tracheal aspirate**
>
> **Endoscopic technique**
> Endoscope (cleaned and disinfected)
> Fibreoptic or video endoscope of at least 1 metre length
> Guarded aspiration catheter*
> Endoscopic light source
> 10–20-ml sterile saline in a syringe
>
> **Percutaneous (transtracheal) technique**:
> Transtracheal kit
> Commercially available kit†
> OR
> 12–14-Gauge intravenous catheter (7.5-cm) or 12-gauge needle (7.5-cm) or nesting trochar
> Polypropelene catheter (5Fr–6Fr dog urinary catheter)‡
> Clippers with a fine (No. 40) blade
> Small gauze swabs (4 × 4) soaked in chlorhexidine (4%) scrub solution§
> Small gauze swabs (4 × 4) soaked in surgical spirit (alcohol)
> Mepivacaine 2%**: 2–3 ml drawn up in a 2–3-ml syringe with a 23–25-Gauge needle
> 30–40-ml sterile saline in a syringe
> Surgical gloves
>
> **Required for both techniques**
> Sterile plain sample pot or tube
> Sample tube containing EDTA
>
> **Optional for percutaneous technique**
> Further mepivacaine 2%**: 4–5 ml drawn up in a 5-ml syringe
>
> **Optional for both techniques**
> 50% Ethanol cytological fixative solution
> Sedation
> Twitch
>
> *EMAC700 (double) or EMAC800 (triple); MILA International Inc., Florence, KY, USA.
> †TW1228 (adults) or TW1628 (foals); MILA International Inc., Florence, KY, USA.
> ‡5Fr × 56-cm polypropylene catheter; Kendall Sovereign, Tyco Healthcare Group, LP, Mansfield, MA, USA.
> §Hibiscrub; Mölnlycke Health Care, Dunstable, UK.
> **Intra-epicaine; Arnolds Veterinary Products, Shrewsbury, UK; Carbocaine-V; Pfizer Animal Health, New York, NY, USA.

laboratory. Keep the samples refrigerated whilst in transit to prevent sample degradation. Improved cytological results will be achieved by placing the cytology sample in an equal volume of 50% ethanol cytological fixative solution rather than EDTA.

Percutaneous technique (transtracheal aspirate)

The percutaneous technique is performed by introducing a sterile catheter into the trachea by means of a large-bore needle or cannula placed in the midcervical region, just above the strap muscles, and lavaging the tracheal lumen with a small volume of sterile fluid, followed by sample aspiration. The site should be prepared by surgically clipping the overlying hair in a 5 × 5-cm region immediately overlying the midcervical trachea. This area is then aseptically prepared, and the skin overlying the trachea at the puncture site is anaesthetised using 2 to 3 ml of injectable local anaesthetic solution injected subcutaneously. The procedure may be performed using commercially available transtracheal aspiration kits or a large-bore catheter, introducer needle or nesting trocar as an introducer and a polypropylene catheter as the flushing catheter.

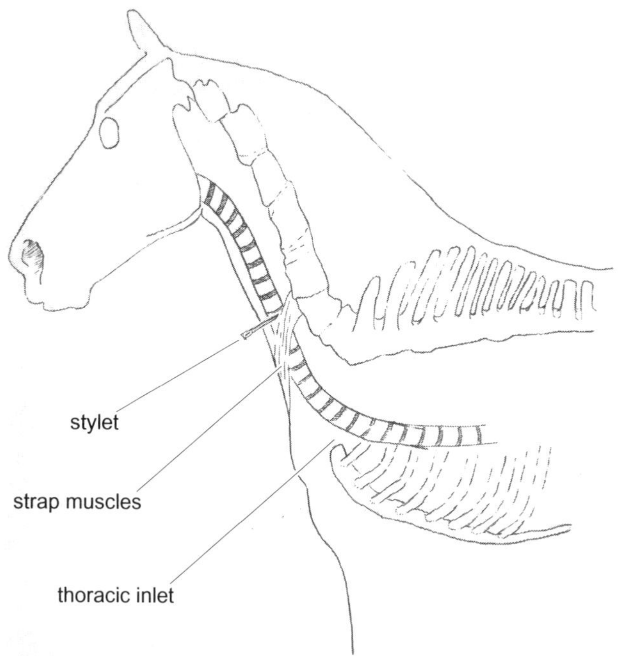

Figure 1.115 The stylet is introduced in the mid-cervical region, just above the strap muscles.

After the skin overlying the trachea is blocked and aseptically prepared, the introducer needle or catheter is placed through the skin using sterile technique. After passing through the skin, the tip of the introducer can be moved carefully until it is positioned between two tracheal rings (Figure 1.115), and then the introducer is passed through the tracheal wall and approximately 2 cm into the lumen of the trachea (Figure 1.116). The flushing catheter is then passed through the introducer into the trachea, guiding the catheter toward the cranial thorax by angling the introducer needle in that direction. Some patients may cough when the flushing catheter is introduced, and this response may be lessened by instilling 3 to 5 ml of mepivacaine rapidly through the introducer needle into the trachea prior to placing the flushing catheter.

The flushing catheter is advanced to the level of the thoracic inlet, and then 30 to 40 ml of sterile saline solution is instilled through the flushing catheter and immediately aspirated using the same syringe as was used for instillation (Figures 1.117 and 1.118). If fluid is not readily obtained, then the catheter should be carefully repositioned in the

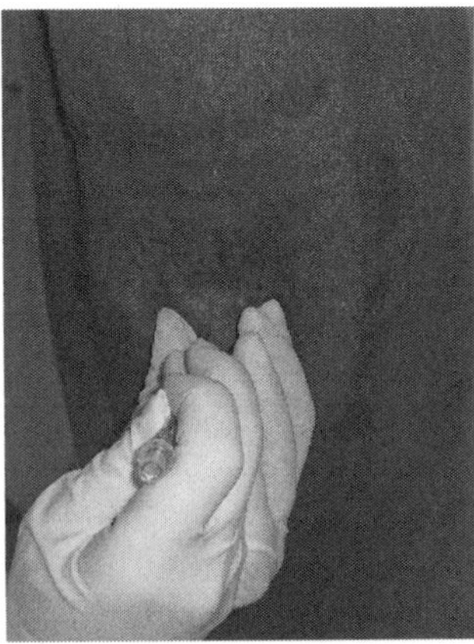

Figure 1.116 Insertion of introducer needle through the skin and tracheal wall. The trachea is stabilised laterally using the thumb and forefinger of the free hand. ©Harold C. McKenzie III 2006.

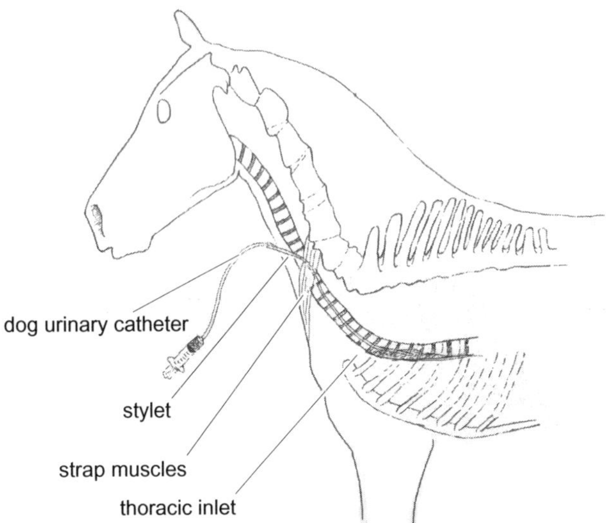

Figure 1.117 After the fluid has been instilled, the polypropelene (dog urinary) catheter is slowly advanced and withdrawn whilst aspirating, until the end is in the pool of fluid at the thoracic inlet and fluid is obtained.

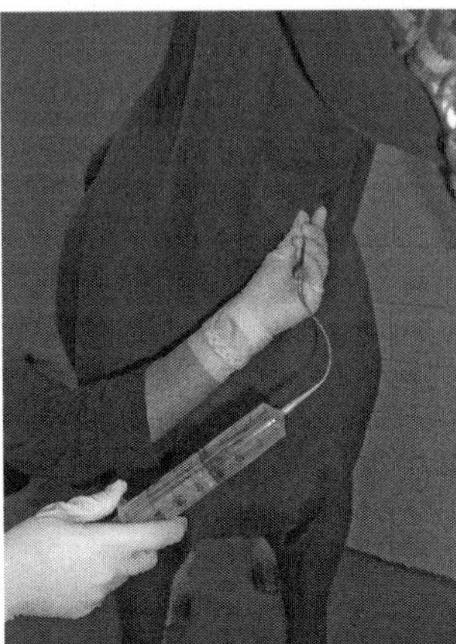

Figure 1.118 Aspiration of instilled fluid from trachea via the aspiration catheter, which has been inserted via the introducer needle. ©Harold C. McKenzie III 2006.

trachea by advancing and withdrawing it gradually whilst repeatedly attempting to aspirate a sample. If no fluid is obtained, a second aliquot of sterile saline may be instilled via the flushing catheter and aspiration again attempted. Upon completion of aspiration, the flushing catheter should be carefully withdrawn through the introducer. After the flushing catheter is withdrawn, the introducer may be removed. Bandaging of the site is generally not required unless evidence of subcutaneous emphysema is noted.

References

1. Darien BJ, Brown CM, Walker RD, et al.: A tracheoscopic technique for obtaining uncontaminated lower airway secretions for bacterial culture in the horse. Equine Vet J 22:170-173, 1990
2. Sweeney CR, Sweeney RW III, Benson CE: Comparison of bacteria isolated from specimens obtained by use of endoscopic guarded tracheal swabbing and percutaneous tracheal aspiration in horses. J Am Vet Med Assoc 195:1225-1229, 1989
3. Krpan MK: Transtracheal aspiration in the horse: a photo essay. Mod Vet Pract 65:A19-A22, 1984

1.34 Bronchoalveolar lavage

Harold McKenzie

The primary utility of bronchoalveolar lavage (BAL) is in the collection of samples of respiratory secretions from the small airways and alveoli for cytological analysis. The utility of BAL samples for culture is limited due to the inherently nonsterile nature of this technique, as a result of the requirement that the lavage tube or endoscope be passed through the upper respiratory tract en route to the lung. BAL is easily performed in the standing adult horse using either an endoscopically guided technique or an unguided technique. As most cases presenting with an indication for BAL are suffering from diffuse disease, the unguided technique is sufficient, because it has been demonstrated to yield diagnostically useful samples in diffuse lung disease.[1] For horses with suspected focal pathology within the lungs, the guided approach is indicated, as this will allow for visual detection of the affected region and targeting of the lavage to the affected area.[2,3]

Equipment needed

The equipment needed is given in Box 1.39. Adequate sedation is required for performing BAL, and this can be achieved using xylazine (0.3 to 0.5 mg/kg IV), although the addition of butorphanol (0.02 to 0.04 mg/kg IV) is helpful due to its antitussive effects. A dilute local anaesthetic solution is used to provide topical anaesthesia in the trachea and bronchi, and this should be prepared prior to initiation of the BAL procedure. The lavage itself is performed using 240 to 300 ml of sterile buffered saline solution. For the

Box 1.39. Equipment for bronchoalveolar lavage

Required for unguided technique
Bronchoalveolar lavage catheter*
5-ml syringe (empty)

Required for guided (endoscopic) technique
Endoscope (cleaned and disinfected)
Fibreoptic or video endoscope of at least 2 metres length
Endoscopic light source

Required for both techniques
Sedation
5–10-ml mepivacaine 2%† diluted into 50-ml of sterile buffered saline in a 60-ml syringe
4–5 syringes (60-ml) filled with 60 ml of sterile buffered saline
Sterile plain sample pot or tube
Sample tube containing EDTA

Optional for both techniques
50% ethanol cytological fixative solution
Twitch

*Examples include 3.0-mm ID × 11-mm OD × 244-cm length BAL lavage catheter; Bivona, Smiths Medical International Ltd., Hythe, Kent, UK.
†Intra-epicaine; Arnolds Veterinary Products, Shrewsbury, UK; Carbocaine-V; Pfizer Animal Health, New York, NY, USA.

unguided BAL, a BAL catheter is used, and this catheter should be cleansed and disinfected prior to performing the procedure.

Unguided (BAL catheter) technique

After the patient is adequately sedated (5 to 10 minutes following administration of the sedatives), the procedure may be performed. Additional restraint using a nose twitch is helpful in most cases. Three people are required to perform the procedure, with one restraining the patient, another passing the lavage catheter and the third operating the lavage catheter and infusing the lavage solution and aspirating the sample.

The lavage catheter is inserted into the trachea via the ventral meatus, with care being taken to ensure that the catheter is neither placed into the oesophagus nor retroflexed into the oropharynx. When the catheter is passed into the tracheal lumen, there is little or no resistance to passage and the patient will typically cough. Upon entering the trachea, the dilute local anaesthetic solution is gradually infused through the lavage catheter as it is advanced, with the last 10 ml being infused after the catheter is securely wedged in the bronchial tree. Whilst maintaining pressure on the catheter to keep it wedged, the balloon on the catheter tip is inflated with 5 ml of air to provide a seal within the airway lumen.

The entire volume of lavage solution is then infused into the lung via the catheter, followed by immediate aspiration using 60-ml syringes to infuse the lavage solution. The yield of lavage fluid may range from nil to 60% to 70% of the volume infused, with a 30% to 50% yield being typical. Following sample collection, the catheter balloon tip should be deflated and the catheter withdrawn from the patient. The samples obtained should be pooled and submitted immediately for cytological analysis. If submission must be delayed, a 5-ml aliquot of the lavage sample may be combined with an equal volume of 50% ethanol cytological fixative in a sterile vacuum collection tube, which provides optimal preservation of cellular morphology. Alternatively, a 2- to 3-ml aliquot of sample may be placed in an EDTA vacuum collection tube, although this does not offer ideal sample fixation. Failure to fix the sample by either means will lead to cellular deterioration within 30 to 60 minutes of sample collection.

Guided (endoscopic) technique

Performing BAL using the guided technique requires a 2-metre or longer flexible fibreoptic endoscope or video endoscope. The fluid is injected down, and aspirated from, the endoscope biopsy channel. The procedure is performed in much the same way as described above, with the difference that there is no cuff on the endoscope to provide a seal within the airway, which may result in slightly lower lavage fluid yields. The endoscope may be directed to areas exhibiting inflammation or drainage, increasing the sensitivity of this technique in cases of focal disease.

References

1. Fogarty U: Evaluation of a bronchoalveolar lavage technique. Equine Vet J 22:174-176, 1990
2. Ito S, Hobo S, Eto D, et al.: Bronchoalveolar lavage for the diagnosis and treatment of pneumonia associated with transport in Thoroughbred racehorses. J Vet Med Sci 63:1263-1269, 2001
3. McKenzie HC: Bronchial lavage for the treatment of focal pneumonia. Presented at the 23rd Annual ACVIM Forum, Baltimore, Maryland, 2005, pp 136-138

1.35 Pleurocentesis

Harold McKenzie

Pleurocentesis can be performed in cases where the presence of pleural fluid is suspected or where fluid has been detected within the pleural space on ultrasonographic examination. This technique allows for the sterile collection of pleural fluid for cytological examination and culture.

Equipment needed

The equipment needed is listed in Box 1.40.

Procedure

Selection of the site for pleurocentesis is ideally based upon ultrasonographic examination, as this allows for the con-

Box 1.40. Equipment for pleurocentesis

Required

Catheter for centesis

- Trocar catheter*
- Bitch catheter
- Teat cannula†

Three-way stopcock (three-way tap)‡
Clippers with a fine (No. 40) blade
Small gauze swabs (4 × 4) soaked in chlorhexidine (4%) scrub solution§
Small gauze swabs (4 × 4) soaked in surgical spirit (alcohol)
Mepivacaine 2%**: 5 ml drawn up in a syringe with a 23–25-gauge needle
Surgical gloves
No. 15 scalpel blade

Optional

Ultrasound machine with a 3–7.5-MHz sector, linear array or linear probe
One-way valve††
Valved chest tube adapter‡‡
7.5-cm (3-inch) wide stretchy adhesive dressing (Elastoplast§§/Elastikon***)
Twitch
Sedation

*Examples include 24Fr–28Fr × 41 cm, Pleur-Evac thoracic catheter; Genzyme Corp., Fall River, MA, USA.
†Udder infusion catheter; Jorgensen Labs, Loveland, CO, USA.
‡Vygon, Ecouen, France.
§Hibiscrub; Mölnlycke Health Care, Dunstable, UK.
**Intra-epicaine; Arnolds Veterinary Products, Shrewsbury, UK; Carbocaine-V; Pfizer Animal Health, New York, NY, USA.
††Examples include Heimlich chest drain valve; Global Veterinary Products, New Buffalo, MI, USA.
‡‡Centesis valve/chest tube adapter, Item No. 175450; MILA International Inc., Florence, KY, USA.
§§Beiersdorf AG, Hamburg, Germany.
***Johnson and Johnson, New Brunswick, NJ, USA.

firmation of the presence of fluid within the pleural space, as well as the identification of structures to be avoided when performing the procedure. Alternatively, the procedure is best performed in either the sixth or seventh intercostal space at a level approximately 10 cm dorsal to the olecranon. Care should be taken to avoid the lateral thoracic vein when performing the procedure (Figure 1.119). The chosen site is clipped and aseptically prepared, followed by infiltration of the area with local anaesthetic solution. The insertion site is opened by making a stab incision to provide a point of entry through the skin. A trocar catheter, bitch catheter or teat cannula is passed through the stab incision and directed around the cranial border of the rib caudal to the intercostal space being entered, ensuring that it avoids the intercostal blood vessels that lie at the cranial extent of the intercostal space adjacent to the caudal aspect of the more cranial rib. Some resistance will be encountered when passing through the intercostal muscles and the parietal pleura, and this is overcome by steady pressure. If additional force is required, use one hand to control the depth of penetration of the trocar, in order to minimise the risk of penetrating too deeply and injuring the lung or the heart. Once the pleural space is entered, one must take care to avoid inadvertent aspiration of air into the pleural cavity, although in cases where pleural fluid is present, the fluid will typically flow spontaneously from the trocar. This risk may be minimised by placing a three-way stopcock onto the catheter or cannula prior to passing it through the thoracic wall (Figure 1.120).

A sample of fluid is collected using a Luer tip syringe, and aliquots of the fluid are placed into EDTA and plain vacuum collection tubes for cytological examination and culture, respectively. Samples should be refrigerated until submitted to the diagnostic laboratory. In cases where large amounts of fluid are present, the trocar catheter may be sutured into place using a Chinese finger trap suture to allow for ongoing drainage. The catheter should be plugged in between drainage episodes or a one-way valve should be fitted to allow fluid to drain whilst preventing air aspiration. Alternatively, a valved chest tube adapter can be used, which allows for active aspiration and evacuation of fluid from the pleural space using a 60-ml syringe without the need for disconnecting the syringe from the catheter.

The potential complications of pleurocentesis include ipsilateral and contralateral pneumothorax, which is usually minimal if precautions are taken, although suction should be available when performing the procedure to allow rapid removal of any aspirated air from the pleural cavity. Other complications include potential trauma to the intercostal vessels, lung, heart and diaphragm.

Normal values for pleural fluid are given in the Appendix (see Table 19.13).

1.36 Evacuation of pneumothorax

Harold McKenzie

Pneumothorax is suggested by the presence of an area of absent breath sounds in the dorsal thorax on auscultation and tympanic sounds on thoracic percussion.

Equipment needed

The equipment needed is given in Box 1.41.

Procedure

This finding is best confirmed using thoracic radiography (Figures 1.121 and 1.122) or thoracic ultrasonography (Figure 1.123). The evacuation of pneumothorax is performed in much the same way as described for pleurocentesis (see Chapter 1.35); however, the site of catheter placement should be more dorsal, typically at the level of the point of the shoulder (Figure 1.124). Small amounts of air may be aspirated using a 7.5-cm 18-gauge spinal needle or a teat cannula. A three-way stopcock or centesis valve

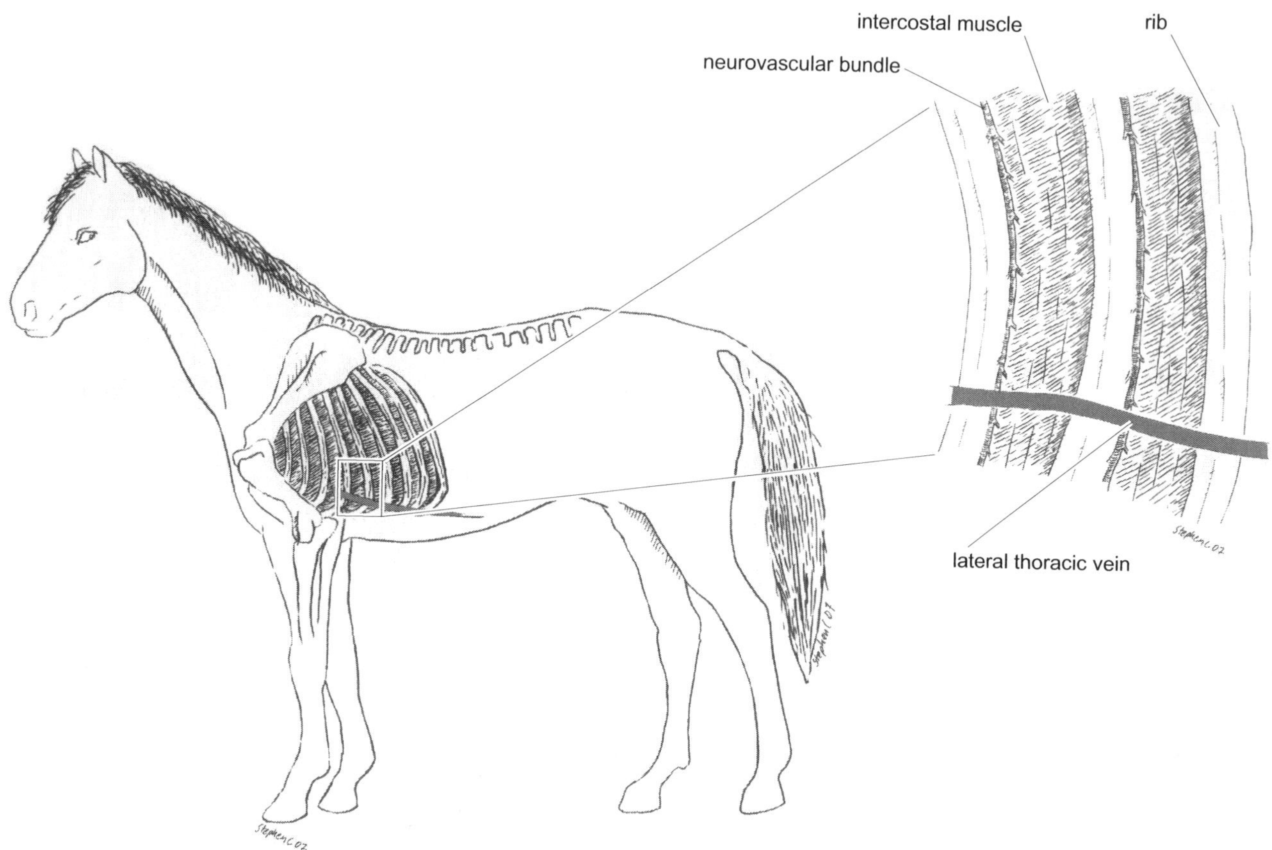

Figure 1.119 Site for placement of thoracic drain for removal of pleural effusion, just above (and avoiding) the lateral thoracic vein. The chest drain is tunnelled forward from the skin over the middle of the rib to the intercostal muscles just in front of it. This means that the tissues form a seal or partial seal when the chest drain is removed.

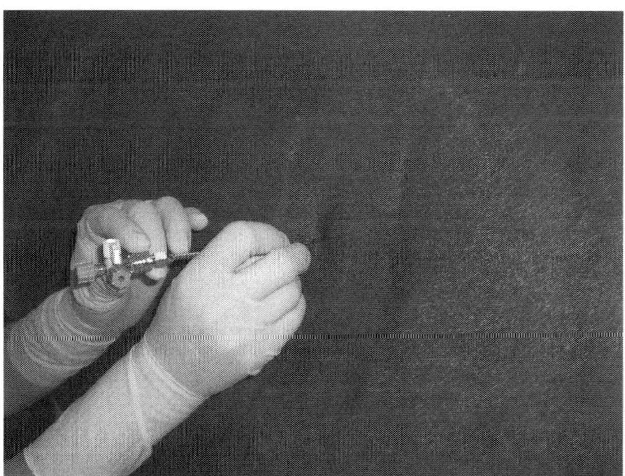

Figure 1.120 Pleurocentesis using a teat cannula and three-way stopcock. ©Harold C. McKenzie III 2006.

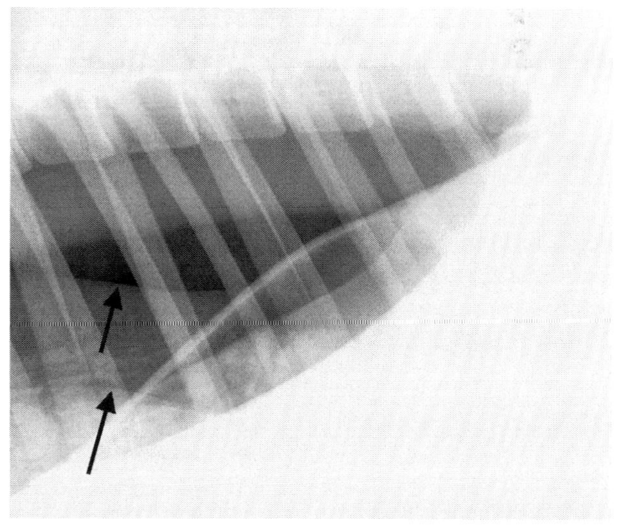

Figure 1.121 Caudo-dorsal thoracic radiograph showing bilateral pneumothorax in an adult horse. The air is seen as radiolucent above the dorsal margins of both lung lobes (*black arrows*), which have been pushed ventrally. ©Kevin Corley 2003.

Box 1.41. Equipment for evacuation of pneumothorax

Required
Thoracic catheter

- Indwelling thoracic trocar catheter*
- 18-Gauge spinal needle (7.5-cm) or a teat cannula

Method to confirm pneumothorax

- X-ray machine capable of 80–90 kV and 40 mA-s with grid
- Ultrasound machine with a 3–7.5-MHz sector, linear array or linear probe

Clippers with a fine (No. 40) blade
Small gauze swabs (4 × 4) soaked in chlorhexidine (4%) scrub solution†
Small gauze swabs (4 × 4) soaked in surgical spirit (alcohol)
Mepivacaine 2%‡: 5 ml drawn up in a syringe with a 23–25-gauge needle
Surgical gloves
No. 15 scalpel blade

Optional
Three-way stopcock (three-way tap)§
One-way valve**
Centesis valve††
7.5-cm (3-inch) wide stretchy adhesive dressing (Elastoplast‡‡/Elastikon§§)
Twitch
Sedation

*Examples include 24Fr–28Fr × 41 cm, Pleur-Evac thoracic catheter; Genzyme Corp., Fall River, MA, USA.
†Hibiscrub; Mölnlycke Health Care, Dunstable, UK.
‡Intra-epicaine; Arnolds Veterinary Products, Shrewsbury, UK; Carbocaine-V; Pfizer Animal Health, New York, NY, USA.
§Vygon, Ecouen, France.
**Examples include Heimlich chest drain valve; Global Veterinary Products, New Buffalo, MI, USA.
††Centesis valve/chest tube adapter, Item No. 175450; MILA International Inc., Florence, KY, USA.
‡‡Beiersdorf AG, Hamburg, Germany.
§§Johnson and Johnson, New Brunswick, NJ, USA.

should be placed on the needle or cannula prior to insertion, in order to prevent further aspiration of air into the pleural cavity. Once the needle or catheter is placed, the air is removed using a 60-ml Luer tip syringe for suctioning air from the chest. The syringe can be left in place on the stopcock, with the valve being alternately opened to allow air from the pleural space to be suctioned into the syringe and then opened to the air to allow the syringe contents to be expelled.

Unfortunately, using a needle or cannula does not allow for ongoing evacuation of air from the thorax as these devices cannot be left indwelling. For this reason, an indwelling thoracic trocar catheter is usually preferred (Figures 1.125, 1.126 and 1.127). The catheter should be

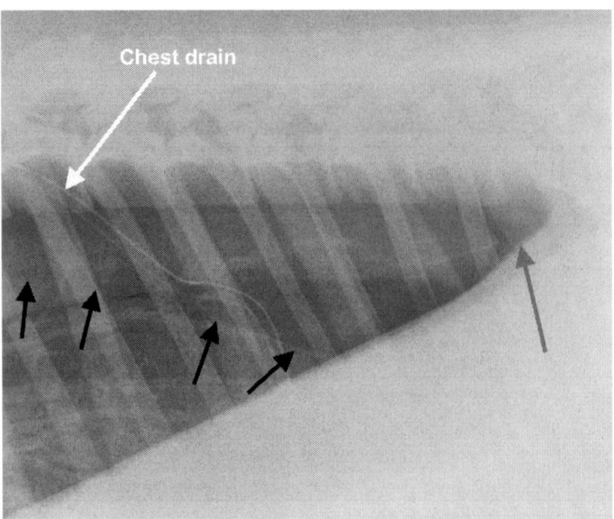

Figure 1.122 Caudo-dorsal thoracic radiograph showing bilateral pneumothorax in an adult horse. The dorsal margin of one lung lobe is greatly displaced ventrally (*black arrows*). There is a very small amount of air in the very caudodorsal margin of the other hemithorax (*grey arrow*). The horse has a chest drain in place. ©Kevin Corley 2001.

sutured in place (as for an abdominal drain, Figure 1.19) and fitted with a one-way valve, as described for pleurocentesis. The thoracic catheter should be protected with stretchy adhesive dressing (Figure 1.128). Catheters may be required bilaterally, as some horses have a complete mediastinum.

1.37 Lung biopsy

Harold McKenzie

Percutaneous lung biopsy is most useful in the evaluation of diffuse pulmonary disease but may be of utility in cases where a specific abnormality is detected and localised using ultrasonography.[1]

Equipment needed

The equipment needed is given in Box 1.42. A manual biopsy needle (Tru-Cut style) is typically used, although automated biopsy devices may also be utilised, thereby decreasing the likelihood of user error.[1] Automated biopsy instruments are also associated with a decreased frequency of complications.[2]

Procedure

The site of biopsy collection is influenced by the pattern of pulmonary disease being investigated, as cases with diffuse disease are best sampled in the seventh-through-eighth intercostal space at a level approximately 8 cm above the elbow joint, whilst the site used for biopsy of focal lesions will be based upon ultrasonographic guidance. Adequate restraint is required to perform this procedure, and this typically consists of intravenous sedation (xylazine ± butorphanol) combined with application of a nose twitch. The biopsy site should be clipped and aseptically prepared, followed by local analgesia using 5 ml of local anaesthetic. A

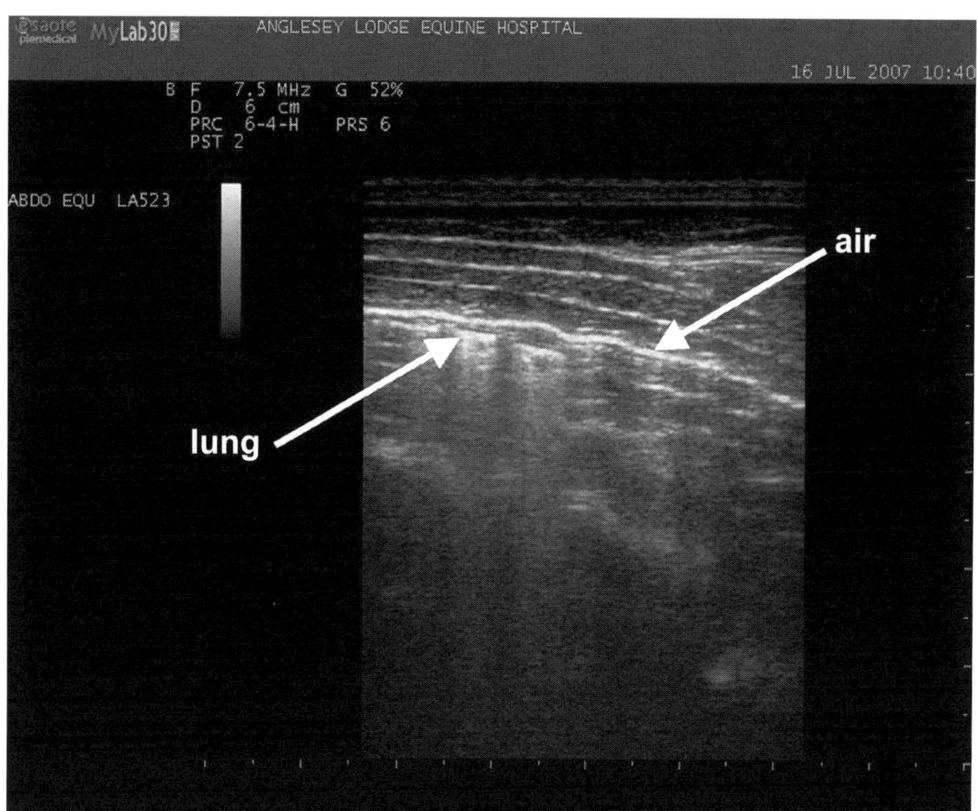

Figure 1.123 Thoracic ultrasound at the junction between the dorsal surface of the lung and air in the pleural space. The lung could be seen to be moving with the respiratory efforts, whereas the air (*bright white continuous echoic line*) was static. ©Kevin Corley 2007.

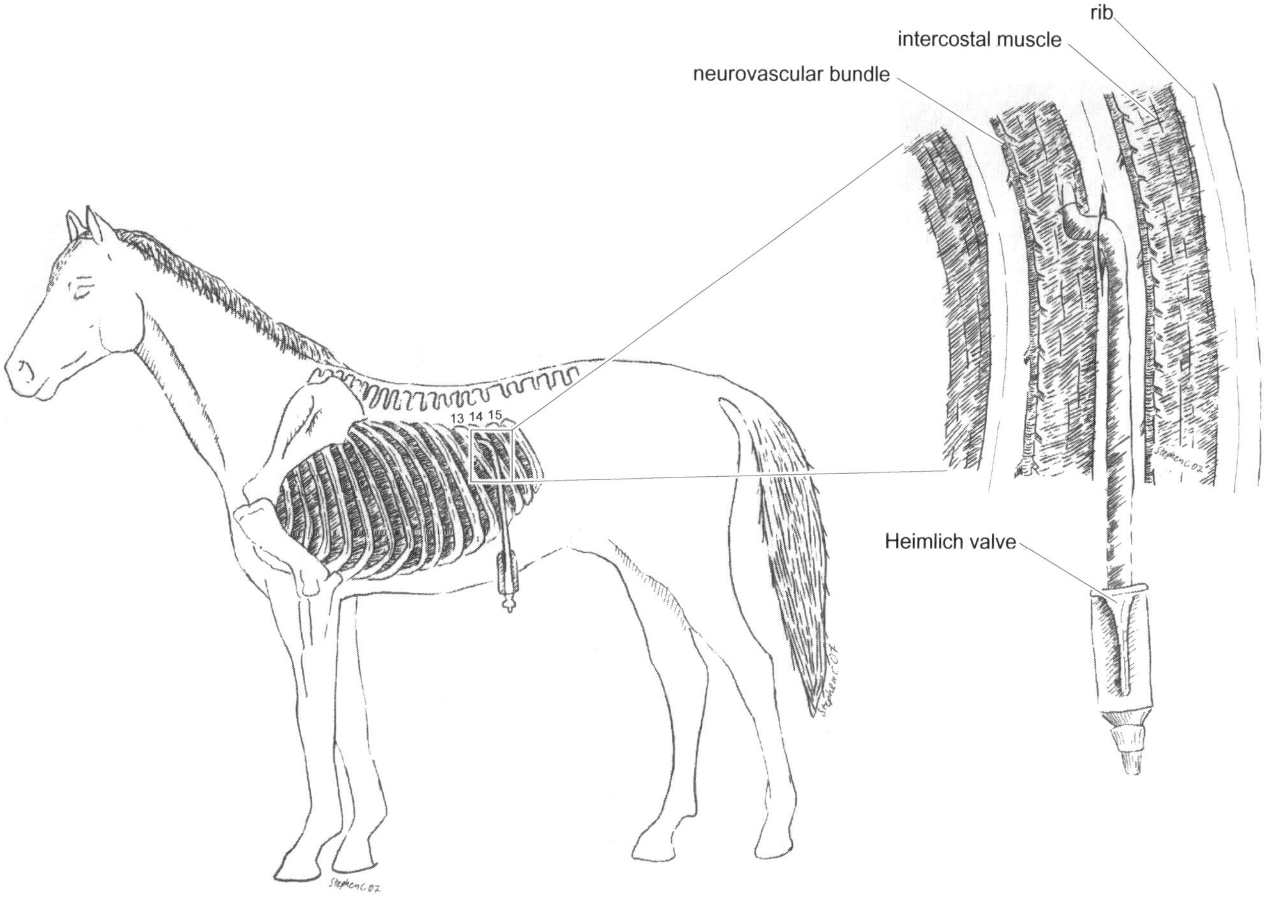

rib
intercostal muscle
neurovascular bundle
13 14 15
Heimlich valve

Figure 1.124 Site for evacuation of pneumothorax. The chest drain is tunnelled forward from the skin over the middle of the rib to the intercostal muscles just in front of it. This means that the tissues form a seal or partial seal when the chest drain is removed. The neurovascular bundle runs at the caudal edge of each rib, and is avoided by this technique.

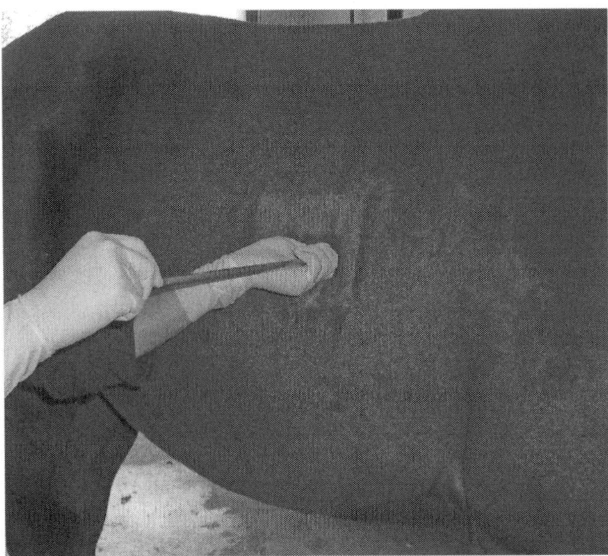

Figure 1.125 Insertion of a thoracic trocar catheter for evacuation of pneumothorax. ©Harold C. McKenzie III 2006.

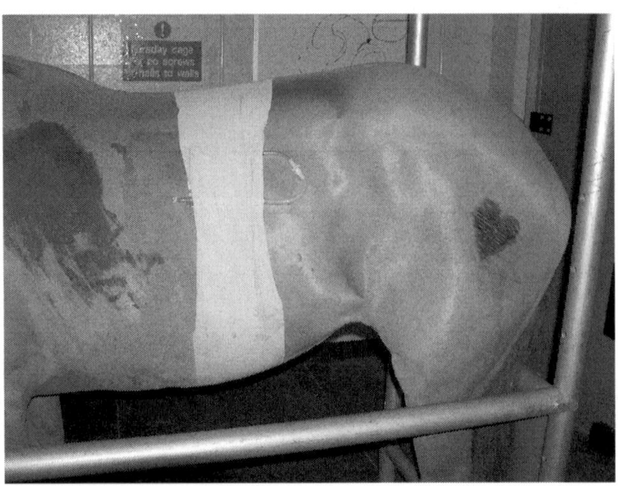

Figure 1.128 Indwelling chest tube for intermittent evacuation of pneumothorax. The tube has a Heimlich valve and is+B138 protected with stretchy adhesive dressing. ©Kevin Corley 2004.

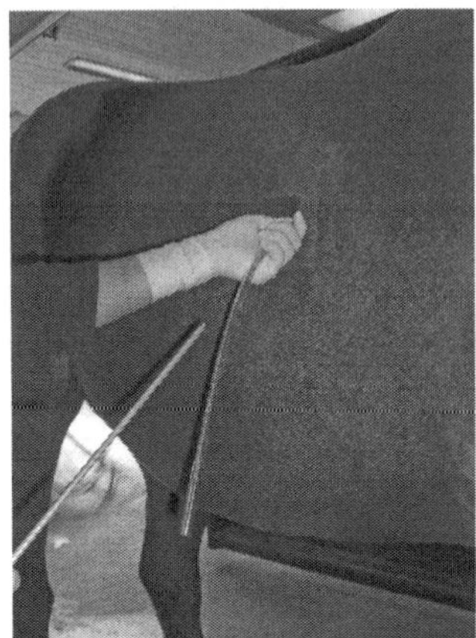

Figure 1.126 Trocar removed from the thoracic catheter. ©Harold C. McKenzie III 2006.

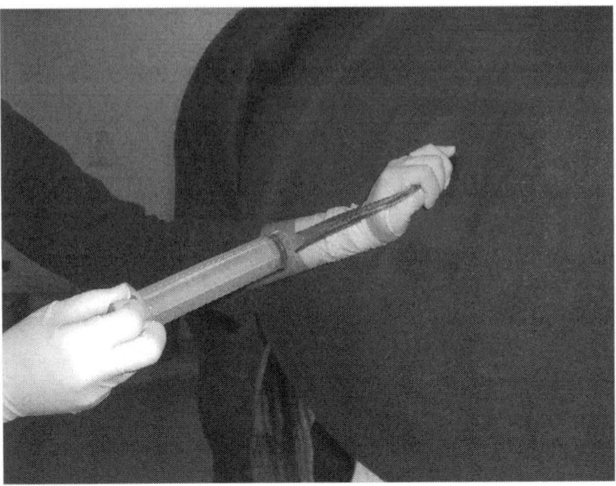

Figure 1.127 Aspiration from the thoracic catheter. ©Harold C. McKenzie III 2006.

Box 1.42. Equipment for lung biopsy

Required

Biopsy instrument

- 14-Gauge, 15-cm manual biopsy needle (TruCut)*
- Automated biopsy device†

Sample pot containing 10% neutral buffered formalin
Two 25-gauge needles
Sedation
Clippers with a fine (No. 40) blade
Small gauze swabs (4 × 4) soaked in chlorhexidine (4%) scrub solution‡
Small gauze swabs (4 × 4) soaked in surgical spirit (alcohol)
Mepivacaine 2%§: 5 ml drawn up in a syringe with a 23–25-gauge needle
Surgical gloves
No. 15 scalpel blade

Optional

Ultrasound machine with a 3–7.5-MHz sector, linear array or linear probe
Tongue depressor
Sterile sample pot, if culture of a biopsy specimen is required
Skin stapler**
Twitch

*Baxter Healthcare, Deerfield, IL, USA.
†Examples include Vet-Core biopsy needle; Global Veterinary Products, New Buffalo, MI, USA; Pro-Mag 2.2; US Biopsy Engineered Products, Franklin, IN, USA.
‡Hibiscrub; Mölnlycke Health Care, Dunstable, UK.
§Intra-epicaine; Arnolds Veterinary Products, Shrewsbury, UK; Carbocaine-V; Pfizer Animal Health, New York, NY, USA.
**Auto Suture Appose ULC 35W; United States Surgical, Tyco Healthcare Group, Norwalk, CT, USA.

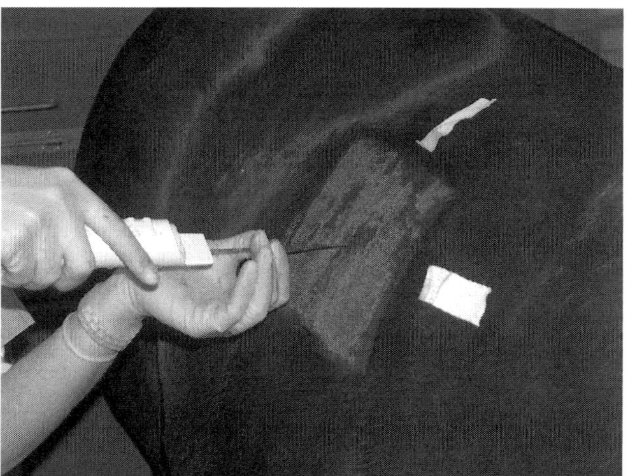

Figure 1.129 Insertion of an automated lung biopsy device. ©Kevin Corley 2005.

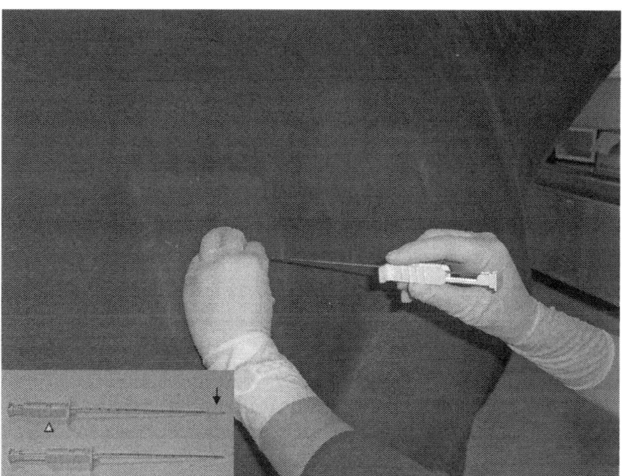

Figure 1.130 Insertion of manual lung biopsy device. The inner portion is advanced (black arrow - inset) when the biopsy device is at the desired depth, then the inner portion is maintained in position while the outer portion of the device is advanced. This action is responsible for the collection of the tissue sample. Following completion of sampling the device is removed from the patient. ©Harold C. McKenzie III 2006.

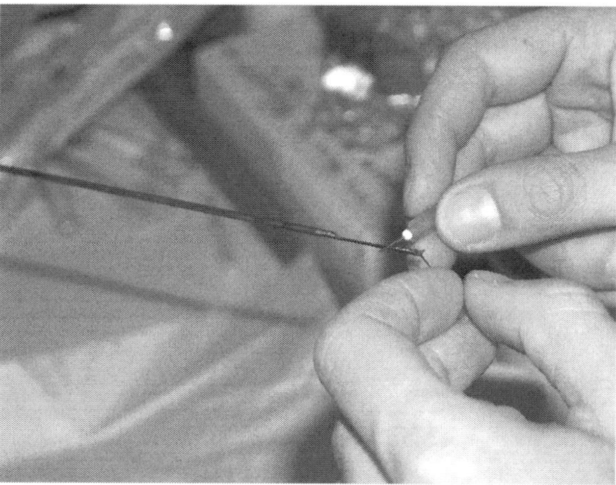

Figure 1.131 Careful removal of the sample from the open biopsy instrument using 25-gauge needles. ©Kevin Corley 2005.

small stab incision is made at the insertion site to allow the biopsy device to be easily inserted.

The biopsy device is inserted through the skin and directed around the cranial border of the rib caudal to the intercostal space being entered, ensuring that the trocar avoids the intercostal blood vessels that lie at the cranial extent of the intercostal space adjacent to the caudal aspect of the more cranial rib. The device should be inserted 2 to 3 cm beyond the body wall before the inner portion of the device is advanced, followed by advancement of the outer portion of the device or firing of the automated device (Figure 1.129). It is important when using the manual device that the inner portion of the device be held firmly in place when advancing the outer segment, as this movement is responsible for the sectioning of the tissue and retention of the sample within the biopsy device (Figure 1.130). This is not a concern with the automated devices, which simply require activation in order to collect a biopsy specimen. Following biopsy collection, the device is withdrawn and the biopsy sample is carefully placed into 10% buffered formalin solution for fixation, using a 25-gauge needle to tease the biopsy from the device with minimal trauma to the biopsy sample (Figure 1.131). The biopsy can be affixed to a tongue depressor by pinning with needles to minimise artifactual changes associated with fixation.

The most frequent complications of percutaneous lung biopsy in the horse include epistaxis secondary to low-grade pulmonary haemorrhage and tachypnoea. Less common complications include respiratory distress, pneumothorax, severe pulmonary haemorrhage, collapse and death. Treatment of severe haemorrhage consists of supportive care, intranasal oxygen administration, blood transfusion and possibly administration of ε-aminocaproic acid (EACA) or tranexamic acid (see Chapter 8.2).

References

1. Savage CJ, Traub Dargatz JL, Mumford EL: Survey of the large animal diplomates of the American College of Veterinary Internal Medicine regarding percutaneous lung biopsy in the horse. J Vet Intern Med 12:456-464, 1998
2. Venner M, Schmidbauer S, Drommer W, et al.: Percutaneous lung biopsy in the horse: comparison of two instruments and repeated biopsy in horses with induced acute interstitial pneumopathy. J Vet Intern Med 20:968-973, 2006

1.38 Sinocentesis

Jennifer O. Stephen

Sinocentesis is a useful diagnostic and therapeutic procedure for paranasal sinus disease. It may be used in the frontal sinus (Figure 1.132), and caudal and rostral maxillary sinuses (Figure 1.133). When performed as a diagnostic procedure, both compartments of the maxillary sinus should be sampled. In young horses (<3 years), care should

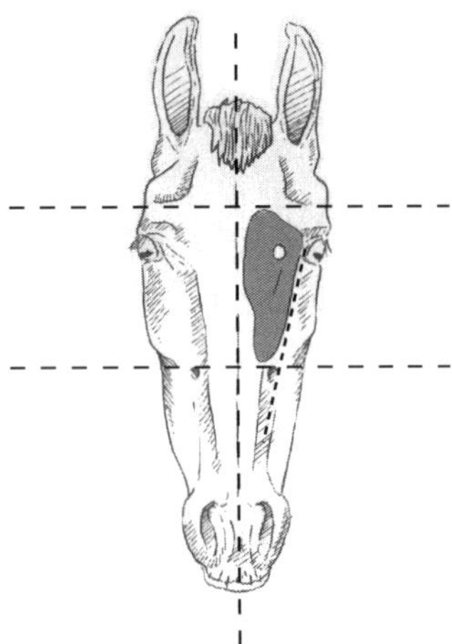

Figure 1.132 Left frontal sinus (*shaded grey*). The left and right sinuses are separate. The caudal margin is a line drawn through the middle of the zygomatic arches. The lateral margin is a line drawn from medial canthus of the eye to the nasomaxillary notch. The rostral extent of the sinus lies on a line drawn between the midpoints of the medial canthus to the nasomaxillary notch on each side. The site for trephination marked as a clear circle.

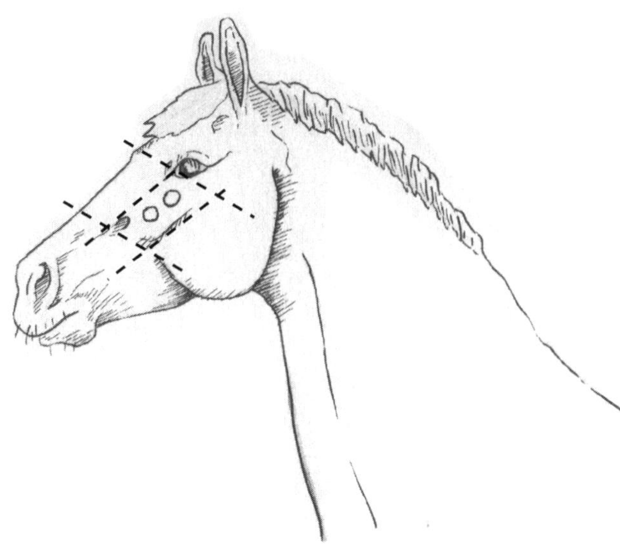

Figure 1.133 Maxillary sinus. The dorsal margin is a line drawn from the medial canthus of the eye to the nasomaxillary notch. The ventral margin is facial crest. The caudal limit is at a line drawn through the middle of the eye to the facial crest. The rostral limit is at the end of the facial crest. The sites for trephination of the rostral and caudal sinuses are marked (*clear circles*).

be taken to avoid the tooth root apices, particularly if performing technique on the rostral maxillary sinus.

Equipment needed

The equipment needed is listed in Box 1.43.

Sites for sinocentesis[1]

- *Frontal sinus* (Figure 1.132): 60% of the distance in a lateral direction from the midline to the medial canthus and 0.5 cm caudal to the medial canthus
- *Rostral maxillary sinus* (Figure 1.133): 50% of the distance from the rostral end of the facial crest to the level of the medial canthus and 1 cm ventral to a line joining the infra-orbital foramen and medial canthus
- *Caudal maxillary sinus* (Figure 1.133): 2 cm rostral and 2 cm ventral to the medial canthus

Technique

Sinocentesis is performed with the horse under standing sedation. The skin should be clipped and aseptically prepared over the selected site. Place a small bleb of local anaesthetic and make a 0.5- to 1-metre incision through the skin. A Steinmann pin, of around 2-mm diameter (large enough to accommodate the end of an extension set/catheter to allow lavage), is put in a Jacob's chuck. Press the end of the pin firmly into the bone and rotate until the sinus is penetrated. The bone in horses with chronic disease may be very thin so care should be taken not to push too hard and to limit the extent of pin exposed to 2 cm (3/4 inch) to avoid damage to underlying structures. If samples cannot be collected, 20 to 30 ml of warm saline may be infused and aspirated, or the sinus should be lavaged and the nasal discharge examined for purulent material. The site is left to heal by secondary intention.

Box 1.43. Equipment for sinocentesis

Required

Steinmann pin (2-mm [5/64-inch] diameter)*
Jacob's chuck†
Sedation
Clippers with a fine (No. 40) blade
Small gauze swabs (4 × 4) soaked in chlorhexidine (4%) scrub solution‡
Small gauze swabs (4 × 4) soaked in surgical spirit (alcohol)
Mepivacaine 2%§: 2–3 ml drawn up in a syringe with a 23–25-gauge needle
Surgical gloves
No. 11 scalpel blade
14-Gauge catheter
20–30-ml sterile saline in a syringe
Sterile sample pot

Optional

Twitch
Fluids for sinus lavage
Fluid extension set
Fluid pressure bag

*Many suppliers, including Animal Orthopaedics, Inc., Bremen, IN, USA.
†Many suppliers, including Veterinary Instrumentation Limited, Sheffield, UK.
‡Hibiscrub; Mölnlycke Health Care, Dunstable, UK.
§Intra-epicaine; Arnolds Veterinary Products, Shrewsbury, UK; Carbocaine-V; Pfizer Animal Health, New York, NY, USA.

Reference

1. Ruggles AJ: Endoscopic examination of normal paranasal sinus disease in 16 horses. Vet Surg 229:508, 1993

1.39 Lumbosacral spinal fluid collection

Martin Furr

Collection of cerebrospinal fluid (CSF) from the lumbosacral (LS) space can be performed in the standing, sedated horse. This is an advantage over collection from the atlanto-occipital (AO) space (see Chapter 1.40), which requires the patient to be anaesthetised. However, the likelihood of sample contamination with blood is increased with collection from the LS space. This technique is also harder to perform than collection from the AO space. The analysis of CSF is discussed in Chapter 14.1.

Equipment needed

The equipment needed is listed in Box 1.44.

Procedure

The technique of CSF collection from the LS space is well described in the literature.[1] Horses can be restrained in a set of stocks (as is the author's preference), or restrained in the open. Stocks are advisable as they provide a degree of protection from reflexive kicks during the procedure. A nose twitch is applied and the horse sedated. Combinations of xylazine (250 mg IV) and butorphanol (5 mg IV) for the 450-kg horse provide a good degree of sedation with a minimum degree of unsteadiness. Alternatively, detomidine (5 to 10 mg IV) can be used.

The optimum site is the point on midline that is intersected by a line drawn between the cranial borders of the tuber sacrale (Figure 1.134). The site should be clipped and scrubbed, and the subcutaneous tissue infiltrated with local anaesthetic. Following this, a small stab incision can be made with a number 15 blade. The stab incision prevents dulling of the spinal needle. A spinal needle is then inserted and stabilised at the skin surface using one hand, and the needle is advanced with the opposite hand. The needle should be advanced steadily, not with jerking movements, and the operator must ensure that the needle is advanced straight down, without lateral or cranial-caudal deviations. It is sometimes useful to have an assistant stand well behind the horse and ensure that the needle is advancing perpendicularly to the horse's back. If not, the needle should be withdrawn almost to the surface and redirected. If it is not withdrawn to the surface, the needle will follow the previous needle path. The LS space will be encountered at a depth of about 5 to 6 inches in most average-sized horses. As the needle approaches the space, increasing resistance will be felt, and then the resistance will abruptly decrease as the needle penetrates the ligamentum flavum. This is felt by the operator as a "pop" and is usually a good indication

Box 1.44. Equipment for collection of spinal fluid from the lumbosacral space

Required

- 18-Gauge spinal needle 20 cm (8 inches) long*
- Sedation
- Twitch
- Clippers with a fine (No. 40) blade
- Small gauze swabs (4 × 4) soaked in chlorhexidine (4%) scrub solution†
- Small gauze swabs (4 × 4) soaked in surgical spirit (alcohol)
- No. 15 scalpel blade
- Mepivacaine 2%‡: 2–3 ml drawn up in a syringe with a 23–25-gauge needle
- Surgical gloves
- Four or five 5–10-ml syringes (empty and sterile)
- Sample pot

Optional

- Stocks to restrain the horse

*1808; MILA International, Florence, KY, USA.
†Hibiscrub; Mölnlycke Health Care, Dunstable, UK.
‡Intra-epicaine; Arnolds Veterinary Products, Shrewsbury, UK; Carbocaine-V; Pfizer Animal Health, New York, NY, USA.

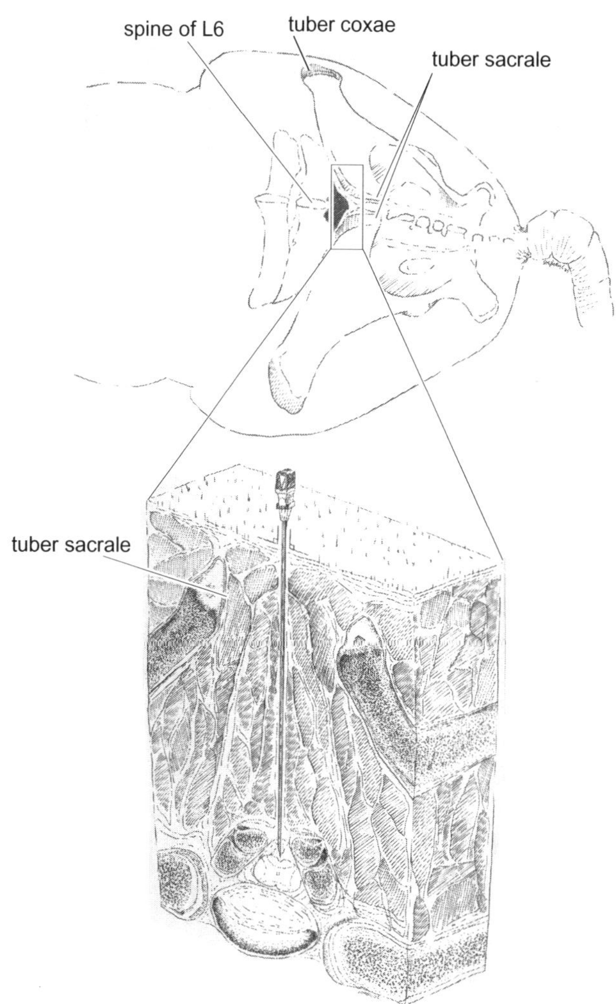

Figure 1.134 Anatomy of the site for collection of fluid from the lumbosacral space. The optimum site is the point on midline that is intersected by a line drawn between the cranial borders of the tuber sacrale.

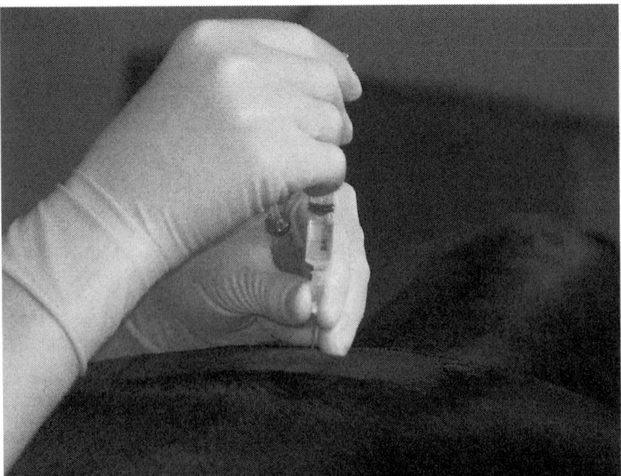

Figure 1.135 The plunger of the syringe is gently withdrawn to allow fluid to flow into the syringe. ©Kevin Corley 2006.

that the membranes have been penetrated and the needle is well positioned. Penetration of the membranes is often accompanied by a reaction from the horse, which may be no reaction at all, restlessness, a tail flick, stomping of the foot or tightening of the caudal muscles. Occasionally, a very violent reaction can be seen; however, with proper sedation and a sharp spinal needle, these reactions are thankfully rare. Persons restraining the horse should be made aware that these are possible, though.

Once the dura has been penetrated, the stylet can be removed and CSF may be collected by gentle aspiration using a 5- or 10-ml syringe (Figure 1.135). If negative pressure is felt, then the needle should be advanced and collection attempted again. Any time the needle is moved, the stylet should be in place and properly seated. Strong suction should be avoided as it leads to blood contamination, and may occlude the needle with membranes or epidural fat.

If no fluid can be retrieved and the operator has confidence that the needle is properly placed, then the needle can be advanced by 1 mm at a time, with fluid collection attempted again until fluid is recovered. Alternatively, the needle can be rotated 90° at a time, with collection attempts repeated. Also, the horse's head can be raised and held up for a few minutes, and the jugular veins can be occluded to increase intracranial pressure and promote CSF movement caudally. If the needle contacts bone without feeling the characteristic "pop" or at a depth less than expected, the needle should be removed and redirected cranially or caudally, until a proper needle depth is achieved or the space is penetrated.

When the sample is collected, the CSF should be withdrawn slowly with gentle aspiration. If the sample has blood contamination, several syringes of CSF should be withdrawn and discarded. If the syringes become progressively more clear, then it is likely the haemorrhage is iatrogenic. If the blood contamination remains uniform throughout the sample, it is most likely truly representative of the CSF. If gross blood is recovered, the needle should be removed and a fresh needle used for a second attempt. Clear fluid can be recovered in these circumstances, although not in all cases. It should be recognised also that it may not be possible to enter the LS space in some animals, due to calcification of the ligaments, etc.

Aftercare for horses following an LS spinal tap is minimal. The site should be kept clean and dry and observed for swelling or discharge. Phenylbutazone or similar analgesics are rarely necessary but may be useful if a horse had multiple attempts.

Normal values for CSF analysis are given in the Appendix (see Table 19.14).

Reference

1. Mayhew I: Collection of cerebrospinal fluid from the horse. Cornell Vet 65:500-502, 1975

1.40 Atlanto-occipital cerebrospinal fluid collection

Martin Furr

The technique of atlanto-occipital (AO) cerebrospinal fluid (CSF) collection has been previously described.[1] The procedure is technically very easy. However, it does require that the horse be anaesthetised. This may or may not be advisable in all cases, and the benefits of collecting the fluid versus the risks of general anaesthesia must be considered on a case-by-case basis. In most cases, an AO CSF sample can be collected quickly following short-acting injectable anaesthesia (see Chapter 4).

Equipment needed

The equipment needed is listed in Box 1.45.

Procedure

After the horse is anaesthetised, the poll is clipped and aseptically prepared, and the horse's head is flexed to open up the AO space. A spinal needle is inserted at the point at which a line drawn between the cranial borders of the atlas intersects the midline (Figure 1.136). The needle is directed toward the lower jaw and advanced until the dura is penetrated, usually at a depth of about 2 to 2.5 inches in the mature adult horse. It is important to ensure that the needle is advanced in the median plane, as it is possible to miss laterally if the needle is angled. Resistance to advancing the needle will increase as the needle penetrates the nuchal ligament and then will abruptly decrease, resulting in a characteristic "pop". The pop is more noticeable at the AO space than at the lumbosacral (LS) space, and needle advancement should cease immediately once it is felt. The stylet can then be withdrawn (Figure 1.137) and fluid collected (Figure 1.138). If no fluid is present, the stylet should

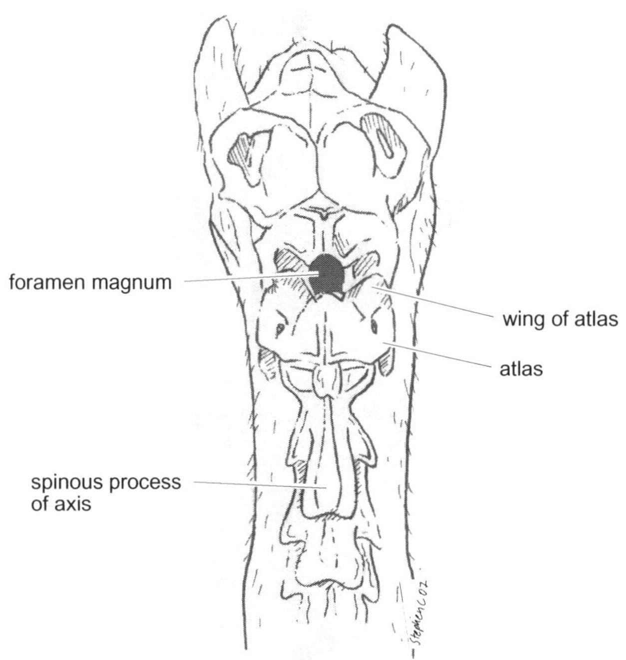

Figure 1.136 Anatomy of the site for collection of fluid from the atlanto-occipital space. The needle is inserted at the midline point along a line drawn between the cranial borders (wings) of the atlas.

Box 1.45. Equipment for collection of spinal fluid from the atlanto-occipital space

Required

18-Gauge spinal needle 9 cm (3.5 inches) long*
General anaesthesia requirements (see Chapter 4)

- Induction and recovery box
- Anaesthetic agent (usually ketamine and an α_2-agonist)
- Jugular catheter

Clippers with a fine (No. 40) blade
Small gauze swabs (4 × 4) soaked in chlorhexidine (4%) scrub solution†
Small gauze swabs (4 × 4) soaked in surgical spirit (alcohol)
Surgical gloves
Sample pot

*511114; Becton Dickinson (http://catalog.bd.com).
†Hibiscrub; Mölnlycke Health Care, Dunstable, UK.

be replaced and the needle advanced in 1-mm steps, attempting collection between each advancement.

Follow-up care after an AO CSF collection is minimal. Nonsteroidal anti-inflammatory drugs can be given if there is neck soreness. It is advisable to keep the horse is a stall and feed from a hay net for 1 to 2 days. This prevents the horse from putting its head down to graze, which appears to increase the degree of neck soreness following an AO puncture.

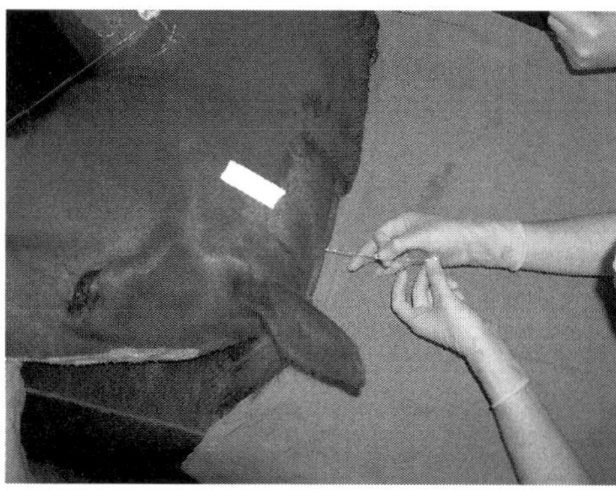

Figure 1.137 After a characteristic "pop" is felt, the needle should not be advanced any farther, and the stylet removed. ©Kevin Corley 2006.

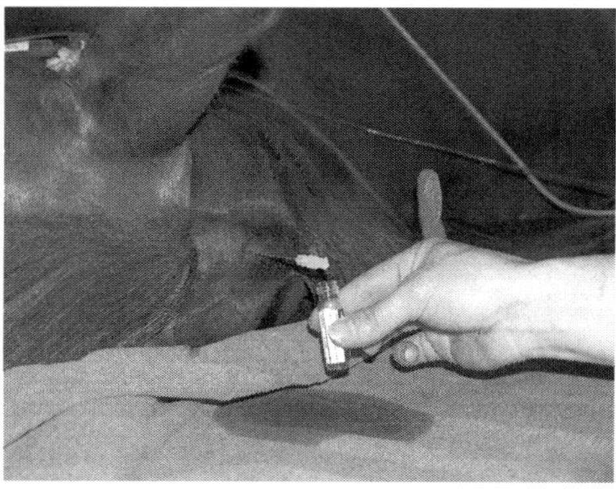

Figure 1.138 The fluid is collected via gravity flow. ©Kevin Corley 2006.

Normal values for CSF analysis are given in the Appendix (see Table 19.14).

Reference

1. Mayhew I: Collection of cerebrospinal fluid from the horse. Cornell Vet 65:500-502, 1975

1.41 Epidural injection and catheterisation

Lydia Donaldson

Caudal epidural injection and catheterisation are used to create anaesthesia or analgesia of the tail, perineum, external genitalia and pelvic viscera and/or hind leg and caudal abdomen, respectively.

Equipment needed

The equipment required is listed in Box 1.46.

Procedure

The needle is passed through the skin, subcutaneous tissue, intervertebral space and interarcuate ligament between coccygeal vertebrae 1 and 2 (C1-C2) and into the epidural space at the level of the cauda equina (Figure 1.139).

The appropriate intervertebral space is identified by raising and lowering the tail whilst feeling for the midline

Box 1.46. Equipment for epidural injection and catheterisation

Required
Epidural needle or catheter kit

- 18-Gauge spinal or epidural needle 5–9 cm (2–3.5 inches) long*
- Epidural catheter kit†

Clippers with a fine (No. 40) blade
Small gauze swabs (4 × 4) soaked in chlorhexidine (4%) scrub solution‡
Small gauze swabs (4 × 4) soaked in surgical spirit (alcohol)
Mepivacaine 2%§: 2–3 ml drawn up in a syringe with a 23–25-gauge needle
Surgical gloves
Drug to be injected (see Table 6.2)

For epidural catheter
7.5-cm (3-inch) wide stretchy adhesive dressing (Elastoplast**/Elastikon††)
Sterile gauze swabs (4 × 4)

Optional
Sedation
Twitch

*511114 or 405025; Becton Dickinson (http://catalog.bd.com).
†9203, Epidural pain management kit; MILA International, Florence, KY, USA.
‡Hibiscrub; Mölnlycke Health Care, Dunstable, UK.
§Intra-epicaine; Arnolds Veterinary Products, Shrewsbury, UK; Carbocaine-V; Pfizer Animal Health, New York, NY, USA.
**Beiersdorf AG, Hamburg, Germany.
††Johnson and Johnson, New Brunswick, NJ, USA.

depression between the dorsal spinous process of the last immovable vertebra (usually C1) and that of the first movable vertebra (usually C2). The location is approximately 5 cm cranial to the first long tail hairs. An area approximately 10 × 10 cm is clipped and aseptically prepared. The position of the intervertebral space is again identified (Figure 1.140). Local anaesthetic is infiltrated into the skin, subcutaneous tissue and interspinous soft tissue. The anaesthetised area is enlarged to either the left or right if an epidural catheter is to be placed and maintained for any length of time. The horse should stand squarely to help identify the midline and facilitate true direction of the needle on that plane.

If a single injection is to be made, the needle is placed into the caudal epidural space by inserting it into the skin overlying the palpable space. The successful angle of insertion depends on the anatomy of the horse and the relative positions of the skin puncture and the space between the vertebrae. This is found by starting at approximately a 90° angle and advancing until the interarcuate ligament or bone is encountered. In the latter case, redirecting the needle, usually to a lesser angle, is necessary until the space is identified. The change in resistance to the advancing needle created by interarcuate ligament may not be perceptible. The depth of insertion of the needle is used to estimate the needle tip location. This varies with needle angle, subcutaneous fat and individual horse's anatomy. In the average horse, the interarcuate ligament is approximately 3 to 4 cm deep to the skin. If the hanging drop technique is to be used to identify the negative atmospheric pressure of the epidural space, a drop of sterile saline or the medication to be administered is placed in the hub of the needle

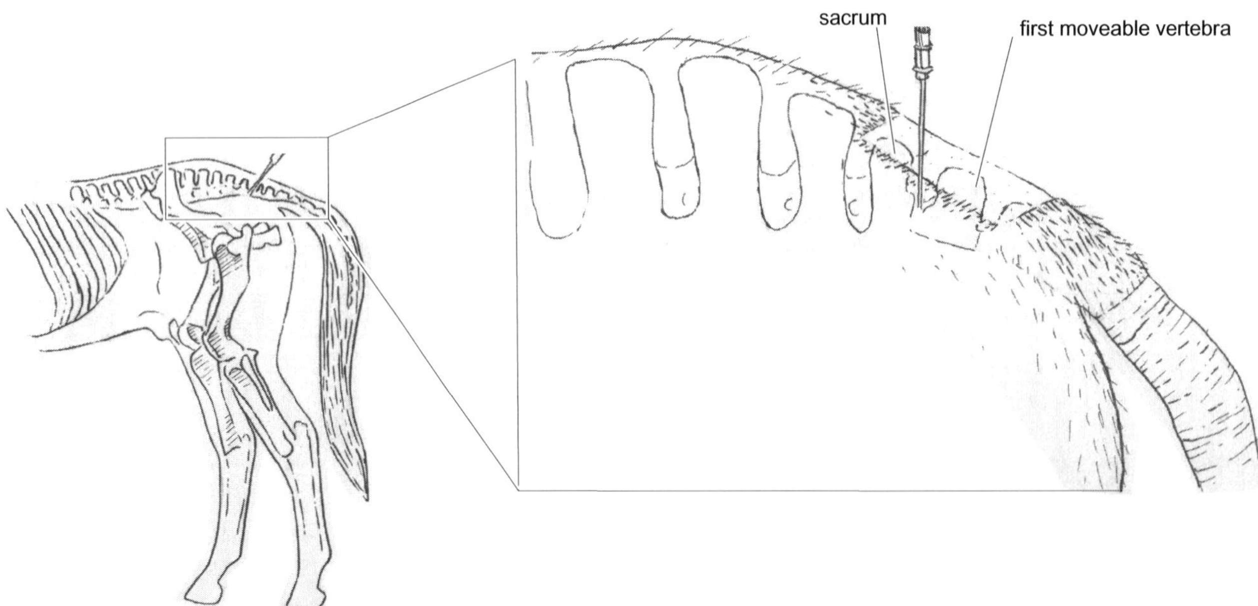

Figure 1.139 Anatomy of the site for epidural injection and catheterisation. The needle is passed through the skin, subcutaneous tissue, intervertebral space and interarcuate ligament between coccygeal vertebrae 1 and 2 (C1-C2) and into the epidural space at the level of the cauda equina.

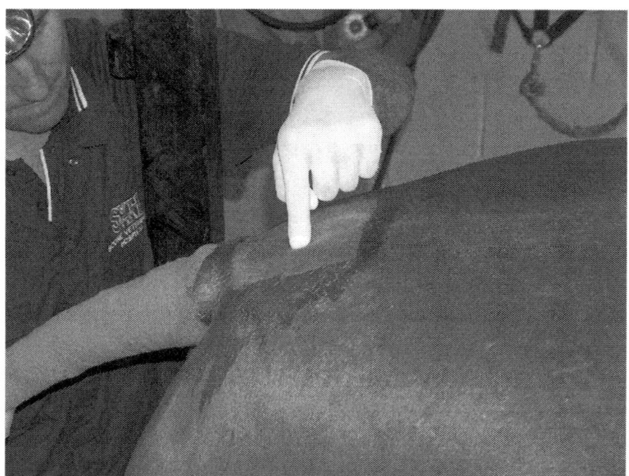

Figure 1.140 The appropriate intervertebral space is identified by raising and lowering the tail while feeling for the midline depression between the dorsal spinous process of C1 and C2. ©Kevin Corley 2004.

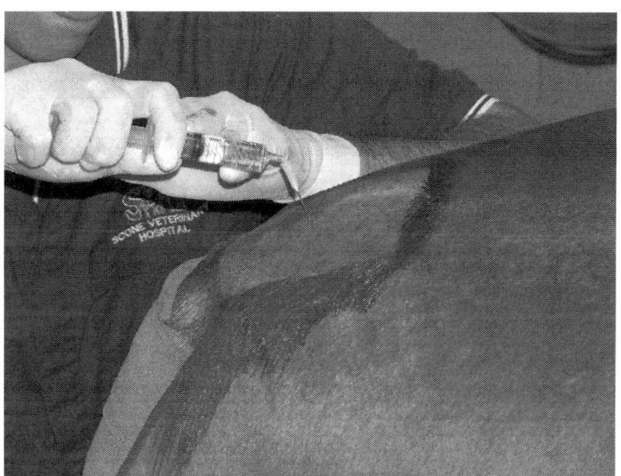

Figure 1.141 The hanging drop technique. A drop of sterile saline or the medication to be administered is placed in the hub of the needle after removing the stylet, if present, and the needle advanced until the drop is sucked into the epidural space. ©Kevin Corley 2004.

after removing the stylet, if present, and the needle is advanced until the drop is sucked into the epidural space (Figure 1.141). A simpler approach is to advance the needle until the floor of the vertebral canal is encountered. As the needle passes past nerve roots, the tail should twitch. The needle must be withdrawn slightly to place the needle tip freely in the epidural space.

If a catheter is to be placed, a skin incision is made with a surgical scalpel because the curved tip of the needle will not slide easily through the skin. The needle is then advanced as described above. A grating feeling may be noticed as the needle passes through denser connective tissue. Placing the needle at a less steep angle to the skin will allow the catheter to more easily slide out of the curved

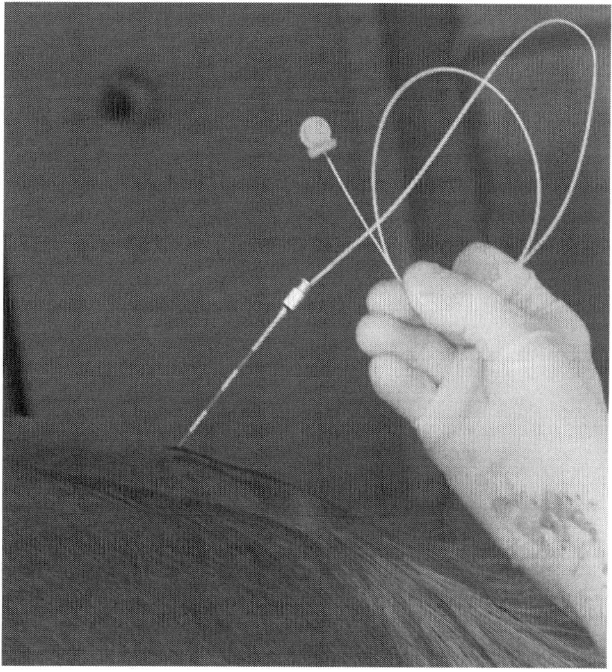

Figure 1.142 An 18-gauge 8.89-cm Hustead epidural needle and a 20-gauge 91.8-cm medical grade Teflon catheter seated in the coccygeal epidural space of a horse. ©Lydia Donaldson 2006.

needle tip. This will require skin puncture more caudad in the palpable indentation to successfully pass through the intervertebral space (Figure 1.142). Many epidural catheter choices are available commercially. A 20-gauge catheter with stylet is the easiest to advance through an 18-gauge thin-walled epidural needle. Most catheters are marked in centimetres to identify the length of catheter inserted beyond the end of the needle.

The absolute test for correct placement is that the catheter will advance. Some redirection and retraction of the needle may be needed to free the tip of the catheter as it passes out of the needle. Partially withdrawing the catheter stylet before advancing the catheter around the curve in the needle will facilitate stylet removal later. Care should be taken to direct the catheter craniad as indicated by the flat surface of the hub of the epidural needle. Once the catheter enters the epidural space, it may slide forward as intended, but it can also turn caudad or wind in circles or knots. For this reason, it is prudent to only introduce enough catheter to prevent it from sliding or being pulled out inadvertently (approximately 5 cm).

The needle is pulled off the catheter externally and the catheter stylet removed. To minimise the chance of unplanned removal and possible potential for descending infection, the catheter is tunneled 2 to 3 cm under the skin from the site of entry. This is most easily done by making a second small skin incision to either side. The epidural needle should be passed from this to the catheter exit, taking care not to cut the catheter. Insert the free end of the catheter, retrograde through the needle and pull the

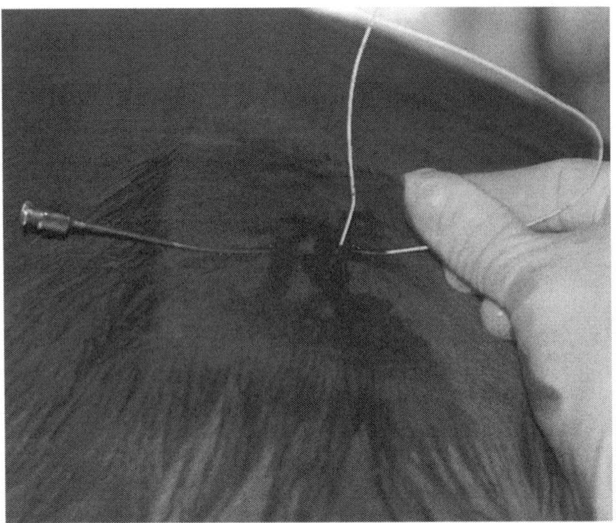

Figure 1.143 An 18-gauge 8.89-cm Hustead epidural needle being used to tunnel a 20-gauge 91.8-cm medical grade epidural catheter under the skin for security after caudal epidural placement. ©Lydia Donaldson 2006.

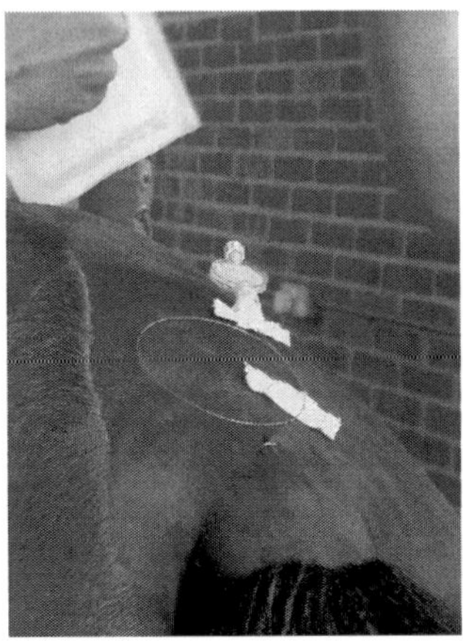

Figure 1.144 Epidural catheter in place, with filter and injection cap. ©Kevin Corley 2002.

needle and catheter through the subcutaneous tunnel to the new exit port (Figure 1.143).

The excess catheter length should be trimmed, an injection port fitted to the free end (Figure 1.144) and the catheter secured with tape tabs and staples or sutures. The catheter site should be lightly bandaged for protection.

Injections should be done slowly, particularly initially. Rapid injection of preservative free morphine and morphine with detomidine has precipitated muscle tremors, transient excitement and recumbency from which the horses immediately recover.

Final confirmation of successful needle or catheter placement is indicated by little resistance to injection (Figures 1.145 and 1.146) and clinical evidence of anaesthesia or analgesia.

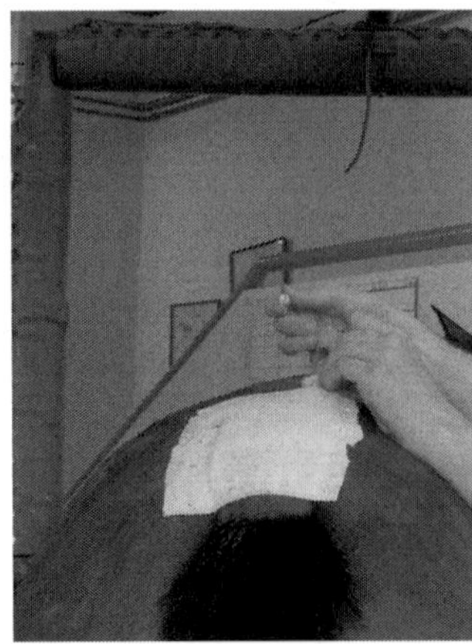

Figure 1.145 Injecting into an epidural catheter. ©Kevin Corley 2002.

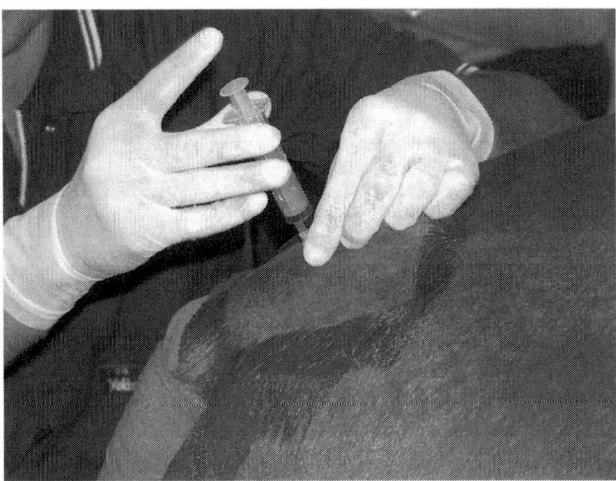

Figure 1.146 Injecting into the epidural space, via a needle. There should be very little resistance to injection. ©Kevin Corley 2004.

1.42 Urinary catheterisation

Anna Hollis

Catheterisation of the male

Equipment needed

The equipment needed is listed in Box 1.47.

Procedure

In the adult male, a low dose of acepromazine (0.05 to 0.1 mg/kg IM or slow IV) is the most reliable at relaxing the penis but is associated with a very small risk of causing paraphimosis.[1] If acepromazine is deemed unsuitable, for example, in the breeding male, an α_2-agonist will usually produce penile relaxation. However, this is less predictable than the use of acepromazine.

Following penile relaxation, the glans and external urethral orifice should be cleaned with dilute povidone-iodine (or chlorhexidine) solution. If an assistant is present, the

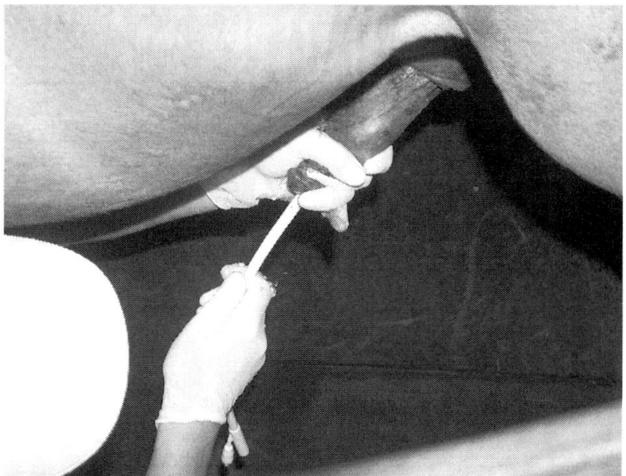

Figure 1.147 Placement of a Foley catheter into the bladder of a gelding. ©Kevin Corley 2004.

Box 1.47. Equipment for urinary catheterisation in the male

Required
Horse urinary catheter*
K-Y Jelly†
Examination gloves
Dilute povidone-iodine or chlorhexidine solution
Small gauze swabs (4 × 4)
Surgical gloves
Sedation
Catheter-tipped 60-ml syringe
Sterile sample pot

Optional
Twitch
Stocks to restrain the horse

*Examples include Portex Horse Catheter, Portex Ltd., Kent, UK.
†Johnson and Johnson, New Brunswick, NJ, USA.

assistant can hold the body of the penis in gloved hands. The person passing the catheter should wear sterile gloves and identify the external urethral orifice. The catheter is lubricated with sterile K-Y Jelly and introduced aseptically into the external urethral orifice (Figure 1.147). This should be passed along the urethra for the full length of the catheter. There may be a slight increase in resistance as the catheter passes round the ischial arch, although the catheter should still pass easily. The stylet can then be removed. Urine does not always flow down the catheter, and its position can be checked by attaching a catheter-tipped syringe to the urethral catheter and applying gentle suction.

Urethral catheterisation is associated with a small risk of introducing infection, so absolute sterility must be maintained during the procedure.

Box 1.48. Equipment for urinary catheterisation in the female

Required
Horse urinary catheter*
K-Y Jelly†
Examination gloves
Dilute povidone-iodine or chlorhexidine solution
Cotton wool or small gauze swabs (4 × 4)
Surgical gloves
Tail bandage (or rectal sleeve and zinc oxide tape)
Catheter-tipped 60-ml syringe
Sterile sample pot

Optional
Sedation
Twitch
Stocks to restrain the horse

*Examples include Portex Horse Catheter, Portex Ltd., Kent, UK.
†Johnson and Johnson, New Brunswick, NJ, USA.

Catheterising the female

Equipment needed

The equipment needed is listed in Box 1.48.

Procedure

The tail should be bandaged or placed in a rectal sleeve secured with zinc oxide tape. The vulva should be cleaned with dilute povidone-iodine solution. Sterile gloves should be worn, and a lubricated hand gently introduced along the ventral surface of the vestibule. The external urethral orifice may be located by introducing a sterile, lubricated finger along the midline, ventral aspect of the vestibule. This is usually found approximately 10 to 12 cm from the vulval lips beneath the vestibulovaginal fold. The orifice of the urethra is large and a lubricated finger can be gently inserted into the urethra. Once located, a sterile catheter can be aseptically introduced by running the catheter underneath the finger locating the orifice. The urethra is short, and once the catheter has entered the bladder the stylet is removed. Urine does not always flow down the catheter, and its position can be checked by attaching a catheter-tipped syringe to the urethral catheter and applying gentle suction.

Urethral catheterisation is associated with a small risk of introducing infection, so absolute sterility must be maintained during the procedure.

Reference

1. Taylor P, Clarke K: Sedation, analgesia and premedication, in: Handbook of Equine Anaesthesia. Edinburgh, WB Saunders, 2003, pp 15-31

1.43 Endoscopy of the bladder and ureters

Anna Hollis

Endoscopy of the bladder is useful for identification of a source of blood in the urine (urethra, bladder, right ureter or left ureter), identification of urinary calculi, to confirm if there is urinary output out of the ureters from each individual kidney, to diagnose bladder neoplasia and to determine the extent of trauma, if present.

Equipment needed

The equipment needed is listed in Box 1.49.

Procedure

The endoscope should be cold sterilised prior to use to avoid the risk of introducing infection. The solution should be introduced into the biopsy channel by aspirating a small amount of fluid into the channel. Following cold sterilisation, the endoscope should be handled with sterile gloves and thoroughly rinsed with 1 to 2 L sterile saline, including the biopsy channel.

The end should be lubricated with K-Y Jelly (taking care not to cover the lens), and it is introduced into the urethra in the same way as a urinary catheter (see Chapter 1.42). The urethra and bladder can be visualised, as well as the ureters where they enter the bladder. To optimise visualisation, predraining the bladder by placement of a urinary catheter may be desirable. Alternatively, the bladder can be manually drained via tubing introduced down the biopsy channel of the endoscope. Distending the bladder with air will allow a more thorough examination. Orientation in the bladder is possible by visualising a pool of urine at the ventral midline. The mucosa should be pale and salmon-pink and becomes reddened with cystitis or urethritis. Calculi are normally readily visualised.

To visualise the ureteral openings, the endoscope should be slowly withdrawn to the bladder trigone. The orifices will be visualised as two small openings either side of the dorsal midline, at approximately 2 and 10 o'clock.[1] Urine samples can be collected from each individual ureter using sterile polyurethane tubing narrow enough to travel down the biopsy portal of the endoscope. Tubing used for transendoscopic tracheal washes is suitable and can be carefully advanced into the ureter. Urine is produced in pulses and can be collected by applying gentle suction to the tubing with a syringe. Urine production from each kidney can be subjectively assessed by watching the ureters; however, normal values of the number of pulses per minute are not established.

Evaulation of the urethra is easiest as the endoscope is gradually withdrawn from the animal. Gentle distension with air will aid visualisation.

Endoscopic examination of the urinary tract is associated with a small risk of introducing infection, necessitating absolute sterile technique during the procedure.

Box 1.49. Equipment for endoscopy of the bladder and ureters

Required

Endoscope

- At least $1\frac{1}{2}$ metre long for males, diameter less than 12 mm

Cold sterilising solution*
2 L sterile 0.9% sodium chloride solution
Surgical gloves
K-Y Jelly†
Examination gloves
Dilute povidone-iodine or chlorhexidine solution
Cotton wool or small gauze swabs (4 × 4)
Tail bandage (females only)

Optional

Sterile polyurethrane tubing for collecting urine samples‡
5–10-ml syringes for collecting urine samples
Sterile sample pot(s)
Biopsy instrument
Sedation
Acepromazine (males only)
Twitch
Stocks to restrain the horse
Horse urinary catheter§

*Examples include Cidex OPA solution; Advanced Sterilisation Products (www.sterrad.com).
†Johnson and Johnson, New Brunswick, NJ, USA.
‡EDC190, EDC220 or EDC1603; MILA International, Florence, KY, USA.
§Examples include Portex Horse Catheter; Portex Ltd., Kent, UK.

Reference

1. Schott H, Varner D: Urinary tract, in: Equine Endoscopy, ed 2. St. Louis, Mosby, 1997, pp 187-203

1.44 Endometrial biopsy

Anna Hollis

Endometrial biopsies may be part of breeding soundness examination and allow detailed cytology to be performed.

Equipment needed

The equipment needed is listed in Box 1.50.

Procedure

This procedure should be performed whilst the mare is in oestrus. A commercially available biopsy instrument is introduced through the cervix in a sterile manner. A vaginal speculum allows visualisation of the cervix and may make the process easier than manual palpation. The biopsy is usually taken from the base of a uterine horn, and for breeding purposes, one biopsy is usually considered representative of the whole uterus. If a particular area is of

Box 1.50. Equipment for endometrial biopsy

Required
Vaginal speculum
Uterine biopsy instrument*
Sterile rectal sleeve
K-Y Jelly†
Dilute povidone-iodine or chlorhexidine solution
Cotton wool or small gauze swabs (4 × 4)
Sample pot containing 10% neutral buffered formalin
Sterile sample pot
Tail bandage (or rectal sleeve and zinc oxide tape)

For rectovaginal technique
Rectal sleeve
Obstetrical lubricant

Optional
Sedation
Twitch
Stocks to restrain the horse
Ultrasound machine with a 5–7.5-MHz Linear rectal probe

*Examples include 141700, uterine biopsy instrument 60 cm; Kruuse, Marslev, Denmark; uterine biopsy punch; Veterinary Instrumentation, Sheffield, UK.
†Johnson and Johnson, New Brunswick, NJ, USA.

interest, the biopsy can be performed concurrent with ultrasonographic examination per rectum, which requires two operators. Alongside cytology, these biopsy samples should be cultured to maximise the information gained.[1]

There are two techniques for obtaining a uterine biopsy: rectovaginal and vaginal.[2,3] Both techniques require the tail to be bandaged or placed in a rectal sleeve and the vulva to be thoroughly cleansed with dilute povidone-iodine or chlorhexidine solution.

Rectovaginal technique

The rectovaginal technique involves passing the sterile biopsy instrument, with its jaws closed, into the vagina with a sterile, gloved, lubricated hand. The instrument is guided through the cervical canal into the body of the uterus. The hand is then withdrawn. With a rectal sleeve and lubricant, the hand is placed into the rectum and the uterus, with the biopsy instrument, located per rectum. The instrument can then be guided to the uterine wall per rectum, and the jaws of the instrument opened with the operator's second hand. The endometrial wall is guided into the jaws of the instrument per rectum, and the jaws closed. The biopsy instrument is withdrawn with the jaws closed.

Vaginal technique

The vaginal technique involves passing the sterile biopsy instrument, jaws closed, into the vagina with a sterile, gloved, lubricated hand. The instrument is carried through the cervix and advanced into the uterine body. The jaws of the instrument are opened, and the instrument guided laterally until the endometrium is reached. The jaws are then closed and the instrument withdrawn.

With both techniques, a gentle tug will be required to take a biopsy. Once obtained, the sample is placed into 10% neutral buffered formalin. If culture is desirable, a sample should also be placed into a plain container. Uterine biopsy is associated with a small risk of introducing infection, so sterile technique is essential.

References

1. Nielsen JM: Endometritis in the mare: a diagnostic study comparing cultures from swab and biopsy. Theriogenology 64:510-518, 2005
2. Reiswig JD, Threlfall WR, Rosol TJ: A comparison of endometrial biopsy, culture and cytology during oestrus and dioestrus in the horse. Equine Vet J 25:240-241, 1993
3. Kenney RM: Cyclic and pathologic changes of the mare endometrium as detected by biopsy, with a note on early embryonic death. J Am Vet Med Assoc 172:241-262, 1978

1.45 Uterine lavage

Anna Hollis

Lavaging the uterus may be performed to obtain cellular material or as a technique to aid cleansing the uterus by removing fluid, pus and debris.

Equipment needed

The equipment needed is listed in Box 1.51.

Procedure

This may be performed in the suitably restrained, conscious mare but may require sedation in some animals. The tail should be bandaged or placed in a rectal sleeve, and the vulva thoroughly cleansed with dilute povidone-iodine or chlorhexidine solution.

Obtaining cellular material

To obtain cellular material, a sterile, gloved, lubricated hand should guide a sterile insemination pipette into the uterus. The hand should be removed from the vagina and inserted per rectum with a lubricated rectal sleeve. Then 60 ml of phosphate-buffered sterile saline should be infused via the insemination pipette and the uterus massaged per rectum.[1] This technique may require two operators. The fluid is then aspirated back with a syringe attached to the pipette. This is centrifuged at 400*g* for 10 minutes, and the cell pellet resuspended in 1 ml of phosphate-buffered saline. This fluid is placed on slides, which are dried and stained.[2] This technique has the potential to introduce infection, so sterile technique must be maintained. Evaluation of uterine lavage samples is discussed in Chapter 13.1.

Box 1.51. Equipment for uterine lavage

To obtain cellular material
Sterile AI pipette
60-ml phosphate-buffered solution OR 5–10 L sterile saline or isotonic fluids
60-ml sterile syringe
Sterile sample pot
Diff-Quik* or other stain

To aid cleansing of the uterus
Sterile stomach tube
5–10L warm water with a small amount of povidone-iodine added OR with electrolytes added to make it isotonic
Jug
Funnel

For both techniques:
K-Y Jelly†
Sterile rectal sleeve (or rectal sleeve and surgical gloves)
Cotton wool or small gauze swabs (4 × 4)
Dilute povidone-iodine or chlorhexidine solution
Tail bandage (OR rectal sleeve and zinc oxide tape)

Optional
Sedation
Twitch
Stocks to restrain the horse

*Available from many suppliers, including Dade Behring (www.dadebehring.com).
†Johnson and Johnson, New Brunswick, NJ, USA.

For uterine cleansing

To aid cleansing of the uterus, a sterile stomach tube can be introduced into the uterus with a sterile, gloved, lubricated hand. Large volumes of very dilute povidone-iodine solution (5 to 10 L) are introduced into the stomach tube with a container and funnel (Figure 1.148). The fluid from the uterus is then allowed to drain through the stomach tube via gravity into a suitable container. This can be repeated several times until the draining fluid appears relatively clear.

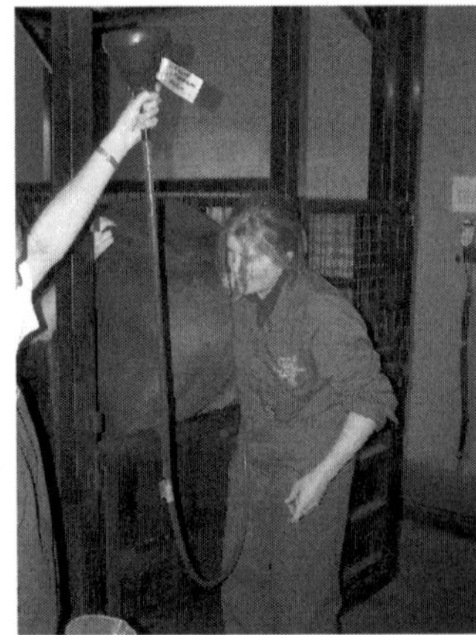

Figure 1.148 Fluid is poured into the uterus via a stomach tube and funnel. ©Kevin Corley 2004.

References

1. Ball B, Shin S, Patten V, et al: Use of low-volume uterine flush for microbiologic and cytological examination of the mare's endometrium. Theriogenology 29:1269-1283, 1988
2. Card C: Post-breeding inflammation and endometrial cytology in mares. Theriogenology 64:580-588, 2005

1.46 Renal biopsy

Anna Hollis

Where abnormalities have been detected on ultrasonographic examination of the kidneys, renal biopsy can be an invaluable tool for definitive diagnosis of the disease process and can provide important prognostic information. However, renal biopsy is not generally necessary in the evaluation and treatment of patients with acute renal failure where prerenal causes are suspected.

Equipment needed

The equipment needed is given in Box 1.52.

Procedure

Ideally, the patient's haemostatic status should be evaluated prior to biopsy (the animal should have a normal number of platelets and, if available, the activated partial thromboplastin time and prothrombin time should be checked).[1]

Where bilateral renal disease is suspected, it is preferable, for practical reasons, to perform biopsies of the right kidney. However, penetration of the spleen to gain access to the left kidney does not appear to be associated with major complications.[2] Although blind renal biopsy techniques have been described,[3] it is generally accepted that renal biopsy should be performed under ultrasound guidance.[2] The procedure is invariably associated with the formation of perirenal haematomas in the horse and may be associated with fatal haemorrhage.[2]

Biopsies may be performed in the standing animal with the infusion of local anaesthetic into the skin and abdominal wall, and sedation is not normally required. The area should be clipped and the kidney imaged ultrasonographically. Following confirmation of an appropriately clipped area and location of the kidney, sterile preparation of the area should be performed. Local anaesthetic should be infused into the skin and abdominal musculature directly overlying the kidney in question. A full sterile preparation should then be performed. A sterile sleeve filled with contact gel can be placed over the ultrasound probe. These are commercially available, although a sterile rectal sleeve works equally well. A stab incision is made into the skin and abdominal musculature with a number 10 or 15 scalpel

Box 1.52. Equipment for renal biopsy

Required

Biopsy instrument

- Automated biopsy device*
- 14–18-Gauge, 15-cm manual biopsy needle (TruCut)†

Ultrasound machine

- For right kidney of adult: 3–5-MHz sector or linear array probe
- For left kidney of adult: 2.5–3-MHz sector or linear array probe
- For foal kidneys: 5-MHz sector or linear array

Sterile ultrasound probe cover
Mepivacaine 2%‡: 10 ml drawn up in a syringe with a 23–25-gauge needle
Sample pot containing 10% neutral buffered formalin
Two 25-gauge needles
Clippers with a fine (No. 40) blade
Small gauze swabs (4 × 4) soaked in chlorhexidine (4%) scrub solution§
Small gauze swabs (4 × 4) soaked in surgical spirit (alcohol)
Surgical gloves
No. 11 or No. 15 scalpel blade

Optional

Sterile sample pot, if culture of a biopsy specimen is required
Skin stapler**
Sedation
Twitch
Antimicrobials

*Examples include Vet-Core biopsy needle; Global Veterinary Products, New Buffalo, MI, USA; Pro-Mag 2.2; US Biopsy Engineered Products, Franklin, IN, USA.
†Baxter Healthcare, Deerfield, IL, USA.
‡Intra-epicaine; Arnolds Veterinary Products, Shrewsbury, UK; Carbocaine-V; Pfizer Animal Health, New York, NY, USA.
§Hibiscrub; Mölnlycke Health Care, Dunstable, UK.
**Auto Suture Appose ULC 35W; United States Surgical, Tyco Healthcare Group, Norwalk, CT, USA.

blade. The biopsy instrument is introduced and imaged ultrasonographically as it passes towards the kidney. A 14- to 18-gauge automated biopsy needle, with a minimum length of 15 cm, is preferred. This allows biopsy with one hand and manipulation of the ultrasound probe in the other hand. The hilus and caudal pole of the kidney should be avoided to avoid major blood vessels.[2] The needle can be ultrasonographically imaged entering the kidney and a sample taken. The sample should be carefully teased from the biopsy needle using one or two 25-gauge needles, placed in neutral buffered formalin and submitted for histopathological examination. The horse should be kept as still and quiet as possible following sample collection to aid the formation of a blood clot. Trace haematuria is often detected following renal biopsy, but gross haematuria is a cause for concern and should be closely monitored. If bilateral renal biopsy is to be performed, at least 24 hours should pass between the two biopsies.

Antibiotic cover is not routinely given, as long as sterility is strictly maintained throughout the procedure. However, the potential for introducing infection makes antibiotic cover a reasonable decision. If this is desirable, a sensible choice would be an antibiotic that is excreted in high concentrations in the urine, such as penicillin. Haemorrhage is a potential complication of renal biopsy in the horse. This may occur even with ultrasound-guided biopsies. If haemorrhage does occur, supportive therapy should be provided (see Chapter 8.2).

References

1. Traub-Dargatz JL, McKinnon AO: Adjunctive methods of examination of the urogenital tract. Vet Clin Equine 4:339-358, 1988
2. Barrat-Boyes S, Spensley M, Nyland T, et al.: Ultrasound localization and guidance for renal biopsy in the horse. Vet Radiol 32:121-126, 1991
3. Bayly WM, Paradis MR, Reed SM: Equine renal biopsy: indications, technique interpretation and complications. Mod Vet Pract 61:763-768, 1980

1.47 Bone marrow biopsy

Roger Smith

Bone marrow biopsy may be used to obtain cells both for diagnosis of haemopoietic disorders and for recovery of stem cells for the use in treatment of tendon injuries. For stem cells, following aspiration of bone marrow, the mesenchymal stem cells need to be recovered and expanded prior to autologous implantation. There are commercial companies who offer this service.*

Equipment needed

The equipment needed is given in Box 1.53.

Procedure

The horse is first sedated with a combination of α_2-agonist and opiate (e.g., detomidine HCl and butorphanol). A 10-cm-wide band overlying the sternum is clipped and scrubbed with surgical scrub (e.g., chlorhexidine) and surgical spirit.

The sternum is examined ultrasonographically to identify the three most caudal sternebrae by the appearance of their intersternebral spaces (Figures 1.149 and 1.150). The position of these intersternebral spaces is marked on the adjacent hair with a marker pen (Figure 1.151). The area of the sternum is prepared aseptically and local anaesthetic

* VetCell BioScience Limited, London, UK (www.vetcell.com).

Box 1.53. Equipment for bone marrow biopsy

Required

11-Gauge 10-cm (4-inch) Jamshidi needle*
Ultrasound machine

- 5–10-MHz linear probe

Sterile ultrasound probe cover
Sedation
Mepivacaine 2%†: 10 ml drawn up in a syringe with a 23–25-gauge needle
20-ml syringe
Two 5-ml syringes
$1\frac{1}{2}$-ml heparin (5000 units/ml)‡
Sterile sample pot
Two 25-gauge needles
Clippers with a fine (No. 40) blade
Small gauze swabs (4 × 4) soaked in chlorhexidine (4%) scrub solution§
Small gauze swabs (4 × 4) soaked in surgical spirit (alcohol)
Surgical gloves
No. 11 scalpel blade

For sending bone marrow for stem cell recovery

Transport pack
Sodium citrate blood tubes

For cytological evaluation of bone marrow

Microscope slides

Optional

Twitch
Stocks to restrain the horse

*Cardinal Health, Dublin, OH, USA; also available from Veterinary Instrumentation, Sheffield, UK (Catalogue No. BMBJV8) and other suppliers.
†Intra-epicaine; Arnolds Veterinary Products, Shrewsbury, UK; Carbocaine-V; Pfizer Animal Health, New York, NY, USA.
‡Multiparin; TechnoPharm, Dublin, Ireland.
§Hibiscrub; Mölnlycke Health Care, Dunstable, UK.

placed at the predicted aspiration entry points to aspirate bone marrow from the second and third most caudal sternebrae.

Prior to aspiration, syringes are preloaded with heparin (to give a final concentration of 625 IU/ml bone marrow). Commonly, a 20-ml syringe is preloaded with 0.5 ml of a 5000 IU/ml heparin solution into which 9.5 ml bone marrow is aspirated.

The area is then scrubbed a final time before a small stab incision is made through the skin. The Jamshidi needle is introduced through the stab incision and advanced until it contacts with the ventral surface of the sternebra in the midline (Figure 1.152). The index finger is placed 2 cm from the skin surface on the needle shaft and the needle gradually advanced using rotating movements until the

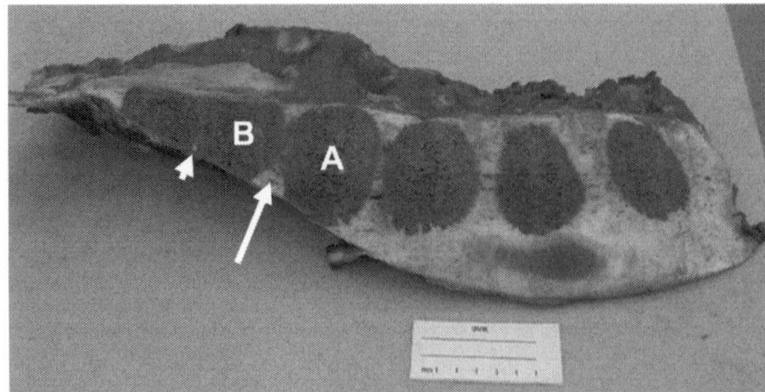

Figure 1.149 Longitudinal sections of sternae (caudal to the left) showing the variation of anatomy that can be present. Usually, there is a smaller intersternebral space between the most caudal two sternebrae (*short arrow*) and a more prominent space seen ultrasonographically as a V-shaped defect (*long arrow*; Figure 1.150). The sternebrae marked "A" and "B" are those aspirated routinely because the most caudal one is thin and there is an increased risk of penetration, and the more cranial sternebrae are covered by a bony prominence. ©RKW Smith, Vetcell Bioscience Ltd and The Royal Veterinary College, 2005.

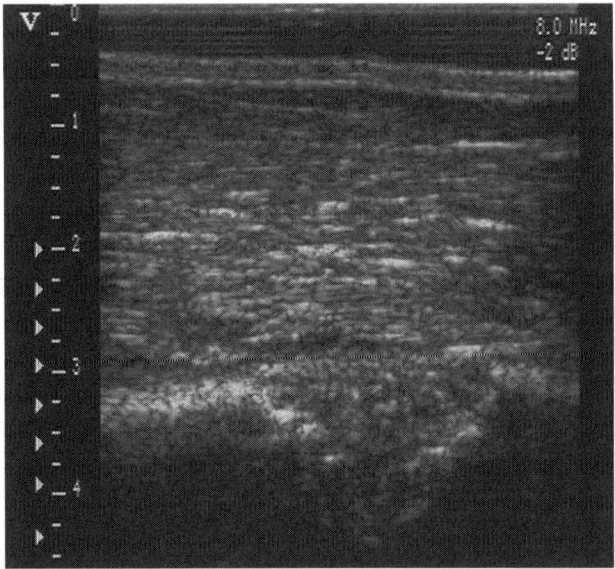

Figure 1.150 The ultrasonographic appearance of the intersternal space between sternebrae A and B shown in Figure 1.149. This space is usually level to the caudal aspect of the elbow. ©RKW Smith, Vetcell Bioscience Ltd and The Royal Veterinary College, 2005.

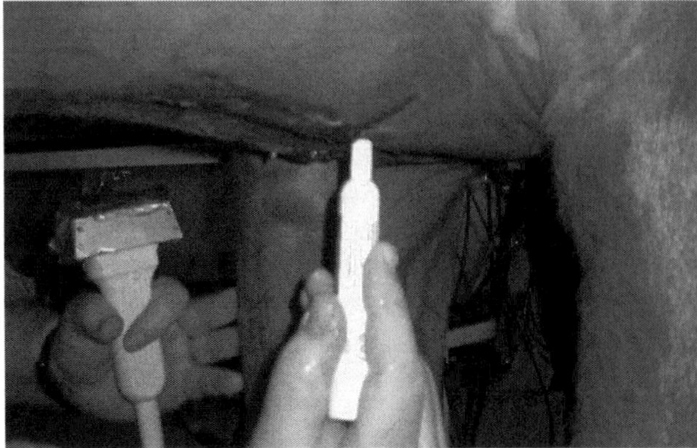

Figure 1.151 Marking the intersternebral space between the two sternebrae to be aspirated with a marker pen. ©RKW Smith, Vetcell Bioscience Ltd and The Royal Veterinary College, 2005.

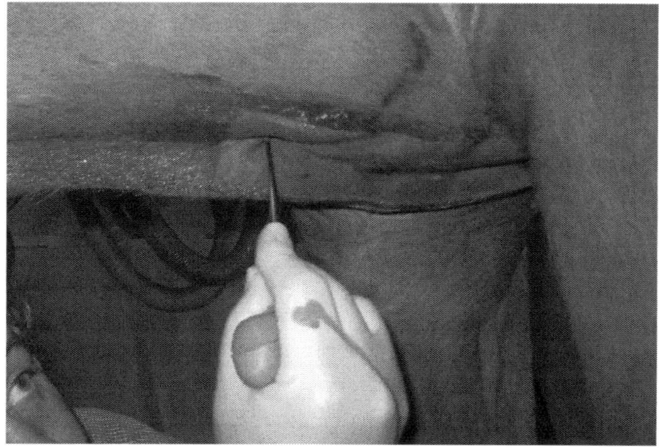

Figure 1.152 Insertion of Jamshidi needle. The index finger should be placed 2 cm from the skin surface once the Jamshidi needle makes contact with the ventral surface of the bone to prevent over-insertion of the needle. ©RKW Smith, Vetcell Bioscience Ltd and The Royal Veterinary College, 2005.

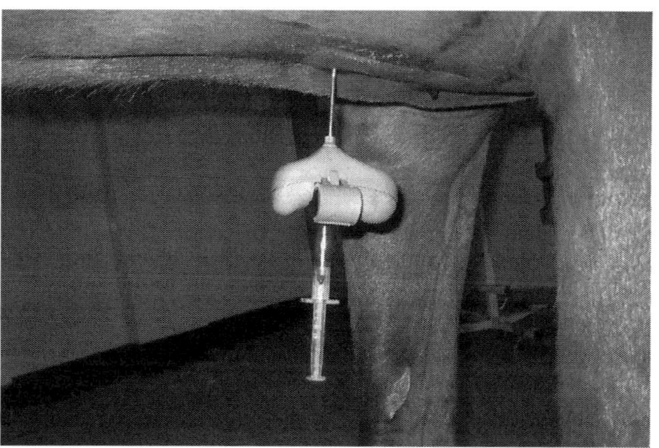

Figure 1.153 Successful aspiration of bone marrow. ©RKW Smith, Vetcell Bioscience Ltd and The Royal Veterinary College, 2005.

index finger is against the skin surface. This ensures the needle does not penetrate the deep surface of the sternebrae.

The central trocar is removed from Jamshidi needle. Bone marrow does not initially flow spontaneously from the needle: it requires gentle aspiration with an attached syringe. This is usually, but only initially, associated with a small amount of discomfort to the horse, usually manifested by a slight guarding of the abdomen. Thereafter, bone marrow flows easily into the syringe (Figure 1.153) and is spontaneously shed from the needle when the needle is disconnected.

If collecting for cytological evaluation, smears should immediately be made of the bone marrow (Figure 1.154).

If collecting for recovery of bone marrow, the bone marrow samples are gently agitated in the syringe to ensure adequate mixing of the anticoagulant with the marrow (bone marrow clots extremely quickly). The samples are then transferred immediately to prechilled shipping containers. One or more samples are also obtained without heparin and transferred immediately to sodium citrate

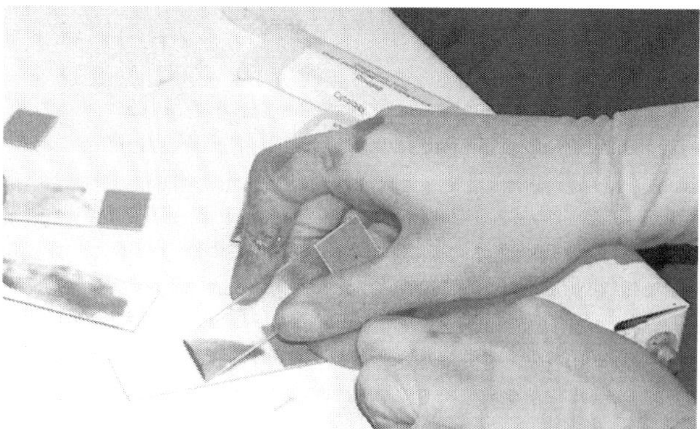

Figure 1.154 Preparing a smear of bone marrow for cytological evaluation. ©Kevin Corley 2003.

glass blood tubes. These samples are used to derive bone marrow supernatant used to resuspend mesenchymal stem cells for implantation. The second, more cranial, sternebra is then aspirated in the same fashion.

Once the Jamshidi needle is withdrawn, the portals can continue to bleed but pressure is usually all that is necessary to stop this haemorrhage. Closure is unnecessary.

1.48 Regional anaesthesia of the eye

Mary Utter

Ocular examination of a horse with a painful eye, or one that is fragile enough to raise concerns about globe rupture with pressure on the lids, can be facilitated by performing an auriculopalpebral nerve block. This block provides akinesia of the orbicularis oculi muscle, which is responsible for eyelid closure, but eyelid sensation persists. In addition, this block may be useful for diagnostic procedures including corneal culture and cytology, as well as for placement of subpalpebral lavage systems (see Chapter 1.49) and any other procedure in which a firmly closed lid would be prohibitive.

Equipment needed

The equipment needed is given in Box 1.54.

Technique

Auriculopalpebral nerve block

The auriculopalpebral is a branch of the facial nerve. Its palpebral branch can be palpated in two places, just lateral to the dorsalmost border of the zygomatic arch, and on the zygomatic arch caudal to the bony process of the frontal bone (Figure 1.155). Injection of 1 to 1.5 ml of 2% lidocaine (lignocaine) hydrochloride at either of these sites should result in paralysis of the superior lid within several minutes, and this paralysis may last several hours. Corneal dessication typically does not result from this temporary inability to blink due to resultant ptosis. In addition to these two sites, the palpebral nerve may be blocked just anterior to the base of the ear, although it cannot be palpated at this site. Two percent mepivicaine may be used

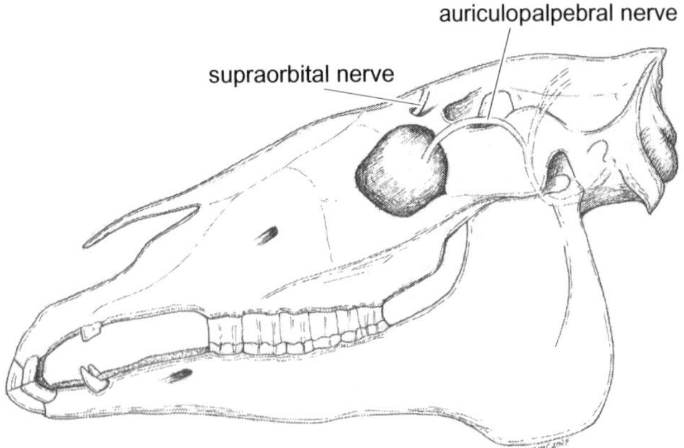

Figure 1.155 Anatomy of the auricopalpebral and supraorbital nerves.

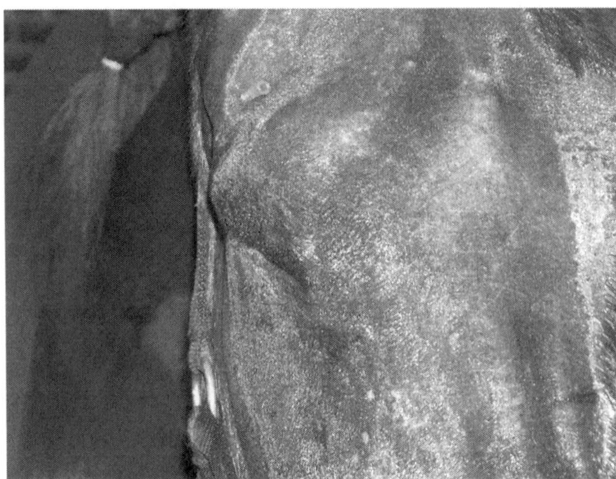

Figure 1.156 Needle placed for an auricopalpebral nerve block. ©Kevin Corley 2003.

> ### Box 1.54. Equipment for regional anaesthesia of the eye
>
> **For auricopalpebral and trigeminal nerve branch blocks**
>
> 25-Gauge needles (2–3)
> Local anaesthetic
>
> - Mepivacaine 2%*
> - Lidocaine (Lignocaine) 2%†
>
> 2–3-ml syringes
>
> **Optional**
>
> Small gauze swabs (4 × 4) soaked in chlorhexidine (4%) scrub solution‡
> Small gauze swabs (4 × 4) soaked in surgical spirit (alcohol)
> Sedation
> Twitch
>
> **For anaesthesia of the cornea and conjunctiva**
>
> Topical ophthalmic anaesthetic
>
> - Proxymetacaine (proparacaine)§
> - Amethocaine (tetracaine)**
>
> *Intra-epicaine; Arnolds Veterinary Products, Shrewsbury, UK; Carbocaine-V; Pfizer Animal Health, New York, NY, USA.
> †Ligno plain 2% sterile injection; Jurox PTY Ltd., Rutherford NSW, Australia.
> ‡Hibiscrub; Mölnlycke Health Care, Dunstable, UK.
> §Minims Proxymetacaine 0.5%, Chauvin, Chauvin Pharmaceuticals Ltd., Surrey, UK; Ophthetic, Allergan, Inc., Irvine, CA, USA.
> **Mimins Tetracaine; Chauvin Pharmaceuticals Ltd., Surrey, UK; Pontocaine; Sanofi-Aventis, Paris, France.

instead of lidocaine (lignocaine); it has a similar onset and slightly longer duration of action.

To perform the auriculopalpebral block, a 25-gauge needle without a syringe attached is gently pushed through the skin adjacent to the nerve (Figure 1.156). The needle is held in one hand and the skin tented with the opposite hand to facilitate needle placement. Placement of the needle typically elicits head tossing, and thus one must be careful not to inadvertently stab another site on the horse or oneself, or drop the needle, if this occurs. Prior to performing the block, clearing the floor of bedding directly in front of the horse, or moving the horse to an area where a dropped needle may easily be located, may save time and frustration should the needle wind up on the ground instead of in the horse's head. Once the needle is positioned through the skin, the hub should be grasped with the opposite hand to prevent movement of the needle under the skin, and a non–Luer-Lock 2- to 3-ml syringe containing the anaesthetic should be attached, and the anaesthetic injected. If the anaesthetic proves difficult to inject, even blowing the syringe backwards off the needle and spraying anaesthetic (possibly in one's face), the needle has most likely been placed intradermally and should be redirected deeper so that it is truly subcutaneous. Repeatedly redirecting the needle whilst injecting (which is sometimes done to facilitate diffusion of the anaesthetic) is not recommended, as this practice could lead to breaking the needle off subcutaneously if the horse jerks the head. Once the anaesthetic has been injected, the needle and syringe should be withdrawn together. There is typically no need to massage the injection site to achieve a good auriculopalpebral block.

Lidocaine (lignocaine) is acidic and is reported by humans receiving a skin block to briefly burn on injection. Studies with humans show that buffering lidocaine (lignocaine) with sodium bicarbonate to achieve a solution with a more physiological pH results in less pain on injection without a loss of anaesthetic effect. Buffered lidocaine is used in small animals for local blocks but typically not in horses.

Blocks of the ophthalmic branches of the trigeminal nerve

Anaesthesia of the eyelids can be achieved by blocking the appropriate sensory branch of the trigeminal nerve (Figures

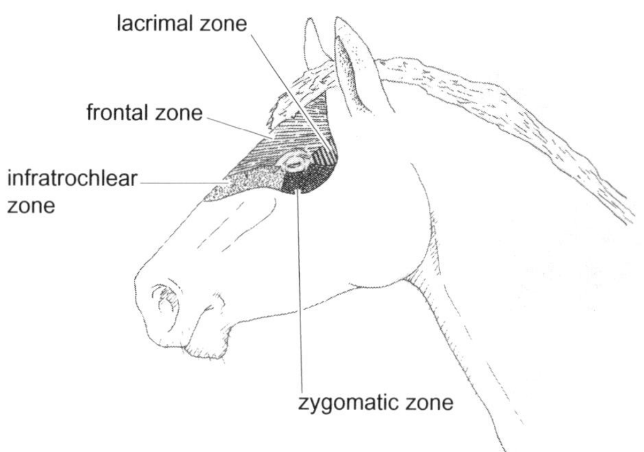

Figure 1.157 Approximate areas of desensitisation with a block to the frontal, infratrochlear, lacrimal and zygomatic nerves (side view).

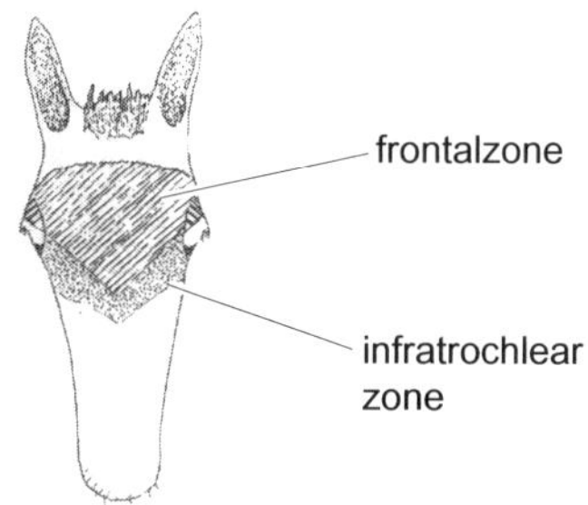

Figure 1.158 Approximate areas of desensitisation with a block to the frontal, infratrochlear, lacrimal and zygomatic nerves (front view).

1.157 and 1.158). The frontal nerve innervates the nasal and central superior lid and can be blocked at the supraorbital foramen, which can be palpated as a depression nasal to the narrowest aspect of the supraorbital process of the frontal bone. This is commonly called a supraorbital block, but it is called a frontal block as well. To perform the supraorbital block, a 25-gauge needle is placed into or just over the supraorbital foramen, and then 1 to 1.5 ml of anaesthetic is injected. It is not necessary for the needle to enter the foramen to achieve a good block. The supraorbital block is most commonly used to anaesthetise the superior lid prior to placement of a subpalpebral lavage. The temporal superior lid is innervated by the lacrimal nerve, which can be blocked along the temporal aspect of the orbital rim. The infratrochlear nerve innervates the nasal aspect of the inferior lid as well as the medial canthus, and it can be blocked at the palpable trochlear notch, on the medial aspect of the orbital rim. These three nerves (frontal, lacrimal and infratrochlear) are branches of the ophthalmic branch of the trigeminal nerve. The temporal inferior lid is innervated by the zygomatic nerve, a branch of the maxillary branch of the trigeminal nerve. The zygomatic nerve can be blocked along the ventrolateral orbital rim. Depending on the intended site of placement of an inferior subpalpebral lavage, the zygomatic or infratrochlear nerve should be blocked.

Anaesthesia of the cornea and conjunctiva

Anaesthesia of the cornea and conjunctiva (including palpebral and bulbar conjunctiva, as well as that overlying the nictitans) can be achieved by topical application of amethocaine (tetracaine) or proxymetacaine (proparacaine). These topical anaesthetics are most easily administered by drawing a small volume (0.5 to 1 ml) into a syringe with a 25-gauge needle, breaking the needle off at the hub by rocking the needle back and forth several times within the needle's cap (partially placed over the needle to catch it as it falls off) and squirting the anaesthetic onto the ocular surface. The nictitans can be anaesthetised by injection of lidocaine (lignocaine) or mepivicaine into its base, either through the inferior lid or directly into the nictitans after lowering the inferior lid to expose it. Duration of topical anaesthesia using amethocaine (tetracaine) or proxymetacaine (proparacaine) has not been definitively established in the horse. For proxymetacaine, the maximal anaesthetic effect occurs for about 5 minutes in cats and 15 minutes in dogs, and the duration of effect is about 25 minutes in the cat and 45 minutes in the dog.

1.49 Placement of a subpalpebral lavage catheter

Mary Utter

The subpalpebral lavage (SPL) system is indicated for topical ophthalmic medication of horses that will not allow medication otherwise, due to profound squinting or head tossing, and when globe fragility precludes manipulation of eyelids to gain access for topical therapy. One of the most common reasons for treatment failure amongst horses that are treated at home, and then referred in to hospital, is inability to administer topical medication.

Equipment needed

The list of equipment needed is given in Box 1.55. Commerical SPL kits contain a trochar, Silastic tubing, Luer adapter (catheter), fixing eyelets and an injection cap (Figure 1.159). Two commercial SPL kits are available, one with a 14-gauge trochar and 18-inch tubing and one with a 12-gauge trochar and 36-inch tubing. The shorter tubing is often insufficient to reach the withers in a larger horse (e.g., warmblood or Thoroughbred with a long neck), and it can be difficult to reach the injection port to administer medications when the shorter tubing is used in a patient that elevates the head and neck in anticipation of treatment.

Site for placement

The SPL may be placed in either the superior or inferior lid (Figures 1.160 and 1.161). Two factors contribute to the

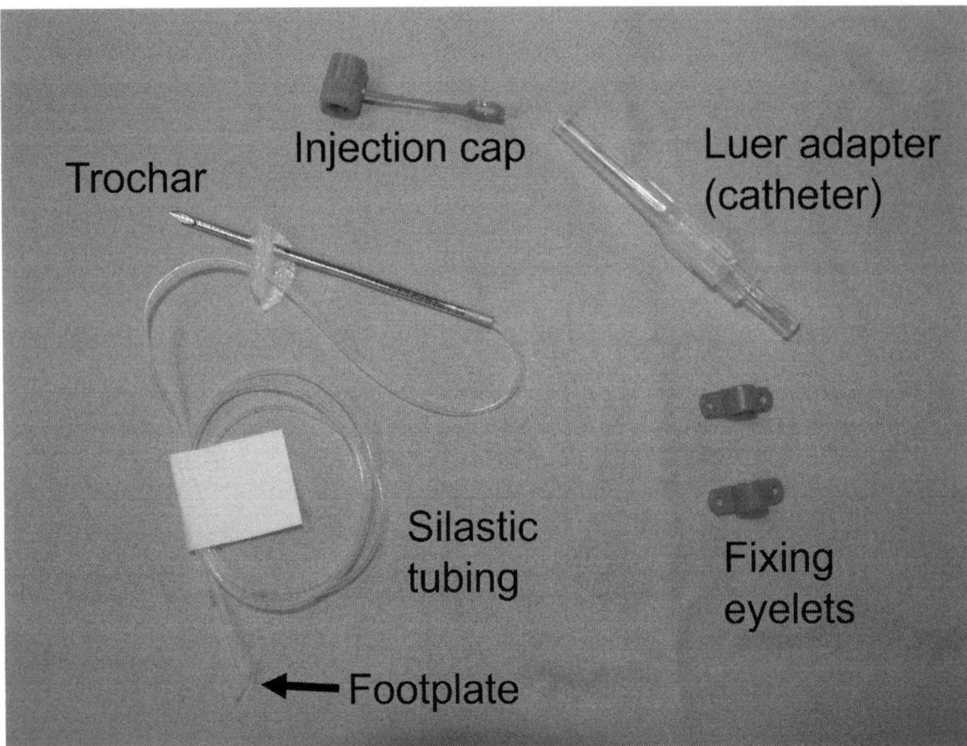

Figure 1.159 Parts of a commercial subpalpebral lavage catheter kit. ©Kevin Corley 2007.

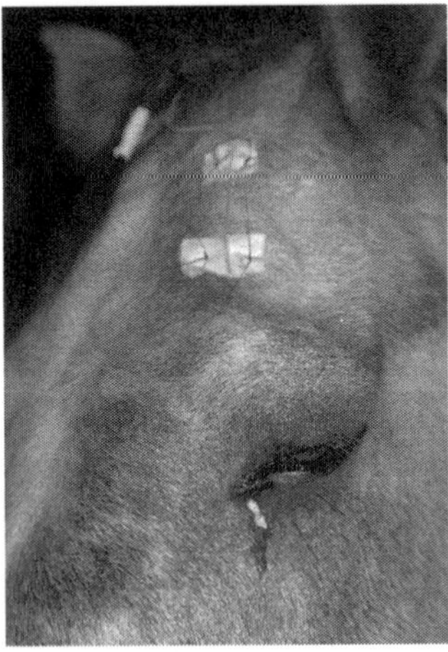

Figure 1.160 A subpalpebral lavage catheter placed in the upper eyelid. ©Mary Utter 2007.

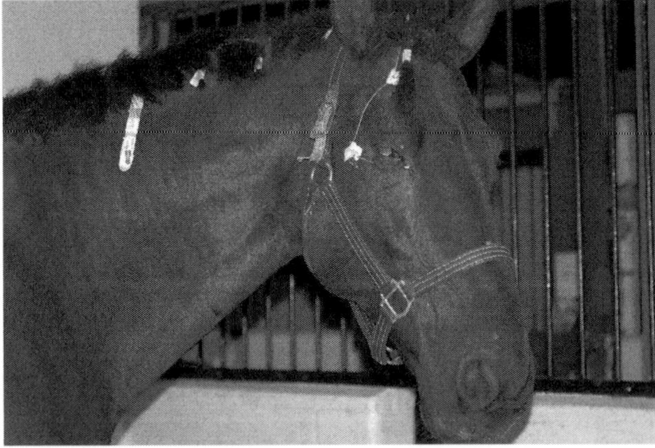

Figure 1.161 A subpalpebral lavage catheter placed in the lower eyelid. Note how the tube is taken back through the braids (plaits) in the mane, and the injection port is supported by being taped to a tongue depressor. ©Mary Utter 2007.

decision regarding which lid: location and character of the lesion, and temperament of the patient. First, placement of the SPL is recommended through the lid that exhibits the least blepharitis and that overlies the smallest proportion of any corneal lesion. For example, an inferior lid SPL placement might be recommended in the case of a melting ulcer located in the superior cornea, just adjacent to the dorsal limbus, thereby avoiding surface contact with the ulcer of the gloved hand or the trochar used to insert the lavage through the lid. Second, temperament of the horse may contribute to a decision to place the SPL in the inferior lid, in patients for which it would prove challenging to replace any of the butterfly sutures holding the SPL tubing in place on the face, should a suture break, due to difficulty handling or restraining such a patient. An example might be a foal that has not been frequently handled, is not halter-broken and might be unduly stressed by resuturing the tubing to the face. If the butterfly suture breaks in an inferior-lid SPL, there is no risk of the SPL footplate slipping and causing an SPL ulcer, as this would require footplate migration against gravity. If a suture breaks in a superior lid SPL, however, footplate migration onto the

Box 1.55. Equipment for placement of a subpalpebral lavage catheter

Required

SPL kit* including Silastic tubing with footplate, trochar
Sedation
Local anaesthetic

- Mepivacaine 2%†
- Lidocaine (Lignocaine) 2%‡

2–3-ml syringes
25-Gauge needles (2–3)
1 : 20 dilution of povidine-iodine solution (NOT SCRUB) with saline—to prepare lid skin and the conjunctival surface
Tongue depressor
Surgical gloves
Zinc oxide tape
Rubber bands for braiding the mane
Eye wash for testing the catheter
Topical ophthalmic anaesthetic

- Proxymetacaine (proparacaine)§
- Amethocaine (tetracaine)**

Optional

20-Gauge catheter (only necessary if catheter not provided in SPL kit)
Sterile injection port (only necessary if catheter not provided in SPL kit)
Twitch

*Subpalpebral Eye Lavage Kit, Item No. 6612; Mila International, Florence, KY, USA.
†Intra-epicaine; Arnolds Veterinary Products, Shrewsbury, UK; Carbocaine-V; Pfizer Animal Health, New York, NY, USA.
‡Ligno plain 2% sterile injection; Jurox PTY Ltd., Rutherford NSW, Australia.
§Minims Proxymetacaine 0.5%; Chauvin Pharmaceuticals Ltd., Surrey, UK; Ophthetic, Allergan, Inc., Irvine, CA, USA.
**Mimins Tetracaine; Chauvin Pharmaceuticals Ltd., Surrey, UK; Pontocaine; Sanofi-Aventis, Paris, France.

corneal surface can easily cause an ulcer that can be difficult to resolve.

Procedure

Adequate sedation is mandatory to place an SPL. It is typical for a higher dose of sedative than is expected to be required to achieve adequate sedation due to most patients' intense dislike of eyelid manipulation and of finger insertion between an eyelid and a painful cornea. Even a patient in five-point stance may toss the head skyward and react profoundly to insertion of even a finger under the eyelid, and this response must be avoided when inserting the large gauge trochar under the lid. Intravenous detomidine alone or in conjunction with torbugesic typically provides adequate sedation. A typical 1000-lb horse may require 5 to 8 mg of each drug for adequate sedation. Use of a nose twitch is recommended to guarantee adequate restraint and thus to prevent inadvertent lid, conjunctival or corneal laceration by the bevelled end of the trochar, or injury to the veterinarian placing the SPL, should the patient toss the head whilst the trochar is being inserted through the lid.

Start by performing an auriculopalpebral (motor) block (see Section 1.48), which is useful for an inferior SPL as well as a superior one, to paralyse the orbicularis muscle and thereby prevent strong blepharospasm from compromising access to the conjunctival fornix. Perform a frontal (also called supraorbital) (sensory) block to anaesthetise the site through which the SPL trochar will pass. For a superior SPL, a supraorbital block (see Section 1.48) is typically sufficient to provide anesthesia of the intended SPL trochar site. For an inferior SPL, however, a local block using 1 to 1.5 ml local anaesthetic is required. Then numb the cornea and conjunctiva with a topical anaesthetic, and prepare the lid skin, cornea and conjunctival surface by squirting dilute povidine-iodine solution onto the lid in question and the ocular surface. This can be accomplished by drawing the 1:20 dilute povidone-iodine solution into a 20-ml syringe with a 25-gauge needle and then breaking the needle off at the hub, allowing a fine stream of solution to be directed onto the lid, conjunctiva and cornea.

The adequacy of sedation and local anaesthesia should be tested by inserting a finger under the lid through which the SPL will be placed and pushing down on that finger, through the lid, with a finger on the opposite hand. If the patient tolerates this, insertion of the SPL trochar will most likely be easily tolerated as well.

Once the patient is adequately sedated and blocked, and the external lid and ocular surface is prepared with dilute povidine-iodine, open the SPL kit, ensure that the patient is restrained with a nose twitch and don sterile gloves. Have an assistant hold the opened SPL kit ready or place it within easy reach. Pick up the SPL trochar in the dominant hand, and use the opposite hand to open eyelids as needed to allow insertion of the SPL trochar, guided by the index finger, to the conjunctival fornix. It is mandatory that the trochar pass through the eyelid at the depth of the conjunctival fornix, no closer to the lid margin, to prevent footplate movement over the cornea and subsequent corneal ulceration. In a moment of truth, push the trochar through the skin, such that about half the needle has gone through the eyelid. This may require a strong push, with a feeling that periosteum has been penetrated (Figure 1.162).

With the nondominant hand, guide the end of the SPL tubing through the length of the trochar, pull the trochar the remaining distance through the lid and off the tubing, and set the trochar down. Pull the tubing the remainder of the way through the eyelid. Place one butterfly about 25 cm from the wound where the SPL tubing exits the skin, and place a single interrupted suture using 2–0 nonabsorbable suture through the butterfly tape on either side of the tubing. Ensure that this butterfly is well adhered to the tubing, so that the tubing does not slip toward the lid, dislodging the footplate. Place a second butterfly about 25 cm

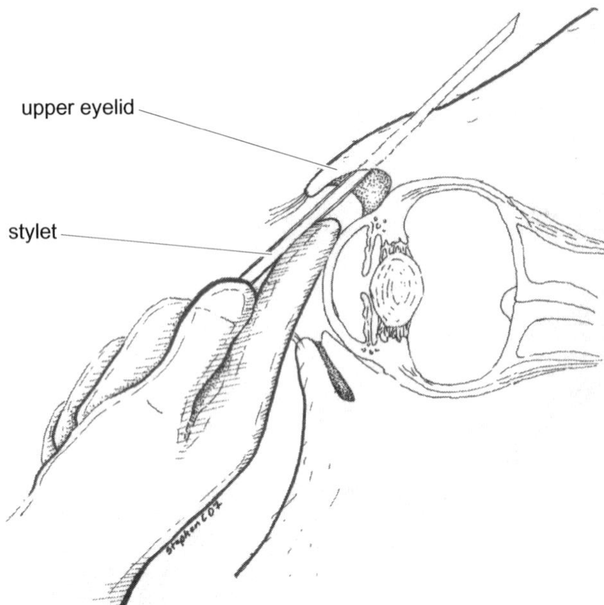

Figure 1.162 Passing the trochar through the upper eyelid. The trochar is pushed through the eyelid at the depth of the conjunctival fornix, to prevent footplate movement over the cornea and subsequent corneal ulceration.

down the tubing from the first, as a backup in case the first breaks (see Figures 1.160 and 1.161). Braid the forelock and the mane in three to five places along the neck, and weave the SPL tubing through the base of the braid to secure it to the neck (see Figure 1.161). Make sure there is plenty of slack in the tubing, so that flexing and extending the neck does not place tension on it. Place a 20-gauge catheter into the tubing by backing the stylet out of the catheter just a small distance, to prevent lacerating the SPL tubing with the stylet, and inserting the catheter into the tubing up to the catheter hub. Remove the stylet. This will provide stability for the end of the tubing. Screw an injection cap onto the catheter. Use white tape to secure a tongue depressor to the braid farthest down the neck and to secure the end of the SPL tubing, with the catheter inserted and closed off with an injection cap (see Figure 1.161).

Test the patency of the SPL by injecting sterile saline or eyewash slowly through the injection port and tubing until it appears through the palpebral fissure and runs down the face. The SPL should be checked every time medication is injected through it to ensure that the tubing has not slid through the butterfly, allowing the footplate to rub on the cornea, and to ensure that medication is directed through the tubing onto the cornea, rather than being injected subconjunctivally.

Medication is typically administered using 0.2 ml of each solution, and for frequent (i.e., more frequently than four times daily) administration, each dose may be injected into the tubing, pushing the dose of medication closest to the footplate out of the tubing onto the eye. When medication frequency is relatively low (i.e., four or fewer times daily), then each medication may be pushed through the tubing onto the cornea using a small amount of air; this avoids having medications mix and sit in the tubing for prolonged periods of time. With a sensible patient, it is reasonable to allow small paddock turnout even with the SPL in place, rather than restricting activity to stall rest with hand walking as is typical for more rambunctious patients, but only with willingness to accept the risk that the SPL will be damaged or dislodged and may need to be replaced (e.g., if the patient rolls and breaks the tubing, or catches it on a fence or foot.).

1.50 Regional analgesia of the limb

Jennifer O. Stephen

The use of specific nerve blocks in the diagnosis of lameness is well documented. However, regional analgesia may also be useful in the hospital setting for the provision of analgesia during standing surgical procedures, during anaesthesia, whilst performing regional limb perfusions or in the acute or chronic management of pain. Local analgesia has been used in some arthroscopic procedures to avoid the expense and potential risks of general anaesthesia.[1] In recent years, there has been much debate over the specific structures that may be desensitised by certain perineural blocks, particularly the palmar-digital nerve block. However, for the purposes described above, this debate is less relevant; the horse should be blocked at a point proximal to the site of pain. Likewise, the quantity of anaesthetic used is less important when blocking for pure analgesia rather than for diagnostic purposes. Slightly larger volumes to ensure a complete block has been performed are acceptable.

General procedure for placing nerve block

Suitable restraint of the horse must be provided. At least two competent people are required. Both should stand on the same side of the horse. When placing a block for analgesia, the horse may be sedated if necessary. Placement of a twitch prior to needle insertion may also be helpful. Blocks may be performed with the horse weight bearing or non–weight bearing as preferred. The site for injection should be clean. Some clinicians recommend clipping hair; however, no significant difference in postscrub bacterial population has been identified.[2] In certain breeds, especially draft and cobs, it may be essential to clip so anatomical landmarks may be identified. It is important to remember that at certain sites inadvertent synovial penetration may occur. At these sites, a full 5-minute aseptic preparation should always be completed. As small a gauge needle as possible should be used (bearing in mind that smaller needles carry the risk of breaking off in the limb if the horse behaves poorly). It is vital that the needle is introduced quickly and firmly. The needle can be inserted in a proximal or distal direction. Once the syringe is attached, the clinician should draw back to avoid injecting into a vessel. If injecting the anaesthetic is very difficult, the needle may be intradermal, and redirection slightly deeper should be attempted. Depending on the agent used, the block is tested 3 to 5 minutes after injection by pressing a dull object (such as a pen) over the area that should be desensitized. Some horses will react to visual stimuli, giving a false-negative result; blindfolding these horses or shielding their eye may be helpful. Once the procedure has been performed, it is important to remember to clean off any residual antiseptic from the nerve block site and to consider applying a wrap to minimise any local irritation and reaction to the block.

Types of nerve block

- *Point block (perineural anaesthesia):* Blocking a specific nerve at a specific site. Blocks the nerve and its branches distal to the injection.
- *Line block:* Produced by infiltrating the anaesthetic along a line. Numbs the nerve branches crossing that line.
- *Ring block or field block:* Injecting anaesthetic in complete or partial circle around the limb. Needle is inserted perpendicular to the long axis of the limb and local anaesthetic injected as the needle is advanced forming a clear SQ bleb.

Perineural analgesia of the limb

Unless stated otherwise, all of these blocks are performed at the same sites on both the medial and lateral sides of the limb. The volume of local anaesthetic required is approximate and refers to the amount used per site. Nerve blocks should always be tested before applying a painful stimulus. The equipment needed and the volume of anaesthetic for each site is given in Box 1.56.

Analgesia of pastern and foot

Abaxial sesamoid block

The anaesthetic should be deposited subcutaneously.
Site: Vascular bundle should be easily palpated on the abaxial side of each sesamoid. Place needle over this, at level of the base of the sesamoid (Figure 1.163).

Analgesia of fetlock (fore limb)

Low four-point block

Site: The palmar nerves are located between the deep digital flexor tendon and the suspensory ligament. Care must be taken whilst blocking these to avoid the tendon sheath. Block about a handsbreadth above the fetlock joint, slightly higher than the buttons of the splint. Aim the needle so it is kept fairly superficial, just subcutaneous and parallel to the tendons (Figure 1.164).

The palmar metacarpal nerves emerge laterally and medially just below the button of the splint. The needle should be at 90 ° to the limb so that the point of the needle arrives directly under the button of the splint.

Cutaneous sensation to the fetlock joint is also provided by the dorsal branch of the median and ulnar cutaneous antebrachial nerves. These may be blocked by leaving a bleb of anaesthetic subcutaneously as the needle is withdrawn after the palmar metacarpal block.

Box 1.56. Equipment for perineural analgesia of the limb

For all blocks
Local anaesthetic

- Mepivacaine 2%*
- Lidocaine (Lignocaine) 2%†

Small gauze swabs (4 × 4) soaked in chlorhexidine (4%) scrub solution‡
Small gauze swabs (4 × 4) soaked in surgical spirit (alcohol)
Appropriate size syringes for the amount of local anaesthetic to be deposited

Abaxial sesamoid block
25-Gauge 2.5-cm (1-inch) needles
3–5 ml of local anaesthetic per site

Low four-point and low six-point blocks
22-Gauge 2.5-cm (1-inch) needles
3 ml of local anaesthetic per site

High four-point block
22-Gauge 2.5-cm (1-inch) needles
5 ml of local anaesthetic per site

Ulnar nerve block
20-Gauge 3.75-cm ($1\frac{1}{2}$-inch) needle
10 ml of local anaesthetic

Median nerve block
20–22-Gauge 3.75-cm ($1\frac{1}{2}$-inch) needle
10 ml of local anaesthetic

Medial cutaneous antebrachial nerve block
22-Gauge 2.5-cm (1-inch) needle
5 ml of local anaesthetic

Tibial nerve block
1 ml subcutaneous bleb
20-Gauge 3.75-cm ($1\frac{1}{2}$-inch) needle
15–25 ml of local anaesthetic

Superficial and deep fibular nerves (peroneal) block
1 ml subcutaneous bleb
20-Gauge 5.0-cm (2-inch) needle
10–15 ml of local anaesthetic

*Intra-epicaine; Arnolds Veterinary Products, Shrewsbury, UK; Carbocaine-V; Pfizer Animal Health, New York, NY, USA.
†Ligno plain 2% sterile injection; Jurox PTY Ltd., Rutherford NSW, Australia.
‡Hibiscrub; Mölnlycke Health Care, Dunstable, UK.

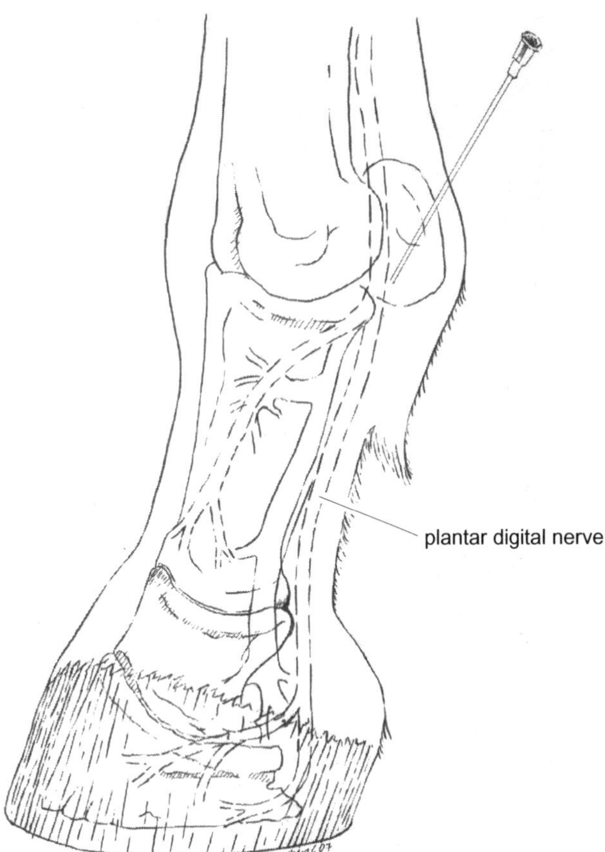

Figure 1.163 Abaxial sesamoid nerve block: The needle is placed over the neurovascular bundle at the base of the sesamoid. The block can be done with the limb weight-bearing (as illustrated), or with the leg held in flexion.

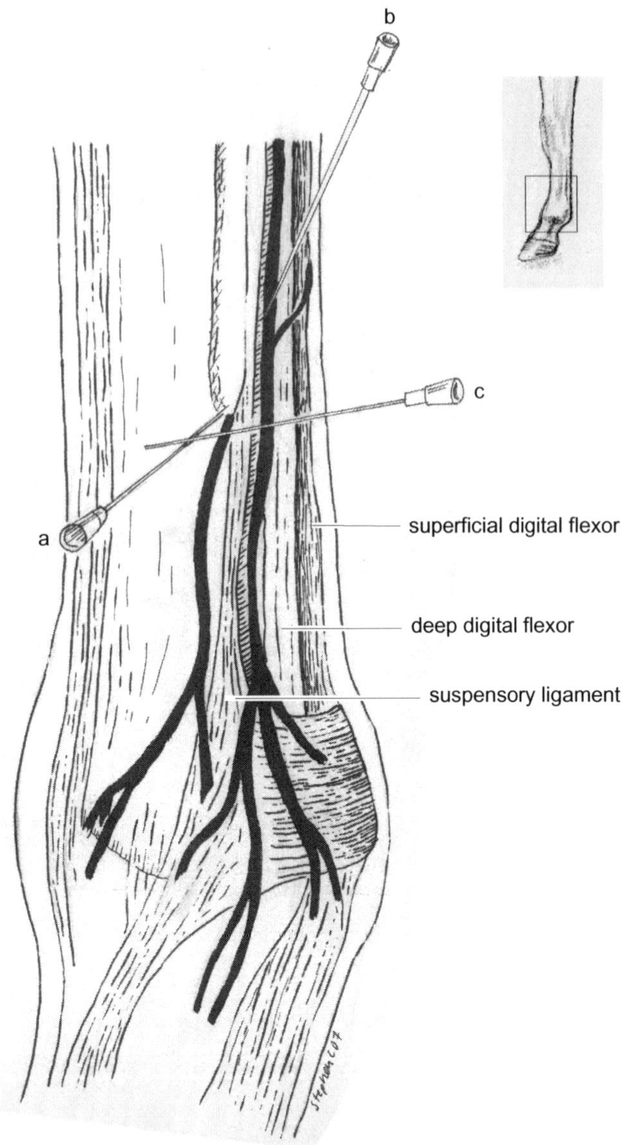

Figure 1.164 Low four-point nerve block: The first needle (**a**) is placed just below the button of the splint bone, to block the palmar metacarpal (plantar metatarsal) nerve. The second needle (**b**) is placed between the deep digital flexor tendon and the suspensory ligament, to block the lateral palmar or plantar nerve. This illustration demonstrates the lateral side of the leg. The medial blocks are performed in the same positions, on the medial side. Low-six point nerve block: For the hind limb, an additional needle (**c**) is used to place a dorsal subcutaneous ring block on both the lateral and medial sides.

Analgesia of the fetlock (hind limb)

Low six-point block

The addition of a dorsal ring (field block) is a necessary adjunct in the hind limb due to the medial and lateral dorsal metatarsal nerves, caudal cutaneous sural nerve and the saphenous nerve, which provide sensation over the dorsal fetlock (Figure 1.164). Otherwise, the technique is as for a four-point block.

Analgesia of the limb distal to the carpus and hock

High four-point block

Sites: Lateral and medial palmar (plantar) nerves subcutaneously, 2 cm distal to the carpometacarpal (tarsometarsal) joint, between the superficial and deep tendons (Figure 1.165).

Palmar metacarpal (plantar metatarsal) nerves course along the axial surface of the splint bone, between this and the suspensory ligament (Figure 1.165). The needle should touch the palmar (plantar) cortex of the cannon bone. Inadvertent penetration of carpometacarpal (tarsometarsal) joint is a potential complication of this block. To produce complete analgesia of dorsum of limb, it is necessary to also complete a circumferential SQ ring block.

In the hind limb, a dorsal ring block should be added, as described for the low six-point block.

Analgesia of the distal antebrachium and carpus

Ulnar nerve block

Palpate the groove between the flexor carpi ulnaris and extensor carpi ulnaris (ulnaris lateralis) muscles 10 cm (4 inches) above the accessory carpal bone on the caudal aspect of the forearm (Figures 1.166 and 1.167). Insert the needle perpendicular to the skin to the hub. Inject 10 ml

Figure 1.165 High four-point nerve block: This is carried out 2 cm distal to the carpometacarpal joint. Injections are placed over the palmar metacarpal (plantar metatarsal) nerves (**1**), on the axial surface of the splint bones on both the lateral and medial side, and subcutaneously over the lateral and medial palmar (plantar) nerves (**2**), between the superficial and deep flexor tendons. High six-point nerve block: For the hind limb, a dorsal subcutaneous ring block is performed, as for the low six-point block (Figure 1.50.2).

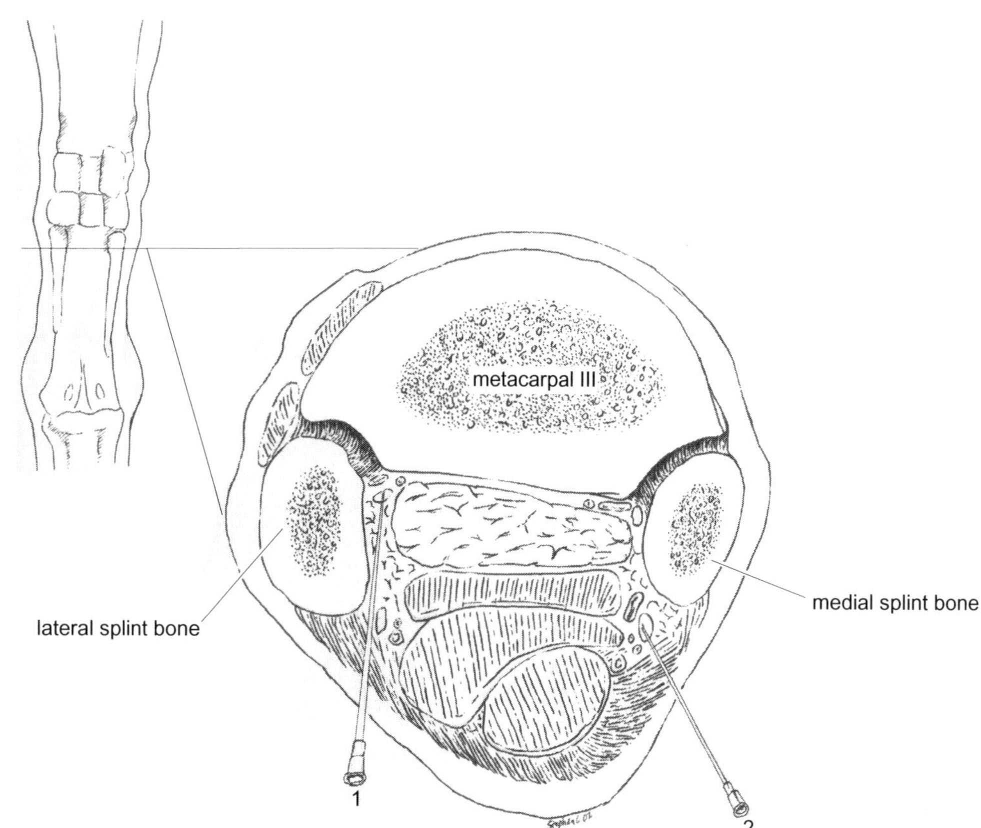

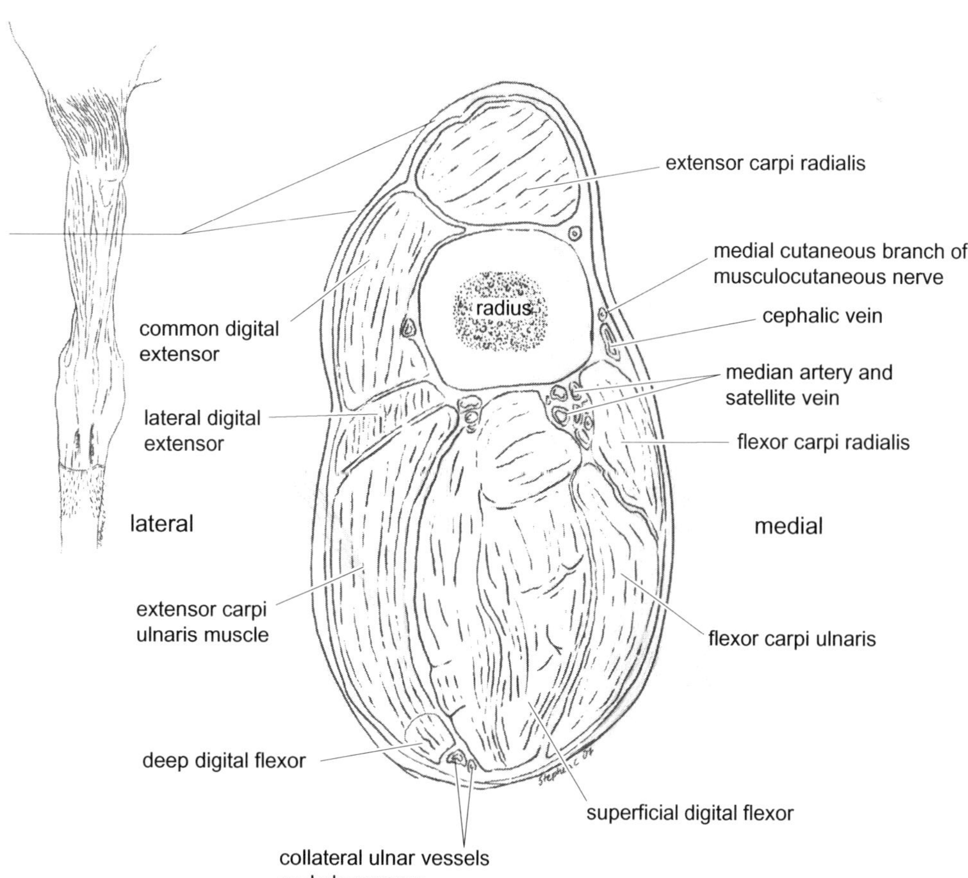

Figure 1.166 Cross section of the forearm of the horse, illustrating the anatomy of the median and ulnar nerves. The median nerve runs in a neurovascular bundle (containing the median artery), deep to the flexor carpi radialis. The ulnar nerve runs superficially caudally, between the deep and superficial digital flexor muscles.

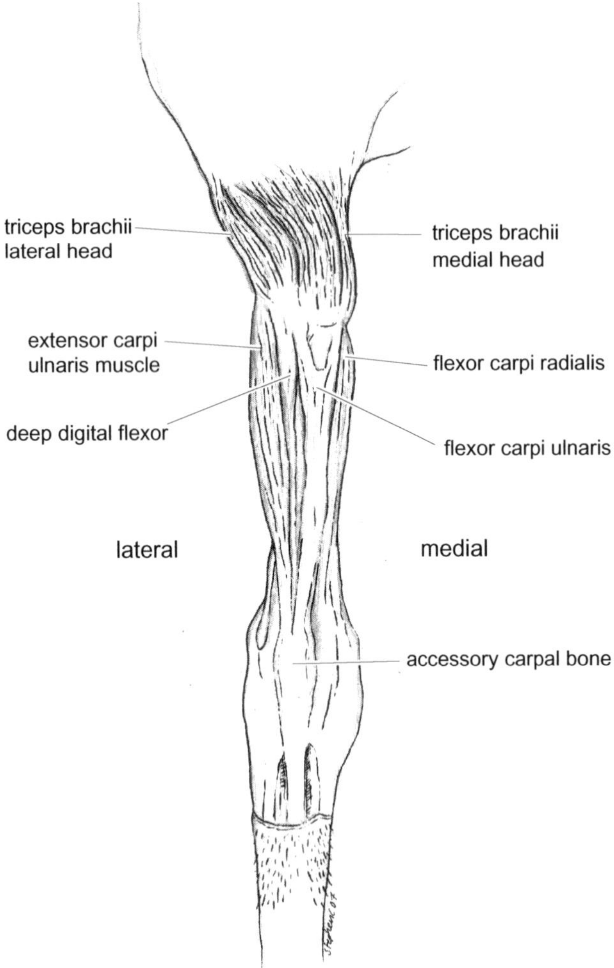

Figure 1.167 Anatomy of the caudal aspect of the fore limb, illustrating the position of the muscles that need to be identified to perform the median and ulnar nerve blocks.

as the needle is withdrawn. NB the nerve is in deep fascia, so if a bleb appears, you are too superficial. If the needle contacts the nerve, the horse may strike forward.

Median nerve block

Location is caudal, medial aspect of the radius, 5 cm distal to the elbow joint, cranial to the caudal border of the flexor carpi radialis (Figures 1.166 and 1.167). Insert needle to the hub along the caudal aspect of the radius. Aspirate, if there is blood in syringe, redirect, and then inject 10 ml anaesthetic. Keep the needle close to or against the caudal aspect of the radius to avoid the median artery and vein. Placement of a superficial bleb of anaesthetic in the skin may be beneficial before this is attempted.

Medial cutaneous antebrachial nerve block

This nerve may be blocked on the medial aspect of the limb as it courses across the lacertus fibrosis before it branches. The nerve is just subcutaneous. Alternatively, the two branches may be blocked (Figure 1.168). Anaesthetic should be injected subcutaneously cranial and caudal to the cephalic vein and cranial to the accessory cephalic vein at about halfway between the carpus and elbow on medial aspect of limb.[3]

Hind limb: Tibial and fibular (peroneal) block

Tibial nerve

The nerve is located on the medial side of the limb about 4 inches above the point of the hock between the common calcaneal tendon and the deep digital flexor tendon (Figure 1.169). The nerve may be palpated by lifting the leg and palpating cranial to the common calcaneal tendon with the thumb and forefinger. The nerve is around 6 mm in diameter and will be located just caudal to the deep digital flexor tendon.[2] The block is performed with the horse standing. The needle may be directed to the nerve from the lateral or medial aspect of the leg. Firstly, place a 1-ml subcutaneous bleb. Insert the needle to the area of the nerve and inject with local anaesthetic.

Superficial and deep fibular nerves (peroneal)

Palpate the septum between the long and lateral digital extensor muscles 4 inches above the tarsus on the lateral aspect of the leg (Figure 1.169). Desensitise skin in this area. Insert a 20-gauge, 50-mm (2-inch) needle between the long and lateral digital extensor muscles to penetrate down to the tibia. Aspirate and inject 10 to 15 ml of local anaesthetic to anaesthetise the deep peroneal nerve. Retract needle and inject 10 to 15 ml of anaesthetic superficially (between 6 and 25 mm deep to the skin) to desensitise the superficial peroneal nerve.

Deep pain will be abolished if these nerves are blocked; however, superficial sensation may persist on the medial aspect and occasionally on the plantar aspect of the limb. A circumferential ring block will completely abolish skin sensation.[4]

References

1. Elce YA: Arthroscopic removal of dorsoproximal chip fractures of the proximal phalanx in standing horses. Vet Surg 31:195-200, 2002
2. Hague BA, et al.: Evaluation of bacterial skin flora before and after aseptic preparation of clipped and nonclipped arthrocentesis sites in horses, Vet Surg 26:121, 1997
3. Stashak TS: Examination for lameness, in Stashak TS (ed): Adams Lameness in Horses, ed 5. Baltimore, MD, Lippincott Williams and Wilkins, 2001, pp 113-183
4. Bassage LH: Diagnostic analgesia, in Ross MW, Dyson SJ (eds): Diagnosis and Management of Lameness in the Horse. St. Louis, WB Saunders, 2003, pp 93-124

1.51 Bandaging of the limb

Louise L. Southwood

Bandaging of the limb, particularly the distal limb, is one of the most commonly performed procedures in hospital-

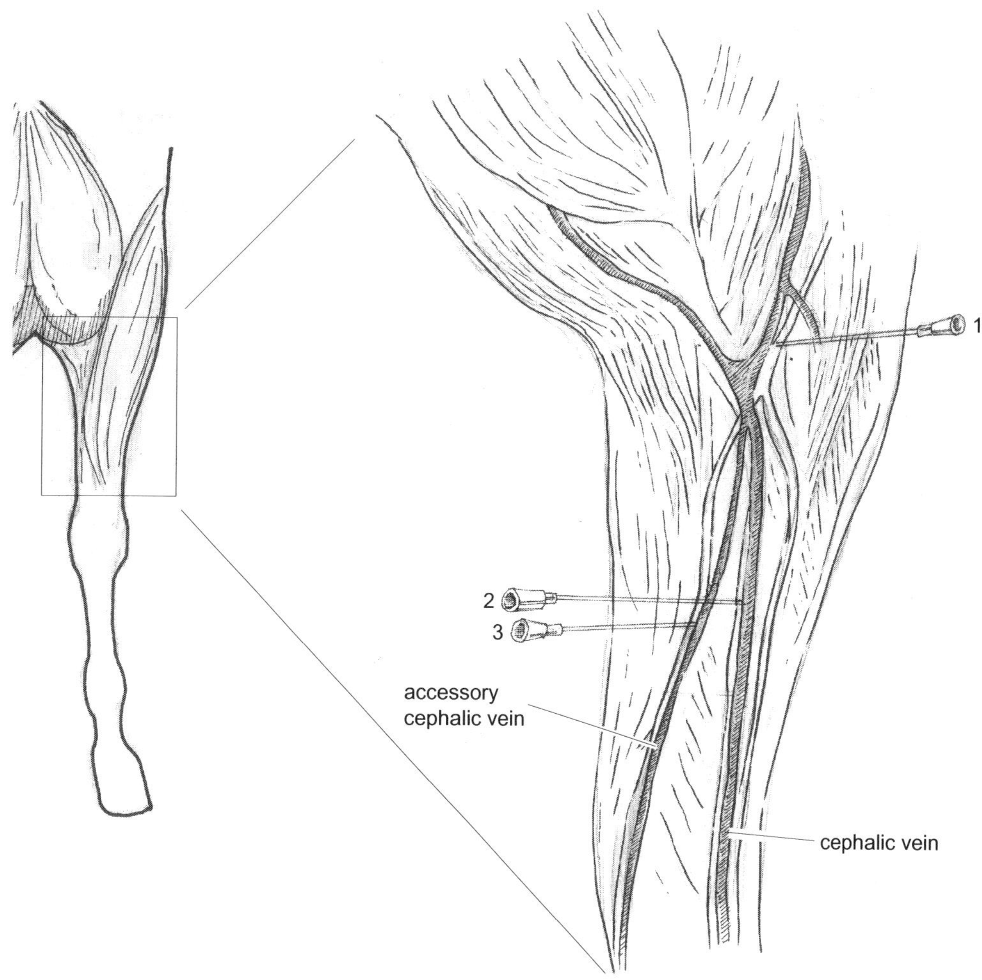

Figure 1.168 Medial cutaneous antebrachial nerve block: This nerve may be blocked on the medial aspect of the limb as it courses across the lacertus fibrosis before it branches (**1**). The nerve is just subcutaneous. Alternatively, the two branches may be blocked (**2** and **3**).

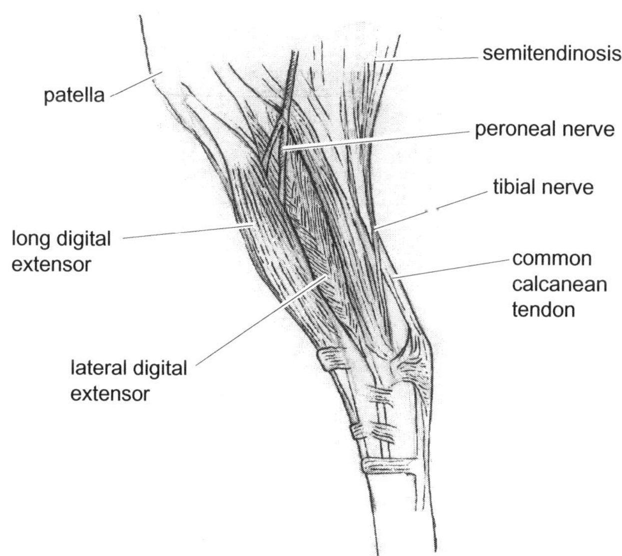

Figure 1.169 Tibial and peroneal nerve blocks: Anatomy of the left crus of the horse, lateral view. The tibial nerve is located on the medial side of the limb about four inches above the point of the hock between the common calcaneal tendon and the deep digital flexor tendon.

ised horses. Bandages are important for reducing oedema formation and haemorrhage in horses with injuries and protection of a surgical site or laceration from contamination and further trauma. They provide a favourable environment for wound healing and immobilisation of wound edges to facilitate healing. Bandages with a wet-to-dry dressing can be used to enhance wound debridement. They can also be used for protection of the distal limb during transport following discharge from the hospital and reduction of distal limb oedema formation ("stocking up") in horses confined to a stall. Bandages are used in conjunction with a splint or cast to provide stability for fractures. Figures 1.170, A–D, 1.171, A–H and 1.172, A–E, show bandaging of three clinical cases that have been included to illustrate some of the principles of limb bandaging.

Equipment needed

A variety of different bandaging materials can be used. Some commonly used examples are given in Box 1.57.

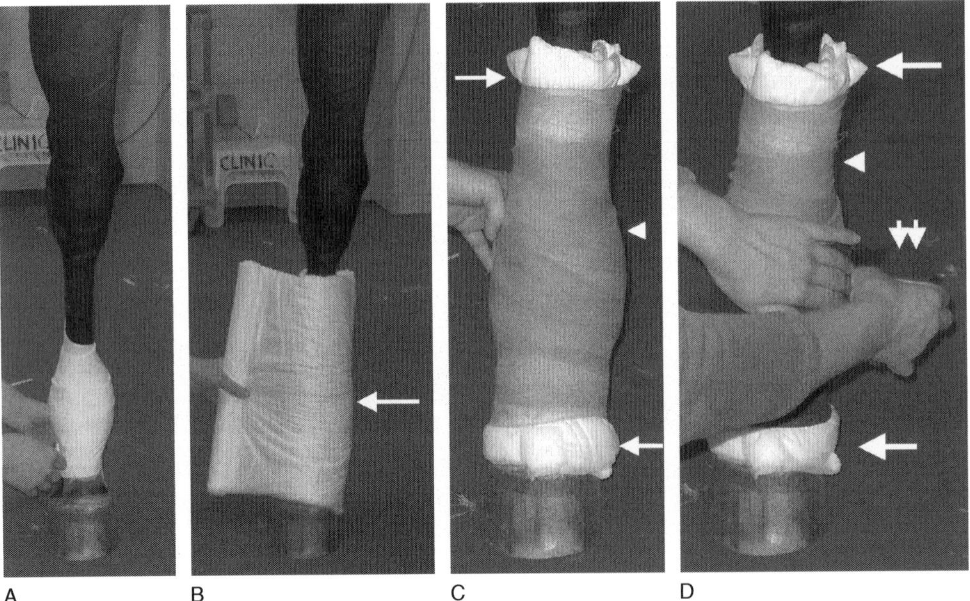

Figure 1.170 A-D A distal or lower limb bandage that was used to cover the surgical wounds, provide support, and reduce joint effusion and periarticular swelling following fetlock arthroscopy. The figure illustrates primary and secondary dressing. The distal limb bandage extends from the most proximal aspect of the metacarpus or metatarsus to the coronary band. The figure demonstrates the primary dressing applied directly over the wound consisting of a sterile nonadherent semiocclusive dressing secured in place with a soft sterile conforming gauze (**A**) and the secondary dressing with combine cotton (*arrow,* **B**), 6-inch brown open weave bandage (*arrowhead,* **C**) and, finally, elastic cohesive bandage material (Vetrap, *double arrows,* **D**). Note that the bandage material is applied firmly and evenly in an overlapping spiral pattern to prevent slipping and that there is at least 2 cm of padding at the proximal and distal aspect of the bandage to prevent injury from the gauze and elastic cohesive material (*arrows,* **C** and **D**). A stretchy adhesive bandage (Elastoplast/Elastikon) can be applied to the proximal and distal aspect of the bandage to prevent soil, straw or shavings from getting under the bandage. ©Louise Southwood 2005.

Box 1.57. Commonly used materials for bandaging of the limb

Possible materials

Padding (cotton wool [roll cotton], sheet cotton or combine cotton)*†
6-inch open weave bandage (Kling)‡
Elastic cohesive bandage (Vetrap)§
7.5-cm (3-inch) wide stretchy adhesive dressing (Elastoplast**/Elastikon††)
Duct tape‡‡

If there is a wound

Soft sterile conforming bandage§§***†††‡‡‡

- Nonadherent semiocclusive dressing§§§****††††
- Petroleum impregnated gauze‡‡‡‡

*Roll Cotton; Henry Schein Inc., Melville, NY, USA; Cotton Wool 500 g; Robinson Healthcare, Worksop, UK.
†Redi Roll (16 × 36 inch); The Franklin-Williamson Co., Lexington, KY, USA.
‡Jorgensen Laboratories Inc., Loveland, CO, USA.
§3M, St. Paul, MN, USA.
**Beiersdorf AG, Hamburg, Germany.
††Johnson and Johnson, New Brunswick, NJ, USA.
‡‡Duct Tape; Henkel Consumer Adhesives, Avon, OH, USA.
§§Soffban; Smith and Nephew, Largo, FL, USA; Soff-ban; BSN Medical Ltd., Brierfield, England.
***Under Cast Padding; The Kendall Company, Mansfield, MA, USA.
†††Specialist Cast Padding; Johnson and Johnson, Somerville, NJ, USA.
‡‡‡Sof-Kling; Johnson and Johnson, Arlington, TX, USA.
§§§Melolin; Smith and Nephew, Largo, FL, USA.
****Telfa nonadherent dressing; The Kendall Company, Mansfield, MA, USA.
††††Release nonadherent dressing; Johnson and Johnson, Arlington, TX, USA.
‡‡‡‡Aquaphor; Beiersdork, Norwalk, CT, USA.

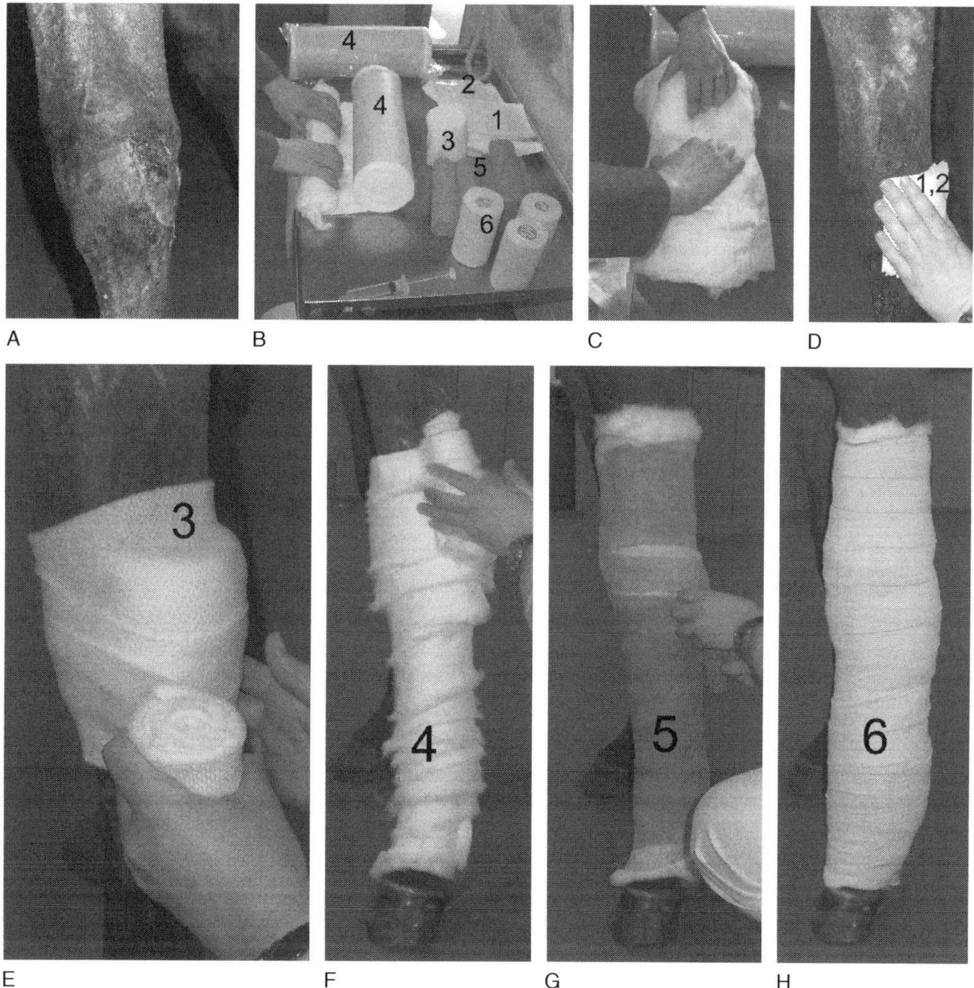

Figure 1.171A-H A full limb bandage that was used to provide a favourable environment for wound healing, wound protection, as well as wound edge immobilization for a 7- to 8-cm-diameter wound on the lateral aspect of the carpus (**A**). Materials that were used for the bandage (**B**) were (1) a sterile nonadherent semiocclusive dressing, (2) small (4 x 4) gauze swabs to increase absorption, (3) soft sterile conforming gauze, (4) roll cotton, (5) 6-inch Brown open weave bandage and (6) stretchy adhesive bandage (Elastoplast/Elastikon). The roll cotton is re-rolled to remove the paper and then split in half to facilitate bandaging (**C**). The wound is initially covered with the sterile nonadherent semiocclusive dressing and the 4 × 4 gauze swabs (**D**) and the soft sterile conforming gauze (primary dressing, **E**). Roll cotton is used as padding and is applied in an overlapping spiral pattern from the coronary band to below the elbow (**F**) followed by 6-inch brown open weave bandage (**G**). For additional stiffness and to provide immobilization, an additional layer of roll cotton and brown cling was applied. Finally, elastic adhesive bandage material (Elastoplast/Elastikon) was applied also in a snug overlapping spiral pattern (**H**). The elastic adhesive bandage was not applied to the proximal (*top*) aspect of the bandage because this particular horse had developed some skin irritation from repeated use of adhesive bandage material. It is important to carefully place a hole in the elastic bandage material over the accessory carpal bone to prevent pressure necrosis of the skin in this area. ©Louise Southwood 2005.

Avoiding problems and treating bandage "bows"

It is important to apply the bandage appropriately to prevent complications such as wound dehiscence and contamination, splint slipping and rotating, or a "bandage bow". A "bandage bow" is usually peritendinous swelling and inflammation and can occur from a bandage that is applied with excessive or uneven pressure, or as a result of a bandage slipping. While most of the damage is usually peritendinous, occasionally tendonitis can occur with diffuse hypoechogenicity along the periphery of the tendon associated with fluid between fibre bundles (Dr. Virginia Reef, personal communication). A "bandage bow" should be treated with cold-hosing, phenylbutazone (2.2 mg/kg PO or IV every 12 hours for 3 to 7 days), and bandaging.

Procedure

Bandages consist of two major parts: (1) primary dressing that is applied directly over the wound and (2) secondary dressing that is applied over the primary dressing (Figures 1.170, A–D, 1.171, A–H and 1.172, A–E). If there is no wound, then the primary dressing is unnecessary. The primary dressing consists of a sterile, usually nonadherent semiocclusive dressing applied to the wound and secured in place using soft, sterile conforming gauze (Figures 1.170,

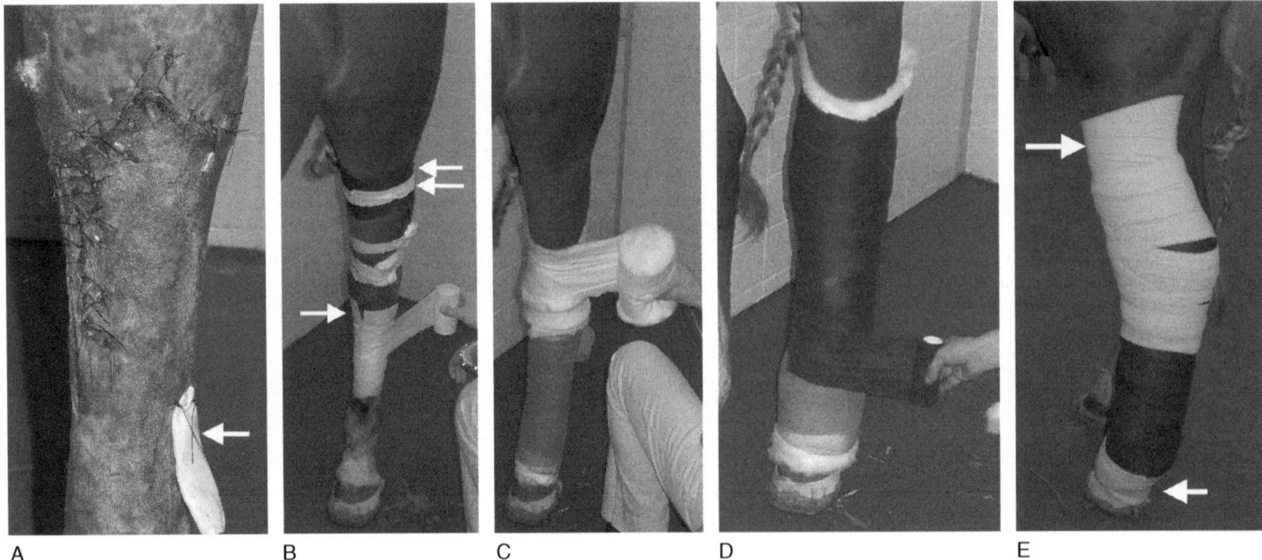

Figure 1.172A-E A tarsal bandage was applied to control moisture and provide wound edge immobilisation of a tarsal wound (**A**). Note that a drain was placed because of the large dead space (*arrow*). A semiocclusive nonadherent dressing (*arrow*) was kept in place with sterile soft conforming gauze (**B**). Regional limb perfusion was performed on this horse prior to bandaging and the tourniquet was still in place (*double arrow*). Multiple layers of roll cotton and 6-inch brown open weave bandage were used (**C**) as for the carpal bandage (Figure 1.171, G). A nonadhesive cohesive bandage (Vetrap) was then applied snugly in an overlapping spiral pattern (**D**). Note that the bandage material is applied so that the flexor tendons are pulled medially. There is also 1 to 2 cm of padding at the proximal (*top*) and distal (*bottom*) aspects of the bandage so that the brown open weave bandage and Vetrap are not in contact with the skin. A stretchy adhesive dressing (Elastoplast/Elastikon) is applied at the top and bottom of the bandage to prevent slipping or dirt, straw, shavings and faecal material getting under the bandage (**E**). ©Louise Southwood 2005.

A, 1.171, E and 1.172, B). Semiocclusive nonadherent dressings are coated with perforated polyethylene and allow movement of moisture away from the wound. While semiocclusive dressings provide a good environment for wound healing, they can dry out the wound. Petrolatum-impregnated gauze can be used as an alternative to keep the wound moist. Nonadherent dressings can be removed without disrupting cells and immature collagen on the wound surface. Semiocclusive nonadherent dressings should be used when managing granulating or epithelialising wounds.[1]

If the wound is still in the debridement phase of healing (days 1 to 3), a wet-to-dry dressing can be used. A wet-to-dry adherent dressing consists of fine mesh gauze that is saturated in sterile saline (± an antiseptic solution) and covered with a dry secondary bandage (see below). When the primary adherent dressing is removed, the top layer of the wound is also removed and the wound gradually debrided.[1] Occlusive dressings, which are manufactured polymers, can be applied during the early phase of healing prior to wound coverage with granulation tissue (days 2 to 6).[1] While occlusive dressings are reported to provide a more suitable environment for migration and proliferation of fibroblasts and epithelial cells, wounds dressed with occlusive dressing have more exudate, exuberant granulation tissue and delayed healing.[2,3] Wound dressings and topical treatments are discussed further in Chapter 16.

Padding is then applied over the primary dressing (secondary dressings) and can consist of roll cotton (cotton wool), sheet cotton or combine cotton. Roll cotton is less expensive than combine cotton and tends to slip less compared to sheet and combine cotton. Combine cotton, however, is easier to apply than the other types of cotton (Figure 1.170, B). Roll cotton is the best to use when a heavy bandage with multiple layers or under splints is needed to provide immobilisation (Figure 1.171, F and 1.172, C). Roll cotton should be separated either longitudinally into two approximately 6-inch full-thickness pieces or two half-thickness 12-inch pieces to facilitate wrapping the limb (Figure 1.171, C). Approximately 1 to 2 cm of padding should be applied to ensure that boney prominences are protected. The amount of padding used will depend on the amount of wound drainage and the degree of immobilisation needed. Whenever applying padding, the palmar or plantar aspect of the distal limb should be wrapped in a lateral-to-medial direction (i.e., pulling the tendons medially; Figures 1.170, B–D, 1.171, F–H and 1.172, C and D), and whilst there is probably no scientific basis to this technique, it is important to a client to see that their veterinarian can bandage a limb "properly". Padding should be applied evenly and snugly. Nonsterile open weave bandage is then applied to keep the cotton in place (Figures 1.170, C, 1.171, G and 1.172, C). An elastic bandage (such as Vetrap [3M] or Elastoplast/Elastikon) is then applied (Figure 1.170, D). While it is expensive and unnecessary to apply an elastic adhesive bandage (Elastoplast/Elastikon) over the full length of the bandage, it can be useful to secure the proximal (top) and distal (bottom) aspects of the bandage to prevent slipping or dirt, straw, shavings and faecal material getting under the bandage and near the wound (Figure 1.172, E). If the purpose of bandaging is to cover a clean, dry wound only, for example, following suture removal 10 to 14 days postarthroscopy, elastic adhesive bandage material can be applied directly over the primary dressing in an overlapping spiral pattern with enough elastic adhesive bandage adhered to the skin so that the bandage does not slip and so that there is a seal proximal and distal to the wound.

Reusable bandages

Reusable bandages are an alternative to disposable bandages. Reusable bandages consist of cloth cotton padding ("quilts") and soft elastic nonadherent bandage applied over the cloth and secured in place with Velcro. These bandages are also called "stable bandages" or "standing wraps" and can be used on the distal limb. Reusable bandages are useful for horses that develop distal limb oedema in a stall or during transport following discharge from the hospital. They require washing between patients and when soiled with haemorrhage or wound drainage, and they need to be changed at least once a day. It is difficult to obtain the same amount of pressure with reusable bandages that can be obtained with disposable bandages. Reusable bandages may be a good alternative to disposable bandages when a distal limb needs to be bandaged for an extended period of time.

Distal limb bandages

Distal limb bandages extend from the coronary band to just below the carpus or tarsus (Figure 1.170, A–D). If the wound is very distal on the limb, for example, the pastern or coronary band, the hoof should be cleaned and the hoof wall and sole included in the bandage. The entire hoof should be covered with duct tape or other impermeable material to prevent wicking of urine and faeces into the bandage. The foot can be bandaged using similar principles to bandaging of the limb; however, it is important to place an impermeable and durable material, such as duct tape or a used 5-L fluid bag over the sole of the hoof.

Full limb bandages

The upper limb can be more challenging to bandage. The carpus can be bandaged using padding either over the carpus alone or along the full length of the limb from the coronary band to just below the elbow (Figures 1.171, A–H). The padding component of the secondary bandage can be roll cotton (Figure 1.171, F) or stacked combine cotton. When the latter is used, the distal limb is wrapped with combine cotton and then a second combine cotton is stacked proximally and slightly overlapping to cover the carpus. Stacking is used to prevent slipping. Following application of a padded carpus bandage, a release hole should made in the elastic bandage over the accessory carpal bone to prevent pressure necrosis of the skin in this area. Some clinicians also recommend making a hole over the distal medial radius to prevent pressure necrosis of the skin overlying the bony prominence created by the distal radial physis. Care should be taken when incising the bandage material over the accessory carpal bone to not cut through the skin because these wounds can take a long time to heal. Carpal bandages often slip, and if the bandage slips, the release hole over the accessory carpal bone should be extended proximally to prevent excessive pressure on the skin over the bony prominence of the accessory carpal bone or the bandage can be replaced.

The carpus can also be bandaged using nonadherent primary wound dressing, conforming gauze, and then an elastic adhesive dressing (Elastoplast/Elastikon) is applied in a figure-of-eight pattern, to cover a wound on the dorsal carpus following arthroscopic surgery, for example.

Tarsal bandages can be applied similarly to carpal bandages; however, the main difference is to avoid placing excessive pressure over the gastrocnemius tendon and the point of the hock (Figures 1.172, A–E). When applying a primary dressing to the hock region, the conforming gauze should be applied in a figure-of-eight pattern around the point of the hock, with the crossing of the eight over the cranial aspect of the hock and leaving the point of the hock out of the bandage.[1]

Splints

Splints (see Chapter 1.52) can be applied over a bandage following placement of the elastic component of the secondary dressing. Splints should be applied snugly over 2 to 3 cm of padding using nonelastic tape. It is important that the splints do not extend beyond the bandage or are well padded if they do extend beyond the bandage, because they can rub the skin or cause pressure sores.

Monitoring and maintenance

The horse should be monitored for signs of lameness, haemorrhage or wound drainage through the bandage and swelling proximal or distal to the bandage, and the bandage should be changed immediately if any of these signs are observed. All bandages should be changed at least twice a week in hospitalised horses. If the wound has extensive drainage, the bandage may need to be changed daily.

References

1. Stone WC: Drains, dressings, and external coaptation, in Auer JA, Stick JA (eds): Equine Surgery. Philadelphia, WB Saunders, 1999, pp 104-113
2. Dyson M, Young S, Pendle CL, et al.: Comparison of the effects of moist and dry conditions on dermal repair. J Invest Dermatol 91:434, 1988
3. Howard RD, Stashak TS, Baxter GM: Evaluation of occlusive dressings for management of full-thickness excisional wounds on the distal portion of the limbs of horses. Am J Vet Res 54:2150, 1993

4. Bramlage LR: Emergency first aid treatment and transportation of equine fracture patients, in Auer JA, Stick JA (eds): Equine Surgery, ed 2. Philadelphia, WB Saunders, 1999, pp 635-638

1.52 Application of splints

Jennifer O. Stephen

Fractures of the limbs, luxations, lacerations of supporting structures, lacerations of major peripheral blood vessels and severe tendon injuries are all examples of orthopaedic injuries that require immediate stabilisation if successful treatment is to be possible and for the welfare and safety of the horse. Most of these injuries will, of course, be seen in the field and may be associated with significant problems in getting the horse to a safe environment for treatment. For transportation to be achieved without compromising the outcome of the case, it is important that correct coaptation is applied (Box 1.58). A complete discussion of emergency first aid and splint application is covered in the musculoskeletal section (see Chapter 15.9).

Equipment needed

The equipment needed is listed in Box 1.59. Splints should be placed over bandages (see Chapter 1.51).

The type of splint that is applied is determined by the location of the fracture. There are four biomechanically important regions in the fore limb and four in the hind limb (Figure 1.173).

Splinting the fore limb: region 1

A dorsal splint should be applied from the toe to distal carpus (Figure 1.174).

Splinting the fore limb: region 2

A full limb Robert Jones bandage (Box 1.60) should be applied with caudal and lateral splints (Figure 1.175).

Box 1.58. Objectives for first aid of a fractured limb

1. Stabilise the limb; this will not only prevent further injury but also plays a major part in relieving the anxiety that accompanies an uncontrollable limb in the horse.
2. Keep the skin intact; prevent a closed fracture from becoming an open fracture.
3. If the fracture is open, try to prevent further contamination.
4. Prevent soft tissue trauma, protect the vascular supply of the limb and prevent neural damage.
5. Minimise any further damage to the bone ends (fragment eburnation).

Box 1.59. Equipment for splinting of the limb

Splint
Anything suitable that is available

- PVC pipe
- Broom handle (broomstick)
- Twitch handle
- Board from a hay pallet

Fixing the splint to the leg

- 7.5-cm (3-inch) wide stretchy adhesive dressing (Elastoplast*/Elastikon†)
- Duct tape‡

For Robert Jones bandage
10–12 rolls 500 g (1 lb) of cotton wool (roll cotton)§
20–25 cotton conforming bandages 15 cm (6 inch)
4–6 rolls 7.5-cm (3-inch) wide stretchy adhesive dressing (Elastoplast/Elastikon)
Duct tape

Optional
Soft sterile conforming bandage**
Low adherent absorbent dressing††

*Beiersdorf AG, Hamburg, Germany
†Johnson and Johnson, New Brunswick, NJ, USA.
‡Duck Tape; Henkel Consumer Adhesives, Avon, OH, USA.
§Roll Cotton; Henry Schein Inc., Melville, NY, USA; Cotton Wool 500 g; Robinson Helathcare, Worksop, UK.
**Soffban; Smith and Nephew, Largo, FL, USA; Soff-ban, BSN Medical Ltd., Brierfield, England
††Melolin; Smith and Nephew, Largo, FL, USA.

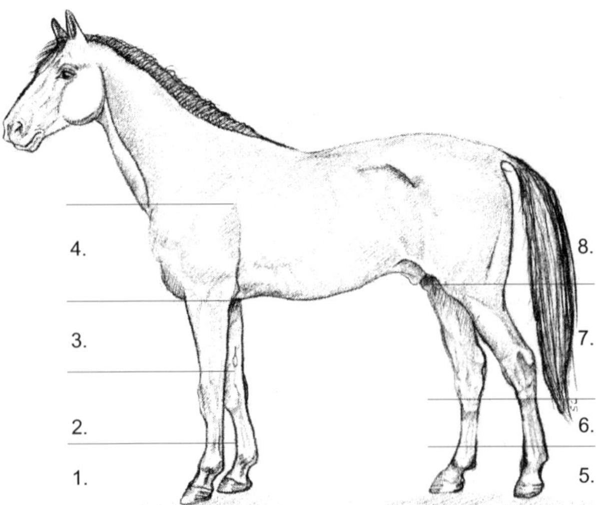

Figure 1.173 Biomechanically important regions of the fore limb and hind limb for splinting; 1. Distal to the distal quarter of the metacarpus. 2. Distal metacarpus to distal radius 3. Distal radius to the elbow. 4. Elbow to distal scapula. 5.Distal to distal quarter of the metatarsus. 6. Distal metatarsus to tarsus. 7. Tarsus to stifle. 8. Proximal to the stifle.

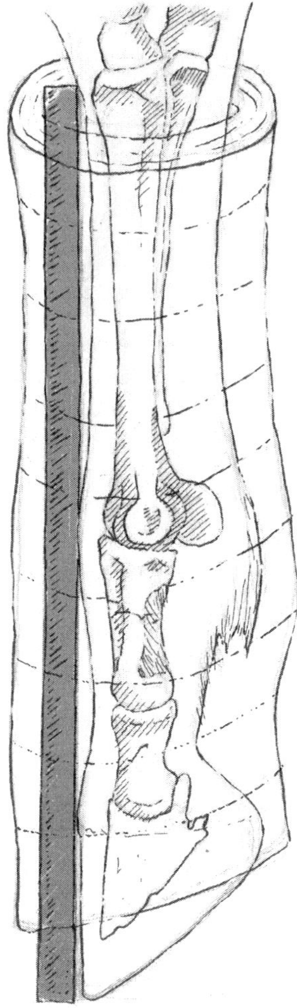
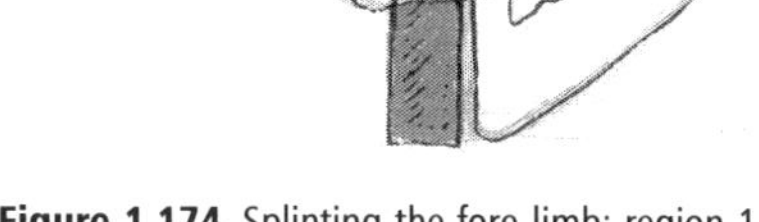

Figure 1.174 Splinting the fore limb: region 1.

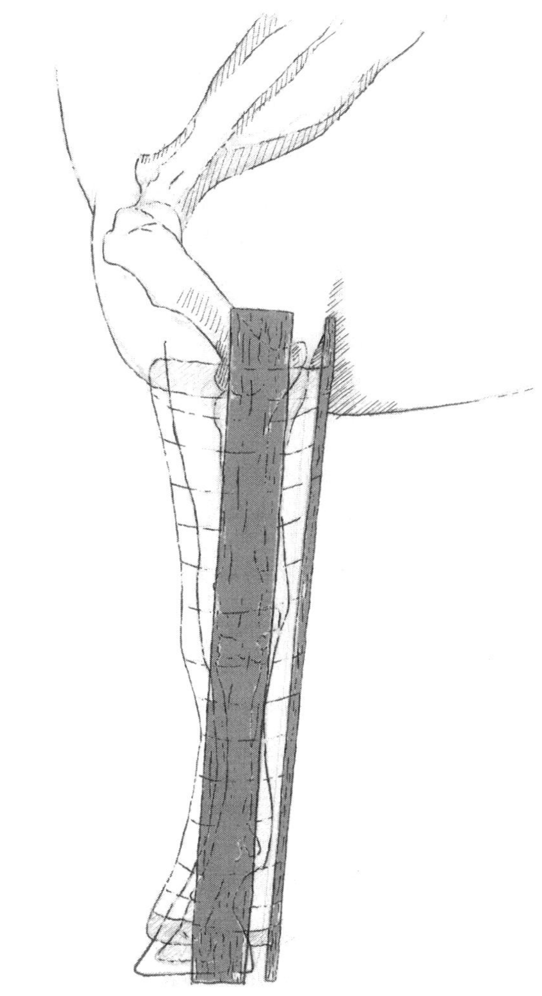

Figure 1.175 Splinting the fore limb: region 2.

Box 1.60. Applying a Robert Jones bandage

1. Fix a suitable dressing over any open wounds with soft sterile conforming bandage.*
2. Begin to apply cotton wool. The bandage should be applied from distal to the coronary band to the most proximal extent of the limb. The cotton wool should be wrapped firmly and smoothly around the limb. Tearing the roll longitudinally to make two 15-cm (6-inch) pieces can help to produce an even bandage.
3. Once three layers of cotton wool have been applied to the entire length of the limb, a conforming cotton bandage should be placed with enough pressure to hold the cotton in place. The bandage should be applied with even tension and overlap itself by 50% on each turn. As with all bandages, 2–3 cm (1 inch) of cotton wool should be left unbandaged proximally and distally to avoid pressure points.
4. Cotton wool/conforming bandage layers are then built up until the limb is three times its original diameter in the front limb or two times the original diameter in the hind limb (at least 4–6 layers). Each layer of bandage should be about 1 inch thick. If too thick a layer is used or if all the padding is placed without conforming layers, the padding will shift and compact, rendering the bandage ineffective and possibly failing to immobilise the injury.[1] The tension with which the conforming bandage is applied may be increased with each layer. The bandage should form a firm, even, tubular cylinder.
5. The final layer is secured with elastic bandage (Elastoplast†/Elastikon‡) or adhesive nonelastic tape (duct tape). At this point, flicking the bandage with the fingers should sound like flicking a ripe melon.
6. Secure suitable splints on to bandage if required.

*Soffban; Smith and Nephew, Largo, FL, USA; Soff-ban; BSN Medical Ltd., Brierfield, England.
†Beiersdorf AG, Hamburg, Germany
‡Johnson and Johnson, New Brunswick, NJ, USA.

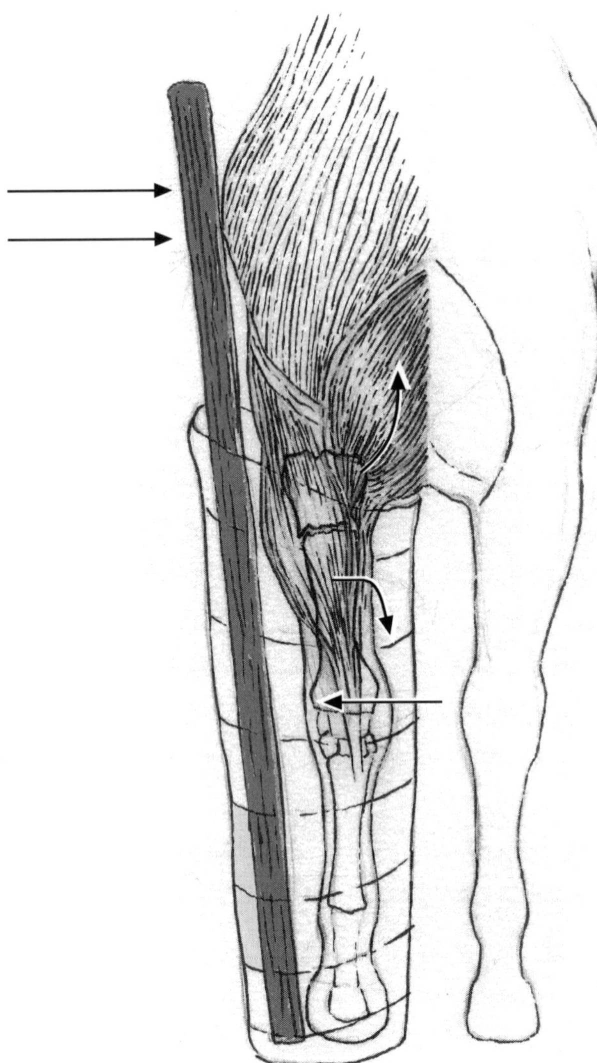

Figure 1.176 Splinting the fore limb: region 3.

Splinting the fore limb: region 3
A full limb Robert Jones bandage should be applied with splints caudally to the elbow and laterally to the withers (Figure 1.176).

Splinting of the fore limb: region 4
A simple full limb bandage should be applied with a caudal splint.

Splinting the hind limb: region 5
A dorsal splint should be applied, toe to tarsus.

Splinting the hind limb: region 6
Full limb Robert Jones bandage with caudal and lateral splints to tuber-calcis.

Splinting the hind limb: region 7
Full limb Robert Jones bandage and metal frame (Figure 1.177).

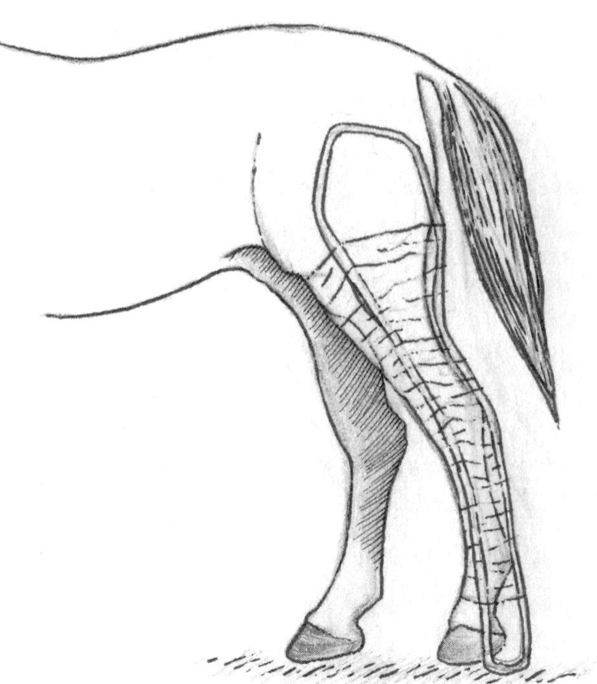

Figure 1.177 Splinting the hind limb: region 7.

Splinting the hind limb: region 8
Useful splinting is not possible.

Reference

1. Bramlage LR: Current concepts of emergency first aid treatment and transportation of equine fracture patients. Comp Cont Educ Pract Vet 5:S564-S574, 1983

1.53 Application of a tourniquet and regional limb perfusion

Jennifer O. Stephen

A tourniquet may be necessary for certain orthopaedic operations, for regional limb perfusion or, rarely, for emergency haemostasis.

Equipment needed

The equipment needed is listed in Box 1.61.

Application of a tourniquet

Prior to the application of a tourniquet, an Esmarch bandage is used to push blood proximally. An Esmarch is a 10-cm-wide strip of thin rubber bandage. The bandage is wrapped around the limb beginning at the coronary band, overlapping each turn by about half its width. When the tourniquet is being applied for orthopaedic surgery, the bandage is continued until it is above the proposed surgical site. Once the Esmarch has been placed, an assistant should keep it secure whilst the tourniquet is placed. Tourniquets

Box 1.61. Equipment for application of a tourniquet and regional limb perfusion

Required
Esmarch bandage*
Tourniquet

- Commercial inflatable tourniquet
- Surgical tubing

For regional limb perfusion
Antibiotics (see Chapter 6.3)

- Adult doses—made up to 20–60 ml with balanced electrolyte solution
    - Gentamicin: 500 mg to 1 g total
    - Amikacin: 500 mg to 1 g total
    - Ceftiofur: 4 mg/kg
    - Vancomycin: 300 mg total
    - Enrofloxacin: 1.5 mg/kg (may result in perivascular oedema and mild cellulitis)
- Foal doses—made up to 10 ml with balanced electrolyte solution
    - Gentamicin: 50 mg to 250 mg total
    - Amikacin: 50 mg to 250 mg total
    - Ceftiofur: 4 mg/kg

Catheter or butterfly needle

- 20 Gauge† for adults
- 22 Gauge‡ for foals

Injection cap
Instant bonding glue (cyanoacrylate adhesive)§

*7134–12; Tetra Medical Corp., Niles, IL, USA.
†IC2001; MILA International, Florence, KY, USA.
‡IC2201; MILA International, Florence, KY, USA.
§Nexaband; Abbott Laboratories, North Chicago, IL, USA; Superglue, Loctite; Henkel Consumer Adhesives, Avon, OH, USA.

are usually placed above the carpal or tarsal joints. For surgery involving the fetlock joint or distal to the fetlock, the tourniquet may be placed over the proximal metacarpal or metatarsal region. A commercial inflatable tourniquet may be used, or several turns with rubber surgical tubing. The Esmarch bandage is then removed.

In trauma cases, it may be difficult or inappropriate to place a tourniquet. Alternative methods of haemostasis include direct ligation, application of a bandage and packing of the wound defect.

Regional limb perfusion

When using a tourniquet for regional limb perfusion, a catheter should be placed in an appropriate superficial vein *prior* to application of tourniquet. The vein should be one that drains the site of injury or infection, at a point close to this site. The catheter may be secured with instant

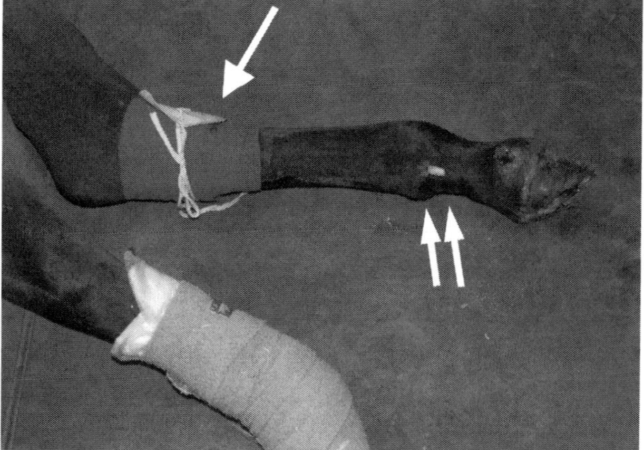

Figure 1.178 Esmarch bandage (*single arrow*) placed below the hock for regional perfusion of the distal limb, in a weanling with a coronary band abscess. A catheter (*double arrows*) has been placed in the plantar digital vein, for instillation of antibiotics. ©Kevin Corley 2007.

bonding glue. The catheter should be maintained in place throughout the procedure, until after the tourniquet has been removed. The Esmarch bandage is started proximal to the venous access point or both proximal and distal to the catheter if the site is more proximal on the limb. The Esmarch bandage itself may be used as the tourniquet for this procedure (Figure 1.178). Several different antimicrobials may be used (Box 1.61 and see Chapter 6.3). The antimicrobial drug should be diluted to 20 to 60 ml in adult horses and 10 ml in foals and injected slowly through the catheter. The tourniquet is maintained for 15 to 20 minutes and then released. Regional limb perfusion is discussed in more detail in Chapters 6.3 and 15.8.

Complications

Application of a pneumatic tourniquet at 600 mm Hg for 120 minutes caused localised acidaemia, increased serum potassium concentrations in the tourniqueted limb vein and reduced haematocrit values compared to control limb.[1] Tourniquet release produced a return to normal values within 10 to 15 minutes.

Arterial hypertension in excess of 200 mm Hg has been observed after tourniquet application. Pain is hypothesised to be the most likely cause of this. Pain will increase in intensity and duration after removal of the tourniquet. Local anaesthetic nerve blocks (see Chapter 1.50) proximal to the tourniquet, removal of the tourniquet or increasing the depth of anaesthesia can be used to counteract this.[2]

References

1. Scott EA, Riebold TW, Lamar AM, et al.: Effect of a pneumatic tourniquet application to the distal extremities of the horse: blood gas, serum electrolyte, osmolality and haematological alterations. Am J Vet Res 40:1078, 1979

2. Muir WW: Complications: Induction, maintenance and recovery phase of anaesthesia, in Muir WW, Hubbel JAE (eds): Equine Anesthesia: Monitoring and Emergency Therapy. St. Louis, Mosby–Year Book, 1991, p 431

1.54 Bandaging of the head

Louise L. Southwood

While bandaging of the head is often unnecessary, when it is necessary, it is imperative that it is performed well to prevent complications associated with dislodgment as well as to provide adequate wound protection and support. A poorly bandaged head can cause respiratory tract obstruction associated with slipping and occlusion of the nares, distress associated with the horse being unable to see because the bandage has moved and is covering the eyes and, most important, wound complications, such as haemorrhage, dehiscence and infection. Bandaging of the head is used to protect the wound from contamination, provide support and a favourable environment for wound healing and apply pressure to prevent haemorrhage and oedema formation. Types of head lesions that may require bandaging include postoperative sinus surgery or a traumatic sinus wound, postoperative ocular surgery or ocular lacerations and aural lesions. Bandaging is not necessary in many cases of head wounds or injury because of the excellent blood supply, solid underlying bony support providing immobilisation and minimising wound tension and relatively clean location compared to the distal limb.

Equipment needed

Types of bandages that can be used include (Box 1.62) (1) 6-inch stockinet, (2) antimicrobial impregnated adhesive drapes, (3) a light sterile primary dressing with a small piece of adhesive elastic bandage material applied with cyanoacrylate adhesive, (4) sterile primary dressing with adhesive elastic bandaging material applied to create pressure at the wound site and (5) stent bandages. Additionally, the head can be protected with a soft helmet or, specifically, the eye can be protected with an eye protector during recovery from general anaesthesia (Figure 1.179).

Procedure

Horses having had sinus surgery or repair of head wounds, for example, often have a 6-inch stockinet placed over the head and neck with holes made for the eyes and ears. Stockinet can be used to cover the wound for recovery from general anaesthesia and during the early postoperative period. This type of bandage protects the wound from gross contamination and mild trauma, such as the horse occasionally rubbing the wound, and is economical to use and easy to change as needed. Stockinet can also be used in combination with other bandages (see below). Antimicrobial adhesive drapes can also be applied to head wounds for protection from contamination during recovery from general anaesthesia. A nonadherent semiocclusive dressing

Box 1.62. Commonly used materials for bandaging of the head

Possible materials

6-inch stockinet*
Antimicrobial impregnated adhesive drape†
7.5-cm (3-inch) wide stretchy adhesive dressing (Elastoplast‡/Elastikon§)
Instant bonding glue (cyanoacrylate adhesive)**
Sterile gauze swabs (sponges)††
Nonadherent semiocclusive dressing‡‡§§***
Padding (cotton wool [roll cotton], sheet cotton or combine cotton)†††‡‡‡
6-inch open weave bandage (Kling)§§§
Elastic cohesive bandage (Vetrap)****
Soft sterile conforming bandage††††‡‡‡‡§§§§*****

Head and eye protection

Soft helmet†††††
Eye protector‡‡‡‡‡

*Jorgensen Laboratories Inc., Loveland, CO, USA.
†Loban 2; 3M, St. Paul, MN, USA.
‡Beiersdorf AG, Hamburg, Germany.
§Johnson and Johnson, New Brunswick, NJ, USA.
**Nexaband; Abbott Laboratories, North Chicago, IL, USA; Superglue, Loctite; Henkel Consumer Adhesives, Avon, OH, USA.
††For example, Versalon All-Purpose Sponges; The Kendall Co., Mansfield, MA, USA; Econopak; General Econopak Inc., Philadelphia, PA, USA.
‡‡Melolin; Smith and Nephew, Largo, FL, USA.
§§Telfa nonadherent dressing; The Kendall Company, Mansfield, MA, USA.
***Release nonadherent dressing; Johnson and Johnson, Arlington, TX, USA.
†††Roll Cotton; Henry Schein Inc., Melville, NY, USA.
‡‡‡Redi Roll (16 × 36 inch); The Franklin-Williamson Co., Lexington, KY, USA.
§§§Jorgensen Laboratories Inc., Loveland, CO, USA.
****3M, St Paul, MN, USA.
††††Soffban; Smith and Nephew, Largo, FL, USA.
‡‡‡‡Under Cast Padding; The Kendall Company, Mansfield, MA, USA.
§§§§Specialist Cast Padding; Johnson and Johnson, Somerville, NJ, USA.
*****Sof-Kling; Johnson and Johnson, Arlington, TX, USA.
†††††Head Bumper; Shank's Veterinary Equipment Inc., Milledgeville, IL, USA.
‡‡‡‡‡Equine Eye Saver; Jorgenson Laboratories, Loveland, CO, USA.

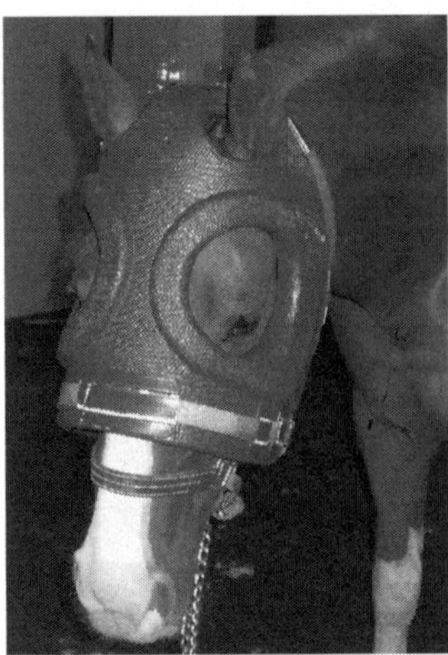

Figure 1.179 A soft helmet can be used to protect the horse's head during recovery from general anaesthesia, for example, following sinus surgery. ©Dr. Elizabeth Davidson, New Bolton Center, University of Pennsylvania, 2005.

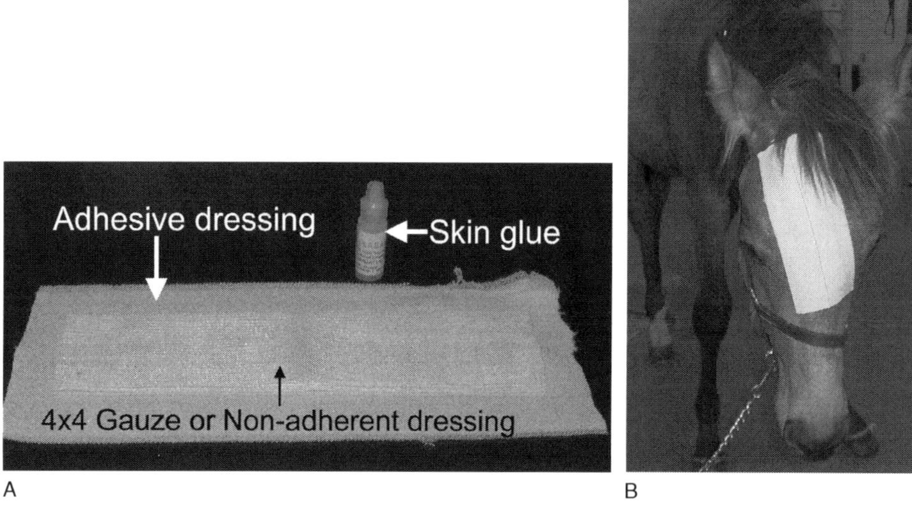

Figure 1.180 A-B The wound can be covered with a small piece of nonadhesive dressing or gauze swab (sponge) and an adhesive bandage (Elastoplast/Elastikon). Cyanoacrylate adhesive can be used to keep the Elastoplast/Elastikon in place. It is important to cut the nonadhesive semiocclusive primary dressing or gauze sponge so that it covers the wound only, leaving at least 2 to 3 cm of adhesive bandage around the edge (**A**). This type of bandage can be used to cover clean, dry wounds where minimal swelling is anticipated, such as following an aseptic elective surgical procedure (**B**). The bandage can be made as large or as small as necessary to cover the wound. The bandage should not need to be removed for approximately 10 to 14 days, because the cyanoacrylate adhesive makes the bandage difficult to change. If this type of bandage is used and it becomes necessary to remove the bandage prior to the cyanoacrylate adhesive loosening, the section of the bandage covering the wound can be cut out and a similar replacement bandage applied over the remaining adhered first bandage. ©Louise Southwood 2005.

and/or sterile gauze swabs (sponges) are placed directly over the wound followed by application of the antimicrobial adhesive drape over the primary dressing. These bandages should be removed soon after recovery because they are impermeable and can cause wound complications, such as infection, associated with accumulation of blood, sweat and wound drainage. Antimicrobial adhesive drapes may also become dislodged if the skin is not completely dry. The use of an adhesive will help keep the antimicrobial adhesive drape in place; however, it can make the bandage difficult to remove postoperatively. Antimicrobial adhesive drapes are expensive compared to stockinet bandages and are generally not replaced following removal postrecovery from general anaesthesia.

Similarly, the wound can be covered with a small piece of nonadhesive semiocclusive primary dressing or gauze swab (sponge) (large enough to cover the wound) and then an adhesive bandage (Elastoplast/Elastikon) applied over the top with cyanoacrylate glue (Figure 1.180, A and B). The three types of bandages discussed so far protect the wound from contamination but do not provide wound immobilisation, pressure or support.

Head wounds can be bandaged using a primary dressing and an elastic adhesive bandage (Figure 1.181). This type of bandage can be used to cover the wound as well as apply pressure to prevent haemorrhage and oedema formation, such as, following an enucleation or a traumatic wound. A nonadhesive semiocclusive dressing and/or gauze swabs (sponges) are placed over the wound or in the eye socket

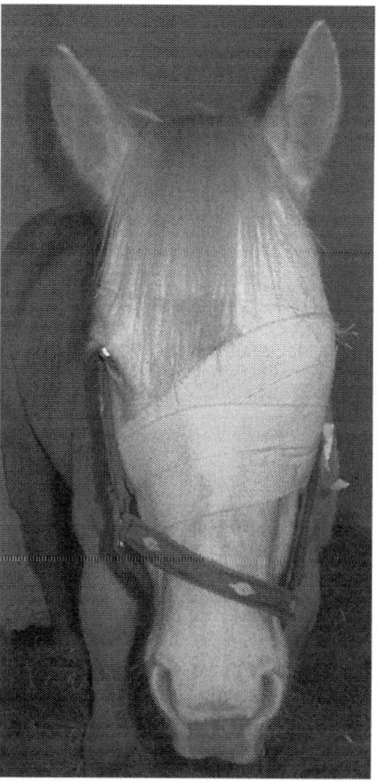

Figure 1.181 Head wounds can be bandaged using a primary dressing and an elastic adhesive bandage. The horse in the figure had an enucleation. Gauze sponges were placed in the eye socket to apply pressure to the wound to control haemorrhage and oedema formation, and to reduce deadspace. Nonadhesive bandaged material (brown open weave bandage (Kling) was wrapped once around the head to avoid having a large surface area of adhesive bandage to remove from the skin and hair. The adhesive bandage material (Elastoplast/Elastikon) was then applied. It is important to have the adhesive bandage in contact with the skin so that the bandage does not slip. ©Louise Southwood 2005.

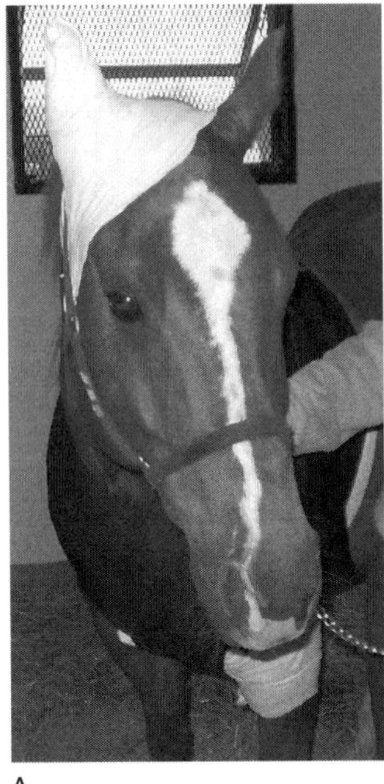
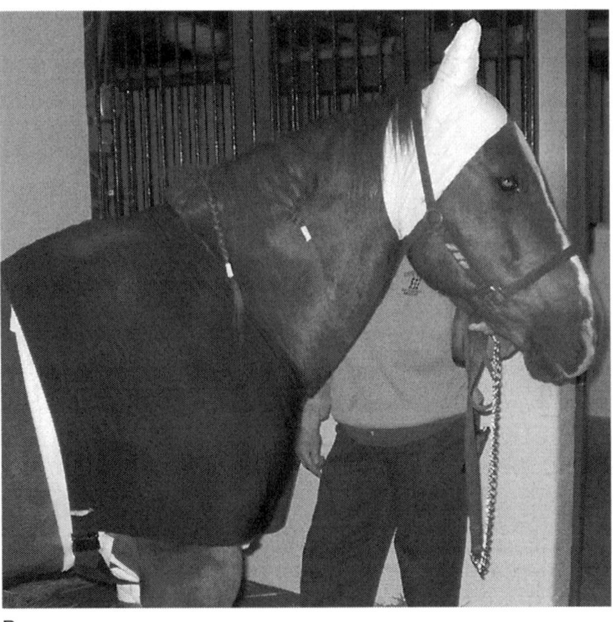

A B

Figure 1.182 A-B This horse's ear was bandaged following sarcoid removal. Front (**A**) and side (**B**) views. Also note that the thoracic wall was bandaged using gauze, elastic adhesive bandage material and a commercially available product following sarcoid removal in this location. ©Louise Southwood 2005.

in the case of enucleation. Gauze swabs (sponges) are useful for applying pressure to the wound to control haemorrhage and oedema formation and to reduce deadspace. Nonadhesive bandaged material can be wrapped once around the head to avoid having a large surface area of adhesive bandage to remove from the skin and hair. The adhesive bandage material is then applied. It is important to have the adhesive bandage in contact with the skin so that the bandage does not slip.

Stent bandages can be used to protect small wounds from contamination and can be used to reduce the tension at the wound edges. A stent bandage can be made with rolled gauze swabs (sponges) or gauze bandage material. An appropriate number of sponges or amount of bandage material should be used so that the stent bandage is not too large or too heavy for the wound. The stent bandage is sutured over the wound using number 2 (5 metric) nylon interrupted sutures or by placing loops with number 2 (5 metric) nylon on either side of the stent bandage and using umbilical tape threaded through the loops in a "shoelace" pattern to keep the bandage in place. The latter technique makes replacement of the stent bandage simple because the stent does not need to be sutured in place each time it is replaced.

Aural lesions can be challenging to bandage and can be best accomplished by inserting rolled gauze into the ear and then bandaging around the ear using a light primary dressing and then an elastic adhesive bandage (Figures 1.182, A and B). The bandage can be extended to include the head and/or neck. Excessive bandaging can make the horse rub the ear and remove the bandage.

1.55 Muscle biopsy

Nicola Menzies-Gow

A muscle biopsy is useful in the diagnostic evaluation of all forms of muscle disorder.[1] It allows the morphologic, biochemical and physiological properties of the myofibres to be examined with minimal complications.[2] The commonest indications are to differentiate the cellular infiltrate in myositis, to confirm a diagnosis of equine motor neuron disease (EMND), to confirm ongoing myopathic changes in cases of chronic rhabdomyolysis and to differentiate polysaccharide storage myopathy (PSSM) and equine polysaccharide storage myopathy (EPSM) as specific myopathies underlying chronic rhabdomyolysis.

Muscle biopsy site

The optimal site for biopsy depends on the suspected diagnosis. For chronic rhabdomyolysis, EPSM and PPSM, the middle gluteal is commonly used for a needle biopsy and the *semimembranosis* or *semitendinosis* for a surgical biopsy. To make a diagnosis of EMND, a surgical biopsy from the *sacrocaudalis dorsalis medialis* (tail head muscle) is required. If the muscle disorder is more localised, then a surgical biopsy from the affected region is most appropriate.

Equipment needed

The equipment needed is listed in Box 1.63.

Needle biopsy

The horse should be adequately sedated and restrained. The biopsy is taken from the middle gluteal muscle, midway

Box 1.63. Equipment for muscle biopsy

Needle biopsy
Modified Bergstrom 6-mm biopsy needle*

Surgical biopsy
Curved haemostats
Tongue depressor or piece of cardboard
Skin stapler† or 2-0 nonabsorbable suture on a straight needle‡

For both techniques
Mepivacaine 2%§: 5 ml drawn up in a syringe with a 23–25-gauge needle
No. 15 scalpel blade
Clippers with a fine (No. 40) blade
Small gauze swabs (4 × 4) soaked in chlorhexidine (4%) scrub solution**
Small gauze swabs (4 × 4) soaked in surgical spirit (alcohol)
Sedation
Surgical gloves
Fixative

- Sample pot containing 10% neutral buffered formalin
- Liquid nitrogen container

Optional
Twitch

*Kruuse, Marslev, Denmark.
†Auto Suture Appose ULC 35W; United States Surgical, Tyco Healthcare Group, Norwalk, CT, USA.
‡628H, Ethilon Nylon; Ethicon, Somerville, NJ, USA.
§Intra-epicaine; Arnolds Veterinary Products, Shrewsbury, UK; Carbocaine-V; Pfizer Animal Health, New York, NY, USA.
**Hibiscrub; Mölnlycke Health Care, Dunstable, UK.

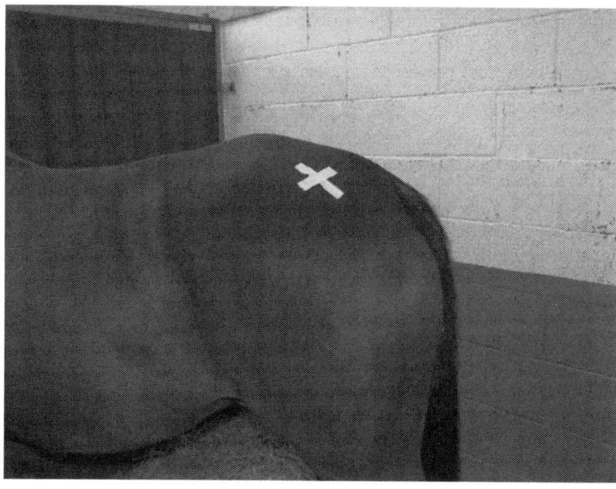

Figure 1.183 Site for surgical biopsy of gluteal muscle, midway along a line from the tuber coxae to the base of the tail. ©Kevin Corley 2007.

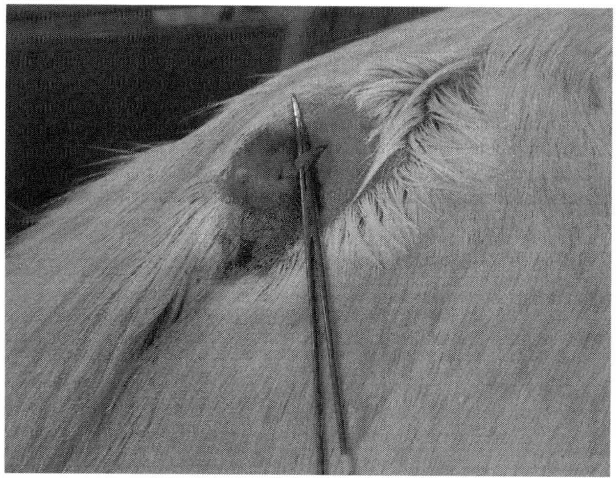

Figure 1.184 A surgical biopsy from the *sacrocaudalis dorsalis medialis* muscle (tail head muscle). ©Nicola Menzies-Gow 2002.

along a line from the *tuber coxae* to the base of the tail (Figure 1.183), using a stainless steel biopsy needle.[3] The biopsy site is clipped and aseptically prepared. Local anaesthesia is achieved by subcutaneous infiltration of local anaesthetic agent such as mepivacaine. Intramuscular infiltration should be avoided, as it will disrupt the histological appearance of the biopsy specimen. A small incision should be made using a scalpel through the skin and underlying fascia at the biopsy site. The stylet should be removed, the biopsy needle inserted at 90 ° to the skin into the gluteal muscle to a depth of approximately 8 cm and four to eight quick cuts are made. The largest possible biopsy specimen can be obtained by ensuring that the window in the biopsy needle is facing dorsally and angling the needle dorsally once inserted to engage more muscle into the window.[1] The stylet is then used to remove the muscle biopsy specimen from biopsy needle and the specimen should be fixed in 10% buffered formalin or frozen by immersion in liquid nitrogen. In general, frozen sections appeared to be better suited for studying myopathies because many histopathological features of skeletal muscle were obscured by formalin fixation. The skin incision may be sutured if necessary. Complications rarely occur.

Surgical biopsy

The advantage of a surgical biopsy over a needle biopsy is that a much larger biopsy specimen is obtained. The skin overlying the muscle of interest is clipped and aseptically prepared. For a *semimembranosis* or *semitendinosis* biopsy, the region adjacent to the *tuber ischii*, proximally or distally, 5 cm lateral to the tail is used. For a tail head muscle biopsy, the region lateral to the tail head is used (Figure 1.184). Local anaesthesia is achieved using an inverted "L" block. A scalpel incision is made through the skin, followed by blunt dissection onto the muscle. Two parallel scalpel incisions are made running in the direction of the muscle fibres approximately 2 cm in length and 1 cm apart. Using curved haemostats, the section of muscle between the parallel incisions is bluntly dissected free and elevated. It is essential that the muscle strip is undermined; otherwise, muscle contraction results in artefact and poor orientation of the fibres.[4] Both ends of this section are then cut using the scalpel. Careful handling of the ends of the muscle sample also decreases artefact.[4] The biopsy specimen should be placed on a piece of cardboard or tongue depressor to prevent contracture artefact and fixed in 10% buffered formalin or frozen by emersion in liquid nitrogen.[5] In general, frozen sections appeared to be better suited for studying myopathies because many histopathological features of skeletal muscle were obscured by formalin fixation. The skin incision is then closed using staples or sutures. Complications are minimal but include include swelling, infection and scarring of the biopsy site.

References

1. Ledwith AN, McGowan C: Muscle biopsy: a routine diagnostic procedure. Equine Vet Educ 16:62-67, 2004
2. MacLeay JM: Diseases of the musculoskeletal system, in Reed SM, Bayly WM, Sellon DC (eds): Equine Internal Medicine, ed 2. Philadelphia, WB Saunders, 2004, p 469
3. Snow DH, Guy PS: Percutaneous needle biopsy in the horse. Equine Vet J 8:150-155, 1978
4. Valentine BA: Equine polysaccharide storage myopathy. Equine Vet Educ 15:254-262, 2003
5. Divers TJ, de Lahunta A, Hintz HF, et al.: Equine motor neuron disease. Equine Vet Educ 13:63-67, 2001

1.56 Suture materials and suture patterns for skin closure

Jennifer O. Stephen

Suture materials

Type

For skin closure, a nonabsorbable monofilament suture is usually used. Nylon*, polypropylene† and polybutester‡ are suitable.[1] Subcuticular tissues are apposed using a synthetic absorbable suture such as polyglactin 910§ or polydioxanone**.

Size

Equine skin: 2–0 (3 metric) to 2 (5 metric)
Equine subcuticular tissue: 3–0 (3 metric) to 4–0 (4 metric)

Suture placement

The goal is accurate apposition of the skin edges with minimal interference to their blood supply.

- The strength of a wound is dependent on the tissue's ability to hold the suture rather than the strength of the suture.[2]
- Sutures should be placed more than 0.5 cm from the edge of a severely traumatised wound.[3]
- Maximum holding strength is obtained when sutures are 0.5 cm apart.[3]
- For wounds under tension, it is better to increase the number of sutures than to increase suture material size.
- Sutures should be tied with sufficient tension to appose skin edges.
- Proper use of bandages/casts will help to support suture lines.

Knots

- The square knot is most secure (Figure 1.185).
- Use a surgeon's knot (Figure 1.186) only where tension dictates necessary.
- A minimum of three throws is required to secure knots in commonly used skin sutures.
- An additional two or three throws should be added at beginning or end of a continuous pattern.[1]

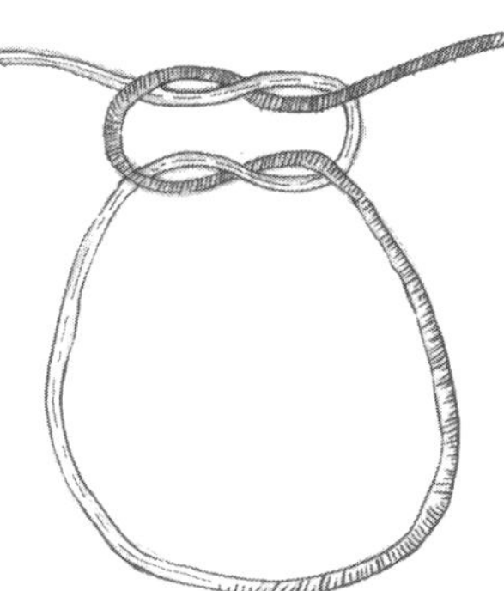

Figure 1.185 Square knot: Tension must be kept equal on the two sides as the knot is tied.

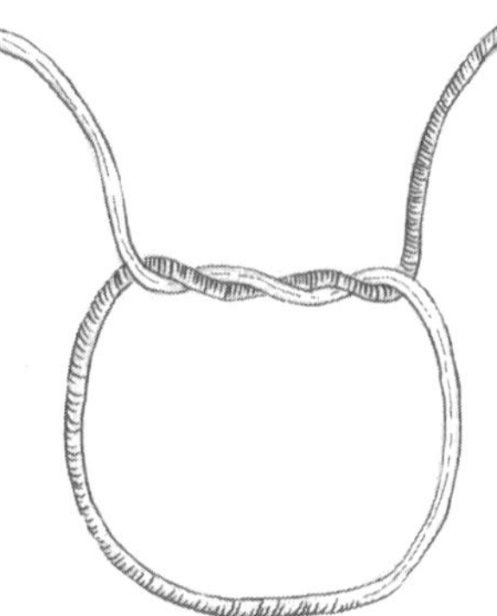

Figure 1.186 Surgeon's knot: This takes longer to tie and places more suture material in the wound than a square knot. It is a good choice where knot security is needed.

* Ethilon Nylon; Ethicon, Somerville, NJ, USA.
† Prolene; Ethicon, Somerville, NJ, USA.
‡ Novafil, Syneture; United States Surgical, Tyco Healthcare Group, Norwalk, CT, USA.
§ Vicryl; Ethicon, Somerville, NJ, USA.
** PDS II; Ethicon, Somerville, NJ, USA.

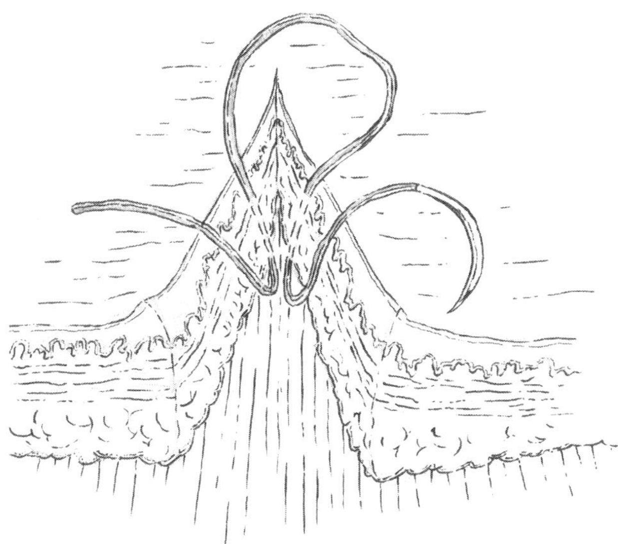

Figure 1.187 Subcuticular pattern: First knot. The first bite from deep subcutaneous tissue to just ventral to the dermis (deep to superficial), and the second bite is reversed (superficial to deep).

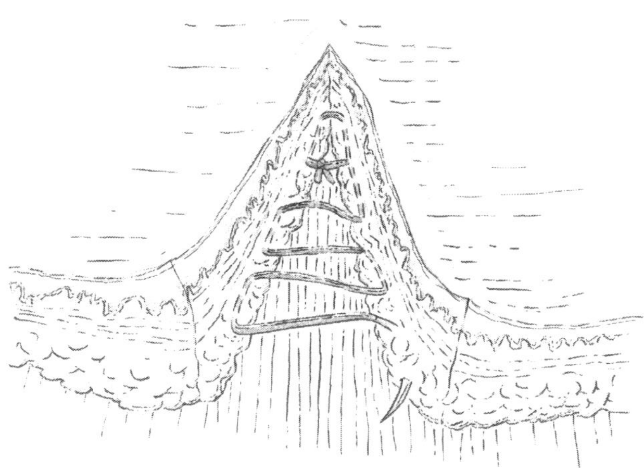

Figure 1.188 Subcuticular pattern: The suture is extended by taking repeated horizontal bites on opposite sides of the wound.

Suture patterns

Subcuticular

Techniquc

The first knot is buried by taking first bite from deep subcutaneous tissue to just ventral to the dermis (deep to superficial), and the second bite is reversed (superficial to deep) (Figure 1.187). This is tied off, and the suture is extended by taking repeated horizontal bites on opposite sides of the wound (Figure 1.188). The final knot (Figure 1.189) is tied deeply; then the free end is buried by inserting the needle through skin away from wound and cutting off the suture under tension.

Advantages

- Helps to give a good result; approximates the skin margins
- Closes dead space

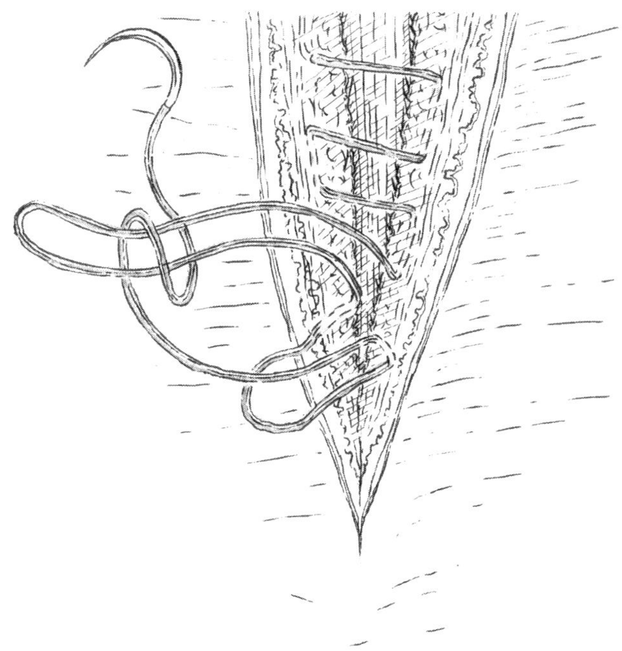

Figure 1.189 Subcuticular pattern: Tying the final knot. The free end of the suture is tied around the penultimate loop as shown, and then the knot is buried deeply.

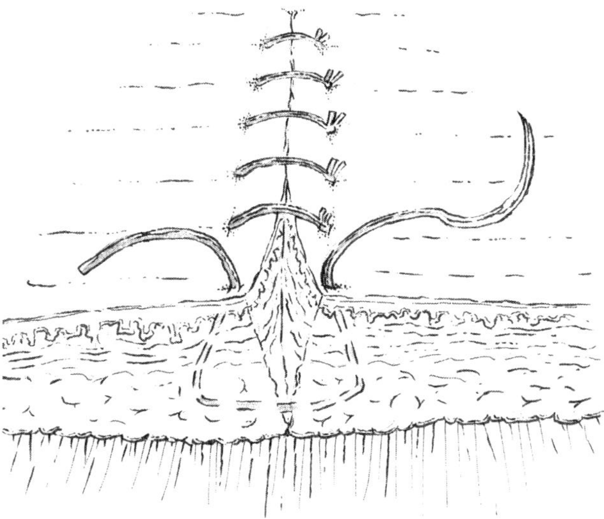

Figure 1.190 Simple interrupted pattern: The needle is passed through the skin at a slight angle, so that slightly larger bites of the dermis are taken.

Simple interrupted

Technique

The needle is directed perpendicularly to the wound. Ideally, these sutures are placed with a cutting needle and swaged suture.[4] A single "bite" through equal amount of tissue is taken on both sides of the wound. The needle should pass through the skin at a slight angle, so that slightly more dermis is taken in the bite, (Figure 1.190). This will evert the edge slightly and give flatter scar after suture removal.[4] The knot is preferably offset to one side

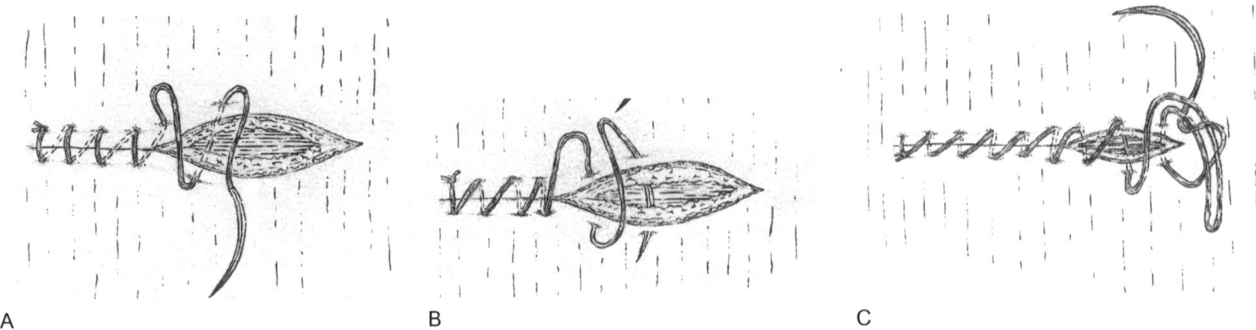

Figure 1.191 Simple continuous pattern: The suture may be advanced above (**A**) or below (**B**) the skin. To make the final knot, the free end of the suture is tied around the penultimate loop as shown (**C**).

of the wound to avoid irritation. Ends should be left long enough to allow easy removal; consider the temperament of patient.

Advantages

- Good tissue apposition (if applied correctly)
- Good alignment of skin edges
- Allows tissue mobility
- Can vary tension on each suture
- Minimal impact on blood supply to wound edges
- Reasonable cosmetic result
- Single sutures may be removed if wound drainage becomes necessary.

Disadvantages

- May cause inversion of wound if excessive tension placed on knot
- Uses large amount suture material
- Slow to place
- Minimal holding power under stress

Simple continuous

Technique

The technique is similar to that for simple interrupted, but the suture is tied only at the beginning and end of the suture (Figure 1.191). The suture may be advanced above or below the skin.

Advantages

- Quick to place
- Provides the most uniform support
- Provides a good seal (if no tension on tissue)

Disadvantages

- May reduce microcirculation to wound edges
- Single failure in the suture disastrous
- Prolongs the inflammatory phase of wound healing[2]
- Increases oedema[2]
- Less strong than simple interrupted
- Gives a less cosmetic result than simple interrupted

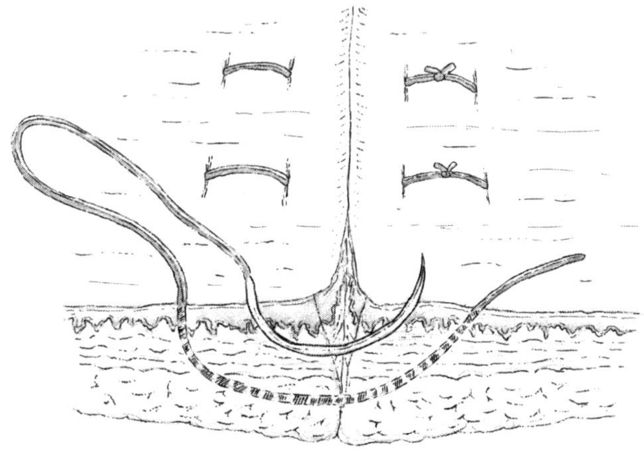

Figure 1.192 Vertical mattress pattern: The basic pattern of suture placement is far-far-near-near.

Vertical mattress

Technique

The needle is directed perpendicular to the skin edge. The basic pattern of suture placement is far-far-near-near (Figure 1.192). The second reversed bite (near-near) splits the thickness of the skin.

Advantages

- Prevents inversion and gapping of wound
- Tension relief suture
- Versatile; can be used with simple interrupted in sites with a lot of tension, "echelon suture pattern"[3] (Figure 1.193) or with quills or stents (Figure 1.194)
- Obliterates dead space
- Minimal impact on blood supply to wound edges
- Gives good cosmetic result (due to slight eversion of skin edges)
- Stronger than horizontal mattress pattern

Disadvantages

- Slow to place and must be placed accurately
- Requires skin at margins of wound to be healthy

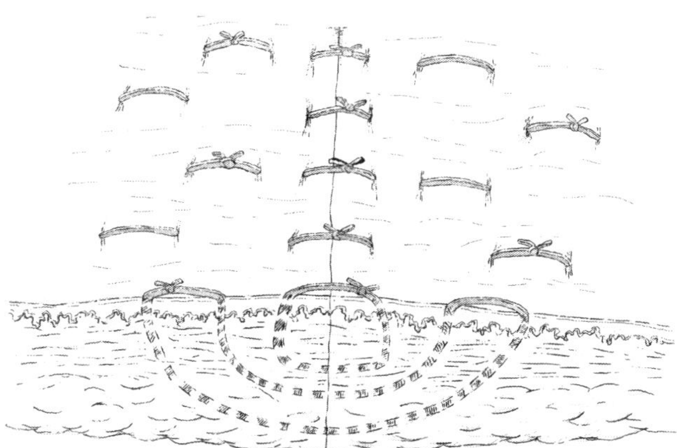

Figure 1.193 "Echelon" suture pattern: This is an adaptation of the vertical mattress suture, in areas with a lot of tension.

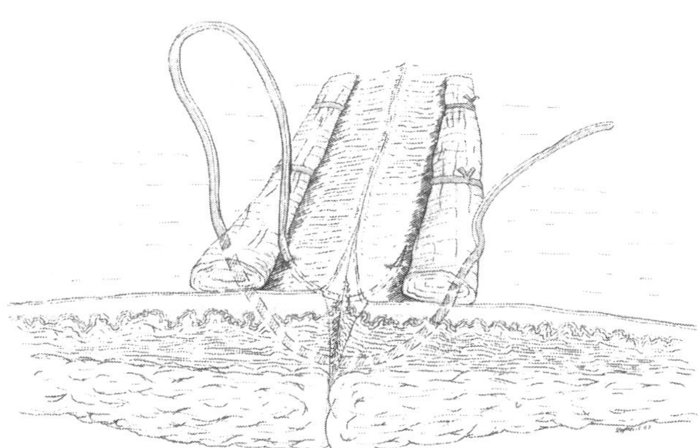

Figure 1.194 Vertical mattress pattern with stents: Sutures looped over a stent (gauze bandage) can be combined with appositional skin suture patterns, in areas of extreme tension.

Horizontal mattress

Technique

This suture technique starts with a similar pattern to the simple interrupted pattern. After the first bite is taken, the needle direction is reversed and a second bite is taken back across the wound. The two ends are then tied (Figure 1.195).

Advantages

- Tension relief
- Can be modified to appose V-shaped flap; see corner suture
- The knot is kept away from the wound.
- May be used with quills (Figure 1.196) or stents

Disadvantages

- Excessive scar formation due to eversion and gapping of skin (not an appositional suture)
- Reduced blood supply to wound edges, potential for skin strangulation; this risk is reduced if stents are used.

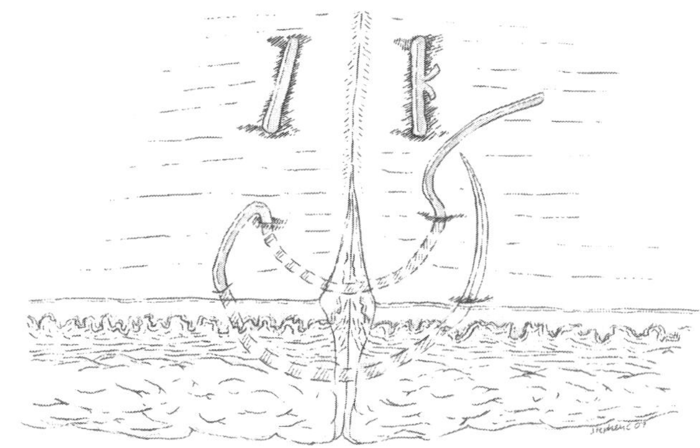

Figure 1.195 Horizontal mattress pattern: This pattern starts in the same way as a simple interrupted pattern. After the first bite is taken, the needle direction is reversed and a second bite taken back across the wound.

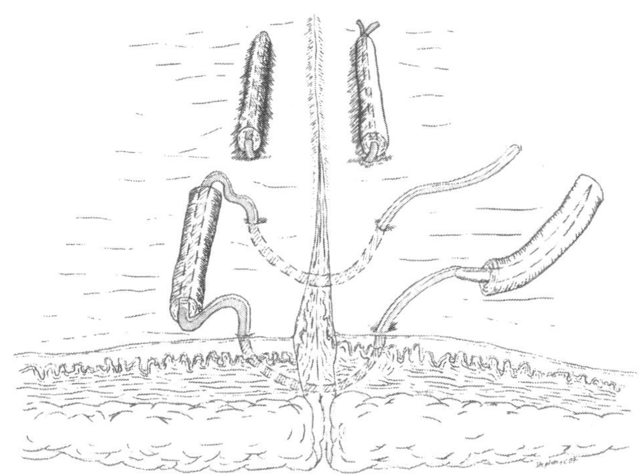

Figure 1.196 Horizontal mattress pattern with quills: The quills are threaded onto the suture between bites, and before the knot is tied. This pattern is used to relieve tension across a wound or incision.

Corner suture (three-point or half-buried mattress suture)

Technique

Essentially, this is a modified horizontal mattress suture (Figures 1.197 and 1.198). The bite that passes through the tip of the flap is placed wholly in the dermis.

Advantages

- Closes point of V-shaped wound with a reduced incidence of tissue necrosis at the tip
- Can be used to convert a V-shaped wound into a Y-shaped wound for closure (Figure 1.198)

Cruciate

Technique

The needle is passed perpendicularly across wound then brought diagonally back over wound to take second bite proximal and parallel to first (Figure 1.199). The suture ends, which are now on opposite sides of the wound, are then tied.

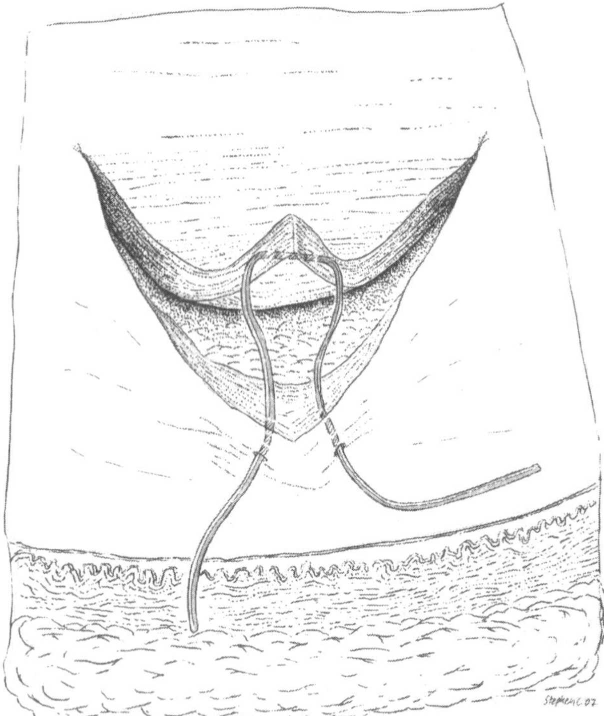

Figure 1.197 Closing a "V-shaped" flap or wound. The bite that passes through the tip of the flap is placed in the dermis.

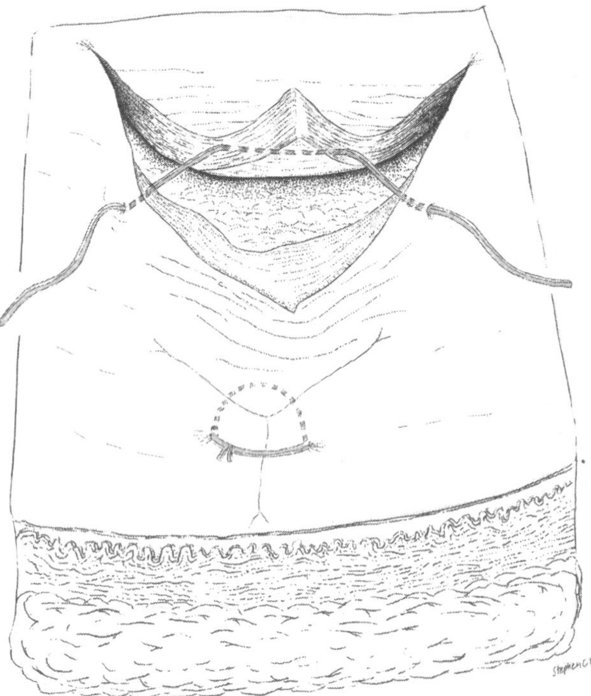

Figure 1.198 Converting a "V-shaped" flap or wound to a "Y-shaped" deficit, to aid closure and ease tension.

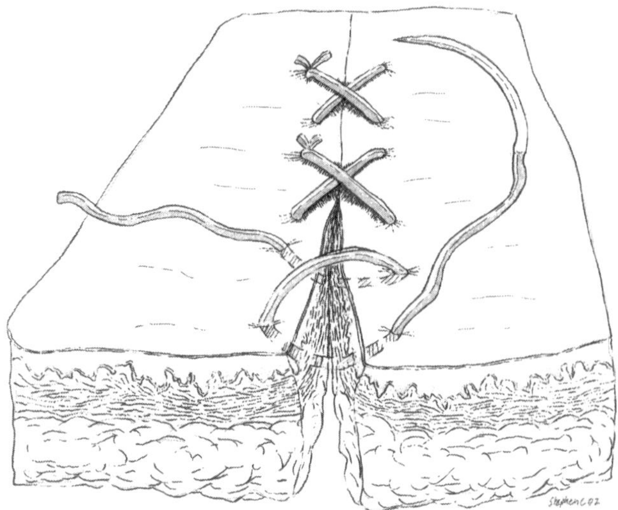

Figure 1.199 Cruciate suture pattern.

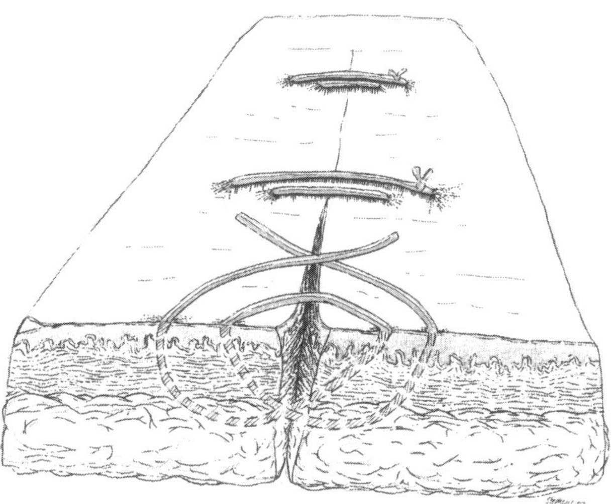

Figure 1.200 Far-near-near-far suture pattern.

Advantages

- Minimal effect on blood supply to wound edges
- Faster than simple interrupted
- Tension suture; provides strength

Disadvantages

- May cause skin inversion
- There may be gapping of skin between sutures

Far-near, near-far

Technique

The far component relieves tension and the near component apposes the skin edges (Figure 1.200).

Advantage

- Higher tensile strength than vertical/horizontal mattress patterns

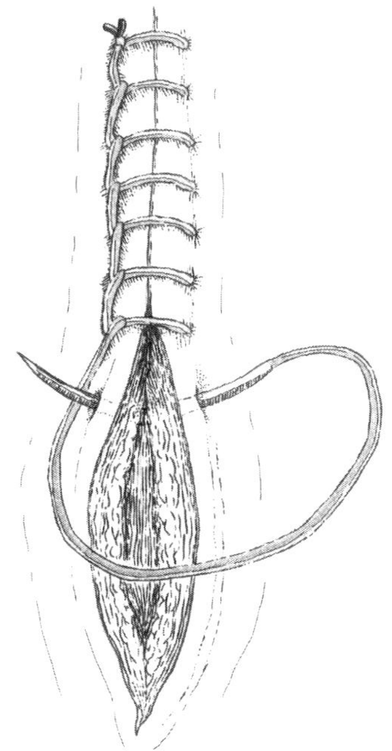

Figure 1.201 Continuous interlocking suture pattern. Also called blanket stitch or Ford interlocking pattern.

Disadvantage
- Large amount of suture material in the wound

Continuous interlocking (blanket stitch, Ford interlocking)
Technique
Technique consists of a series of parallel bites, each taken in the same direction. The needle passes above the unused suture following each bite (Figure 1.201).

Advantages
- Greater security if partial failure of suture line
- Even tension relief along wound

Disadvantages
- Large amount of suture used
- May cause pressure necrosis
- Slow to remove

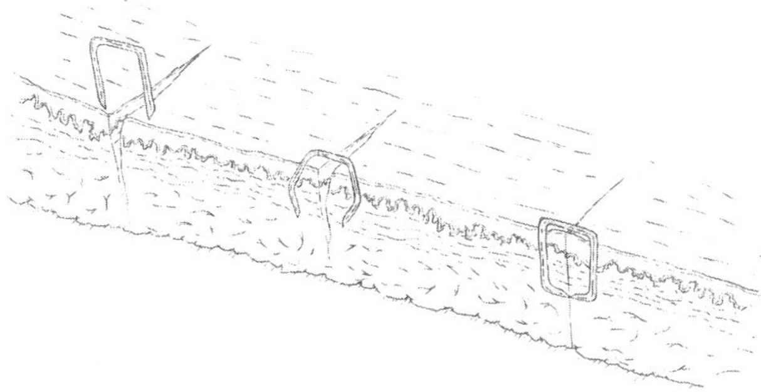

Figure 1.202 Skin staples. The staple forms a rectangular pattern, which results in good skin apposition.

Skin Staples
Technique
The arrow on the instrument is aligned midline on wound. The instrument is then pressed down firmly, and the trigger is pulled to release a single staple (Figure 1.202).

Advantages
- Horses can generally tolerate placement without local anaesthetic.
- Very quick
- Good apposition
- Inert

Disadvantages
- Will not work if there is any tension on wound
- Must be able to oppose the skin edges manually

References

1. Blackford L: Suture materials and patterns, in Auer JA, Stick JA (eds): Equine Surgery, ed 3. St. Louis, Saunders Elsevier, 2005, pp 187-202
2. Bailey JV: Principles of reconstructive plastic surgery, in Auer JA, Stick JA (eds): Equine Surgery, ed 3. St. Louis, Saunders Elsevier, 2005, pp 254-268
3. Stashak TS: Selection of suture materials and suture patterns for wound closure, in Stashak TS (ed): Equine Wound Management. Philadelphia, Lea and Febiger, 1991, pp 52-67
4. Swaim SF, Henderson RA: Wound management, in Swaim SF, Henderson RA (eds): Small Animal Wound Management. Baltimore, Williams and Wilkins, 1997, pp 13-51

2

Procedures in the neonatal foal

Kevin Corley

2.1 Nasotracheal and orotracheal intubation
2.2 Cardiopulmonary resuscitation
2.3 Mechanical ventilation
2.4 Restraint of the neonatal foal
2.5 Placing an indwelling nasogastric tube
2.6 Jugular vein catheterisation
2.7 Indirect blood pressure measurement
2.8 Collection of arterial blood gas/arterial catheterisation
2.9 Placement of a urinary catheter
2.10 Ultrasonography of the umbilicus

2.1 Nasotracheal and orotracheal intubation

Intubation is relatively straightforward in the foal. Nasotracheal intubation has the advantage of being safe in the conscious foal, because it is possible for the foal to damage the tube with its teeth after orotracheal intubation. Orotracheal intubation is technically easier, and allows the passage of a large bore tube, offering less resistance to airflow.

Equipment required

Intubation is achieved with the use of 55-cm-long, cuffed endotracheal tubes.* The internal diameter of the tube should be matched to the size of the foal (Table 2.1).

Table 2.1. Matching the size (internal diameter) of endotracheal tube to the weight of the foal

Weight of foal	Typical breeds	Typical sizes for nasotracheal intubation	Typical sizes for orotracheal intubation
20–35 kg	Premature foals	7 mm	9 mm
	Pony foals	9 mm	10 mm
35–50 kg	Arab	8 mm	9 mm
	Larger pony breeds	9 mm	10 mm
	Premature foals		
45–60 kg	Thoroughbred	9 mm	10 mm
	Warmblood	10 mm	12 mm
60–80 kg	Draft breeds	12 mm	12 mm
			14 mm

Smaller tubes are easier to pass but provide more resistance to airflow.

* Jorgenson Laboratiories, Loveland, CO, USA.

Nasotracheal intubation

In the conscious or lightly sedated foal, the foal should be standing or in sternal recumbency. The head should be extended, so that the head is in line with the neck. This allows a straight line through the nares and the larynx to the trachea. Intubation is easiest if the nondominant hand is held just under the end of the mandible, to extend the head. The fingers of this hand can be used to direct the end of the tube into the ventral meatus. In the unconscious or heavily sedated foal, place the foal flat on the ground, with the head extended, so that the ventral neck is parallel to the lower jaw. The tube should be held so that it curves downwards. One hand should be used to push the tip of the tube medially and ventrally in the nares, into the ventral meatus. The other hand is used to smoothly advance the tube (Figure 2.1). When the tube reaches the nasopharynx, gentle rotation in either direction can help it slip through the larynx and into the trachea. There is little resistance to advancing the tube, once the end is past the trachea.

Orotracheal intubation

Place the foal flat on the ground, with the head extended, so that the neck and jaw are in a straight line. The tongue should be gently pulled forward and to the side with one hand (Figure 2.2); this helps to stabilise the larynx. The tube is held so that it curves downwards and is smoothly advanced over the tongue, in a midline position. When the end of the tube is in the oropharynx, gentle rotation in either direction can help it slip through the larynx and into the trachea. There is little resistance to advancing the tube, once the end is past the trachea.

Checking that the tube is correctly placed

It is vital to check that the tube has successfully passed into the trachea and did not enter the oesophagus. Compress

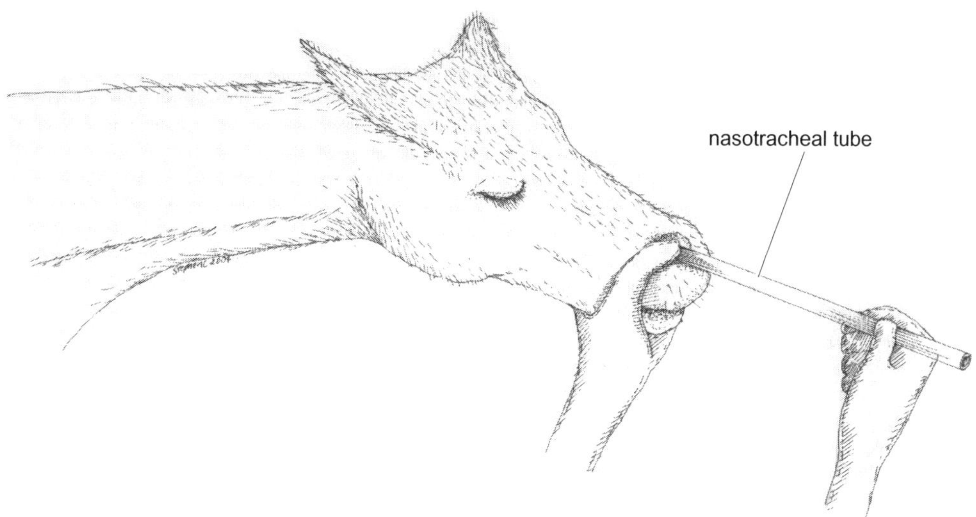

Figure 2.1 Nasotracheal intubation. The thumb of one hand is used to guide the tube ventrally and medially, into the ventral meatus, whilst the other hand advances the tube.

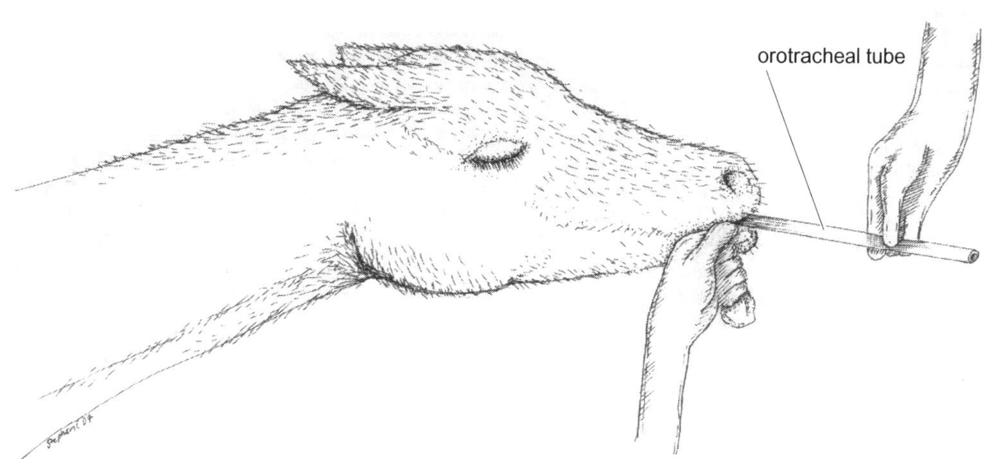

Figure 2.2 Orotracheal intubation. One hand gently pulls the tongue forward, whilst the other hand is used to advance the tube over the tongue to the oropharynx.

the thorax and simultaneously feel for expired air at the proximal tube end. The thoracic wall should also rise when the first breath is given. If the tube has entered the oesophagus, it can often be felt in the cranial neck just dorsal to the caudal larynx or proximal trachea. Once the tube is in place, the cuff of the tracheal tube should be gently inflated.

Strategies for difficult intubations

Tubes passed via the nose can stick at the caudal nasal passage, in the region of the ethmoid turbinates. The tube should be slightly withdrawn, gently rotated and gently advanced. If this is unsuccessful, the tube should be withdrawn, and replaced in the ventral meatus to check it is correctly ventral and medial. If this is not successful, the tube should be placed in the opposite nostril. Most tubes that will pass down the ventral meatus will pass through the caudal nares into the nasopharynx. There is a congenital condition, choanal atresia, where there is a membrane across the caudal aspect of the nares blocking the passage of both the tube and air. The condition can be unilateral or bilateral. Foals with bilateral choanal atresia should have an emergency tracheotomy performed. Orotracheal intubation can also be used in these foals, but this risks damage to the tube and loss of the airway, if the foal is conscious.

During cardiac arrest, if two swift attempts at nasotracheal intubation have proved unsuccessful, orotracheal intubation should be attempted. Occasionally, it can prove hard to pass the tube into the trachea, and the tube continually ends up in the oesophagus. This is most common when there is little muscle tone in the oropharynx. Unfortunately, this occurs most frequently when intubating during cardiopulmonary arrest. Gently occluding the proximal oesophagus, just dorsal to the larynx, by applying

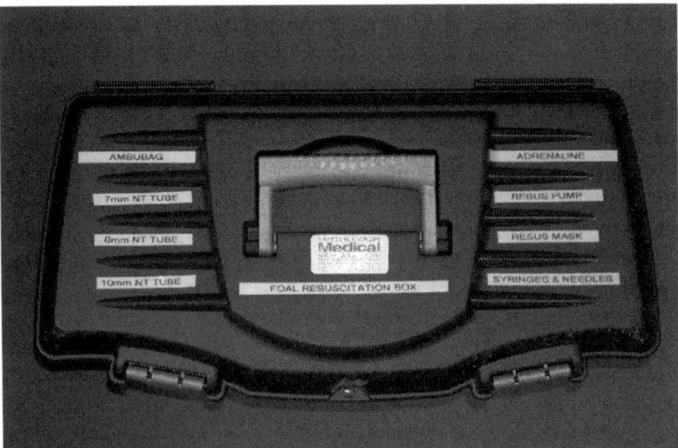

Figure 2.3 Equipment for CPR should be kept in a dedicated box. The contents of the box should be regularly checked, and replaced if necessary. ©Kevin Corley 2004.

pressure to this area either side of the neck can help prevent this. Adjusting the angle of the head relative to the neck can also help a tube pass into the trachea. If necessary, a semistiff wire with a smooth rounded end can be passed into the trachea to use as a guide for the tube. An endoscopic biopsy instrument is suitable for this, if the wire is first passed through the tube. Placement of the wire in the trachea can be checked by rattling the proximal trachea and feeling the wire within it, palpating the oesophagus and confirming the wire is not there, or checking placement by endoscopy or radiography. Keeping a firm hold on the wire, the tube is passed over the wire and into the trachea. If none of these techniques results in successful intubation, a tracheotomy should be considered.

For cardiopulmonary resuscitation, a mask and pump is an alternative to intubation. Mouth-to-nose resuscitation can also be successful.

Box 2.1. Equipment for cardiopulmonary resuscitation

Required
Nasotracheal tube* (see Table 2.1)
5-ml syringe to inflate nasotracheal tube cuff
Self-inflating resuscitation bag†
Small pen torch (flashlight)
Epinephrine (adrenaline) bottle‡
Five 2-ml sterile syringes
20-Gauge 1-inch needles

Additional equipment for newborn foals
Bulb syringe
Clean towels

Equipment that should be available if possible
Oxygen cylinder and flow valve
Steel 14-gauge 1–1.5-inch needles
Four 1-L bags of lactated Ringer's solution
Fluid administration set
14-Gauge IV catheter
End-tidal carbon dioxide monitor
Electrical defibrillator

For stud farms without resident veterinarians
Suitable facemask together with a resuscitation bag or pump§

*Cook Veterinary Products, Bloomington, IN, USA.
†"The Bag" Disposable Resuscitator Adult 840043; Laerdal, Wappingers Falls, NY, USA.
‡Epinephrine injection 1 : 1000; Butler, Dublin, OH, USA.
§C.D. Foal Resuscitator; McCulloch Medical Products, Glenfield, New Zealand.

2.2 Cardiopulmonary resuscitation

The key to successful cardiopulmonary resuscitation (CPR) is a disciplined, ordered approach. The mantra "**Airway, Breathing, Circulation**" is especially important in resuscitation of the newborn foal, because respiratory arrest (rather than cardiac arrest) is almost always the primary problem.

Equipment needed

Keeping the equipment in a dedicated box (Figure 2.3), in a readily accessible place, is essential to allow rapid initiation of CPR. The equipment should be checked before the foal season, after each use and at regular intervals. The equipment recommended for CPR is given in Box 2.1.

The first 20 seconds

The first thing to do is to decide whether CPR is appropriate for this foal. Thereafter, this short time is dedicated to preparing the foal for CPR. The foal should be placed in lateral recumbency on a hard, flat surface. If any of the ribs are broken, the side with the broken ribs should be placed against the ground. If ribs are broken on both sides, the side with more cranial ribs (3, 4 and 5) broken should be placed on the ground. The head should be extended, so that the nose is in a straight line with the trachea.

In the **newborn foal**, the nares and mouth should be cleared of membranes as a priority during this time. Vigorous towel drying should also be started, which acts as a strong stimulus to the foal to start breathing.

Airway

If an endotracheal tube is available, it should be placed as soon as possible. As a rule, no more than two attempts should be made at nasotracheal intubation, before orotracheal intubation is attempted. These techniques are described in Chapter 2.1. The endotracheal tube should be attached to a self-inflating resuscitation bag (Ambu bag).

If an endotracheal tube is not available, or the expertise to use it is not available, the next best option is a pump and mask. The mask should be fitted over the foal's muzzle, to include both nostrils and form a reasonable seal. If possible, a second person should gently occlude the proximal oesophagus, to prevent air being forced into the stomach, which will hinder movement of the diaphragm. The oesophagus is best occluded dorsal to the trachea, just caudal to the larynx. For people with medium-sized to large hands, the fingers can be used on one side of the neck, and the thumb of the same hand on the other side of the neck. The fingers and thumb are gently pressed together on the tissue dorsal to the trachea, to occlude the oesophagus.

Mouth-to-nose resuscitation

If neither an endotracheal tube nor a pump and mask are available, it is possible to perform mouth-to-nose resuscitation. One hand should be used to cup the chin and occlude the down nostril. The other hand should occlude the proximal oesophagus, as described above. The head and neck should be straightened as far as possible to give good access to the airway, but the head should not be lifted (Figure 2.4). The resuscitator should watch to check that the thorax rises as he or she blows into the foal's nostril.

Breathing

The breathing rate should be **10 to 20 breaths per minute**. This is the same, whichever method is used to provide air into the lungs. If possible, the resuscitation bag or pump should be connected to an oxygen supply. However, this is not essential, and CPR should not be delayed or interrupted to connect the oxygen.

Circulation

If, after 30 to 60 seconds of supported ventilation the foal has a heart rate less than 40 beats per minute, thoracic compressions should be started. If the heart rate is between 40 and 60 beats per minute, supported ventilation should be continued for another 30 to 60 seconds and then the heart rate rechecked. If it has decreased or not changed during this period, thoracic compressions should be started.

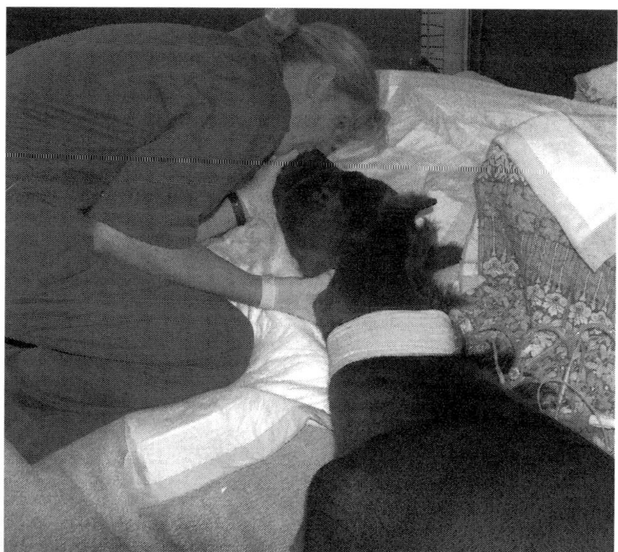

Figure 2.4 Mouth-to-nose resuscitation. The mouth is placed over the uppermost nares. One hand occludes the lower nares, whilst the other hand occludes the oesophagus. ©Kevin Corley and Jane Axon 2004.

The foal should be on a hard surface in lateral recumbency for thoracic compressions. If the foal is being cared for on a foal mat, it needs to be moved to the floor prior to thoracic compressions. The best position for the resuscitator to adopt when performing thoracic compressions is as follows: The resuscitator should kneel down, close to the foal's backbone at the level of the thorax (Figure 2.5). The resuscitator should place his or her hands at the highest part of the thorax, about one handwidth behind the triceps mass. The hands are placed flat on the thorax, one hand on top of the other. The resuscitator should lean forwards so that his or her shoulders are directly over his or her hands. The resuscitator should then transfer his or her weight forward, to put firm even pressure on the hands, keeping the elbows locked, and aim to compress the chest. The hands should travel through approximately 3 to 5 cm as they compress the chest (Figure 2.5). The aim is for fast compressions, in the region of **90 to 120 compressions per minute**. An effort should be made not to put any pressure on the thorax in the brief gap between compressions. Performing thoracic compressions is extremely tiring. If more than one person is available, they should take turns at thoracic compressions every 2 to 3 minutes. If only one person is available, he or she should perform 15 thoracic compressions, followed by 2 breaths. If two people are performing the CPR, the two resuscitators should perform breathing and compressions at the same time, at the appropriate rates. Thoracic compressions should not be interrupted for a breath.

If available, an electrogardiograph (ECG) should be connected to the foal. The base-apex lead position (lead I, with one arm lead on the jugular groove, and the other just above or behind the heart, and the leg leads anywhere on the neck) is quick to attach and suitable for determining the rhythm of the heart.

Drugs

Epinephrine (adrenaline) is the most useful drug in resuscitation of the foal. It should be given if the heart rate remains very low (<40 bpm) or absent after 2 minutes of full CPR (thoracic compressions and breathing). The dose is **0.01 to 0.02 mg/kg IV** (**0.5 to 1.0 ml per 50 kg body weight**) when using standard 1 mg/ml (1:1000) epinephrine. This dose should be repeated every 3 to 5 minutes until a regular heart rate has returned, or it has been decided that CPR has been unsuccessful. If venous access is not possible, epinephrine can be injected into the trachea (below the cuff of the endotracheal tube, if present). The dose for intratracheal epinephrine is 0.1 to 0.2 mg/kg (5 to 10 ml per 50 kg body weight). Intracardiac injection should be avoided.

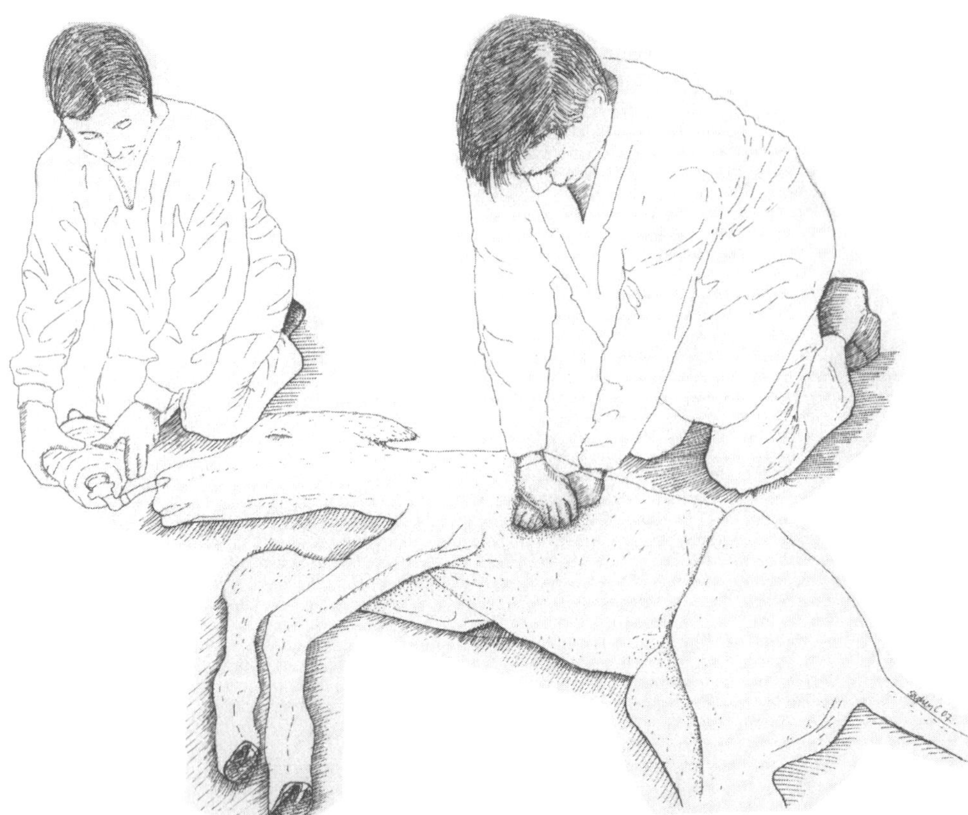

Figure 2.5 Positive pressure ventilation and thoracic compressions in a foal. Thoracic compressions are delivered by kneeling with the shoulders over the hands. The hands are at the highest point of the foal's thorax, just behind the triceps mass. Thoracic compressions should not stop during delivery of breaths.

Other drugs have a much more minor role in CPR of foals and are rarely used in acute resuscitation. Fluid therapy (bolus of 10 ml/kg crystalloids) may be helpful in restoring the circulation. The following drugs are contraindicated in resuscitation of the newborn foal: **atropine, calcium** and **doxapram.**

Defibrillation

If ventricular fibrillation is recognised, undulating electrical activity with no discernable complexes, electrical defibrillation is appropriate. Electrical defibrillation may also be used on a foal in asystole that does not respond to thoracic compressions and epinephrine injection. The dose is **2 to 4 J/kg** (**100 to 200 J per 50 kg**), increasing the energy by 50% with each defibrillation attempt.

Monitoring CPR

The effectiveness of CPR can be monitored in several ways. A positive (normal) pupillary light response suggests that an adequate circulation is being maintained. A dilated, fixed pupil is a poor prognostic sign. The strength and consistency of a peripheral pulse can also be felt to monitor thoracic compressions, but this is difficult during resuscitation.

If available, end-tidal carbon dioxide (CO_2) tension represents the best way to monitor the effectiveness of cardiopulmonary resuscitation. Tensions greater than 15 mm Hg indicate good perfusion and portend a good prognosis, whereas tensions persistently lower than 10 mm Hg indicate ineffective CPR and a poor prognosis.

When to stop

If started, thoracic compressions should be stopped when there is a regular heart beat of greater than 60 bpm. Ventilatory support should be stopped when there is regular, spontaneous breathing at a rate greater than 15 breaths/min. It is important not to stop ventilatory support too early. Intermittent support may be required before it can be completely withdrawn. A spontaneous heartbeat should start instantly when thoracic compressions are stopped. However, there may be a lag between stopping ventilatory support and spontaneous breathing, due to decreased blood CO_2 tensions. This lag period should not be greater than 30 seconds; after this time, if there are no spontaneous breaths, ventilatory support should be restarted.

If there is no return of spontaneous circulation after 15 minutes of full CPR, the outlook is hopeless.

An overview of CPR is given inside the back cover.

2.3 Mechanical ventilation

Mechanical ventilation is a therapy that is undertaken on relatively few foals, as it is only available at a few hospitals. However, with good patient selection and correct application, mechanical ventilation is both a clinically and financially worthwhile therapy.

Indications

Foals that are candidates for mechanical ventilation fall into two broad groups. Group 1 consists of conditions where there is a failure of neurological control of breathing, and Group 2 consists of conditions where there is primary lung pathology (Box 2.2). Generally, foals that fall into group 1 present with hypercapnia and a relatively normal alveolar-arterial oxygen gradient. Group 2 foals often present with hypoxaemia that is variably accompanied by hypercapnia.

The prognosis between these two groups is markedly different. Group 1 foals have a good to excellent prognosis (greater than 80% discharge rate from the hospital[1,2]), provided mechanical ventilation is instituted early. Group 2 foals have a much more guarded prognosis. The timing of institution of mechanical ventilation is vital to success in both groups. There has been a tendency in some clinics to reserve mechanical ventilation for moribund patients, with inevitable poor outcomes.

Equipment needed

The equipment required for mechanical ventilation is given in Box 2.3. If ventilating using cylinders of compressed air and oxygen, these will have to be replaced fairly frequently. A "J" size (6400-litre) compressed air cylinder may only provide 6 to 8 hours of ventilation, depending on the ventilator settings. The respiratory and circulatory systems need to be monitored closely during mechanical ventilation.

Preparation for mechanical ventilation

Nasotracheal intubation (see Chapter 2.1) is greatly preferred for ventilation. Use of a nasotracheal tube (as opposed to an orotracheal tube) allows mechanical ventilation without sedation or anaesthesia. Foals that are showing jerky muscular movements as part of their disease process (most often, foals with perinatal asphyxia syndrome) may require sedation for mechanical ventilation. The largest-diameter nasotracheal tube that it is possible to pass should be employed (see Chapter 2.1). The relative ease of placing and maintaining a nasotracheal tube means that tracheostomy is only very rarely utilised to ensure an airway. The foal should be maintained in sternal recumbency on a soft mat, if possible. This is to promote equal ventilation of both lungs. If an active humidifier/warmer is being used in

Box 2.2. Underlying disease conditions in foals that are candidates for mechanical ventilation

Group 1

Conditions where there is a failure of neurological control of breathing

- Perinatal asphyxia syndrome
- Botulism
- Prematurity
- Avermectin (usually moxidectin) toxicity

Group 2

Conditions of primary lung pathology

- Infectious pneumonia (bacterial or viral)
- Acute lung injury
- Acute respiratory distress syndrome
- Neonatal respiratory distress syndrome

Box 2.3. Equipment needed for mechanical ventilation of the foal

Required

Critical care ventilator with synchronised intermittent mandatory ventilation (SIMV) and pressure support (PS) modes

- Many ventilators are suitable.
- Examples of ventilators that have been used for foal ventilation include:
  - Siemens Servo 900C
  - Puritan-Bennett 840
  - Bird 6400 ST
  - Newport Breeze E150
  - Bear 1000

Sterile ventilation circuit tubing
Active humidifier, or heat-moisture exchange (HME) filters
Nasotracheal tube (see Table 2.1)
Oxygen supply, with suitable connectors to attach to the ventilator
Compressed air supply (compressor or cylinders), with suitable connectors to attach to the ventilator
Blood gas analyser
Blood pressure monitor

Equipment that should be available if possible

End-tidal carbon dioxide monitor
Blood lactate analyser
Suction—manual aspirator* or suction machine with suction catheter (catheter width no wider than half the internal size of the nasotracheal tube)

Helpful, if available

Continuous (indwelling cannula) blood gas analysis
Pressure-flow loop analyser
Cardiac output monitor

*For example, RES-Q-VAC; Repro-Med Systems Inc., Chester, NY, USA.

the circuit, the circuit should be prewarmed if possible to reduce "rain-out". Use of heat-moisture exchange (HME) filters prevents the problems associated with maintaining an active humidifier.

Connecting the foal to the ventilator

Initial settings for ventilation should be chosen, and dialled into the ventilator, prior to attaching the foal. Examples of initial settings are given in Box 2.4. The most commonly used mode for ventilation in the foal is synchronised intermittent mandatory ventilation (SIMV) with pressure support, which is described in Box 2.5.

The exact way to connect the circuit to the ventilator will depend on the make of ventilator, but is likely to be similar to the description that follows. There is one port on the ventilator marked "To Patient" or "Main Flow to Patient" or "Inspiratory Port". This port is connected to the active humidifier (if used) by a short length of tubing (Figure 2.6). The port marked "From Patient" or "Expiratory Port" should be attached to an HME filter (Figure 2.7). If a water trap is incorporated into the expiratory arm, the bottle should be attached (Figure 2.6). The circuit should then be connected. The inspiratory part of the circuit is attached to the "To Patient" port (without an active humidifier) or to the output of the active humidifier, and the expiratory arm of the circuit is attached to the "From Patient" port. If used, the fluid collection caps should be fitted to the centre of each arm of the circuit. If there is a proximal pressure sensor on the ventilator, the tubing from this should be connected to the pressure port on the Y-piece of the circuit. If the ventilator has a temperature sensor, this should be

Box 2.4. Example of initial settings for mechanical ventilation in the foal

Mode	SIMV-PS
Minute volume	160–240 ml/kg/min
Tidal volume	6–8 ml/kg
SIMV breaths per minute	20–30
PEEP	5–10 cm H_2O
Pressure support	10 cm H_2O
Trigger sensitivity	–2 cm H_2O
I:E ratio	1:2
FiO_2	Usually start with 1.0 Rapidly try to decrease below 0.6

Aim for

- Improved arterial blood gas results
- Plateau pressures below 30 cm H_2O
- As low FiO_2 as possible
- Good ventilator–patient synchrony

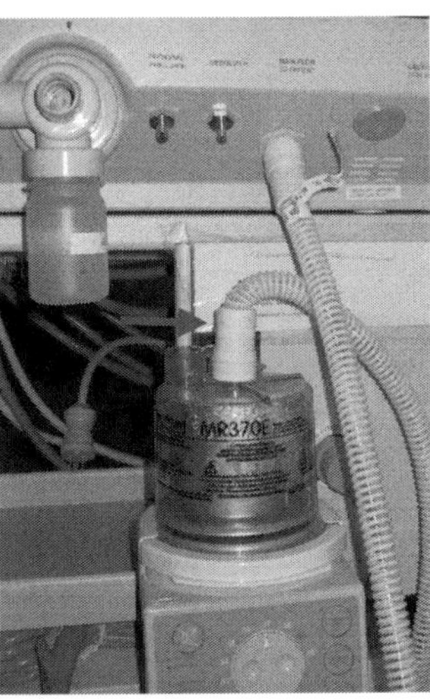

Figure 2.6 Connecting the inspiratory arm of the ventilator circuit to an active humidifier. The water trap bottle on the expiratory arm is also illustrated. ©Harold McKenzie III 2006.

Box 2.5. Description of foal-ventilator interactions in the synchronised intermittent mandatory ventilation with pressure support (SIMV-PS) mode

SIMV period

During this period, the machine waits for the foal to trigger a breath (by generating a negative pressure less than the trigger sensitivity). If the foal triggers a breath, a full mechanical breath is delivered according to the settings on the ventilator. After the breath is delivered, the machine switches to the spontaneous period for the rest of the ventilation cycle. If the foal makes no sufficient respiratory effort during the entire SIMV period, a full mechanical breath is delivered at the end of the SIMV period without a foal trigger.

Spontaneous period

During this period, respiratory efforts by the foal result in supported spontaneous breathing, rather than full mechanical breaths. In SIMV without pressure support, the only support is that the oxygen concentration that the foal breathes in from the circuit may be greater than room air. However, there is some extra work of breathing to overcome the resistance of the circuit.

Pressure support—the foal triggers the breath, set by the trigger sensitivity. During this breath, the ventilator applies a set pressure. When the inspiratory flow reaches a predetermined (usually not user controlled) percentage of the peak flow, the ventilator switches into expiration and the pressure is switched off. In many ventilators, this switch to expiration occurs at 25% of peak flow. The breath rate is used as a safety feature in pressure support, as a time-gate to prevent the ventilator being stuck in inspiration if there is a leak in the circuit and flow does not decelerate. If pressure support is used together with positive end-expiratory pressure (PEEP), it is added to PEEP during inspiration.

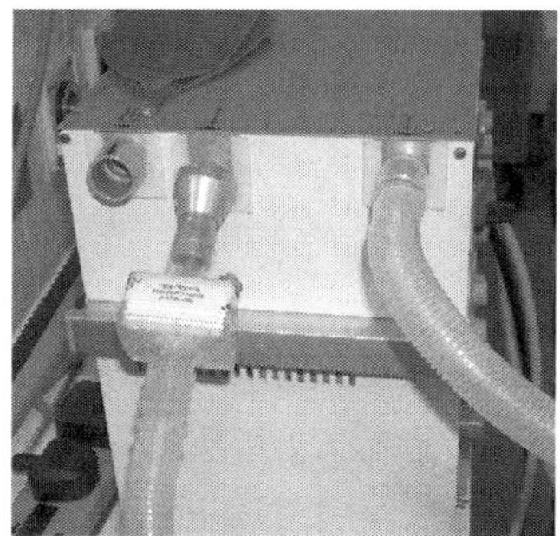

Figure 2.7 A heat-moisture exchange (HME) filter attached to the expiratory arm of the ventilator circuit. ©Kevin Corley 2006.

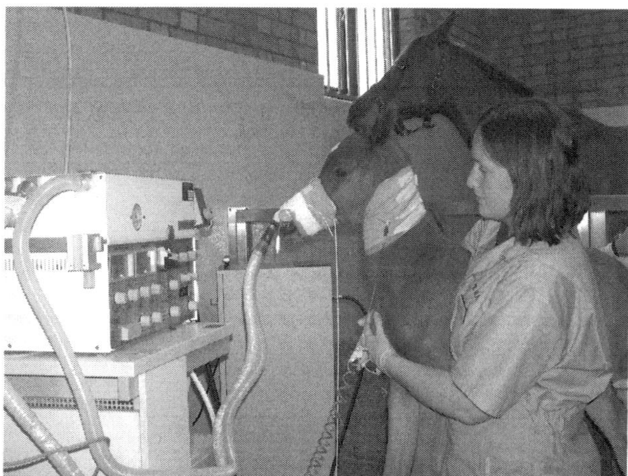

Figure 2.8 A foal standing with assistance whilst being ventilated. This foal is being ventilated with reverse-ratio pressure-controlled ventilation (see Box 2.8). ©Kevin Corley 2005.

Box 2.6. Monitoring and maintenance in foals maintained on mechanical ventilation

Essential monitoring
- Patient response and physical examination
- Thoracic auscultation
- Arterial blood gas tensions
- Blood pressure
- Blood lactate concentration
- Culture respiratory secretions
- Thoracic radiographs

Additional monitoring if available
- End-tidal carbon dioxide concentration
- Pulse oximetry
- Ventilator flow-pressure loops

Regular maintenance
- Regular deflation/reinflation of the cuff
- Respiratory toilet
- Nasotracheal tube exchange

connected to the temperature port in the Y-piece, and to the humidifier and humidifier discharge, if appropriate. If an end-tidal CO_2 monitor is being used, this should then be attached to the port in the Y-piece (if present). For side-stream CO_2 monitors, the clear plastic adapter should be attached to the end of the Y-piece. The ventilator circuit should then be attached to the nasotracheal tube in the foal.

Adjusting the ventilator to the foal

Choosing the optimum settings for ventilation of an individual foal is achieved by a combination of observing the effects on the cardiorespiratory system and the patient's respiratory efforts. Parameters to monitor are given in Box 2.6.

Achieving patient–ventilator synchrony is extremely important to effective mechanical ventilation. If the patient attempts to breathe out during the inspiratory phase of a mechanical breath or breathe in during the expiratory phase, this leads to a phenomenon known as "bucking" the ventilator. This prevents an adequate tidal volume being delivered and causes patient discomfort. Often, the ventilator will briefly alarm for high pressure during a patient "buck", as the opposing efforts of the patient and ventilator greatly increase the pressure in the circuit. Strategies for improving patient–ventilator synchrony are given in Box 2.7. Sedation to improve synchrony is rarely required, and foals will tolerate ventilation when fully conscious (Figure 2.8).

Box 2.7. Strategies for improving ventilator–patient synchrony

Change the frequency of ventilator-delivered breaths
- Most often, increasing the frequency helps synchrony.
- The tidal volume should be changed appropriately to maintain the desired minute volume.

Change the mode of ventilation
- Synchronised mandatory intermittent ventilation is usually the best-tolerated mode in foals.
- Occasionally, a switch from volume-cycled ventilation to pressure-cycled ventilation can improve synchrony.

Change spontaneous period duration in SIMV mode
- Changing the duration of the spontaneous period within the ventilation cycle (usually increasing the spontaneous period) can help patient synchrony.

Change the flow profile of the mechanical breath
- Occasionally, changing from a square flow profile to an accelerating profile can help.

Sedate the foal
- This is rarely required, and is the action of last resort to improve synchrony.
- Possible sedatives include
  - Propofol, constant rate infusion, to effect
  - Midazolam 0.2–1.0 mg/kg/hr constant rate infusion

Box 2.8. Strategies for improving arterial blood gas tensions during ventilator treatment

To decrease arterial carbon dioxide tension (target 35–55 mm Hg)

- Increase expired minute volume.
  - Increase frequency of machine-delivered breaths.
  - Increase tidal volume.
  - Possible side effects
    - Increased intrathoracic pressure causing decreased cardiac filling
    - Increased plateau pressures and barotraumas
- Decrease deadspace ventilation.
  - Decrease distance between ventilator circuit and nares.
  - Increase positive end-expiratory pressure (PEEP) to recruit alveoli.
  - Avoid excessive PEEP, which will result in further increases in $PaCO_2$.
  - Possible side effects
    - PEEP increases intrathoracic pressure causing decreased cardiac filling.

To increase arterial oxygen tension (target 70–120 mm Hg)

- Increase fraction of inspired oxygen (FIO_2).
  - Possible side effects
    - Prolonged (>48–72 hours) $FIO_2 > 0.6$ may result in oxygen toxicity (oxidative damage to the lung tissue).
- Increase positive end-expiratory pressure (PEEP).
  - Helps gas exchange in the alveoli
  - Possible side effects
    - PEEP increases intrathoracic pressure causing decreased cardiac filling.
- Institute reverse-ratio ventilation.
  - Allows longer for gas exchange in the alveoli
  - Initially change I:E ratio to 1:1. Can be changed to 2:1, if necessary
  - I:E ratios of greater than 1 : 1 are best tolerated in pressure-controlled ventilation.
  - In volume-controlled ventilation, deep sedation may be necessary.
  - Possible side effects
    - Can have profound negative effects on cardiovascular system

Changing the ventilator to improve arterial blood gas tensions is always a compromise between the beneficial and harmful effects of increasing gas exchange. In general, ventilator settings that improve gas exchange are detrimental to the circulation. Therefore, in addition to monitoring the respiratory response, cardiovascular variables should also be monitored (Box 2.6). Strategies for reducing CO_2 tension or improving arterial oxygenation of the blood are given in Box 2.8.

Maintenance

The disease process can be very dynamic in critically ill foals, and this can mean that ventilator settings may need to be frequently changed to maintain optimum ventilation. Therefore ventilated foals should be intensively monitored (Box 2.6). Ventilated foals also require some routine maintenance. The cuff should be deflated and reinflated at least every 6 hours to prevent pressure necrosis of the tracheal lining. In foals with an exudative respiratory disease, regular respiratory toilet is necessary to remove respiratory secretions, improve ventilation and prevent tracheal tube obstruction. The frequency of respiratory toilet depends on how much secretions are being produced, and the thickness of the secretions, but it may not be necessary in every patient. A long catheter (either a dog urinary catheter or a specifically designed suction catheter) should be placed down the nasotracheal tube and intermittent suction applied to remove the respiratory secretions from both the tube and the airway just beyond it. Suction should not be applied for more than 5 to 10 seconds at a time, as it inhibits inspiratory movements. Percussion or coupage (see Chapter 18) prior to suctioning the airway helps loosen secretions ready for aspiration.

Weaning

Weaning from mechanical ventilation should be considered if the FIO_2 is less than 0.40, the arterial oxygen tension is greater than 70 mm Hg, the CO_2 tension is less than 55 mm Hg and the foal is making good respiratory movements. As the foal improves, the frequency of mechanical breaths in SIMV mode can be reduced to move the foal towards more spontaneous breaths and weaning. If available, pressure support (PS) or continuous positive airway pressure (CPAP) ventilation should be provided, after stopping machine delivered breaths. Both these modes provide some support to reduce the work of breathing and ease the transition to spontaneous ventilation. If these are not available, the alternative is to remove the foal from the ventilator and supply supplementary oxygen through a T-piece connected to the nasotracheal tube or by extubating and providing intranasal oxygen. For PS, the pressure should be set at 10 cm H_2O and the peak end-expiratory pressure (PEEP) at 5 cm H_2O or less. The amount of PS is gradually reduced, and the foal is disconnected from the machine when it reaches 5 cm H_2O or less. For CPAP, the PEEP level should be initially set at 5 cm H_2O and gradually reduced.

It is important to continue to intensively monitor the cardiorespiratory system of foals that have been mechanically ventilated in the first 48 to 72 hours after weaning has been completed, as foals are particularly prone to relapses or further pathological changes during this period.

References

1. Wilkins PA, Palmer JE: Mechanical ventilation in foals with botulism: 9 cases (1989-2002). J Vet Intern Med 17:708-712, 2003
2. Palmer JE: Ventilatory support of the critically ill foal. Vet Clin North Am Equine Pract 21:457-486, vii-viii, 2005

2.4 Restraint of the neonatal foal

Proper restraint of the neonatal foal is the key to safety when carrying out procedures. For most procedures, it is easiest and safest to restrain the foal in lateral recumbency. Straightforward procedures, such as jugular venous blood collection, can be done with the foal standing or in sternal recumbency.

Restraint of the standing foal

The degree of restraint applied to the foal needs to be matched to the temperament of the animal. In almost all situations, one person is required to hold the foal whilst another performs the procedure. In a few foals, more than one person is required for the restraint. However, in many foals, increasing restraint can lead to increased resistance. Foals often show "passive resistance", where they will sink down (or "play dead") as restraint is applied. A novice clinician could interpret this behaviour as collapse.

Restraining a foal in a standing position is often best achieved against a wall. Methods of restraint include one or all of the following depending on which part of the foal is being examined (Figure 2.9).

1. The foal is held with one arm around the midneck of the foal, preventing it moving forward. This can be fairly gentle restraint.
2. The tail is held firmly at its base. The fingers of the hand holding the tail should be closest to the foal, with the thumb on top of the tail. Pulling the tail vertically up and forward can increase the degree of restraint. This decreases, but does not eliminate, the ability of the foal to kick backwards with its hind limbs.
3. If the foal is held around the neck with one arm, and at the base of the tail with the other, the body can be used to confine the foal against the wall.
4. To increase control of the head and front of the foal, the handler should reach around the foal's neck, and grasp the ear on the opposite side of the head. In the recalcitrant foal, firmer grasping of the ear or twisting of the ear can be used to increase control.
5. In the really recalcitrant foal, both ears can be held and twisted if necessary. This should only be done in extreme situations, such as administering sedation, when none of the other techniques have been successful.

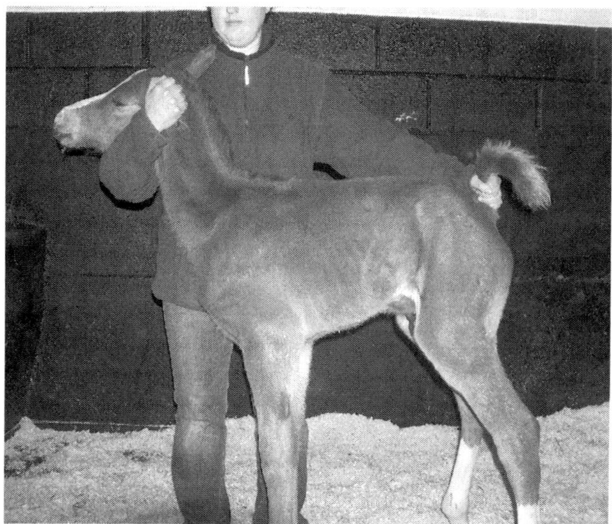

Figure 2.9 Restraint of the recalcitrant standing foal. The tail is held firmly at its base, and the head is controlled by holding the ear on the opposite side from the handler. ©Kevin Corley 2007.

Laying down a foal

There are many techniques for laying down a foal.

In smaller foals, it may be possible to physically lift them up and place them on their side. There are not many foals in which the weight of the foal is sufficiently low for one person to safely lift. The handler or handlers stand next to the flank of the foal on the side to which it is to be laid down. They reach over the foal to grasp the elbow and stifle of the leg next to them (the bottom leg). They then lift the foal up and place it on its side. It is important to closely coordinate the efforts of two people. In this lifting technique, the head of the foal is in danger of striking the ground. A third person is useful to protect the head, if available.

It is possible to lay down a foal with one person without lifting the foal. The handler stands next to the flank of the foal on the side to which it is to be laid down. There must be space and a suitable surface behind the person for the foal to lie down. One hand is placed on the base of the tail, as it joins the body. The other hand is placed on the bridge of the foal's nose. The foal's nose is pushed away from the handler, towards the tail. The head should be brought around so that the nose is almost touching the flank of the foal on the opposite side to the handler. At the same time, the tail is gently but firmly pushed away from the handler, to try to curve the lower spine. The idea is to bend the foal into a C-shape. The handler then places a knee under the chest of the foal and pulls the foal towards him or her. The handler should slowly sink down, so that the foal is pulled over into his or her lap. Although this technique is usually successful, it can be less than graceful!

Restraint in lateral recumbency

Many procedures can be carried out in neonatal foals restrained in lateral recumbency without sedation. However, older foals, that are not debilitated, may require sedation to aid in laying down and restraint. One possible combination for this is diazepam (0.05 to 0.1 mg/kg IV), xylazine (0.2 to 0.6 mg/kg IV) and butorphanol (0.2 mg/kg IV). If this does not provide sufficient sedation, further small increments of diazepam and xylazine can be added.

The method of restraint for lateral recumbency depends on the number of people available. For procedures on the cranial half of the animal, adequate restraint of most foals can be achieved with one person holding the foal. The handler sits just behind the backbone of the foal at the level of the withers. One leg is extended beneath the neck of the foal and the other leg is placed over the body of the foal, so that minimal contact is made with the thorax. The foot can be used to prevent the hind limbs coming forward (Figure 2.10). The arm nearest the head of the foal is passed under the head, and the hand wraps round to hold the chin. The other hand is rested on the side of the face, just below the ear, and is available to hold the ear if required. The other person, who is performing the procedure, should kneel down so that both fore limbs of the foal are held between his or her legs. It is important for this person to get his or her knees above the level of the carpus on the foal to ensure proper control of the fore limbs. If an additional handler is available, he or she can kneel with the foal's hind limbs between his or her legs, ensuring that his or her knees are proximal to the hocks on the foal.

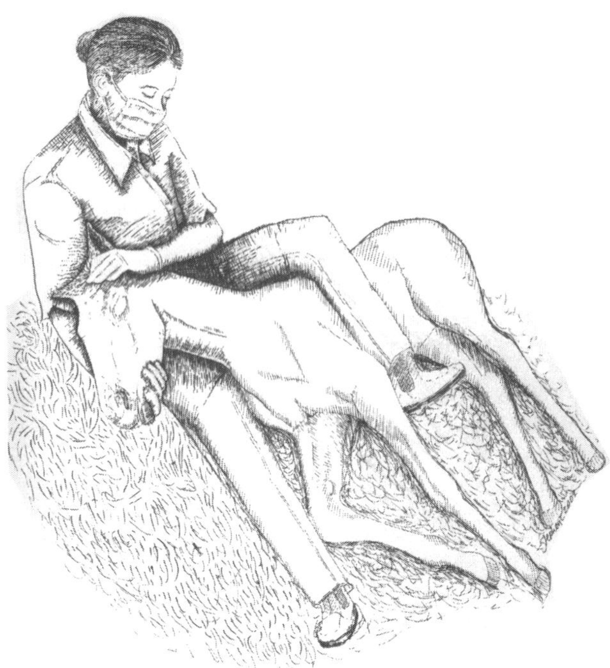

Figure 2.10 Restraint of the foal in lateral recumbency. One leg is extended beneath the neck, whilst the other is placed over the thorax. The leg over the thorax prevents the hind legs coming forward.

For techniques involving the caudal end of the foal, such as urinary catheterisation, control of the hind limbs is essential. This may involve a further handler kneeling behind the foal and grasping the cannon bone of the uppermost hind limb with both hands. The leg is flexed and held as close to the body of the foal as possible. The person performing the procedure kneels with the lower hind limb between their legs. Although this is necessary for access to some parts (such as the prepuce and penis) this person should be aware of the danger of being kicked by the upper hind limb if it slips from the grasp of the handler. In other cases the handler may have to control both hind limbs, either by holding them both together between their knees, or by holding the uppermost leg and controlling the lower leg with their knees.

Restraint in sternal recumbency

To restrain a conscious foal in sternal recumbency takes two or three handlers. One of these may be the person performing the procedure. The foal is first placed in lateral recumbency, as described above. The fore limbs are flexed at the carpus and held next to the body, to allow the foal to be rolled into sternal recumbency. One handler kneels next to the shoulder of the foal, supporting it. One hand is placed either around the chest, or to cup and support the chin. It is possible for this person to perform a procedure at the cranial half of a quiet foal, such as placing a nasogastric tube. The second handler is responsible for the hind end of the foal. Usually, they will kneel with both hind limbs between their legs, ensuring that their knees are proximal to the hocks on the foal. This may need to be adapted, depending on the procedure to be performed.

2.5 Placing an indwelling nasogastric tube

Placing an indwelling nasogastric tube is a way to ensure adequate nutrition in a foal with good gastrointestinal activity but uncoordinated or poor swallowing or nursing activity. It is also a way to supplement foals with nutrition, when they are not receiving adequate milk from the dam.

Equipment needed

Narrow flexible nasogastric tubes are preferred for this purpose, because they are less likely to cause pharyngitis and allow the foal to nurse with the tube in place. Twelve French polyurethane feeding tubes designed for foals are commercially available and are recommended. The equipment needed for nasogastric intubation is given in Box 2.9.

Placement

It is easiest to place a feeding tube with the foal held in sternal recumbency. It is also possible to place a tube with a foal standing and restrained against a wall (see Chapter 2.4). Before placing a tube, it should be measured against (but not actually touching) the side of the foal

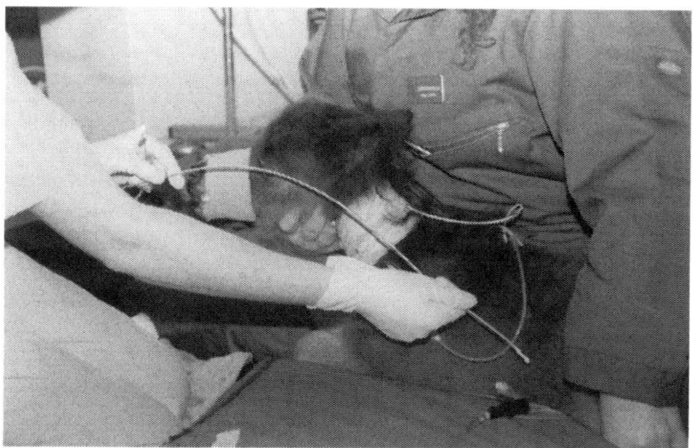

Figure 2.11 Measuring the length of the nasogastric tube to place in the foal. The distal end should be caudal to the base of the heart, preferably at the level of the stomach. ©Kevin Corley 2003.

Box 2.9. Equipment for placing an indwelling nasogastric tube

Required

12Fr polyurethane foal feeding tube*
7.5-cm (3-inch) wide stretchy adhesive dressing (Elastoplast†/Elastikon‡)
Two tongue depressors
Zinc oxide tape
Bandage scissors

Helpful

Endoscope (9-mm diameter or smaller)
OR
X-ray machine and plate

*12Fr × 108-cm Nasogastric Feeding Tube (NG1243); MILA International Inc, Florence, KY, USA.
†Beiersdorf AG, Hamburg, Germany.
‡Johnson and Johnson, New Brunswick, NJ, USA.

(Figure 2.11). The distal end should be placed over the caudal thorax at the level of the stomach or the oesophagus caudal to the base of the heart. The length required for the tube to reach the stomach or distal oesophagus should be estimated by bending the tube to the approximate pathway of the thoracic and cervical oesophagus and the nasal cavity and marking the point level with the nares.

Two tongue depressors, wrapped together with zinc oxide tape, should be prepared in advance as a fixing device for the nasogastric tube. The tongue depressors need to be prepared by measuring them alongside the maxilla of the foal. They should be long enough to reach the facial crest of the foal, when the curved end overlaps the nares (Figure 2.12). If the tongue depressors need to be shortened, they should be shortened to the same length by making a new curve at the cut end and ensuring there are no sharp edges. The two tongue depressors are placed together and covered in tape to make a smooth, padded support for the feeding

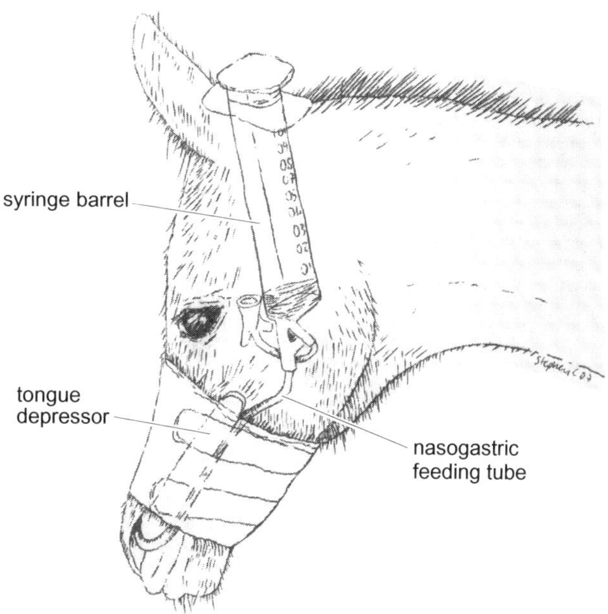

Figure 2.12 How to fix an indwelling nasogastric feeding tube to the foal. The tube is taped along the edge and one curve of zinc oxide tape–covered tongue depressors. The curve is used to redirect the tube so that it points caudally into the nares. The tube and tongue depressors are then secured to the foal's muzzle with elastoplast.

tube. This is then put to one side until the tube is successfully passed. A single layer of stretchy adhesive dressing should be placed around the foal's muzzle, just caudal to the nares. This should be placed tight enough so that there are no folds or parts not in contact with the foal but not too tight to prevent the foal from easily opening its mouth.

Prior to placement, the distal part of the feeding tube should be dipped in water, or lightly coated with K-Y jelly, to provide lubrication. One arm should be passed over the foal's poll round the opposite side of the foal's head, to cup the foal's chin with the hand. This hand can then be moved to guide the feeding tube into the nares with one finger, whilst still restraining the foal with the rest of the hand and the arm. The other hand should be used to gently pass the feeding tube. If there is a curve to the tube, it should be passed so that the arc of the curve is pointing dorsally. The hand holding the foal's chin is used to direct the tube into the nostril and into the ventral meatus, which is ventral and medial. The tube is passed until it reaches the oropharynx (very approximately 15 to 17 cm in the 50-kg Thoroughbred foal). If the tube meets resistance before this point (at approximately 8 to 12 cm in the 50-kg Thoroughbred foal), it is likely to be caught on the ethmoid turbinates and should be withdrawn and redirected to the ventral meatus.

Once the tube is in the oropharynx, it should be twisted through 180° and gently advanced until resistance is met. At this point it is important to get the foal to swallow the tube, which can be assisted by one of two methods. The first method is to very gently move the tube forwards and backwards to come into contact with the oropharynx, which stimulates a swallowing reflex. The second method is to place a gloved finger (which can be from the restraining hand) into the mouth to stimulate a suckling reflex. These methods can be combined. When the foal swallows, the tube must be advanced a short way, without great force. If no excessive resistance is met, the tube should be advanced until the premarked spot is level with the nostril. It is best to temporarily fix the tube to the foal at this point by folding it back along the muzzle. Zinc oxide tape should be wrapped around the muzzle over the tube and the pre-placed stretchy adhesive dressing. Once the tube is temporarily fixed to the foal, it should be confirmed that the tube was correctly placed into the oesophagus.

Checking the placement of the tube

There are four ways to check that the tube has been correctly placed. The first two are the most reliable but also the most expensive and time-consuming.

The first method is to take a lateral thoracic radiograph of the foal. Commercially available feeding tubes are usually radiopaque and the tube (or end of the tube) can be imaged extending caudal and dorsal to the carina of the trachea and the base of the heart. Radiography allows confirmation that the end of the tube has not double-backed within the oesophagus (a possible complication if there is no stylet or if the stylet does not reach the distal end of the tube).

The second method is endoscopy of the nasopharynx. An endoscope with a suitably small diameter (9 mm or less for a 50-kg Thoroughbred foal) is required. The endoscope is passed via the ventral meatus of the opposite nostril into the nasopharynx. This may be done in a well-restrained conscious foal. A correctly placed tube can be seen crossing the nasopharynx entering the oesophagus just dorsal or dorsilateral to the arytenoids.

The third method is to palpate the tube within the oesophagus. The oesophagus runs dorsal to the trachea and can be palpated in the proximal neck caudal to the larynx. The oesophagus is soft and flexible and cannot be differentiated from the other soft tissues that surround it. However, when the tube is in the oesophagus, it can be felt as a firm, round object. With experience, this method can be as accurate as endoscopy.

The fourth method is to auscultate over the stomach whilst rapidly injecting a small amount of air (approximately 5 ml) into the tube. If the tube is correctly placed, a bubbling sound will be heard in the stomach. With experience, this method can be reasonably accurate.

It is possible that despite appearing to be correctly placed a tube checked by any method other than radiography could be double-backed within the oesophagus. This can be tested for by injecting a small amount of water (only after correct placement has been confirmed). If there is significant resistance to injection of this water, it is likely that the tube is kinked or double-backed. When this has occurred, the stylet may also be very difficult to remove. If it is suspected that a tube has kinked or double-backed, it should be withdrawn very rapidly about 10 cm and then readvanced very slowly and steadily. If this is not successful, the tube will need to be completely removed and the procedure started again. Tubes that have kinked once will often kink again and may need to be replaced.

Fixing the tube to the foal

Once the feeding tube is correctly placed, it needs to be securely fixed. Prior to this, the tube that is outside the foal should be held as straight as possible in front of the foal and the stylet removed. The tube is then curved back alongside the muzzle of the foal. The distance of the tube from the nostril that is equivalent to the length of one long edge and one curved end of the tongue depressor should be estimated. This is done by laying the tongue depressor alongside the tube that extends out from the nose. The tube is then fixed to the tongue depressor starting with the part that is furthest from the nostril. This part of the tube is attached to one long edge of the tongue depressor, using zinc oxide tape (Figure 2.12). The tube closest to the nostril should then be carefully taped along the whole curve of tongue depressor, so that it travels back along the opposite straight edge for approximately 5 mm ($\frac{1}{5}$ of an inch) (Figure 2.12). It is important to get the tube exactly on the edge of the tongue depressor and to tape it well. Otherwise, the tube may kink (Figure 2.13). Not taping the tube to the curve will allow the tube to be easily displaced from the oesophagus (Figure 2.14). Once the tube is fixed to the tongue depressor, the tongue depressor is laid alongside the strip of stretchy adhesive dressing that has already been applied to the foal's muzzle. The tongue depressor should be positioned with the tube on the ventral side to avoid the end of tube going near the eye (Figure 2.15). The part of the tongue depressor where the tube leaves the tape and enters the nostril should be positioned so that there is virtually no untaped tube visible outside the nasal cavity (Figures 2.12 and 2.15). The tongue depressor should then be fixed in place by wrapping round the foal's muzzle with stretchy adhesive tape on top of the previously placed elastoplast. Many brands of stretchy adhesive tape will begin to peel back from the corners with time, and this can be avoided by placing short strips of zinc oxide tape over the corners of the end.

Testing and using the tube

Once permanently fixed, the tube should be tested and then is ready for use. The tube is tested by gently injecting a small amount (approximately 5 ml) of water. There should be minimal resistance to injection. If there is great resistance to injection, it is likely that the tube has become kinked. The part outside the nostril should be carefully examined for kinks, unwrapping the tape if necessary. If this does not reveal the kink, the thorax should either be radiographed or the tube should be rapidly

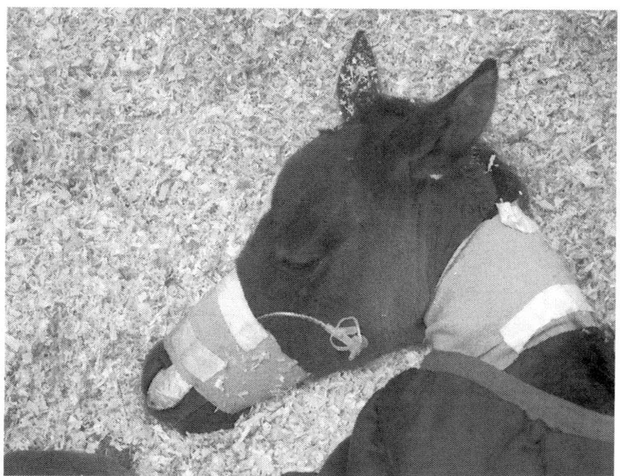

Figure 2.13 Incorrectly placed nasogastric feeding tube in a foal. The tube has been inadequately taped to the curve of the tongue depressors, causing it to kink. ©Kevin Corley 2003.

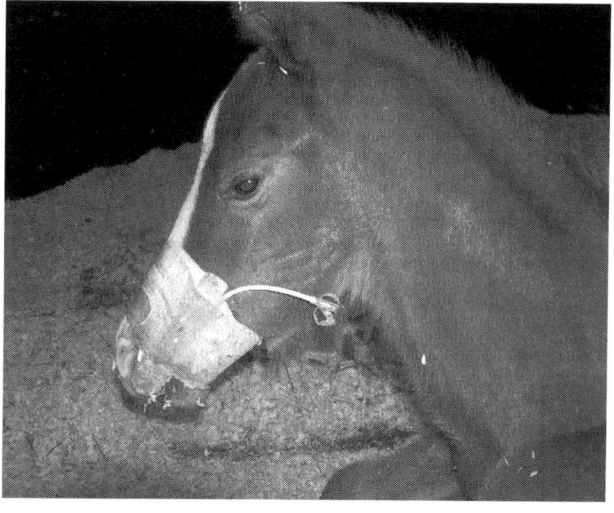

Figure 2.15 Correctly placed nasogastric feeding tube in a foal. ©Kevin Corley 2007.

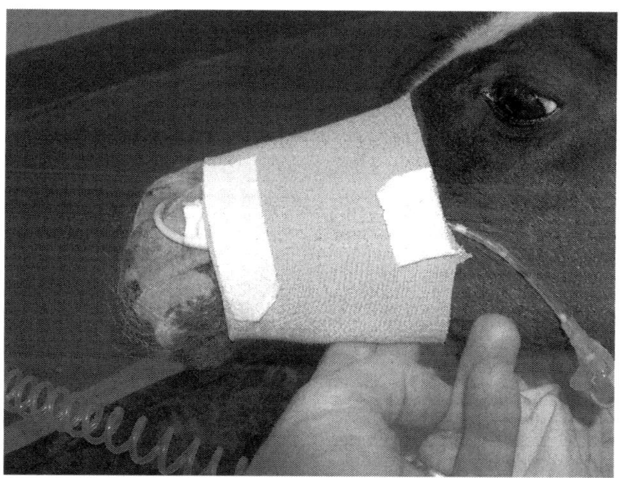

Figure 2.14 Incorrectly placed nasogastric feeding tube in a foal. The tube has not been taped to the curve of the tongue depressors. The tube will tend to straighten and start to come out of the nares. The exposed loop of tube is also in danger of being caught on something and pulled out. ©Kevin Corley 2006.

withdrawn 10 cm and then gently replaced, as described above.

It is best to give nutrition and fluids via the tube by gravity rather than injecting with a syringe. Enteral feeding bags are commercially available* and are very useful. Alternatively, fluid bags and administration sets may be used (or reused). However, fluid sets typically have smaller bores than enteral feeding sets and delivery of the fluids or nutrition may be very slow. A further alternative is to use the barrel of a 60-ml catheter tip syringe connected to the feeding tube and fill this with milk (Figure 2.12). The disadvantage of this open system is that it is less hygienic and also liable to end up with the foal handler covered in milk if the foal is at all active.

When starting a foal on nutrition, it is important to use small amounts to begin with and then gradually transition the foal to the desired final intake. The tube should also be aspirated prior to each use to check for excess gastric residual fluid. For further information on feeding via a nasogastric tube, see Chapter 5.2.

2.6 Jugular vein catheterisation

Jugular vein catheterisation is fairly straightforward in the foal. There are two main types of catheter that are used in foals: over-the-needle and over-the-wire. In general, catheters placed by the over-the-wire method are less likely to cause damage to the intima of the vein and are more suitable for long-term (>2 day) use. Preparation of the site is the same for both types of catheter.

Equipment needed

The equipment needed for jugular catheterisation is listed in Box 2.10.

Restraint

Foals should be catheterised in lateral recumbency. Standing foals are difficult to catheterise with expert restraint. Sudden movements of the foal can lead to contamination of the catheter or failure to place the catheter altogether. With the foal restrained in lateral recumbency (see Chapter 2.4), the person placing the catheter should kneel so that both fore limbs of the foal are held between his or her legs. It is important for this person to have his or her knees above the level of the carpus on the foal to ensure proper restraint.

* Flexiflo Gravity Feeding Set; Ross Products, Abbott Laboratories, IL, USA; Enteral Feeding Bag; Plasco Engineered Products, Columbus, MS, USA.

Box 2.10. Equipment for placing a jugular catheter in the foal

Suitable catheters

7Fr double-lumen (14-gauge/18-gauge) 20-cm (8-inch) over-the-wire catheter*
16-Gauge single-lumen 20-cm (8-inch) over-the-wire catheter†‡
16-Gauge, 13-cm (5.25-inch) over-the-needle polyurethane catheter§
16-Gauge, 7.5-cm (3-inch) over-the-needle polyurethane catheter**

Other required equipment

Clippers with a fine (No. 40) blade
Drape or disposable incontinence pad††
Small gauze swabs soaked in chlorhexidine (4%) scrub solution‡‡
Small gauze swabs soaked in surgical spirit
Mepivacaine 2%§§: 2 ml drawn up in a 2–3-ml syringe with a 23–25-gauge needle
Surgical facemasks
Surgical gloves
No. 15 scalpel blade
2-0 Nonabsorbable monofilament suture on a straight needle***
High-flow extension set†††, if not supplied with catheter
1 (2 for two-lumen catheter) 10-ml syringe of 0.9% sterile saline (±5 units/ml heparin)
Injection cap(s) (if not supplied in catheter kit)
7.5-cm (3-inch) wide stretchy adhesive dressing (Elastoplast‡‡‡/Elastikon§§§)
Zinc oxide tape
1 Sterile small gauze swab (4 × 4)
Bandage scissors

*CV-17702; Arrow International Inc., Reading, PA, USA.
†CV-04301; Arrow International Inc., Reading, PA, USA.
‡1610; MILA International, Florence, KY, USA.
§1611; MILA International, Florence, KY, USA.
**1603; MILA International, Florence, KY, USA.
††6427; PHS Incontinence pads (75 × 57 cm); National Veterinary Services, Stoke-on-Trent, UK.
‡‡Hibiscrub; Mölnlycke Health Care, Dunstable, UK.
§§Intra-epicaine; Arnolds Veterinary Products, Shrewsbury, UK; Carbocaine-V; Pfizer Animal Health, New York, NY, USA.
***628H, Ethilon Nylon; Ethicon, Somerville, NJ, USA.
†††8590; MILA International, Florence, KY, USA.
‡‡‡Beiersdorf AG, Hamburg, Germany.
§§§Johnson and Johnson, New Brunswick, NJ, USA.

Preparation

Hair should be removed from a rectangle 15 cm long and 10 cm wide over the jugular groove, in the middle to cranial part of the neck. A drape or disposable incontinence pad should be placed underneath the neck of the foal, over the leg of the person restraining it. The area should be aseptically prepared. The vein is raised, and the site for catheterisation is identified. This should be in the middle of the prepared area, directly over the jugular vein. Any superficial skin vessels that traverse the jugular groove should be noted and avoided. A small (1 ml) bleb of mepivacaine is placed subcutaneously at the site of catheterisation. Mepivacaine should also be placed where the catheter extension set will be sutured to the foal approximately 3 to 4 cm dorsal to the catheterisation site. Ideally, the person placing the catheter and all those restraining the foal should put on surgical facemasks at this point.

The clipped area should be given a full surgical scrub. Some clinicians drape the catheter site with a four-point draping technique, at this point. The procedure should always be done with sterile surgical gloves.

Placing the catheter

For ease of description, the dominant hand will be assumed to be the right hand. However, no special adaptations are needed for left-handed people, other than using the left hand where the description says right, and vice versa. For right-handed people, it is generally slightly easier to place the catheter in the right jugular vein of the foal, and for left-handed people, the left jugular vein. However, either vein is easily catheterised with either hand.

Placing an over-the-wire catheter

The technique varies according to the make of catheter used. However the following technique will work for most over-the-wire catheters. This description is based on placing an Arrow catheter.

Once the sterile gloves have been put on, the catheter kit is checked. The J-wire assembly is carefully removed (Figure 2.16) and the wire withdrawn so that the end is level with the end of the plastic nozzle. The wire is placed on top of all other elements except the introducer needle. In some kits it may be necessary to remove an injection port from the end of the catheter to allow passage of the wire at this point. The introducer needle is taken from the catheter set and held between the thumb and forefinger of the right hand. People with larger hands may also choose to take the J-wire arrangement into the right hand at this time. In this

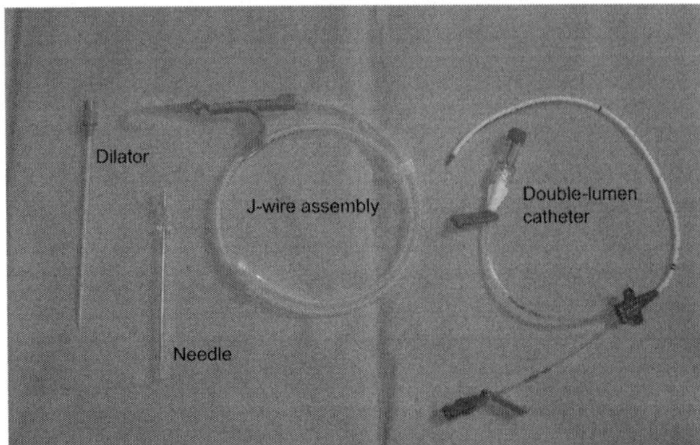

Figure 2.16 Parts of a double-lumen over-the-wire catheter. ©Kevin Corley 2007.

case, the circular plastic holding the J-wire is held by the middle and fourth finger flat against the palm.

The knuckle of the left first finger is used to raise the vein, within the surgically prepared area. The needle is held parallel to the jugular vein, pointing caudally and with the bevel up (so that the sharp tip is nearest the foal). The needle should be at 35° to the skin of the foal. The point of the needle is pushed through the skin, at the site where mepivacaine was placed, and the needle slowly advanced until blood is seen in the hub of the needle. At this point, the needle is flattened towards the neck of the foal, so that it makes an angle of approximately 5° to 10°. The needle is then advanced an additional 1 to 2 cm. The left hand is then moved to carefully hold the needle in position. The thumb and forefinger are used to do this, whilst the back of one of the other fingers keeps the vein raised to prevent aspiration.

The J-wire assembly is taken into the right hand. The nozzle is inserted into the needle carefully, making sure that the needle position is unaltered (Figure 2.17). A common error at this point is to push the needle through and out of the vein as the J-wire assembly is attached. The wire is advanced, using the thumb slide (just behind the nozzle on the J-wire assembly). If the needle is correctly placed the wire will run easily. If the wire stops advancing after 6 to 7 cm (or the length of the needle), the needle has probably come out of the vein. Using excessive force to advance the wire may cause it to enter the tissue planes, and it will either advance a small amount or kink or both. When this happens, the skin over the point of the needle can be seen to move as the wire is forced out of it. If the wire does not pass freely from the end of the needle, it should be removed and the position of the needle checked and altered. Once 10 cm of the wire has passed into the vein, the wire may be advanced more rapidly. One technique of advancing the wire more rapidly is to disconnect the nozzle of the J-wire assembly from the needle, grasp the exposed wire between the thumb and forefinger of the right hand and advance it. The wire should be advanced to the point where 5 to 10 cm is protruding from the end of the needle. The wire should then be held with the left hand temporarily at an angle away from the skin of the foal. The plastic coil assembly should be pulled from the end of the wire. The wire should be held in one or the other hand until it is removed to prevent it either touching the foal or slipping completely into the vein.

Holding the end of the wire with the right hand, the needle should be withdrawn with the left hand (Figure 2.18), until it is free of the foal. The wire below the needle is then held, and the needle completely removed. The needle can then be passed to an assistant for disposal. The wire is held at an angle from the foal's skin. The tissue dilator (which is light blue hard plastic in Arrow catheter kits) is then threaded onto the wire. The right hand is used to advance the dilator and push it through the skin into the vein. There can be considerable resistance to passage of the dilator through the tissue planes. Keeping the dilator at an angle of 5° to the foal's neck whilst rotating it from side to side can help it advance. The dilator should be advanced to the hub and then withdrawn. The dilator is removed completely from the wire in a similar way to removing the needle.

Removing the catheter from the tray without contaminating it can be challenging. Grasping the catheter in the middle to lift it up minimises the risk of this. The catheter should be placed in the palm of the right hand with the end held between the thumb and forefinger. The wire should be held vertically up at almost 90° to the foal's neck close to its free end. The catheter is then carefully threaded onto

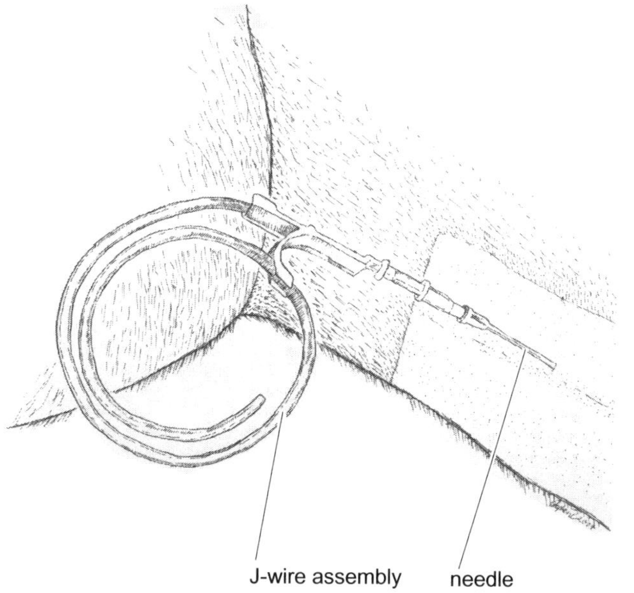

J-wire assembly
needle

Figure 2.17 The needle has been placed into the jugular vein. The J-wire assembly is attached to the needle, and the wire is advanced into the vein.

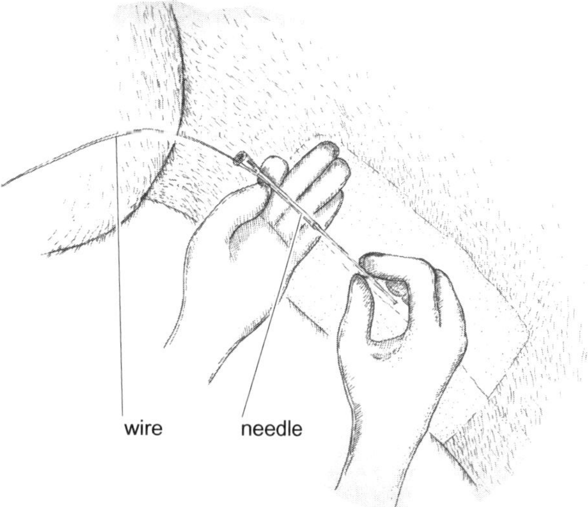

Figure 2.18 Leaving the wire in the vein, the needle is removed from the vein and slid off the end of the wire. It is important not to let go of the wire at any time during catheter placement.

the wire. In double-lumen catheters, the wire should be fed into the most distal hole. It may be necessary to slightly pull the wire out of the vein, so that the wire emerges from the catheter port. In Arrow double-lumen catheters, the wire will emerge from the brown port. Once the wire emerges from the proximal end of the catheter, the wire is held with the left hand and not withdrawn any farther. The catheter is held near its tip and threaded onto the wire and through the skin into the vein. There may be a small amount of resistance as the catheter first enters the skin. The catheter is seated all the way down so that its hub is against the skin of the foal (Figure 2.19).

The author's preferred option at this point is to suture the hub of the catheter to the foal, before any further manipulations are done. The wire is withdrawn a small way (approximately 5 cm) and grasped by a nonsterile assistant at the very end (still at virtually 90° to the foal's neck). Using 2–0 nonabsorbable monofilament suture on a straight needle, the catheter hub is sutured to the foal's skin. The author prefers a cruciate pattern. The person placing the catheter then holds the catheter extension at the portal, and the nonsterile assistant pulls out the wire and discards it. A sterile sample of blood for culture and blood for clinicopathological analysis may be withdrawn at this point. The port(s) of the catheter should be flushed with saline or heparinised saline. The port(s) of the catheter should then be connected to a primed fluid set or covered with an injection cap.

The extension set(s) are then sutured to the foal's skin, 3 to 4 cm above the catheter hub. The positioning of the suture on the extension sets is important, as placing it cranially or caudally to the hub can result in the extension sets kinking. The easiest method to secure the extension sets to the skin is to first place a zinc oxide tape "butterfly" (Figure 2.20) on the extension set, just behind the port. The butterfly is then stitched to the skin either side of the extension set. It is advisable to wrap the whole catheter assembly. This is done by placing a sterile gauze swab over the catheter hub and entry hole and wrapping stretchy adhesive dressing round the neck to completely cover the catheter and swab. It is important to lay the stretchy adhesive dressing on the neck gently so that it does not result in occlusion of venous return. Exit holes for the extension ports should be made.

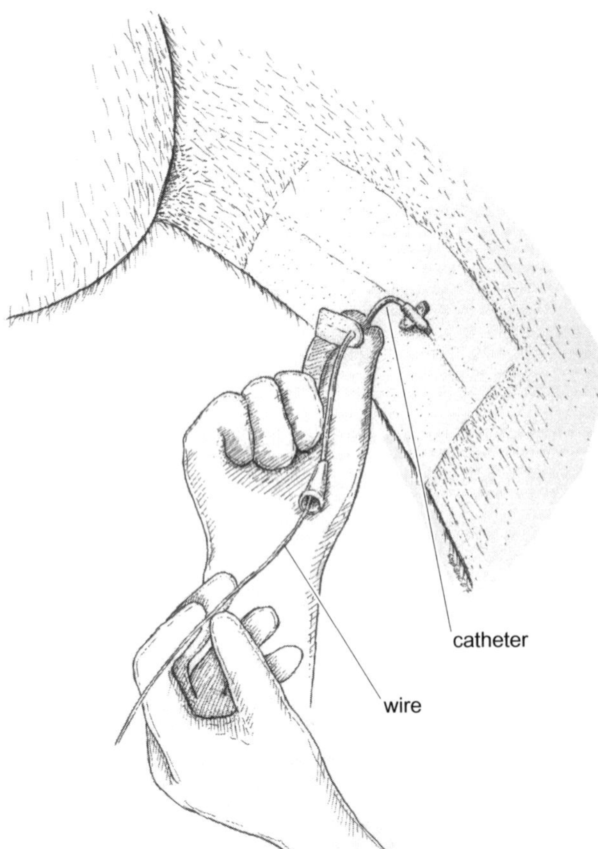

Figure 2.19 The catheter is threaded onto the wire. The wire is fed out through the catheter, until it can be grasped beyond the catheter hub. Holding the wire in place, the catheter is then slid forwards into the vein.

Placing an over-the-needle catheter

Preparation including placement of local anaesthetic is as previously described. Once the sterile gloves have been put on, the catheter is set up and checked. The catheter and stylet should be picked up together and the catheter gently eased approximately 2 to 3 mm off the stylet, and then replaced so that the stylet is firmly against the catheter hub. For some catheter makes, it may be necessary to make a small stab incision through the skin over the middle of the jugular vein. The back of the left hand is used to raise the vein, within the surgically prepared area.

The catheter is held between the thumb and first two fingers of the right hand, pointing back towards the hand, at about a 30° angle to the wrist and forearm. The bevel of the stylet is turned so that the point of the stylet is closest to the foal's skin. The stylet point is rested on the foal's skin in the middle of the raised jugular vein. The catheter and stylet are held parallel to the jugular vein, at approximately 45° to the neck of the foal. The stylet point is pushed through the skin (or stab incision) and into the middle of

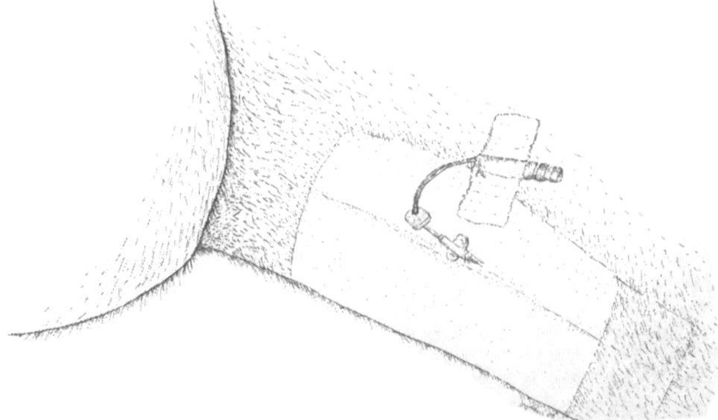

Figure 2.20 The catheter is sutured to the skin of the foal. The hub can be fixed with a cruciate suture, and the extension set fixed with a "butterfly" made out of zinc oxide tape. The butterfly is then sutured, either side of the extension set, to the skin of the foal.

the lumen of the raised vein. The catheter is held in position and the port of the stylet is examined for blood coming back (may take several seconds), indicating correct placement. If blood is not seen, the catheter should be withdrawn to almost out of the skin and readvanced into the vein. If blood is seen, the catheter is flattened towards the foal's neck to an angle of 5° to 10°. The whole catheter and stylet assembly is then advanced an additional 0.5 to 1.5 cm. The port of the stylet is again examined for blood coming back. If there is no blood, the catheter should be withdrawn by approximately 1 to 2 cm and advanced at a flatter (lesser) angle, ensuring that it is in line with the jugular vein.

When blood is seen in the stylet port after this second advancement, the left hand is used to hold the stylet by its end. It is important not to move the stylet relative to the foal from this point until the catheter is slid into position. Holding the catheter hub firmly with the right hand, the left hand is used to completely remove the stylet. An extension set or injection cap is immediately connected to the catheter. The catheter hub is sutured to the foal's skin using 2–0 nonabsorbable monofilament suture on a straight needle. The author prefers a cruciate pattern. The catheter may be wrapped, as described for the over-the-wire catheter, above.

Catheter care

Catheters in neonatal foals are prone to infection and thrombophlebitis and should be monitored carefully. Twice-daily monitoring for heat or swelling is essential. The vein should also be monitored for any heat, swelling or hardness.

If movement of the foal results in any part of the catheter shaft (below the hub) being exposed, it should be resutured to prevent this. This type of movement of the catheter results in bacteria being collected from the skin of the foal and brought into the catheter tract through the skin or the vein.

If there is resistance to flow (or occlusion errors on an electronic pump), the catheter should be very carefully inspected. Extension sets may move and kink underneath the wrapping. Another site where it is common for catheters (especially over-the-needle catheters) to kink is just below the hub as the catheter enters the skin. If this occurs, it is necessary to replace the catheter.

If an over-the-wire catheter needs to be replaced for a reason other than infection of the skin or infection or thrombophlebitis of the vein, it is possible to do an over-the-wire exchange. For this, the skin around the existing catheter is surgically prepared, leaving the catheter in place. The wire is then passed down the existing catheter. The catheter is removed over the wire, leaving the wire in place, and catheterisation proceeds as described above. If the same size of catheter (or smaller) is being placed, it will not be necessary to use a tissue dilator.

Catheters that are removed because of suspected infection should be submitted for bacterial culture.

Box 2.11. Equipment for indirect blood pressure measurement in the foal

Required

Automated oscillometric noninvasive blood pressure machine

- With neonate mode (and neonate hose, if required)

No. 4 neonatal cuff (7–13 cm) (bladder width 52 mm)—soft cuffs are preferred

2.7 Indirect blood pressure measurement

Indirect blood pressure measurement is very straightforward in the neonatal foal, with a small amount of equipment. New blood pressure monitors are relatively expensive, but second-hand machines from human hospitals or clinics are widely available and more economical.

Equipment needed

The equipment needed for indirect blood pressure measurement is listed in Box 2.11.

Placement of the cuff

The coccygeal artery is accurate for blood pressure measurement for most machines. The dorsal metatarsal artery is not as accurate as the coccygeal artery in some machines.[1] The centre of the bladder of the cuff should be placed over the artery. It is marked by an arrow on some makes of cuff or lies between the two hosepipes on models that have two hosepipes.

Coccygeal artery

The coccygeal artery is located on ventral midline of the tail. Measurements are most accurate when the cuff is placed as close to the base of the tail as possible. The cuff should be orientated so that the hose runs away from the body of the foal (Figure 2.21). The cuff should be reasonably tight before taking a measurement.

Dorsal metatarsal artery

The dorsal metatarsal artery runs on the lateral side of the hind limb, for the first half to two-thirds of the cannon bone distal to the hock. It lies caudal and parallel to the edge of the cannon bone (Figure 2.22). It is fairly superficial and can usually be identified by its pulse. It is important that the foal does not move its leg during a measurement, so this site is only really suitable in recumbent foals. The hoof may be lightly restrained to try to prevent movement during the reading.

Taking a measurement

Measurements are made by the machine. Many machines have the option of a manual measurement or automated measurements repeated after a set interval. Measurements

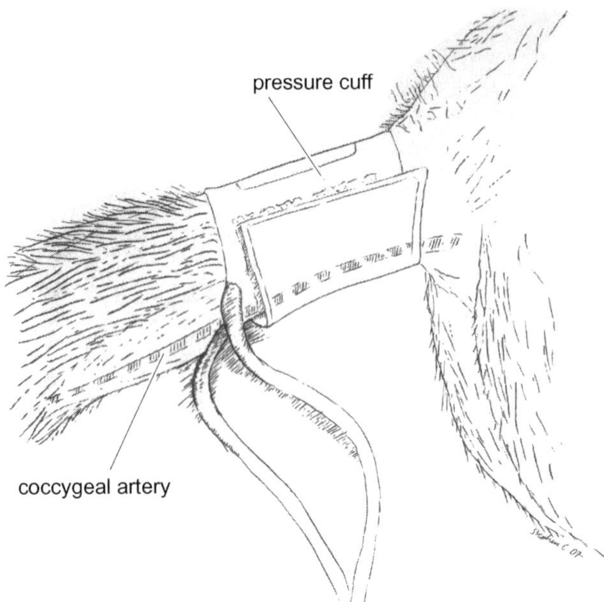

Figure 2.21 Indirect blood pressure cuff over the coccygeal artery.

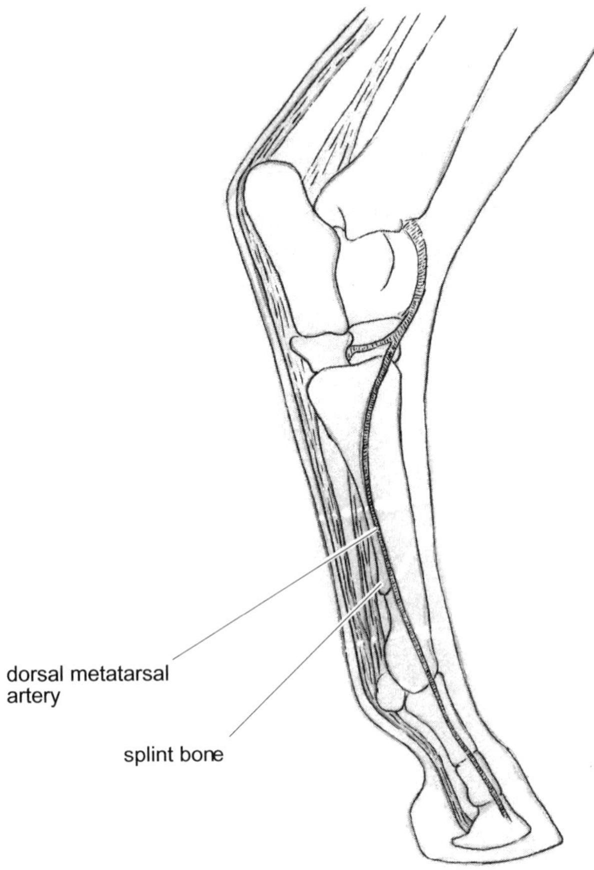

Figure 2.22 Anatomical location of the dorsal metatarsal artery.

of mean arterial pressure are the most accurate by this methodology.[2] Measurements of diastolic pressure are also sufficiently accurate for clinical use, but measurements of systolic pressure are not accurate.[2]

Troubleshooting

Failure to get a measurement

This is the most common problem. A stepwise approach is necessary, with an attempt to take a measurement after each step:

1. Reposition the cuff.
2. Check the patient clinically—if it is likely to be extremely hypotensive, the machine may not work.
3. Check the patient does not have a gross cardiac dysrhythmia, which may interfere with the machine working.
4. Remove the cuff from the foal, and check that it is inflating when the machine is activated; if not, check the system and cuff for leaks.
5. Check the cuff for a slow leak (may be necessary to immerse it in water).
6. Place the cuff on a different artery.
7. Check that the machine is reaching a sufficient starting pressure above your estimated systolic pressure for the patient.
8. Replace the cuff.
9. Check that the machine is working by using a larger cuff around your own upper arm, or trying it on another patient.
10. Try another machine.

Inconsistent measurements

Inconsistent measurements are also reasonably common with the indirect method. The steps to rectify this problem are as follows:

1. Make sure that the foal is not moving during the measurement.
2. If the machine gives a readout of pulse rate, check this against the foal's heart rate. Discard readings where the pulse rate does not closely match that of the foal.
3. Reposition the cuff.
4. Check the patient clinically—if it is likely to be extremely hypotensive, the machine may not work consistently.
5. Check the patient does not have a gross cardiac dysrhythmia, which may interfere with the machine working.
6. Perform five measurements one after another. If three or more measurements for mean pressure are within 5 to 8 mm Hg of each other, this is probably close enough to the real mean pressure to make clinical decisions.
7. Try a new cuff.
8. Try a different machine.

References

1. Giguère S, Knowles HA Jr, Valverde A, et al.: Accuracy of indirect measurement of blood pressure in neonatal foals. J Vet Intern Med 19:571-576, 2005

2. Nout YS, Corley KTT, Donaldson LL, et al.: Indirect oscillometric and direct blood pressure measurement in anesthetized and conscious neonatal foals. J Vet Emerg Crit Care 12:75-80, 2002

2.8 Collection of arterial blood gas/arterial catheterisation

The dorsal metatarsal artery is the most easily catheterised artery in the foal. It is also the author's preferred site for collection of arterial blood for gas analysis. Some clinicians prefer the median artery for collection of arterial blood, and the technique for this will also be described.

Equipment needed

The equipment needed for arterial blood collection and arterial catheterisation is listed in Box 2.12.

Box 2.12. Equipment for arterial blood collection and arterial catheterisation

For both techniques

Clippers with a fine (No. 40) blade
Small gauze swabs soaked in chlorhexidine (4%) scrub solution*
Small gauze swabs soaked in surgical spirit

For arterial blood gas collection

1–3-ml blood gas syringe

- Commercial syringe with lithium heparin pellet†
- 2–3-ml syringe flushed with sodium heparin solution

25-Gauge, 1.6-cm ($\frac{5}{8}$-inch) needle (for collection from the dorsal metatarsal artery)
23-Gauge, 1.6-cm ($\frac{5}{8}$-inch) needle (for collection from the median artery)

For arterial catheterisation

20-Gauge, 4.5-cm (1.75-inch) polyurethane Seldinger-technique arterial catheter‡
Short, narrow extension set
Mepivacaine 2%§: 1 ml drawn up in a 2–3-ml syringe with a 23–25-gauge needle
Surgical gloves
Instant bonding glue (cyanoacrylate adhesive)**
Injection cap or three-way tap
Clean (nonsterile) small gauze swabs
Zinc oxide tape
Self-adherent bandaging tape††
5 ml syringe filled with 0.9% sterile saline with 5 units/ml heparin

*Hibiscrub; Mölnlycke Health Care, Dunstable, UK.
†Available from many suppliers, including QS-50, Radiometer, Brønshøj, Denmark; Blood Gas Monovette, Sarstedt (www.sarstedt.com), Newton, NC, USA; and Nümbrecht, Germany.
‡RA-04020; Arrow International Inc., Reading, PA, USA.
§Intra-epicaine; Arnolds Veterinary Products, Shrewsbury, UK; Carbocaine-V; Pfizer Animal Health, New York, NY, USA.
**Nexaband; Abbott Laboratories, North Chicago, IL, USA; Superglue, Loctite; Henkel Consumer Adhesives, Avon, OH, USA.
††Vetrap; 3M Products, St. Paul, MN, USA.

Dorsal metatarsal artery (blood collection)

The dorsal metatarsal artery runs on the lateral side of the hind limb, for the first half to two-thirds of the cannon bone, distal to the hock. It lies parallel to, and on the caudal edge of, the cannon bone (Figure 2.22). The hair should be removed over the artery, in a rectangle of approximately 6 to 8 cm × 3 to 4 cm. The artery can often be seen just beneath the skin and can be identified by its pulse.

Blood collection

The foal should be restrained in lateral recumbency (see Chapter 2.4). The person collecting the blood can support the hoof of the upper hind limb between his or her knees but cannot really help restrain the foal. Ideally, there should be two people to restrain the foal (Figure 2.23). The collection leg should be held with a slight bend in the stifle and hock joints. If the collection leg is held too tight or in too straight a position, it can reduce the flow through the artery.

It is not necessary to perform a full surgical scrub for blood collection from the artery. Repeated sampling is often necessary and the skin can react to the scrub solution, becoming hard and scaly and making sampling difficult. A quick scrub with surgical spirit is an alternative, but this may cool the skin over the artery and make the artery much less apparent. If the skin over the artery is grossly contaminated, it should be cleaned before blood collection.

Some clinicians choose to place local anaesthetic over the artery prior to collection. The author only does this when a foal has reacted several times. Placing local anaesthetic over the artery makes it harder to palpate and harder to obtain blood from. Instead, the skin over the site of needle entry is pinched hard between the thumb and forefinger of the left hand, and only relaxed just before the needle is pushed through the skin. In most foals, this provides adequate skin analgesia for sample collection.

It is important to have a clear idea of the course of the artery. This allows the needle to be held absolutely in line with the artery when it is inserted. The needle should be inserted pointing towards the hock at a flat angle (10° to 20°) to the skin of the foal. People with smaller hands often opt to remove the needle from the syringe for insertion into the foal. This allows greater control of the needle and visualisation of the pulsing nature of the blood to confirm that it is arterial. However, it risks moving the needle out of the artery when the syringe is attached and results in some blood spillage. The author keeps the needle attached to the syringe. Prior to use, the syringe barrel is withdrawn a short way and replaced to break any seal.

Just prior to inserting the needle, the author uses one hand to grasp just above the hock. This helps restrain the leg in case of a withdrawal response to the needle insertion. The needle is inserted with the bevel up in one swift move-

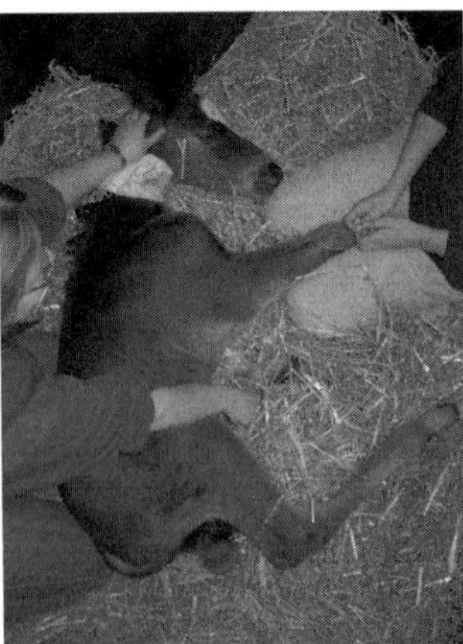

Figure 2.23 Foal restraint for collection of a blood sample from dorsal metatarsal artery. One person controls the front legs, whilst a second person controls the lower hind leg. The person performing the procedure controls the upper hind leg, and takes the sample from it. ©Kevin Corley 2007.

ment. A small amount of pressure is placed to withdraw the barrel of the syringe (if attached) (Figure 2.24). A successful stick results in blood being drawn freely into the syringe or coming out of the unattached needle (Figure 2.25). It is common not to successfully insert the needle into the artery on the first attempt. The needle may be withdrawn a small way and redirected to the left or right. If the needle is completely withdrawn from the skin, the skin should be pinched prior to reinsertion.

If it proves impossible to find the artery, the other leg may be tried or the median artery. If the leg is very cold, warming the leg (with a moderately hot water bottle) can be extremely useful. In foals that are very hypotensive, this technique can be very difficult. Usually in this situation, reversing the hypotension is more of a priority than obtaining an arterial blood sample.

Normal values for arterial blood gases are given in the Appendix (see Table 19.10).

Median artery (blood collection)

The median artery runs on the caudomedial side of the radius, caudal to the cephalic vein and deep to the flexor carpi radialis muscle (Figure 2.26). The artery can be identified by its pulse by pressing the fingers fairly firmly towards the caudal part of the medial radius in the mid antebrachium. Blood collection is similar to that from the dorsal metatarsal artery, except as follows. The foal should be in lateral recumbency, with the hind limbs controlled (see Chapter 2.4). The person collecting the blood can hold the lower fore limb, from which the blood will be collected, between his or her legs. The upper fore limb is either folded at the elbow and carpus and held against the body of the foal or drawn forwards so that it is controlled away from the other fore limb. The area over the median artery is clipped and may be given a quick alcohol scrub. Local anaesthetic may be used but is rarely necessary. Blood is collected by directing the needle at 90° to the artery,

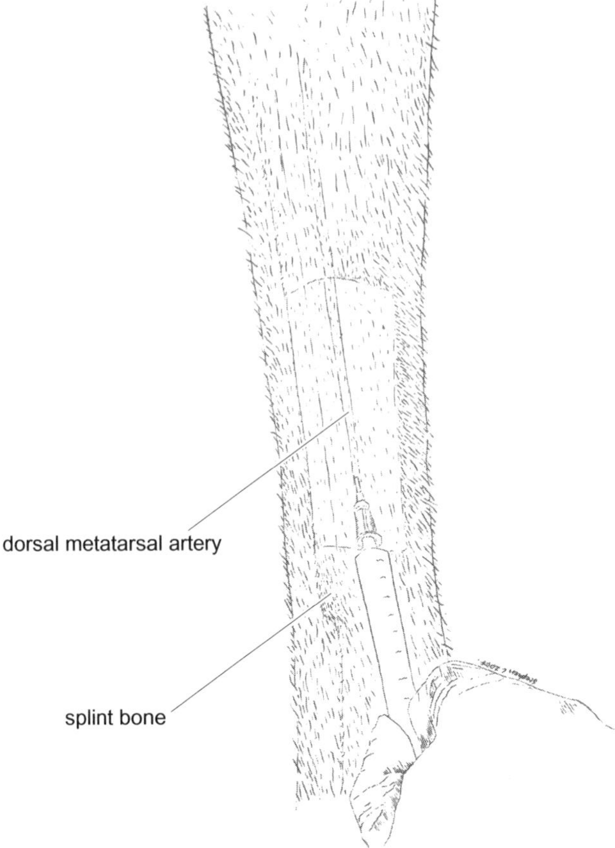

Figure 2.24 Location of the dorsal metatarsal artery, and orientation of the syringe for arterial blood collection.

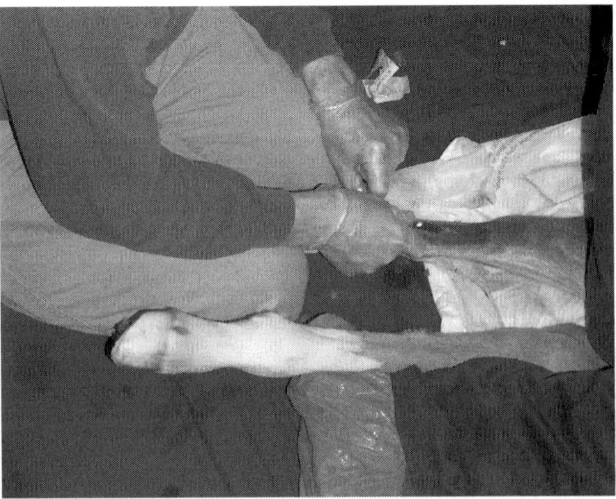

Figure 2.25 Collection of blood from the dorsal metatarsal artery. ©Kevin Corley 2004.

through the muscle into the artery. Specifically designed arterial blood gas syringes can be extremely useful for this technique as the blood will "flash" into the syringe when the needle is inserted into the artery.

Normal values for arterial blood gases are given in the Appendix (see Table 19.10).

Dorsal metatarsal artery (catheterisation)

This is similar to blood collection from the dorsal metatarsal artery, and restraint is performed in the same manner. The area is clipped as described but is aseptically prepared. The site for catheter entry should be chosen carefully. The catheter is placed pointing up the leg, towards the hock. The whole of the catheter is placed in the straight part of the artery as it courses along the bone, before it starts to curve as it approaches the hock. The entry site is therefore as distal as possible along the artery but where it can still clearly be seen superficially. Any transversing skin vessels should be avoided.

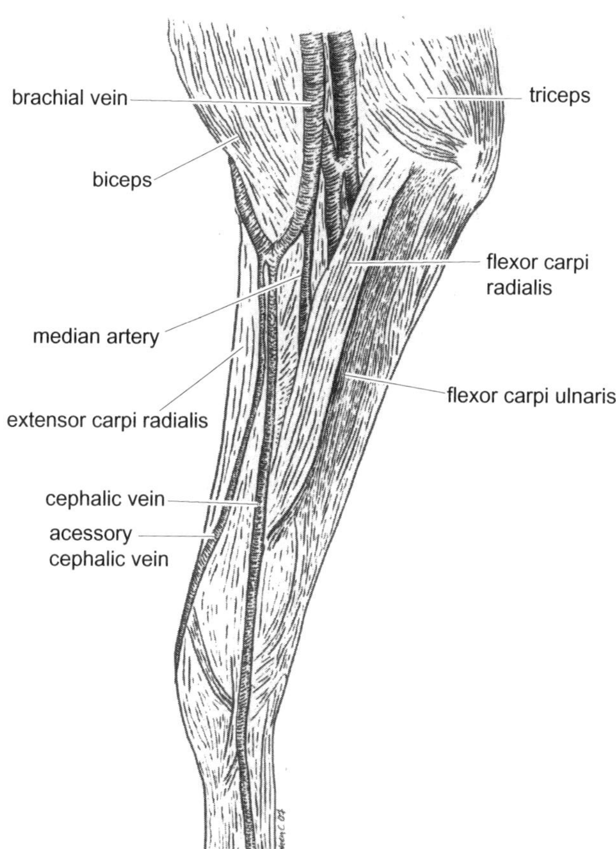

Figure 2.26 Anatomical location of the median artery.

The artery is palpated and a small bleb of local anaesthetic is placed subcutaneously. The area is given a full surgical scrub. The person placing the catheter puts on surgical gloves and is handed the catheter. The recommended human radial artery catheter* is inserted via the Seldinger technique. It consists of the following parts: wire assembly joined to the needle stylet, catheter over the needle and wire advancer (Figure 2.27).

An injection cap or three-way tap should be open, ready and within reach. It is very important to have a clear idea of the course of the artery, and therefore it is palpated at several places along its length. This allows the catheter to be held absolutely parallel to the artery when it is inserted. Holding the wire assembly with the dominant hand, the tip should be inserted through the area of local anaesthetic, pointing towards the hock. The whole assembly is advanced at a flat angle (10° to 20°) through the skin of the foal. As soon as blood is seen in the flash hub, the wire assembly is held very still and the nondominant hand is used to advance the wire by pushing forward the wire advancer. The wire assembly is still held still. The nondominant hand is used to smoothly advance the catheter forward off the wire assembly and into the artery (Figure 2.28). Once the catheter hub is snug against the skin of the foal, the whole wire assembly and stylet are quickly removed and replaced with an injection cap or three-way tap. If the catheter is correctly placed, blood should spurt out of catheter hub as soon as the stylet is removed.

Securing the arterial catheter

Maintaining arterial catheters in foals can be difficult, especially in foals that are active or have seizure activity. The following method of securing the catheter has been successful for the author. The catheter hub is immediately affixed to the skin of the foal with a small amount of Superglue on either side. It may be necessary to swab away blood from the skin, before using the Superglue, to ensure that it sticks. The catheter hub is supported by two rolled-up gauze swabs (4 × 4), placed on either side (Figure 2.29). Depending on the contour of the leg, a rolled-up gauze swab placed between the injection cap and the leg can help keep the catheter straight. The catheter and swabs should be secured with zinc oxide tape wrapped around the leg at

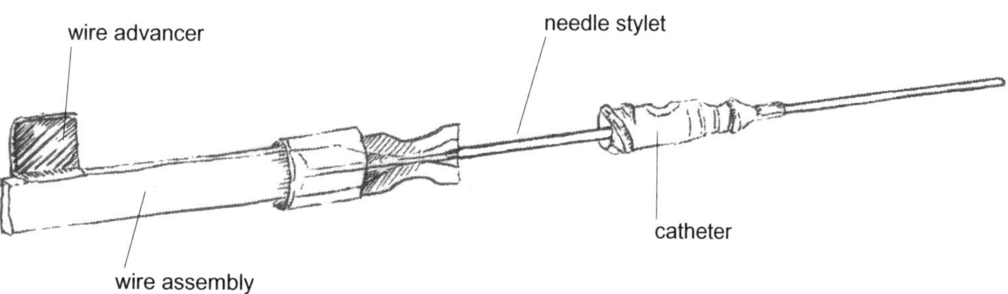

Figure 2.27 Parts of a Seldinger technique arterial catheter.

* RA-04020; Arrow International Inc., Reading, PA, USA.

the level of the catheter hub. The whole assembly should be wrapped with self-adhesive bandaging tape. The catheter should be flushed with the heparinised saline. If being left for extended periods, a "heparin lock" can be useful, if heparin is not contraindicated in the patient. For a "heparin lock", a small amount (<0.3 ml) of undiluted (25,000 units/ml) heparin is injected into the catheter, through the injection cap, to sit in the catheter whilst not in use.

2.9 Placement of a urinary catheter

Placement of a urinary catheter serves several functions in the foal. Firstly, it allows for monitoring of urination. The hourly amount and specific gravity of urine are extremely important for assessing the adequacy of fluid therapy and circulatory support in haemodynamically unstable foals. Secondly, in foals with renal concerns, continuous collection of urine allows feedback on the effectiveness of treatments. It also allows measurement of endogenous creatinine clearance. Finally, in recumbent foals, it keeps the foal clean and dry.

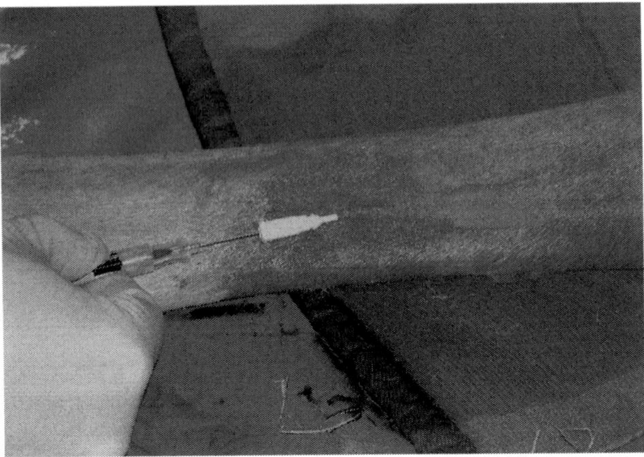

Figure 2.28 The arterial catheter has been slid into place off the needle after a flash of blood was obtained and the wire was advanced. ©Kevin Corley 2004.

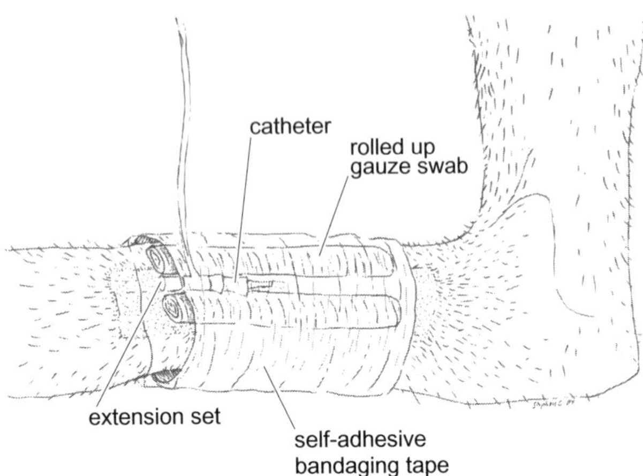

Figure 2.29 Securing an arterial catheter. Rolled-up gauze swabs are placed either side of the catheter hub. The catheter and swabs are secured with zinc oxide tape wrapped round the leg at the level of the catheter hub. The whole assembly should be wrapped with self-adhesive bandaging tape.

It is possible to introduce infection with a urinary catheter. Strict asepsis during placement with good hygiene whilst the catheter is maintained can help to minimise the risk of this.

Equipment needed

The equipment needed for urinary catheterisation is listed in Box 2.13.

Male foal

For most foals, two people are required to pass a urinary catheter, in addition to those restraining the foal. The foal should be restrained in lateral recumbency (see Chapter 2.4), with the hind limbs apart and the uppermost hind limb securely held. One person should put on examination (nonsterile) gloves. This person should firmly hold the shaft of the penis in one hand, approximately 7 to 12 cm caudal to the opening of the preputial skin. The other hand

Box 2.13. Equipment for urinary catheterisation of the foal

For male and female foals
Cotton wool
Chlorhexidine (4%) scrub solution*
Sterile water for irrigation or sterile saline
Surgical gloves
10-ml syringe filled with sterile saline
Urine drainage collection bag†
Sterile K-Y Jelly‡
Empty, sterile, 60-ml catheter-tipped syringe

Additional equipment for male foals
12Fr, 55–64-cm-long Foley catheter with a 10-ml balloon§

Additional equipment for female foals
12Fr, 33-cm-long Foley catheter with a 10-ml balloon§
A resterilised wire from a feeding tube**
OR a sterile narrow (4Fr) dog urinary catheter

Optional
2-0 nonabsorbable monofilament suture on a straight needle††
Zinc oxide tape
7.5-cm (3-inch) wide stretchy adhesive dressing (Elastoplast‡‡/Elastikon§§)
Bandage scissors

*Hibiscrub; Mölnlycke Health Care, Dunstable, UK.
†74.5220.005; Sarstedt, Drinagh, Co. Wexford, Ireland.
‡Johnson and Johnson, New Brunswick, NJ, USA.
§Porges SAS, France.
**12Fr × 108-cm Nasogastric Feeding Tube (NG1243); MILA International Inc, Florence, KY, USA.
††628H, Ethilon Nylon; Ethicon, Somerville, NJ, USA.
‡‡Beiersdorf AG, Hamburg, Germany.
§§Johnson and Johnson, New Brunswick, NJ, USA.

is then placed near the preputial opening and used to gently pull the preputial skin caudally to try and expose the penis head. It can be difficult to expose the penis head in some foals, either because the preputial opening is not very large or because it is difficult to identify and firmly hold the shaft of the penis under the skin.

Once the penis head is exposed, it should be held firmly so that the urethral process and opening is exposed and so that there is not undue pressure on the urethra (to allow passage of the catheter). This is most easily achieved with two hands (Figure 2.30). The head of the penis should then be cleaned with cotton wool soaked in chlorhexidine scrub solution by the person putting in the catheter. The chlorhexidine should be thoroughly washed off with cotton wool soaked in sterile water or saline. This person should then open the surgical glove packet, to create a small sterile area for preparation of the catheter. A small amount of K-Y Jelly is squeezed out onto the open glove packet. The Foley catheter packet is either partially opened so that the catheter can be removed sterilely or handed to an assistant to open. The sterile gloves are then put on.

The end of the Foley catheter is rolled in the blob of K-Y Jelly on the glove packet to lubricate it. This end is then carefully placed into the urethral opening in the centre of the urethral process. The catheter is fed into the urethra as far as it will go. The foal may slightly raise its tail or struggle as the tip of the catheter passes the ischium. Once the catheter is passed into the foal as far as possible, the balloon of the Foley catheter should then be filled with sterile saline (Figure 2.31). Often, urine will flow out of the end of the catheter at this point.

If a Foley catheter with a 10-ml balloon is used, it will self-retain in almost all foals. However, if a catheter with a smaller balloon is used or a struggling foal is catheterised, it may be prudent to suture the catheter in place. This is best achieved by placing a zinc oxide tape "butterfly" on the catheter just in front of the penis, and suturing this to the skin.

Further steps (checking and connecting the catheter to a drainage bag) are the same between male and female foals and are described after the section on female foals, below.

Female foal

It can be difficult to pass a urinary catheter in a female foal, particularly a small one. The foal should be restrained in lateral recumbency (see Chapter 2.4), with the tail held up away from the vulva. The hind limbs should be restrained by a dedicated person if possible. This allows the angle separating the hind limbs to be varied between catheterisation attempts, which can help the catheter to pass if it is proving difficult. The perineum and external vulva should be cleaned with cotton wool soaked in chlorhexidine scrub solution. The chlorhexidine should be thoroughly washed off with cotton wool soaked in sterile water or saline. The surgical glove packet should be opened to create a small sterile area for preparation of the catheter. A small amount of K-Y Jelly is squeezed out onto the open glove packet. The Foley catheter and the wire or dog urinary catheter packets are either partially opened so that the contents can be removed sterilely, or handed to an assistant to open. The person putting in the catheter should then put on the sterile gloves.

The person placing the catheter should carefully feed the sterile wire or dog urinary catheter into the lumen of the Foley catheter, to stiffen the catheter, The person putting the catheter in should thoroughly lubricate the end of the forefinger of the dominant hand and the tip of the Foley catheter in the blob of K-Y Jelly. The lubricated finger is then gently inserted into the vagina until the pelvic bones are palpated (Figure 2.32). Occasionally, the urethral opening can be palpated, in which case the end of the finger should be positioned over this opening. This finger is very

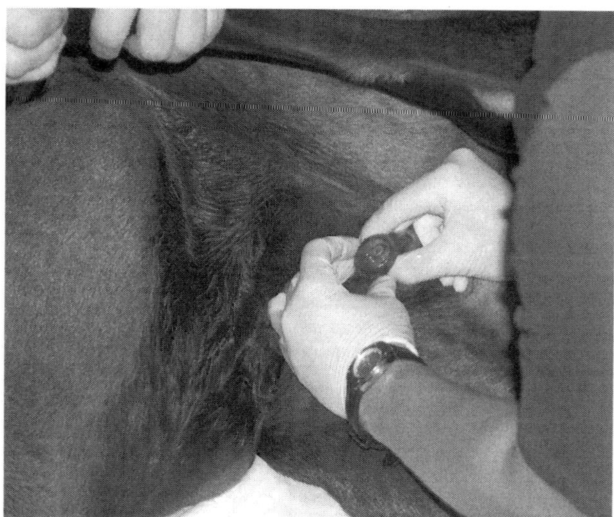

Figure 2.30 Holding the penis of a foal for insertion of a urinary catheter. Care should be taken not to occlude the urethra to allow passage of the catheter. ©Kevin Corley 2004.

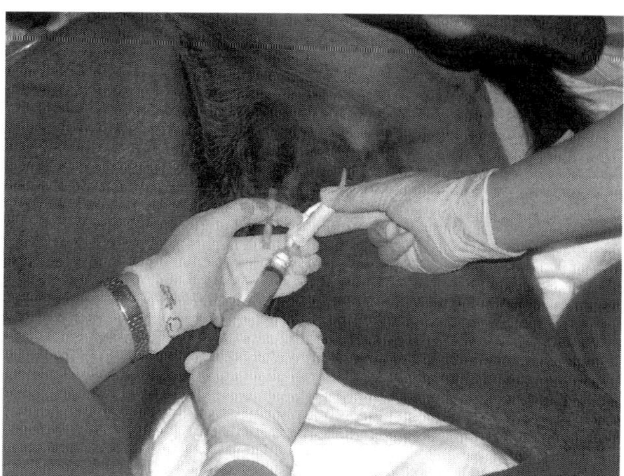

Figure 2.31 Filling the balloon of the Foley catheter, after it has been passed into the bladder, in a male foal. ©Kevin Corley 2004.

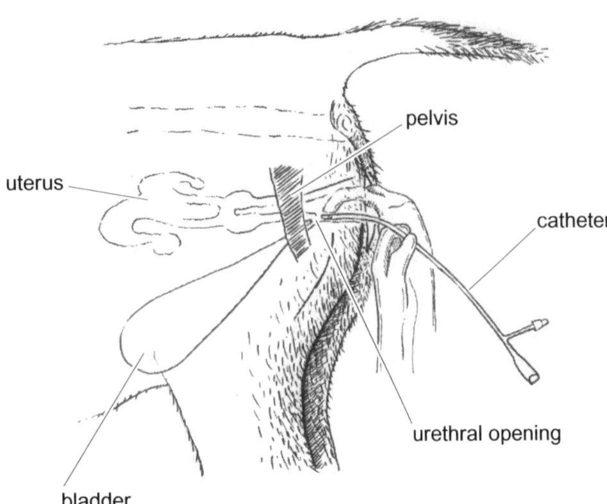

Figure 2.32 Schematic drawing illustrating placing a urinary catheter in a female foal. The catheter is passed along the ventral aspect of a lubricated finger inserted into the vulva, which directs the catheter downwards and into the urethral opening.

slightly curled ventrally. The catheter is then passed ventrally underneath this finger, which gently presses it into the midline ventral floor. The idea is for the catheter to pass into the urethra and on into the bladder (Figure 2.32). If this occurs, most of the catheter will be able to be gently passed forward. Once the catheter is passed into the foal as far as possible, the balloon of the Foley catheter should then be filled with sterile saline (shown in the male in Figure 2.31). If resistance to passing the catheter is felt after having been advanced 1 to 4 cm beyond the end of the finger, the catheter is almost certainly against the cervix and should be withdrawn. Changing the angle between the hind limbs (separating them or bringing them closer together) can help the catheter pass into the urethral opening, if it does not pass the first time.

Checking and connecting the catheter

The catheter should be checked by aspirating with a 60-ml catheter-tipped syringe. This sample can be used for bacterial culture and analysis if sterility has been maintained during the procedure. If the urine has not already started flowing, aspiration with a syringe should start urine flow (if there is any in the bladder). The catheter should be connected to a drainage bag with a one-way valve and a relief valve (Figure 2.33). A fluid-giving set and an empty 1-L fluid bag can be used in place of a surgical drainage bag but do not contain an antireflux valve and the sterile system needs to be opened to empty it. A surgical drainage bag is not necessarily more expensive than a fluid-giving set.

If the foal is able to get up on its own, the urine bag should be fixed to the foal's leg to avoid it standing on it when it gets up (Figure 2.34). A layer of stretchy adhesive dressing (Elastoplast) is placed just above the hock. The urine collection bag is taped to this with zinc oxide tape.

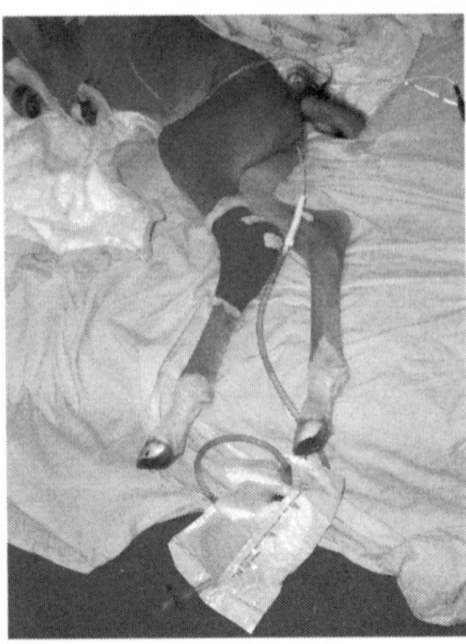

Figure 2.33 Connection of the urinary catheter to a surgical drainage bag to form a closed system in a female foal. ©Kevin Corley 2004.

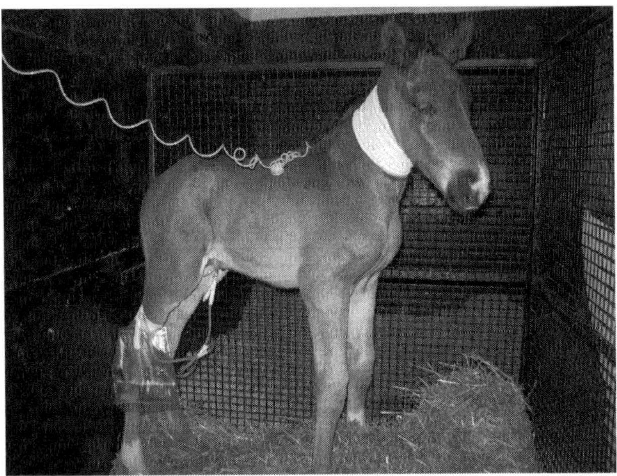

Figure 2.34 Closed urine collection system in an ambulatory colt foal. The catheter is stitched to the skin just in front of the prepuce. The bag is taped just above the hock. ©Kevin Corley 2007.

Stitching the zinc oxide tape to the Elastoplast with thick suture avoids the urine bag falling off when full.

2.10 Ultrasonography of the umbilicus

Ultrasonography of the umbilicus is indicated in any foal with an abnormality of the external umbilicus, including swelling, heat, persistent wetness or dripping urine or pus. It is also indicated in foals less than 3 weeks old with fever, leucocytosis or leucopenia, irrespective of the appearance of the external umbilical stump.

Equipment needed

Most ultrasound machines used in veterinary practice are suitable for imaging the umbilical structures of the foal, including those routinely used for reproductive scanning of the mare. The best images are obtained with 10- to 12-MHz probes, but diagnostic images can usually be obtained with probes of 5 to 8 MHz. Linear and curvilinear probes are suitable for scanning the umbilicus (Box 2.14).

Ultrasonographic examination

This is most easily done in a well-restrained standing foal (see Chapter 2.4). If the foal is unable to stand, it can be imaged in lateral recumbency. If imaging a lively foal in a standing position, it is a good idea to tie a piece of bandage material around the wire of the probe and loop this around the wrist of the operator, to prevent a dropped ultrasound probe hitting the floor.

It is occasionally possible in fine-coated foals to obtain an acceptable image without clipping, but a better image is obtained if the hair is removed. The hair should be clipped from the umbilical stump cranially to the xiphisternum along the midline (approximately 5-cm-width clip) and caudally from the external umbilical stump to the prepuce or mammary gland. This area should be thoroughly cleaned and covered with ultrasound coupling gel. The probe is held in a transverse position across the body of the foal. The angle of the probe should be adjusted slowly to try and create the most circular profile possible of the vessel being examined.

> **Box 2.14. Equipment for ultrasound of the umbilicus**
>
> **Required**
>
> Ultrasound machine with a linear or curvilinear probe, rated between 5 and 12 MHz
> Clippers with a fine (No. 40) blade
> Cotton wool or gauze swabs soaked in surgical spirit
> Ultrasound contact gel

The internal umbilical structures consists of the right and left arteries and the urachus, which are caudal to the external stump, and the vein, which is cranial to the stump. The right and left umbilical arteries travel caudally with the urachus towards the bladder and then separate to run either side of the bladder. These arteries become the round ligaments of the bladder. The umbilical vein travels along the cranial midline towards and into the liver (Figure 2.35).

If the internal umbilical stump containing the arteries cannot be immediately imaged, it is a good idea to place the probe caudally and to try to image the bladder. The bladder is recognised as a large echolucent (black) structure (Figure 2.36). The arteries course along either side of the bladder. The probe should be moved slowly cranially, and the arteries can usually be imaged at the apex of the

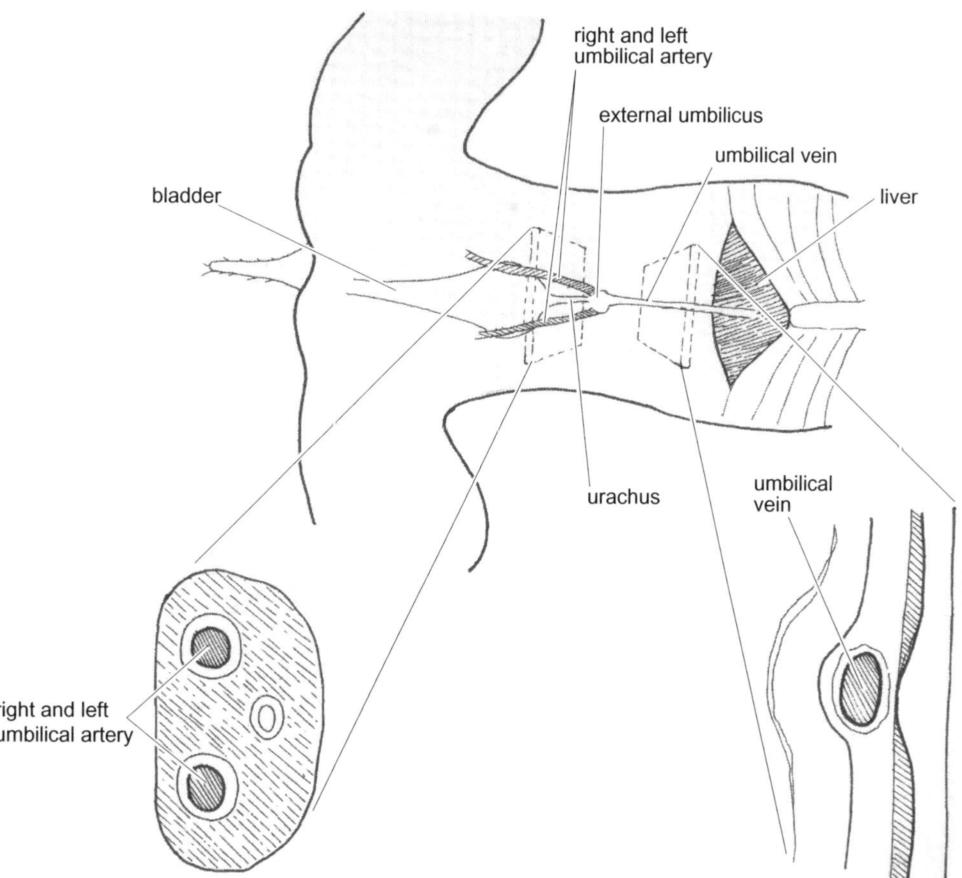

Figure 2.35 Schematic diagram showing the anatomy of the internal umbilical structures of the foal.

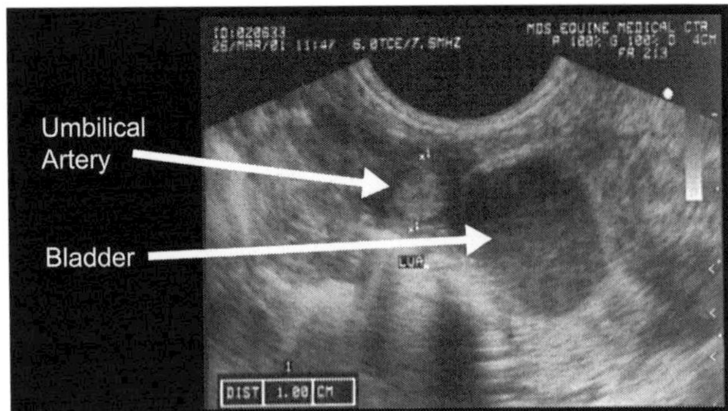

Figure 2.36 Ultrasonogram of the bladder apex and the left umbilical artery. ©Kevin Corley 2000.

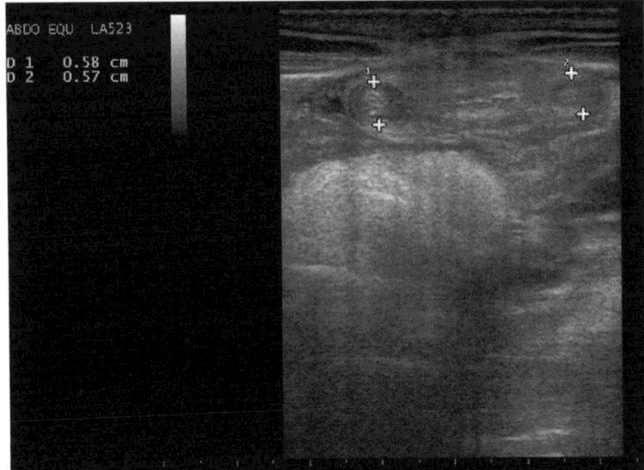

Figure 2.37 Ultrasonogram of the internal umbilicus, showing normal umbilical arteries (and their measurements), and a slightly enlarged urachus. ©Kevin Corley 2007.

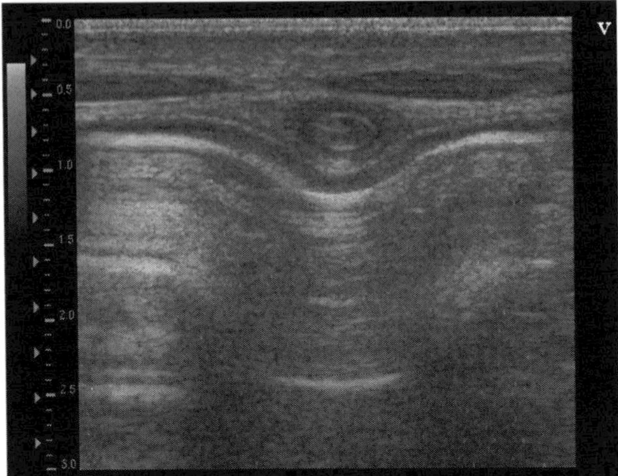

Figure 2.38 Ultrasonogram of the internal umbilical vein, showing normal structures. ©Kevin Corley 2006.

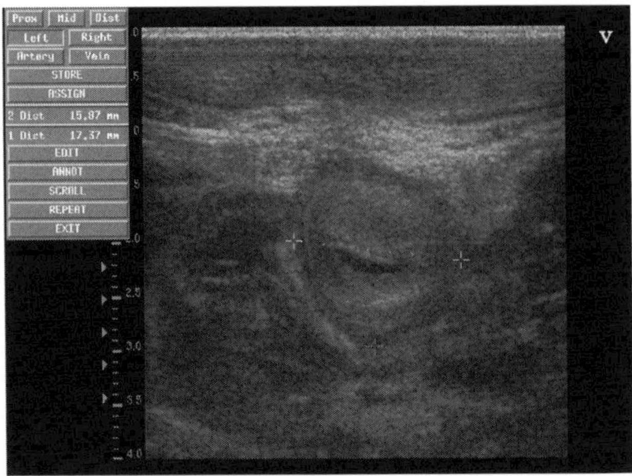

Figure 2.39 Ultrasonogram of an infected umbilical vein, with a diameter of 15.8 to 17.3 mm. ©Kevin Corley 2004.

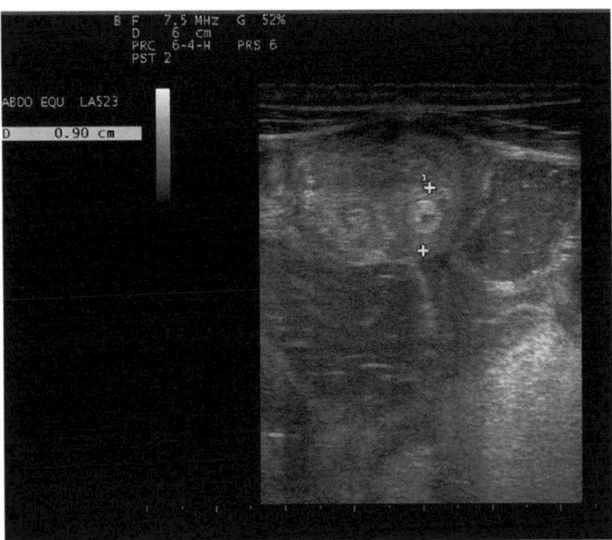

Figure 2.40 Ultrasonogram of an infected umbilical artery. Note the hypoechoic lesion in the centre of the artery, and the thickened arterial wall. The internal umbilicus was removed at surgery, and *E. coli* was cultured. ©Kevin Corley 2007.

bladder and the internal umbilical structure followed forward to the umbilical stump. The umbilical vein is most easily imaged immediately cranial to the stump, on the midline. It may be traced from here cranially towards the liver.

Normal umbilical arteries have a mean diameter of 8.5 mm (range, 5 to 14 mm) (Figure 2.37). The umbilical vein is slightly ovoid in shape and has a maximum diameter of 6 mm at the cranial and caudal ends and of 5 mm in the midsection (Figure 2.38). Increases in diameter and an area of hypoechogenicity in the core are signs of infection in the internal umbilical structures (Figures 2.39 and 2.40).

3

Hospital design and organisation

3.1 Designing and building an equine hospital
3.2 Diagnostic imaging
3.3 Biosecurity for equine hospitals: Protecting the patient and the hospital
3.4 Hospital forms

3.1 Designing and building an equine hospital

Tim Greet

Introduction

People develop equine hospital facilities for various reasons. In the majority of instances, it is to allow the provision of high-quality diagnostic, medical and surgical services from premises to which clients are encouraged to bring their horses and ponies. This is clearly highly efficient from the veterinary point of view, obviating the need for less effective delivery of such services on a peripatetic basis. However, some may also consider it as a necessary investment to maintain or improve the quality of horse work undertaken, or even as a means to increase veterinary business and therefore income. Whatever the reason, more and more private practices and academic institutes have built or modernised their equine facilities to hospital standards in recent years.

The use of the word "hospital" to describe a clinic has for some time implied a certain standard of facility and carried a special meaning within the veterinary profession; in fact, in the United Kingdom, the phrase "veterinary hospital" is protected by the Royal College of Veterinary Surgeons (RCVS). The name can only be used to describe those premises having achieved that standard when examined through an appropriate inspection process. At the time of writing, veterinary hospitals are to be classified in Tier Three of the new RCVS Practice Standards. Not every equine clinic is developed to such a standard and nor does it need to be; it is very much a matter of "horses for courses." Furthermore, the structure of the building and available facilities should be designed to satisfy its use. A clinic that specialises in artificial insemination clearly has vastly different needs from that of a high-volume surgical facility.

The intention of this chapter is to describe the process of design and the development of a building to house equine diagnostic, surgical and medical facilities such as might be found in larger private practices or any large referral hospital. This is not intended to be a blueprint for the ideal hospital—merely to provide an approach to thinking about the various issues that must be considered before undertaking such a development. These are very much my thoughts, and certainly others may have quite different views about design and function.

The concept and the site

Before any time is spent on designing a hospital, it is imperative that adequate thought is directed at the *raison d'être* of the building. Critical issues such as the geographical and physical location of the site in relation to access roads, including major transport routes if referral cases are to form a significant element of the caseload, must be addressed at the outset. The planning authorities will demand that the planners are involved at a relatively early stage to ensure success once a planning application has been submitted, and it is sensible to do so. Inevitably, the impact of the hospital on the local environment will be a priority in their minds, and therefore this must be to the fore in the mind of the design team. However, with a moderately supportive local planning department and a scheme carefully thought out in advance, there is a high chance of permission being granted. Equestrian business is one of the few success stories in the rural environment these days, and veterinary hospitals can provide much needed local employment.

Should an architect be engaged for the project? The answer for a structure of any significant size is almost certainly going to be "yes". However, even if such a person is experienced in designing veterinary or even equine hospital buildings, the veterinary team will have to have done much of the spade work in terms of deciding how the building and site should operate, before best use can be made of architectural expertise.

In an ideal world, the hospital should be located in a rural setting and sufficiently divorced from surrounding habitation to avoid the creation of a nuisance. This chapter is based on the assumption that you are working from a blank sheet of paper. Of course, in reality, that is seldom the case, and there may be a necessity to work with preexisting buildings, or the size or shape of the available space, or the nature of the land in some parts of the site, may dictate the overall scheme of the hospital site plan. However, the general principles of hospital design still apply under such circumstances, and adapting generic suggestions made here to a particular local circumstance is perfectly valid.

One of the most important matters to be attended to at an early stage is to write brief notes on the thinking behind each aspect of the building and a description of how each element of the site is intended to function after the building is completed. Each room should be identified by purpose, size, specific requirements, intended contents and its relationship to the rest of the site. It is inevitable that some aspects of structure or function will be changed or will evolve during, or even after the building process. However, committing such ideas to paper or to a computer screen from the start ensures that each item is carefully thought out and integrated into the greater scheme of the project. Such notes will form the basis for a permanent portfolio that will include the final architects' plans, standard operating procedures for every aspect and function of the site and all health and safety matters. It is also useful to photograph carefully each aspect of the site, before, during and after completion of the project. Much architectural work is carried out using computers these days, and it may be possible to integrate the necessary site survey, the architects' plans and drawings and the photographs into a user-friendly guide to the whole project.

Car and lorry parking

The entrance must take note of the type of access road and allow adequate visibility for vehicles entering and leaving the site. A gate is essential to provide security and prevent the escape of loose horses, but it must not impede the flow of traffic during working hours. Ideally, the gate should be set back from the road to allow the longest horse box (goose-necked trailer) (and they seem to be getting ever larger these days!) to pull off the road safely when the gates are shut (Figure 3.1). Automatic gates that can be left open during the working day and opened from a distance (e.g., from within the reception area) to admit patients out of hours are ideal. It is sensible to think about some sort of security camera system, which may include the use of additional dummy cameras as well as a video link, to identify any miscreants. Specialist security firms abound around the country and a reliable one should be contacted to give you advice in this regard. These days, the use of Webcams linked to the hospital server can provide all the surveillance needs of the most complex hospital design. These can be linked via the server to computers at various points in the hospital or even to a distant site.

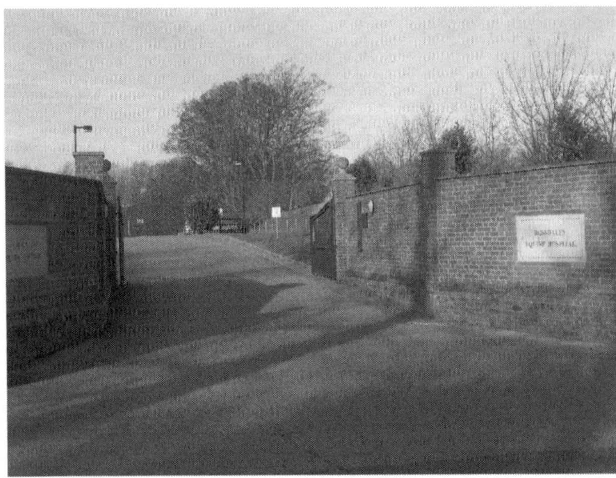

Figure 3.1 Gates sited back from the road, allowing lorries to pull off the road when the gates are shut. ©Tim Greet 2006.

Numerous clearly visible signs distributed around the site warning of camera surveillance will add to the sense of security. Standard operating procedures regarding opening, closing and locking of the gates should be allied to a protocol for admitting and discharging patients at unsocial hours of the day and night, and on weekends and holidays. Some clients may wish to leave trailers on the premises. Such requests should be given careful thought and only allowed with adequate disclaimers in case of theft. Parking should be under the scrutiny of the security camera system as theft of equine transport is not a rare occurrence!

The car and lorry (horse trailer or horse float) park needs to be situated conveniently for the buildings but preferably not far from the gates; it is absolutely counterproductive to have vehicles driving all over the site, particularly if there are horses being walked or trotted about. In this regard, you need to think carefully about the flow of people (staff and visitors) as well as horses and their handlers. The type of client likely to be visiting the hospital will dictate the type of loading ramps to be used. In a large referral hospital, it is wise to have easy access for both side-loading and rear-loading boxes (Figure 3.2, A and B). The provision of walls to a ramp will also help with horses and ponies that are difficult to load. Remember that you will need a gently sloping ramp for orthopaedic emergencies that must be close to both radiographic and surgical facilities.

In addition, consideration must be given to service vehicles that will have to visit the site on a regular basis, including the muck removal lorry. It should be borne in mind that the muck pit must not be situated too distant from the stables but must also be easily accessible by road; removal

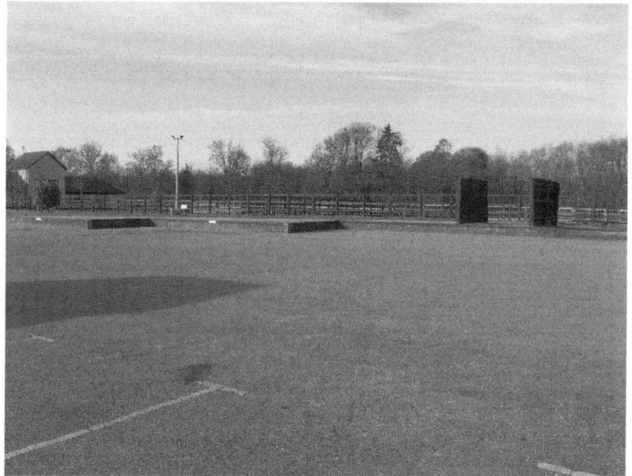

A

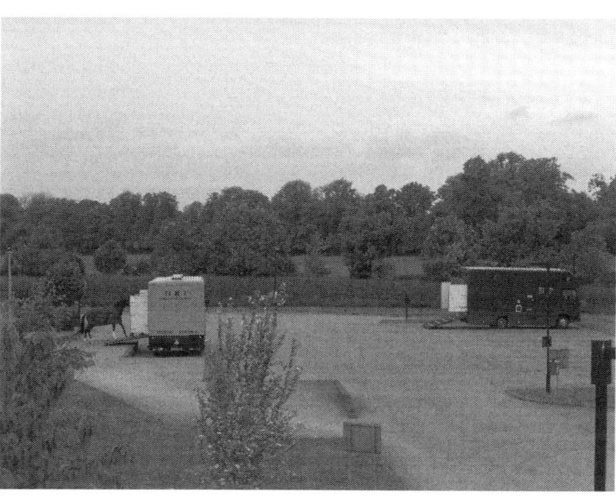

B

Figure 3.2A-B Loading ramps allowing unloading of both side loading and end loading lorries. ©Tim Greet 2006.

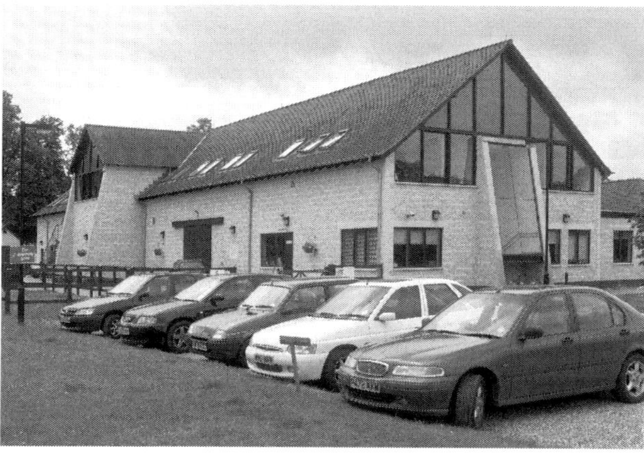

Figure 3.3 Visitors car park. ©Tim Greet 2006.

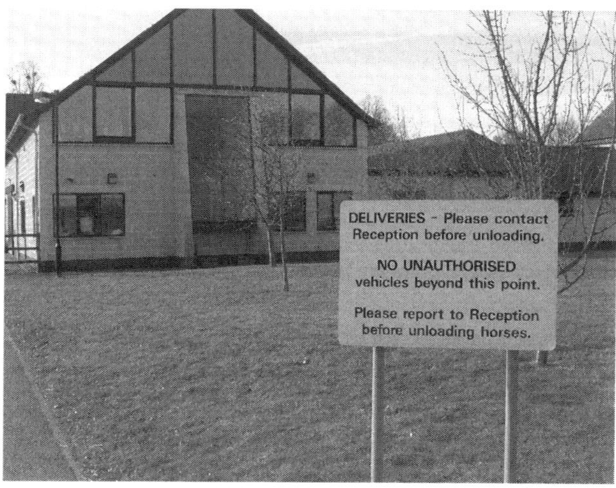
DELIVERIES - Please contact
Reception before unloading.
NO UNAUTHORISED
vehicles beyond this point.
Please report to Reception
before unloading horses.

Figure 3.4 A sign asking clients and delivery vans not to unload before reporting to reception. ©Tim Greet 2006.

of both clinical and nonclinical waste is another major requirement, and the site for storage of this material, similarly, must not be too far from the hospital or the access road. Also, the supply of drugs, medical gases and other materials and car parking for those providing technical support for the veterinary and other equipment must be taken in to consideration. An overflow car park for visitors attending lectures or other meetings in the hospital might prevent unwanted vehicles from obstructing access to the buildings (Figure 3.3).

There should be lighting in the car and lorry park, which could be automatically triggered by a light sensor or a time switch. This lighting must extend to the doors of the hospital as it is essential to ensure safety of staff and clients at night or when the ambient light is poor. The lights around the hospital doors can be triggered by heat sensors.

Clear signs in the car and lorry park area should indicate the location of hospital reception. There should also be a sign instructing clients to come to reception before unloading their horse (Figure 3.4). It should warn drivers that vehicles may not come closer to the hospital building except by special arrangement. Signs offering health and safety advice about the dangers of horses to people or at least to children and disclaimers about theft may be considered unattractive in the forecourt of your high-class building but are probably useful in the event of an accident or if something were to be stolen.

Buildings

Stabling and the yard

Stabling can be built readily employing "off the peg" designs or be designed individually to suit a particular need. If the hospital deals with many larger breeds of horses or has a high throughput of mares and foals, a number of larger stalls will be required. In any case, most hospitalised horses are confined with minimal exercise and may easily become bored, so good-sized stalls are advisable. In an ideal world, it is best for hospitals to have stalls of differing sizes to accommodate the various sizes and needs of individual patients.

If sick foals are commonly dealt with, it may be advisable to create a specialised foal unit, with large stalls using a moveable barrier to separate mare and foal, thus allowing critical care nursing of the foal. Examples of different barrier arrangements are shown in Figure 3.5, A–E. Consideration must be given as to how the foal will be nursed in this situation. Some sick foals must be kept warm, and the use of a heated water bed can be very valuable (Figure 3.5, A). Access to laboratory and medical support is also important. A foal unit should be kitted out with enough cupboard space to stock everything that might be needed in an emergency, including an oxygen supply and a ventilator. An inventory of all items should be prepared and checked carefully before each breeding season, when supplies should be replenished and the unit cleaned and prepared for the action to come.

Critical care of adult horses is equally important and access to the laboratory, stores of intravenous fluids and other drugs is essential. Critical care stalls should be heated, and infrared heat lamps or heat panels can be used (Figure 3.6). It is important that large volumes of intravenous fluids can be administered without the horse needing to be held. This can easily be accommodated by using a swivelling hoist mechanism in the roof and flexible tubing. It is beneficial to have some heating in the fluid store so that time is not needlessly wasted when a horse requires intravenous fluids in an emergency. Critical care stalls should be within easy reach of the anaesthetic rooms and the surgical suite, as frequently sick postoperative patients will be moved from anaesthetic recovery directly into a critical care stall for supportive therapy.

Critical care stalls must be very easy to wash down and clean as these stables are often occupied by the sickest patients, and infectious agents such as *Salmonella* spp. are an occupational hazard when nursing such animals. Some sort of impervious flooring is preferable to concrete, but flooring is a very critical issue that will be dealt with later in the chapter. Each hospital should be able to steam clean and disinfect stables suspected of harbouring infectious agents, and routine cleaning and disinfection should be carried out on a regular basis, in any case. Standard operating policies for using and cleaning critical care stabling are mandatory, as is the consideration of health and safety issues in nursing such patients.

Every hospital must have isolation facilities, and the RCVS hospital regulations stipulate their minimum standard. However, the management of patients with potentially contagious or zoonotic infections requires considerable thought. Without question such a facility must be sited away from other stables. In fact, in our hospital, we are lucky enough to have premises some 2 miles from the hospital site and we keep our isolation patients there. There is always a dilemma between keeping potentially "infectious" patients away from other horses yet easily accessible to the nursing staff and all the support systems that such patients sometimes require. Inevitably, some compromises must be made, but they should only be allowed bearing the worst-case scenario in mind.

Other issues regarding the stables include the type of bedding to be used. My preference is for dust-free materials such as paper or clean shavings. However, we have straw bedding in our foal unit, as that is what most brood mares are used to. In some stables, we have rubber flooring that can be used without bedding. This can be useful for some patients with long bone fractures whether or not the injured limb is supported in a cast. Bedding, particularly long straw, can wrap around limbs, particularly when they are in a cast, and thus interfere significantly with locomotion. In addition, such a rubber floor is much less likely to cause abrasion to the solar surface of fibreglass casts.

Some fracture patients are best managed by tying the horse up to a bar fixed to a stable wall (Figure 3.7). This must be fixed to allow the horse to gain access to feed and water mangers without difficulty and is only intended to prevent horses from lying down or, more importantly, from having to stand up and compromising the fractured limb. Such patients then are also better managed on rubber flooring. We have several stables so equipped.

Some horses with severe lameness are best managed in a stable with a soft floor or bedding, which can pack into the sole and frog of the weight-bearing limb to reduce the risk of "overload" laminitis. So the use of a stable with a sand floor or a readily compressible bedding material such as peat or sawdust can be very valuable in such instances.

Generally speaking, hay is fed via a net suspended from the stable wall, although in some hospitals, horses are fed from the floor; this is certainly advisable in some clinical situations (e.g., after laryngoplasty). A fixed or removable manger can be used for feeding. Whilst provision of automatic watering devices might be seen as labour saving, it does not allow assessment of water consumption by the patient, which may be vital in some situations. Manually filled water mangers are therefore preferred.

Somewhere near the stables, an equipment store should be built. This can cater for tractors, mowers, yard vacuum cleaners and a range of equipment used for mucking out and maintenance of the stable yard. There must also be a tack room that should be sited where stable staff can monitor horses and people coming and going from the yard. This should house all the tack, rugs, stable bandaging and any other equipment required to run a hospital yard. It should have adequate heating for the winter months and a place to make tea and coffee and to wash hands. Like all parts of the hospital, it must be connected to the telephone; thought should be given to placing an external bell to draw the attention of stable staff to incoming telephone calls when they are in the yard.

Siting the muck pit correctly is quite critical, as mentioned above, and its position may depend upon the method used to muck out the stables. For example, it is much easier for it to be situated at a site distant to the stabling if a tractor and trailer rather than muck sacks are to

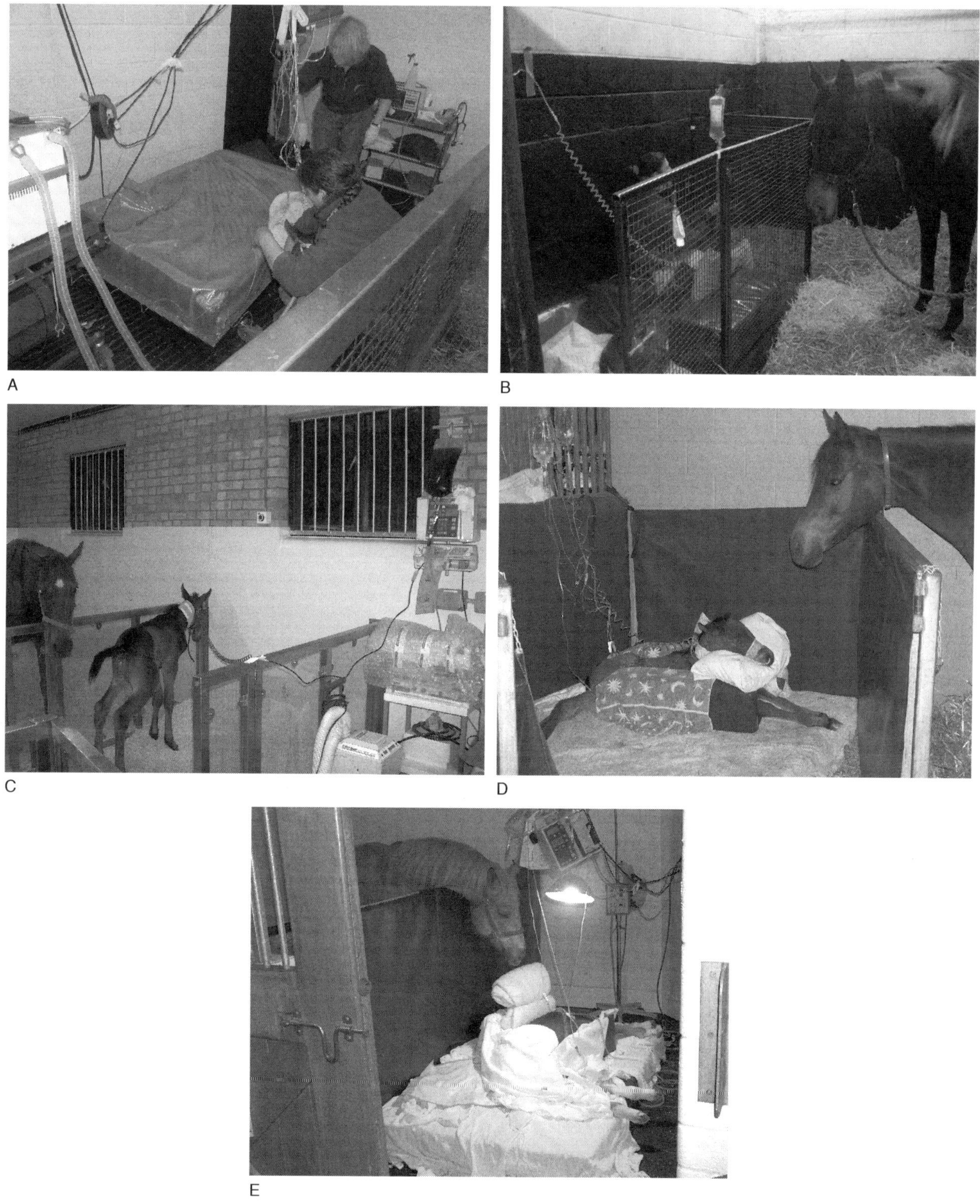

Figure 3.5 Arrangements for separating mares and foals, during treatment of the foal at Rossdale and Partners, Newmarket, UK (**A**), Anglesey Lodge Equine Hospital, The Curragh, Ireland (**B**), the Royal Veterinary College, London, UK (**C**), Scone Veterinary Hospital, Scone, NSW, Australia (**D**) and Cornell University, Ithaca, NY, USA (**E**). ©Tim Greet 2006 (**A**) and ©Kevin Corley 2007 (**B–E**).

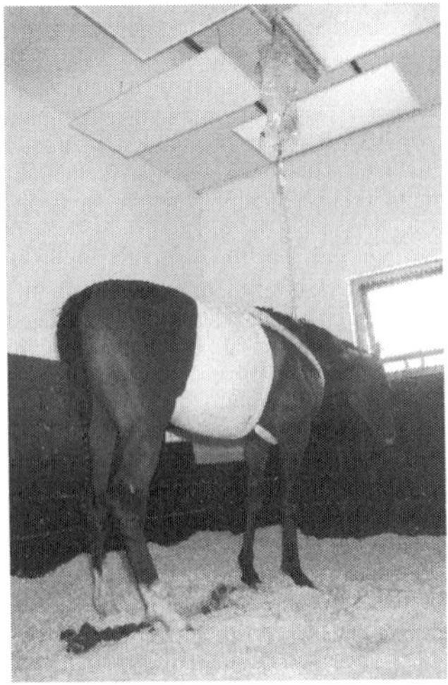

Figure 3.6 An intensive care patient receiving fluids. Note the ceiling-mounted heating panels and fluid hangings. ©Tim Greet 2006.

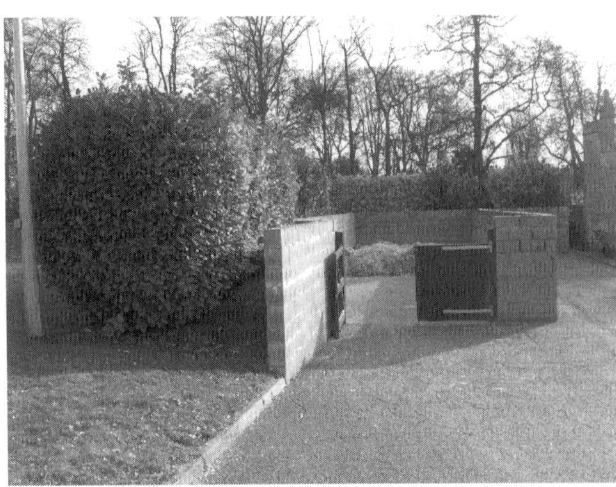

Figure 3.8 The muck pit can be screened with trees and bushes, to prevent environmental pollution by bedding material, and to improve the aesthetic appearance. ©Tim Greet 2006.

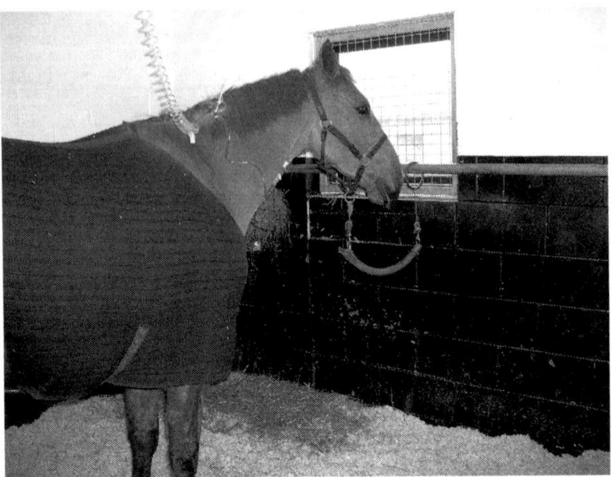

Figure 3.7 In-stall rail for tying-up fracture patients, to prevent them lying down. ©Tim Greet 2006.

be used. You must also consider the prevailing wind and how exposed is the site, to avoid paper and other bedding material blowing around. Screening the pit by planting trees or shrubs and covering the pit with a net will both help to improve its aesthetic appearance and reduce environmental pollution by bedding material (Figure 3.8).

Health and safety issues have a very high priority when running an equine hospital, and both employees and clients must be catered for. So, for example, a risk assessment must be carried out for the filling and emptying of the muck pit and potential hazards identified and neutralised where possible. All of these must be included in written standing operating procedures and shown to the relevant employees.

Other areas to be considered when designing the yard include trot up areas, a lunge ring and possibly a ménage to allow horses to be ridden safely. It is an advantage to have flood lighting associated with these areas to allow their use when the ambient light level is low. Exercising some colic patients on a lunge line is standard practice in our hospital, and often happens during the hours of darkness.

If the routine work of the hospital involves many racehorses, access to a gallop would also be very useful. Trotting up areas may be indoors or outdoors but should at least have a flat firm surface of sufficient size to allow trotting in a straight line, and in 10- to 20-metre circles. Access to a soft surface for trotting is also very useful, as is somewhere with a slope to assess both lame horses and those suffering from neurological disorders.

The hospital

The reception and client waiting area

These areas are of great importance as they influence the first impression that any client has of the hospital. They must be strategically positioned at the very entrance to the hospital area, in such a way that all visitors and clients have no choice but to report there, before doing anything else. It is also useful if the reception staff can monitor all arrivals and departures from the hospital site, and having a clear view of the car and lorry park is a distinct advantage. This is probably an area that will need to accommodate an expansion in staff numbers as the hospital becomes busier, so ensure there is the potential to increase the available desk space to allow for such an increase. Obviously, there needs to be plenty of electrical sockets and Internet access.

The waiting area for clients with surgical or medical patients need not be too large, as in most situations clients can be dispatched home once the patient has been admitted and the clinician has explained the proposed course of action, risks and likely prognosis. As mentioned later, in an ideal world, the lameness department may be sited separately from the surgical and medical units. In such a situation, a separate larger waiting area can accommodate clients who might spend much of the day waiting for the results of a lameness investigation.

It is good public relations to provide tea, coffee and biscuits in the client waiting areas. Many people leave home at a very early hour and travel a significant distance to come to the hospital. Although many modern horse boxes have every conceivable facility and some clients might choose to wait in their box, there will have to be an interface between client and staff at some point, and this should be as positive an experience for the client as possible. Being shown some consideration by the hospital staff invariably makes a good impression. Conversely, rude staff may result in clients refusing to come back to the hospital no matter how skilled the veterinary attention might be. A good selection of current equestrian magazines is a useful distraction for clients who might have to wait longer than intended. There should be space enough for moderately comfortable seating, particularly for clients who have to await the results of lameness investigations.

For a variety of reasons, it is useful to have a museum of various anatomical bits and pieces. Firstly, they can be amusing for clients to look at. Secondly, they can provide useful props when explaining to clients about proposed operations or certain injuries. Finally, a set of equine bones is also very useful for surgeons or radiologists as an *aide memoire*, when making a surgical plan or interpreting a radiographic image. In fact, an articulated set of bones is very valuable in many clinical situations.

The reception area should be the hub of communications in the hospital, and a reliable telephone and paging system must be based there. In our hospital, there are television screens connected to cameras in the operating theatres so that the reception staff knows where the surgical team might be found at any time. Closed circuit cameras surveying the gate and lorry park also feed into a television screen and 24-hour video-recorder in the reception area. As the sentinel post for the whole site, there should be large windows allowing clear vision towards the gate and driveway, and desks should face the windows to ensure the best chance of identifying visitors as they arrive or depart (Figure 3.9). There needs to be clear signposting in the car and lorry park to the reception area. It is most undesirable having people meandering around the site who have not booked in first at reception. Nowadays, it should be standard practice to create an electronic file for each case and for appropriate indemnity forms to be signed at the very outset of any procedure.

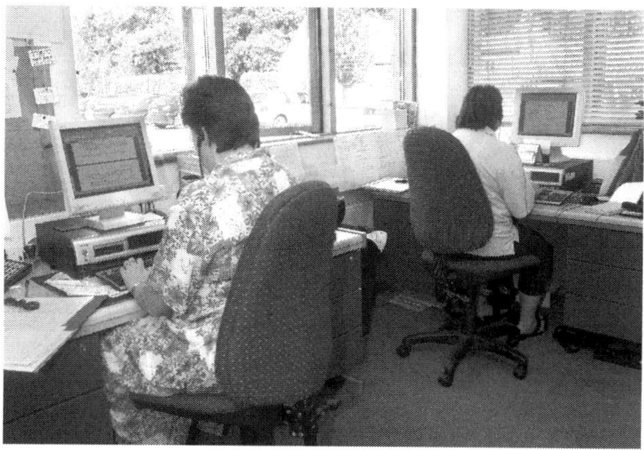

Figure 3.9 The reception office should face the front of the site, and the car park and horse unloading area in particular. ©Tim Greet 2006.

The nurses' base and the main clinical area

Close to the stables and the nerve centre of veterinary operations is the nurses' base. This is where the records of inpatients are kept, daily treatments are determined and appropriate drugs drawn up, and also where medicines, bandages and equipment required to minister to all categories of patient will be stored. Provision must be made for several large sinks, space for a refrigerator, washing and drying machines and plenty of cupboards to house the plethora of instrumentation necessary to deal with all situations that are likely to occur. It is from here that the effective perioperative management of the surgical patients is delivered and coordinated. It is also a very convenient site to locate a small hospital laboratory, which is best kept in an adjacent room. It should have several telephone connections and access to the Internet.

In our hospital, we keep a white board on the back of a door and a wall that identifies all the stables, the nature and name of the patients they house, their medications, proposed investigations or surgical treatment, clinician involved, expected date of departure and any other information relevant to the management of that case. This board becomes the focus of twice-daily clinical fora, where cases and treatments are discussed and courses of action decided. It also allows a regular check on clinical progress and on the all-important communication with client and referring veterinary surgeon, which is essential to the efficient running of any modern equine hospital. Needless to say, the board is frequently updated and is the source of information for all staff dealing with the patients, and this information is relayed daily to the reception staff so that updates are available to keep concerned owners informed. The level of communication will depend on the individual case, but it is important that all staff who might find themselves giving out information to clients must do so accurately and speak with "one voice". Mixed messages are a recipe for client confusion and dissatisfaction.

There is also merit in having a closed circuit televisual or Webcam connection between the nurses' base and foal or adult critical care, and isolation stalls, if funds allow. This accommodates distant monitoring (and recording if necessary) of either sick patients or for conditions such as narcolepsy that occur so intermittently that it would be impractical to provide nursing staff to observe the patient continuously.

The main clinical area should be close to the nurses' base. It needs to be floored with a nonslip and easily cleaned material (see later). At least one set of stocks should be available for general use. The design of these is discussed later. The addition of separate clinical rooms will allow the examination of several horses simultaneously. It is important that the central clinical area is large enough to allow horses to pass without danger and to enter any additional rooms without disturbing the examination of other horses. Our clinic hall is just about adequate for our needs at approximately 12.5 × 6 metres. The additional rooms should certainly be no less than 4 metres square, and significantly larger if stocks are to be installed. One of these rooms can be equipped with a high rolled steel joist from which a hoist can be suspended. Such an arrangement can then be used to suspend a horse in slings for orthopaedic or neurological problems. However, one disadvantage of this arrangement is that such patients can clutter up one of the busiest areas in the hospital, often for several days or longer. It might therefore be more suitable to set up a beam in one of the outside stables away from the examination area but hopefully close enough to allow convenient administration of intensive care to the patient if necessary.

These additional rooms are invaluable to allow the examination of patients preoperatively, the changing of bandages, the treatment of sedated foals if joint lavage or cast or splint application is necessary and a whole range of other activities that are best carried out with ready access to medicines, bandage materials, etc. Of course, such rooms could also be set up with stocks to allow ultrasound examinations, extracorporeal shock wave therapy and an additional location for endoscopy. It is important to consider where such equipment is to be stored to remain convenient for use but without cluttering the clinical area. Thus, an additional room can be used as an equipment store.

The layout of these rooms and the central clinical area is one of the most critical in the whole design of the hospital. As mentioned previously, it is very useful to consider the design process in several stages. Firstly, the intended uses of the area should be listed, and potential conflicts of interests, duplication of function and, most importantly, the flow of horses and staff worked out. This must be considered in the context of the whole site. Next, it is important to determine the most effective size for each individual room. Most veterinary surgeons have great difficulty in visualising the available space from architects' plans or drawings, and the process is facilitated by considering it in life size. Thus, the rooms should be mapped out in full size in a large open space like a car park, paddock or any convenient piece of ground. This technique is also very valuable when designing the operating theatres, standing surgical rooms and other areas where horses and equipment must be accommodated together in a way that maximises efficiency. In that instance, it is helpful to know the size of operating tables, anaesthetic machines, ventilators and any other bulky equipment such as radiographic generators that might be used in the space. Visiting other successful hospitals is also highly recommended as a source of good ideas. There is no point in reinventing the wheel, although individual working methods will vary considerably and necessitate differing building requirements.

The anaesthetic stalls and surgical facilities

The central clinical area should also be close to the anaesthetic rooms, as this allows ready transfer of patients following a preanaesthetic check to the stall where general anaesthesia is induced. In our hospital we have designed these areas to be adjacent parallel oblong spaces (Figure 3.10). Thus, at one end we have the examination stalls; next a large clinic hall with stocks; next to that are three anaesthetic stalls; next to that an anaesthetic hall; next to that two operating theatres; and next to that cleaning, sterilising, instrument and theatre equipment storage, changing rooms, trolley lay up and scrub up areas. This arrangement works very well and has been based on the concept of "nonsterile" horses entering at one end and "nonsterile" people from the opposite end. They meet up in the middle, where both are hopefully as "sterile" as possible! It is vital to consider the flow of "dirty" to "clean" to "aseptic" and to designate each area with its own code for dress and degree of cleanliness/asepsis. Following this approach, the interrelationship between connecting areas can be identified and incorporated into the building design. As mentioned earlier, it is very valuable to mark out the individual spaces in full size to assess how they will function when the building has been constructed. Time spent considering such details at an early stage will pay dividends in the long run.

Very few equine hospitals employ environmental positive pressure ventilation systems in the operating theatre as has become standard in many human hospitals. The cost and impracticality of incorporating such a system have precluded its use in all but a few equine hospitals around the world. It is my view that such an omission can be accommodated without compromising the patient to any extent, provided sufficient attention is paid to the other major principles involved in aseptic surgery.

In our hospital, we have created three padded anaesthetic rooms, to deal with our throughput of general anaesthetic patients (currently between 750 and 800 per annum). The largest one in the middle is designed to allow induction of general anaesthesia with a bolus of ketamine after sedation with an α_2-agonist and with the anaesthetist and a nurse in the stall as the patient falls to the floor. The horse is then intubated and administered a mixture of oxygen and anaesthetic gas. This approach seems to work well, although clearly other systems, such as using a gate to trap the patient whilst a mixture of guaiphenesin is administered prior to a bolus of anaesthetic agent, work equally well. This stall measures approximately 4.5 × 4 metres, which is adequate for all types of equine patient using our

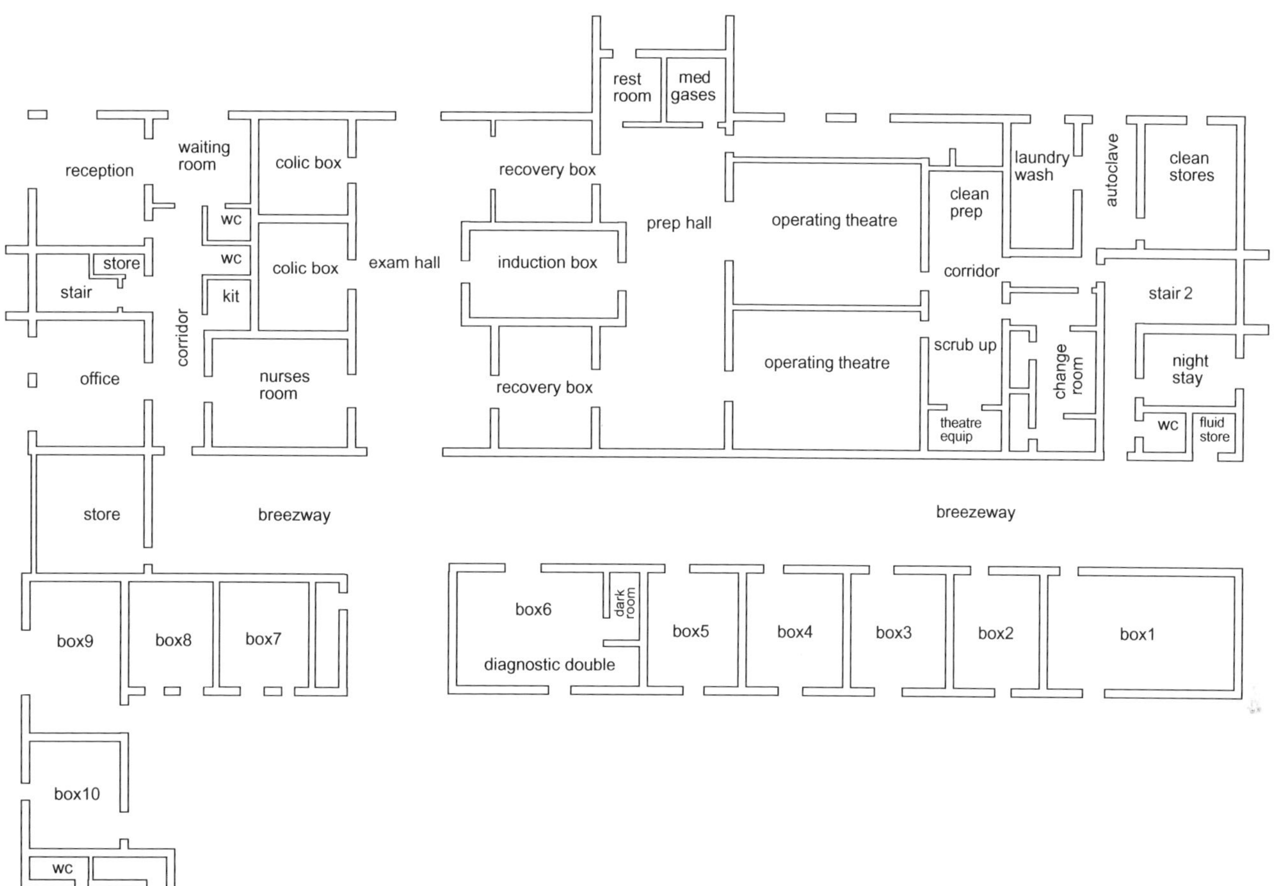

Figure 3.10 Architectural plan for the ground floor level of Rossdale and Partners Hospital. Redrawing of original architectural plan for clarity. ©Tim Greet and Stephen Cahalan 2007.

system of inducing general anaesthesia. We have two smaller rooms that are used for recovery from anaesthesia. These measure 4 × 3.5 metres, which is adequate for the recovery of all our patients. They have both been equipped with a rope recovery system in the manner described by Wilderjans[1] (Figure 3.11, A and B). We use that system to recover all patients except foals and horses over 700 kg. Each of the stalls is equipped with lights which can be dimmed, heat lamps, convex mirrors and viewing ports in each of the two doors ("out" to the clinic hall and "in" to the anaesthetic hall). The walls and the floor are lined with padded mats*. I have used it for almost 30 years in different centres and found it to be eminently suitable for the purpose. It is safe and relatively easy to keep clean, provides good nonslip support for the feet and is relatively resistant to damage by hoof or shoe (which we wrap with duct tape).

The number and sophistication of the operating rooms will depend on the likely throughput of surgical cases and the type of patient. It is my view that invariably the dirtiest item in an equine operating theatre is the patient, and that keeping the throughput low is most likely to assist in preserving the cleanest environment. We therefore use one theatre solely for horses requiring fracture repair and all arthroscopic procedures, except the treatment of septic synovitis; thus this theatre is used less frequently than the other. We feel adopting this approach ensures that the main orthopaedic theatre is less likely to harbour microorganisms that might result in resistant nosocomial infections. Clearly it is essential to work tirelessly to avoid such infections, and a rigorous protocol for theatre cleaning under normal circumstances, and when the presence of infectious agents is suspected, is enforced vigorously. Both theatres measure 6 × 5.5 metres, which is barely adequate to deal with the variety of surgical procedures we undertake. The theatre is certainly cluttered when both arthroscopy and fluoroscopy are in use simultaneously.

The orthopaedic theatre allows for no incidental light, thus allowing the best visibility of television or fluoroscopic screens at all times. The other theatre has high windows that allow for reflected light from outside the building and is a less harsh environment to work in for long periods. We have piped-in music from a CD player as an option to help create a relaxing atmosphere for the surgical team.

* Linatex Ltd, Yateley, UK.

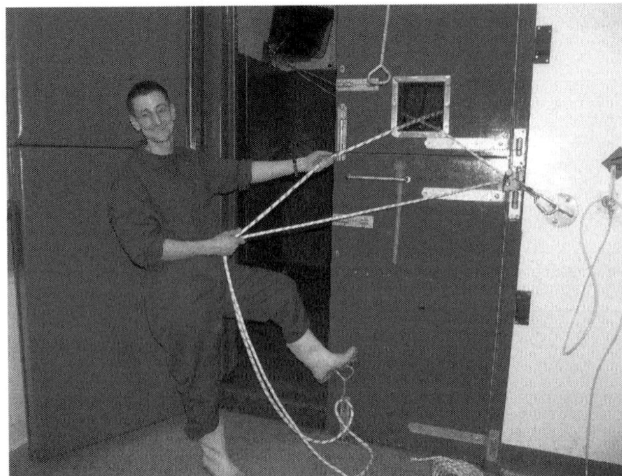

A

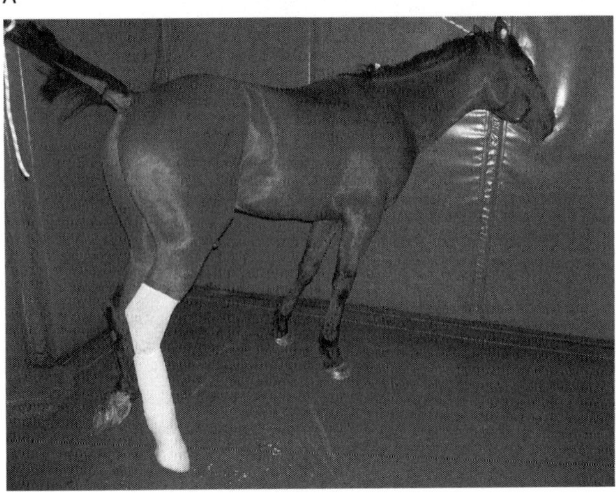

B

Figure 3.11A-B Pulley and rope system for assisted recovery of horses from anaesthesia. ©Tim Greet 2006.

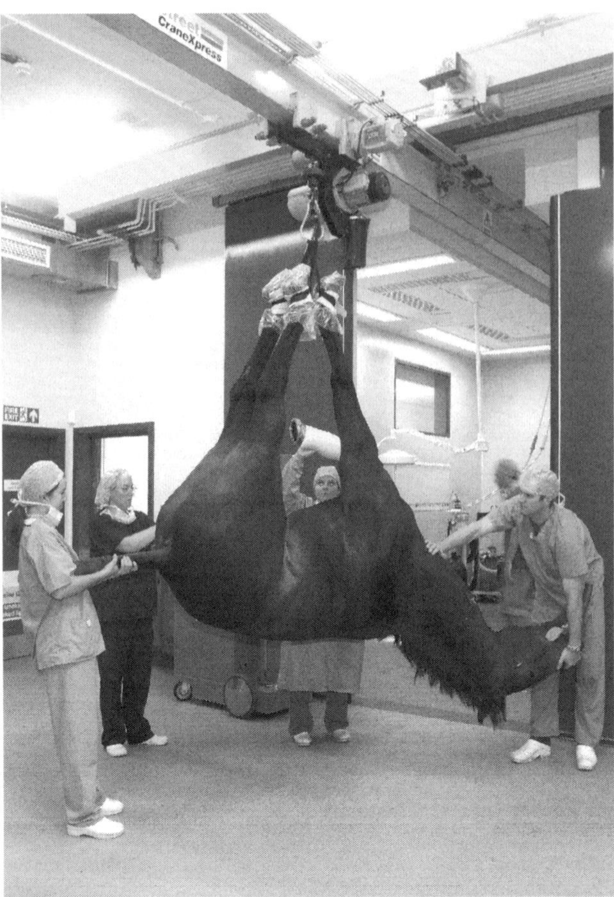

Figure 3.12 A moving beam allows the use of both theatres and all three anaesthetic boxes. ©Tim Greet 2006.

In both theatres the floors are easy to clean, comfortable to walk on and smooth surfaced, to allow easy movement of trolleys and other equipment. There is a trapdoor in the floor at one end of the most used theatre, which is sited to allow the emptying of intestinal contents or other bodily waste directly into the main drain; the system is equipped with a flush toilet mechanism that can be supplemented by using a fire hose if a particularly heavy load has to be disposed of, such as when a large colon is emptied.

Theatre lighting is a critical issue and one that we got badly wrong in our hospital. The difficulty is that with a necessarily high ceiling, it is difficult to finding robust ceiling mounted operating lights that can cover all possible areas of surgical interest. We had two put up in each theatre but they are neither robust nor particularly effective. We are just in the process of considering additional lighting, probably using wall-mounted lights. The down side of this plan is that it will inevitably add further clutter to the theatre.

With three anaesthetic stalls and two operating theatres, it is important to have complete flexibility when moving horses backwards and forwards between areas. This is achieved in our hospital by a moving rail that travels up the anaesthetic hall and can connect to a beam in each of the anaesthetic stalls and operating theatres (Figure 3.12). By this means, horses can be moved suspended by hobbles from the induction, or indeed any anaesthetic stall, to either theatre, and back again. There are two hoists, both of which can run the system. In the anaesthetic hall, there is a small nurses' office with a sink and fridge, which allows the theatre team to make a cup of tea or coffee and a snack and to relax between patients. There is a strict dress code so that all personnel must remove their outdoor clothes and wear scrub suits. This is relaxed only for transient visitors and workpersons, for whom clean boiler suits and disposable "cover shoes" are provided.

In the anaesthetic hall there are lockable cupboards for anaesthetic agents and other drugs and for all the equipment required to run a modern operating theatre. We use piped anaesthetic gases that are supplied from a medical gas room, which is located next to the office at the end of the anaesthetic hall. The medical gas room is serviced from outside the building, and an alarm system is installed to ensure the gas never runs out. Piped gas suitably monitored is a great space saver, and keeping clutter to a minimum in theatre is a worthy ambition, whatever the number of surgical cases. However, portable canisters systems are very practical and simple to use with either "to and fro" or "circle" anaesthetic machines. In our system, we also have piped oxygen to our anaesthetic stalls to facilitate anaesthetic recovery. A scavenging system is employed wherever anaesthetic gases are used.

There are a number of simpler configurations that are very practical for anaesthetic/operating room combinations. The simplest involves two adjacent rooms with a single beam running between the two; however, this configuration is rather limited and really only suited to a low throughput hospital. A relatively simple amendment is to have two anaesthetic stalls side by side connected by a "U"-shaped beam that can run from each anaesthetic room to a single operating theatre. This provides an induction and recovery stall allowing a significantly greater throughput, as inevitably the limiting factor in speed of throughput is anaesthetic recovery time. A variation on the overhead beam is to use a mobile operating table as the means of transporting the patient from the anaesthetic room to the theatre and back. This system works very well with lighter operating tables on wheels that turn easily, but can be quite an ordeal if the table or patient is heavy or the floors uneven. A hoist is still required at each end of the system to lift and position the patient. More complicated systems will probably require a three-phase electrical supply.

One critical issue to be considered at an early stage in the building design is the height of the roof. This, in areas where horses are to be hoisted by their legs under general anaesthesia, must be of sufficient height to allow the largest horse to be suspended by hobbles and a karabiner to a hook, chain, block and tackle and the beam, which in turn must be suspended from the roof. Thus, it is imperative to ensure adequate clearance to allow the effective hoisting of even draft horses if they should require surgery in the hospital. Similarly, the hoist must be able to lift at least 1000 kg (2200 lb) or preferably 1500 kg (3300 lb). Advice about hoisting systems should be sought from a specialist firm at an early stage, as this will have a major impact on building design.

There are a number of operating tables suitable for equine use, and in some hospitals an individually designed table is used. The first hydraulic tables were heavy and usually formed part of the anaesthetic room floor, moving on rails to a hydraulic ram in the theatre floor or, worse still, from a pit in the theatre floor. These theatres were extraordinarily difficult to keep clean and a potential source of infection to the patients. The tables were also very unwieldy and cumbersome to work around. Inflatable operating tables were also popular in smaller clinics or as a backup in larger hospitals. Whatever operating table is employed, it is critical to ensure adequate padding and limb positioning stands to avoid postoperative muscular or nervous dysfunction, which was the bane of general anaesthesia 30 years ago (Figure 3.13). Of course, intraoperative fluids, monitoring arterial pressure and supporting this by medication and, most importantly, a reduction in surgical time have all helped to make a major improvement in anaesthetic morbidity and mortality. Nevertheless, the CEPEF study[2] clearly highlighted that almost 1% of "healthy" patients (i.e., not patients with colic or major long bone fractures) succumb to this process despite our best efforts. So this element of hospital design should receive considerable attention to ensure that this unfortunate statistic is kept to the very minimum.

One other issue that should be considered in relation to an operating table is whether there may be a requirement to carry out laparoscopy on an anaesthetised horse. This usually requires the table to be tilted so that the patient can assume the Trendelenburg position (i.e., the end of the table holding the horse's hind quarters is elevated to approximately 35°, allowing the intestines to fall cranially away from the inguinal and pelvic regions, which are usually the areas of interest). This either necessitates a table that has an inbuilt tilting device† or the hoist or some other device must be able to be attached to elevate the table to create the same effect.

When designing our hospital, one area about which much thinking time was spent was the scrub up and surgical trolley laying-up room. I had operated in too many clinics over the years where the scrub up sinks and trolley lay-up areas were squeezed in to the theatre or an adjacent toilet, almost as an afterthought! In fact the scrubbed and gowning surgeon and the laying up of sterile instruments represent arguably the most sacrosanct processes in the whole cycle of surgery and should be allocated a separate area that is devoid of unnecessary people and a space that is large enough to allow unhindered gowning and sterile instrument preparation for surgery. This must be a "no go" area for most of the theatre staff during the process of preparing for surgery. It should be accessed from the changing rooms and toilets by the surgeons, but "nonsurgeons" should, in an ideal world, use a second door leading to a corridor that avoids the scrubbing and trolley lay-up area and enter the operating theatre by the patient entrance or a side door.

As mentioned above, storing equipment in the operating theatre is undesirable for several reasons, including attempting to maintain a sterile or at least a clean environment. Therefore, commonly used items, such as fluoroscopy machines, radiographic generators and arthroscopy stacks, should be housed in an adjacent equipment store. Equipment housed in theatre should be kept to an absolute minimum and probably only consist of an anaesthetic

† For example, Haico Telgte II surgery table; Haico, Loimaa, Finland.

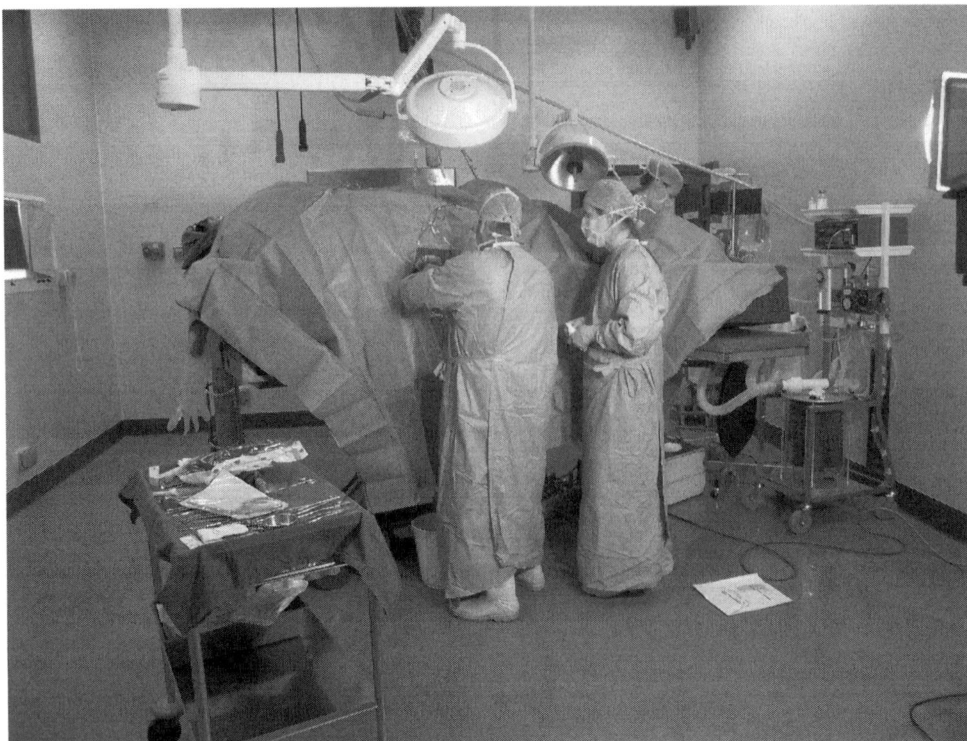

Figure 3.13 Horse positioned on the operating table for spinal process resection. ©Tim Greet 2006.

machine and a ventilator, but nothing else. Surgical instruments should be kept in a separate store. The position of this should be determined by constructing a flow chart of sterile instruments coming from a store, being laid-up on a surgical trolley, removed after use from the theatre, cleaned, repacked, resterilised and then returned to their correct place in the instrument cupboard. This process should be followed for sterile gowns and gloves (best stored near or in the scrubbing area), drapes, swabs, scalpel blades and other disposable instruments, arthroscopy and AO instruments, plus all the other equipment required to perform any conceivable operation successfully. Careful consideration of the cycle of sterilisation, use, cleaning, repacking, re-sterilisation and storage should be applied to ensure a logical and effective maintenance of theatre asepsis whilst preserving convenience for the nursing staff. This must also apply to all disposable materials and to clinical and nonclinical waste.

During the design process, we found it very useful to enact on paper common scenarios, such as the delivery of materials, anaesthetic gases and the removal of waste materials. These activities should be incorporated into the proposed flow diagram, to ensure the process works efficiently. This also allows the creation of detailed standard operating procedures for the various processes involved in theatre work, and such local rules should be extended to the management of various anaesthetic problems including cardiac and respiratory arrest, the disposal of the carcases of horses that are euthanised or have died in theatre (or indeed anywhere in the hospital), the protocol for visitors, the cleaning and disinfection of the various areas and the use of chemical and gas sterilising equipment if appropriate, as well as autoclaves. In fact, all possible situations should be examined and considered, including the steps necessary to deal with power failure whilst surgery is being undertaken or what to do if the hoist is unable to function. In all cases, a risk assessment for staff should be made and all health and safety issues should be incorporated into the health and safety dossier for the hospital.

Vehicular access

It is important that the dead-horse removal vehicle can gain access to all parts of the site from where dead horses may need to be collected. In our hospital, we have made the clinic hall in the hospital building itself and all the stables easily accessible. Furthermore, our overhead beams from the anaesthetic stalls extend out over the clinic hall area to allow dead horses to be loaded directly onto a truck. We also have easy access for vehicles to our euthanasia area (see later).

Specialised examination rooms

Already described are generic rooms close to the clinical examination area, which could be used for almost any type of procedure. However, in larger units it may be preferable to divert patients that are to be examined for lameness and other nonsurgical problems to a site distant from the hustle and bustle of the perioperative areas. There is nothing quite so alarming to the average horse or pony owner than to bring their much loved animal to a battle zone, full of refluxing colic patients or horses with severe epistaxis! Much better that lameness cases should be examined in a separate area, preferably close to a waiting room that is well equipped to deal with clients who may have to wait a number of hours, for example, whilst a lengthy "nerve-blocking session" is conducted, followed by diagnostic imaging.

Radiography rooms

Certainly a specially designed radiography unit is a high priority for most hospitals with a large lameness throughput, whether a mobile generator or gantry mounted tube head is to be used. Equipping the area where the horse stands with a low platform allows the radiographic tube head to go low enough to obtain good images of the distal limb. The room should offer enough space for horse, support staff and radiographic equipment to be accommodated safely. Some clinicians prefer the use of stocks for radiography, but I believe that a well-restrained and preferably sedated patient is more easily imaged without such encumbrance. Whether digital or more traditional radiography is to be used there needs to be a convenient arrangement of image processing equipment and preferably multiple screens available away from clients, whether they are involved in holding the horse or not. This is essential to allow clinicians to inspect and consult over the images without having to answer a multiplicity of questions from the owner. In an ideal world, there should also be a separate consulting room, to allow a discreet explanation of the radiological findings and perhaps other diagnostic or prognostic issues, which are better discussed confidentially. Horse owners tend to exhibit a natural curiosity about other peoples' animals, and public discussions over potentially sensitive matters, which are almost inevitable in a busy unit, convey an "unprofessional" impression to clients.

It is not the purpose of this chapter to describe the precise requirements for individual radiography suites (which are discussed in Chapter 3.2), save to say that the regulations regarding ionising radiation must be stringently observed and the design should be coordinated with health and safety issues to the fore, under the guidance of the radiation protection officer. This equally applies to rooms involved in gamma scintigraphy (Figure 3.14) or to stables in which such patients are housed. Visible local rules must be available throughout such areas and should be read by all staff. Obviously a number of warning signs must also be clearly displayed for the benefit of clients and staff alike.

The precise physical requirements of radiographic areas will depend upon whether a gantry-mounted tube head (Figure 3.15), or a mobile or portable radiographic generator, is to be used. These days, many larger hospitals are equipped with gantry-mounted tube heads, and an increasing number employ cassette-based or direct digital radiography (Figure 3.16). It is also important to sort out whether the equipment requires a three-phase electrical supply, and then to ensure that the necessary connections are installed.

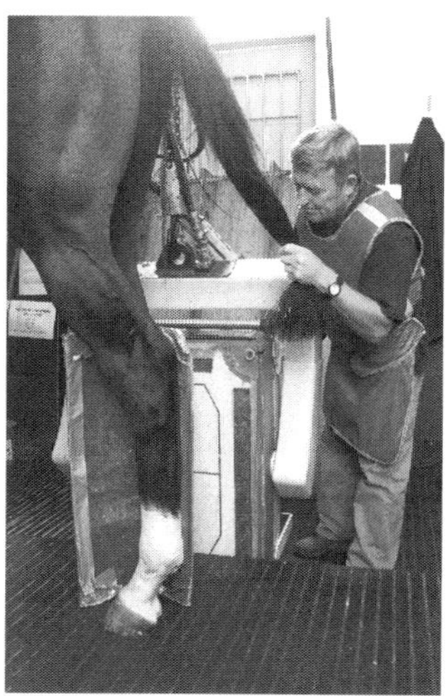

Figure 3.14 Using the gamma scintigraphy camera. ©Tim Greet 2006.

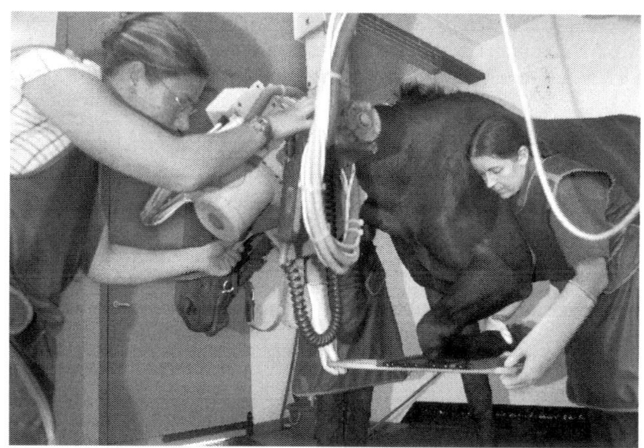

Figure 3.15 Using a gantry-mounted radiographic tube head. ©Tim Greet 2006.

In smaller hospitals, it may be more convenient to duplicate the use of the radiography room to accommodate a variety of imaging modalities, and even in larger hospitals, rooms suitable for endoscopy are equally useful for ultrasonography procedures or even as a standing surgery room. They should be equipped with a good set of stocks (see later) and, if to be used interchangeably for these various procedures, should have variable lighting available to cater for relative darkness required during imaging, whilst ensuring adequate brightness necessary for surgical procedures.

The flooring should always be nonslip (see later) and the walls easily cleaned. Adequate cupboard space should be available to accommodate the ancillary equipment and the drugs and disposable materials that such procedures entail.

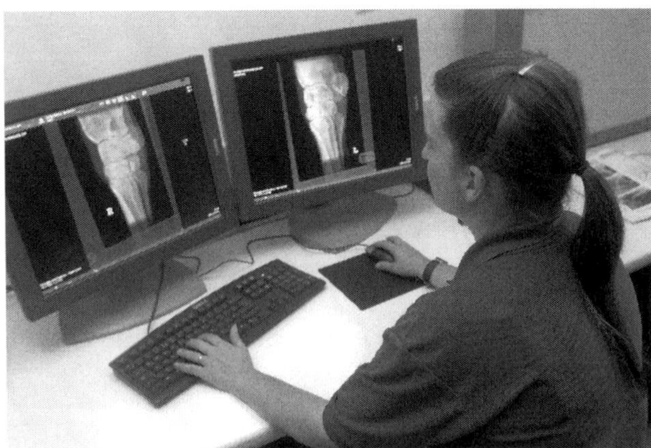

Figure 3.16 Manipulating digital radiographic images on a computer workstation. ©Tim Greet 2006.

A sink is also usefully situated in this area and of course plenty of electrical sockets. There should also be a conveniently located and easily accessible equipment store in which the various types of imaging apparatus can be stored safely away from the examination area. Requirements for buildings or rooms housing magnetic resonance image (MRI) and computed tomography (CT) units are discussed in Chapter 3.2.

Rooms for performing nerve blocks

A specific room in which regional or intrasynovial analgesia can be performed safely is a great asset if many lame horses are to be examined. This needs to have a nonslip floor and plenty of work top and cupboard space to store needles, syringes, local anaesthetic agents, clipping and scrubbing materials, twitches, sedatives and any other equipment necessary to carry out such procedures safely and effectively. In my view, in addition to the usual high-quality lighting required in any room in which detailed examination of a patient is to be undertaken, extra lighting located about 0.6 metre (2 feet) above floor level greatly facilitates the insertion of needles in the distal limb. Having a door that can be locked from the inside, or a warning light visible outside the stall, prevents unwanted visitors at a critical time with a fractious or nervous patient.

Farriery area

Lighting fitted at a low level is also a very useful addition in the forge or farriery area. A viewing stall or computer workstation is useful for viewing radiographs taken to determine foot balance. If a hospital forge is to be built, it is advisable to design this in conjunction with the farriers(s) who will use it. Obviously the specific requirements, for example, for whether a coal or gas-fired forge, or other electrical equipment is to be installed, will depend on the individual farrier. Many farriers are happier these days working from the back of a van and require minimal equipment to be provided by the hospital. However, in all cases there must be sufficient space to work safely all around a horse (Figure 3.17), and it may be necessary to provide an area sufficient in size to allow several horses to be shod safely at one time.

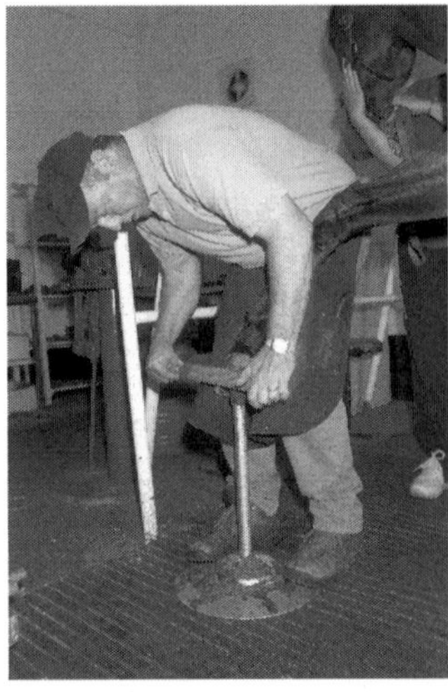

Figure 3.17 A farrier working in a dedicated room (forge room) in the hospital. ©Tim Greet 2006.

The pharmacy

There is massive bureaucracy associated with the use of veterinary medicines, which necessitates accountability and traceability, and therefore recording of all medicines administered to horses. The recording of batch numbers of all prescription-only medicines has become required in European countries. This is in addition to maintaining a register for dangerous drugs and the provision of lockable cupboards for safekeeping of such pharmaceutical products.

Although a central pharmacy is a logical way to try to satisfy the recording, safekeeping and effective distribution of medicines to the rest of the hospital site, clearly this is an area that must also be accessed from the outside by delivery vans. The easiest way to record the use of batch numbers is by bar code at the time of delivery, so this system should be put in place when constructing a new hospital. Internet access is also essential in this area, as the ordering of many medicines is now done most conveniently “online”.

It is difficult to predict how things might progress in the future, but many European regulatory authorities have accepted that any veterinary surgeon may dispense to another’s prescription, so there may well be commercial advantage to ensuring the pharmacy is of the highest quality and accessible to members of the general horse-owning public. However, I hesitate to suggest that this additional business merits another waiting room!

The laboratory

The hospital laboratory may simply be a room or even part of a room near the nurses’ base (see earlier). However, in more modern hospitals there is a tendency to reserve this area for the most simple and acute testing of blood or other fluids for cell counts. More sophisticated haematological, biochemical, microbiological or pathological investigations are carried out elsewhere in a specialised laboratory area.

The laboratory area should house its own administration and staff to ensure reliable reporting of results. There will need to be computer access, and Internet availability is advantageous. Clearly the laboratory rooms themselves require enough bench or floor space to accommodate whatever type of laboratory equipment is desired. Thought should also be given to possible expansion as more tests become achievable within practice laboratories in future. Separating haematology and biochemistry from cytology and histology makes sense from both a management and a health and safety point of view. Bacteriology and mycology should also ideally be housed in a separate space to reduce the risk of accidental culture of organisms from the environment.

Health and safety issues are important in this part of the hospital and appropriate advice must be taken at an early stage in the planning, to accommodate such apparatus as a fume cupboard with an extractor hood, to allow the processing of histological sections and the handling of microbiological samples with a potential risk to the health of the technician. This is another area where it makes sense to mark up in actual size the larger pieces of equipment to be installed, to give an accurate idea of the necessary room size and the flow of laboratory samples and personnel. A separate microscope room is useful as it allows careful examination of histological sections in a quiet environment.

In some hospitals there may be a good reason for having the post-mortem facility close to the laboratory—for example, if it is likely that many pathological samples are to be collected. This is particularly useful in hospitals that have a large surgical throughput or deal with breeding mares and foals, where prompt pathological investigations are often a necessity.

Offices and staff facilities

It is very easy when designing a hospital to concentrate all your efforts on producing a high-quality building to cope with its equine needs. In the process of "future proofing" the operating and examination facilities, it is very easy to overlook the requirements of the staff. Very commonly a significant miscalculation takes place regarding the increase in staff numbers that is almost inevitable with the development of a hospital. I am speaking from personal experience here because we had no idea of the explosion in staff numbers when we built our hospital. Not only does this impact on the provision of office space, but it also concerns toilet facilities, car parking and even adequate space for coffee breaks and lunch. Clearly there may be a local café or a public house nearby, but quite often equine hospitals are erected miles away from any local habitation. Providing facilities to ensure a happy working environment is key to the success of the whole venture. Some hospitals actually provide a canteen with catering facilities. We do this in a small way but do not provide daily staff meals.

Adequate numbers of offices are required to accommodate veterinary surgeons, nurses, secretaries, accounts staff, receptionists, grooms and the inevitable students and other visitors, which most equine hospitals seem to attract. Careful thought should be given, not only to their location within the structure of the buildings but also upon their method of interaction. Thus it is logical to have secretarial and accounts staff located near one another, and with an excellent system for communication, preferably "online". The revolution in electronic and other forms of communication has really opened up tremendous possibilities for reporting, accounting, record keeping and almost every process necessary to ensure the hospital functions most efficiently.

We have provided flats and "bedsits" in our hospital for the nurses and interns. However, it is also valuable to consider supplying such accommodation for students. We set up an extern programme many years ago, which encourages both undergraduates and young visiting veterinary surgeons to stay in the hospital. This provides free labour at all hours and, equally importantly, free accommodation for young people who come to learn about equine clinical work. It has been undoubtedly one of our most successful ventures. They are able to cook in our kitchen areas, which is valuable when they are on call when we are very busy. I am sure in the years to come practices will find an ever more important role in educating young veterinary surgeons and providing accommodation should form part of this arrangement.

Seminar and meeting rooms

The modern equine hospital has an important role as a teaching centre. This may not appear obvious at first sight, but educating a variety of types of person should form one of the cornerstones of a successful modern veterinary business. Firstly, there is the training of the hospital's employees. This can range from young veterinary surgeons and students, veterinary nurses and trainees, to a range of other support staff. Next is the education of clients. Client evenings are becoming increasingly popular amongst a horse- and pony-owning population, hungry for more detailed information. This not only endows the clients with a better understanding of veterinary procedures; it is a valuable marketing tool, promoting the latest practice services. The same is true for hospitals offering a referral service. There is nothing like offering a CPD evening with a glass of wine to encourage more referred cases, and this can be geared to promoting a particular service or individual. Hospitals also tend to make ideal venues for the meeting of local veterinary groups. All of this provides invaluable good public relations and continuously keeps the hospital's name to the forefront in the area.

Such rooms clearly can be multifunctional, providing a lecture theatre, board room and discussion forum for the veterinary surgeons (Figure 3.18). Having an adjacent kitchen area is very useful to allow the provision of food and drink, and facilities for washing up and storing cutlery, glasses and crockery. Depending on the intended use of the room, it is valuable to purchase a number of comfortable seats which can be stored easily and set out for each meeting. A boardroom table is a luxury, but extraordinarily valuable for serving food at meetings, as well as a place around which to sit during partners meetings.

Modern audiovisual aids are fantastic, and a digital projector and high-quality screen are very worthwhile investments. However, it is useful to retain a 35-mm slide projector, as the world has not entirely "gone digital" yet—just mostly!

The library

Every hospital should have a good library, which is an essential resource in an environment that is based upon scientific knowledge. Not only is it important in the education of young members of staff, but it is vital for the lifelong learning process to which all members of the veterinary and allied professions must be committed.

There should be a catalogue of all books and this must be kept up to date as new editions are added. The library shelves should be labelled clearly and books kept in their appropriate sections.

The greatest problem with all libraries is the loss of books. Whilst there are clever electronic methods of tagging each book and installing alarm systems much as used in many shops these days, most hospitals rely upon the honesty of the library users. Each of our books is covered in tape with the hospital name embossed and we have large signs instructing library users that books must not be removed. Other methods of discouraging the disappearance of library contents include the provision of a photocopier in the room, to allow copying of papers, and having all journals bound reduces the instinct to remove a single issue. These days access to the Internet is also very valuable in a library as so much material is available online. We have no telephone in our library, to maintain it as quiet an area as possible, although it can frustrate the hospital paging system!

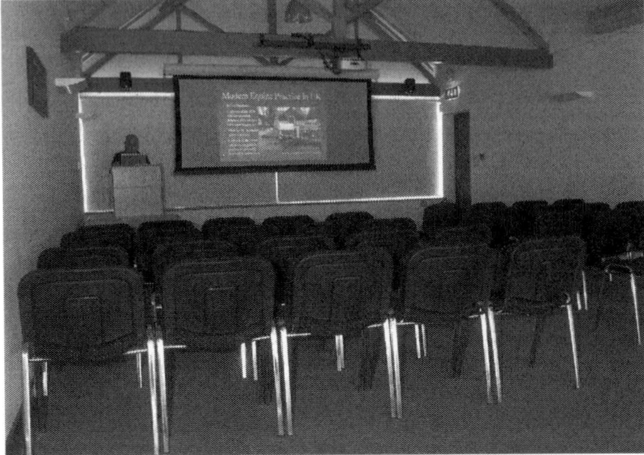

Figure 3.18 A seminar room equipped with a digital projector is a very useful asset. ©Tim Greet 2006.

In our hospital library, we also have slide-copying equipment available for staff to make presentations. However, it is mainly used as a haven for quiet study in a hospital environment that in most other areas is almost permanently in a state of organised chaos!

Miscellaneous items

A killing area and facilities for a post-mortem examination

Whilst many horses may be euthanised by injection, both in the operating theatre or in a stable, and collected by lorry from there (see earlier), we prefer where possible to walk horses out to a killing area. This allows us to destroy a patient using a free bullet quickly and efficiently in complete safety. The area is surrounded by high walls and lined with wood to prevent ricochet. There is an area in front of the killing zone which is also shielded from public view, where the vehicle used for collection of carcasses can park and which allows us an opportunity to perform a simple post-mortem examination. It is important that this area be situated at a distance from other stables to avoid the sound of gunshots disturbing other patients. Clearly it should not be sited close to human habitation for the same reasons. An important additional consideration in this area is a powerful hose to wash down the inevitable blood and bodily fluids that accumulate, and good drainage is essential.

We have a more sophisticated post-mortem room elsewhere. This is designed to allow horses to be hoisted from the back of the truck on to an easily cleaned and well-drained floor. There are also tables to allow more detailed dissection of specific areas of the horse or to carry out the post-mortem examination of a foal or even a placenta. It is useful to have a band saw available to allow splitting of heads or necks, and instrument cupboards must be able to store the variety of saws and other cutting and dissecting equipment, preservatives and containers of all sizes in which to collect specimens and samples destined for laboratory. There should also be hoses available in the dissecting room, and there must be adequate space to store bins for the discarded limbs and organs. A separate anteroom should allow space for changing into protective clothing and a store for more vulnerable items such as tape recorders and paper for making notes of any examination carried out.

Flooring in the hospital

There is arguably no more important consideration in any hospital than the flooring. As mentioned earlier, specialised padded flooring is used in the anaesthetic stalls, of which several types are available. They are all expensive but selecting one is not a great challenge. Floors for the reception and offices are a routine matter and even those used for the theatres and ancillary areas are relatively straightforward. The problem areas are those required for clinical examination and various imaging modalities. Over many years we have tried an endless variety of surfaces, none of which has provided the perfect solution. If cost is an issue, there is little better than rough concrete, which is hard wearing and relatively nonslip, except when covered with obstetrical lubricant, more of which later. However, when constructing an expensive building full of all the latest "high-tech" equipment, where the fees are not insignificant and clients' expectations are high, most veterinary surgeons naturally want to install an impressive, attractive-looking floor.

The ingredients for a successful floor are given in Box 3.1. I am unaware of any flooring material of this type that can reliably pass the "obstetrical lubricant test". I have also seen several floor surfaces that turn into a skating rink when covered with surgical spirit. In areas that are constantly used and cleaned, tiles tend to lift and water seeps underneath them. Poured on surfaces initially work well but are usually not very hard wearing, tending to suffer marked erosion in places, which eventually leads to complete failure of the surface. We are currently using this sort of pour-on "rubber mix" in our stalls attached to the clinic hall where they have a large throughput of patients for preanaesthetic preparation, bandage changes and a variety of other treatments. This is probably the third floor of this type we have had installed during a 9-year period! It is constantly being repaired or patched.

At one stage, we used a number of rubber mats that we had professionally laid and joined by what was claimed to be an impervious seal. These seals invariably failed and water and debris penetrated beneath the mats that was unsightly in appearance and, far more importantly, a hazard to health. Such a potential harbour for infectious organisms has been indicted as the cause of an outbreak of salmonellosis in a veterinary hospital.[3] Great care must therefore be taken, when using mats or tiles as flooring, to ensure the seal between them and to walls is genuinely impervious and durable.

We have a large clinic hall and it was felt that we must have a light-coloured surface that would not appear "visually oppressive", so we used grey tiles. This floor is now so marked and discoloured after less than 10 years that I am sure we should have used a darker colour. Having said that, the floor tiles have raised circular profiles for extra grip, which is fairly good except when covered with obstetrical lubricant. It also receives very heavy use and has worn well.

As you will realise from the above, flooring requires significant consideration. You should make extensive enquiries as there are always new products on the market. Make sure you see them in use. A good track record on a floor that receives heavy use over a prolonged period is the best recommendation for a good floor material. I think they are hard to find and usually expensive.

Above all it is important to avoid covering any floor surface with obstetrical lubricant, as catastrophic human injuries can result from a fall. All staff should be made fully aware of the risks and that they should be vigilant in cleaning up promptly any lubricant which might spill on the floor during a procedure.

Box 3.1. Ideal properties of flooring for hospitals

1. Nonslip
2. Hard wearing and resistant to hoof or equine shoe damage
3. Easy to clean
4. Comfortable for staff and clients to walk on
5. Look that is clean and "professional"

Stocks

The restraint of equine patients in stocks is one of the most important management aids when performing veterinary work on horses. However, one encounters quite differing opinions within the profession about when such equipment is most valuable and even more so about their construction. As I have mentioned, I do not consider stocks to be particularly helpful for restraining horses for equine radiography, nor for regional or intrasynovial analgesia. However, they are unquestionably helpful during diagnostic ultrasonography and endoscopy.

There is a basic dilemma in the construction of stocks. They need to be strong enough to be safe for the patients and personnel and yet they should be able to be dismantled easily in an emergency—for example, should a horse collapse or become trapped in stocks, to ensure equine safety. Stocks that can readily be dismantled encourage the use of the area for other purposes, affording greater flexibility for using the building.

There are a whole variety of "off the peg" designs that can provide for the intended purpose. We have used our own design for many years, based on an idea from steel scaffolding, which is strong and light, but I would not say that it is ideal for all our needs.

We are just in the process of designing a new standing surgery area and we intend to have stocks with short posts to allow clear visibility of the television monitor for laparoscopic surgery. So the specific design of the stocks will depend upon their most common use.

Drains

An equine hospital needs an excellent drainage system. There are always great challenges to whatever arrangement one employs. Consideration must be given to the system in the operating theatres, for example. We opted not to have a drain in our orthopaedic theatre and rely on using a "squeegee" type of mop to clean the floor. By contrast, in the other theatre we use the sump in the floor at the anaesthetic hall end of the theatre to drain debris and for floor cleaning directly into the main drain. There is a central drain in the anaesthetic hall, which is a little small for the purpose and takes a long time to clear water, but we have another sump under large sinks at one end of the anaesthetic hall that is more efficient although the floor flows down to the central drain. There are marginal drain channels along both sides of our clinic hall that need to be cleared out on an almost daily basis or they become blocked.

The drains throughout any hospital are always vulnerable, because inevitably they have to cope with large volumes of fluid and debris. So it is imperative that adequate traps are incorporated to avoid blockage and it is equally important that they are emptied regularly depending on an assessment of their loading. Like so many routine elements within an equine hospital, regular drain management is fundamental to the effective working of the hospital and a rigorous protocol should be written and adhered to. Employment of staff dedicated to this type of apparently mundane work is absolutely essential.

Generators

The continued supply of power to vital hospital equipment must be ensured under all circumstances. In particular, maintaining electrical supply to overhead hoists, operating tables, lights and vital electronic surgical and monitoring equipment must be catered for by some backup system. The nature of this ancillary power will depend upon the size of the hospital, the throughput of emergency cases in particular, the reliability of the local grid supply and the available money to spend on this equipment. We have a large diesel generator that is wired to kick in automatically when the main supply fails. This without question affords peace of mind and allows the staff to focus on the job in hand, during a power cut, instead of having to worry about finding, starting and attaching an alternative source of supply. However, even this sort of support must never be taken for granted and should be tested regularly to ensure it is working and an adequate supply of fuel must be on hand and the tank topped up regularly. In fact, it is useful periodically to run a drill, much as you would do in the event of a fire, just to ensure that all the members of staff know what to expect in case of power failure. This must also be written clearly in the standard operating procedure book that covers all of the major issues in the hospital.

A treadmill

A treadmill is the most practical way of assessing causes of respiratory obstruction at exercise. However, it is only probably justified in hospitals associated with centres with large numbers of performance horses and racehorses in particular or in referral hospitals that see significant numbers of such cases as a second opinion. The specific requirements for a building to house such a piece of apparatus will depend to a large extent on the nature of the treadmill. However, in addition to providing a building of adequate size to accommodate the horse, treadmill, equipment and staff, it is important that consideration be given to the volume of noise that is inevitably generated when a horse gallops on a treadmill. Such specifications are beyond the scope of this chapter and advice should be sought from the manufacturer if a treadmill is to be incorporated into the hospital design.

Conclusions

Designing and then building a successful purpose built hospital can be one of the most satisfying nonveterinary activities with which an equine veterinary surgeon ever becomes involved. However, as anyone who has ever built anything will be only too painfully aware, there are always potential problems in the building process, and frustrations with builders and architects alike can cause sleepless nights and major additional expense. Therefore, a clear vision of your carefully considered intentions at the outset of the project is absolutely essential and must be discussed fully with first architect and then builder. They will be able to assess the practicalities and costs of delivering the building and provide options available to achieve your ambition. If the design team and builder are fully in sympathy with the vision, a successful outcome at a reasonable cost is much more likely. By contrast, changing the plan during the building process is almost always a recipe for dissatisfaction and unnecessary expenditure. The finest architects and builders in the land cannot be expected to understand the needs of equine patients, and a detailed brief to the architect at the outset necessitates much careful thought about all aspects of the project.

References

1. Wilderjans H: Advances in assisted recovery from anaesthesia of horses with fractures, in BEVA Equine Specialist Meeting, Royal College of Physicians, London, UK, 2000
2. Johnston GM, Eastment JK, Wood JLN, et al.: The Confidential Enquiry into Perioperative Equine Fatalities (CEPEF): mortality results of Phases 1 and 2. Vet Anaesth Analg 29:159-170, 2002
3. Tillotson K, Savage CJ, Salman MD, et al.: Outbreak of *Salmonella infantis* infection in a large animal veterinary teaching hospital. J Am Vet Med Assoc 211:1554-1557, 1997

3.2 Diagnostic imaging

3.2.1. Facilities and equipment for diagnostic imaging

Renate Weller, Fiona M. Ripley and Nick Bolas

Introduction

Diagnostic imaging plays a central role in the workup of both internal medicine and surgical cases encountered in an equine hospital: In our referral hospital, the workup of more than 90% of the surgical cases and more than 60% of the medicine cases includes at least one diagnostic imaging procedure. While the exact percentage may vary between hospitals depending on the specific caseload, diagnostic imaging equipment will be used on a daily basis in any clinical setting; hence careful planning is essential to optimise work flow and avoid frustration of staff.

Equine radiography

When designing a radiography room, it is vital that careful consideration is given to the equipment that will best suited for your requirements, how to make best use of your budget, the room dimensions and also the practicalities involved in taking good radiographs.

Room Dimensions and Design

Getting the correct room dimensions is the first step in the making of an efficient, user-friendly radiography suite. When first considering the size of the room, there are certain variables that should be taken into consideration: the size and type of equipment that will be used, the distance that is required between the x-ray machine and the animal to acquire diagnostic and correctly exposed images and the large variety in size of horses that will be imaged. Depending on the x-ray system used one, two or three rooms may be required: the main room where the pictures are taken, a room for developing the films and, if a high-end system is used, a generator room. If the main room is large enough, the generator and the control console of the x-ray unit can be in the same room as long as adequate lead shielding is provided. If a conventional film based system is used, a separate dark room is necessary while the laser scanner and work station necessary for computerised radiography can be in the main room.

The main room should provide enough space for the x-ray unit to be manoeuvred around the horse and allow for taking all common views without having to move the horse, whilst still providing for enough space to move the x-ray tube out of reach of the horse. If the room is used for taking the radiographs only, a room size of 8 × 8 metres should provide ample space. This space needs to be increased depending on how much of equipment is stored in there.

If a ceiling mounted x-ray unit and plate holder are going to be installed, then a strong, high ceiling is essential. Some radiographic studies are performed with the horse under general anaesthesia, such as intraoperative radiographs or myelography. If these are to be performed, a system that allows the x-ray equipment to move into the normal operating theatre, such as an extension of a ceiling mounted hoist, is required. Myelography can be performed independent of an operating theatre, if there is a stall for recovery from general anaesthesia adjacent to the radiography room. A hoist to lift the horse onto the table for myelography may also be required.

The room should be well drained for the purposes of easy cleaning and should the patient urinate. The floor should be level and nonslip even when wet. While rubber floors work well with ceiling mounted x-ray systems, some of them make the use of mobile systems difficult because the wheels cannot move freely due to the softness of the rubber or the surface contour or because the wheels get stuck in gaps between adjoining rubber mats. Care should be taken to choose a rubber floor that has sealed gaps to ensure a hygienic environment.

Wide doorways of no less than 175 cm are advisable when designing a radiography suite (Figure 3.19). Although 120 cm is the standard width for stable doors, remember that the patients are often sedated or are perhaps injured and require more room to move. Also, they are entering a completely foreign environment and may require some persuasion to enter the room. Therefore, wider doorways are far more inviting and safer.

The most common site of lameness in the horse is the foot; hence, this is the most commonly radiographed area. Unfortunately, many x-ray systems do not go low enough to the ground to allow for the beam to be centred on the foot. If this is the case, either the horse has to be raised or the x-ray machine lowered. The easiest option is to put the horse's foot or both feet on a block. Alternatively, the whole horse can stand on a ramp-like elevation of the floor or the x-ray machine can be sunk into a groove into a recess in the floor. Depending on the method used, stocks may be beneficial. Conventional stocks usually have the disadvantage that the posts get in the way; ceiling mounted stocks get rid of this problem but cannot be used in conjunction with ceiling mounted x-ray systems. A viewing window made of lead glass is useful since it allows people to observe what is going on while not actually being exposed to radiation. This is popular for owners and useful for students and others who wish to learn about radiography.

Power points and light switches also have to be considered. These should be nonperturbing if possible, water

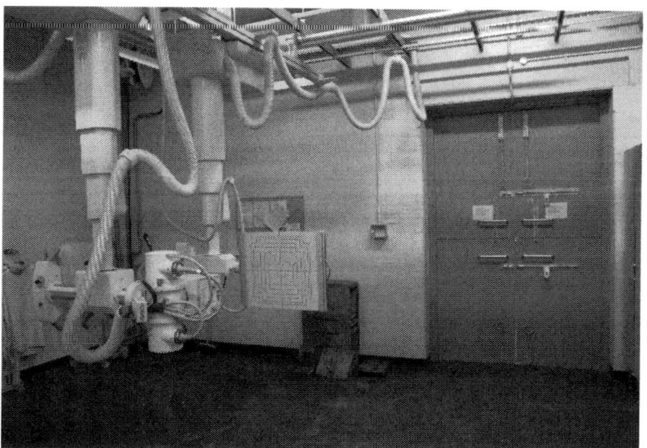

Figure 3.19 Equine radiography suite with a ceiling-mounted x-ray machine and plate holder. ©Renate Weller 2007.

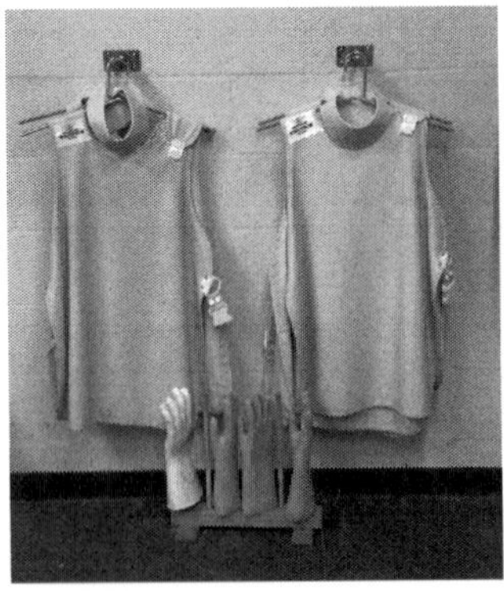

Figure 3.20 Correctly stored lead gowns, thyroid shields and gloves. ©Renate Weller 2007.

tight and covered. If using portable x-ray units, make sure that you have enough power points all around the room to avoid having long electric cables stretching around the patient. Some x-ray units (especially high-end generators) require three-phase power. Light switches should allow for the light to be dimmed, as this makes it easier to see the collimated area. For the same reason, windows should be small or covered up. If possible, a lockable cupboard should be installed within easy reach of the radiography suite to store sedation. This allows further doses of sedative to be administered easily and quickly.

Specially designed racks and hangers should be used for the correct storage of lead aprons, lead gloves and thyroid shields (Figure 3.20). Lead aprons should never been crumpled up or folded because this leads to cracks in the lead lining. The rack has to be well secured and strong to cope with the weight of the lead.

It is also very useful to have a broom and shovel should the patient pass faeces. A good, well-maintained farriery kit should also be kept close at hand for the swift removal of shoes and trimming of feet prior to feet radiographs. A bucket and wire brush is also useful for cleaning the feet prior to imaging.

Radiography equipment

Mobile x-ray units

Mobile x-ray units come in different sizes and configurations. Small, portable x-ray units are mainly used in ambulatory practice and can be a very useful piece of equipment in any size of equine practice or hospital. They are essential for on-farm radiography, for radiography of patients that are unable to move to the x-ray room or where it is clinically contraindicated to walk them that distance, and of those that will not tolerate the large ceiling mounted units. There are a wide range of portable x-ray units on the market that range in price and power. Prices will start at very approximately £5000 (7,500 Euro; 9000 US Dollars; 11,500 Australian Dollars) for new units. The areas that you will be able to image will depend on the machine purchased, but most machines will cope with distal limbs without any difficulty. However, portable machines will struggle with areas with a greater body mass such as chests and thoracic vertebrae. In such cases, a larger, more powerful unit will be required.

Larger mobile units are mounted on wheels. They have an inbuilt generator with control box and the x-ray tube mounted on an extending, movable arm. These are commonly used in hospitals for bedside radiographs and thus are often available second-hand for a relatively cheap price.

Along with the mobile x-ray machine, you will require x-ray machine stand, an extension cable and a circuit breaker. The units should be purchased with service contracts and require servicing once per annum.

Ceiling-mounted x-ray units

Ceiling-mounted units are much larger than the mobile units and can cope with much higher exposures, making them invaluable when imaging areas of high radiographic density. Although large, the ceiling mounted units are very manoeuvrable, enabling one to image any part of the body. The units are mounted on a telescopic column on a gantry system attached to a strong ceiling (see Figure 3.19). They are usually custom-made and require professional installation. In these units, the generator is separate from the x-ray tube and is ideally housed in a separate room. Special consideration should be given on how to use the room to its full potential by ensuring that the machine has full movement in all directions and as far around the room as possible. It is important that the x-ray beam may be directed along horizontal, vertical and intermediate planes, centred to a range of locations. This will make the imaging far more time efficient, as it will reduce the movement of the (often sedated) horse. Thought should also be put in to where the machine should be stored when not in use, so that it is out of the way of horses entering the room and also doorways.

To complement the ceiling mounted x-ray unit, a plate holder (see Figure 3.19), also mounted from the ceiling, can be installed. This plate holder works in unison with the x-ray unit and is a great asset when imaging areas that require higher exposures. It is usually combined with either a stationary or, preferably (although much more expensive), moving grid. The plate holder is ideal to image areas such as vertebrae and chests with minimum exposure of personnel. Careful consideration should also be given as to where the plate holder should be stored when not in use as, like the ceiling-mounted x-ray unit, they are fairly large pieces of equipment and are expensive to replace if accidentally damaged.

Conventional film/screen radiography

Many practices still use conventional film/screen combinations. This involves chemical processing of the exposed film, which requires a dark room adjacent to the x-ray suit with an automatic processor or a series of tanks for manual processing. In addition to the processor the dark room needs to be equipped with a red light, a storage cabinet for the unexposed films, a scriber to label films and a lightproof, lockable door. The developed films are put in envelopes, and since veterinarins are legally required to keep radiographs for a minimum of several years (regulations differ in different countries), thought should go into how much storage room is required. A light box needs to be available for viewing the films; double-screen boxes allow comparison of films by hanging them next to each other, and in-built shutters help to improve viewing quality by blinding out the parts of the image that are not of interest. A hot light is strongly recommended to enable viewing of areas that would be otherwise overexposed.

Computerised radiography

Computerised radiography has become more popular over recent years. With these systems, films are replaced by fluorescent screens. These screens are read, after exposure by conventional x-ray systems, in a special laser scanner. The digitised image is displayed on a screen. While these systems are relatively expensive to buy, they have several advantages: Computerised radiography allows images to be viewed on a computer screen and can be manipulated in a way that aids the interpretation of the radiographs. The contrast and brightness can be altered and there is also the potential to zoom in and out and magnify images. Quality of the original images can be improved by post acquisition collimation and contrast enhancement. Images can then be archived or saved on to storage media and transported digitally to other practices or hospitals, making for an improved and more efficient service. It is still possible to print the radiographs. However, the printer needs to be purchased separately and the film is expensive to buy. Initially, teething problems can be experienced whilst exposures and algorithms are established but once set up, digital radiography can prove an invaluable system in the modern equine hospital.

Direct digital radiography

New systems have been developed that record x-rays without a cassette. These systems employ an imaging plate in place of the cassette, and the radiographs are immediately displayed on a screen on a desktop computer or laptop. Older versions of this technology work by converting the x-ray to visible light in the imaging plate [using either a gadolinium oxysulphide (GdO_2S) or caesium iodide]. This light is then converted to a digital image using a CCD (charge-couple device, commonly used in digital cameras) or a CMOS (complementary metal oxide semiconductor) image sensor. Newer systems convert the x-ray directly to electricity using an amorphous selenium layer or a cadmium telluride layer. These newer systems may provide greater detail and sharpness than the systems that depend on generation of a light signal.

There are two major advantages of direct digital radiography over computerised radiography. The major one is that the image is displayed immediately and can be immediately checked for diagnostic quality. This comes into its own for survey radiographs of animals for sales or prepurchase examination (especially when this is performed away from the hospital premises and therefore the radiographic processor), as it will greatly shorten the total time required for the production of a complete set of diagnostic radiographs. The second advantage is that the image quality is probably superior to that of computerised radiography, and both soft tissue and bony lesions can be imaged in a single exposure. It is not yet proven that this improved quality leads to improved ability to diagnose equine lesions.

The major disadvantage of the direct digital system is the cost. These systems are expensive to purchase or lease. Typical lease deals are around £900 (€1250; US$ 1550; AS$ 2000) per month. The imaging plates are a relatively large part of this expense and are relatively fragile. The necessity of placing the imaging plate in close proximity to a horse increases the chance of it being damaged during normal use.

Protective lead clothing

Lead (Pb) protective clothing is the most important accessory to be purchased for radiography. There is a great range of lead aprons on the market. Aprons vary from single sided aprons to double sided aprons to aprons that come in two parts. There is also a range of the thickness in lead offered (0.20 mm Pb offering 94% protection, 0.35 mm Pb offering 97% protection, 0.50 mm Pb offering 99% protection).

Lead aprons are heavy and are commonly associated with neck and back pain. Therefore, it is very much worthwhile investing in aprons that distribute the weight more evenly, such as the two-piece suits. These are, however, often more expensive, so often a compromise has to be made. It is best, however, to try and avoid compromising on staff protection. Lead aprons should be checked periodically for cracks and defects in the lead. To reduce damage to the aprons, they should be hung up on very strong, specially made coat hangers in a rack firmly attached to the wall (see Figure 3.20). Thyroid shields and lead gloves should also be purchased. Cotton inner gloves protect the lead gloves from perspiration that can cause damage to the gloves, and prolong their useful life.

Cassette and cassette holders

Except for direct digital systems, cassettes and cassette holders are a vital part of the radiography equipment. A holder is required for the imaging plate of direct digital systems for many views. Cassettes usually come in the following standard sizes: 18 cm × 24 cm, 24 cm × 30 cm, 35 cm × 43 cm. The type of cassette depends on the type of radiography system, conventional or digital. Regardless of the type of system, it is very beneficial to have at least four cassettes in each size. The cassettes that are required for the digitised system are more expensive than conventional film/screen combinations but, if cleaned and maintained, will last several years. A strong shelf or cupboard for the safe storage of the cassettes should be provided.

If conventional film/screen combinations are used, it is advisable to have medium and high detail combinations available. High detail combinations (like the ones used in human mammography) provide excellent detail but require higher exposures and are mainly used for radiographing feet in the horse. Medium combinations are a good compromise between exposure and detail and provide diagnostic images of other regions of the horse. Grids are another means of improving detail by reducing scatter radiation, hence optimising image quality; yet again, the use of a grid increases exposure values and requires exact positioning. If grids are used in conjunction with a computerised radiography system care has to be taken to choose a grid that does not cause interference with the orientation of the laser scanner reading the cassettes. This needs close collaboration between the manufacturers of the computerised radiography and the x-ray system.

The type of cassette holder required can vary between practices, depending on the setup of the radiography room and the machine used. Some holders come in the form of blocks with groves in them that sit on the ground holding the cassette (Figure 3.21). These are useful for foot and pastern radiographs. Handheld cassette holders are versatile and suitable for many views taken in equine practice. They should be lightweight and have long handles to keep hands away from the primary beam (Figure 3.22). Many of the commercially available handheld cassette holders are not ideal for equine use, and a friendly farrier might be persuaded to make made-to-measure holders. Ideally these should be made out of lightweight, strong material, such as aluminium. A long handle should be fitted, allowing 360° rotation of the cassette but remaining in position once the x-ray shot has been aligned. In designing the holder, it is important to include the weight of the cassette and any grids used in calculating the required resistance to rotation once placed in position. The handle should come from the centre of the back of the cassette holder and should have no protruding or sharp attachments that could injure the horse or handler. The handle should be long enough to allow the handler to keep their hands well away from the primary beam, whilst allowing for a firm and steady hold. Ideally, there should be a small clip at the opening of the cassette holder to secure the cassette in place, to avoid the cassette falling out and spooking the horse. Wall-mounted cassette holders can also be used, but these can be awkward in practice, as one has to move the horse to the holder as opposed to the holder to the horse.

Blocks

Blocks can be very useful when positioning horse to acquire different views, especially of the feet and distal limbs. Again, these can be homemade and whilst wood is acceptable, sometimes the grain of the wood can appear on the radiograph. Perspex and aluminium are therefore preferable to wood but obviously harder to make oneself. Commonly used for equine radiography are the tunnel block and the "Oxspring" block (Figure 3.21).

The tunnel block is rectangular, about 10 cm high, and has a recess underneath to hold a 24 × 30-m plate. This block can be used for a number of different projections. One of the most common is the weight-bearing lateromedial view of the feet. Very often the x-ray system cannot get low enough to the ground to centre on the distal interphalangeal joint. Raising one foot on the block allows this view to be taken. Ideally, the horse would be stood on two tunnel blocks, with one under the foot of interest and one under the contralateral foot. This allows more natural weight bearing and a more diagnostic image. The second projection for which the tunnel block can be used is

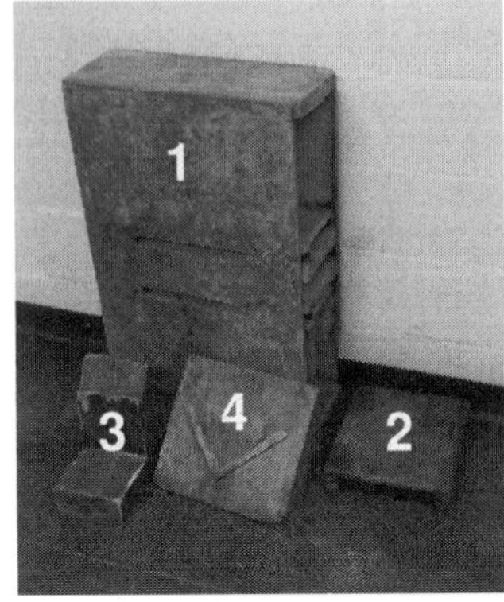

Figure 3.21 A range of blocks used in equine radiography (1 = rectangular block for lateromedial projections of horses' feet with slots to hold the plate, 2 = tunnel block, 3 = Oxspring-block, 4 = V-block for oblique projections). ©Renate Weller 2007.

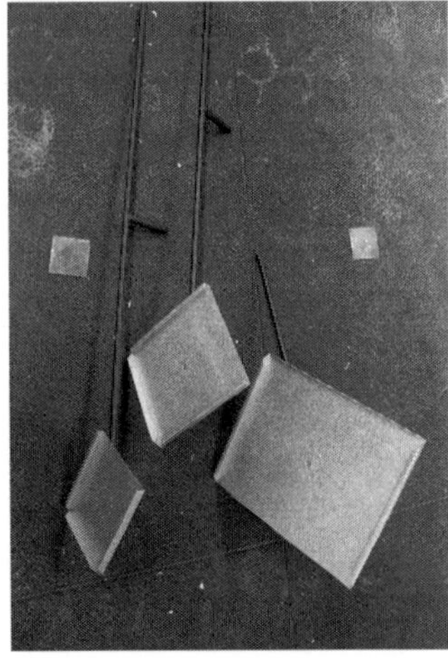

Figure 3.22 A range of lightweight plate holders with a 360° swivel handle. ©Renate Weller 2007.

the palmaroproximal-palmarodistal oblique ("skyline" or "flexor" view) of the navicular bone.

The tunnel block can also be used for the dorsoproximal-palmarodistal oblique projection of the distal phalanx ("upright pedal bone view") or the navicular bone ("navicular view"). With this block, however, the beam will hit the cassette at an oblique angle that causes the structures to appear elongated on the film. To avoid this distortion, a "Hickman" or "Oxspring" block can be used for these projections. This block allows for positioning the foot at a 60°/65° angle to the horizontal beam (Figure 3.21).

Additional equipment

It is very useful to have an adjustable stand for the horse's head for a number of reasons. When the horse is sedated, a head stand will help steady the horse and reduce swaying. It is also helpful when imaging heads and necks where the straightness and stability are vital. A rope head-collar should also be purchased for head and neck radiographs to avoid any metal artefacts that may overlay the bony structures.

If is not only useful to have a wall chart will all the different exposures displayed next to the x-ray system and a log book to record all the exposures taken, but, in many countries, it is a legal requirement. A radio or CD player provides not only entertainment for staff but also masks the sounds when the x-ray machine is moved that otherwise often startle horses.

It is also useful to have a rack on the wall to store the film badges when not in use to ensure that they do not go missing and that they are used when imaging is in progress; these should not be stored in the imaging room itself, but close by, to avoid incidental exposure.

Scintigraphy

Scintigraphy is the only radiographic imaging modality that visualises function rather than morphology. Whilst it is usually very sensitive and allows for imaging early disease process, it provides poor anatomical detail. In human medicine, a large variety of radiopharmaceuticals are available to target specific organs. In the horse, the vast majority of scintigraphic examinations are performed to assess musculoskeletal disorders. The radiopharmaceutical of choice to target skeletal tissue is phosphonate coupled with a metastable form of technetium (Tc), e.g., ^{99m}Tc methylendisphosphonate. Tc is a gamma ray emitter with a half-life of 6 hours (long enough to get to the bone and be imaged, short enough for the patient to be able to go home after 2 days) and an energy of 140 keV (high enough to be picked up by a scintillation camera, low enough to be safe to use).

The radiopharmaceutical can either be bought from a local hospital or generated on site. On-site generation has the advantage that the amount and timing of the radiopharmaceutical is under the control of the user. The disadvantages, however, are that careful quality control is necessary (otherwise done by the hospital), a controlled area has to be assigned and permission has to be acquired to keep not only Tc but also radioactive molybdenum (the mother isotope from which Tc is generated). It is usually much easier to come to an agreement with a local hospital. The half-life of the Tc isotope and the dose required for a horse means that the supplying hospital should be no further than 1 hour's drive away. Ideally, the hospital should be able to provide the radiopharmaceutical at any day of the week when notified the day before; in reality, however, many hospitals are only willing to deliver on the days when their own requirements are low. The radiopharmaceutical needs to be delivered by an authorised courier displaying the appropriate warning signs (exact requirements vary in different countries) in a lead container.

Scintigraphic examination of a whole horse can last more than 2 hours, so the bone phase scanning should be started no later than 3 PM; hence injection should be no later than 12 NOON. Delivery of the radiopharmaceutical should be timed accordingly. Once delivered, the lead container is opened in a controlled area. To minimise exposure to personnel, the radiopharmaceutical should be drawn up behind a lead glass screen with a lead-shielded syringe. This is best done with the glass vial still in the container using a needle long enough to reach the bottom of the glass vial. Lead syringe shields are clumsy to use, but those with a lead glass window at least allow visualisation of the drug has being drawn up. It is advisable to have two sizes (5 ml and 10 ml) of syringe shield available as the amount of radiopharmaceutical varies according to the size of the horse. The drawn-up syringe is carried to the horse in a lead-lined box and injected via an intravenous catheter (usually one of the jugular veins is used; for neck scans, the cephalic or ventral thoracic can also be used). Needles, syringe and gloves used for the procedure have to stay in the controlled area, ideally in a lead-lined cabinet, for a minimum of 48 hours.

Lead protective clothing should be worn during the actual scanning procedure. Because most studies take some time, lightweight two-piece suits are ideal to minimise discomfort and the risk of back pain. Hangers and hooks should be provided to ensure appropriate storage of the lead clothes. Latex (or equivalent) gloves and overshoes should be worn in the scanning room and in the horse's stable. The feet of the horse should be covered, e.g., with old fluid bags, while the horse is in the stable to avoid contamination of the feet through urine. The bags need to be removed when the horse leaves the stable to avoid contamination of the premises. Needles, syringes, bags and gloves used for the procedure have to stay in the controlled area, ideally in a lead-lined cabinet for a minimum of 48 hours. The scanning room as well as the stable has to be marked as controlled area by putting up the appropriate signs stating what was injected, when and by whom.

The scintigraphy signal is captured by a scintillation detector. Gamma cameras are the most commonly used detectors, but point counters are still available. These cameras come in different shapes and sizes. For the horse, a rectangular camera with large field of view is ideal (at the moment, 60 cm × 40 cm is the maximum field commercially available) (Figure 3.23). These are, however, expensive and smaller; circular cameras are usually much cheaper, especially when bought second hand from a human hospital. Different collimators to suit different radioisotopes and different applications are available. For musculoskeletal work in horses, a general purpose, mid–energy level collimator is recommended.

Gamma cameras are heavy (around 500 kg) and therefore are best mounted on a modified forklift system or from a hoist from the ceiling. Either mounting system can be driven manually or motorised. Ceiling mounted systems sometimes have the tendency to vibrate hence introducing motion artefacts, whilst forklift mounted systems are often more cumbersome to manoeuvre around the horse.

The crystal in the gamma camera is sensitive to sudden changes in temperature, and in many cases a simple measure such as covering the camera with an old horse rug or duvet will prevent the crystal from cracking when cold air flows into the room. If room is not an issue, the most elegant solution would be to operate a double-door system.

The room for scintigraphic examination needs to be large enough to house the gamma camera, its controls and the workstation to run the camera, with some space for blocks and lead shields. It usually also houses a lead-lined cabinet for storing disposables for 48 hours and the workbench with lead glass shield for drawing up the radiopharmaceutical. A cabinet to hold sedation drugs, disposable gloves and overshoes is also recommended as well as room for buckets for catching urine and manure, a shovel, a broom and a container with sawdust. A handle for the urine bucket maximises the distance between hands and radioactive urine. This can be made of a broomstick and a metal ring.

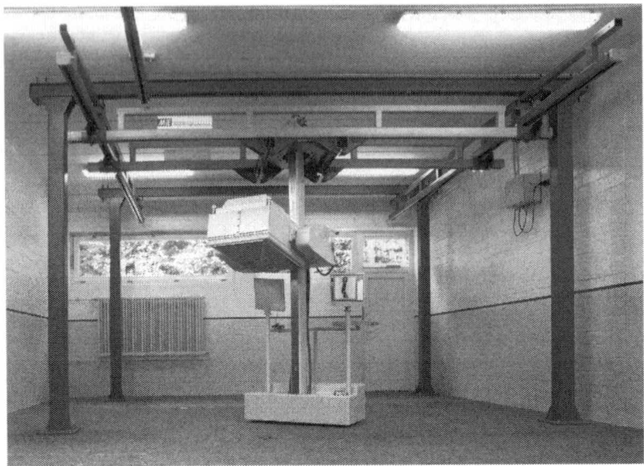

Figure 3.23 Ceiling mounted rectangular gamma camera (courtesy of MIE Inc., Germany).

Shields for masking out the bladder can be made by covering an old tennis or squash racket with some lead sheets from the DIY store. Some stands for shielding the other leg(s) during acquisition can be made by covering pieces of guttering with lead or by recycling old lead gowns.

To obtain images of the feet, the gamma camera needs to be sunk into a pit, the horse needs to be elevated or the feet need to be put on a block. The pit has to be built to the specifications of the camera manufacturer. If money is not an issue, a two-camera system can be installed, with one camera entirely dedicated to imaging of feet. Most scintigraphic facilities for horses do not have stocks because they hinder movement of the camera around the horse. However, some hospitals have developed systems around stocks and found them useful.

Some examinations, such as the back and sacroiliac region, require a prolonged image acquisition time to obtain a high-count number and diagnostic images. These high counts (in the region of a few million) can only be achieved under general anaesthesia, to avoid loss of image quality due to movement. This necessitates an anaesthetic induction and recovery stall with a hoist adjacent to the scanning room, and a custom-made table.

Ultrasonography

Ultrasonography is the diagnostic imaging modality of choice to visualise soft tissue. There is huge variety of scanners and probes (more properly called transducers) on the market, ranging from small portable units with a single transducer to large multitransducer units. Recommended transducer types and frequencies for various applications are given in Box 3.2. The higher the frequency, the greater is the detail but the lower is the tissue penetration.

Ultrasonography is the least demanding imaging modality when it comes to room requirements and additional equipment. Ultrasonography can be performed in any examination room. However, the ability to reduce light (especially sunlight) in the room is extremely advantageous to clearly viewing the image on the screen. Some clinicians find stocks useful for restraining the horse. When not in use, the ultrasound machine should be stored away safely in a designated corner or walk-in cabinet and covered to protect it from dirt and dust. High-end machines often come with a separate workstation for image archiving and manipulation for which a small desk area has to be provided. Clippers (best fixed to the wall) and a sink are essential for skin preparation prior to ultrasonographic examination. A cabinet can be useful to store coupling gel, stand-offs and transducers that are not used every day. Before the room is built, it is worth checking out whether there are any radiotransmitting stations in the vicinity that may cause interference. If this is the case, the screening of the ultrasound room with a metal mesh to create a Faraday cage (electromagnetic shielding cage) has to be considered.

Box 3.2. Ultrasound transducer types and frequencies recommended for common applications in horses

Examination of	Transducer	Frequency
Mare reproductive tract	Linear rectal probe	5–7.5 MHz
Scrotum and testes	Linear probe	5–10 MHz
Adult horse right kidney	Sector or linear array	3–5 MHz
Adult horse left kidney	Sector or linear array	2.5–3 MHz
Transrectal	Sector or linear rectal probe	5–7.5 MHz
Adult bladder	Rectal linear array	5–7.5 MHz
Foal kidneys	Sector, linear array or linear	5 MHz
Adult horse GI tract	Sector or linear array	2.5–3.5 MHz
Transrectal	Linear rectal probe	5–8 MHz
Adult Liver	Sector or linear array	3.5–7.5 MHz
Foal GI tract	Sector or linear array	5 MHz
Foal internal umbilicus and bladder	Sector, linear array or linear	5–12 MHz
Adult heart	Sector or phased array	2.5–3.5 MHz
Foal heart	Sector or phased array	3–7.5 MHz
Adult lungs	Sector, linear array or linear	3–7.5 MHz
Foal lungs	Sector, linear array or linear	3–10 MHz
Joints (except the stifle)	Sector, linear array or linear	5–10 MHz
Stifle joint	Sector or linear array	2.5–5 MHz
Tendons and ligaments	Linear probe	7.5–12 MHz
Muscles	Sector, linear array or linear	5–10 MHz
Pelvis (ilium)	Sector, linear array or linear	2.5–5 MHz
Eye	Linear array or linear	6–12 MHz

Computed tomography

Conventional radiographs depict a three-dimensional object as a two-dimensional image. Their main limitation is that overlying tissues are superimposed on the image. Computed tomography (CT) overcomes this problem by scanning thin slices of the body with a narrow x-ray beam that rotates around the body, producing an image of each slice as a cross section of the body. X-ray slice data are generated using an x-ray source that rotates around the object; x-ray sensors are positioned on the opposite side of the circle from the x-ray source. Many data scans are progressively taken as the object is gradually passed through the gantry. They are combined together by the mathematical procedure known as tomographic reconstruction.

Another limitation of the conventional radiograph is its inability to distinguish between two tissues with similar density. CT can differentiate between tissues of similar density because of the narrow x-ray beam and the use of "windowing". The information acquired by CT is stored on computer as digital raw data and an image can be displayed on a video monitor or printed onto x-ray film. The image is made up of a matrix of thousands of tiny squares, or pixels. Each pixel has a CT number (measured in Hounsfield units) attributed to it. The CT number is a measure of absorption of the initial x-ray beam by the tissues at each point in the body. This varies according to the density of the tissues. The denser the tissue, the higher is the CT number (Figure 3.24).

Air	Fat	Water	Muscle	Bone
-1000HU	-300HU	0H	-50HU	>200H

Figure 3.24 Hounsfield units of various body tissues for computed tomography. ©Renate Weller 2007.

Ideally, the image would be displayed with a different shade of grey for every different CT number. However, the human eye is much more limited in distinguishing shades of grey, so a system of windowing is used. The radiographer selects the range of CT numbers to be displayed and all the numbers within this range are spread over the grey scale of the human eye.

The benefits of CT do not come without a price. Firstly, CT is considerably more expensive than conventional radiography. Secondly, the radiation dose from CT is much greater than for conventional radiography. Thirdly, in the horse, it requires general anaesthesia with its associated risks. In the adult horse, CT is limited to head, legs and cranial part of neck due to size of gantry opening. Very recently a CT system has been developed that allows for scanning heads in the standing, sedated horse (Figure 3.25).

CT has proved to be useful for the diagnosis of head problems in the horse, especially for the evaluation of fracture configuration, cysts, abscesses and tumours of the jaws, sinuses, nasal cavity and orbits. For detection of brain

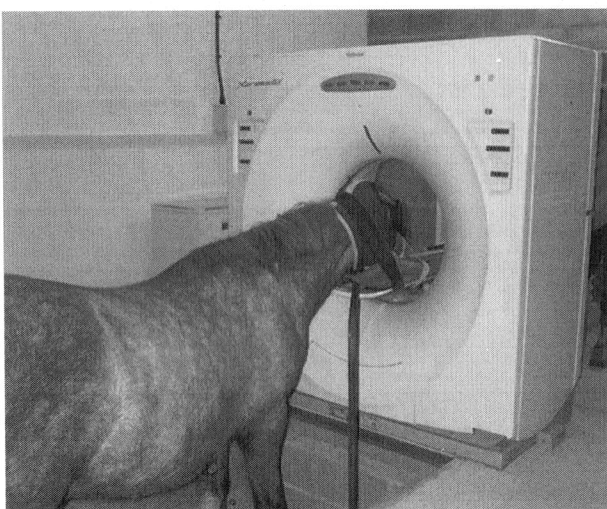

Figure 3.25 CT scanner for scanning heads in the sedated horse (courtesy of Alistair Nelson, Rainbow Equine Clinic, UK).

tumours, CT scanning with intravenous contrast can be used, but this technique is less sensitive than magnetic resonance imaging (MRI). CT has also been used for the evaluation of dental disease, the diagnosis of the causes of chronic sinusitis and imaging of the hyoid apparatus, the temporomandibular and atlanto-occipital joints. In the horse, CT is restricted to the cranial part of the neck by the size of the gantry opening. CT has been found useful in the diagnosis of osteomyelitis, fractures of vertebral body and changes in the facet joints, and contrast-enhanced CT has been shown to be useful in the diagnosis of cervical stenotic myelopathy.

CT is the method of choice for the evaluation of subchondral bone disease (e.g., occult subchondral osseous cyst-like lesions of the equine tarsocrural joint and osteochondritis dissecans–like lesions of the proximal phalanx). CT has also been shown to aid in diagnosis of navicular syndrome, osteoarthritis and osteomyelitis. CT enables the thorough assessment of complex fractures, because of its ability to reconstruct the area of interest in multiple planes. It is widely used in research for bone density measurements (e.g., to assess the effect of training on third metacarpal bone in racehorses). CT angiography allows the mapping and evaluation of blood vessels in three dimensions. In foals and small-breed horses, the use of CT can be extended to the proximal part of the limbs, the back, the thorax and abdomen.

To date, there is no horse-specific CT scanner on the market; rather, CT scanners developed for humans are modified to allow docking of a table sturdy enough support the weight of a horse (human tables are too small and limited to 200 kg maximum weight). One system* includes a table that slides over the base of the human table. This table supports the weight of the horse but uses the motor from the human table to move the horse in and out of the scanner. Recently, another method has been developed that allows for scanning of the horse in recumbency as well as scanning the horse's head in the standing, sedated horse. This system positions the horse on the opposite side of the human table. The table for the anaesthetised horse docks onto the human table with a simple bolt connection (similar to the connection between a trailer and a car). To allow the motor of the human table to pull the weight of the horse, the table moves on air hovers, thus reducing friction to a minimum. For CT scans of the head of the standing sedated horse, the horse stands in a pit in front of the CT scanner (3 m × 1 m). In this pit, there is a platform on hovers that connects to the human table of the CT scanner. The horse is walked into the pit over a ramp and stood on the platform. The horse is heavily sedated and its head is placed on the end of the human table, supported by a cradle used for infant scanning and fed into the CT by the moving the human table and therefore the platform on hovers. While this system is very cost effective, it is not commercially available and the different components have to be bought separately and put together. Second-hand CT scanners from human hospitals can often be bought for much less money than new or refurbished systems.

The table used for CT scanning has to allow for the horse to be put in lateral as well as in dorsal recumbency. The most space-saving option for this is to have a table base to which extensions for the head and legs can be added as required. To keep the horse stable in dorsal recumbency, appropriate support brackets have to be available to clip onto the sides.

The CT scanners made by the major manufacturers (GE, Hitachi, Philips, Siemens, Toshiba) are all similar in dimension (approximately 2 metres wide, 2 metres high, 3.5 metres long, including patient table). Large-bore scanners have a gantry opening of up to 85 cm, which allows the scanning of horse legs proximal to carpus and tarsus and the neck to C4-C5, depending on the size of the horse. Another factor to consider is the distance between the isocentre (the area where the actual scanning takes place) and the outside of the gantry. The shorter this distance, the easier it is to position a horse.

Depending on the table design, a CT room should be a minimum of 8 × 6 metres to not only make room for the CT scanner and the table but also allow easy movement of the horse on the table and the anaesthetic equipment. A knock down/recovery stall and a control room are required next to the CT room, as well as space for the CT generator and, if the hover system is installed, for the compressor producing air for the hovers.

Equine Magnetic Resonance Imaging

Like CT, MRI is a tomographic imaging modality that represents a three-dimensional object as a series of two-dimensional slices and hence avoids superimposition of

* Universal Medical Systems Inc., Ohio, USA.

structures. The underlying technical principle of MRI is, however, completely different. MRI is based on the physical phenomenon of nuclear magnetic resonance. Nuclear magnetic resonance describes the physical phenomenon that all atoms that contain odd numbers of nucleons have an intrinsic magnetic moment. The most common molecule in the body is hydrogen and the nucleus of hydrogen is composed of an unpaired proton. It is this proton that plays a major part in the generation of the MRI signal. The direction of the magnetic moment of these protons is randomly distributed in nature. If those protons are put in the field of stronger magnet, the tiny spins of the hydrogen atoms align themselves with the magnetic field. If a third, perturbing magnetic field is introduced to this system, the aligned spins are aligned afresh, depending on the strength and duration of the perturbing field. When this perturbing field is suddenly turned off, the spins begin to wobble before gradually realigning themselves to their original vector in the magnetic field. Whenever a magnetic vector spins, it induces a current in a nearby coil, and this is the principal by which the signal is detected from the realigning magnets. The realigning of the magnets is called the *relaxation* and occurs in two different ways: T1 and T2 relaxation. Depending on the application, the emphasis is put on one or the other and results in "T1-" or "T2-weighted" images.

MRI has all the advantages of a tomographic imaging modality without involving ionising radiation. So far it has not yet been possible to establish any damaging effect on the body.

The major application in the horse is the evaluation of foot-related problems. Over the last few years, a series of studies have demonstrated that MRI is an excellent diagnostic tool in the diagnosis of soft tissue problems (especially ligaments and tendons, such as the deep digital flexor tendon or collateral ligaments in the foot). It has been used for the assessment of fractures and subchondral bone pathology but is inferior to CT in the visualisation of bone pathology. It allows for detection of cartilage damage in clinical circumstances and has been used as a research tool to assess cartilage metabolism. It has been used in the diagnosis of brain tumours and abscesses in horses. As for CT, many more organs and tissues can be examined in foals or miniature breeds than in mature horses.

Based on the strength of the magnet (expressed in Tesla [T]), MRI systems can be grouped into two categories: high-field systems with superconducting magnets (>1 T) and low-field systems with permanent magnets (<1 T). High-field systems have a tubular, gantry-based configuration, whereas low-field systems have a sandwich configuration ("C" or "U" shaped). A stronger magnetic field produces a stronger signal; hence high-field scanners can produce higher resolution pictures in a shorter time than low-field scanners. Low-field systems, however, make access for horses easier and are much cheaper to buy and maintain. Low-field systems have been specially configured for use in the standing horse† (usually referred to as "standing MRI") (Figure 3.26). Standing MRI is a relatively new imaging tool that, unlike the traditional MRI system, does not require the animal to be anaesthetised.

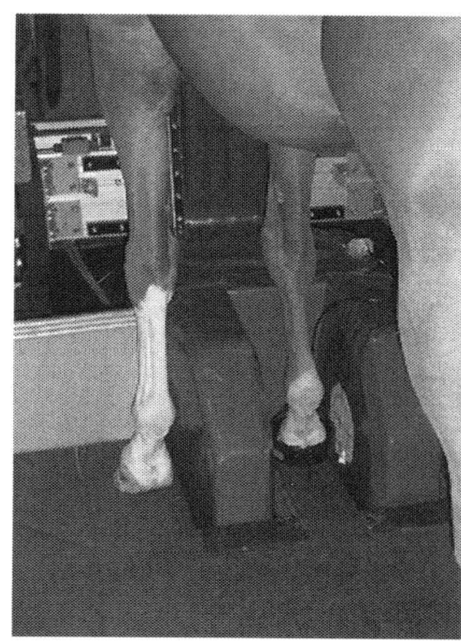

Figure 3.26 Low-field MRI system for scanning of standing horses (courtesy of Hallmarq Ltd, UK).

High-field magnets are very expensive to buy new and currently cost approximately £500,000 (€750,000; US$ 900,000; AS$ 1,200,000). Recommissioned systems may be adequate and are cheaper. Maintenance costs for high-field magnets may also be high. Compared to CT, MRI also requires more technical expertise in operating and troubleshooting, and most human hospitals employ MRI physicists to ensure smooth operation of their MRI system(s).

In addition to the magnet itself, coils have to be purchased. Because there are no equine-specific coils on the market, human coils need to be adapted. Human torso array and extremity coils will probably be of best use in equine MRI. There is a selection of coils on the market, but again it may be worth purchasing recommissioned coils as again they are very expensive. A lockable cabinet for safe storage of the coils should be provided.

For gantry-based systems, the animal has to be anaesthetised and an adjoining recovery stall, with hoist, will be required with an MRI-compatible table. Due to the limited market demand for such tables, they have to be specially made. MRI-compatible anaesthesia equipment will also have to be purchased.

Building an MRI facility

In planning a hospital facility for equine MRI, three concerns must be addressed: planning for the scanner, for the horse handling and for the operator.

Scanner

The main component of an MRI imaging system is the magnet. This may be a large superconducting system or a smaller permanent magnet. In each case, the magnetic field

† Hallmarq Veterinary Imaging, Guildford, Surrey, UK.

will be strongest at the opening of the magnet and will rapidly fall off with distance. Magnetic fields do not create ionising radiation and pose no known biological hazards, but do create important safety concerns. The most severe is the risk of magnetic objects being attracted to the magnet with sufficient force to cause injury. Many patients have been killed in human MRI systems by gas cylinders, surgical instruments and other flying metal objects, and the hazard must be taken extremely seriously, particularly in the veterinary environment with less rigorously trained operators and common metal objects such as farriery tools and horseshoes. A secondary risk is posed by magnetically operated switches in cardiac pacemakers and other metallic surgical implants. The international safety standard is set at a field strength of 5 G (0.5 mT)—warnings are required above this field strength and individuals with pacemakers and implants must stay outside the 5-G line.

The only feasible protection against the static field is distance, so the building must be planned so that any public space is outside the 5-G isocontour in all directions. External sources of magnetic interference must be kept sufficiently far from the scanner. One manufacturer recommends a minimum distance of 1 metre for small fixed objects such as steel-reinforcing bars in concrete, up to 5 metres for cars in a car park and further still for objects such as trains, electrical substation transformers and power lines. Special care is needed if the scanner is close to any instrumentation that is sensitive to magnetic fields such as electron microscopes, nuclear scintigraphy cameras or other MRI systems.

An MRI system transits and receives radiofrequency (RF) signals and must be enclosed in a completely screened room in order to prevent external interference from degrading the images. Note, though, that this room does not block the static magnetic field in any way. The screened room, or Faraday shield, is made of copper or thin steel plates bonded to chipboard panels. It completely surrounds the scanner, with special seals on any doors or windows. Penetrations such as drains, air conditioning and access for ventilation and monitoring equipment must also be carefully screened and require special attention during room design. Manufactures of RF screens typically supply and install the shield based upon drawings provided by the client or client's design team.

Lighting must be incandescent and cannot be under the control of a dimmer (which generates electrical interference), so two or more separate circuits are recommended to allow for changes in room illumination. Electrical installations, such as circuits for lighting and power outlets, within the MRI shielded room must be adequately filtered on entry to the room to avoid RF interference. The necessary electrical line filters are normally installed as a component part of the RF shielded room.

Room temperature control is particularly critical for permanent magnet-based systems. For the standing equine MRI system, the manufacturers specify a range of no more than ±2° C, 24 hours a day/365 days a year. Such regulation requires a close control, industrial-grade air conditioning system. Consideration should be given to the location of the air conditioning unit, ductwork routes and service area required for the maintenance of the system during the design of the MRI room and adjacent areas.

In addition to the magnet, any MRI system will require space for the electronic parts. These will generally be two units: a computer rack and an operator station. The computer rack will generate a considerable amount of heat (for example, 5 kW for the Hallmarq system) and must be well ventilated to prevent overheating. The operator console may be inside (standing systems) or outside (superconducting systems) the screened room. The MRI system is typically supported and monitored for performance via Internet links, so a suitable network connection must be provided close to the computer rack. A telephone is convenient for the operator, but it is often impractical to electrically filter a telephone connection into the room, so the location of a phone and the type of connection should be discussed with the MRI system manufacturer while planning the facility.

Access routes to and through the building for the delivery of the system must be given careful consideration with regards to the physical dimensions of the scanner and its packaging, imposed loads on the building structure, specification of lifting equipment, turning circles and protection to internal finishes. In some cases the best option is to build the room with a removable section of wall that can be replaced once the system is installed and removed again if the system has to be dismantled.

Horse handling

For safe horse handling, the room must be sufficiently large. The manufacturer recommends a room size of 5 m × 7 m (16 ft × 24 ft) for the standing equine MRI scanner. Ideally, there should be at least two doors to provide an escape route in case of emergency.

If any horse is to be anaesthetised, then convenient access to the knock-down and recovery areas is crucial, and the room must be large enough to accommodate the recumbent horse in any desired position around the magnet, together with anaesthetic equipment and technicians. Since some anaesthetic equipment may be magnetic, sufficient space should be allowed for this to be secured well outside the 5-G line, or outside the room with appropriately shielded access.

The floor of the MRI room should be easy to clean and sterilise. Rubber stable mats or other forms of nonslip plastic flooring are in common use. Drainage is difficult as any drains would have to penetrate the screened room, so it is common for the room itself to be undrained but for the floor to slope slightly toward the door. Floor cleanings are then swept outside the room to a nearby drain. Similarly, providing a water supply inside the room requires special attention to the screening of the incoming pipe work and is often forgone in favour of a hosepipe outside the room.

Operator

The operator of a superconducting system will invariably be outside the magnet room, whilst for the standing system, the use of specially shielded monitor allows the operator to be inside the room which reduces the staff costs of running the scanner. The monitor screen, keyboard and mouse must be located in convenient positions with good visibility of the horse and the ability to move quickly in case of emergency. It is common for the operator to prefer a high, barstool-type operating position for convenience and safety. Shelf space should be provided nearby for notebooks and pens and for books as the interpretation of MRI is complex and often aided by reference texts.

Storage and workspace must also be provided for animal care equipment (drugs, syringes, swabs, clinical waste disposal) and for MRI equipment (spare coils, test equipment). Archived images are often stored to CD or DVD, and secure storage should be provided off-site as protection in case of fire, flood or theft. A range of pads, sand bags and ropes is necessary for optimal positioning of the horse.

Archiving image data

Diagnostic imaging has undergone considerable changes over the last decade in human and veterinary medicine, largely caused by advancements in information technology. Fast computers, necessary for computing complex algorithms and with the ability to process and store vast amounts of data in small spaces, have become readily available (and affordable). This has led to a shift from conventional imaging methods, such as film-based x-ray systems towards digital imaging modalities.

Image data require large amounts of memory, and many digital systems require daily backup of images on tape, CD or DVD. A more efficient and space-saving solution is provided by picture archiving and communication systems (PACS). Until recently, cost-efficient PACS were only available for large hospitals. In the last few years, however, custom-tailored systems affordable for smaller practices and hospitals have come on the market. These systems allow for central storage of large quantities of image data from any DICOM-compatible imaging modality and easy retrieval to different computers (on-site or off-site). DICOM files not only store the image data itself but also information about the patient such as patient identification number, date of examination, breed, age, name, etc. The stored data can be searched according to each of the included parameters.

A PACS usually consists of a server for data storage and a workstation with dedicated software to retrieve and manipulate images. A network infrastructure has to be installed to allow for sending data from the various imaging modalities to the server and to the workstation. To ensure safe backup, the server should be housed remote from the scanning facilities. The workstation should be placed for convenient access because it allows for displaying all images of a patient simultaneously. This not only facilitates reporting of studies but also allows quick and easy access to images for showing to clients. Most PACS also interlink to billing and clinical record systems, which can make workflow more efficient.

Website addresses of suppliers of diagnostic imaging equipment are given in Box 3.3.

3.2.2. Radiation safety

Renate Weller

Introduction

Diagnostic imaging plays a central role in the equine hospital. The majority of imaging modalities available for horses involve ionising radiation and therefore pose a potential health hazard to staff, owners and animals. Ionis-

Box 3.3. Some suppliers of imaging equipment

Radiography/computed tomography/magnetic resonance imaging/ultrasonography/ scintigraphy

GE Healthcare: www.gehealthcare.com
Hitachi Medical Systems: www.hitachimedical.com
Philips Medical Systems: www.medical.philips.com
Siemens Medical Solutions: www.medical.siemens.com
Toshiba Medical Systems: www.medical.toshiba.com
Esaote-Piemedical: www.esaote-piemedical.com
BCF Technology: www.bcftechnology.com

Horse-specific CT and MRI systems

Universal Medical Systems: www.veterinary-imaging.com
Hallmarq Veterinary Imaging: www.hallmarq.net

Computed radiography systems

Agfa Health Care: www.agfa.com/healthcare
Fujifilm Medical Systems: www.fujimed.com
Kodak: www.kodak.com/global/en/health

Direct digital radiography systems

Idexx Laboratories Inc: www.idexx.com
Afp Imaging Corp: www.afpimaging.com
Eklin Medical Systems: www.eklin.com

Horse-specific scintigraphy systems

Bartec Medical Imaging Solutions: www.bartectechnologies.com
Hermes Nuclear Diagnostics: www.hermesmedical.com
Medical Imaging Electronics: www.mieamerica.com

Veterinary-specific PACS

Eklin Medical systems: www.elinc.net
Visbion, Vision in Biomedicine: www.visbion.com

Table 3.1. Units of radioactivity

For illustration purposes, the units have been compared to rainfall.

Quantity	Unit	Old unit	Rainstorm equivalent
Activity	Becquerel (Bq) (1 decay per second)	Curie (Ci)	Amount of rain falling
Absorbed dose	Gray (Gy) (1 J/kg)	rad	Amount of rain hitting you
Dose equivalent	Sievert (Sv)	rem	How wet you get

ing radiation acts at cell level by changing molecule configurations, leading to cell death and/or mutations. Health effects of radiation are divided into two categories: threshold effects and nonthreshold effects. Threshold effects (e.g., sterility, death) appear after high levels of radiation exposure, which cause enough cells to be damaged to make the effect apparent. Nonthreshold effects (e.g., cancer) can occur at any level of radiation exposure, but the risk of harmful health effects generally increases with the amount of radiation absorbed.

Ionising radiation is encountered in equine hospitals in the form of x-rays from closed sources (radiography, fluoroscopy and computed tomography) or gamma-rays from open sources (radiopharmaceuticals used in nuclear medicine, most commonly technetium 99m for musculoskeletal scintigraphy). There is considerable confusion when is comes to units associated with ionising radiation; however, a basic understanding of these is essential when performing equine diagnostic imaging. A short summary is given in Table 3.1.

Principles of minimising radiation exposure

Although it is almost impossible to avoid exposure of staff to ionising radiation in equine diagnostic imaging, this should be reduced to a minimum by optimising building setup, equipment and procedure.

Basic principles to minimise radiation hazard are given in Box 3.4. This is obviously down to clinical judgement and should follow the principles of evidence-based medicine.

Regulatory requirements

The specific regulatory requirements differ between countries but usually follow the recommendations of the International Commission on Radiological Protection (ICPR publication No. 60). Work with ionising radiation requires prior notification by the regulatory body. A prior risk assessment is commonly required and is done in cooperation with a radiation protection advisor, a radiation specialist recognised by the regulatory body. Written local rules for each imaging section should be drawn up in consultation with the radiation protection advisor. These should be accessible for all members of staff (they are often displayed in or just outside the imaging room) and have to be easily understood. The main person responsible for observing the rules is the principal of the veterinary practice. Manufacturers and installers of equipment are to ensure that the equipment is designed and installed in a way to meet regulations and that appropriate instructions for its use are provided. However, if the veterinary practice self-installs second-hand equipment, the responsibility lies with the practice principal and should be done in consultation with the radiation advisor.

Box 3.4. Basic principles to minimise radiation hazard

- No procedure should exceed the legal dose limits. These are based on the recommendations of the International Commission on Radiological Protection (ICPR).
- Each procedure should follow the ALARA principle = As Low As Reasonably Achievable
- Diagnostic imaging procedure should only be performed if
  - There is a clear clinical indication.
  - The outcome of the procedure is likely to change prognosis and/or therapy of the patient.
  - No alternative diagnostic procedure (not involve ionising radiation) is available that provides the same information (for example, ultrasonography or blood tests).

Monitoring and safety testing

Monitoring the exposure of all staff involved in diagnostic imaging on a regular basis is key in minimising radiation hazard. This is done by providing each individual with a dosemeter (usually in the form of film-badges). These should be worn on the trunk (and not be moved when protective clothing is put on) and have to be exchanged and read by an approved dosemeter service in regular intervals (usually once a month). Radiation levels in imaging rooms can be monitored by mounting dosemeters on fixed positions and read in regular intervals depending on the workload.

Each procedure has to be recorded. The records should include patient identification, date, area examined, exposures/dose used and quality of the resulting radiographs. The use of a hardbound book for each modality is recommended to avoid pages going missing. Technical equipment as well as protective clothing has to be safety tested before it is taken into use and subsequent safety tests have to be performed and the results recorded on a regular basis (usually annually or more frequently) by a competent person according to the local rules.

Training

All staff involved in equine diagnostic imaging have to have adequate training in the theory and practice of each diag-

Box 3.5. Areas to train staff as regards radiation hazard

- Health hazards associated with ionising radiation. Especially people without any previous medical training tend to have a rather light-hearted attitude towards ionising radiation ("what I cannot see, cannot harm me").
- Radiation physics: different kinds of ionising radiation and how these relate to shielding and the inverse-square law
- Horse handling and constraining horses for the procedure
- Practical training on how the equipment is used (normally done best without a horse present until the operator is familiar with the equipment)

nostic imaging modality. Staff should have an understanding of the topics described in Box 3.5.

Radiography

Room requirements

A designated room must be provided for radiography. It is desirable but not essential that the room is used for radiography only; however, when radiography is undertaken, the room must not be used for any other purposes. The room has to be of adequate size to ensure that personnel involved in radiography can be a minimum of 2 metres away from the beam axis during exposure. Walls subjected to primary beam should have a lead equivalent of 2 mm (double brick), and walls subjected to scatter radiation, a lead equivalent of 0.5 mm (single brick). Doors and windows have to be shielded adequately by lining them with lead sheets and using x-ray–resistant glass.

Warning signs and lights must be provided at each entrance to an x-ray room. The warning sign should incorporate the radiation symbol and a legend (e.g., "X-rays—do not enter when light is on"), the warning light should be connected to the x-ray circuit to come on automatically when x-rays are taken. Windows should be equipped with blinds and the light switch should incorporate a dimmer to dim the light sufficiently to line up the primary beam with the plate and to collimate the primary beam to a minimum.

Radiography outside a designated room

Some situations require the use of x-rays outside the designated x-ray rooms, such as in a stable or in an operating theatre. In this case, a controlled area has to be established where access is restricted and the area can be overseen by the radiographer at any time during the procedure. The controlled area has to be demarcated such as by the use of cones or tape and portable signs. The direction and collimation of the primary beam (often difficult due to light levels) has to be considered carefully.

Equipment

X-ray machines for referral level equine radiography have to have powerful generators to be able to produce the high exposures necessary for diagnostic images of the proximal anatomy of the horse. The maximum output of an x-ray machine is often described by its maximum kV and mA-s; however, the maximum mA is of interest because this determines the time component of an exposure. Because horses are usually radiographed while standing, the time of an exposure has to be kept to a minimum to avoid movement blur.

It is the manufacturers' responsibility to ensure that new x-ray machines comply with radiation regulations. If, however, a second-hand x-ray machine is installed, the principal of the practice has to ensure that these regulations are met. The features of particular importance to radiation safety are the light beam diaphragm (borders and alignment), exposure accuracy, beam filtration and radiation leakage. The exposure button should be either situated outside the x-ray room, behind a suitable screen/wall or on a cable that extends more than 2 metres from the primary beam axis. To obtain radiographs of diagnostic quality of the proximal anatomy of the horse, the use of a grid is often necessary; this is best incorporated in a ceiling or stand-mounted plate holder. Grids require increased exposure and their use should be considered carefully.

Each x-ray room should have its own set of lead gowns, gloves and thyroid protectors and should be equipped with appropriate storage facilities. Lead gowns should not be folded or crumbled up because this can result in a crack in the lead lining, but instead hung up over large-diameter bars or on hangers. Please be aware that lead clothing is designed to provide protection from scattered radiation and does not shield against the primary beam. Protective clothing should be checked visually for obvious defects before each use and thoroughly examined annually.

The fastest film/screen combinations that still result in diagnostic-quality radiographs should be used to minimise exposure time and the risk of movement blur. Film processing facilities should be adjacent to the x-ray room and be maintained carefully to avoid wasted exposures. Computerised facilities have the advantage to allow for correction of (especially overexposed) radiographs, thus reducing the need for repeat exposures.

Suitable plate holders for a range of different sized plates should be available and handholding of plates avoided.

Procedure

The procedure should only be carried out with trained personnel and clear guidelines have to be set out on how the procedure is performed. These have to be in writing and accessible to all staff. Nobody under 18 years old or pregnant is allowed in the room during a study. It is an advisable policy not to allow any clients in the x-ray room. This ensures that only trained people are present and also saves one from asking (potentially embarrassing) questions about age and pregnancy. Laypersons must only assist with restraint and not with the technical part of the study. They should give their informed consent.

The number of people present in the room should be reduced to a minimum, and equipment such as free-standing plate holders used whenever possible. If a horse is properly restrained, there should be no need for more than one person in the room during exposure (the one holding the horse). All persons present have to wear protective clothing and should stand at least 2 metres away from the primary beam. This, however, is often not achievable in equine radiography, especially if the horse is not sedated.

The use of a horizontal x-ray beam is common in equine radiography, and the direction and the distance of the x-rays have to be considered carefully because they carry on beyond the plate. It is generally advisable to choose positions so that the x-ray beam is pointing towards a brick/concrete wall rather than a door or wooden division. If this is not possible, a thick (>2-mm) lead beam stop should be placed behind the plate.

Whenever possible, free-standing or wall-mounted plate holders should be used. Some radiographs, such as a lateromedial projection of the stifle, however, require somebody to handhold the plate. In this case, a large plate should be used and held by a corner with lead gloves as far away from the primary beam as possible. It is not acceptable to have any body part within the primary beam. High exposures are necessary for radiographing the upper limb, thorax and spine of the horse. This often results in high energy scatter radiation backfiring from the horse, which has to be taken into account. To reduce scatter, the primary beam should be minimised to leave an unexposed border on all edges of a radiograph.

Horses are radiographed while conscious and standing. Thus, in addition to the radiation hazard, the horse itself poses a health hazard during the procedure. Proper restraint of the animal is essential to minimise both of these by making the horse more manageable and keeping the horse still during setup and acquisition, thus reducing the need for repeated studies. It is generally advisable to sedate the horse at the onset of the study rather than trying to proceed with manual restraint only. This often results in an agitated horse and increased exposure times, putting personnel and equipment unnecessarily at risk. The area of interest should be prepared carefully before the examination (e.g., removal of shoes) to avoid repeat exposures.

Fluoroscopy

For fluoroscopy, all the regulations for conventional radiography apply. Fluoroscopy should not be used as a substitute for conventional radiography and should only be used in the anaesthetised horse. Screening times should be limited to the minimum necessary for a diagnostic examination. Vertical beams should be used whenever possible, and care should be taken to direct the beam towards a brick wall or lead screen when a horizontal or angled beam is employed. Additional personnel (e.g., anaesthetists) should only stay within the room if absolutely necessary.

Computed tomography

All regulations for conventional radiography apply to computed tomography (CT). CT should only be undertaken when clinically required and should not be used as a substitute for conventional radiography. No personnel should be in the scanning room during the procedure; if, however, the presence of a member of staff is necessary, that person has to wear protective clothing and should stand behind a protective screen.

CT is mainly performed in the anaesthetised horse, and remote anaesthetic monitoring is required.

Nuclear medicine

Regulations

There is a wide range of different radiopharmaceuticals used in human medicine for diagnostic and therapeutic purposes, each of which requires different details of handling based on the type of emitted radiation (α, β, γ rays), half-life and magnitude of radiation. Equine nuclear medicine mostly involves the use of technetium 99m for musculoskeletal applications ("bone scanning"). Technetium 99m is a γ-ray emitter (140 keV) and has a half-life of 6 hours.

The holding and disposal of radioactive substances are tightly controlled and the regulatory requirements differ between countries. Before commencing working with radioactive material, the appropriate authorities have to be consulted. Written arrangements including detailed instructions on the handling of the radiopharmaceutical, the radioactive horse and waste, as well as a contingency plan to minimise the spread of exposure in case of spillage, have to be provided. Monitoring equipment suitable for contamination monitoring in and outside the scanning area is required and is usually provided in form of a portable Geiger counter.

Radioactive substances have to be accounted for, and the type of radiopharmaceutical, source, date, time, activity and way of disposal have to be recorded. Radioactive substances may only be acquired from authorised sources. For many equine hospitals, this will be the nearest human hospital. Special regulations apply to the transport of radioactive substances, and it is usually advisable to employ a commercial, authorised courier.

Procedure

In an equine hospital, it is often necessary to distinguish between the area where a horse is injected with the radiopharmaceutical (stable or scanning room), where the actual scan is performed (scanning room) and where the horse is housed after injection (stable). All areas have to be labelled, indicating the radiation source and the date/time of injection and/or date/time it is safe to enter. The scanning room and stable should not be entered a minimum of 48 hours after injection. Horses should be watered and fed at the door but not mucked out.

Equipment for safe handling of the radiopharmaceutical has to be provided: a lead glass screen and lead-shielded syringes of different sizes (usually 5 ml and 10 ml) for drawing up the radiopharmaceutical and a lead-lined box for carrying the syringe to the site of injection. Goggles, protective clothing, gloves and overshoes are advisable in case of spillage. All equipment has to be labelled with the radiation symbol. Injection of the radiopharmaceutical should be performed through an intravenous catheter.

Technetium is eliminated from the body via the urinary tract. This results in a massive uptake in the bladder, which can mask lesions in the proximity and often interfere with hind limb and back studies. Some authors recommend the injection of a diuretic prior to scanning; care has to be taken that this takes place well in advance of the scan (a minimum of 1 hour is recommended), so as not to cause the horse to urinate on the way from the stable to the scanning room or in the scanning room itself. Bladder catheterisation in a radioactive horse is not an acceptable procedure because it puts the person performing the procedure in close proximity of radioactive urine and spillage usually cannot be avoided. To avoid spreading radioactive urine and avoid getting false-positive results by radioactive urine on the skin/hoof surface, horses' feet should be wrapped in plastic bags (e.g., used intravenous fluid bags) between injection and scanning and removed before the horse leaves the stable. Care has to be taken by the person removing the bags to avoid contamination, and adequate protective clothing (aprons/coveralls, gloves and overshoes) should be worn at any stage. If contamination occurs in the stable or in the scanning room, the clothes have to be left there for a minimum of 48 hours.

Horses undergoing scintigraphy are best sedated, and a bucket with a long handle should be provided to catch urine, which has to remain in the scanning room for a minimum of 48 hours. When performing a scintigraphic study of the hind limb, the bladder can be masked with the aid of a lead-lined squash or tennis racket during acquisition. To ensure images of diagnostic quality, the contralateral leg should be shielded. This is often done by person holding a lead gown between the legs. This is not advisable, because it requires another person close to the source of radiation and also increases the risk of this person getting kicked by the horse. An alternative are free-standing leg shields that are easily made by lining a piece of plastic guttering with lead foil, both available from DIY stores. Acquisition times should be kept to a minimum (<2 minutes per area) to reduce exposure and movement blur. This is largely facilitated by adequate sedation. Most scintigraphy software offers motion correction facilities, which can correct for certain amounts of movement, hence reducing the need of repeat acquisitions. There has to be a clear clinical indication for performing a scintigraphic study, and the area of interest should have been narrowed down through clinical examination prior to the study. Whole horse scans should be avoided because these are rarely diagnostic and involve very long exposure times for everybody involved. Following the administration of a radiopharmaceutical, further investigations (with the exception of emergencies) should be delayed for a minimum of 48 hours.

The use of lead gowns during a study has been controversially debated for years; however, recent findings suggest that there is a significant reduction in personnel exposure with the use of lead gowns.

3.2.3. Endoscopic equipment

Jennifer O. Stephen

Equipment

Endoscopes for general use in equine practice should have a 7- to 9-mm outside diameter, ability to move the tip in four directions, air and water flushing systems and a high-quality image.

Two types of flexible endoscope are used in equine practice: fiberoptic endoscopes and video endoscopes. In fiberoptic endoscopes, the image is generally transmitted through optical glass fibres to an eyepiece. These are easy to use in ambulatory practice for diagnostic purposes but difficult to use in surgical procedures and obviously unsuitable for high-speed treadmill examinations.

Video endoscopes produce high-quality images, allow images to be captured and recorded and are excellent for client communication and staff/student training. There are two types of video endoscopes. In one, an external video camera is attached to the eyepiece of a fibreoptic endoscope to allow the image to be displayed on a monitor. A device called an endocoupler maintains the mechanical and optical connection between the scope and the camera. Couplers of 32 to 35 mm are suitable for use with rigid endoscopes; 22 to 28 mm works best with flexible gastroscopes and colonoscopies.[1] The other type of video endoscope, the video image endoscope, has an electronic microchip called a charged coupling device (CCD) in the tip of the endoscope. Cells in this device convert light into electronic charges, producing a much clearer image than conventional fibreoptic systems.

Light sources

Halogen or xenon light sources are available. Halogen light sources are cheap and portable, making them very suitable for ambulatory practice. Xenon light sources produce higher-intensity "whiter" light, giving more accurate representation of true colour.

If using a video system, the type of light source you can use is dependent on the type of camera you have. Auto-exposure cameras control the light sensitivity and can be used with any light source. Non–auto-exposure cameras do not and must be used with an auto-exposure light source.

In order to be able to use the endoscope for a variety of purposes, a light source that also provides an air/water pump should be selected.

Image recording equipment

Various equipment is available for recording endoscopy images. New units generally have a computer system and the ability to store images and movie clips to the hard disk. There is also the option to download the image and movie files to various media, depending on the model, often including writable DVD and/or CD and USB memory sticks. One disadvantage of these systems is that with heavy use, the internal hard disk can become full very quickly. Some systems crash and will not operate when the hard disk is full. This can be prevented by regular archiving of images and clearing them from the hard disk.

Older units may not have an image storage system. Generally, these units have a video output (NTSC or PAL), and this can be connected to a digital video recorder (hard disk recorder), DVD recorder or video recorder. Still images may be recorded at the time of the examination with a digital video recorder or with an image capture device*, although these have largely been superseded and are generally only available second-hand.

Scope size

A scope for general use should have a 7- to 9-mm outside diameter. The length and outer diameter of a scope will determine the clinical procedures for which it can be used. The maximum outer diameter for examination of respiratory tract in foals is 9 mm; in adults, up to 12 mm may be used. However, a 12-mm examination of the bronchial tract may be limited and there may be difficulty in accessing the guttural pouches. The minimum length of scope for a complete examination of the respiratory tract is 1 metre.

For gastroscopy, a 2.5- to 3-m-long endoscope is required. In order to image the pyloric antrum, a length of 2.8 to 3 metres is required in a 450-kg horse. To pass through the pylorus into the very proximal duodenum, a 3-metre scope is required. Because of the high prevalence of lesions in the pyloric antrum,[2] a full gastroscopy should include this region, and therefore 2.8- to 3-metre endoscopes are recommended.

Endoscopy of the female urinary tract can be achieved with a 1-metre scope, and the male urinary tract with a 1.6-metre endoscope. For these examinations, the narrower the endoscope, the better. Endoscopes of 12 mm and wider may be difficult to pass up the male urethra.

Purchasing a second-hand endoscope

The scope should be laid out on a table. Turn the controls and ensure that the tip of the scope moves in synchrony with the controls. Delay in movement suggests damage to the angulation cables. Next, check the light transmission fibres by holding the tip of the scope to a light, look at the end of the light guide probe that plugs into the light source. This should be evenly illuminated, if greater than 30% of this area is dimmed the scope may need to be replaced.[1] Keeping the tip pointed at a light look through the eyepiece. Broken fibres will show up as black dots, determine if these interfere unacceptably with the image for your purpose. Inspect the outside of the scope for any holes or damage and perform a leak test on the instrument with a hand-held leak tester. Major damage may be done to scopes by water leakage.[1] Finally, check that the biopsy channel is patent by passing an instrument through it. If any problems are encountered, consult a service facility to determine the costs of repair prior to negotiation of purchase.

Website addresses of manufacturers of diagnostic imaging equipment are given in Box 3.6.

* For example, Sony Mavicap; Sony Corporation, Minato-ku, Tokyo, Japan.

Box 3.6. Some suppliers of endoscopy equipment and accessories

Olympus:	www.olympusamerica.com, www.olympus-europa.com/endoscopy/ and www.keymed.co.uk
Fujinon Inc.:	www.fujinonendoscopy.com
Karl Storz:	www.karlstorzvet.com
VES Vet Vision:	www.vesvetvision.com
EV Veterinary:	www.ev-veterinaryproducts.co.uk
Pentax:	www.pentaxmedical.com
N. Stenning & Co:	www.nstenning.com.au
Inline systems:	www.inline.com.au
MILA International:	www.milaint.com
Cook Medical:	www.cookmedical.com

References

1. Burns J: Endoscopic instrumentation, in Slovis NM (ed): Atlas of Equine Endoscopy. St. Louis, Mosby, 2004, pp 3-27
2. Murray MJ, Nout YS, Ward DL: Endoscopic findings of the gastric antrum and pylorus in horses: 162 cases (1996-2000). J Vet Intern Med 15:401-406, 2001

3.3 Biosecurity for equine hospitals: Protecting the patient and the hospital

Helen Wheeler Aceto and Barbara Dallap Schaer

Introduction

Between 1975 and 1995, the incidence of hospital-acquired infections (HAIs) in the United States increased by 36.1%, and the U.S. Centers for Disease Control and Prevention (CDC) report that approximately 90,000 people die annually from HAIs.[1–3] HAIs represent a risk to the hospitalised patient and hospital personnel and, depending on the environmental persistence of the organism, potentially to the facility. Annual health care costs in hospitalised humans have increased dramatically in recent years due in part to HAIs.[4,5] Moreover, in the United States, up to 70% of the bacteria that cause HAIs are currently resistant to at least one of the antimicrobials commonly used to treat them.[6] As a result, HAIs are often difficult to treat and associated with increasing morbidity and mortality, prolonged hospital stays and concomitantly higher costs.[5,7,8] In one U.S. state alone, a 2004 study revealed that HAIs were responsible for $2 billion in extra hospital charges and an additional 205,000 days of hospitalisation.[9] In many instances, HAIs are still underreported, often incorrectly recorded as a procedural complication. Attention to infection reporting and nosocomial infections in human hospitals has resulted in renewed interest in biosecurity* and infection control programmes (ICPs) in both human and veterinary medicine. An effective ICP, complete with compliance evaluation, infection reporting and patient[10] and environment surveillance,[11] will result in decreased HAIs.[12–14]

Defining an infection as hospital acquired (as opposed to community acquired) has been an evolving process in the human medical field. There is extensive literature describing development of these definitions, formalized by organizations such as the CDC[15] and the World Health Organization (WHO).[16] This process is markedly less well developed in veterinary medicine, and it is not always straightforward or even particularly appropriate to adapt definitions developed for human HAIs to the veterinary patient (Table 3.2). Determining whether or not a particular infectious problem is truly hospital acquired may not be so simple, and particular characteristics of the infectious organism may play a role in modifying the definitions for veterinary patients. There is a paucity of information regarding rates of HAI in individual veterinary hospitals and even fewer coordinated multicentre efforts that might enable veterinary hospitals interested in developing an ICP to better assess and manage infection risks or determine how well they are performing. However, just like human hospitals, veterinary facilities that provide care to hospitalised animals are undoubtedly places where contagious disease-causing organisms, a greater proportion of which will be multidrug resistant than is found in the general

* In general, the term "biosecurity" connoted preventing the introduction of a disease agent into a population, while "biocontainment" referred to controlling the spread of an introduced agent. Dunowska et al.[14] note that in a dynamic situation such as occurs at a veterinary hospital, it is, however, difficult to separate the two, and a more broad definition of "biosecurity" (used interchangeably with "infection control") "to encompass all practices intended to prevent (limit) the introduction and spread of infectious diseases within a group of equine patients and their human care givers" is appropriate.

Table 3.2. Simplified guidelines for surveillance of nosocomial infections

Type of nosocomial infection	Simplified criteria
Surgical site infection	Any purulent discharge, abscess or spreading cellulitis at the surgical site during the month after the procedure
Urinary infection	Positive urine culture (one or two species) with at least 10^5 bacteria/ml, with or without clinical signs
Respiratory infection	Respiratory symptoms with at least two of the following signs appearing during hospitalisation: • Cough • Purulent nasal discharge • New infiltrate on thoracic radiograph consistent with infection
Gastrointestinal infection	Gastroenteritis must fulfil one of two criteria: 1. Acute onset of diarrhoea (liquid stools for >12 hours) with or without vomiting or fever and no likely noninfectious causes 2. Patient has at least *two* of the following signs with no other recognized cause: nausea, vomiting, abdominal pain or headache *and* at least *one* of the following a. Enteric pathogen cultured from faecal sample b. Enteric pathogen detected by routine or electron microscopy c. Enteric pathogen detected by antigen or antibody assay on blood or faeces d. Evidence of an enteric pathogen detected by toxin assay e. Diagnostic single antibody titre (IgM) or 4-fold increase in paired sera (IgG) for pathogen
Vascular catheter infection	Inflammation, lymphangitis or purulent discharge at the insertion site of the catheter
Septicaemia	Fever or rigours and at least one positive blood culture

Nosocomial infections are infections acquired during hospital care that are not present or incubating at the time of admission. In human medicine, infections occurring more than 48 hours after admission are usually considered nosocomial. However, because incubation period varies with pathogen and to some extent the patient's underlying condition, each infection must be assessed individually for evidence linking it to hospitalisation.

Adapted from Ducel G, Fabry J, Nicolle L (eds): Prevention of Hospital-Acquired Infections: A Practical Guide, ed 2. Geneva, World Health Organization, 2002; available at http://www.who.int/csr/resources/publications/drugresist/whocdscsreph200212.pdf; accessed June 9, 2006; and Garner JS, Jarvis WR, Emori TG, Horan TC, Hughes JM: CDC definitions for nosocomial infections, in: Olmsted RN (ed): APIC Infection Control and Applied Epidemiology: Principles and Practice. St. Louis, Mosby, 1996, pp A1-A20. Available at http://www.dhh.louisiana.gov/offices/publications/pubs-249/20050427NosocomialInfectionDefinitions.pdf; accessed June 9, 2006.

community, are present in high numbers and able contact susceptible patients.[17–22] As in human medicine, there are certainly both medical and economic consequences to the occurrence of HAIs in veterinary settings. The latter includes increased length of hospital stay, increased treatment costs, possible indemnification and legal costs, loss of future business, etc. As large referral hospitals become more common and advances in veterinary medicine allow us to treat more critical cases, the potential vulnerability of our patient population increases and HAIs will inevitably gain in importance in veterinary hospitals. Veterinarians must therefore take an active role in developing infection control strategies that protect the hospitalised patient, the personnel who take care of them and the entire veterinary facility. Appropriate ICPs are integral to providing optimal patient care, ensuring a safe working environment for hospital employees and protecting the hospital from financial loss and possible litigation.

Compared to infection control practices in human medicine, the development of such practices in veterinary medicine is in its infancy and their application is far from universal.[23] Over the last few years, increasing attention has, however, been paid to infection control in equine medicine.[12–14] In October 2003, a small meeting conducted by the Dorothy Russell Havemeyer Foundation, Inc. was dedicated to the topic of nosocomial infection and biosecurity in equine hospitals. The topics discussed at that meeting are collected in a 2004 issue of the *Veterinary Clinics of North America: Equine Practice*, and the resulting volume is an excellent resource for those involved in biosecurity and infection control for equine practices in general and equine hospitals in particular.[24] To further the initiative started by that first meeting, a second Dorothy Havemeyer Foundation, Inc. workshop was conducted in September 2006.[25]

Although there is no "one-size-fits-all" programme that can be used interchangeably for all veterinary facilities, this chapter briefly describes the areas and functions that must be considered when developing and implementing an ICP. It draws on our own experience at the University of Pennsylvania's George D. Widener Hospital for Large Animals but also owes a great deal to the proceedings of the Havemeyer Foundation workshops and the practices of others;[12,14,24–27] much detailed practical information can be found in the associated references. The extent to which an individual equine clinic implements biosecurity practices (whether by necessity, choice or capacity) is contingent on a number of factors including size and character of caseload, facility size and design, personnel and economic issues, level of risk aversion, etc.

Biosecurity: Why we need it; lessons from outbreaks

While little information exists on the endemic infections that occur commonly at low levels in equine hospitals, reports of nosocomial outbreaks in large-animal veterinary teaching hospitals are abundant in the literature. These reports only serve to underscore the need for an effective biosecurity programme. Among such outbreaks, salmonellosis is by far the most common.[18,28–45] However, methicillin-resistant *Staphylococcus aureus* (MRSA)-associated infections,[46–50] clostridial enterocolitis,[51–54] outbreaks of strangles caused by *Streptococcus equi*,[13,55] herpesvirus myeloencephalitis,[56,57] equine influenza,[13,55] equine viral arteritis,[58] equine infectious anemia[59,60] and a possible outbreak of infections caused by *Serratia* spp.[61] have all been reported.

Such outbreaks may result in temporary suspension of certain hospital services or complete closure of a facility.[12–14,28,31,36,44,57,59] In the case of a large-animal teaching hospital, facility closure has far-reaching implications for the student body, hospital personnel and the equine community, none of which should be underestimated. For example, in 2004 the George D. Widener Hospital experienced an outbreak of salmonellosis that resulted in closure of the hospital to all admissions for 85 days.[28] Although some services (e.g., laboratory and ambulatory services, along with those conducted at sites separate from the main hospital complex) remained in operation, the outbreak resulted in severe disruption to the educational process of students and house officers (residents and interns), delays in clinical research and a complete lack of referral services to the large-animal community. In the case of any outbreak, but particularly one leading to hospital closure, there is a large expense associated with decontamination and remediation often necessary in such circumstances.[12–14,28,62] This expense, combined with that of any accompanying decrease in revenue, can be substantial and pose a very serious financial burden to the affected facility. Additionally, deleterious impacts on client (and staff) confidence can have long-term effects on the business and financial health of any facility that has suffered an outbreak of infectious disease. Although an active ICP had been in place at the Widener Hospital prior to the outbreak, the organism responsible (*Salmonella enterica* serotype Newport MDR-AmpC) had developed specific features that significantly contributed to the scope and magnitude of the problem. These included profound multidrug resistance [in addition to a plasmid-mediated *ampC* β-lactamase gene ($bla_{CMY\text{-}2}$) encoding resistance to extended-spectrum cephalosporins, the outbreak strain also harboured an extended-spectrum β-lactamase (ESBL) gene $bla_{SHV\text{-}12}$[63]] and stubborn environmental persistence. As part of the existing ICP, environmental surveillance for *Salmonella* had been in place at the Widener Hospital for more than a decade prior to 2004 and an Infection Control Committee was charged with developing and overseeing those policies and procedures designed to limit infection risks. It was, however, very apparent that these mechanisms failed to protect the hospital from a serious disease outbreak. There were a number of reasons for this. Perhaps chief among them, and one of the most important lessons learned, was the fact that no individual was dedicated to monitoring infection status in the hospital or ensuring that surveillance and infection control protocols were both appropriate and effectively implemented in response to changing threats. Although not in itself causal, a heavy caseload, a large proportion of which are emergency and critical cases (in our case, up to 25% of admissions), compounded the problem of inadequate oversight. As a result, rather than having a nimble, proactive, highly responsive ICP, the ability to both recognise and respond to nosocomial infection issues was sluggish at best.

There is ample evidence demonstrating the continued evolution of infectious organisms that can threaten veterinary facilities. Moreover, equine populations, particularly racehorses and other performance animals, exist as large metapopulations. "Metapopulations" are defined as a number of subpopulations that are apparently discrete and separated in space but in fact are loosely connected through mixing such as occurs at racing or other competitive events.[64] Intuitively, different populations between which there is the greatest amount of mixing are the most likely to suffer spread of contagious disease.[65] However, the pattern of contacts also has a major influence on disease spread. The contact structure of equine populations involved in athletic activities generally has the characteristics of a small-world network (the network of contacts has a short average pathlength and high clustering).[64] As a result, directly transmitted infections can spread through these populations with relative ease and rapidity, and disease agents that would tend toward extinction in homogeneously mixing populations may persist and become endemic in a small-world network.[64] The network structure of horse populations and the degree of mixing that occurs mean that even up to an international level, horses suffer inherent risks of contacting contagious disease agents. This risk is probably only exceeded by that of humans.[65] A recent outbreak of equine herpesvirus myeloencephalitis centred in Florida, in which the index case was identified as a horse shipped from Germany via New York to Florida for competition, and where veterinary clinics as well as sporting/boarding venues were affected, illustrates these issues well.[66] The continued evolution and emergence of infectious organisms, and the constant threat of introduction or reintroduction of these agents to the hospital via patients, necessitate a very proactive and evaluative ICP. As equine hospitals are themselves nodes in the contact network, the role of the hospital in disseminating infectious agents to the rest of the equine population should also be borne in mind when considering the need for biosecurity.

In light of our experience at the Widener Hospital and the sure knowledge that, as a hospital, we will be faced with constant challenges from infectious and possibly highly contagious agents, a full commitment to biosecurity was made. A Director of Biosecurity was charged with developing a long-term biosecurity plan for the hospital with the assistance of a Biosecurity Advisory Committee that includes representatives from all clinical, diagnostic and critical support (nursing, housekeeping, animal attendants and facilities) services. We point this out because no matter what size the clinic, the need to engender support at all administrative levels and to involve and inform *all* hospital personnel in the process is important to success in implementing and, more challengingly, sustaining any biosecurity efforts. Proper hygiene practices, patient segregation, personnel segregation, patient and environmental surveillance and handling of patients at high risk for infectious disease are cornerstones of an effective programme.[12–14] Vigilant, sometimes daily, data analyses are also critical to provide relevant and timely information with regard to hospital and patient status. Biosecurity, in the form of an effective ICP, benefits both the patient and the hospital and provides an opportunity to educate both the public and veterinarians in training.

Infection control programme: Overview

A successful biosecurity programme addresses areas of hygiene, patient surveillance, patient contact and education of veterinarians, staff, referring veterinarians and clients, along with house officers and students in the case of teaching institutions.[12–14] Broadly speaking, any programme can be divided into several major components, each of which will achieve its aims by focusing on different aspects of patient monitoring and management. It is worth pointing out that no aspect of biosecurity exists in isolation and there is considerable cross-over between different components of an ICP.

Largely, the goals of any biosecurity programme are optimisation of patient care and ensuring a safe or "healthy" hospital for personnel and patients alike. More specifically, objectives are to minimize HAIs, develop strategies for accurate infection reporting and play an active role in responsible antimicrobial use.[67–69] As the size and caseload of a hospital increase, the effort directed toward managing potential problems must also increase. In addition to overall size, the type of case admitted influences infection risk. Hospitals that offer high-level, complex care to critically ill patients should raise their infection control efforts concomitantly. Resources permitting, the ideal approach is to have an individual (or individuals) dedicated to biosecurity. In smaller hospitals, this needs to be someone with authority and access to budgetary decisions, such as a senior partner. In a university setting with a large caseload consisting of a variety of species, appointing a designated Biosecurity Officer with specialized training in epidemiology or infectious disease to oversee the programme is ideal, although the training of the individual and associated staff may vary depending on the size and scope of the hospital. In large university hospitals, it is highly desirable for the Biosecurity Officer to be a veterinarian with minimal to no clinical obligation; this eliminates conflict of interest regarding patient status, allowing them to make difficult or unpopular decisions about the disposition of specific patients without bias. However, this is clearly impracticable in smaller hospitals, and the person overseeing biosecurity needs to be aware of their potential bias. Removing patient-related clinical duties also promotes the mind-set of "the hospital as a patient" for that individual and allows a broader focus on the entire hospital population rather than on specific patients. Nevertheless, all decisions must balance the needs of the hospital with those of the individual patient and must also take into account any impact on client relations. Educating clients to the risks of hospitalisation, including infection and how an ICP is integral to providing the highest-quality patient care, is key to good client relations. If it is anticipated that specific actions such as moving a case to isolation may be negatively perceived by the client, the attending clinician and, if necessary, the Biosecurity Officer should be prepared to explain why such actions are being taken. Smaller hospitals have the advantage that there is generally much better communication between veterinarians managing cases, and patterns of infection or resistance may be noted without specific data collection and analysis. However, it is not adequate or safe to rely solely on "coffee-table" talk to alert the hospital of potential biosecurity problems, and conscious daily efforts to monitor, review and maintain biosecurity need to be introduced. These should include obtaining objective data, rather than relying on clinical impression (Box 3.7). In either case, it should be the responsibility of the individual(s) tasked with overseeing the programme to adjust the focus of surveillance and any associated testing based on developments in the hospital, literature and knowledge of active outbreaks in the hospital referral area, and for ensuring that staff and clinicians alike are cognisant of the ICP and their role(s) in it.

Box 3.7. Development and implementation of a biosecurity programme: Focus on small to medium-sized clinics

1. Appoint a senior member of the practice to be in charge of infection control.
2. Review incidence of the following:
   a. Contagious disease-causing agents, such as *Salmonella*, *Streptococcus equi equi*, EHV-1, EIA, etc., in your hospitalised patients and practice referral area
   b. Incisional infections and other HAI in your patients
   c. MDR bacterial infections; collate available antimicrobial susceptibility profiles
3. Collect information on a, b and c above, prospectively.
4. Designate an isolation area for hospitalised patients suspected of infection with *Salmonella*, *S. equi equi*, EHV-1, EIA, etc., and develop policies to support this area.
5. Review available facilities and personnel; determine whether to accept horses that may require isolation (e.g., acute diarrhoea, known or suspected strangles, acute neurological disease, abortions). Even if you decide against accepting such cases, isolation facilities are still needed for horses that develop these or other infections during the course of routine hospitalisation, e.g., certain MDR bacterial infections.
6. Review types of case treated and group into broad risk categories. Based on facilities and personnel, assess practicality of segregating horses from different risk categories in separate areas of hospital.
7. Review facilities and traffic patterns (animal and human) with infection control in mind; where practical, make any necessary changes.
8. Based on incidence of contagious diseases and HAI in the population, design a prospective surveillance plan. May involve targeted collection and submission of samples for bacterial culture from patients and hospital environment. Even if size and character of caseload do not warrant an active surveillance program, you must still closely monitor patients and results of clinical submissions for infection problems. *Have an action plan should evidence of problems be detected, e.g., criteria that automatically trigger an investigation and what your response will be.*
9. Review antimicrobial use in your hospital; follow prudent use guidelines[67–69]; if necessary, set specific policies based on incidence and nature of MDR infections.
10. Develop protocols and schedules for cleaning and disinfection, waste disposal, maintenance of surfaces to ensure that they remain sealed and cleanable, etc.
11. Educate your veterinarians, all staff and your clients to the need for vigilance and in the infection control policy you have developed.
12. Regularly review the data you are generating and the adequacy of the policy.

For additional details on specific topics, see main text.
HAI, hospital-acquired infection(s); MDR, multidrug resistant.

Monitoring and surveillance

An effective surveillance programme is absolutely essential to a successful ICP; surveillance of both the hospital's patients and environment are necessary for success.

Patient surveillance

Patient monitoring and surveillance constitutes a cornerstone of infection control. Surveillance data and identification of patients at risk, both for disease transmission and nosocomial infection, essentially direct many other biosecurity efforts in a hospital. Patient monitoring should include collection of data with respect to infectious organisms and encompass collection and collation of data regarding HAIs. Acquired infections include catheter-associated thrombophlebitis, anaesthetic- or ventilator-associated pneumonia and surgical site infections. Incidence of MRSA or vancomycin-resistant *Enterococcus* (VRE) infections should also be determined and carefully monitored. Depending on the level of care the hospital provides, and the types of cases admitted, it may be necessary to conduct routine patient surveillance of particularly problematic infectious organisms. In a referral hospital setting, monitoring and evaluation of multidrug resistant infections and trends in microbial resistance in isolates derived from clinical submissions should be part of the biosecurity effort. Clearly, ensuring a good working relationship between those individuals involved in biosecurity and the diagnostic laboratory is essential to success. At the Widener Hospital, although routine surveillance is focused on *Salmonella* (see later), data are collected and collated on other agents of concern and on the antimicrobial sensitivity profiles of selected organisms, including *Staphylococcus aureus*, *Escherichia coli*, *Klebsiella*, *Enterococcus*, and *Enterobacter* spp. Using software developed for the management of microbiology laboratory data and analysis of antimicrobial susceptibility test results can help provide close to real-time trend analysis (enabling rapid notification of the appearance of new organisms or sudden shifts in microbial populations) and enhance the use of laboratory data for the complex question of guiding therapy, assisting with infection control and characterising resistance epidemiology. There are many examples of such software, but the WHO's Windows-based WHONET software[70] has a veterinary module and is available for free download at http://www.who.int/drugresistance/whonetsoftware/en/.

Although there are many infectious organisms to consider in the hospitalised equine patient (Table 3.3), in a large equine hospital, especially those that regularly treat the critically ill, monitoring patients and the environment for *Salmonella* can offer a reasonable assessment of the efficacy of an ICP (particularly with respect to containment and hygienic practices) and provide a basis for appropriate patient and personnel segregation. The rationale for using *Salmonella* as a biosensor in this way is first and foremost precedent; *Salmonella* has been and continues to be a problem organism for many large-animal hospitals. In addition, its persistence in the hospital environment, relative ease of detection, relative resistance to disinfectants, ability to spread on fomites, propensity to exhibit multidrug resistance and infectious nature all help make *Salmonella* the focus of ICP in many large-animal hospitals.[12,14,27,40] Using *Salmonella* as a general biosensor does not preclude initiating investigation of other organisms, and part of a proactive biosecurity programme should be to determine trigger points for the initiation (and just as important the cessation) of testing for other/additional organisms. An example of such a trigger point would include indications of an epidemiological link between likely HAIs and specific procedures or areas of the hospital, such as a particular operating room and incisional infections. It goes without saying that developing these protocols requires collection of baseline data, without which it is not possible to assess the likelihood that particular infections are HAIs, determine whether there has been an increase in such infections or evaluate the efficacy of any interventions. That being said, for the remainder of this discussion, biosecurity efforts aimed at minimizing nosocomial spread of a gastroenteric organism such as *Salmonella* will serve as a model for organizing an ICP in a large-animal hospital.

In addition to microbiological monitoring and surveillance, monitoring the clinical status of patients can be useful in rapidly identifying and containing potential problems. Changes in patient status that might trigger additional testing and/or increasingly stringent isolation procedures designed to contain potential problems are most easily managed by use of specific algorithms (see section on Patient Handling and Figure 3.27).

Hospitals providing colic surgery or admitting animals with colitis should consider routine patient surveillance for *Salmonella* shedding. At the outset, faecal cultures for detection of *Salmonella* could be used on the whole patient population to determine the overall incidence of shedding and identify groups of patients that are at higher risk for shedding *Salmonella*. Identification of patients as "high-risk" directs biosecurity and any related testing efforts (both of which can be costly) towards the proper sector of the patient population. Based on shedding incidence, patients and, where possible, the personnel who care for them can be segregated according to risk, and appropriate barrier precautions for each patient category can be developed.[71] Any correlation of shedding with particular clinical signs can be used to refine algorithms for patient management.

With respect to patient surveillance, animals in high-risk patient groups should be monitored for the duration of their stay. If surveillance relies only on information gathered at admission or during early hospitalisation, the risk of the patient to the hospital may be underestimated. In the case of *Salmonella*, monitoring is by means of faecal

Table 3.3. Equine contagious and zoonotic diseases of nosocomial importance

Disease	Agent and incubation period	Mode of transmission	Clinical signs in horses	Clinical signs in humans	Diagnostic testing	Disinfection	Biosecurity and precautions for personnel
Anthrax*	*Bacillus anthracis.* 1–7 days	Direct contact (cutaneous), aerosol (pulmonary), possibly vector, e.g., horseflies (cutaneous), ingestion of undercooked contaminated meat by humans (GI)	Horses very susceptible, can present as acute enteritis with signs of colic, usually very rapid progression, septicaemia, fever, haemorrhagic enteritis, depression, death	Cutaneous (most common), pruritic macule leading to black eschar. Pulmonary, febrile respiratory disease rapidly fatal. Intestinal, febrile GI disease.	High level of bacteraemia on smears of blood or aspirated oedema fluid. Culture and ID possible but fluorescent antibody testing of smears of froth, blood or splenic aspirate safer for personnel.	Anthrax spores resistant to heat, drying and many disinfectants. Spores killed by 2% glutaraldehyde or 5% formalin.	Complete protection (gloves, boots, protective coveralls respiratory and eye protection) required when handling suspects. Avoid necropsy of infected or suspect cases beyond blood collection. Unopened carcass decomposes rapidly and spores are destroyed. Burn or deep bury carcass.
Clostridial enteritis†	*Clostridium difficile* neonatal foals, adults primarily during or immediately after antimicrobial therapy and *Clostridium perfringens* neonatal foals. *C. difficile* most important in terms of nosocomial infection. 8–24 hours	Faecal-oral spread by direct contact, environmental contamination, on fomites, via humans on hands, etc. Public health risk of equine clostridial infections uncertain.	Acute colitis, abdominal pain, diarrhoea of varying severity, may be accompanied by dehydration, fever, toxaemia and leukopaenia.	Sudden onset abdominal discomfort, diarrhoea, nausea; vomiting and fever usually absent. Generally self-limiting, short duration but may be more severe disease; necrotising enteritis, sepsis. *C. difficile* common cause of antimicrobial-associated and nosocomial diarrhoea. *C. perfringens* more frequently foodborne.	Culture <u>and</u> toxin detection in faecal samples, blood culture.	Vegetative form killed by exposure to air, spores resistant to many disinfectants but can be reduced by thorough cleaning with a detergent followed by disinfection with diluted (1 : 10) bleach solution.	Isolation of confirmed cases with protective clothing (boots, barrier gown, gloves). Strict hand hygiene. Minimize stress especially dietary. Judicious use of antimicrobials. Consider routine examination for *C. difficile* and toxins A and B in foals and with antimicrobial-associated diarrhoea.
Dermatoses • Dermatophytosis (ringworm)	*Trichophyton equinum* most common; also *T. mentagrophytes Microsporum equinum* (*M. canis and M. gypseum*). 4–14 days	Direct contact or indirect contact with fomites—saddle blankets, grooming equipment, etc.	Round, hairless, scaly skin lesions.	Circular or annular lesions with scaling, occasionally erythema, itching.	Direct exam of hair, culture, histology of biopsy. Wood's lamp unreliable for equine dermatophytosis.	Diluted (1 : 10) bleach (sodium hypochlorite) solution	Gloves, strict hygiene, disposal or disinfection of grooming and other equipment.
• Dermatophilosis (rain rot)	*Dermatophilus congolensis.* Less than 7 days	Direct contact. Trauma and biting insects aid in spread.	Exudative crusted skin lesions, hair in "paintbrush" clumps.	Rare zoonosis. Afebrile, acute to chronic pustular to exudative dermatitis.	Cytology—Gram stain of crust, histology, culture.		For dermatophilosis also minimize exposure to excessive moisture, employ insect control/repellents.
Ectoparasites • Acariasis (mange), zoonotic scabies	Sarcoptes, psoroptes, chorioptes, demodex (rare in horses) and other mites. 1–2 weeks after infestation.	Highly contagious by direct contact with infected animal. Also transmitted on fomites.	Intense pruritis, alopecia, crusting may be lichenification of skin. Location depends on mite involved.	Resolves spontaneously not transmitted between humans.	Physical examination	Most effectively controlled by treating infested animal with acaricides.	Gloves, boots and protective clothing. Do not share equipment. Discard or disinfect equipment used on infected animal.

• Pediculosis	Biting or chewing lice *Werneckiella (Damalinia) equi* or sucking lice *Haematopinus asini.* Obligate parasite, all stages on horse, egg to egg development time 4–5 weeks.	Direct contact but can possibly spread on blankets and other equipment.	Itching and skin irritation leading to scratching, rubbing, and biting. Most common locations affected are head, mane and ventral neck area.	Nonzoonotic	Physical examination	As above, treat with insecticides such as pyrethrins	Separate grooming equipment, blankets etc. Lice can live 2–3 weeks off host, but a few days more typical. Eggs may continue to hatch over 2–3 weeks in warm weather. Rigorously clean and disinfect areas that housed infested animals.
Equine herpesvirus infection (equine rhinopneumonitis)*†	Eight different types, EHV-1 and EHV-4 of major concern in horses. Incubation 2–10 days. Abortions occur 2–12 weeks after infection, usually between 7 and 11 months of gestation.	Direct contact, aerosol (up to 35 feet), fomites.	EHV-1 inapparent to mild respiratory disease with fever, to abortion in mares, to rapidly progressing, often fatal, neurological disease (ascending paralysis). EHV-4 rhinopneumonitis primarily horses <3 years of age.	Nonzoonotic	PCR or virus isolation from nasopharyngeal secretions or white blood cells.	Easily killed by many disinfectants including 1% bleach, 70% ethanol, iodine-based disinfectants, quaternary ammonium disinfectants, peroxygen disinfectants, phenolics, etc.	Isolation for EHV-1 infection, monitor temperature of surrounding animals, submit samples for testing if fever (≥38.6° C) develops. Proper disposal of aborted foetuses and related material. EHV-4 barrier precautions, no sharing of equipment.
Equine infectious anaemia (EIA, swamp fever)*†	Lentivirus, related to other important lentiviruses including HIV but not zoonotic. 1–3 weeks but may be as long as 3 months	Primarily via transfer of contaminated blood by biting insects (most often tabanids) or fomites contaminated with blood.	Intermittent fever, depression, inappetance, weight loss, oedema, thrombocytopaenia, transitory or progressive anaemia. No therapy.	Nonzoonotic	AGID (Coggins test); for animals testing positive a second confirmatory test recommended. Other ELISA tests available.	Diluted (1:10) bleach solution, 70% ethanol, 2% glutaraldehyde peroxygen disinfectants, phenolics.	Proper handling and disposal of biohazard material. Strict insect-proof isolation until testing confirmed. Due to lifelong infection risk, consider euthanasia for positive animals.
Equine influenza*†	Orthomyxovirus A Usually 1–3 days, range 18 hours to 5, or rarely 7, days. Most frequently diagnosed and economically important viral respiratory disease of the horse.	Respiratory route; aerosol, direct contact with infected secretions. Survives and may spread on fomites for several hours. Highly contagious, despite careful hygiene horses sharing same air space likely to become infected.	Acute, febrile, respiratory disease. High fevers, coughing, nasal discharge common; as are depression, anorexia, weakness. Occasionally pneumonia or other complications.	Although influenza A viruses can infect humans, equine-lineage viruses have very limited zoonotic risk. Recently, however, transmission of equine-lineage H3N8 virus has caused influenza in dogs in the United States.	Virus isolation from nasopharyngeal swab collected as soon as possible after onset of illness, or paired serology. Directigen Flu-A test can be used "stallside".	Easily killed by many disinfectants—see EHV above.	Isolation. Avoid sharing equipment. Strict hand hygiene. Maintain isolation until no symptoms and body temperature normal for ≥5 days. Consider vaccination of contact animals to control an outbreak.

Table 3.3. *Continued*

Disease	Agent and incubation period	Mode of transmission	Clinical signs in horses	Clinical signs in humans	Diagnostic testing	Disinfection	Biosecurity and precautions for personnel
Equine viral arteritis (EVA)*†	Arterivirus, equine arteritis virus. Average 7 days, range 2 to 13 days.	Respiratory from acutely infected horse, direct contact or via relatively close contact, e.g., adjacent stall, limited spread on fomites. Venereal from acute or chronically infected stallion.	May be subclinical or only transient oedema, or acute fever, depression, dependent oedema especially limbs, scrotum and prepuce in stallions, conjunctivitis, nasal discharge, abortion.	Nonzoonotic	Virus isolation or PCR from nasal secretions, conjunctival swabs or buffy coat. Paired serology. Virus isolation from semen of infected stallions	Easily killed by many disinfectants—see EHV above.	Isolation of cases. Quarantine close contacts for at least 21 days after last clinical case, 30 days used in some previous outbreaks.
Multidrug-resistant bacterial infections or infections caused by organisms with antimicrobial resistance of concern†	Various including *Salmonella*, MRSA, *E. coli*, *Klebsiella*, *Enterobacter*, *Enterococcus* (VRE and non-VRE), *Pseudomonas*, *Acinetobacter*, organisms resistant to extended spectrum beta lactams, etc.	Multiple including faecal-oral, by direct contact with infected animals, via humans, or on fomites, in some cases aerosol. For some organisms, e.g., MRSA, *Salmonella* animals and/or humans can be inapparent carriers.	Depending on organism, many different clinical presentations, e.g., GI, respiratory, catheter-related, or surgical site infections, septicaemia (especially in foals), etc. Nosocomial cases may occur as low level endemic infections or in epidemic outbreaks of varying severity.	Many have zoonotic potential. Clinical signs depend on organism involved.	Culture and sensitivity. Regular monitoring required to assess incidence and detect changes that may require investigation or intervention. Additional molecular ID may be necessary if a nosocomial problem is suspected.	Often susceptible to many disinfectants. Regular cleaning and disinfection controls environmental load. If nosocomial problem identified additional cleaning and disinfection of specific areas may be required. Conduct of disinfectant kill-curves may aid in control.	Judicious use of antimicrobials. Barrier precautions or possibly isolation for confirmed cases (organism dependent). Strict hand hygiene. Maintenance of good, regular hygienic practices for equipment and environment.
Rabies (not a nosocomial problem but an important zoonotic disease)*	Rhabdovirus of genus *Lyssavirus*. Few days to several years, most cases apparent after 1–3 months.	Contact (saliva, CSF, neural tissue). Mucous membranes or compromised skin, bites, cuts, etc.	Wide range of possible clinical signs. Progression of encephalic signs may be aggression (furious form, more common), or depression (paralytic, dumb form). Average survival from onset of clinical signs 5 days, maximum 10 days.	Early signs of malaise, fever, headache, pruritis at site of virus entry. Progressive anxiety, confusion, abnormal behaviour. Encephalitic or paralytic form can occur. Death usually in 2–10 days.	No definitive antemortem test. Brain from suspect animal must be submitted to an approved laboratory for rabies testing.	Lipid solvents (soap solutions, acetone), 2% bleach, 2% glutaraldehyde, 45%–75% ethanol, iodine-based or quaternary ammonium disinfectants. Inactivated by sunlight, limited environmental survival.	Clearly label as rabies suspect. Strictly limit number of personnel involved in managing suspect animal. Record all in-contact personnel. Clearly label any laboratory specimens as rabies suspect. Full barrier precautions including gloves, boots, protective clothing, face shield. Promptly submit necropsy samples using approved methods.

Rhodococcus equi infection	*Rhodococcus equi*, incubation period uncertain, often insidious onset.	Environmental exposure (soil), aerosol, contact, rarely via wound contamination.	Most often respiratory but other body systems can be involved. Most commonly fever, coughing, increased respiratory rate and effort, mucopurulent nasal discharge, pyogranulomatous pneumonia. Primarily foals 1–6 months old.	Rare human infection, only in the severely immunocompromised, appears to be via environmental exposure. Slowly progressive granulomatous pneumonia.	Culture of tracheobronchial aspirate or other samples. PCR can be valuable but best used in conjunction with culture. Radiographs useful.	70% ethanol, 2% glutaraldehyde, phenolics, and formaldehyde.	Shed in faeces, prompt removal of manure and good hygiene limits accumulation. Frequent hand washing. Uncertain infection risk but consider barrier precautions on affected foals (at least up to 72 hours after starting antimicrobial therapy) if susceptible foals housed in same area.
Rotavirus infection†	Rotavirus group A. 12–24 hours.	Faecal-oral, highly contagious, spreads readily on fomites or other contaminated material.	Variable severity of diarrhoea in foals from mild to life threatening	Nonzoonotic	Shed in faeces of foals for several weeks after diarrhoea ceases. Where introduction a concern, test faecal swab using faecal antigen test, e.g., Virogen Rotatest, Rotazyme	Phenolics are virucidal even in presence of organic material.	Isolate. Full barrier precautions. Proper sanitation and disinfection of contaminated material and equipment. In general, without other explanation, e.g., typical foal heat, diarrhoeic foals should be considered infectious and possibly contagious until proven otherwise. Good hygiene critical.
Salmonellosis†	Various *Salmonella enterica* 12–72 hours in humans, possibly similar in debilitated horses, incubation in the healthy exposed animal variable and uncertain.	Contact with faeces from an infected animal, most commonly ingestion, possibly via inhalation. Readily spread on fomites, in feed, water or via vermin, birds, insects. Good environmental survival, can be very difficult to control.	Inapparent, to fever, leukopaenia, severe diarrhoea, to septicaemia. Anorexia and depression common.	Most common equine zoonosis. Inapparent, to self-limiting but often severe gastroenteritis (diarrhoea generally much more prominent than vomiting), can be invasive leading to septicaemia.	Faecal culture (sensitivity for MDR), gastrointestinal reflux may also be cultured. Consider additional molecular ID if a nosocomial problem is suspected.	2% bleach, 70% ethanol, 2% glutaraldehyde, iodine-based disinfectants, phenolics, peroxygen disinfectants and formaldehyde.	Isolate confirmed cases. Strict hygiene. Prompt cleaning of all areas contaminated with faeces. Gloves, frequent hand washing, protective clothing, boots or footwear that can be easily cleaned, face mask/shield with pipe-stream diarrhoea.

Table 3.3. *Continued*

Disease	Agent and incubation period	Mode of transmission	Clinical signs in horses	Clinical signs in humans	Diagnostic testing	Disinfection	Biosecurity and precautions for personnel
Staphylococcosis†	*Staphylococcus* sp Methicillin (oxacillin) resistant *S. aureus* of special concern	Direct contact most important, particularly hand-to-nose transfer. Purulent discharge from infected sites very infectious. Aerosol less important but can occur with coughing or snorting.	Inapparent nasal carriage (including of MRSA), to thrombophlebitis, other suppurative draining lesions.	Subclinical, can be nasal carriers of MRSA and spread to other animals or people. Clinical may be suppurative lesions, usually skin (impetigo, boils). Gastroenteritis associated with toxin ingestion sudden onset nausea, cramps, vomiting.	Standard culture with speciation to identify *S. aureus* because MRSA strains in horses can be very weakly coagulase positive and may be misidentified. Sensitivity, Oxacillin resistant = MRSA	2% bleach, 70% ethanol, 2% glutaraldehyde, iodine-based disinfectants, quaternary ammonium disinfectants phenolics, peroxygen disinfectants	Gown, gloves, boots strict hand hygiene. Surgeon-type facemask may help limit hand-to-nose transfer in personnel. Consider isolation with full barrier precautions for MRSA positive animals.
Strangles†	*Streptoccocus equi* 3 to 15 days	Direct contact, also spread on fomites contaminated with infected secretions.	Abrupt onset fever, mucopurulent nasal discharge, acute swelling and subsequent abscessation of submandibular, retropharyngeal lymph nodes. May be metastatic spread, purpura haemorrhagica or other complications	Nonzoonotic	PCR and aerobic culture of nasal/pharyngeal wash or swab, pus from abscesses ± guttural pouch/upper airway endoscopy especially in suspected carriers	Quaternary ammonium disinfectants, 1% bleach, 70% ethanol, iodine-based disinfectants, phenolics.	Isolation. Fever occurs 2–3 days before nasal shedding; promptly isolate febrile horses in an outbreak. Good hygiene and sanitation, careful cleaning or disposal of contaminated equipment or other material.
Vesicular stomatitis*†	Rhabdovirus of genus *Vesiculovirus.* 3–7 days	Direct contact or aerosol, insect vectors (sand flies, black flies). In endemic areas, oral examination prior to admission may prevent introduction during outbreaks.	Excess salivation, fever, vesicles on mucous membranes of mouth, epithelium of tongue, coronary band.	Infection rates in exposed humans are low. Manifest as fever, headache, myalgia, rarely oral blisters. Recovery usually in 4–7days.	Standard test for VSV antibodies is virus neutralisation, complement fixation or ELISA can also be used.	2% sodium carbonate, 4% sodium hydroxide, 2% iodophor disinfectants, chlorine dioxide.	Vector control, gloves, protective clothing including facemask, strict hand hygiene.

*World Animal Health Organisation (OIE) listed diseases. Some of these diseases are reportable at the national level in animals and/or humans. They may also be notifiable at a regional level. Check with your government veterinarian or public health veterinarian for a current listing of reportable diseases in your area.

†Agents that have been linked to nosocomial outbreaks of disease.

Isolation and Barrier Flow Chart

Definitions

- **Leukopenia**: less than 4000 WBC per µl
- **Fever**: multiple temperature spikes greater than 39.2° C (102.5° F) in a 24 hour period
- **Diarrhea**: liquidy faeces retaining no shape in the bedding passed more than twice in a 12 hour period
- **Barrier**: "tape-off" the patient witr disposable boots, gowns, gloves, and 2% Virkon-S® dip tub stall side

- **Culture Series**: Series of three faecal cultures (gastrointestinal reflux can be used in absence of faeces) submitted on consecutive days to the microbiology lab; submit first culture within 24 hours of symptom onset.

*** **A POSITIVE CULTURE IN THE PRESENCE OF CLINICAL SIGNS MANDATES ISOLATION!!**

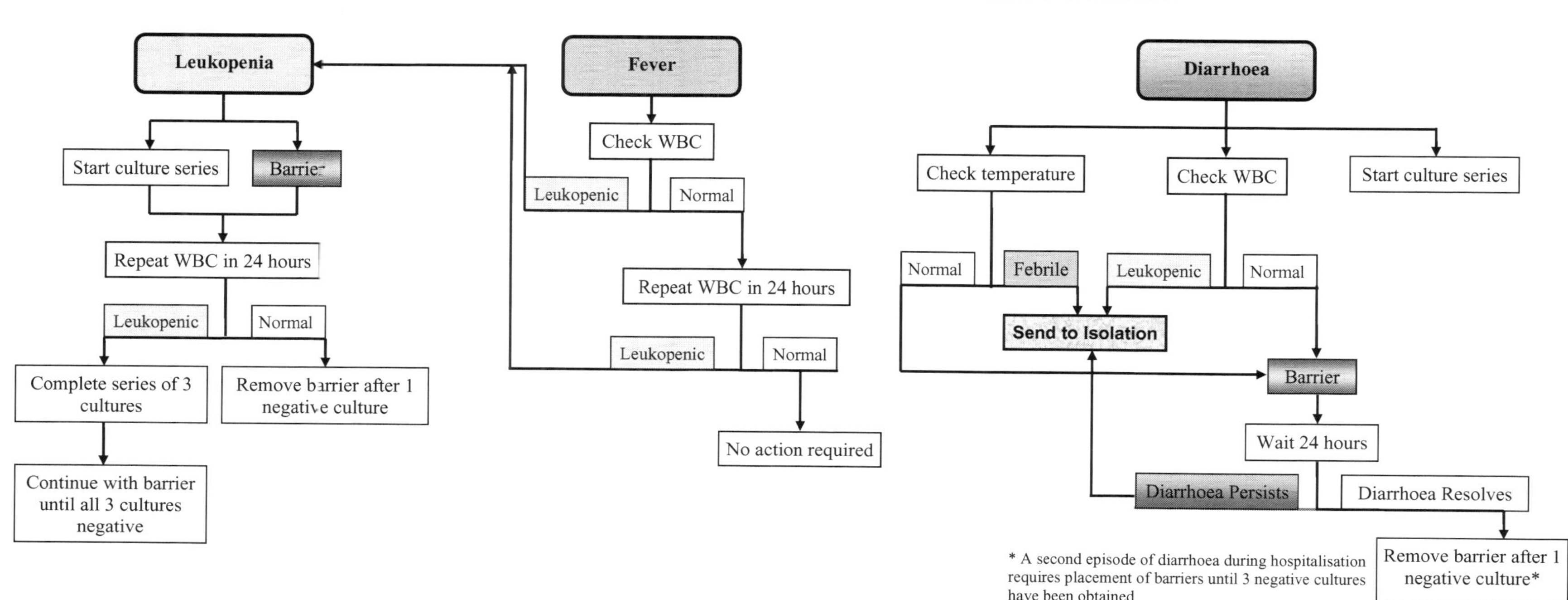

Figure 3.27 Example of an algorithm for the management of equine patients with clinical signs suspicious for salmonellosis. For additional examples of algorithms, see reference 27. ©Helen Aceto 2007.

culture. Surveillance data from the Widener Hospital serve to illustrate how the information can be used to adjust protocols in order to optimize the benefit-to-risk ratio and control costs. Samples collected at admission and during hospitalisation (twice weekly for high-risk colic, ICU/NICU, isolation and bovine patients and once weekly for all other patients) from more than 6500 inpatients over 2 years revealed that only 1.3% of elective patients and non-gastrointestinal emergency admissions were detected as positive for *Salmonella*. In equine colic patients and those admitted with either diarrhoea and/or fever as their presenting complaint, rates were 9.8% and 20.7%, respectively. Similar results have been obtained at other institutions.[12,35,40] Only 16% of *Salmonella*-positive equine colic patients were detected at admission. Based on these data, surveillance protocols were changed so that an admission sample is still collected from all low- to medium-risk patients, but they are no longer subject to in-hospital surveillance; should their clinical status change, testing could potentially recommence (see later). High-risk patients continue to be sampled at admission and twice weekly during hospitalisation.

Environmental surveillance

Monitoring of the hospital environment is also critical to a successful biosecurity programme. While this does mean that areas should be closely monitored to ensure proper hygienic practices and control clutter that might impede proper cleaning, it does not always imply microbiological testing of the environment. Nevertheless, we have found environmental sampling useful in determining which patient populations, traffic patterns and protocols present a risk for hospital contamination, and in assessing how well our containment efforts are performing. Assigning direct clinical relevance to environmental surveillance data, however, requires great caution. If undertaken, high-traffic areas, treatment areas and facilities that house high-risk patients should be the focus of environmental surveillance. Overall, in a large-animal hospital, environmental monitoring based on culturing for *Salmonella* appears to be an effective way of evaluating an ICP.[11,12] Currently, monitoring can only effectively be done by means of standard culture procedures but more sophisticated techniques with faster turnaround times such as real-time polymerase chain reaction may be available for both environmental and patient samples in the future. However, prior to full implementation, care should be exercised to ensure that any new tests are properly validated and that information is available on the test's characteristics and performance (e.g., sensitivity and specificity) when used in the manner in which it will ultimately be applied.

A successful protocol for environmental surveillance may include sampling using electrostatic wipes,[11] followed by culturing techniques designed to select for *Salmonella* and identify small numbers of organisms on surfaces rather than in faecal samples (see footnote*). We have found it both useful and instructive to divide high-traffic areas into hand and foot collection sites. Depending on the type of area and associated exposure, samples from large spaces of similar risk may be pooled and then further evaluated based on the results obtained. Careful analysis of environmental cultures can play a role in modifying biosecurity practices, including directing disinfection protocols, determining patient segregation and traffic and optimising personnel traffic and utilization.

Microbiological and other testing techniques

Surveillance tests and strategies should be under constant review. Critical evaluation of the microbiological techniques used for patient and environmental surveillance must be performed periodically. In particular, reevaluation of the techniques employed should occur if there is a widely perceived or proved increase in the incidence of infectious disease in the face of negative test results. Depending on prevailing patterns of infectious disease in the referral population or particular HAI concerns, it is possible that more sensitive or specific surveillance techniques could be implemented, either in a targeted or a more general fashion. In other words, if the "hospital's clinical presentation" does not match culture information or if the surveillance protocols in place will not adequately address changing infection threats, further investigation and/or implementation of new procedures may be warranted.

Patient handling

Hospitalised patients are not the same as the general population. Animals in hospital are more likely to shed or acquire an infectious agent than are those in the general population because they are more likely to be under stress, may be less able to respond immunologically, have altered

* Environmental samples for detection of *Salmonella* are cultured using the WHO/ISO technique. Briefly, the samples collected on Swiffer disposable cloths[11] (Procter and Gamble, Cincinnati, OH, USA) are placed in a Whirl-Pak bag to which 100 ml of buffered peptone water (BPW) is added. Samples in BPW are then incubated at 37° C for 24 hours. The preenriched samples are subsequently inoculated into Rappoport-Vassiliadis (RV) broth and incubated for a further 24 hours at 42° C, followed by subculture onto DCA (deoxycholate-citrate-agar), MacConkey and XLD (xylose-lysine-deoxycholate) plates. The RV broth is then reincubated and a second subculture is performed after 48 hours. In all cases, plates are incubated overnight at 37° C. This technique is extremely sensitive for small numbers of *Salmonellae* but may not be available or cost-effective in a smaller hospital setting. However, similar techniques with high sensitivity and specificity have been described.[11,72] Organisms isolated by this technique and presumptively identified as *Salmonellae* are subject to serogrouping. For epidemiological purposes, selected isolates undergo further analysis including antimicrobial susceptibility testing, serotyping and pulsed-field gel electrophoresis (PFGE).[63,72]

nutrition, have disturbances to their normal flora, may be receiving antimicrobials and are concentrated in close proximity with other animals that have similar risk factors. Moreover, animals in a hospital come from different places, so every patient admission is essentially admixing animals from separate populations, thereby providing an opportunity to introduce infectious organisms to potentially naïve individuals. However, as already mentioned, not all hospitalised patients are at equal risk of shedding or acquiring infectious agents. Patients should therefore be divided into risk categories (most conveniently designated as low, medium or high). Once this has been determined, rational strategies for appropriate patient segregation can be developed. During this process strict attention should be paid to animal and human traffic flow. Application of barrier precautions and subsequent limits on traffic (including clients/visitors) should be based on risk. The outline plan presented below is arguably a close to ideal situation, but personnel and facility restrictions at individual clinics may limit the degree to which patients can be segregated. In these circumstances, those responsible for biosecurity must choose the most logical, risk-averse approach that is not cost-prohibitive. In this context, risk category may be defined in two manners: risk *to the hospital* from the patient or risk *to the patient* of hospitalisation.

Patients requiring intensive care should be considered at higher risk for contracting infectious diseases and may be more susceptible to all types of HAIs. As a result, implementation of rigorous barrier precautions and personnel segregation in this area are advisable. In addition to providing for proper hand hygiene, such as alcohol-based hand sanitisers, precautions might include dedicated clothing and shoes (Box 3.8). If possible, personnel involved in the management of patients in intensive care should not participate in treating isolated patients or those at high risk for shedding contagious organisms such as *Salmonella*—for example, horses with colic.

Patients admitted with the complaint of colic should be segregated in one facility/area, while those with diar-

Box 3.8. Practical tips for isolating equine patients at small to medium-sized clinics

- **Designate an isolation area.**
  - If possible, designate isolation stall(s) away from high traffic areas. When occupied, limit access by placing barrier around stall or between it and other areas of the hospital; something as simple as cones and tape can work.
- **Always try to deal with isolated patients last.**
  - If separate personnel are not an option, always try to move from low to high risk and attend to isolated patient(s) last. If clothes get dirty despite barrier precautions, change/launder before working with other cases.
- **Always wash hands.**
  - Wear disposable gloves and a disposable plastic gown. Even when gloves are used **you must still wash hands**. Alcohol-based hand sanitizers can be readily placed stallside and are effective provided hands are not visibly dirty. Dirty hands **must** be washed with soap and water.
- **Provide waterproof footwear and use a disinfectant foot dip.**
  - Place waterproof footwear (rubber overboots are ideal, but they must be easy to get on and off) and foot dip containing disinfectant in front of isolated stall. Change disinfectant daily or sooner if dirty. Most disinfectants will not work if high levels of organic material—e.g., shavings, straw, dirt or feces are present. Dilute bleach (2%–4%) is cheap and effective but readily inactivated in the presence of organic debris so *must* be changed regularly. Other types of disinfectant can also used, e.g., peroxygen-based such as Virkon-S (DuPont Animal Health Solutions, Sudbury, UK).
- **Clean other stalls before that of the isolated patient.**
  - Clean isolated stall(s) last; use completely different set of tools (pitchfork, shovel, broom, etc.) or ensure that equipment is thoroughly cleaned and disinfected before using elsewhere. Clean with detergent and brush to remove gross debris, immerse equipment's head in bleach solution (2%–4%), wipe down handles, drying in sun is helpful.
- **Do not share buckets and feed tubs or *any* other equipment.**
  - Make sure that the same bucket, feed tub and any other equipment stay with the isolated patient and do not get used for other horses. After discharge, thoroughly clean and disinfect equipment before reusing or, if necessary, discard.
- **Carefully dispose of materials that come into contact with isolated patient(s).**
  - Key to containment is limiting environmental contamination. Provide receptacles for separate disposal of gloves, gowns and any materials used in treatment of isolated patient(s). Remove feces as often as possible to minimise contamination of soil and non-cleanable surfaces in stall. Collect feces, used bedding and uneaten feed separately. Avoid placing manure in an area allowing direct drainage into any water system. Ideal disposal method for feces, bedding and feed is proper composting. Field spreading with prolonged exposure to sunlight may be acceptable as long as areas will not be used for feed or animals for at least 30 days.

The above instructions can also be adapted for the client who needs to isolate a horse at home, but some understanding of layout and animal management practices at the client's stable is necessary to ensure that the information provided is appropriate.

rhoea or suspected enterocolitis should be admitted directly to isolation. Although these animals all have increased rates for shedding *Salmonella* and could be handled by personnel dedicated to caring for both groups of patients, physical separation is highly desirable because colic patients are at increased risk for infection due to disturbances in normal gastrointestinal function. Barrier precautions for isolated and colic patients should include disposable gowns (gowns are essential with infected foals because of the intimate physical contact involved in handling them), gloves, waterproof dedicated footwear and foot baths[73,74] or mats[75,76] located at stall and area entrances. Additional baths or mats may be placed at areas that function as "choke-points" or have the effect of concentrating foot traffic. Proper maintenance of footbaths and mats is critical to their efficacy[73–76] and includes monitoring disinfectant levels, timely changing of disinfectant and minimising organic contamination and exposure to the elements such as sunlight and rain. Patients in high-risk categories should have dedicated equipment that remains in their space. Complete personnel segregation between the highest-risk and lowest-risk patients may not be practical based on manpower and facility limitations in all but the largest hospitals. Environmental surveillance data demonstrate that proper use of barrier precautions effectively contains *Salmonella* (when present) to a specific area (Aceto et al., unpublished observation) and suggest that limited cross-over of personnel can safely occur provided all protocols are carefully followed. However, as every movement between areas carries a potential risk of spread, separation of personnel responsible for handling low-medium and high-risk cases should be maintained wherever possible and particularly when known infections are present.

Biosecurity precautions in low- or medium-risk patient populations may be minimal (e.g., footmats at entrances, attention to hand and general hygiene) and should be based on incidence of infectious disease in this population. If possible, low-risk patients should be housed separately from those at higher risk of developing HAIs secondary to hospitalisation and, when practical, personnel segregation should also be implemented. If allowed by facility layout, elective cases (low risk) should be housed separately from those patients on antimicrobials (parenteral or enteral) for more than 72 hours and nongastrointestinal emergencies (low to medium risk), and they should certainly be segregated from critical patients and any patients presenting for colic or diarrhoea or other conditions requiring isolation (high risk).

For emergency admissions, presenting complaint and a good history may well dictate how a patient should be handled; even in the absence of any obvious clinical signs. For example, if an animal is admitted from a facility where there is a known or suspected outbreak of a contagious disease, it should be treated as a suspect contact and housed accordingly. Tests and clinical monitoring appropriate to the condition of concern should be initiated and could be something as simple as increased frequency of measuring rectal temperature. In the case of diseases such as infection with equine herpesvirus that may be spread by aerosol, it is prudent to also increase clinical monitoring of other animals housed in the same area, even when that is the isolation facility. Obvious clinical signs such as diarrhoea and abscesses in the region of the retropharyngeal lymph nodes,[77] when accompanied by either an appropriate or uncertain history, should mandate that cases be isolated.

In terms of infection threat to the hospital, the most difficult patient to handle is the unknown threat or unrecognised case. These are patients incubating a contagious disease that have no suspect history and no clinically apparent disease at presentation. There may be no way to identify this animal at admission, but a proactive infection control programme that includes daily updates on patient clinical status and promotes heightened awareness of infection risks among all staff involved in patient management should be capable of rapidly identifying potential problems and limiting spread. In this context, algorithms that trigger increased testing, implementation of barrier precautions or movement of patients to isolation facilities can be useful tools for managing patients and promoting hospital safety for all patients and personnel. Figure 3.27 shows a typical example of an algorithm developed to ensure consistent handling of *Salmonella* suspects. Algorithms must be evidence-based, prominently posted and strictly adhered to, with no exceptions.

Hand hygiene and disinfection protocols

The importance of excellent hygiene and overall cleanliness cannot be overemphasised. Strict hand hygiene and rigorous routine cleaning and disinfection should be stressed. Hand hygiene is of critical importance when treating neonatal foals, where there is frequently extensive handling, including of their mucous membranes. To promote proper hand hygiene, ready access to hand washing facilities or hand sanitisers should be available at all times. Increased hand washing or sanitising with alcohol-based products has been demonstrated to reduce the incidence of HAIs in human medicine,[78] and preliminary studies suggest that hand sanitisers are also effective in veterinary hospitals.[79] As many veterinary facilities (particularly animal housing areas) were not constructed with infection control in mind, ready access to hand washing facilities is not always available. In order to correct this fundamental system error,[80] alcohol-based hand sanitisers should be prominently located throughout the facility; we place them on every stall door, in every treatment and procedure area and in all animal handling areas. In smaller hospitals, with well-trained staff, individual hand sanitisers kept on the belt are an alternative. The need for personal responsibility[80] and use of proper technique in hand hygiene (such that if hands are visibly dirty or contaminated with proteinaceous material, including blood or other body fluids, they *must* be properly washed with soap and water; otherwise, hand sanitisers are acceptable) should be repeatedly emphasised to all personnel and clients as well. Hand washing is necessary even when gloves are required in patient handling. Careful choice of sanitising products and/or availability of emollients may improve compliance and prevent the development of dermatitis that can compromise integrity of skin on the hands and inhibit effective cleansing.[78,81]

In a veterinary hospital where faecal material and respiratory or other secretions are abundant, frequently defy containment and may represent a nosocomial risk, cleanliness of treatment spaces, animal housing, procedure areas and operating rooms is absolutely crucial. At a minimum, cleaning and disinfection protocols should include four steps: (1) detergent to remove organic debris (critical to the efficacy of most disinfectants), (2) rinsing, (3) drying (optimum; or at a minimum water removal, as application of disinfectant to a water-logged area may result in dilution to the point of inefficacy) and (4) disinfectant application. Some, but not all, disinfectants require rinsing. Drying after cleaning and disinfection is always beneficial to pathogen control.

In areas of high concern, multiple disinfectant steps may be useful (Box 3.9). Care must be taken to ensure that the properties of the detergent and disinfectant are compatible and that disinfectants are properly diluted. Disinfection protocols should be frequently reviewed and altered based on evidence gathered through patient and environment surveillance. Bacterial resistance is a constant threat, and kill-curves directed towards organisms of concern may be periodically warranted. Consideration should also be given to the effect of disinfectants on equipment, personnel and the environment. A particular disinfectant may be more costly at the outset but overall might be a prudent choice because of minimal destruction of equipment. If prolonged use of a disinfectant is found to damage surfaces, an alternative should be sought, as loss of surface integrity defeats the object of maintaining sealed, cleanable surfaces in potentially critical areas. There are several valuable resources covering the properties and use of disinfectants.[14,27,82–87]

Due to the presence of specialised equipment and environmental controls such as air handling equipment, ICUs can be particularly challenging to effectively disinfect.[62] Particular care needs to be paid in these areas to patient and environmental monitoring, as well as to enforcement of all biosecurity protocols. Not only are the ICU patients at more risk for HAIs, but contamination can result in costly decontamination and disruption of much needed care. Because the urgent nature of procedures performed on critical patients may occasionally result in disordered biosecurity protocols, more frequent disinfection may be needed and increased surveillance during times of high patient occupancy should be considered.

Facility evaluation

All aspects of the hospital must be evaluated with infection control in mind.[12,14] In a large-animal hospital, this means a wide assessment of the infrastructure including, but not limited to, manure handling, feed and water delivery, waste disposal, flooring, ventilation systems, hospital data systems and isolation facilities. In animal housing and clinical spaces, the goal should be to have cleanable, nonporous surfaces in as many areas as possible; this may be as simple

Box 3.9. An example of an effective, broad application, cleaning and disinfection protocol

Steps in cleaning and disinfection

1. Have all material safety data sheets (MSDS) for cleaning and disinfection materials available and follow instructions for proper mixing, disposal and personal protective equipment, e.g., gloves, eye protection, etc.
2. Remove all visible organic material, e.g., bedding and manure prior to cleaning.
3. Clean surfaces with an anionic detergent (7.5 g/L; 2 oz per US gallon of water). Mechanical disruption (scrubbing) of surfaces is often necessary to remove biofilms and stubborn organic debris, especially in animal housing areas.
4. Rinse with clean water.
5. Allow to dry or at least ensure that the bulk of surface water is removed.
6. Apply a dilute solution (2%–4%) of bleach and allow at least 15 minutes contact time. Alternatively, particularly on sensitive surfaces, a quaternary ammonium disinfectant can be employed (dilution rates vary by product). Bleach and quaternary ammonium disinfectants can also be used sequentially with rinsing in between but should NEVER be mixed because of possible chlorine gas formation.
7. Rinse thoroughly with clean water and allow the treated area to dry as much as possible.
8. In contaminated or high-risk areas, careful spraying with a peroxygen disinfectant such as 2% Virkon-S (DuPont Animal Health Solutions, Sudbury, UK) should be used as a final decontamination step. Allow at least 10 minutes contact time.
9. Rinse with clean water (not always necessary but feed tubs, water buckets etc., should be rinsed).
10. Drying is important to achieving maximum effect, so allow the area to dry as much as possible before rebedding or reintroducing animals. If postcleaning environmental samples are being collected, the area must be completely dry.

For more detailed information about disinfectant properties and uses, see references 14, 24, 27 and 81.

as ensuring that wood surfaces are properly sealed and painted or as involved as installing complex monolithic flooring systems. Critical evaluation of the hospital environment is essential. Noncleanable surfaces in high-risk patient areas provide a threat to the care of all animals, but particularly the critically ill. A significant consequence of segregating patients by risk, as opposed to how ill they are, is the potential inability to provide appropriate patient care in an isolation facility or areas designated to house other high-risk patient groups (e.g., horses with colic, foals). Strict patient segregation aims to protect all of the patients and the hospital itself, but it also means that isolation and other facilities for housing high-risk patients must have the ability to care for the critically ill equine patient. Depending on the patient population of the hospital, this may include the ability to ventilate a patient, provision of climate control and possible availability of a sling/hoist system.

Education and awareness

Despite the paucity of data in some areas and the difficulties in defining HAIs in a veterinary setting, there is no doubt that, as with hospitalised humans, nosocomial infections in equine patients are an inherent risk of hospitalisation. It is essential that these potential risks are properly conveyed to clients when their animals are admitted to the hospital. In addition, people working with animals in a hospital are likely to be exposed to a variety of infectious agents, including those with zoonotic potential, even when this not apparent. Education and awareness of zoonotic and contagious diseases of importance and the routes of transmission by which causative organisms spread from animal to animal, animal to human, or human to animal are the keys to reducing infection risk, preventing outbreaks of disease and protecting human health. Training and education should be integral to any programme so that EVERYONE has awareness of these dangers and understands their specific responsibilities in maintaining high standards of hygiene (particularly hand and foot hygiene) and reducing risk whenever possible.

Infectious/zoonotic diseases of the hospitalised horse

Table 3.3 lists equine contagious and zoonotic diseases of greatest nosocomial importance. Disease description, clinical signs, mode of transmission, testing, disinfection and suggested protective measures (barrier precautions, housing recommendations) are briefly described. In many instances, known positive animals should be isolated; which implies full barrier precautions (footbaths, boots, gloves and gowns or other protective clothing, scrupulous hand hygiene, no shared equipment) in a dedicated isolation facility or segregated section of a larger facility with strictly controlled human and animal traffic. In the case of some zoonotic diseases, additional personal protective equipment such as eyewear or face shields is required. As many zoonotic organisms, including *Salmonella* (which, in addition to being one of the most important nosocomial infections capable of causing serious disease outbreaks in equine hospitals, is also the most common equine zoonosis), can be spread by the oral route, people should not be permitted to eat or drink in animal housing or clinical areas.

Based on routes of transmission, all means of spread must be considered. In the case of faecal-oral spread, in addition to general cleanliness, hand and foot hygiene and preventing contamination of feed and water sources, rodent control, bird control and even insect control must be taken into consideration and included in a comprehensive biosecurity programme.

For zoonotic diseases, the *Compendium of Veterinary Standard Precautions* provides details on preventing zoonotic disease in veterinary personnel[88] and includes a model infection control plan for veterinary practices.[89] As with all zoonoses, if personnel suspect they have been exposed to a zoonotic disease, they should consult their health care provider as soon as possible.

Some contagious and zoonotic equine diseases are considered exotic to Europe and North America. Although beyond the scope of this chapter, persons involved in biosecurity should be aware of these diseases and remain vigilant for emerging zoonotic and contagious disease threats.

Concluding remarks

The needs of the hospital as a "patient" are best met by making evidence-based decisions. Biosecurity efforts are most effectively directed through collection and critical evaluation of *data*. Efforts and resources can be wasted by making decisions based solely on clinical impression. The implementation of an effective biosecurity programme must be focused on the principles of hygiene, patient contact, education and awareness, and surveillance. Concerns regarding HAIs can only be appropriately addressed by allowing data to direct protocols. It is essential to appreciate that just as disease-causing organisms evolve and change, evidence-based evolution of biosecurity protocols is inevitable and necessary if we are to keep pace with infection threats, optimise the benefit-to-risk ratio and cost-effectiveness of the programme and ensure ongoing success.

The appearance of increasingly resistant organisms in community as well as hospital settings, combined with the mobility of our animal populations, makes it likely that the risk of introduction of infectious agents capable of causing outbreaks of disease will increase over succeeding years, as will the appearance of HAIs that are increasingly difficult to treat. All equine facilities, but particularly veterinary hospitals, must consider developing a biosecurity programme to protect them against such events. A demonstrably effective biosecurity programme improves the quality of the facility by optimising patient care, reducing HAIs, protecting personnel and clients from zoonotic agents, providing educational opportunities, limiting financial losses and liability and restoring confidence to staff and clients. Written plans, careful data management, attention to detail, good communications and a persistent message are imperative to success.

Implementation and, more importantly, long-term maintenance of an ICP are not without problems. Acceptance of biosecurity requires commitment to dealing with a variety of fundamental issues across many constituencies including, but not limited to, education, communication, cost, data management, impact on patient care and legal liability. Nevertheless, even in a relative short period, it is possible to effect major changes in attitude and behaviour with respect to biosecurity that are ultimately to the benefit of patients, hospital and personnel alike.

References

1. Burke JP: Infection control: a problem for patient safety. N Engl J Med 348:651-656, 2003
2. Jarvis WR: Infection control and changing health-care delivery systems. Emerg Infect Dis 7:170-173, 2001
3. Weinstein RA: Nosocomial infection update. Emerg Infect Dis 4:416-420, 1998
4. Roberts RR, Scott RD II, Cordell R, Solomon SL, Steele L, Kampe LM, Trick WE, Weinstein RA: The use of economic modeling to determine the hospital costs associated with nosocomial infections. Clin Infect Dis 36:1424-1432, 2003
5. Kollef MH, Fraser VJ: Antibiotic resistance in the intensive care unit. Ann Intern Med 134:298-314, 2001
6. Anonymous: National Nosocomial Infections Surveillance (NNIS) System Report, data summary from January 1992 through June 2004, issued October 2004. Am J Infect Control 32:470-485, 2004
7. Stosor V, Peterson L, Postelnick M, Noskin G: *Enterococcus faecium* bacteremia: does vancomycin resistance make a difference? Arch Intern Med 158:522-577, 1998
8. Abramson MA, Sexton DJ: Nosocomial methicillin-resistant and methicillin susceptible *Staphylococcus aureus* primary bacteremia: at what costs? Infect Control Hosp Epidemiol 20:408-411, 1999
9. Anonymous: Pennsylvania Health Care Cost Containment Council (PHC4) Research Brief Issue No. 5, July 2005. Hospital-acquired infections in Pennsylvania. Available at http://www.phc4.org/reports/researchbriefs/071205/default.htm. Accessed May 25, 2006
10. Morley PS: Surveillance for nosocomial infections in veterinary hospitals. Vet Clin North Am Equine Pract 20:561-576, 2004
11. Burgess BA, Morley PS, Hyatt DR: Environmental surveillance for *Salmonella enterica* in a veterinary teaching hospital. J Am Vet Med Assoc 225:1344-1348, 2004
12. Smith BP, House JK, Magdesian KG, Jang SS, Cabral RJ Jr, Madigan JE, Herthel WF: Principles of an infectious disease control programme for preventing nosocomial gastrointestinal and respiratory tract diseases in large animal veterinary teaching hospitals. J Am Vet Med Assoc 225:1186-1195, 2004
13. Traub-Dargatz JL, Dargatz DA, Morley PS, Dunowska M: An overview of infection control strategies for equine facilities, with an emphasis on veterinary hospitals. Vet Clin North Am Equine Pract 20:507-520, 2004
14. Dunowska M, Morley PS, Traub-Dargatz JL, Van Metre DC: Biosecurity, in Sellon DC, Long MT (eds): Equine Infectious Diseases. St. Louis, MO, Saunders Elsevier, 2006, pp 528-539
15. Garner JS, Jarvis WR, Emori TG, Horan TC, Hughes JM: CDC definitions for nosocomial infections, in Olmsted RN (ed): APIC Infection Control and Applied Epidemiology: Principles and Practice. St. Louis, Mosby, 1996, pp A1-A20. Also available at http://www.dhh.louisiana.gov/offices/publications/pubs-249/20050427NosocomialInfectionDefinitions.pdf. Accessed June 9, 2006
16. Ducel G, Fabry J, Nicolle L (eds): Prevention of Hospital-Acquired Infections: A Practical Guide, ed 2. Geneva, World Health Organization, 2002, available at http://www.who.int/csr/resources/publications/drugresist/whocdscsreph200212.pdf. Accessed June 9, 2006
17. Boerlin P, Eugster S, Gaschen F, Straub R, Schawalder P: Transmission of opportunistic pathogens in a veterinary teaching hospital. Vet Microbiol 82:347-359, 2001
18. Dargatz DA, Traub-Dargatz JL: Multidrug resistant *Salmonella* and nosocomial infections. Vet Clin North Am Equine Pract 20:587-680, 2004
19. Dunowska M, Morley PS, Traub-Dargatz JL, Hyatt DR, Dargatz DA: Impact of hospitalisation and antimicrobial drug administration on antimicrobial susceptibility patterns of commensal *Escherichia coli* isolated from the feces of horses. J Am Vet Med Assoc 228:1909-1917, 2006
20. Ogeer-Gyles JS, Mathews KA, Boerlin P: Nosocomial infections and antimicrobial resistance in critical care medicine. J Vet Emerg Crit Care 16:1-18, 2006
21. Ogeer-Gyles J, Mathews KA, Sears W, Prescott JF, Weese JS, Boerlin P: Development of antimicrobial resistance in rectal *Escherichia coli* isolates from dogs hospitalised in an intensive care unit. J Am Vet Med Assoc 229:694-699, 2006
22. Koterba A, Torchia J, Silverthorne C, Ramphal R, Merritt AM, Manucy J: Nosocomial infections and bacterial antibiotic resistance in a university equine hospital. J Am Vet Med Assoc 189:185-191, 1986
23. Smith BP: Evolution of equine infection control programmes. Vet Clin North Am Equine Pract 20:521-530, 2004
24. Bain FT, Weese JS (eds): The Veterinary Clinics of North America: Equine Practice—Infection Control. Vet Clin North Am Equine Pract 20(3):December, 2004
25. Traub-Dargatz JL, Bain FT, Paul Morley PS, Scott Weese JS, Dargatz D, Kirby A: Summary of the 2006 Estes Park Workshop On Infection Control in Equine Hospitals and at Equine Events: conducted by the Dorothy Havemeyer Foundation. Available at http://havemeyerfoundation.org/Documents/Dorothy_Havemeyer_Inf_Control_Workshop_Summary_Final_Version.doc. Accessed November 21, 2006
26. Ontario Veterinary College: Infection Control Manual; Veterinary Teaching Hospital, 2004. Available at http://www.ovc.uoguelph.ca/vth/documents/InfectionControlManual2005update.pdf. Accessed November 21, 2006
27. Colorado State University: General Biosecurity Standard Operating Policies and Procedures (Draft): James L. Voss Veterinary Teaching Hospital, 2006. Available at http://www.

csuvets.colostate.edu/biosecurity/biosecurity_sop.pdf. Accessed January 02, 2007

28. Aceto H, Rankin SC, Dallap BL, Dolente B, Munro DS, Benson CE, Smith G: An outbreak of *Salmonella enterica* serotype Newport at a veterinary teaching hospital. Proceedings of the 109th Annual Meeting of the US Animal Health Association, Hershey, PA, November 2005, pp 563-566. Available at http://www.usaha.org/meetings/2005/2005_USAHA_Proceedings.pdf. Accessed November 26, 2006
29. Baker JR: An outbreak of salmonellosis involving veterinary hospital patients. Vet Rec 85:8-10, 1969
30. Bauerfiend R, Wieler LH, Weiss R, Baljer G: Comparative plasmid profile analysis of *Salmonella* typhimurium var. Copenhagen strains from a *Salmonella* outbreak in hospitalised horses. Berl Munch Tierarztl Wochenschr 105:38-42, 1992
31. Castor ML, Wooley RE, Shotts EB, Brown J, Payeur JB: Characteristics of *Salmonella* isolated from an outbreak of equine salmonellosis in a veterinary teaching hospital. Equine Vet Sci 89:236-241, 1989
32. Dorn CR, Coffman JR, Schmidt DA: Neutropenia and salmonellosis in hospitalised horses. J Am Vet Med Assoc 166:65-67, 1975
33. van Duijkeren E, Sloet van Oldruitenborgh-Oosterbann MM, Houwers DJ, van Leeuwen WJ, Kalsbeek HC: Equine salmonellosis in a Dutch veterinary teaching hospital. Vet Rec 135:248-250, 1994
34. Dunowska M, Patterson G, Traub-Dargatz JL, Hyatt DR, Morley PS: Recent progress in controlling *Salmonella* in veterinary hospitals. Proceedings of the 50th Annual Convention of the American Association of Equine Practitioners, Denver, CO, 2004. International Veterinary Information Service Document No. P1461.1204. Available at http://www.ivis.org/proceedings/AAEP/2004/Dunowska/chapter.asp?LA=1. Accessed January 25, 2007
35. Ernst NS, Hernandez JA, MacKay RJ, Brown MP, Gaskin JM, Ngyuen AD, Giguere S, Colahan PT, Troedsson MR, Haines GR, Addison IR: Risk factors associated with fecal *Salmonella* shedding among hospitalised horses with signs of gastrointestinal tract disease. J Am Vet Med Assoc 225:275-281, 2004
36. Hartmann FA, Callan RJ, McGuirk SM, West SEH: Control of an outbreak of salmonellosis caused by drug-resistant *Salmonella* anatum in horses at a veterinary hospital and measures to prevent future infection. J Am Vet Med Assoc 209:629-631, 1996
37. Hird DW, Pappaioanou M, Smith BP: Case control study of risk factors associated with isolation of *Salmonella* saintpaul in hospitalised horses. Am J Epidemiol 120:852-864, 1984
38. House JK, Mainar-Jaime RC, Smith BP, House A-M, Kamiya DY: Risk factors for nosocomial *Salmonella* infection among hospitalised horses. J Am Vet Med Assoc 214:1511-1516, 1999
39. Kim LM, Morley PS, Traub-Dargatz JL, Salman M, Gentry-Weeks C: Factors associated with *Salmonella* shedding among equine colic patients at a veterinary teaching hospital. J Am Vet Med Assoc 187:256-257, 2001
40. Morley PS, Dunowska M, Hill A: Surveillance for *Salmonella* shedding in large animal patients. Proceedings of the American College of Veterinary Internal Medicine Forum, Minneapolis, MN, 2004, p 881
41. Palmer JE, Benson CE, Whitlock RH: *Salmonella* shed by horses with colic. J Am Vet Med Assoc 218:740-748, 1985
42. Paré J, Carpenter TE, Thurmond MC: Analysis of temporal and spatial clustering of horses with *Salmonella* krefeld in an intensive care unit of a veterinary hospital. J Am Vet Med Assoc 209:626-628, 1996
43. Schott HC II, Ewart SL, Walker RD, Dwyer RM, Dietrich S, Eberhart SW, Kusey J, Stick JA, Derksen FJ: An outbreak of salmonellosis among horses at a veterinary teaching hospital. J Am Vet Med Assoc 218:1152-1159, 2001
44. Tillotson K, Savage CJ, Salman MD, Gentry-Weeks CR, Rice D, Fedorka-Cray PJ, Hendrickson DA, Jones RL, Nelson AW, Traub-Dargatz JL: Outbreak of *Salmonella* infantis infection in a large animal veterinary teaching hospital. J Am Vet Med Assoc 211:1554-1557, 1997
45. Ward MP, Brady TH, Couëtil LL, Liljebjelke K, Maurer JJ, Wu CC: Investigation and control of an outbreak of salmonellosis caused by multidrug resistant *Salmonella* Typhimurium in a population of hospitalised horses. Vet Microbiol 107:233-240, 2005
46. Cuny C, Kuemmerle J, Stanek C, Willey B, Strommenger B, Witte W: Emergence of MRSA infections in a veterinary hospital: strain characterization and comparison with MRSA from humans. Eurosurveillance 11:44-47, 2006. Available at http://www.eurosurveillance.org/eq/2006/01-06/pdf/eq_1_2006_44-47.pdf. Accessed June 10, 2006
47. Middleton JR, Fales WH, Luby CD, Oaks JL, Sanchez S, Kinyon JM, Wu CC, Maddox CW, Welsh RD, Hartmann F: Surveillance for *Staphylococcus aureus* in veterinary teaching hospitals. J Clin Microbiol 43:2916-2919, 2005
48. Seguin JC, Walker RD, Caron JP, Kloos WE, George CG, Hollis RJ, Jones RN, Pfaller MA: Methicillin-resistant *Staphylococcus aureus* outbreak in a veterinary teaching hospital: potential animal-to-human transmission. J Clin Microbiol 37:1459-1463, 1999
49. Weese JS, Rousseau J, Willey BM, Archambault M, McGeer A, Low DE: Methicillin-resistant *Staphylococcus aureus* in horses at a veterinary teaching hospital: frequency, characterization, and association with clinical disease. J Vet Intern Med 20:182-186, 2006
50. Weese JS, Archambault M, Willey BM, Hearn P, Kreiswirth BN, Said-Salim B, McGeer A, Likhoshvay Y, Prescott JF, Low DE: Methicillin-resistant *Staphylococcus aureus* in horses and horse personnel, 2000-2002. Emerg Infect Dis 11:430-435, 2005
51. Båverud V, Gustafsson A, Franklin A, Lindholm A, Gunnarsson A: *Clostridium difficile*-associated with acute colitis in mature horses treated with antibiotics. Equine Vet J 29:279-284, 1997
52. Båverud V: *Clostridium difficile* diarrhea: infection control in horses. Vet Clin North Am Equine Pract 20:615-630, 2004
53. Madewell BR, Tang YJ, Jang S, Madigan JE, Hirsch DC, Gumerlock PH, Silva J Jr: Apparent outbreaks of *Clostridium difficile*-associated diarrhea in horses in a veterinary medical teaching hospital. J Vet Diagn Invest 7:343-346, 1995
54. Weese JS, Staempfli HR, Prescott JF: A prospective study of the roles of *Clostridium difficile* and enterotoxigenic *Clostridium perfringens* in equine diarrhoea. Equine Vet J 33:403-409, 2001

55. Hirsch DC: Hospital-acquired (nosocomial) infections. In Smith BP ed. Large Animal Internal Medicine (3 ed), St. Louis, Mosby, 2002, pp 1363-1370
56. Reed SM and Toribio RE: Equine herpesvirus 1 and 4. Vet Clin North Am Eq Pract 20:631-642, 2004
57. Anonymous: Colorado State Veterinary Teaching Hospital implements precautionary suspension of elective equine admissions. CSU press release October 31, 2006. Available at http://agnews.colostate.edu/index.asp?page=news_item_display&news_item_id=478302186. Accessed October 31, 2006
58. Collins JK, Kari S, Ralston SL, Bennett DG, Traub-Dargatz JL, McKinnon AO: Equine viral arteritis at a veterinary teaching hospital. Prev Vet Med 4:389-397, 1987
59. Irish Department of Agriculture and Food: Equine infectious anaemia—note for industry/private veterinary practitioners, 2006. Available at http://www.agriculture.gov.ie/index.jsp?file=animal_health/EIA/EIA.xml. Accessed December 8, 2006
60. ProMED-mail: Equine infectious anemia—Ireland (04), 2006. Available at http://www.promedmail.org/pls/askus/f?p=2400:1202:6860253557122756098::NO::F2400_P1202_CHECK_DISPLAY,F2400_P1202_PUB_MAIL_ID:X,34718. Accessed December 8, 2006
61. Colahan PT, Peyton LC, Connelly MR, Peterson R: *Serratia* spp. infection in 21 horses. J Am Vet Med Assoc 185:209-211, 1984
62. Luftman HS, Regits MA, Lorcheim P, Czarneski MA, Boyle T, Aceto H, Dallap BL, Munro DS, Faylor K: Chlorine dioxide gas decontamination of the University of Pennsylvania's George D. Widener Large Animal Hospital intensive and neonatal care units. Appl Biosaf 11:144-154, 2006
63. Rankin SC, Wichard JM, Joyce K, Stephens L, O'Shea K, Aceto H, Munro DS, Benson CE: Detection of a bla_{SHV} extended-spectrum β-lactamase in *Salmonella* Newport MDR-AmpC. J Clin Microbiol 43:5792-5793, 2005
64. Wood JLN, Newton JR, Daly J, Park AW, Mumford JA: It's all in the mix: infection transmission in populations. Equine Vet J 35:526-528, 2003
65. Christley RM, French NP: Small-world topology of UK racing: the potential for rapid spread of infectious agents. Equine Vet J 35:586-589, 2003
66. Florida Department of Agriculture and Consumer Services Press Release, December 19, 2006. Available at http://www.doacs.state.fl.us/press/2006/12192006.html. Accessed January 17, 2007
67. Morley PS, Apley MD, Besser TE, Burney DP, Fedorka-Cray PJ, Papich MG, Traub-Dargatz JL, Weese SJ: Antimicrobial drug use in veterinary medicine. J Vet Intern Med 19:617-629, 2005. Available at http://www.acvim.org/uploadedFiles/Consensus_Statements/Antimicrobial.pdf. Accessed June 10, 2006
68. American Veterinary Medical Association: Judicious therapeutic use of antimicrobials, 2005. Available at http://www.avma.org/reference/jtua/default.asp. Accessed January 24, 2007
69. American Association of Equine Practitioners: Prudent Drug Usage Guidelines, 2001. Available at http://www.avma.org/reference/jtua/equine/jtuaequine.asp. Accessed January 24, 2007
70. WHONET software available at http://www.who.int/drugresistance/whonetsoftware/en/. Accessed November 21, 2006
71. Weese JS: Barrier precautions, isolation protocols and personal hygiene in veterinary hospitals. Vet Clin North Am Equine Pract 20:543-559, 2004
72. Dunowska M, Morley PS, Traub-Dargatz JL, Davis MA, Patterson G, Frye JG, Hyatt DR, Dargatz DA: Comparison of *Salmonella enterica* serotype Infantis isolates from a veterinary teaching hospital. J Appl Microbiol, published online October 30, 2006. Available at http://www.blackwell-synergy.com/doi/full/10.1111/j.1365-2672.2006.03198.x?prevSearch=allfield%3A%28Dunowska+M%29. Accessed November 26, 2006
73. Morley PS, Morris SN, Hyatt DR, Van Metre DC: Evaluation of the efficacy of disinfectant footbaths as used in veterinary hospitals. J Am Vet Med Assoc 226:2053-2058, 2005
74. Stockton KA, Morley PS, Hyatt DR, Burgess BA, Patterson G, Dunowska M, Lee DE: Evaluation of the effects of footwear hygiene protocols on nonspecific bacterial contamination of floor surfaces in an equine hospital. J Am Vet Med Assoc 228:1068-1073, 2006
75. Amass SF, Arighi M, Kinyon JM, Hoffman LJ, Schneider JL, Draper K: Effectiveness of using a mat filled with peroxygen disinfectant to minimize shoe sole contamination in a veterinary hospital. J Am Vet Med Assoc 228:1391-1396, 2006
76. Dunowska M, Morley PS, Patterson G, Hyatt DR, Van Metre DC: Evaluation of the efficacy of a peroxygen disinfectant-filled footmat for reduction of bacterial load on footwear in a large animal hospital setting. J Am Vet Med Assoc 228:1935-1939, 2006
77. Sweeney CR, Timoney JF, Newton JR, Hines MT: *Streptococcus equi* infection in horses: guidelines for treatment, control and prevention of strangles. J Vet Intern Med 19:123-134, 2005. Available at http://www.acvim.org/uploadedFiles/Consensus_Statements/Strangles.pdf. Accessed June 10, 2006
78. Centers for Disease Control and Prevention: Guideline for hand hygiene in health-care setting. MMWR Morb Mortal Wky Rep 51:RR-16, 2002. Available at http://www.cdc.gov/mmwr/PDF/rr/rr5116.pdf. Accessed January 18, 2007
79. Traub-Dargatz JL, Weese JS, Rousseau JD, Dunowska M, Morley PS, Dargatz DA: Pilot study to evaluate 3 hygiene protocols on the reduction of bacterial load on the hands of veterinary staff performing routine equine physical examinations. Can Vet J 47:671-676, 2006
80. Goldmann D: System failure versus personal accountability: the case for clean hands. N Engl J Med 355:121-123, 2006
81. Larson E: Hygiene of the skin: when is clean too clean? Emerg Infect Dis 7:225-230, 2001
82. Dvorak G: Disinfection 101, 2005. Available at http://www.cfsph.iastate.edu/BRM/resources/Disinfectants/Disinfection101Feb2005.pdf. Accessed November 28, 2006
83. Dwyer RM: Environmental disinfection to control equine infections. Vet Clin North Am Eq Pract 20:531-542, 2004
84. Dunowska M, Morley PS, Hyatt DR: The effect of Virkon-S® fogging on survival of *Salmonella enterica* and *Staphylococcus aureus* on surfaces in a veterinary teaching hospital. Vet Microbiol 105:281-9, 2005
85. Patterson G, Morley PS, Blehm KD, Lee DE, Dunowska M: Efficacy of directed misting application of a peroxygen disin-

fectant for environmental decontamination of a veterinary hospital. J Am Vet Med Assoc 227:597-602, 2005

86. Alinovi CA, Ward MP, Couëtil LL, Wu CC: Detection of *Salmonella* organisms and assessment of a protocol for removal of contamination in horse stalls at a veterinary teaching hospital. J Am Vet Med Assoc 223:1640-1644, 2003
87. Ewart SL, Schott HC II, Robison RL, Dwyer RM, Eberhart SW, Walker RD: Identification of sources of *Salmonella* organisms in a veterinary teaching hospital and evaluation of the effects of disinfectants on detection of *Salmonella* organisms on surface materials. J Am Vet Med Assoc 218:1145-1151, 2001
88. National Association of State Public Health Veterinarians, Veterinary Infection Control Committee: Compendium of Veterinary Standard Precautions: Zoonotic Diseases Prevention in Veterinary Personnel, 2006. Available at http://www.nasphv.org/Documents/VeterinaryPrecautions.pdf. Accessed November 21, 2006
89. National Association of State Public Health Veterinarians, Veterinary Infection Control Committee: Model infection control plan for veterinary practices, 2006. Available at http://www.nasphv.org/Documents/ModelInfectionControlPlan.doc. Accessed November 21, 2006

3.4 Hospital forms

Veronica Roberts and Shaun McKane

Documentation of care is an important part of medical treatment. Good documentation helps improve patient care by aiding transfer of information from one provider to another,[1] is important for legal reasons and enables accurate retrospective research and invoicing. A review of reports from human hospitals[2] suggested that improvements in information exchange would help prevent at least some of the incidents reported. The form must be designed in such a way as to include all standard relevant information yet also be flexible enough to enable reporting of facts specific to individuals.[3] Design of a form can have a significant impact on the completion rate of form elements.[2] Therefore, it is essential to design forms that aid the user in completion; with electronic forms some data points can be made mandatory. Ideally, the form should cover only one side of paper and, to standardise information, most data points should be designed as tick boxes or numerical scale data. With electronic forms, a pull-down menu should be used where possible to limit input options and semi-quantitative descriptions. Where comment is required, sufficient space should be given. The layout should follow a logical pattern. A limiting factor in realising the full potential of electronic medical records (EMRs) is physician reluctance to use these applications.[4] However, the use of EMRs should be encouraged to improve legibility, standardise and enforce responses, thereby aiding the processing and review of documents. The advent of the PDA is likely to make the use of electronic records more practical.

Consent forms

All clients should sign a consent form on arrival at the hospital that gives permission for examination, administration of drugs, sedation, anaesthesia and surgery (Figure 3.28). It is advisable at this stage to state the risk of mortality and morbidity from anaesthesia. Permission for euthanasia and post-mortem examination should also be obtained (Figure 3.29), including permission for retention of organs and tissues for clinical research. Following the Royal Liverpool Children's Hospital (Alder Hey) Enquiry[5] into retention of tissues, U.K. National Health Service guidelines are that the consent form should state that organs as well as small tissue samples may be retained. The client should agree that all records of investigation and treatment are the property of the hospital. In Europe, it is the veterinarian's duty to treat the horse as a food-producing animal unless a statutory waiver has been signed to exclude the animal from the food chain. It should be stated that the hospital is not responsible for mortality or morbidity of the inpatient unless staff are proved negligent. The client should agree to cover all costs, and at this stage it may be useful to give an estimate; however, an additional signature to that given for consent should be given for the estimate, due to the difficulty in reaching an accurate figure. Separate consent forms should be obtained, for example, for inclusion of the patient in a clinical trial.

The consent form must be written at a level consistent with a layperson's reading ability and in a format that is readily understandable.[6] Forms that are structured in bullet points and columns and illustrated with diagrams are perceived by the public as easier to read and have been shown to be better received than standard forms.[6] Clients signing a consent form for their horse are essentially performing the same procedure as parents signing a pediatric consent form. In a study of parental understanding of a pediatric consent form,[6] parents who received additional, verbal information showed greater understanding and less anxiety. Parents perceived their own level of understanding to be significantly greater than what was judged to be their real understanding when interviewed. This suggests that simply asking clients if they understand may be insufficient and reinforces the need to reiterate and clarify their understanding of the most important elements before informed consent is obtained.

Record keeping

A standard form should be filled in for every case, detailing the animal's signalment, the client's name and contact details and, where applicable, contact details for the referring veterinary surgeon. This is important not only for hospital administration but for future retrospective research studies. Parameters of critical cases at admission should also be recorded (Figures 3.30 and 3.31).

CONSENT FORM

THE UNIVERSITY OF LIVERPOOL
EQUINE HOSPITAL
Leahurst, Neston
Cheshire, CH64 7TE

Tel : 0151-794 6041
Fax: 0151-794 6034

I am the owner*/am acting on behalf of the owner*, of the animal detailed above. I give my consent to the following at the University of Liverpool Philip Leverhulme Large Animal Hospital:

1. For examination and performance of further investigations as appropriate, for sedation and/or anaesthesia, for the administration of treatment or medications (including agents licensed for use in other species or humans where appropriate).
2. For surgical operation (...) where appropriate.
3. For euthanasia if necessary for humane reasons.
4. For post mortem examination in the event of death or euthanasia.
5. For retention of tissues, organs and DNA for purposes of clinical research. Clinical research is necessary to further our understanding of diseases of horses so that we can improve the treatment and welfare of our patients (please ask if you want to know more about clinical research in this Department)
6. The animal is insured for veterinary fees with .... (the "Insurer"), I can confirm that I have notified them that I have brought the animal to the hospital.
7. I understand that the animal will be cared for by members of Hospital staff and students, and that whilst I can request a particular surgeon treats the animal, this may not always be possible.
8. I understand that all records of investigation and treatment are the property of the Hospital.
9. I agree to pay a deposit of £500 within 24 hours if requested and to pay the Hospital all costs and expenses necessary to treat the animal on presentation of invoice.
10. I agree to collect the animal when requested. Please note that a livery surcharge will be made if the horse is not collected within 48hrs of discharge notification unless prior arrangements have been made.
11. I agree that the Hospital will not be responsible to me if the animal dies whilst it is being treated or if the animal suffers any illness or injury as a result of the treatment, unless the veterinary surgeon or hospital staff are proved negligent.
12. I agree to abide by the regulations of the Equine Passport Scheme.

N.B. All anaesthetics, surgery and other procedures involve some risk to the patient.
All cases may be used for the purposes of teaching, under proper supervision.

SIGNATURE OF OWNER* OR AGENT* *(*Delete as appropriate)* **DATE:** ____________________

_________________________________ **NAME (PRINT):** ________________________________

OF (ADDRESS)____ **POST CODE:** ______ ______

Initial estimate of costs: £ ______________________________ Date: ________________________
This estimate does not constitute a final invoice and actual costs may vary if further diagnostic or therapeutic procedures become necessary.
I am over 18 years of age and accept responsibility for the bill.

I have left a deposit of £_______ in the form of :- Cash [ ] Credit Card [ ] Cheque [ ]

Deposit Received By ___________________________ Signature: ________________________________

Our accounts are due for payment upon presentation. We reserve the right to charge interest at a rate of 8% above Barclays Bank plc base rate on any accounts that are more than 28 days old. In addition you will be held liable for all recoverable collection costs. As members of *The Veterinary Register*, we reserve the right to post debt information with them which will automatically be issued to all other veterinary members. If the event of any dispute, English law applies.

Figure 3.28 Consent form for treatment used at the University of Liverpool. ©University of Liverpool 2006.

EUTHANASIA / DEATH IN HOSPITAL FORM

PLEASE STICK CASE LABEL HERE	**THIS FORM MUST BE COMPLETED BY CLINICAL STAFF DURING ANY DISCUSSION WITH A CLIENT ABOUT EUTHANASIA OR HOSPITAL DEATH, OR WITHIN 24 HOURS OF THE DEATH IF THE OWNER IS TOO UPSET AND NEEDS TIME TO DECIDE**

Please let clients know that their wishes are being recorded for our case records.

	CLIENT EUTHANASIA CHECKLIST ALWAYS Check the Consent Form for signature and deletions re post mortem and tissue retention prior to discussions.	**AGREED? (yes, no or N/A)**
1	Does the client agree to allow us to euthanase their horse (*if relevant*)?	
2	Is the client aware that this may not be classed as humane destruction and therefore that the insurance company ***will not pay out*** for mortality?	
3	Does the owner/insurance company want a full Post Mortem? ***If so, is the owner aware that the cost could be at least £320*** (inc VAT), depending on tests needed and that insurance companies ***will not*** pay this even if they request a PM? Cremation/disposal is charged on top of PM cost.	
4	Does the owner request private cremation? If so, please give estimate of costs from company price sheet (Possibly up ***to £1000)***, Owner to pay company direct, but we can arrange collection.	
5	Does the owner want communal cremation? If so, please let them know the cost for disposal is £235.	
6	If you would like to investigate the cause of death, make sure you ask the client's permission to do so. Please point out this **is not a full PM and there will be no written report, that the client will not be charged, but you must be willing to verbally discuss cause of death. In agreeing this with the owner, *you*** *are responsible and MUST take ownership of the task.*	
7	If yes to 3 or 6, remind the owner that, as already agreed in the Consent Form we may retain tissue and organs for future examination.	
	IF SPECIFIC CONSENT HAS NOT BEEN GIVEN, CLINICIANS *MUST NOT* TAMPER WITH THE BODY. NO P.M. MUST EVER BE PERFORMED WITHOUT THIS BEING CONFIRMED AND AGREED WITH THE OWNER ON THIS FORM	

	CLINICIAN CHECK LIST	
1	**Has permission to euthanase been given by the Insurance Company?**	
2	**Has the body been clearly labelled, with case number, horse name, owner name, cremation company name or Cluttons?**	
3	**Is owner requesting a piece of mane or tail?**	

Clinician to sign: ______________________ **Date:** ______________

PRINT NAME: ______________________ Feb 06/PJG

Figure 3.29 Clinicians' checklist for communications with owners regarding the euthanasia or death of their animal. ©University of Liverpool 2006.

THE PHILIP LEVERHULME EQUINE HOSPITAL, UNIVERSITY OF LIVERPOOL

EQUINE COLIC ADMISSION FORM

Owners name: ………………. V/S name: ………………… Case number: ……………

GENERAL HISTORY

B.I.0.P.: ……………………………… **Pre-Purchase examination?**: Y/N

Horse used for: general riding / racing / eventing / showjumping / breeding / other

Level of work: hours/day ……… novice / intermediate / advanced

Management: private stable / livery stable / racing yard / grass livery / other

Who cares for horse: owner / private groom / professional yard staff / friend

Bedding: shavings / straw / paper / other

Feeding: coarse mix / chaff/ mollychop / alf-alfa / bran / barley / oats / pellets or cubes / hay / soaked hay / silage or horsehage / grass

Worming: frequency: every …………wks / months

PRODUCT used last time: ……………………..

horse wormed in synchrony with others Y/N

Routine dental care? Y / N **by whom**: veterinary surgeon / horse dentist

Vices? none / crib-biting / windsucking / weaving / box-walking

Recent changes in routine or feeding (e.g. sedation for clipping, new hay, box rest, medication started) ………………………………………………………………………

How long since change occurred? ………………… hrs / days

Previous major disease or episodes of colic? Y/N

If "YES" please specify:………………………………………………………………

SHORT-TERM HISTORY

Date and time when colic first observed : ………………………………………………

Duration of colic (hours since last seen normal ie no colic symptoms) …………… hrs

Signs of colic: flank watching / pawing / lying still / kicking belly / rolling / violent rolling / sweating / muscle tremors / salivation / flatulence

Droppings over previous 12 hours : none / scant / normal / diarrhoea

Time of first visit by referring vet: ……………………………………………………

Response to treatment : none / improved / deteriorated / unknown

Time of subsequent visits by referring vet: ……………………………………………..

Decision to refer (approx. time): …………………………………………………………

Figure 3.30 Admission form for recording signalment, history and initial findings for horses with colic. ©University of Liverpool 2006.

CLINICAL EXAMINATION **Case number:** ………………..

Any current lameness present?: RF / LF / RH / LH
Lameness localised to particular area? Foot / fetlock / tendon / knee / hock / elbow/shoulder / stifle / hip
How was this localised? Nerve block / radiographs / scan / swelling / scan / other

Attitude: normal / painful / violent / dull and depressed / unwilling to move
Pain: none / mild / moderate / severe
Body condition: normal / fit / poor / overweight
Other signs: sweating / salivation / muscle fasciculation
Cleanliness of horse: clean clipped / clean unclipped / moderate / filthy

Cardiovascular system
Heart rate: ……………….. beats/min **Pulse quality**: normal / weak / bounding
Mucous membranes : normal /congested / cyanotic / pale / jaundiced / other
Extremities cold? Y/N **CRT:** ……………..… secs
PCV …………….. % **Total protein :** …………… g/litre

Gastrointestinal system
Abdominal distension? Y/N **Auscultation**:

Rectal examination : ……………………………………………………………………
……………………………………………………………………………………
……………………………………………………………………………………

Gastric reflux: Y/N **Volume**: …………… litres

Paracentesis: gross appearance: normal / turbid / sanguinous / gut contents / chylous / no fluid obtained / not performed
WBC: ………x10^9/litre **T.P.**: ……….. g/litre

Diagnostic imaging
Interpretation of any procedures performed: ……………………………………………
……………………………………………………………………………………..

PRE_SURGICAL DIAGNOSIS: (please complete this section)

……………………………………………………………………..
……………………………………………………………………………………..

Medical management: Y/N
Surgical management: Y/N
Outcome (if known at this time) survived/died/euthanased
before surgery/at surgery/after surgery/without surgery

Figure 3.30 *Continued*

Anglesey Lodge Equine Hospital Foal Intensive Care Programme

NEONATAL FOAL ADMISSION FORM

Owner: ____________ **Dam:** __________ **Sire:** ___________ **Date:** ________

Address: ____

Phone number: ________________ **Referring vet:** __________________________

Signalment:

Time since birth (hours)	Colt or Filly (circle one)	Breed	Length of Gestation (days)

Physical examination:

Heart rate	Respiratory rate	Rectal Temperature	Heart Auscultation
Blood Pressure	Mucous Membranes Pale Pink / Dark Pink / Red / Purple / White / Icteric	crt (seconds)	Petechiation Yes / No Ears / Oral mm / other
Neurological Status	Umbilicus	Joints	Eyes and Sclera

History:

(Record full history on separate sheet)

Meconium passed? Yes / No Enema given? Yes / No	Antibiotics given? Yes / No Which:	Fluids given? Yes / No Amount:	Colostrum given? Yes / No How Much:
Birth: Assisted / Unassisted Time taken:	Did foal stand? Yes / No How long after birth:	Did foal nurse? Yes / No How long after birth:	How many foals has mare had previously?

Initial Lab Data:

Blood Culture Submitted Yes / No	White Blood Cell Count	Neutrophil%	Lymphocyte%
pH	Arterial pCO2	Arterial pO2	Haematocrit
Sodium	Potassium	Ionised Calcium	Glucose
Lactate	Creatinine	Urea	**IgG**

Initial Treatment:

Catheter (circle): placed / present 1-lumen / 2-lumen Right / Left Jugular / Cephalic / Saphenous

Litres of Hartmann's given: 1 2 3 4

Litres of Plasma given: 1 2

Rate and amount of glucose given: 20ml/hr 40ml/hr 80ml/hr ________ml in first hour

Figure 3.31 Admission form for recording signalment, history and initial findings for neonatal foals. ©Kevin Corley 2007.

DAILY RECORD SHEET

DATE:
STUDENT:
RESIDENT/CLINICIAN:

STICK CASE LABEL HERE OR WRITE DETAILS
(Ask Office Staff for further sheets if required)

Animal Name:

Owner Name:

Case Number:

TIME	COMMENTS (INCLUDE WOUND HEALING/LAMENESS ASSESSMENT) & TPR		
A.M	T:	P:	R:
S			
O			
A			
	TURN SHEET OVER FOR ADDITIONAL SPACE		

ACTION PLAN – MEDICATIONS (include creams, eye drops, sprays, ointments, vitamins etc)

Generic name	Trade Name	Formulation (liq/paste)	Dose (mgs/ml)	Amount (in mgs)	Vol (mls)	Route	Freq	Time	Time	Time	Time	Time	Time

ACTION PLAN – CASE MANAGEMENT/FEEDING ETC.

****USE INTENSIVE CARE SHEETS IF MAKING MORE THAN 2 CHECKS/DAY****

Figure 3.32 Daily record sheet for hospitalised animals. ©University of Liverpool 2006.

INTENSIVE CARE SHEET

Use this sheet if making more than two checks per day - 1 SHEET PER 24hr (8am - 8am)

STICK CASE LABEL HERE OR COMPLETE:

Horse's name:
Owner's name:
Case Number:

DATE:		DAY#:					
TIME OF EXAM 24hr CLOCK	**CALL IF**	08:00					
Demeanor							
Pain							
Temperature							
Pulse rate and quality							
Resp rate and quality							
Mucous Mmbs							
Cap Refill Time							
Vein							
PCV TP							
Bloodwork - *K+*							
Mg++/Ca++							
Glucose							
Other							
No. of faeces							
Quality of faeces							
Wound Oedema							
Wound Disch.							
GI Motility							
Digital Pulses							
Reflux							
Crystalloids PLAN							
Rate prescribed L/hr							
Current drip rate drop/s							
Litres already hanging							
Litres received last 4hr							
New drip rate drop/s							
Bags fluid added							
Total litres hanging							
Electrolytes added							
Other (Colloids/Prokinetics)							
Food							
Grazing							
Water							
OTHER/COMMENTS							VROBERTS.SMCKANE.MBOWEN

CONTINUE ON REVERSE

Figure 3.33 Sheet for recording data from adult intensive care patients. ©University of Liverpool 2006.

BOX____OWNER__________________

Drug/Treatment	TIME	Date	Date	Date	Date	Date
Amount						
Route						
Frequency						

Drug/Treatment	TIME	Date	Date	Date	Date	Date
Amount						
Route						
Frequency						

Drug/Treatment	TIME	Date	Date	Date	Date	Date
Amount						
Route						
Frequency						

Drug/Treatment	TIME	Date	Date	Date	Date	Date
Amount						
Route						
Frequency						

Drug/Treatment	TIME	Date	Date	Date	Date	Date
Amount						
Route						
Frequency						

Figure 3.34 Simple form for ordering treatments for hospitalised patients. A box is drawn on the sheet against a time at which a treatment should be given, and this box is ticked (checked) when the treatment has been given. ©Anglesey Lodge Equine Hospital 2007.

Anglesey Lodge Equine Hospital Foal Intensive Care Programme

Owner: ____________ Foal: ____________ Date: ____________

TIME												
Position*												
Heart rate												
Temp												
Resp Rate												
mm												
GI Sounds												
Mean BP												
Systolic BP												
Diastolic BP												
Joints												
Umbilicus‡												
Urine Output (ml)												
Urine S.G.												
Faeces												
Blood Glucose												
Lactate												
Intranasal O_2 (L/min)												
Amt milk ordered												
Amount milk fed												
Amount reflux												

*Stand=has stood in last hr / LSR = Left Sternal Recumbency / RSR = Right Sternal Recumbency / LLR = Left Lateral Recumbency / RLR = Right Lateral Recumbency
‡Norm = normal / PU = Patent urachus / Thick = thickened / Pus – leaking pus

Figure 3.35 Sheet for recording data on hospitalised neonatal foals. ©Kevin Corley 2007.

Anglesey Lodge Equine Hospital Foal Intensive Care Programme

Owner: ____________________

DATE____________________

Foal: ____________________

Anglesey Lodge Equine Hospital

Procedure	TIMES
Check Over	1A 2A 3A 4A 5A 6A 7A 8A 9A 10A 11A 12N 1P 2P 3P 4P 5P 6P 7P 8P 9P 10P 11P 12M
	1A 2A 3A 4A 5A 6A 7A 8A 9A 10A 11A 12N 1P 2P 3P 4P 5P 6P 7P 8P 9P 10P 11P 12M
Milk Mare	1A 2A 3A 4A 5A 6A 7A 8A 9A 10A 11A 12N 1P 2P 3P 4P 5P 6P 7P 8P 9P 10P 11P 12M

Cross out and initial under circled procedures when given

Drug	Dose	Route	Frequency	TIMES
				1A 2A 3A 4A 5A 6A 7A 8A 9A 10A 11A 12N 1P 2P 3P 4P 5P 6P 7P 8P 9P 10P 11P 12M
				1A 2A 3A 4A 5A 6A 7A 8A 9A 10A 11A 12N 1P 2P 3P 4P 5P 6P 7P 8P 9P 10P 11P 12M
				1A 2A 3A 4A 5A 6A 7A 8A 9A 10A 11A 12N 1P 2P 3P 4P 5P 6P 7P 8P 9P 10P 11P 12M
				1A 2A 3A 4A 5A 6A 7A 8A 9A 10A 11A 12N 1P 2P 3P 4P 5P 6P 7P 8P 9P 10P 11P 12M
				1A 2A 3A 4A 5A 6A 7A 8A 9A 10A 11A 12N 1P 2P 3P 4P 5P 6P 7P 8P 9P 10P 11P 12M
				1A 2A 3A 4A 5A 6A 7A 8A 9A 10A 11A 12N 1P 2P 3P 4P 5P 6P 7P 8P 9P 10P 11P 12M
				1A 2A 3A 4A 5A 6A 7A 8A 9A 10A 11A 12N 1P 2P 3P 4P 5P 6P 7P 8P 9P 10P 11P 12M

Cross out and initial under circled treatments when given

Fluid	Additives	Initial Flow rate	TIMES
			1A 2A 3A 4A 5A 6A 7A 8A 9A 10A 11A 12N 1P 2P 3P 4P 5P 6P 7P 8P 9P 10P 11P 12M
			1A 2A 3A 4A 5A 6A 7A 8A 9A 10A 11A 12N 1P 2P 3P 4P 5P 6P 7P 8P 9P 10P 11P 12M
			1A 2A 3A 4A 5A 6A 7A 8A 9A 10A 11A 12N 1P 2P 3P 4P 5P 6P 7P 8P 9P 10P 11P 12M
			1A 2A 3A 4A 5A 6A 7A 8A 9A 10A 11A 12N 1P 2P 3P 4P 5P 6P 7P 8P 9P 10P 11P 12M

Circle to order treatments, procedures or fluid rate changes

Write changes in rate under the relevant time and initial

Figure 3.36 Daily sheet for ordering treatments for hospitalised neonatal foals. ©Kevin Corley 2007.

POST-OPERATIVE COLIC INFORMATION SHEET

Circle answers as applicable

Cleanliness of horse pre-op: *clean clipped / clean unclipped / moderately dirty / filthy*

Subcutaneous suture used? *Yes / No*

Stent used? *Yes / No*

Adhesive drape used in recovery? *Yes / No*

Post-op pain (up to day 7)? *None / Moderate / Severe*

DAY	INCISION OEDEMA	WOUND DRAINAGE	INFECTION
DAY 1 *date............*	*Normal / greater normal / severe*	*None / blood / serum / pus*	*Yes / No*
DAY 2 *date............*	*Normal / greater normal / severe*	*None / blood / serum / pus*	*Yes / No*
DAY 3 *date............*	*Normal / greater normal / severe*	*None / blood / serum / pus*	*Yes / No*
DAY 4 *date............*	*Normal / greater normal / severe*	*None / blood / serum / pus*	*Yes / No*
DAY 5 *date............*	*Normal / greater normal / severe*	*None / blood / serum / pus*	*Yes / No*
DAY 6 *date............*	*Normal / greater normal / severe*	*None / blood / serum / pus*	*Yes / No*
DAY 7 *date............*	*Normal / greater normal / severe*	*None / blood / serum / pus*	*Yes / No*
DAY 8 *date............*	*Normal / greater normal / severe*	*None / blood / serum / pus*	*Yes / No*
DAY 9 *date............*	*Normal / greater normal / severe*	*None / blood / serum / pus*	*Yes / No*
DAY 10 *date..........*	*Normal / greater normal / severe*	*None / blood / serum / pus*	*Yes / No*
DAY 11 *date.........*	*Normal / greater normal / severe*	*None / blood / serum / pus*	*Yes / No*
DAY 12 *date.........*	*Normal / greater normal / severe*	*None / blood / serum / pus*	*Yes / No*
DAY 13 *date.........*	*Normal / greater normal / severe*	*None / blood / serum / pus*	*Yes / No*
DAY 14 *date.........*	*Normal / greater normal / severe*	*None / blood / serum / pus*	*Yes / No*

Figure 3.37 Form for monitoring postsurgical colic patients. ©University of Liverpool 2006.

Dr. Lesley Young BVSc PhD DVA DipECVA DVC MRCVS

CARDIOVASCULAR EXAMINATION

GENERAL DETAILS:

NAME: SEX: AGE:

USE : BREED:

HISTORY:

PHYSICAL EXAMINATION:

PULSE RATE: .... QUALITY: ....

RHYTHM: ....

JUGULAR PULSE: .... MEMBRANES: ....

AUSCULTATORY FINDINGS:

LEFT HEMITHORAX

S_1 S_2 S_1 S_2 GRADE: ....

PRECORDIUM: .... PMI: .... RADIATION: ....

PRESUMPTIVE DIAGNOSIS: ....

RIGHT HEMITHORAX

S_1 S_2 S_1 S_2 GRADE: ....

PRECORDIUM: .... PMI: .... RADIATION: ....

PRESUMPTIVE DIAGNOSIS: ....

ECG REST: YES/ NO **ECG EXERCISE:** YES/NO

COMMENTS **COMMENTS**

ECHOCARDIOGRAM: YES/NO

COMMENTS:

FINAL DIAGNOSIS: ....

Figure 3.38 Form for recording the results of a cardiovascular examination. ©Lesley Young 2006.

Respiratory System Clinical Examination Sheet

PLACE CASE STICKER HERE

DATE:
USE:
CLINICIAN:
RESIDENT:
INTERN:

1. HISTORY

Complaint:____

Environment: Stabled ☐ Out at grass ☐ Combination ☐ Bedding: Shavings ☐ Straw ☐

Seasonality of condition: Spring ☐ Summer ☐ Autumn ☐ Winter ☐

Stress Factor: Recently moved ☐ New horses in group ☐ Illness ☐ Training ☐

2. CLINICAL EXAMINATION

	N	S	A
Demeanour			
Posture			
TPR			
Mucous Membranes			
Pulse Quality			
Jugular Pulse			
Hydration Status			
Sign of Pain			

4. LARYNX & TRACHEA

	At Rest		Post Exercise	
	N	A	N	A
Larynx Size & Shape				
Dorsal Musculature				
Slap Test				
Muscular process arytenoids				
Trachea size & shape				
Thoracic inlet palpation				
Laryngeal scarring				
Tracheostomy Scar				

Comments: ____

3. RESPIRATORY EXAMINATION

Cough: Non-productive ☐ Productive ☐ Soft ☐ Harsh ☐ Hacking ☐ Painful ☐

Respiratory Effort: Normal ☐ Insp Dyspnoea ☐ Exp. Dyspnoea ☐ Heave Line ☐

			AT REST					AFTER EXERCISE				
			N	S	A	U	B	N	S	A	U	B
Nasal airflow												
Nostril symmetry												
Nasal Mucosa												
False Nostril												
Breath Odour												
Alar Fold												
Frontal Sinus Percussion												
Max Sinus Percussion												
Submandibular LNs												
Parotid Region												
Discharges	U	B	m/mo/s	ser	muc	mp	haem	mms	ser	muc	mp	haem
Nasal Discharge												
Ocular Discharge												

Comments: ____

Figure 3.39 Form for recording a workup of the respiratory system. ©University of Liverpool 2006.

AUSCULTATION

	LEFT SIDE			RIGHT SIDE				
	Rales	Rhonchi	Pleur F	Rales	Rhonchi	Pleur F	INSP.	EXP.
Cran -V								
Caud -D								

Tracheal Auscultation: Cranial – N ☐ A ☐ **Thoracic Inlet** – N ☐ A ☐

Re-breathing Bag: L-side - Same ☐ Increased ☐ R-side – Same ☐ Increased ☐

Percussion: L-side – Normal ☐ Resonant ☐ Dull ☐ **Delineate Line of Transition on Diagram Overleaf**

R-side – Normal ☐ Resonant ☐ Dull ☐

6. ENDOSCOPY

	AT REST						AFTER EXERCISE					
	N		S		A		N		S		A	
Anatomical structure	L	R	L	R	L	R	L	R	L	R	L	R
Nasal Cavity												
Nasal Conchae												
Nasal Septum												
Nasomaxillary Drainage												
Ethmoturbinates												
Nasopharynx												
Guttural Pouch												
Soft Palate												
Epiglottis												
Arytenoid Cartilages												
Lateral Ventricles												
Larynx												
Trachea												
Bronchi/Carina												
Stertor/Roaring												

Comments: ____________________

____

Laryngeal Hemiplegia: Grade 1 ☐ Grade 2 ☐ Grade 3 ☐ Grade 4 ☐
(see overleaf for grading categories)

7. FURTHER DIAGNOSTIC TESTS

Haematology ☐ ____________________

Nasopharyngeal Swab ☐ ____________________

Tracheal Lavage ☐ ____________________

Bronchoalveolar Lavage ☐ ____________________

Thoracocentesis: Transudate ☐ Modified Transudate ☐ Exudate ☐ Chylous Effusion ☐

Radiography ☐ ____________________

Ventigraphy ☐ ____________________

Arterial Blood Gas Analysis ☐ ____________________

Ultrasonography ☐ ____________________

Lung Biopsy ☐ ____________________

Please record brief findings in spaces provided above

Guidelines to Respiratory Clinical Examination Sheet

Figure 3.39 *Continued*

Key:
2/3/4/6
N = Normal
S = Suspect
A = Abnormal
U = Unilateral
B = Bilateral

3. m/mo/s = Mild/Moderate/Severe (Indicate amount of discharge by choosing the relevant description)
ser = Serous Discharge
muc = Mucoid Discharge
mp = Mucopurulent Discharge
haem = Haemorrhagic Discharge

5. Cran-V = Cranio-ventral lung field
Caud-D = Caudo-dorsal lung field
Rales = Crackles – Detected in COPD and acute obstructive pulmonary disease and pulmonary oedema
Rhonchi = Wheezes – Musical notes that occur in obstructive lower airway diseases inc. COPD, bronchopneumonia
Pleur F = Pleural Friction - Crunching/creaking sounds that may be detected in early pleuritis
INSP. = On Inspiration
EXP. = On Expiration

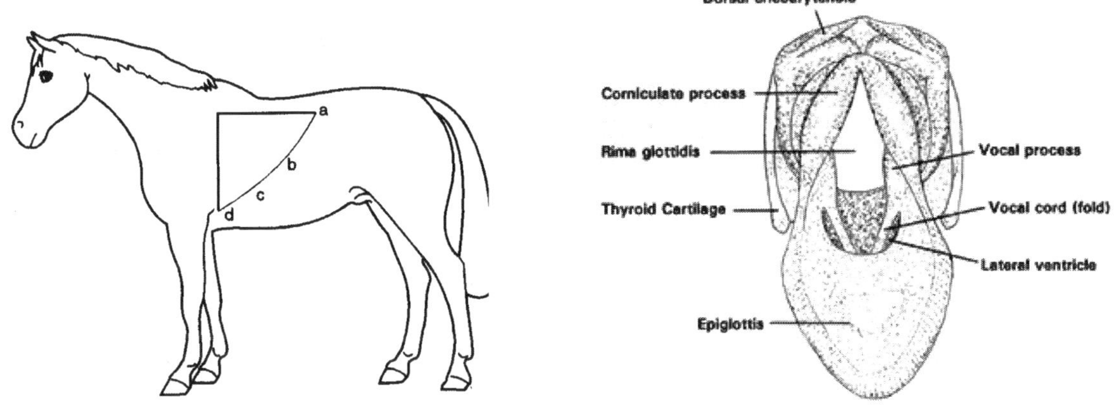

6. Grading Scheme for Laryngeal Anatomy (Annotate Diagram Above)

Grade I: Synchronous full abduction and adduction of left and right arytenoids cartilages.
Grade II: Asynchronous movement such as hesitation, flutters, adductor weakness of the left arytenoids during inspiration or expiration or both, but full abduction induced by swallowing or nasal occlusion.
Grade III: Asynchronous movement such as hesitation, flutters, adductor weakness of the left arytenoids during inspiration or expiration or both, but full abduction not induced and maintained by swallowing or nasal occlusion.
Grade IV: Significant asymmetry of the larynx at rest and lack of substantial movement of the left arytenoids.

7. Arterial Blood Gas Reference Ranges

pH	7.35-7.45
$PaCO_2$	35-45mmHg
PaO_2	> 80mmHg
HCO_3^-	22-26meq/l
Base Excess	-2 to +2 meq/l

Figure 3.39 *Continued*

Leahurst Hospital
University of Liverpool

1 Case number	2.Horse	3. Owner
4.Referring vet		5.Date

6a.Signalmen	Age	Gender	Weight	Breed	Height
	Activity			Type of life	

6b.History

6c	Complaint	Onset
Kery Words	Progress	Event related to complaint

6d.General examination

HR

PassExam	LF			RF			LH			RH			L			Back			R		
	N	S	A	N	S	A	N	S	A	N	S	A	N	S	A	N	S	A	N	S	A

12.AnatPal	7.Superficial palp
Shoes	neck
Feet	fl/wither
Coronet	thorax
Pastern	lumb
Fetlock	sc/glut 1
Met	8.Deep Palpation
Carp/hock	L · Midline · R
Rad/tibia	
Elbow/stifle	
Sch/hip	
13.Susp lgt	9.Muscles
14.Flex.	neck
Distal	fl
Carpus	th
Proximal	lumb
15.Extens.	hl
16.H.Tester	10.Flexions
Toe	LF · DF/VF · LF
Md T-quart	
Lat T-quart	neck
Med.heel	th-lumb
Lat. Heel	11.Conformation
Frog	
Heel/heel	19.Transrectal palpation
17.Toe ext t	genitalia
18.Conform	arteries
20.Summary passive exam	L6-S1
	L5-L6
	Psoas
	L3
	Other

Figure 3.40 Form for recording the results of a complete lameness workup. ©University of Liverpool 2006.

Leahurst Hospital
University of Liverpool

Active	L			R			L			R						
Exam	N	S	A	N	S	A	N	S	A	N	S	A		N	S	A
21.Walk/L													Backwards			
Walk/R													Head elevated			
Balance													Patella			
22.Neuro																
23.Trot str																
Trot/L/Hard													Roller			
Trot/R/Hard													Saddle			
Trot/L/Soft													Other			
Trot/R/Soft																
Hoof tester													26.Summary active ex			
24.Flexion																
Distal																
Carpal																
Proximal																
Abduction																
25.Other tst																
27.Plan of action/(1)Asking the clinical question																
28.Blocks													***32.(1)Refining the clinical question***			
29.x rays																
30.U sounds																
31.Scinti																
33.(2)Search strategy for the best evidence/(3)critical appraising																
34.(4)Clinical application/TTM/Discharge instructions																
35.(5)Self-assessment																

Figure 3.40 *Continued*

LA NEUROLOGIC EXAMINATION

History and complaint:

General Observations: **Standing?** **Recumbent?** **Sweating?**

Mentation/Behavior:

Neck/body symmetry:

Manipulation of neck:

Spontaneous involuntary movements (tremors, myoclonus, myotonia):

CRANIAL NERVE EXAMINATION: (N - normal; AB - abnormal, NE- not evaluated)

Menace:
Pupil size:
Pupil symmetry:
PLR:
Doll's eye:
Pathological nystagmus:

Facial symmetry- expressive:
Facial symmetry- mastication Mm:
Palpebral reflex:
Gag reflex :
Slap test :
Tongue pull :

Reflexes (increased, decreased, normal, not evaluated)

Tail tone ______
Anal ______
Patellar ______
Triceps ______
Withdrawal ______
Other ______

Urinary LMN UMN
Rectal ______
Sweating ______

Cutaneous sensation dermatomes:

Pain sensation dermatomes:

Figure 3.41 Form for recording the results of a neurological examination.

GAIT and PROPRIOCEPTION - Description in terms of Ataxia, Weakness, Dysmetria:

Grading: 0 – No gait deficits / 1 – Deficits barely perceptible, worse with provocations / 2 – Deficits noted at walk / 3 – Deficits noted at rest, walking; nearly falls with head elevation / 4 – Nearly falls at normal gaits

Stance:

Walk:

Sway reaction (standing):
- Left:
- Right:

Hopping (if possible):
- Left
- Right

Sway reaction (walking):
- Left
- Right

Backing:

Elevation of head:

Circling:

Up/down incline:

Trot:

	Ataxia	Dysmetria	Weakness
LF			
RF			
LH			
RH			

ASSESSMENT/COMMENTS:

LESION LOCALIZATION:

DIFFERENTIAL DIAGNOSIS:

DIAGNOSTICS:

- ☐ CSF: L/S A/O
- ☐ Radiographs, myelogram
- ☐ EMG, EEG

Figure 3.41 *Continued*

ABDOMINAL ULTRASOUND

Circle the relevant findings and record all measurements.
State if not visualised/examined.

CASE LABEL

Examination number:

BRIEF HISTORY

____

____

LEFT SIDE

Left kidney			
Size	Reduced	Normal	Increased
Architecture	Normal	Abnormal	
Location	Normal	Abnormal	
Spleen			
Size	Reduced	Normal	Increased
Architecture	Normal	Abnormal	
Echogenicity	Hypoechoic	Normal	Hyperechoic
Location	Normal	Abnormal	
Nephrosplenic space			
	Not visualised	Normal	Displaced colon
Stomach			
Size (<5 rib spaces)	Normal	Distended	
Wall architecture	Normal	Abnormal	
Location	Normal	Abnormal	
Small intestine			
Wall thickness (<4mm)	____mm	Normal	Thickened
Motility	Hypomotile	Normal	Hypermotile
Luminal diameter (<5cm)	_____cm	Normal	Distended
Location	Normal	Abnormal	
Strangulating lesion	Visualised	Not visualised	
Left dorsal colon			
Wall thickness (<4mm)	____mm	Normal	Thickened
Motility	Hypomotile	Normal	Hypermotile
Location	Normal	Abnormal	
Left ventral colon			
Wall thickness (<4mm)	____mm	Normal	Thickened
Motility	Hypomotile	Normal	Hypermotile
Location	Normal	Abnormal	

Figure 3.42 Form for recording the results of an abdominal ultrasound. ©University of Liverpool 2006.

PERITONEAL SPACE

Fluid amount	Normal	Increased
echogenicity	Normal	Increased

RIGHT SIDE

Right kidney			
Size	Reduced	Normal	Increased
Architecture	Normal	Abnormal	
Location	Normal	Abnormal	
Caecum			
Motility	Hypomotile	Normal	Hypermotile
Location	Normal	Abnormal	
Right dorsal colon			
Wall thickness (<4mm)	____mm	Normal	Thickened
Motility	Hypomotile	Normal	Hypermotile
Location	Normal	Abnormal	
Right ventral colon			
Wall thickness (<4mm)	____mm	Normal	Thickened
Motility	Hypomotile	Normal	Hypermotile
Location	Normal	Abnormal	
Duodenum			
Wall thickness (<4mm)	____mm	Normal	Thickened
Motility	Hypomotile	Normal	Hypermotile
Location	Normal	Abnormal	
Liver			
Size	Reduced	Normal	Increased
Architecture	Normal	Abnormal	
Echogenicity	Hypoechoic	Normal	Hyperechoic
Location	Normal	Abnormal	

TRANSRECTAL

Bladder			
Wall thickness	____mm	Normal	Thickened
Wall architecture	Normal	Abnormal	
Calculi	Visualised	Not visualised	
Ureters			
Architecture Left	Normal	Abnormal	
Right	Normal	Abnormal	
Calculi	Left ureter	Right ureter	Not visualised
Aorta			
Blood flow	Normal	Abnormal	
Left kidney			
Width (10-14cm)	____cm	Normal	Abnormal

Figure 3.42 *Continued*

Reproductive Organs

Uterus	Normal	Abnormal
Left ovary	Normal	Abnormal
Right ovary	Normal	Abnormal
Accessory sex glands	Normal	Abnormal

SUMMARY OF ABNORMAL FINDINGS

____

____

____

____

DIFFERENTIALS

____

____

____

PLAN

____

____

____

RECORDS (Please tick)

Pictures	Attached		Stored on computer	
Video	Attached		Stored on computer	

NB – A detailed examination of the reproductive organs warrants a reproductive examination form and should not be recorded on this sheet.

Figure 3.42 *Continued*

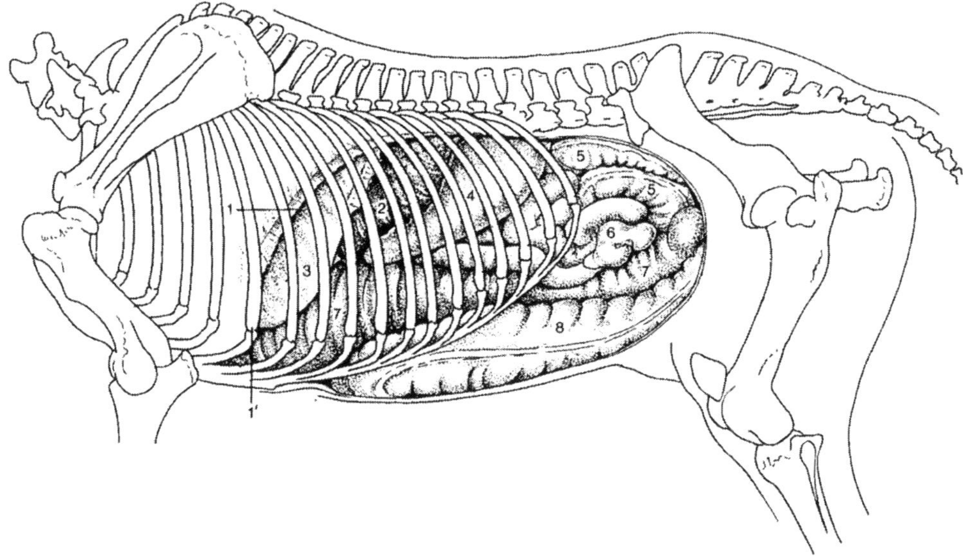

Visceral projections on the left abdominal wall (including the diaphragm).

1, Cut edge of diaphragm; 1′, rib 6; 2, stomach; 3, liver; 4, spleen; 5, descending colon (banded); 6, jejunum (smooth); 7, left dorsal colon; 8, left ventral colon.

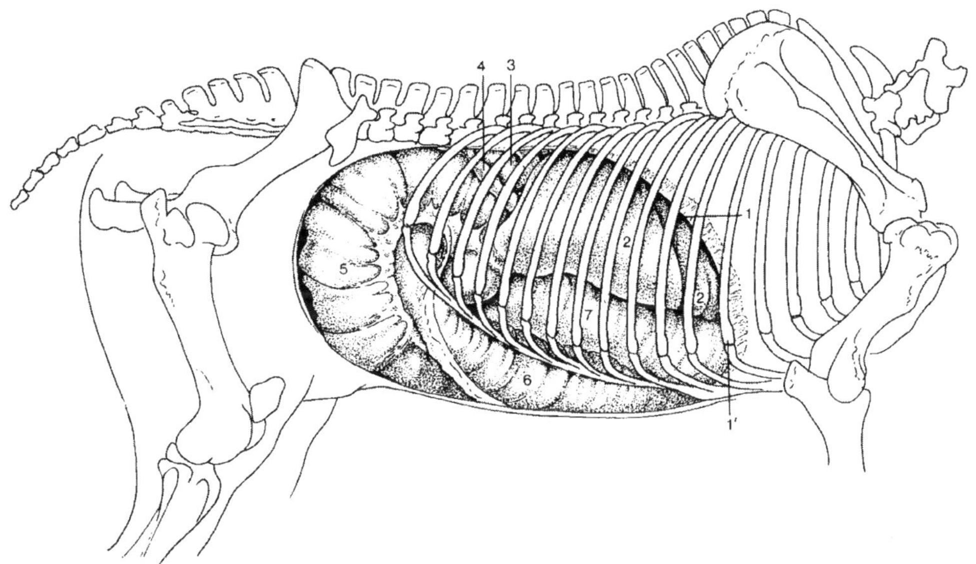

Visceral projections on the right abdominal wall (including the diaphragm).

1, Cut edge of diaphragm; 1′, rib 6; 2, liver; 3, right kidney; 4, descending duodenum; 5, body of cecum; 6, right ventral colon; 7, right dorsal colon.

Figure 3.42 *Continued*

SURGERY REPORT	STICK CASE LABEL HERE OR COMPLETE:
DATE:	**Horse's name:**
SURGEON:	**Owner's name:**
RESIDENT:	**Case Number:**
STUDENT:	

PROCEDURE PERFORMED:

STANDARD SURGERY COSTS		SET PRICE PROCEDURES	
Theatre set up		Hobday	
Surgery time - # hours		Hobday & tieback	
Linear cutter - # firings		Castration - yearling	
Laser treatment - standing		Castration – 2+ years	
Laparoscopic surgery - # hours		Umbilical hernia - simple	
Laparoscopy (standing) set up		Rig inguinal	
Bags fluids (flushing)		Rig abdominal	
Other special consumables (list)		Laparoscopic ovariectomy (bilateral)	
e.g. plates, screws antibiotic beads, hernia mesh		Cataract surgery	
		Others, please list:	

SURGERY REPORT

Post-operative management instructions:

Diagnosis/es:

Signed (Clinician): **Signed (Student):**

Pjg/jan06

Figure 3.43 Surgery report form. ©University of Liverpool 2006.

Progress notes

These may take the form of a structured sheet for daily clinical examination and then further investigation, or a more flexible method of recording, may be employed (Figure 3.32).

Monitoring and treatment sheets

Orthopaedic, surgical, medical, neonatal and intensive care cases all have different requirements so it is advisable to have different forms for at least some of these cases (Figures 3.33 through 3.37). Recording of fluid therapy must allow not only recording of the prescribed fluid rate but also recording of the actual volume received by the horse so that the rate can then be adjusted accordingly. Daily drug regimen should be clearly recorded, including drug name (generic and brand name), dose rate (mg or international units [IU] per kg), dose (total mg), formulation, concentration, volume prescribed, method of administration and dosing interval. It may also be useful to record how many days that drug has been used for. Provision should also be made be for recording drugs given as required, such as sedatives.

Specialist examination forms

These should be employed when considering specific body systems or conditions so that a standardised examination protocol is followed (Figures 3.38 to 3.43).

Discharge instructions and client information sheets

Discharge instructions are extremely important to inform the client (and referring vet, if applicable) what further treatment is required for their horse. These tend to be very disease or condition specific, and the only standard sections are likely to be the headings. However, horses with similar conditions are likely to require similar instructions. Therefore, building up a computer bank of previously written discharge instructions, catalogued by condition, can allow the clinician to alter previous instructions to suit the current animal and save time.

Information leaflets for the client to take home and read are invaluable in increasing client understanding of specific disease processes and of preventative care.

References

1. Horsky J, Kuperman GJ, Patel VL: Comprehensive analysis of a medication dosing error related to CPOE. J Am Med Inform Assoc 12(4):377-382, 2005
2. Marco AP, Buchman RN, Lancz C: Influence of form structure on the anaesthesia preoperative evaluation. J Clin Anesth 15(6):411-417, 2003
3. Lovis CL, Lamb A, Baud R, Rassinoux AM, Fabry P, Geissbuhler A: Clinical documents: attribute-values entity representation, context, page layout and communication. AMIA Annu Symp Proc 396-400, 2003
4. Sittig DF, Kuperman GJ, Fiskio J: Evaluating physician satisfaction regarding user interactions with an electronic medical record system. Proc AMIA Symp 400-404, 1999
5. The Report of The Royal Liverpool Children's Enquiry, 1999
6. Tait AR, Voepel-Lewis T, Malviya S, Philipson SJ: Improving the readability and processability of a pediatric informed consent document; effects on parents' understanding. Arch Pediatr Adolesc Med 159(4):347-352, 2005

4

Anaesthesia

Lydia Donaldson

4.1 General anaesthesia
4.2 Anaesthesia for some specific situations
4.3 Total intravenous anaesthesia
4.4 Standing surgery sedation and anaesthesia
4.5 Postanaesthetic morbidity

When the editors approached me to write a chapter on anaesthesia for the hospitalized horse, their request was for a "very practical discussion" and that I "share my thoughts". The following will, therefore, be that: my thoughts based on my experience. These observations may not apply to all physical layouts and clinical dynamics as most of my practice has been in one location with a limited group of clinicians.

4.1 General anaesthesia

Facilities

To properly perform surgery and general anaesthesia of duration longer than 15 to 30 minutes, a room dedicated to that purpose should be included in the hospital design. Operating room (OR) design is discussed in detail elsewhere in this book but from the perspective of an anaesthetist, the room must be big enough to permit easy navigation around a 17-hand horse in lateral recumbency, all the surgical toys (arthroscopy or laparoscopy cabinet, endoscope, etc), anaesthesia machine and monitor(s).

The decision to include an anteroom for aseptic preparation of the patient is a matter of the surgeon's personal preference. For elective cases, clipping and the initial surgical scrub can often be done before the horse is anaesthetised, thereby reducing recumbency time, which is always an objective of equine anaesthesia. Sometimes this is also possible for emergencies but, more often than not, these cases are clipped and prepped under general anaesthesia. For an anaesthetist, pausing between induction and the OR is awkward. The anaesthetic management choices during this period are (1) to maintain the horse with either an injectable or inhalant anaesthetic, (2) to support (or not) ventilation and oxygenation or (3) how aggressively to monitor. Monitoring with a finger on the pulse has much to be said for it, but if a problem occurs, it would be difficult to specifically identify and document. Many cardiac arrests during equine anaesthesia occur within 30 minutes of induction,[1,2] a period of anaesthetic and physiological flux. Not including a surgical prep stop in the move from induction to the OR minimises the period of limited monitoring and support with, anecdotally, no apparent increase in the incidence of relevant surgical complications.

Induction area

Induction and recovery areas are often and easily the same space. One consideration during hospital construction is to estimate the expected surgical caseload and its distribution over a workweek. If it is anticipated that several surgeries will be done in a day, then the hospital design should include more than one induction/recovery area per OR. The most efficient arrangement of these spaces is to have two induction/recovery rooms open onto one side of the OR. This necessitates either two hoists, one hoist with a track that allows it to be run into both induction/recovery rooms or some other means by which to get the horse onto the surgery table. An equivalent alternative is to have the induction/recovery areas on opposite sides of the OR with a single hoist traversing the OR. In this configuration, the hoist and track could be used to help position a horse during surgery. Whether hoists are OR clean might be debatable.

Hoisting horses by their legs is certainly the easiest way to pick them up and carefully position them on the surgical table. The combination of pulling on limbs designed to bear weight, ventroflexing a thoracolumbar spine designed for minimal movement and collapsing the abdominal viscera into the diaphragm is physiologically worrisome. That we do not recognise problems related to these stresses is probably because they are more subtle than the insult associated with the primary indication for surgery. The ventroflexion and thoracic compression can be reduced slightly by using a bar on the hoist hook to attach the limb hobbles to instead of bringing all four feet to a single point (Figure 4.1).

An alternative to hoisting that has been incorporated in the design of a number of equine hospitals is to build the

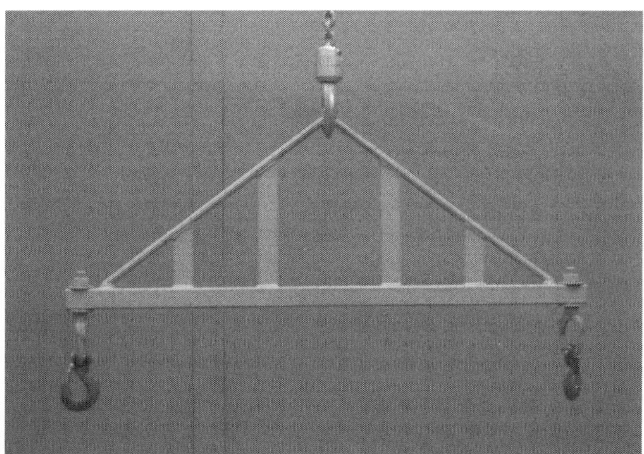

Figure 4.1 Bar on hook and chain of a hoist used to lift horses while putting less stress on its back and legs than if all 4 feet were bunched at the hook. ©Lydia L. Donaldson, 2007.

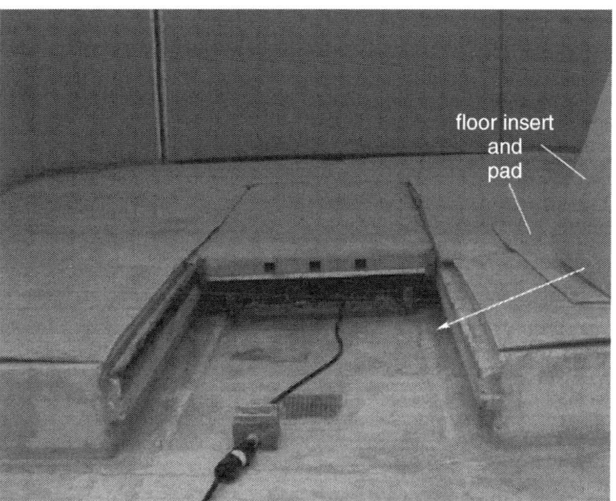

Figure 4.2 Surgery table designed to be part of the induction/recovery floor. ©Lydia L. Donaldson, 2007.

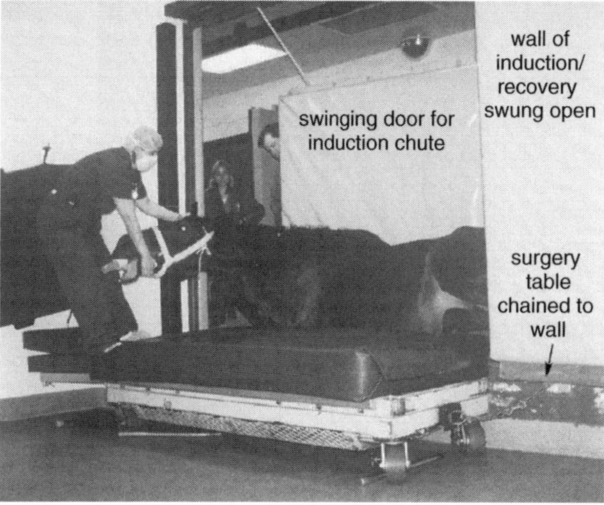

Figure 4.3 Surgery table fastened to the wall beneath the wall/door of the induction/recovery stall in a transitional room between induction/recovery and the OR. ©Lydia L. Donaldson, 2007.

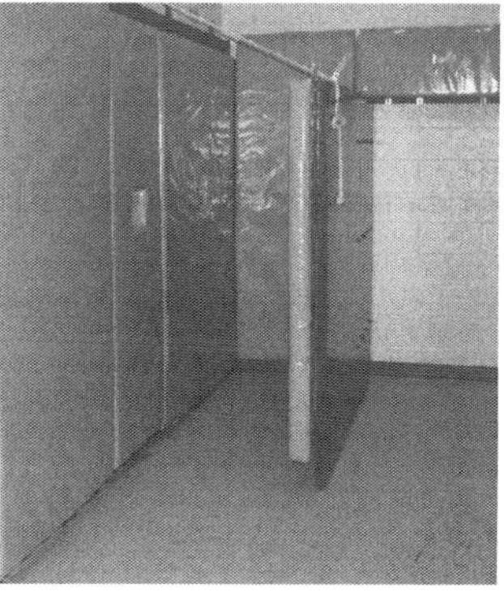

Figure 4.4 Induction space created by a partition hinged on the back wall and secured by a rope over the horse's head. ©Lydia L. Donaldson, 2007.

OR below ground level such that the surgery table surface is level with the floor of induction/recovery. With these systems, the wall between induction/recovery and the OR can be moved away. Once the horse is induced, the wall is opened and the horse is positioned on the surgery table and moved to the OR. One of the oldest of these designs is to have the surgery table as part of the induction/recovery floor (Figure 4.2). Variants of this are to have the table surface be round and rotate out into the OR or the surgery table be an extension of the induction/recovery floor so the horse can be pulled on that surface into the OR. Major problems with these methods are difficulty keeping the OR and surgery table clean of the inevitable dirt associated with recovery and covering the interface between table and floor to create a smooth surface for recovery. To minimise OR contamination, there can be an anteroom between induction/recovery and the OR. In this room, the surgery table can be fastened to the wall beneath the hinged wall, the horse rolled on to the table and table plus horse moved to the OR (Figure 4.3). Such a room can serve as a place to do less sterile procedures such as hoof sole explorations or endoscopic relief of oesophageal obstructions. For the average-size horse, four people—one each on head, tail and pairs of legs—can position the horse properly on the table and can pull the horse off the table into recovery.

Intuitively, induction behind a swinging partition seems safer for all involved. The partition should extend to the surface of the floor to prevent the horses' legs from being caught in compromising positions (Figure 4.4). Most induction techniques result in the horse sitting back and sinking down. Ideally this involves flexion of the hindlegs but often they slide forward in extension leaving the horse in an awkward, potentially stressful position. Rarely, the patellae lock requiring the partition to be open and the tail pulled to shift the horse down. Securing the open end of the swinging partition to the wall with a rope that goes over the horse's head, not across its chest, prevents possible jugular occlusion and/or catheter damage as the horse's head is lowered with sedation and when the horse drops to recumbency. A swinging partition, however, is not necessary and is an additional construction expense. Standing the horse next to the wall, with its hindquarters in a corner, a person on its head and another by its shoulder to help guide it down often works just as well with only slightly added risk to personnel. A third person at the horse's hip contributes that much more persuasion for a controlled drop.

Recovery room

There are as many recovery room designs as equine anaesthesiologists and surgeons. The debates stem, in part, from differences in philosophy on how to let or help horses recover. There is no debate over the need for padded walls and these should be high enough that a tall horse cannot hit the wall above it with lips and teeth (approximately 3 metres). Whether the corners should be square to offer the horse a place to lodge its face as a fifth point of support when it stands or rounded so the horse is carried around the stall without impacting the wall bluntly or occluding its nares in a corner is a matter of opinion. Not having the recovery stall too big (3.5–4 × 3.5–4 m) can discourage early efforts to stand as the horse is confronted with a wall as it moves forward. Smaller recovery areas also decrease the speed of impact with the wall for those horses that insist on standing before they can balance. They do need enough room to lever their head and neck as they pull themselves up over their front legs and get their hind feet under them. Some cushion should be added to the floor to protect from direct trauma and offer some traction. Whether this is merely a layer of rubber, firm or soft, textured or smooth or vinyl covered foam padding and whether the horse is placed on additional mats (approximately 30 cm × 1.5 m × 3 m) for the recumbency phase are some of the variations in use today. Even if head and tail ropes are not going to be used routinely, it would be prudent to put rings approximately 3 metres high on one wall (or the corners of opposite walls spanning one wall) so rope support would bring a horse up against a wall to lean on. Keep in mind that cleaning the recovery area is very important and the easier it is to do, the better it will be done. No one has studied the effect of recovery stall design, floor surface or management on the occurrence of life-threatening injury. Such a study would best be a prospective study over many years and would probably still not control for the infinite number of variables intrinsic to the situation independent of the many management methods. Oxygen should be available for recovery.

Storage

Although perhaps not essential, a small room near the OR dedicated to storage of anaesthesia supplies and extra equipment is something to consider during hospital construction. This is more important with a higher volume surgical load where having spare and a larger selection of endotracheal tubes, rebreathing bags and ECG leads could make the difference in a successful day of surgery and anaesthesia.

Equipment

Surgical table: Positioning and padding

The subtleties of surgical table design are certainly not my bailiwick. The table and its accessories must provide for the ability to position the horse in either lateral or dorsal recumbency without creating unnecessary pressure or tension on any muscle group or nerve. This includes passive stretch on adductor muscles and distal limb innervation and blood supply. Being able to support the legs in some way as best as the surgical or diagnostic procedure permits, regardless of the position, is fundamental. They should be supported in as close to a neutral position as possible. If potentially compromising positions are needed to successfully complete the surgery, intermittent release of the leg from the abnormal position will help protect against muscle or nerve injury and consequent weakness in recovery that could lead to catastrophic injury. Surgical table padding is another subject of debate and opinion. The conclusion to draw from the several studies that have demonstrated the importance of position and padding to intracompartmental muscle pressures[3–5] is that some padding is desirable, but perhaps more important is that the surface be even and smooth and the horse be positioned with care.

Large-animal anaesthesia machines

A summary of the basic equipment recommended for anaesthesia of horses in the hospital setting is listed in Table 4.1. Not all the elements listed are essential, and the costs shown are approximate. Globally, there is a fair selection of large-animal anaesthesia machines available (Box 4.1). All models have their critics and advocates. The non-specialist should choose a unit with a track record (i.e., has been on the market long enough to have gone out of production if it was difficult to operate or dangerous). If equine general anaesthesia is a completely new venture, consultation with an anaesthesiologist on both the purchase and initial use of the equipment is advised.

The basic large animal anaesthesia machine (Figure 4.5) is just an enlarged version of a small-animal circle system. Circle systems should include an oxygen flowmeter, an out-of-the-circle riser vaporiser, an oxygen flush valve and the rebreathing circuit consisting of breathing hoses, a Wye-piece, an inspiratory and an expiratory one-way valve, a CO_2 absorber canister, a rebreathing bag and a pressure relief valve. Ventilators are options. They may be purchased separately or as integral parts of the anaesthesia machine. A machine that can be used with or without a ventilator (Figure 4.6) will allow safer anaesthesia, in that ventilation can be assisted manually with the rebreathing bag if the ventilator malfunctions. The first step in familiarising yourself with an anaesthesia machine is to trace the oxygen flow into and around the circle, identifying each component.

The requirements for an anaesthesia machine to function properly are that the flowmeter(s) allow controlled

Table 4.1. Equine anaesthesia equipment

Equipment	Accessories	Approximate cost new (US$)
Anaesthesia machines		
Large-animal circle system*		$7,000–10,000
—Flowmeter	30-L rebreathing bag	$160
—Out-of-the-circle vaporizer	15-L rebreathing bag	$160
—CO_2 absorber canister	50-mm ID rebreathing hoses	$70
—Two unidirectional valves	50-mm Y-piece	$200
—In-circle manometer	CO_2 absorber	$125/gal
—O_2 flush valve		
—(Drain)		$700–$900
Weanling conversion	Smaller absorber canister and hoses	
Large-animal ventilator*	10–20-L bellows	$8–$12,000
Weanling conversion	Smaller bellows and housing	$900
Small-animal circle system for foals <150 kg	Double CO_2 absorber canister	$3–$4,000
	5-Liter rebreathing bag	$20–$40
	22-mm ID rebreathing hoses 22-mm Y-piece	$5–10
Endotracheal and nasotracheal tubes (NT)	Adults: 26- and 30-mm ID, 100 cm	$150
	20- and 22-mm ID, 90 cm	$90
	Weanlings: 16–18-mm ID, 70–75 cm	$70
	Foals: 10-, 12-, 14-mm ID, 55–57 cm	$50
	NT: 7-, 8-, 9-mm ID, 55 cm	$70
Demand valve	At 50 psi, max flow = 40–160 L/m	$300
Monitors		
Cardiovascular	Monitor	$10,000
	Three-limb ECG leads and cable	$150–$300
	Pressure transducer	$60–$150
	Pressure transducer cable	$200–$400
	Arterial catheter, extension set and three-way stopcock	$3
	Flexible temperature probe	$130
Blood gas analyzer (point of care)		$8,000
Other	Pulse oximeter	$1,000
	Sensors	$75–$200
	Capnograph	$3,000
	Anaesthetic agent	$4,000
Recovery		
	Wall mats	$4,000
	Flooring	$2,000
	Pads (≈30 cm × 1.5 m × 3 m)	$800

*Frequently incorporated as a single unit = $13,000–$18,000.
ID, internal diameter; NT = nasotracheal.

fresh gas flow, the vaporiser deliver an accurate inhalant anaesthetic output, the one-way valves prevent reverse flow in the circle, the carbon dioxide (CO_2) absorber granules* be active and the whole system not leak so badly as to contaminate the operating theatre with anaesthetic gas. In the United States, oxygen (O_2) is supplied as a gas in a variety of sizes of high-pressure cylinders or as a liquid. The latter is only economical for hospitals with a high surgical caseload and a neonatal intensive care unit. In a busy hospital, it might be advantageous to have a small E cylinder of O_2 [2200 pounds per square inch (gauge) (psig), approximately 7000 L] on hand for emergencies that occur beyond the reach of the hospital's built in O_2 outlets, as they are easily transported. However, the main supply of O_2 will be several larger H cylinders (2200 psig, approximately 7000 L) stored in a protected storage area that is easily accessible from the outside of the hospital. Oxygen use is determined by anaesthesia circuit flowmeter settings (3–10 L/min), ventilators settings (respiration rate, tidal volume) and use in recovery (160 L/min per breath by demand valve versus 10–15 L/min insufflation). Ventilators can be driven by any nonflammable, compressed gas, but it is reasonable to use O_2 as its cost is comparable to that of other compressed air, and having a single gas source eliminates the need for additional regulators. In large

*Sodasorb; Grace Darex Packaging Technologies, Cambridge, MA, USA.

Box 4.1. Some large-animal anaesthesia equipment sources

Source	Equipment
BDO Medipass The Netherlands www.veterinarytechnics.com	Circle and ventilator Ventilator
Burtons of Maidstone Ltd. Kent, UK www.burtons.uk.com	Circle SurgiVet circle and ventilator
H.B. Hospitalar Sao Paulo, Brazil www.hbhospitalar.com.br	Circle and ventilator
Hallowell Engineering and Manufacturing Corp. Pittsfield, MA, USA www.hallowell.com	60- and 78-inch transparent breathing tubes Y-piece ± sampling port ET tube brush Vaporizers
JD Medical Distributing Co., Inc. Phoenix, AZ, USA www.jdmedical.com	Circle and ventilator Ventilator Weanling conversion Manufacturer will customise Demand valve
Mallard Medical, Inc. Redding, CA, USA www.mallardmedical.net	Circle and ventilator Ventilator
Matrx/ Orchard Park, NY, USA www.matrxmedical.com	Circle
Miden Medical Tullamarine, Victoria, Australia www.midenmedical.com.au	Circle designed for hospital or field use
Minerve France www.minerve.com.fr	Circle and ventilator
SurgiVet (Smith Medical) MN, USA www.surgivet.com www.smiths-medical.com	Circle and ventilator Ventilator Weanling conversion Bivona endotracheal tubes Monitors Scavenge systems
Dandy Products, Inc. Goshen, OH, USA www.dandyproductsinc.com	Recovery wall pads and floor Mats and pads
Shank's Veterinary Equipment, Inc. Milledgeville, IL, USA www.shanksvet.com	Recovery wall and floor Mats and pads Hobbles

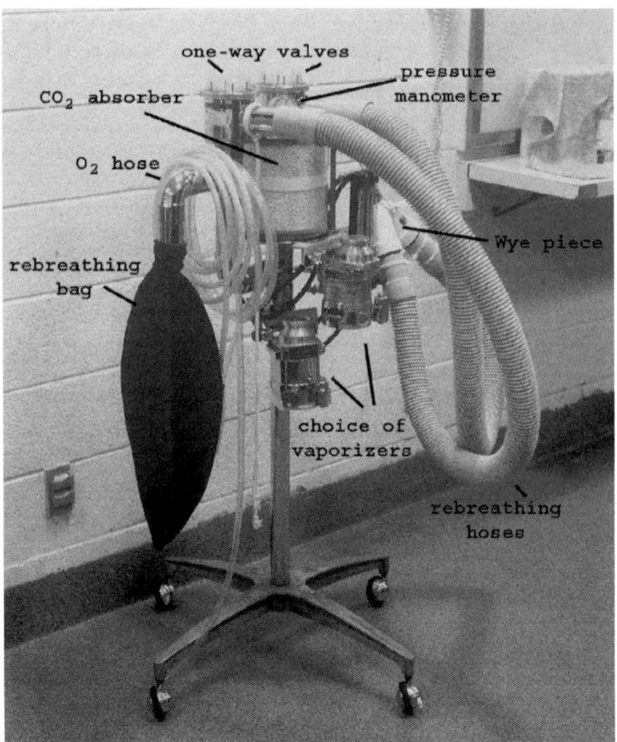

Figure 4.5 Basic large animal anaesthesia circle system with vaporiser(s) outside the circle. ©Lydia L. Donaldson, 2007.

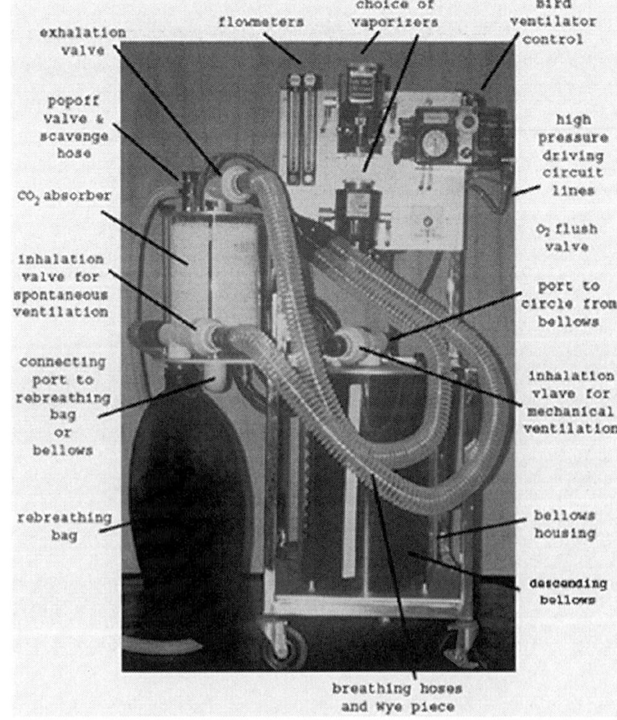

Figure 4.6 Large animal anaesthesia machine designed to be used with spontaneous or mechanical ventilation. ©Lydia L. Donaldson, 2007.

referral centres it might be economical to have an air compressor. Ninety minutes of ventilation-assisted anaesthesia for a 500-kg horse would be expected to consume 5000 to 6000 L of O_2 (i.e., approximately one H cylinder). Oxygen outlets in the hospital should be located in the OR and recovery, perhaps in one stall in the barn, a neonatal intensive care area and a receiving/treatment area. From the high-pressure oxygen source (2200 psig), a regulator reduces the O_2 pressure to 50 psig. Standard flowmeters, ventilators and demand valves are calibrated at this pressure but can be used safely at 60 psig. Regulator pressure indicators and flowmeter function should be visually inspected routinely.

Vaporisers should be cleaned and calibrated by trained personnel annually or biannually depending on use. Many anaesthesia supply companies offer vaporiser cleaning, calibration and repair services. The CO_2 absorber canister should be large enough to accommodate a maximum expired breath (approximately 20 ml/kg) in space around the absorbent granules which are considered to occupy approximately 50% of the entire volume. Small-animal or human machines with double absorber canisters are the best choice for foals weighing less than 150 kg. The absorbent should be changed after about 10 to 12 hours of use and therefore the date and hours of use should be recorded. Crude tests of activity are dye indicator colour change and hard rather than crumbly granules. Palpable heat production during use confirms that the active exothermic reaction of absorber with CO_2 is occurring. The most accurate and expensive method of determining absorber function is to measure inspired CO_2 by capnography. Ideally, in a properly functioning circle system with active CO_2 absorber, there should be no CO_2 in the inspired gases. Due to the accuracy of the monitor and some slight mixing of inspired and expired gases at low fresh gas flows, inspired CO_2 readings may be 1 to 3 mm Hg (0.13–0.4 kPa). It is advisable to change the absorber when the inspired CO_2 begins to rise, as once the absorber begins to change, it exhausts rapidly.

Proper unidirectional valve function is easily tested by breathing into the Wye-piece and watching the valve diaphragms move. If the valves are not transparent, they should be inspected directly to be sure the diaphragm is intact, moves freely and sits evenly to occlude the valve opening. They can then be tested individually by disconnecting and obstructing each limb at the Wye-piece and checking for no flow in the appropriate direction of the intact limb. The rebreathing (reservoir) bag should be inspected for cracks and holes. These most often occur at the neck or along folds. Ideally, the rebreathing bag should be large enough to accommodate the maximum inspiratory (vital) capacity of the animal's lung. For the adult horse, this is approximately 60 ml/kg. Available bags are 15 or 30 L and are sufficient for the standard range of horse sizes. For foals, miniature horses and small ponies (<150 kg), 5-L bags are adequate. Positive pressure leaks in the circle are identified by occluding the Wye-piece, filling the system with oxygen and watching that the rebreathing bag remains inflated for 2 to 3 minutes. Most anaesthetic systems today have pressure manometers in the circle. This allows more accurate leak testing by inflating the system to 20 cm H_2O and watching that this pressure is maintained for several minutes. The manometer also helps guide safe assisted ventilation as excessive positive airway pressure can interfere with venous return and cardiac output and potentially cause barotrauma to the lung. Scavenging of anaesthetic gases actively or passively directs excess breathing circuit gases from the pop-off valve out of the building. Low O_2 flows will result in less excess breathing gas, environmental pollution and waste.

Large-animal anaesthesia ventilator

Even if surgeries are performed under variable rate total intravenous anaesthesia and a vaporiser is never turned on, the horse should be intubated, some fraction of additional oxygen should be administered and the ability to assist ventilation should be available. Hypoxaemia and hypoventilation are well-recognised hazards of equine anaesthesia. This is most reasonably done with an anaesthesia machine that includes a ventilator. No two large-animal anaesthesia ventilator models are quite alike. Therefore, the best approach to ventilators is to choose one and concentrate on becoming fully versed in its logic. The one thing they all have in common is a bellows that is compressed by the influx of gas into an airtight housing around the bellows to force an inspiration. This design is known as "double circuit" in that the gas driving of the ventilator is separate from the gas being delivered to the patient. The practicality of this is that the driving gas should be at a pressure of 50 psig for proper ventilator function. The patient circuit gas pressure, on the other hand, fluctuates with the respiratory cycle and should not exceed 30 cm H_2O (approximately 0.04 psig) during positive pressure inspiration in the normal horse. Thus, keeping these circuits separate is essential. Fortunately, the primary barrier between them is the bellows which is completely compressed during peak inspiration and thus most leaks in it should be pressed closed. High patient circuit pressure due to a crack in the bellows allowing a leak of driving gas during early inspiration has been reported.[6] The other interface of the 2 circuits is a "spill over" valve which is closed by the driving gas during inspiration and opened by the breathing circuit gas overflow during the expiratory pause. Malfunction of this valve is rare, but the possibility is an argument for including a manometer in the large animal breathing circle design for continuous patient circuit pressure monitoring. When using a ventilator, the hose from the bellows is attached to the rebreathing bag port on the anaesthetic circle, the pop-off valve on the circle is closed and the scavenge hose should be moved from the circle's pop-off valve to the overflow (spill over) valve in the patient/bellows circuit of the ventilator.

Academics like to discuss the pros and cons of bellows that ascend versus descend during the expiratory phase of a respiratory cycle (Figure 4.7). The concern stems from the need to be able to identify leaks in the patient circuit. Clearly, a bellows that depends on gas flow into an intact

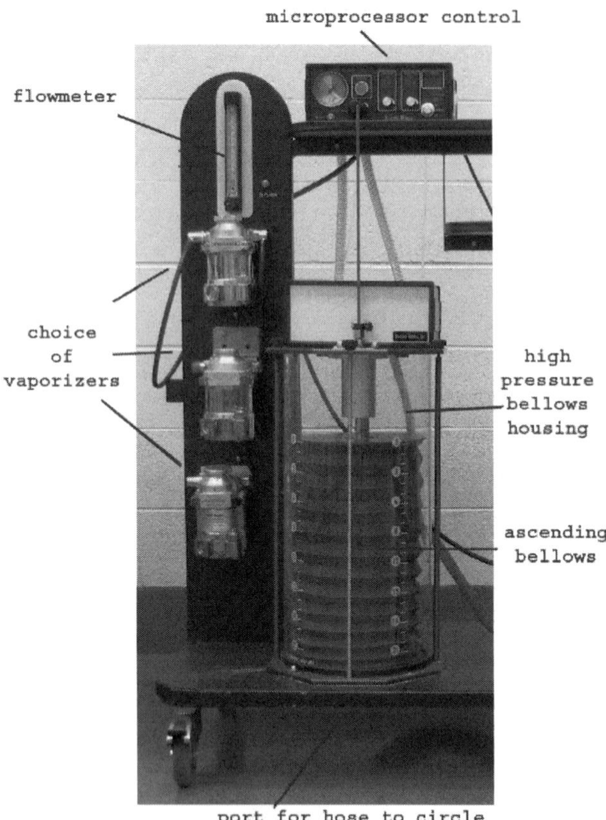

Figure 4.7 Large animal ventilator with microprocessor control and ascending bellows. ©Lydia L. Donaldson, 2007.

patient circuit to ascend to its starting position during expiration will not do so if there is a leak or disconnect. A descending bellows will drop to its starting position due to gravity, regardless of the circuit integrity. However, during inspiration in the presence of a leak, neither bellows will deliver to the expected peak inspiratory pressure. This is more easily detected when using a pressure cycled ventilator as it will not cycle out of inspiratory phase if the preset peak inspiratory pressure is not reached. With a volume-cycled ventilator, the full volume will be delivered out of the bellows but only a portion of it will reach the patient as some will exit the circuit through the leak and the peak inspiratory pressure will be less than before the leak developed. All this discussion serves to illustrate the biggest problem with ventilators: there are numerous systems of control, each with its own logic, which impact not only what can be adjusted but also how malfunctions are manifested.

The objective of mechanical ventilation is to insure the patient breaths well enough to maintain a normal arterial carbon dioxide (and therefore pH) and adequate arterial oxygen (i.e., to prevent respiratory acidosis and hypoxaemia, either of which have profound repercussions on organ function, morbidity and mortality). Minute ventilation (respiratory rate × tidal volume) should be sufficient to clear CO_2 from the lung at the rate it is delivered to the lung from the body by pulmonary arterial blood. Therefore, logical controls on any ventilator would be respiratory rate and tidal volume (Table 4.2, Figure 4.8). Many ventilators have a knob labelled "Respiratory Rate" but some require respiratory rate to be determined by adjusting "Expiratory Time", "Inspiratory Time" and/or "I:E ratio" (the ratio of inspiratory to expiratory duration). Several large-animal ventilators set tidal volume physically by raising or lowering a plate in the bellows housing that restricts the descent or ascent of the bellows, respectively. The housing has calibration marks indicating the approximate tidal volume for each position. Alternately, tidal volume is manipulated by adjusting "inspiratory flow" (speed at which the driving gas enters the bellows housing and therefore speed at which the bellows is compressed and patient circuit gases are driven into the lung) and inspiratory time. The combination of flow (litres/min) and time (minutes) results in volume (litres). The inspiratory time may be a knob on the ventilator control panel so labelled or may be changed by adjusting respiratory rate, expiratory time and/or I:E ratio. The I:E ratio may be directly adjusted or be a function of the other settings. As the inspiratory phase of the respiratory cycle is the period of positive intrathoracic pressure when thoracic viscera other than the lung will be compressed, the general recommendation is that the I:E ratio be 1:2 at the most. Again, learn the logic of the ventilator you choose and how to recognise when it malfunctions. As with the circle breathing system, ventilators should be checked for leaks before every use. One simple way to do this is to fill the bellows, disconnect the ventilator from the anaesthesia circuit while obstructing the end of that connecting hose and turn on the ventilator using settings similar to those you will use on a horse. If there are no positive pressure leaks in the patient circuit, the bellows will remain in its full position. If the ventilator's driving circuit and controls are intact and functional, it will cycle at the set rate, times, pressures and/or ratios. Any visible change in bellows volume will be the equivalent of stretch in the connecting hose as there should be no net flow. If there is a progressive loss of bellows volume, there is a leak.

All of the large-animal ventilators currently available, except the JD Medical LAV2000, are electronically controlled and pneumatically driven. This means they need to be plugged into both an electrical outlet and a 50-psig gas source. The LAV2000 is controlled by a modified Bird Mark 7 servo that uses the driving gas to cycle the ventilator. For most, inspiration is volume cycled (i.e., the inspiratory phase ends when a preset tidal volume has been delivered). The LAV2000's tidal volume is determined by limiting inspiration to a preset peak inspiratory pressure. The significance of these differences is that delivering a fixed volume may lead to excessive pressures, whereas delivering a fixed pressure may not deliver an adequate volume.

Most horses that die during general anaesthesia do so from cardiac arrest.[7,8] In the otherwise healthy horse, this is usually a vagally mediated event (i.e., sinus or atrioventricular [AV] block). In the compromised, often endotoxemic, horse with colic, there may be an early vagal phase

Table 4.2. Control variable choices on large-animal electronic ventilators

Controls	Unit	Normal	Potential effect on:
On-off switch			
Respiratory rate (RR)	breaths/minute	6–12	IT, ET, I : E ratio
Tidal volume (V_T)	litres/breath	10–20 ml/kg bwt of patient	IT, PIP
Minute ventilation (RR × V_T)	ml/kg/min	60–240	RR, V_T
Inspiratory time (IT)	seconds	1.8–3.0*	RR, ET, I : E ratio, V_T, PIP
Expiratory time (ET)	seconds	1.8–6.3*	RR, IT, I : E ratio, V_T
Inspiratory flow (IF)	ml/kg/sec	2–3*	V_T, PIP
I : E ratio		1 : 1–1 : 4	IT, ET, IF, V_T
Peak inspiratory pressure (PIP)	cm H_2O	20–30	V_T, IT, IF

Objectives: normal Pa_{CO_2}, acceptable Pa_{O_2}
Limiting factors: excessive PIP causing cardiovascular compromise, equipment capabilities

*Estimated from studies on horses awake,[123,124] xylazine sedated and during xylazine, diazepam and ketamine anesthesia with and without a nasotracheal tube.[124]

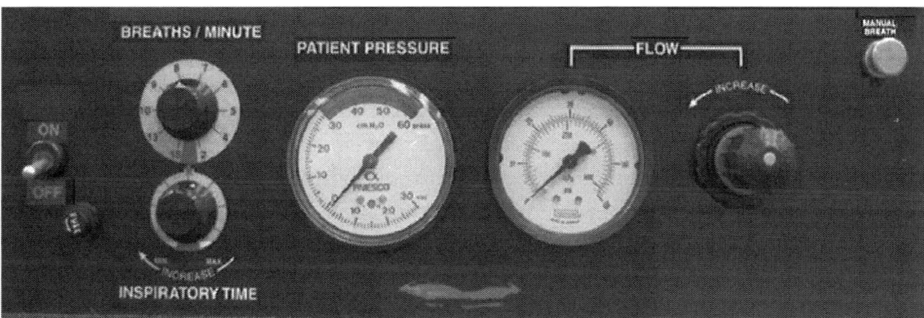

Figure 4.8 Large animal ventilator microprocessor controls. ©Lydia L. Donaldson, 2007. On/off = turns electronic servo on or off; Breaths/Minute = respiratory rate; Inspiratory Time = duration of inspiration (at a set respiratory rate, affects expiratory time and I : E ratio; Patient Pressure = pressure in the breathing circuit; Flow = rate of gas influx into bellows housing compressing the bellows to create an inspiration and generate a pressure in the housing displayed on the accompanying dial; Manual Breath = manually assisted breath independent of the set respiratory rate, i.e., a sigh; Tidal volume (liters) = Flow (liters/second) X Inspiratory Time (seconds)

of AV block or sinus tachycardia, either of which can progress to ectopic ventricular activity and ultimately degenerate to ventricular fibrillation.

Monitoring equipment

Without an electrocardiogram, sudden death during anaesthesia is only that. The mechanism of cardiac arrest cannot be known. Palpation of peripheral pulses is very subjective and cannot identify a cause of irregularities or deficits. Horses also die or are euthanised after general anaesthesia from debilitating myopathy or neuropathy, which are ischaemia–reperfusion injuries. Although maintaining mean arterial blood pressure above 60 mm Hg (8.0 kPa) does not guarantee prevention of myopathy/neuropathy, research[9–11] and the practice of monitoring and supporting blood pressure suggest that maintaining a theoretically adequate perfusion pressure does reduce the incidence.[12] Postanaesthetic lameness has been statistically associated with a mean arterial pressure (MAP) of less than 70 mm Hg (9.33 kPa) for longer than 10 minutes.[13] Thus, monitoring cardiac electrical activity and arterial blood pressure is critical to early detection of problems, which, in turn, allows corrective measures to be taken before a fatal cascade can develop.

Cardiovascular monitors

There are numerous cardiovascular monitors available (Box 4.2). Until recently, most were manufactured for use in humans, were expensive and were not designed to accommodate heart rates less than 30. Many of the older, refurbished human units are perfectly serviceable as long as their ECG and blood pressure cables are still available. In general, these monitors are robust, and investing $3000 to $6000 (£2000–4000; €3000–6000) will purchase a used monitor that will require little repair and continue to perform accurately for decades. It is wise to select a product that has a good track record in equine anaesthesia and to purchase from a company that offers a warranty. A feature

Box 4.2. Some sources of multiparameter monitors

Veterinary	
Cardell	www.sharn.com
SurgiVet	www.surgivet.com
Human	
Criticare Systems	www.csiusa.com
Datascope Corp.	www.datascope.com
Datex-Ohmeda	www.us.datex-ohmeda.com
Protocol Systems	www.monitoring.welchallyn.com
Used	
DRE	www.vetlab.dremed.com
Grady Medical Systems, Inc.	www.gradymedical.com
Whittemore Enterprises, Inc.	www.wemed1.com

to look for in a cardiovascular monitor is display visibility. This includes being able to read it from all angles, in all lighting situations and that the ECG trace display is wide enough to show more than three complexes at the normal equine heart rate of 32 beats/min. Most monitors manufactured for use in human medicine come with a choice of a five-lead or three-lead ECG. The latter may be referred to as defibrillator leads by the vendor, are longer than the standard five-lead sets and are the best choice for horses. Because most electronic ECG monitors display lead II automatically when turned on, it is simplest to read from this setting by placing the right arm and left leg leads in a position that records across the heart and does not interfere with the surgical site. In the past decade, medical equipment manufacturers have begun to target the veterinary market, but cardiovascular monitors designed for small-animal practice may still not accommodate low heart rates.

Direct blood pressure monitoring

Direct blood pressure monitoring with a pressure-to-electronic signal transducer and electronic display is sufficiently more accurate and reliable than the other methods of measuring blood pressure in the horse, in which maintaining muscle perfusion is so critical, to justify the initial expense of the equipment and per-case expense of a catheter, an extension set and a little heparinised saline. It is more expensive than an arterial catheter attached to a simple manometer and a cuff plus sphygmomanometer or Doppler system but really not more expensive than any of the oscillometric indirect blood pressure monitors. Once the initial investment has been made, there is little cost of use and considerably less stress when anaesthetist and surgeon are confident in the measurement technique. The "disposable" transducers designed for single use in human medicine will last more than a year if care is taken to avoid contamination and physical damage. Temperature probes are often included in the monitor package, and knowledge of thermal loss in cases of colic and caesarean section and all foal surgeries will improve patient care.

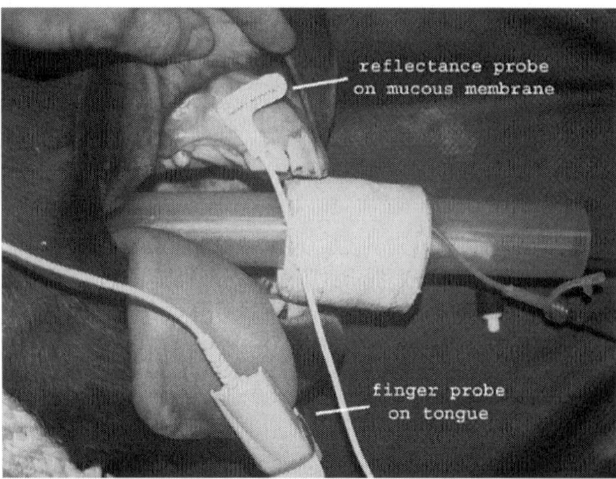

Figure 4.9 Pulse oximetry probes: reflectance probe on gingival mucous membrane and finger probe on tongue. ©Lydia L. Donaldson, 2007.

Blood gas

A blood gas machine is probably next on the list of equine intra-anaesthetic monitoring equipment, particularly if colics and emergency surgeries are undertaken. Although the gold standard, bench top gas analysers are both very expensive as initial investments and to maintain in that they require routine in-house and trained personnel care. There are now several point-of-care blood gas analysers that can be cost effective if the surgical and critical care caseload is high enough. An alternative might be to make arrangements to have blood gas analysis done at a nearby human hospital.

Pulse oximetry, capnography and airway gases

The other variables often monitored are pulse oximetry, capnography and airway gases. To date, pulse oximetry in horses is less reliable than in other species. Part of the problem is finding a site compatible to the probe. There are innumerable probe designs, not all of which are available for all pulse oximeters. Standard human ear or finger clips or reflectance probes can be placed on the tongue, lip, nasal septum, ear or gingival, vulvar or preputial mucous membrane (Figure 4.9), but often these tissues are too thick or pigmented or placement is too unstable to provide a dependable reading. There is sufficient inaccuracy in pulse oximetry reading from the horse such that an Spo_2 reading of less than 93% may not be indicative of arterial haemoglobin O_2 desaturation; conversely, at truly hypoxaemic Pao_2 values (≤60 mm Hg [8.0 kPa], Sao_2 <90%), Spo_2 readings may occasionally be falsely high.[14–17] In practice, if the heart rate reported by the pulse oximeter does not agree with that from the ECG or arterial blood pressure, the Spo_2 reading is less likely to be accurate.[18]

Thus, pulse oximetry is still best used as a first alert of hypoxaemia to be confirmed by arterial blood gas analysis.

Capnography, inspired and expired oxygen and inhalant anaesthetic analysis are luxuries that enable fine tuning but are not essential for good anaesthetic management. In the healthy lung, end expired CO_2 ($ETco_2$) should be the same as arterial CO_2 ($Paco_2$). Even in the healthy anaesthetised horse, the difference between $Paco_2$ and $ETco_2$ tends to be 5 to 10 mm Hg (0.66–1.33 kPa) due to ventilation–perfusion mismatch and deadspace ventilation.[18–21] The greatest advantage to capnography is that it allows breath-by-breath monitoring of ventilation and pulmonary blood flow (i.e., cardiac output). It is an easy guide to adjustments of mechanical ventilation and rapidly detects patient circuit leaks. Because expired CO_2 is dependent on delivery of CO_2 to the alveolus by pulmonary blood, cardiac arrest will cause a precipitous drop in $ETco_2$. Extubation or complete anaesthetic circuit disconnect will result in an even more abrupt drop in $ETco_2$ reading to 0 mm Hg. As mentioned earlier, inspired CO_2 will increase when the absorber is exhausted. Rapid increases in $ETco_2$ are also the first indication of malignant hyperthermia, a life-threatening event that has been reported in horses.[22–25]

Personnel

It is important to have one staff member take primary responsibility for the equipment, supplies and training of other members of the hospital team in anaesthesia. This person should like anaesthesia and not be afraid of the challenges and risks it presents. Pay this person well. Many equine surgeons have a foundation in anaesthesia and an opinion on how they want the anaesthesia to be done and prefer to do the basic training of their anaesthetists themselves. This is certainly understandable as the surgeon is ultimately responsible and must be able to communicate with his or her anaesthetist. Once the basics are mastered by a designated anaesthetist, it is beneficial to send him or her to a university for several days or have an anaesthesiologist visit the practice for a day periodically. The benefits are 2-fold: the technician(s) gain(s) knowledge that will improve the anaesthetic care of your patients and the technician(s) is(are) given a sense of his or her (their) value to the practice. Even if the caseload is light and restricted to elective procedures, it would be wise to have a second person who is well enough trained in the use of the equipment and basic methods that he or she can step in to help. This person should not be used only when the primary anaesthetist is not available but should be scheduled to do an occasional case in order to remain moderately facile in the techniques. If the practice offers 24-hour, 7-days/week service, at least four members of the hospital team should be trained in anaesthesia. Even if the emergency caseload is not high, this allows emergency duty to be distributed to reduce lifestyle stress and, in high-volume practices, to prevent exhaustion and burnout.

Alternately, in a multiple veterinarian practice, an associate veterinarian may be the primary anaesthetist. Ideally, this would be someone with a long-term commitment to the practice who enjoys anaesthesia. In the United States, it is the practice to have interns do the anaesthesia. This only works if there is an experienced, supervising veterinarian or technician who can oversee their training, support their efforts and maintain the equipment and supplies.

Anaesthetic risk

The most comprehensive epidemiological study of perianaesthetic mortality in horses prospectively gathered data from 129 clinics for 41,824 general anaesthetics (Confidential Enquiry into Perioperative Equine Fatalities [CEPEF]). The study found a 1.6% mortality rate for the entire population that broke down into a 0.9% for electives and 7.9% for colics.[8] These numbers are slightly higher than smaller, single-site studies that have reported an overall rate of 0.12% to 0.8% and a colic mortality rate of approximately 6.9%.[2,7,26–28] All give horses a higher risk of death than the 0.10% to 0.43% rate reported for small animals.[29–31] The CEPEF study identified cardiac arrest (33.2%), fractures in recovery (25.6%), myopathy (7.0%), neuropathy (5.5%) and respiratory complications (3.7%) as causes of death for the 328 fatalities in 35,978 anaesthetized horses for non-colic procedures. Of the equine anaesthesia drug choices, only the use of acepromazine* as a preanaesthetic sedative was unambiguously associated with a significantly decreased risk of perianaesthetic mortality.[8] That mortality was lower with total intravenous anaesthesia (TIVA) than with inhalants requires some interpretation because TIVA has traditionally been used for procedures of less than 1 hour duration and longer anaesthesia had a significant negative impact on outcome.[1,8] There were fewer cardiac arrests in horses anaesthetised with isoflurane† compared to halothane‡, although overall mortality was similar.[32]

It is easy to understand why horses with colic are at greater risk. At best, they are in pain and mildly dehydrated and have been given an assortment of drugs to control their pain, behaviour and perhaps gastrointestinal function. At worst, they are in septic shock: hypotensive, relatively hypovolaemic, tachycardic, hypoproteinaemic, haemoconcentrated, hypothermic, tachypnoeic, lactic acidaemic, hypocalcaemic, hypokalaemic and moribund. If these patients make it to induction, they die shortly afterwards and the role that anaesthesia plays is difficult to fully assess. Of perhaps more interest are the other populations at risk of death or complications. My bias is toward the extremes

---

*ACP Injection 10 mg/ml; Novartis Animal Health, Litlington, Herts, UK; PromAce; Fort Dodge Animal Health, Fort Dodge, IA, USA; AceMav; MAVLAB PTY LTD, Slacks Creek, Qld, Australia.

†Vetflurane; Virbac Animal Health Ltd. Bury St Edmunds, Suffolk, UK.

‡Halothane-Vet; Merial Animal Health Ltd, Dublin, Ireland.

of age, mid-to-late term pregnant mares, horses anaesthetised for internal fixation of long bone fractures, horses with cardiac or pulmonary disease and horses debilitated by systemic disease. The last, in many cases, may have chronic pain and cachexia from a septic orthopaedic problem because renal, hepatic and endocrine disease is neither common nor likely to be present in a horse taken to surgery. Neonatal foals did tend to be at increased risk in the large CEPEF study.[8] Subjectively, sinus bradycardia and second- and third-degree block seem to be more common in anaesthetised foals, and life-threatening dysrhythmias have been reported in neonates anaesthetised for ruptured bladder repair.[33–35] The CEPEF study also found horses 14 years and older to be at greater risk of death. A retrospective comparison of 100 horses older than 20 years with a matched population of 2- to 12-years-olds did not identify any greater incidence of death, recovery injury or myopathy, although intraoperative dysrhythmias were more common.[36] Consistent with the 77% to 92% survival rate reported for mares anaesthetised to relieve dystocia,[37–39] the CEPEF study found a higher mortality rate in third-trimester mares.[1,8] Elsewhere, survival to discharge of pregnant mares after exploratory laparotomy was comparable to that of nonpregnant horses.[40,41] Horses anaesthetised for fracture repair have one of the highest mortality rates.[8] Refracture/implant failure during recovery is one of the explanations for this, but it did not account for all of the deaths in this group of horses. As many fractures occur in physically fit horses during strenuous exercise, it may be that postexercise metabolic imbalances, muscle trauma and hydration status in addition to severe pain in an often-uncompromising temperament contribute to perianaesthetic complications.

Thus, although we have a sense of which populations of horses are at greater risk in association with general anaesthesia, the choice of anaesthetic agents and methods of anaesthetic management for horses are relatively limited. Those that are currently most popular have become so by virtue of being both successful and practical. A widely held belief in all anaesthesia practice is that a certain degree of standardisation is important as it reduces error and allows early recognition of unusual, perhaps adverse, responses.

Elective procedures

Horses can be maintained anaestheticsed with intravenous, inhalant or a combination of intravenous and inhalant anaesthetics. The advantage to inhalants is that they are rapidly eliminated and have no active metabolites and therefore recovery is relatively rapid. On the other hand, they are potent cardiovascular and respiratory depressants and recoveries can be explosive. Blood pressure and cardiac output may be higher and the stress response to surgery less under TIVA than under inhalant anaesthesia, but recoveries may be prolonged. Recently, combinations of injectable anaesthetics and inhalants (balanced anaesthesia) have been explored on the premise that smaller doses of each will have fewer of the undesirable side effects of either but will be additive, if not synergistic, to produce good surgical anaesthesia. A summary of drug choices for inhalant-based general anaesthesia is shown in Table 4.3.

Preanaesthetic evaluation

The most important component of the preanaesthetic evaluation is a thorough physical examination. Increasingly, horses are pets and are not required to be exercise tolerant, traditionally a measure of fitness for the stresses of general anaesthesia and surgery. Examples of the physical examination findings that have led me to question the wisdom of elective anaesthesia include frequent, multifocal ventricular premature depolarizations in a Quarter Horse mare, frequent unifocal ventricular premature contractions/complexes in a fit Thoroughbred, aortic and mitral insufficiency in an aged Thoroughbred, atrial fibrillation in an assortment of horses, elevated creatine kinase (CK > approximately 300 U/L) and aspartate aminotransferase (AST > approximately 400 U/L) in horses in training and unexplained fevers in horses otherwise at risk for pneumonia (i.e., younger members of mobile populations such as sales yearlings or racehorses). All these horses were anaesthetised on the condition that the owner was informed of the additional risk for perfusion-related postoperative complications or life-threatening dysrhythmias in the former and postanaesthetic pneumonia in the latter. An effort to categorise some of these preanaesthetic concerns is made in Table 4.4.

As in other species, minimal blood work should include a packed cell volume and total protein as rough estimates of O_2-carrying capacity and hydration status. Ideally, preanaesthetic muscle enzyme (CK and AST) analysis to assess preoperative muscle status would be routine in the population of equine athletes at risk for myopathy. A full chemistry profile is rarely indicated for elective surgeries as renal, hepatic and endocrine diseases are not common, particularly in horses presenting for elective surgery. Renal or hepatic status has little clinically evident impact on inhalant anaesthesia because the clinical effect of intravenous induction agents is largely terminated by redistribution from the brain to other tissues. Even the effects of delayed metabolism and excretion are unlikely to extend beyond the period of inhalant anaesthesia. On the other hand, TIVA should be avoided in horses with hepatic or renal insufficiency, and extra care should be taken during inhalant anaesthesia as hypotension with potential for tissue hypoxia could add insult to marginal organ function. A leukogram and fibrinogen in the truly healthy horse are of little importance to anaesthesia. However, elevated fibrinogen levels may be the only hint of subclinical pulmonary disease. Many anaesthetic agents, endotracheal intubation and mechanical ventilation alter normal pulmonary defense mechanisms[42–44] and contribute to the development of atelectasis in the recumbent horse.[45,46] Administering general anaesthesia to a horse with a brewing respiratory infection invites serious pneumonia or pleuropneumonia.

Table 4.3. Equine inhalant-based anaesthetic drug choices

	Dose (mg/kg unless otherwise indicated)	Comments
Premedication		
IV xylazine or other α_2-agonist	0.5–0.6	≈5 minutes before induction for most horses
IM acepromazine	0.02–0.04	≈30 minutes before induction for anxious horses
IM detomidine	0.02–0.04	≈30 minutes before induction; helpful for unbroken, dangerous horses
IV butorphanol	0.01–0.02	After the α_2-agonist
Induction		
IV ketamine	1.7–2.2	Some horses may not be effectively induced
IV benzodiazepine	0.04–0.08	Midazolam kinetics may be more suitable for short procedures to avoid weak recoveries Gentle relaxation may protect limb fractures
IV guaifenesin	25–100	Titratable
IV thiopental	6–10	Easier to deliver the appropriate dose when added to guaifenesin and infused to effect
Maintenance		
Halothane	MAC = 0.88	Surgical anaesthesia = 1.5–2 × MAC
Isoflurane	MAC = 1.3%	
Sevoflurane	MAC = 2.3%	
IV ketamine	0.2–0.4	Rapid increase in anaesthetic depth; < 10 minutes
IV butorphanol	0.01–0.02	To improve analgesia, every ≈1 hour
IM butorphanol	0.05–0.1	Shortly after induction, every ≈2–4 hours
IM pethidine (meperidine)	0.2–0.4	Every ≈1 hour
IM morphine	0.1–0.2	Every ≈ 90 minutes
CRI* morphine	0.15 mg/kg; 1.7 μg/kg/min	Clinical observations of improved anaesthetic stability not demonstrable experimentally[97]
CRI lidocaine	1–3 mg/kg; 30–50 μg/kg/min	≈25% less inhalant, administer loading dose over 10–20 minutes, discontinue 20 minutes before end of anaesthesia[95,98,204]
CRI ketamine	1.0–2.2 mg/kg; 17–50 μg/kg/min	≈30% less inhalant, slow infusion rate after 1 hour, discontinue ≈10 minutes before end of anaesthesia[92,94,150,205]
CRI medetomidine	5–7 μg/kg; 0.06–0.08 μg/kg/min	≈30% less inhalant[92,93,96]
Recovery		
IV xylazine	0.1–0.2	Give at disconnect, nystagmus or extubation
IV acepromazine	0.004–0.01	Give ≈15 minutes before the end of anaesthesia
IV romifidine	4–10 mg	Give at disconnect

*CRI, constant rate infusion—protocols include administration of a loading dose followed by an infusion which is usually at a constant rate with adjustments in anaesthetic depth made by increasing or decreasing the vaporizer setting of the accompanying inhalant.

No formal study of the incidence of postanaesthetic pulmonary complications has been done in horses, but 12.2% of those treated for pleuritis secondary to pneumonia were postsurgical patients in one report.[47]

Important to the anaesthetic management of any horse is an assessment of its temperament, tractability and trust in humans. Kind, well-mannered horses who accept human instruction are more likely to be less stressed during induction and responsive to reassurance during recovery.

In addition to evaluating the patient, the equipment, OR and induction/recovery should be checked for proper function and supplies (Table 4.5). The O_2 supply and CO_2 absorber status should be checked to be sure they are more than adequate for the expected duration of surgery and recovery. The vaporiser should be full of inhalant, the endotracheal tube cuff, anaesthesia circle and ventilator should have no leaks and all pads should be available and clean. The initial preparation for recovery should be made before the horse is induced.

Table 4.4. Anaesthetic concerns related to preanaesthetic physical examination findings in horses scheduled for elective anaesthesia

PE finding	Concern	Further assessment	Evidence for concern
Heart rate <20	Sinus or third-degree AV block leading to arrest	ECG, echocardiography, atropine challenge	Anecdotal: bradycardia is the most common cause of cardiac arrest during equine anaesthesia
Premature ventricular contractions	Ventricular fibrillation	ECG, echocardiography	Theoretical: altered autonomic control; inhalants sensitize the myocardium
Atrial fibrillation	Ventricular tachycardia and/or fibrillation	ECG, echocardiography	Theoretical: altered autonomic balance may facilitate atrioventricular conduction
Recurrent obstructive airway disease	Hypoxaemia	ABGs, assess pulmonary function and gas exchange	Theoretical: many are hypoxaemic when standing; altered flow characteristics trap alveolar air
Unexplained fever	Postoperative pneumonia or pleuropneumonia	CBC, fibrinogen, repeat temperature, auscult with rebreathing, delay, BAL	Anecdotal and theoretical: anaesthetics disrupt pulmonary defense mechanisms
Elevated CK and/or AST	Postanaesthetic myopathy	Delay until normal > 7 days; assess muscles, kidneys; treat if indicated	Theoretical: anaesthesia and recumbency cause muscle injury
Fit racehorse	Hypotension, myopathy, rough recovery	Delay until out of training 1–2 weeks	Anecdotal: altered autonomic balance, marginal hydration and electrolyte balance, mentally primed to compete
Late pregnancy	Hypoventilation, hypoxaemia, recovery injury	Delay until after foaling	Anecdotal and theoretical: gravid uterus fills abdomen, mare exhausted often old
Neurological deficits	Deterioration of status, inability to stand	Repeated neurological evaluation to establish disease progression	Theoretical: muscle relaxation, positioning, manipulation; altered CNS haemodynamics
Geriatric	Arrhythmias, difficulty standing, borderline renal function	Critically evaluate cardiovascular, renal, musculoskeletal systems	Theoretical: age-associated reduced cardiovascular reserve, sarcopenia

Premedication

The objective of premedication is to calm the horse with minimally compromising drugs before inducing and maintaining anaesthesia with potentially life-threatening ones. Preanaesthetic sedation reduces the dose requirements for induction and maintenance and, depending on the sedative and route of administration, may help calm recovery. The most common practice in the United States is to administer xylazine**, intravenously, after the horse is in the induction stall (i.e., shortly before induction). Any α_2-agonist would serve the purpose and the choice is a matter of personal preference and availability. In many ways, intravenous premedication at induction defeats the purpose stated in the first sentence of this paragraph as bringing a horse out of its stall is likely to cause some apprehension and xylazine is not a "minimally compromising" drug. On the other hand, most horses are tame and only slightly disconcerted in the induction area, and most respond well to relatively small, less-compromising doses of xylazine (0.4–0.6 mg/kg IV). The alternative of administering a premedication before moving the horse out of its stall, where it is at least somewhat acclimated and relaxed, is theoretically better but practically more problematic. If the premedication is an intravenous α_2-agonist, the horse may be too sedated to walk safely to induction. Intramuscular premedication has to be administered at least 15, if not 30, minutes before induction, which can add it to the logistical challenges of co-ordination in an ever-changing day's plan. Thus, an IV α_2-agonist shortly before induction remains the standard in many busy clinics. In light of the finding that acepromazine, alone or in combination with an α_2-agonist, may reduce the risk of anaesthetic complications,[1] perhaps this practice should be revisited. If a horse is particularly worried or unmanageable, IM acepromazine (0.02–0.04 mg/kg) or detomidine†† (0.01–0.02 mg/kg), respectively, can be given in the stall and additional sedation with an α_2-agonist of preference given in induction to achieve the desired level of sedation if necessary.

Although there is some debate about the advantages of adding butorphanol,‡‡ or other opioids, to inhalant anaes-

** Rompun; Bayer Animal Health, Newbury, Berkshire, UK; Chanazine 10%, Chanelle Animal Health, Liverpool, UK.

†† Domosedan; Pfizer, Sandwich, Kent, UK.

‡‡ Torbugesic; Fort Dodge Animal Health, Fort Dodge, IA, USA.

Table 4.5. Preanaesthetic preparation

Action	Comments
Evaluate patient	Even if done the day before look for changes in physical status, additional laboratory work, treatments, scheduled surgery time
Check O_2 supply	H cylinders (≈2200 psi = ≈7000 liters of O_2; to estimate liters remaining = ≈3 × psi)
Check equipment	Inspect for obvious damage, missing parts Fill vaporizer CO_2 absorber (hours of use can be recorded on a piece of tape on the canister) Check circle and ventilator for leaks Turn on monitor; check ECG leads, supplies for arterial catheterisation, blood pressure transducer, etc Set up in OR appropriately for surgical procedure Confirm appropriate padding is available
Check supplies for recovery	Dry floor, O_2 delivery system, ropes, mats, towels, extra syringes etc
Check anesthetic and emergency drugs	Stock anaesthesia supplies, prepare dobutamine solution, confirm availability of in date resuscitation drugs, assorted fluids
Choose endotracheal tube	Most adult horses take a 26-mm ID tube Check cuff for leaks
Draw up premedication and induction agents	Have a little extra sedation and induction agent readily available to use if needed
Communicate with other personnel	Confirm time, position, procedure, any special needs

thesia,[48–50] there is little question that they contribute to standing sedation. Adding a small dose (0.01 mg/kg IV butorphanol) to low-dose α_2-agonist sedation may be the least compromising way to achieve suitable sedation in some horses. The disadvantage to adding an opioid is that they make horses push forward, which requires a strong and determined person on their head to contain them in the induction chute. One way to deal with this while achieving the same overall quality of induction is to accept slightly less than optimal α_2-agonist sedation and administer the opioid with the induction agent. Opioids other than butorphanol may provide better or longer-acting analgesia, be more economical or be more appropriate for some situations. Keep in mind that intravenous administration of morphine§§ and pethidine (meperidine)*** may cause histamine release.

§§ Morphine sulphate injection; Antigen Pharmaceuticals, Dublin 4, Ireland.

*** Pethidine injection 50 mg/ml; Arnolds Veterinary Products, Shrewsbury, Shropshire, UK; Demerol; Abbott Laboratories, Abbott Park, IL, USA; Pethidine injection; Parnell Laboratories, Alexandria, NSW, Australia.

Induction

Ketamine††† (1.7–2.2 mg/kg IV) is by far the most popular induction agent for horses, and the benzodiazepines (BDZs) (diazepam‡‡‡ or midazolam§§§, 0.04–0.08 mg/kg IV) have pretty much replaced guaifenesin**** (25–100 mg/kg IV) as the method of improving muscle relaxation and prolonging the induction phase. An advantage of guaifenesin is that it can be given to effect, and it is therefore more difficult to administer an overdose. On the other hand, the BDZs have few side effects and the effective dose used for induction in horses is small compared to the anticonvulsant dose or the recommended anxiolytic dose used in other species (0.1–0.2 mg/kg). Large doses of either guaifenesin or the BDZs can cause venodilation, reduce venous return and cardiac output and contribute to hypotension. Water-soluble midazolam has more predictable pharmacokinetics than water-insoluble diazepam. Theoretically, this would make it preferable for induction when the expected duration of anaesthesia is short. Where rapid infusion of guaifenesin and a ketamine bolus often makes the horse drop abruptly to the floor, induction with a BDZ plus ketamine is typically gentle: a gradual sinking to the floor. This controlled muscle relaxation is a particular advantage when inducing horses with fractures or other injuries requiring protection from further damage.

The theoretical contraindications for ketamine are situations in which increases in intraocular or intracranial pressure are to be avoided. Near-thickness corneal lacerations or ulcers, and descemetocoels are cases where increased intraocular pressure might cause rupture of the globe. Increased intracranial pressure is rarely a concern in equine medicine but could accompany head trauma, particularly if there is altered mentation or evidence of cranial nerve injury. Traditionally, thiopental†††† has been used as the induction agent for such cases. Guaifenesin infusion followed by thiopental bolus (3–6 mg/kg IV) as is done with ketamine or infusion of a guaifenesin-thiopental mixture (500 ml 5% guaifenesin with 2.5–3 g thiopental for the average horse) to recumbency are the safest methods of induction as opposed to a larger IV bolus (6–10 mg/kg) of thiopental alone.

††† Ketaset; Fort Dodge Animal Health, Fort Dodge, IA, USA.

‡‡‡ Valium; Roche Laboratories, Basel. Switzerland; Diazemuls; Dumex Ltd, Whiddon Valley, Barnstaple, EX32 8NS, UK; diazepam injection; Parnell Laboratories, Alexandria, NSW, Australia.

§§§ Midazolam injection; Antigen Pharmaceuticals, Dublin 4, Ireland.

**** Guaifenesin USP; Boehringer Ingelheim Chemicals, Inc, Petersburg, VA; Guailaxin; Fort Dodge Animal Health, Fort Dodge, IA, USA.

†††† Pentothal; Merial Ltd., Iselin, NJ, USA.

Intubation

Intubation can be done with the horse in lateral or sternal recumbency (Figures 4.10 and 4.11). The former is more popular because it allows intubation while hobbles are being applied for hoisting. A situation when sternal recumbency intubation and cuff inflation might be advantageous would be in the horse with significant gastrointestinal reflux. Securing the airway before the horse's pharynx is placed lower than its stomach may help prevent aspiration. The least expensive and cumbersome speculum for holding the horse's mouth open during intubation is an approximately 5-cm length of approximately 5-cm-diameter PVC pipe placed between upper and lower incisors. The choice of endotracheal tube is determined by the size of the horse's trachea except when nasotracheal or tracheal intubation is required for surgical access. The objective is to reduce the airway diameter no more than necessary and thereby minimise increases in resistance to airflow. This is more important when the horse is allowed to breathe spontaneously. Because ventilation today is mechanically assisted in most horses, the current trend is to opt on the smaller side for an endotracheal tube, to minimise possible pharyngeal or tracheal trauma.[51,52] A 26-mm-internal diameter (ID) endotracheal tube will suffice for the average horse (900–1200 kg) and should be part of the initial purchase of anaesthesia equipment. The luxury of nasotracheal intubation with a special order 18- to 22-mm ID, longer (100–110 cm) tube facilitates oral surgeries and does not seem to hinder assisted ventilation but would not be essential. The tube should be well lubricated before introduction as this may help prevent epistaxis on extubation due to dry mucosa sticking to the tube surface. Endotracheal tube cuffs should be inflated just enough to prevent a leak as an overinflated cuff will cause tracheal mucosal ischaemia and necrosis.[53]

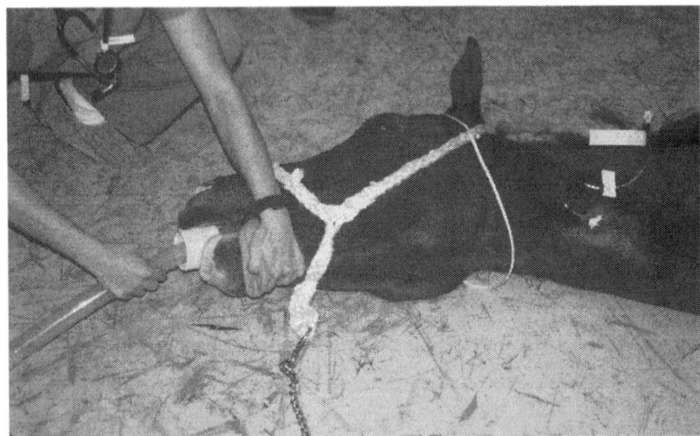

Figure 4.10 Intubation with horse in lateral recumbency. ©Lydia L. Donaldson, 2007.

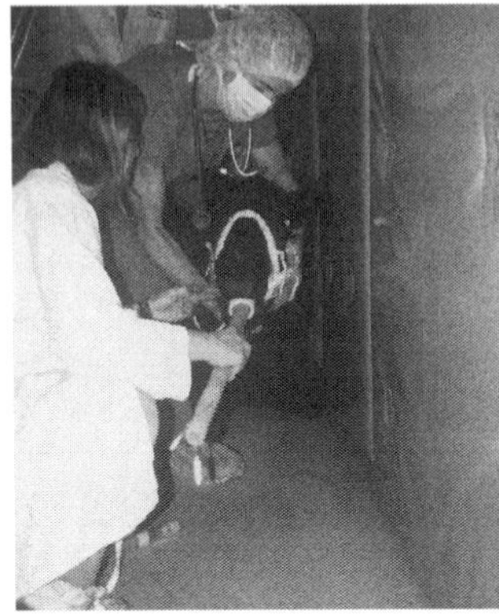

Figure 4.11 Intubation with horse in sternal recumbency. ©Lydia L. Donaldson, 2007.

Maintenance of anaesthesia

Halothane, isoflurane and sevoflurane‡‡‡‡ are the inhalant anaesthetics most commonly used for maintenance of anaesthesia in veterinary species. All are most safely administered with an agent-specific, precision vaporiser. Clinically, the differences among the three are subtle. They all produce dose-dependent cardiovascular and respiratory depression.[54–57] In the horse, halothane depresses cardiac output more and respiratory drive less than do the other two. Heart rates tend to be lower with halothane and vagally mediated bradycardias are more common. Clinically, it seems that dysrhythmias of other origins are also seen more often under halothane, but there is no real evidence to support this other than the CEPEF report that cardiac arrest occurred more often in horses under halothane (30 of 4080, or 0.7%) than isoflurane (13 of 4028, or 0.3%).[32] Whereas in other species, experimentally induced ventricular dysrhythmias in response to infusion of epinephrine occur at lower epinephrine doses under halothane than under isoflurane and sevoflurane,[58,59] the arrhythmogenic infusion rate has been reported to be 1.12 to 1.37 μg/kg/min for halothane-,[60,61] 1.06 μg/kg/min isoflurane- and 1.31 μg/kg/min for sevoflurane-anaesthetised horses.[62] Isoflurane tends to cause greater vasodilation and slightly higher heart rates.[54,63–66] Surgical anaesthesia seems to require a relatively greater expired concentration of halothane with respect to minimum alveolar concentration (MAC) than of isoflurane, and of isoflurane than of sevoflurane.[66,67] Horses were effectively anaesthetised for arthroscopy at end-tidal concentrations of 1.6% to 1.8% for both halothane and isoflurane (vaporiser setting of approximately 2–3% with O_2 flows of 3 L/min) where MAC for halothane is 0.88% and for isoflurane, is 1.31%.[68] Thus, in these horses, surgical anaesthesia was achieved at 1.8 to 2.0 $MAC_{halothane}$ and 1.2 to 1.4 $MAC_{isoflurane}$.[67] A similar qualitative disparity seems to occur with sevoflurane.[66] Horses will be immobile and unresponsive to surgical stimulation and have a slowed but present palpebral reflex on 2.4% to 2.6% end-tidal (vaporiser setting of approximately 3%–4%) (i.e., 0.86–1.1 $MAC_{sevoflurane}$ where MAC = 2.3%–2.8%).[57,69] Table 4.6 attempts to identify the

‡‡‡‡ SevoFlo; Abbott Animal Health, Queenborough, Kent, UK.

Table 4.6. Summary of the subjective differences in the clinical signs of surgical anaesthesia in adult horses under halothane, isoflurane and sevoflurane after xylazine premedication and guaifenesin/ketamine induction

Indicator of depth	Halothane (H)	Isoflurane (I)	Sevoflurane (S)
Eye position*	Central	Slightly medial	Central
Palpebral reflex	Slowed but present	Brisker than H	Quieter than I†
Corneal reflex	Rarely absent	Present	Present
Lacrimation	Present	More than H	Less than I
Nystagmus	Occasionally	Very rare	Rare
MAP (mm Hg)	60–80	60–80	70–90
Heart rate (bpm)	28–32	30–34	29–33
Respiratory rate	6–8	4–6	2–4
$Paco_2$ (mm Hg)	60–70	70–80	70–80
Vaporiser setting (%)	2–3	2–3	3–4
Movement on arousal	Tense neck, wave	Tense neck, flail	Tense neck, paddle

*Evaluate both eyes; frequently one eye will be central and the other slightly medial, and palpebral reflexes may also be different.
†May have intermittent slow spontaneous blink.

subtle differences in clinical indications of surgical anaesthesia seen with these three commonly used inhalants.

A more concrete difference among them is their blood solubility. Theoretically, the induction, depth changes and recovery should be more rapid with sevoflurane due to its lower blood solubility (blood/gas coefficient [B/G] = 0.68). Likewise, isoflurane (B/G = 1.46) should be faster than halothane (B/G = 2.54). This is difficult to appreciate clinically. Nasotracheal induction and recovery of foals anaesthetised with either isoflurane or sevoflurane were similar.[70] Time to standing of adult horses has been reported to be shorter or the same after sevoflurane compared to isoflurane[56,71] and shorter after isoflurane compared to halothane.[56,63,67,72] A fourth inhalant anaesthetic, desflurane,§§§§ is available and, in time, may prove to be the best for horses. It has lower blood solubility (B/G = 0.42) and is less potent (MAC = 7.6%–8.1%).[73,74] It seems to be less of a dose-dependent cardiovascular depressant but equally as respiratory depressant as the others.[74,75] Recoveries are rapid.[73,74]

Because of the large volume of the anaesthetic circle, with or without a ventilator, and size of the patient, high fresh gas flows (6–10 L/min) and vaporiser settings (3%–5% halothane and isoflurane or 4%–7% sevoflurane) are necessary to obtain an immobilisation depth of inhalant anaesthesia before the induction agent anaesthesia has receded. The actual vaporiser setting depends on both the physical status of the horse and its anaesthetic depth at the time the endotracheal tube is connected to the anaesthetic circuit. There are many occasions when 3% isoflurane or halothane (or 5% sevoflurane) will result in a gentle transition from injectable to inhalant without an accompanying profound drop in blood pressure. One way to facilitate the transition is to load the anaesthetic circuit with anaesthetic gas before inducing the horse. This allows the CO_2 absorber and plastic or rubber components of the system to absorb inhalant and reduces the amount they will "steal" from the horse later. To do this, stopper the Wye-piece, close the pop-off valve (*do not forget* to open it when the horse arrives if not using the ventilator) and turn on the O_2 flow at 10 L/min until the bag or bellows fills or a slight pressure registers on the circle's manometer. Turn off the O_2 flow and leave the machine until the horse arrives.

Halothane, isoflurane and sevoflurane depress ventilation dose-dependently. This is one of the arguments for choosing to use a ventilator. Halothane is the least depressant, and a horse in lateral recumbency for a reasonably short (<2 hours) procedure can be expected to breathe well enough at 6 to 10 breaths/min to keep $Paco_2$ between 50 and 70 mm Hg (6.66–9.33 kPa). A similar horse on isoflurane or sevoflurane might only take 3 to 5 breaths/min and allow $Paco_2$ to reach 80 mm Hg (10.66 kPa) or higher.[54–57,68] Typical ventilator settings for an average horse are 6 to 8 breaths/min and a tidal volume of 10 to 20 ml/kg adjusted to a peak inspiratory pressure of approximately 20 cm H_2O (1.96 kPa). If not using a ventilator, manually assisting a breath periodically will help keep $Paco_2$ in a reasonably physiological range but may disrupt respiratory drive and result in a period of apnoea.

Once a surgical plane of anaesthesia is reached, the O_2 flow can be safely reduced to 2 to 3 L/min and the vaporiser setting reduced according to the subjective assessment of anaesthetic depth. Note that in most currently available anaesthesia machines, the vaporiser is outside the breathing circle so reducing the O_2 flow through the vaporiser will reduce the rate of delivery of inhalant to the circle and therefore changes in the circle concentration will be slower than at higher fresh gas flows. The circle inhalant concentration (i.e., dose the horse is breathing) is a function of how fast the inhalant is being brought to the circle by the O_2 from the vaporiser and how fast the horse (and circle

§§§§ Suprane; Baxter Healthcare Corporation, Deerfield, IL, USA.

components) is absorbing it. Anaesthetic uptake by the horse is a function of getting it into the horse's alveoli (effective alveolar ventilation) and removal from the alveoli by pulmonary capillary blood. Thus, cardiac output (pulmonary capillary blood flow) and the distribution of pulmonary blood to ventilated alveoli influence inhalant uptake and ultimately, during recovery, elimination. Theoretically, the O_2 flow can be reduced to just meet the horse's O_2 consumption (approximately 4 ml/kg/min at rest).[76] Without a means of measuring circuit O_2, it may not be safe to decrease the flow to less than 2 L/min. Recognise that the O_2, and inhalant it is carrying, not picked up by the horse are wasted through the pop-off valve and a method of scavenging this gas out of the building needs to be attached to the pop-off valve. This can be as simple as running tubing at least the diameter of the pop-off outlet to a vent in the room. Be sure the vent does not recirculate air to another area of the hospital. There are also various commercial scavenge devices available (Box 4.1).

Hypoventilation and hypotension

The most common problems during maintenance of inhalant anaesthesia of healthy horses are hypoventilation and hypotension. The former is taken care of with a mechanical ventilator. The management of hypotension is multifactorial. Because the measurement of the indices of cardiovascular function that are of real interest (cardiac output and tissue blood flow) is not easily done on client-owned horses, blood pressure is used as an indicator of tissue perfusion. One principle that guides anaesthetic practice is the knowledge that the renal, cerebral and coronary vascular beds lose their ability to autoregulate (i.e., are unable to maintain a minimum required blood flow), when MAP drops below 50 to 60 mm Hg (6.67–8.0 kPa). Additionally, postanaesthetic myopathy has been associated with persistent periods of MAP less than 60 mm Hg (<8.0 kPa).[9–13] Thus, current common practice is to recognise MAP of 60 mm Hg as an absolute limit and to address a decreasing MAP at 70 mm Hg (9.33 kPa). Always the first step in managing hypotension is to assess anaesthetic depth and reduce it if possible because vasodilation and decreased cardiac output are well-documented, dose-dependent effects of the inhalant anaesthetics. The second step is to ensure adequate fluid administration. What is adequate? Every patient is different and the actual volume is unknown. The inhalants decrease vascular tone, thereby increasing the intravascular space. Minimally invasive surgeries cause little blood or tissue fluid loss, but intestinal resection in colic patients will make a significant contribution to hypovolaemia in horses already at risk of intravascular fluid loss. Typically, with elective surgeries, ensuring at least 10 ml/kg/hr and increasing this rate by raising the IV pole or applying pressure to the fluid bag are sufficient. The possible exception would be sinus or nasal procedures where excessive bleeding may occur. In approaching cases where haemorrhage is a likely complication, there should be a plan to control bleeding and either stop the surgery or administer cross-matched or autologous blood. An awake animal will compensate for loss of up to 30% of its blood volume (approximately 80 ml/kg) with only a small drop in MAP, but autonomic reflexes are obtunded by anaesthesia and systolic, diastolic, mean and pulse pressure decrease progressively with acute blood loss.[77] Standard approaches to resuscitation in the face of haemorrhage include 3 L of balanced electrolyte solution/L of blood lost, whole blood transfusion, colloids and hypertonic saline. Shock rates of isotonic fluid administration approach 90 ml/kg/hr.

Most often when faced with a hypotensive horse, the inhalant dose cannot be reduced without the horse waking up. Increasing isotonic fluid administration alone will not bring the MAP above 70 mm Hg (9.33 kPa), so an inotrope is administered (Table 4.7). Dobutamine***** has proven safe and effective. Infusion rates of 1 to 2 μg/kg/min usually raise the MAP in healthy horses under a light surgical plane of inhalant anaesthetic. Failure of MAP to increase at this low infusion rate may indicate excessive anaesthetic depth, α_1-adrenoreceptor block by acepromazine, endotoxaemia or SIRS or be associated with an apparent dobutamine-associated sinus or AV bradycardia or junctional dysrhythmias.[78] Dopamine††††† is the other sympathomimetic frequently used for cardiovascular support with the theoretical advantage of increasing cardiac output with vasodilation (i.e., increasing tissue blood flow), at low doses. Dopamine may be more likely to cause tachycardia and ventricular dysrhythmias.[79–82] For some horses, a single dose of ephedrine‡‡‡‡‡ (0.05–1.0 mg/kg IV) is sufficient to bring up MAP during the induction–maintenance transition phase of instability.[83] Horses that require continual inotropic support may benefit from a slow infusion of calcium (up to 1 ml/kg 23% calcium gluconate§§§§§) as it improves both myocardial contractility and vascular tone in isoflurane-anaesthetised horses.[84,85] Too rapid administration of calcium may cause cardiac dysrhythmias, including cardiac arrest, so care must be taken to give it slowly. Phenylephrine****** infusion titrated to effect and most often in conjunction with dobutamine infusion can help support blood pressure, particularly in horses known to have been given acepromazine within 24 hours before surgery. Phenylephrine is an α_1-adrenergic receptor agonist causing vasoconstriction and may not be the optimal approach to improving muscle blood flow.[82,86] In theory, when phenylephrine increases diastolic blood pressure, myocardial blood flow and cardiac output are improved.

***** Dobutrex; Eli Lilly and Co, Ltd, Basingstoke, UK.

††††† Dopamine HCl; Mayne Pharma PLC, Royal Leamington Spa, Warwickshire, UK; Dopamine HCl; David Bull Laboratories, Melbourne, Australia.

‡‡‡‡‡ Ephedrine sulfate; Bedford Laboratories, Bedford, OH, USA.

§§§§§ Calcium gluconate 23%; many manufacturers including Veterinary Laboratories, Inc., Lenexa, KS, USA.

****** Phenylephrine injection BP; Sovereign Medical, Basildon, Essex, UK.

Table 4.7. Cardiovascular and pulmonary support for anaesthetised horses

	IV Dose	Dilution*	Typical dose/rate†
Atropine L.A. 15 mg/ml	0.015 mg/kg	Not applicable	0.5 ml/500 kg
Glycopyrrolate 0.2 mg/ml	0.003–0.004 mg/kg	Not applicable	5–10 ml/500 kg
Dobutamine 12.5 mg/ml	1–2 μg/kg/min	125 mg/500 ml (250 μg/ml)	30 drops/min ≈1.5 μg/kg/min/500 kg
Calcium gluconate 23% (20.7 mg/ml, 1.06 mEq Ca^{2+}/ml)	5–20 mg/kg 0.2–1.0 meq Ca^{++}/kg	Not applicable Compatible with most electrolyte solutions	Start at 30–40 drops/min, watch for bradyrhythmias/ dyshythmias; can increase rate if none
Phenylephrine 10 mg/ml	0.5–10 μg/kg/min 1–10 μg/kg slow bolus	30 mg/150 ml (200 μg/ml)	30 drops/min ≈1.5 μg/kg/min/500 kg
Dopamine 80 mg/ml	1–20 μg/kg/min	120 mg/500 ml (240 μg/ml)	30 drops/min ≈1.4 μg/kg/min/500 kg
Ephedrine 50 mg/ml	0.05–0.10 mg/kg	Not applicable	25 mg, single bolus; repeat in 5–10 minutes
Epinephrine 1 : 1000 (1 mg/ml)	6–10 μg/kg bolus	Not applicable	3–5 ml/500 kg Foals: 0.1–0.3 ml
Norepinephrine 1 mg/ml	0.1–10 μg/kg/min	10 mg/150 ml (66.5 μg/ml)	20 drops/min ≈0.25 μg/kg/min/500 kg
Lidocaine 2% (20 mg/ml)	0.5–2.0 mg/kg bolus 25–100 μg/kg/min	Not applicable 1.5 g/150 ml (6.7 mg/ml)	50 ml, repeat ×1 = 1 g/500 kg 30 drops/min ≈1.4 μg/500 kg
Albuterol (salbuterol) 0.5% (5 mg/ml)	2 μg/kg inhaled via endotracheal tube	To 1–2 ml	1 mg/500 kg over several breaths

*0.9% NaCl or 5% dextrose.
†Standard administration set–10 drops/ml.
Clinical uses: Atropine–critical bradycardia of sinus or AV origin
Glycopyrrolate–noncritical bradycardia
Dobutamine–low arterial blood pressure; improve cardiac output, high doses may cause tachycardia
Calcium–low arterial blood pressure when response to dobutamine is sluggish
Phenylephrine–low blood pressure; vasoconstriction, improve diastolic blood pressure and coronary perfusion
Norepinephrine–low blood pressure that responds to dobutamine with little increase in pressure and tachycardia
Dopamine–low cardiac output; low doses vasodilate, more dyshythmogenic than dobutamine
Ephedrine–low arterial blood pressure; induces a transient release of endogenous norepinephrine to boost cardiac output
Epinephrine–cardiac arrest
Lidocaine–ventricular dyshythmias; may protect against reperfusion injury
Albuterol–hypoxemia

Occasionally, significant bradycardia (heart rate <20 or persistently <26 beats/min) contributes to the low arterial blood pressure. In situations where the heart rate hovers in the low 20s and MAP in the 60s or lower, particularly when the response to dobutamine is a further decrease in heart rate with sinus or AV block, it is appropriate to administer glycopyrrolate†††††† (2.5–5 μg/kg).[87] Acute drops in heart rate, either sinus or commonly advanced second- or third-degree AV block, should be treated with atropine‡‡‡‡‡‡ (0.015 mg/kg, approximately 7.5 mg/average horse). As cardiac arrest is pending, a sympathomimetic agent (3–5 mg epinephrine,§§§§§§ rapid infusion of dobutamine or dopamine, whichever is readily available) should be in hand in case the situation deteriorates.[88,89] External cardiac compression by the largest person in the OR dropping his or her knees over the left thoracic wall with the horse in lateral recumbency does produce cardiac output.[90] Very rarely, a horse develops atrial fibrillation during general anaesthesia.[91] This may initially be noted by almost beat-to-beat fluctuations in blood pressure that on closer inspection prove to be due to the irregular rate of ventricular systole. These horses generally have no problems, but care

†††††† Robinul; Wyeth Ayerst, Cherry Hills, NJ, USA.
‡‡‡‡‡‡ Atropine sulfate; American Pharmaceutical Partners, Schaumburg, IL, USA.

§§§§§§ Epinephrine injection USP 1 : 1000; American Regent, Inc. Shirley, NJ, USA; Astra Zeneca Adrenaline; Astra Zeneca, North Ryde, NSW, Australia.

must be taken when administering dobutamine and anticholinergics avoided if possible as increasing AV conduction could allow too many of the atrial impulses to reach the ventricles, leading to ventricular tachycardia and perhaps fibrillation.

Balanced anaesthesia

It was the persistent hypotension and assumed hypoperfusion seen with inhalant anaesthesia that stimulated anaesthesiologists to explore balanced anaesthesia. Interest in whether reducing the inhalant component would improve ventilation and oxygenation spurred the search for optimal combinations. For a long time, small doses of ketamine and thiopental have been used acutely to prevent or stop a horse from moving and opioids have been given as adjuncts to inhalant anaesthesia for more painful surgeries, such as fracture repair. Likewise, regional nerve blocks prior to surgical incision and before recovery have been included in the anaesthetic management of very distal limb surgeries such as palmar digital neurectomies and hoof procedures where lack of digital sensation during recovery will not add risk. Over the past 10 years, adding constant rate infusions (CRIs) of guaifenesin, ketamine, BDZs, detomidine, medetomidine*******, morphine, lidocaine††††††† and combinations of these have become popular. Experimental and clinical reports support the theoretical basis for this practice as inhalant requirement is less and blood pressure and cardiac output more acceptable than with inhalant alone.[92–97] Whereas accumulation of α_2-agonists can be incorporated into recovery management strategies, agents that might affect muscle strength and coordination (BDZs, guaifenesin, lidocaine) or cause disorientation (ketamine, opioids) should be administered judiciously toward the end of surgery to avoid any adverse influence on the quality of the horse's effort to stand.[98]

Hypoxaemia

Hypoxaemia is one of the other major dilemmas of equine anaesthesia. Emergency surgery, dorsal recumbency and low pulse pressure (systolic minus diastolic arterial pressure) are statistically associated with poor oxygenation.[99] Relative hypoxaemia, defined as a Pao_2 less than predicted from the concentration of oxygen in inspired gases, is ubiquitous and potentially tissue-threatening hypoxaemia (Pao_2 < 60 mm Hg [<8.0 kPa]) are all too common, particularly in horses with colic. Atmospheric pressure (760 mm Hg [101 kPa] at sea level) is 21% O_2. Anaesthesia rebreathing circles contain 95% to 99% O_2. The partial pressure of O_2 in the alveolus, the source of O_2 for the arterial blood, can be calculated from the inspired O_2 and is approximately 100 mm Hg (13.3 kPa) and 600 mm Hg (80 kPa) on room and anaesthetic circuit, respectively. Typically, Pao_2 averages in the 200 to 400 (26.7–53.3) range in healthy horses anaesthetized for elective procedures.[100,101] As this level of oxygenation is more than adequate for haemoglobin saturation, most horses are not at risk of tissue hypoxia due to inadequate O_2. The inefficiency of O_2 exchange at the lung, however, is indicative of the mismatch of pulmonary blood flow to ventilated alveoli.[102] Not only does atelectasis occur with anaesthesia and recumbency,[45] but cardiac output and pulmonary blood flow distribution fail to deliver blood to all ventilated alveoli.[103] Although early application of mechanical ventilation after induction may partially prevent alveolar collapse,[100,104] it also decreases cardiac output[102] and its influence on oxygenation depends on the individual horse, its physical status, its recumbent position and, in some cases, the surgical site.[100,101,104]

There is no reliable method of improving Pao_2. Efforts are directed at improving cardiac output, supporting open alveoli and encouraging blood flow to ventilated lung. Dobutamine alone, despite increasing cardiac output, does not improve O_2 exchange but rather increases blood flow through existing open pulmonary vascular beds.[105] Positive end-expired pressure (i.e., not letting airway pressure return to 0 cm H_2O at the end of expiration in effort to "hold open" alveoli) sometimes alleviates hypoxaemia but significantly decreases cardiac output and arterial blood pressure.[106–108] Occasional large breaths or sighs to higher peak inspiratory pressures designed to reopen atelectatic alveoli are also not consistently successful. "Recruitment manoeuvres" that are a combination of sighing with PEEP over a series of breaths have gained popularity for managing hypoxaemia in human medicine and show some promise in anaesthetised horses.[109,110] Aerosolized albuterol‡‡‡‡‡‡‡ (salbuterol) injected into the endotracheal tube during inspiration improves oxygenation presumably by dilating small airways and perhaps vascular beds of perfusion-ventilated alveoli.[111] The concern that hypoxaemia would result in tissue hypoxia and increased postoperative morbidity and mortality has not been thoroughly investigated. One small retrospective study concluded that complications and outcome were unaffected by low Pao_2.[112]

Recovery

Controlling the recovery of such volatile and large animals is difficult. There are probably as many methods of recovering horses as there are veterinary anaesthesiologists and surgeons. All are unsubstantiated, personal preference and continually evolving. In the past there was considerable concern that prolonged recovery would increase the chance of myopathy and postoperative pneumonia. With improved monitoring and cardiopulmonary support, the maintenance phase of anaesthesia is more carefully titrated to a physiologically acceptable balance. As a result, the current

******* Domitor; Pfizer, Sandwich, Kent, UK.

††††††† Xylocaine; AstraZeneca Pharmaceuticals LP, Wilmington, DE, USA.

‡‡‡‡‡‡‡ Ventolin; GlaxoSmithKline, Research Triangle Park, NC, USA.

trend is to sedate horses in recovery and to encourage them to remain recumbent until they are more fully able to stand. To achieve this, it has become common practice to administer an α_2-agonist intravenously: 0.1 to 0.2 mg/kg xylazine, 0.001 to 0.002 mg/kg detomidine, 0.008 to 0.02 mg/kg romifidine§§§§§§§.[113,114] If administered at the time of disconnecting from the anaesthesia machine, xylazine will delay extubation and may be no longer effective when the horse actually becomes aware. Alternatively, a slightly larger dose of the α_2-agonist can be given at the first sign of nystagmus or at extubation. A problem with this strategy is that the horse may be too aroused and the sedation less effective. Typically, return to awareness after halothane is slower, which allows xylazine given at the first swallow to effectively calm the horse. After isoflurane, the horse may swallow as it moves to get up, making it difficult to administer anything. Tiny doses of acepromazine (3–5 mg/horse) delay extubation and interest in standing. It should be given about 20 minutes before leaving the OR as the onset is slow even after intravenous administration. Because quiet horses are often completely content to lie in recovery until asked to get up after acepromazine, horses that were particularly anxious preoperatively or did not respond optimally to the α_2-agonist premedication are the logical candidates for acepromazine. Additional sedation with an α_2-agonist may or may not be necessary. Horses needing a perfect, atraumatic recovery (e.g., those with fracture repairs) are candidates for both acepromazine and an α_2-agonist in recovery. In theory, romifidine causes less ataxia and has a longer duration of effect than xylazine, and there is some indication this may be the case at doses of 0.008 to 0.02 mg/kg IV.[113,114] Intramuscular administration of α_2-agonists is also a perfectly reasonable approach to calming recovery but may not give the same degree of control. Opioid analgesia has been reported to contribute to quieter and better recoveries,[115,116] but caution should be taken in redosing just before recovery if the opioid-induced compulsive behaviour seen with higher doses would be detrimental. Intramuscular opioid analgesia for recovery may be best as excitement is less likely after this route of administration. The impact of "balanced anaesthesia" techniques or management of recovery by transitioning to IV anaesthesia from inhalant before allowing the horse to emerge remains to be seen, but information to date is encouraging.[117,118]

Because longer recumbency is expected, O_2 should be supplemented with a demand valve to assist ventilation if the horse is not breathing spontaneously or, if it is breathing, by insufflation at 10 to 15 L/min. Both effectively prevent absolute hypoxaemia in recovery in most horses.[119–121] When connected to a 50-psig oxygen source, a demand valve delivers 100% O_2 into the endotracheal tube at a maximum flow rate of 160 L/min. This effectively ventilates an apnoeic horse when the demand valve is triggered manually but may not meet the normal inspiratory flow of a spontaneously breathing horse,[122] which has been reported to be approximately 220 L/min in the standing horse,[123] approximately 110 L/min through a 22-mm ID endotracheal tube[124] and greater than 300 L/min through a 30-mm ID endotracheal tube[57] in the laterally recumbent, anaesthetised horse. The resulting impedence to inspiratory flow created by the demand valve may distress the semiconscious horse and stimulate it to attempt to stand prematurely. For this reason, in spontaneously breathing recovering horses, insufflating O_2 from a wall-mounted flowmeter with flexible tubing placed well into the endotracheal or nasotracheal tube is perhaps safer.

Partial or complete airway obstruction on extubation is a recognised risk in equine recovery. Dependent nasal oedema due to the head being, at best, level with the heart in lateral recumbency and clearly lower in dorsal recumbency can be managed with intranasal phenylephrine spray******** to induce vasoconstriction and reduce nasal mucosal swelling[125] or placement of a short, uncuffed nasal or nasotracheal tube and securing the endotracheal tube until the horse stands. Nasotracheal or endotracheal tubes also prevent life-threatening complete airway obstruction believed to be due to laryngospasm, presumably in response to pharyngeal inflammation. Upper airway obstruction within 60 minutes of the end of anaesthesia has been associated with longer (>3-hour) anaesthetic periods.[126,127] Complete upper airway obstruction resulting in fatal negative pressure pulmonary oedema has been reported.[128–130]

Physical restraint and assisted recoveries

The use of physical restraint and assistance in recovering horses is a matter of personal preference and somewhat a function of the recovery stall design. Larger recovery stalls allow the average horse to careen forcefully into a wall, and some means of tempering this seems advisable. Carefully applied tension on a head rope as the horse initiates an effort to sternal or stand can discourage premature efforts and can help the horse balance. Adding a tail rope to steady the dancing of a stronger horse or help lift the hindquarters of weaker horses has distinct advantages in some circumstances. The objective of putting the horse on a fairly deep (12 inches) pad for the recumbent phase of recovery may be to protect against myopathy if recovery is prolonged. However, situating the horse on the pad such that its first effort to sternal is thwarted by the pad often encourages the horse to relax back in lateral recumbency to eliminate more anaesthetic before the next attempt, which will, consequently, be more co-ordinated. More awake in sternal, they tend to be more willing to pause and are more organised in their effort to stand (Figure 4.12). Having a large mat in the recovery stall is an argument for using a head

§§§§§§§ Sedivet; Boehringer Ingelheim, Bracknell, Berkshire, UK.

******** Neo-Synephrine Nasal Spray; Bayer Healthcare, Morristown, NJ, USA.

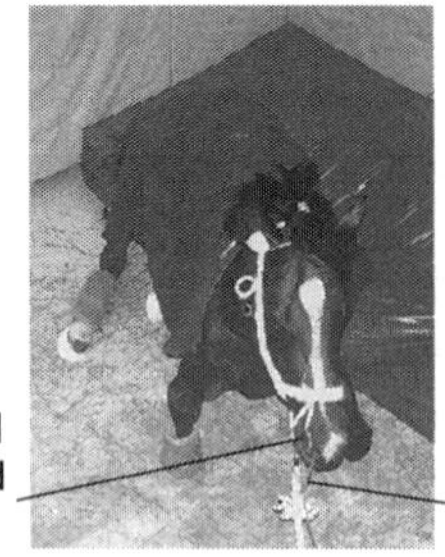

Figure 4.12 Horse in sternal recumbency during recovery. ©Lydia L. Donaldson, 2007.

rope to keep the horse from tripping on it. Several facilities have more elaborate methods for recovering horses: several pool systems,[131,132] an inflatable floor[133] and the Anderson sling[134] have been documented. An online review of assisted recovery is available at www.ivis.org.[135]

Postoperative pain management

Postoperative pain management (see also Chapter 6.2) begins in the preoperative period with nonsteroidal anti-inflammatory agents if nothing else. Painful hind limb procedures can benefit from epidural analgesics (see chapter on pain management). The onset of epidural morphine†††††††† (0.1–0.2 mg/kg) is slow (2 hours) and peak effect may not occur until 6 to 12 hours[136]; therefore, if it is to contribute significantly to postoperative analgesia, it should be administered well before surgery. Adding detomidine (20–30 μg/kg) hastens the onset, but the systemic α_2-agonist effects such as sedation, bradycardia and vasoconstriction are pronounced and will need to be incorporated into management of the induction, maintenance and recovery phases of the anaesthesia. Epidural morphine and systemic detomidine reduce MAC,[137,138] making them valid components of balanced anaesthesia. Intra-articular local anaesthetic can contribute to the anaesthesia if lidocaine or mepivicaine is placed in the joint before surgery and to postoperative pain if injected at the end of the surgery. Intra-articular morphine has been shown to provide postoperative analgesia in other species[139] and to have no adverse effects in the equine joint.[140]

4.2 Anaesthesia for some specific situations

Foals

The most common indications for surgery in equine neonates are ruptured bladders, septic joints, umbilical abscesses and occasionally meconium impactions, diaphragmatic hernias and small intestinal volvulus. Many foals with septic joints or umbilical abscesses are not yet systemically septic. Foals with ruptured bladders and meconium impactions are also at risk of systemic inflammation. They may or may not be hypovolaemic or have electrolyte disturbances depending on the promptness of the diagnosis. Like bladder ruptures, diaphragmatic hernias in foals usually occur during birth, but the impact of the diaphragm defect depends on how many and which abdominal organs are in the thorax and how badly ventilation and visceral perfusion are impacted by the translocation. Foals with small intestinal volvulus are in acute and extreme pain, which often puts them on the surgery table before complete ischaemic insult and the systemic effects of endotoxin release from devitalised small intestine become factors in anaesthetic management. The common anaesthetic choices for neonatal as well as older foals are listed in Table 4.8.

The traditional approach to anaesthesia for the neonate has been to avoid anaesthetics that require hepatic metabolism and renal excretion when possible on the assumption that neither the liver nor kidney is mature. There is some indication that this assumption is correct in the equine neonate,[141,142] but this species, born ready to stand and run, is likely to be more mature physiologically than those born in nests, blind and hairless. Nevertheless, equine neonates are often not given any premedication and are induced with an inhalant anaesthetic by nasotracheal tube (Figures 4.13 and 4.14). In healthy, rambunctious foals for which nasotracheal intubation may be stressful, xylazine (0.3 to 1.0 mg/kg, IV) is helpful. In less robust but ambulatory neonates, a BDZ (diazepam or midazolam 0.05–0.1 mg/kg IV) may facilitate intubation and contribute to a more stable maintenance phase of anaesthesia. BDZ sedation is subtle but clearly apparent in foals less than 2 weeks of age, particularly when combined with butorphanol (0.02–0.04 mg/g IV). In healthy older foals and adults, BDZs cause transient excitement, muscle relaxation and mild clinical anxiolysis most apparent in that the effects of other sedatives and anaesthetics are enhanced.

Oxygen flows and vaporiser settings for induction are relatively high (3 L/min and 3%–5% halothane and isoflurane or 5% sevoflurane, respectively) until recumbency, at which time the vaporiser setting should be reduced (1.5%–2% halothane and isoflurane, 3% sevoflurane) and shortly thereafter the O_2 flow can be turned to a maintenance rate of 1 L/min. Induction with propofol* (2–4 mg/kg IV) after BDZ/butorphanol premedication is an alternative and potentially less stressful for vigorous foals. Positioning of foals on the surgery table is less critical than for adults because of their smaller body mass, but abnormal positions should be avoided. In dorsal recumbency, the hind legs should be supported to prevent excessive abduction. Likewise, deep padding is not necessary, but a fleece pad, a heating pad covered with a towel or light blanket or some comparable arrangement of cushion and thermal support is beneficial. If a nasotracheal tube is used for induction, once the foal is at a somewhat stable anaesthetic plane, this smaller diameter (7–9-mm ID) tube can, but does not need to, be replaced by larger (10–14-mm ID) oral tube. Respi-

†††††††† Duramorph; Baxter Healthcare Corporation, Deerfield, IL, USA.

* Rapinovet; Schering-Plough Animal Health, Union, NY, USA.

Table 4.8. Anaesthetic choices for equine neonates and older foals

	Neonate (<60 kg)	1–2 months (<150 kg)	4–6 months (<300 kg)
Premedication	None	IV xylazine 0.5–1.1 mg/kg	IV xylazine 0.5–1.3 mg/kg
	IV midazolam 0.05–0.1 mg/kg	IV butorphanol 0.01–0.03 mg/kg	IV butorphanol 0.01–0.02 mg/kg
	IV butorphanol 0.01–0.04 mg/kg	IM xylazine 0.8–1.5 mg/kg	IM xylazine 0.5–2.2 mg/kg
	IV xylazine 0.6–1.6 mg/kg	IM butorphanol 0.02–0.04 mg/kg	IM detomidine 0.01–0.02 mg/kg
		IM Acepromazine 0.02–0.04 mg/kg	IM acepromazine 0.015–0.03 mg/kg
Induction	Inhalant By nasotracheal tube	Ketamine 1.8–2.4 mg/kg IV	Ketamine 1.8–2.4 mg/kg IV
	Propofol 1–3 mg/kg IV	Propofol 1–2 mg/kg IV	Midazolam 0.05–0.08 mg/kg IV
		midazolam 0.05–0.1mg/kg IV	
Maintenance	Inhalant	Inhalant	Inhalant
	Propofol ≈1 mg/kg IV repeat bolus CRI*: 0.15–0.3 mg/kg/min	Xylazine/ketamine ≈0.3/0.6 mg/kg IV repeat bolus	Xylazine/ketamine ≈0.3/0.6 mg/kg IV repeat bolus
		Propofol ≈1 mg/kg IV repeat bolus CRI: 0.15–0.3 mg/kg/min	Guaifenesin/ketamine /xylazine (5% G, 1–2 mg/ml K and 0.5–1 mg/ml X) 1–4 ml/kg/min
		Propofol/ketamine CRI: ~0.1–0.15 P and 0.05 K mg/kg/min[149,150]	Propofol/ketamine CRI: ~0.1–0.15 P and 0.05 K mg/kg/min
Recovery	Manual restraint	Xylazine 25–50 mg IV	Xylazine 50–75 mg IV
	Head and tail assist	Manual restraint	Manual restraint
		Head and tail assist	Tail ± head assist

*CRI, constant rate infusion, which, when used as the sole anaesthetic, is not constant but rather adjusted to achieve the anaesthetic level needed. When ketamine (K) and propofol (P) are used together, generally the propofol rate is adjusted over a constant infusion of ketamine. The CRI of ketamine may be slowed during longer procedures and should be discontinued 10 more minutes before propofol depending on the duration of the anaesthesia.

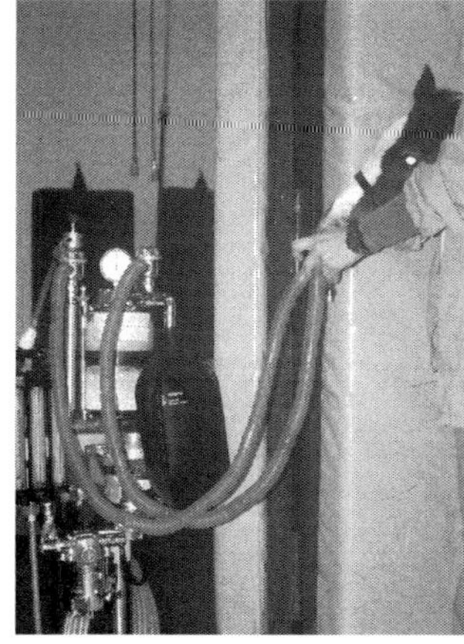

Figure 4.13 Inhalant anaesthesia induction of a young foal. ©Lydia L. Donaldson, 2007.

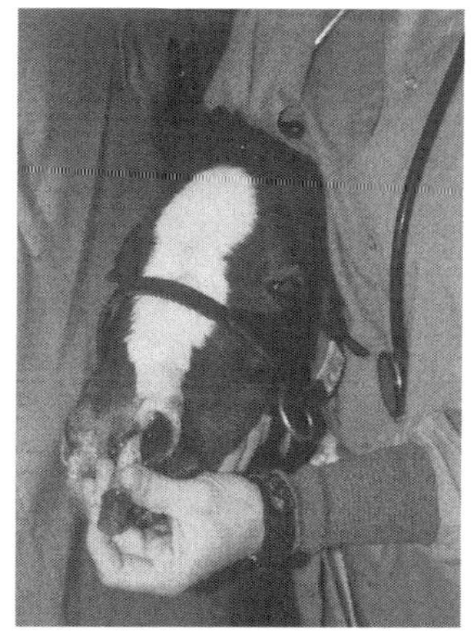

Figure 4.14 Nasal intubation of a foal. ©Lydia L. Donaldson, 2007.

ratory depression is as pronounced as in adult horses but, with the exception of foals with diaphragmatic hernias or sepsis, gas exchange seems to be compromised less by anaesthesia and recumbency. Usually, foals breathe well enough to maintain their $Paco_2$ at less than 60 mm Hg (8.0 kPa) and occasional manual sighs are sufficient ventilatory support. Thus, the purchase of a small-animal ventilator can be postponed until the caseload might warrant it. Systemic blood pressure should be monitored as hypotension is common. However, awake neonate and pediatric mammals have lower arterial blood pressures than adults and an MAP above 50 mm Hg (6.66 kPa) under anaesthesia is considered acceptable. Autonomic balance continues to develop during the early neonatal period,[143,144] which may explain the frequency with which second-degree AV block occurs during neonatal anaesthesia. Life-threatening sinus arrest and third-degree AV block are well documented, particularly with bladder or intestinal manipulation.[33–35] The administration of atropine (0.01–0.03 mg/kg IV), if the bradycardia is profound and abrupt, or glycopyrrolate (0.0025–0.005 mg/kg IV), if it is less pronounced but persistent, is appropriate when faced with these vagally mediated dysrhythmias. Having the surgeon stop manipulating the bowel or bladder may or may not turn off the vagal shower. Likewise, the bradycardia may or may not return with the resumption of surgery. The onset of vagal dominance may not be associated with any apparent surgical stimulus.

Other than an increased incidence of life-threatening, vagally mediated dysrhythmias, the challenge of neonatal equine anaesthesia is that it is harder to find the balance between surgical anaesthesia and acceptable blood pressure. In foals, isoflurane MAC may be the same or lower than that of adult horses.[145] Clinically, it seems as though foals require similar isoflurane concentrations as adults to produce surgical anaesthesia but that this plane of anaesthesia may be accompanied by a greater hypotension. Foals do respond nicely to dobutamine but, consistent with our understanding of the immature cardiovascular system, an increase in heart rate frequently accompanies the increase in blood pressure. As many neonatal foals presented for anaesthesia and surgery may be marginally anaemic, hypoproteinaemic and in the early stages of a systemic inflammatory response, the administration of balanced electrolyte solutions should be more judicious than in comparably sick adults. Although the common practice is to prevent nursing for only 30 minutes before anaesthesia, even healthy neonates are at risk of hypoglycaemia due to limited glycogen stores. This can be prevented by administering 2.5% dextrose in half-strength ($\frac{1}{2}$) lactated Ringer's solution or NaCl.[146] Alternately, 5% dextrose piggy-backed on the hospital's isotonic balanced electrolyte solution and infused at 25% to 50% of the total fluid rate will achieve a similar result with an only moderately hypertonic solution.

Recovering neonatal foals from general anaesthesia involves physical restraint followed by manual assistance on head and tail when they are ready to stand. During recumbency, O_2 insufflation and continued prevention of thermal loss (heating pad, blanket) are important. Foals should be restrained on their first attempt to roll sternal while wildly flailing their legs at or shortly after extubation as they are not ready to stand and most will relax for a period before trying again. As is characteristic of young foals, too much tail and head restraint will trigger passive resistance and they will refuse to support with their legs after making a good, co-ordinated effort to stand. Frequently, healthy foals want to nurse shortly after they stand. Allowing them to suckle while watching to be sure there is normal pharyngeal function usually results in only brief contact, after which the foal is content to lie down quietly.

Often, the biggest challenge in anaesthetising healthy older foals and weanlings is that they resent handling. A small dose of intramuscular α_2-agonist (0.5 mg/kg xylazine) may suffice to tame a 1-month-old for placement of a jugular catheter. A 6-month-old, opinionated weanling may need 2 mg/kg xylazine (0.02 mg/kg detomidine or 0.08 mg/kg romifidine) intramuscularly to permit safe handling. Otherwise, these older foals are similar to adults in their responses to sedatives, analgesics, anaesthetics and inotropes. Induction with just ketamine or ketamine plus a BDZ is most efficient. Propofol after premedication with xylazine, with or without butorphanol, is approximately 3 times more expensive than ketamine and offers no physiological or pharmacological advantage over ketamine in older foals when used for induction only. Maintaining foals less than 100 kg with propofol for very short procedures may be economical in that recovery times, and therefore personnel time, are shorter.[147,148] The use of propofol as a CRI (0.15–0.3 mg/kg/min) may be practical in the younger, smaller individuals or in combination with a CRI of ketamine (0.01–0.15 mg/kg/min propofol and 0.05–0.08 mg/kg/min ketamine).[149,150] Several of the suppliers of large-animal anaesthesia equipment offer methods of reducing the volume of their system to better suit foals that are too big for a small animal (>150 kg) but really too small for the adult (<300 kg) machine. Although a nice idea, this degree of sophistication is certainly not essential as these foals can be managed on the large circuits. The concern in putting a 200-kg weanling on a small-animal machine is that the breathing hoses are smaller than the foal's trachea and therefore add resistance to breathing. The 5-L reservoir bag is also too small to accommodate a maximal tidal breath (approximately 60 ml/kg). The concern in putting a 200-kg weanling on the large-animal circuit is that their normal tidal volume (10–20 ml/kg) may not effectively move expired gases around the large-diameter breathing circle as the expiratory pressure driving flow may be absorbed by rebreathing hose compliance. Thus, the O_2 flow should be kept as high as for an adult (>3 L/min) to encourage gas flow around the circle and minimise rebreathing. Recovery is managed according to the size of the individuals, and sedation with xylazine (50 mg/foal IV) helps prevent excessive purposeless floundering. In medium-sized foals, discouraging them manually until their efforts are strong and co-ordinated and then supporting them on the tail seems to be tolerated better than head support, as well as it being safer for the assistant to be behind the scrambling front legs.

Colics

The anaesthetic challenges that accompany the acute equine abdomen are hypovolaemia due to dehydration and/or extravascular fluid shifts, vasoplegia and myocardial depression due to endotoxaemia and the systemic inflammatory response, decreased thoracic compliance due to abdominal gas distension or intestinal impaction and hypoxaemia due to impaired gas exchange secondary to any of the above. Hypovolaemia should be addressed prior to anaesthesia and surgery[151,152] but the horse's behaviour in response to its abdominal pain and the urgent need to relieve intestinal ischaemia before irreversible pathology develops often make this impossible. The foundation of resuscitation from shock is large-volume isotonic, balanced electrolyte solution administration. If vascular endothelial barrier integrity is not compromised by the disease process, as is often the case with simple large-bowel displacements, isotonic fluids at 15 to 25 ml/kg/hr will usually suffice. Horses with small-intestinal strangulation/obstruction or colon torsion, unless taken to surgery immediately, will be in various stages of systemic inflammation. Hypovolaemia due to intravascular fluid leak will be accompanied by haemoconcentration and hypoproteinaemia. Isotonic fluid retention in the vascular space will be transient, and intravascular fluid volume as well as plasma oncotic pressure may need to be supported by the administration of hypertonic saline and/or a colloid.[151–155] There is some evidence that using these together is more beneficial than either alone.[156–159] Endotoxin and the mediators it releases interfere with normal myocardial and vascular smooth muscle function. For the horse under anaesthesia with compromised bowel, this may mean blood pressure is life-threateningly low and poorly responsive to dobutamine even after aggressive volume expansion and at a borderline plane of anaesthesia. In these cases, increasing the rate of dobutamine infusion usually results in little increase in blood pressure and tachycardia. The latter increases myocardial work when coronary blood flow is potentially inadequate. Adding calcium may improve cardiac and vascular smooth muscle tone, although there is controversy surrounding the administration of calcium in sepsis.[160,161] Blood pressure may be raised to maintain an aortic diastolic pressure well above coronary blood vessel closing pressure (approximately 20 mm Hg [2.66 kPa]) and therefore consistent with myocardial perfusion by the judicious administration of a vasoconstrictor. Infusion of either norepinephrine† or phenylephrine (Table 4.7), particularly when used to complement the positive inotropic support of dobutamine, to effect, will improve blood pressure in the sickest of horses. Problems often arise in these animals when this level of cardiovascular support must be discontinued for recovery. Continuing fluid and inotrope/vasoconstrictor administration during the early, recumbent phase of recovery may allow sufficient systemic recuperation for the horse to survive in the short term. Generally, horses that require norepinephrine to maintain a mean arterial blood pressure above 70 mm Hg (9.33 kPa) do not live to hospital discharge, suggesting that the need for this level of support truly reflects the severity of their disease.

The hypoventilation that is a direct effect of the anaesthetic agents is compounded by dorsal recumbency and gas- or ingesta-filled abdominal viscera as the former places the latter on the diaphragm and dorsal caudal lung lobes. If the source of abdominal pain is a diaphragmatic hernia, the intrathoracic situation is that much worse. Fortunately, rapid decompression of gas-distended intestine, elevation of a heavy colon or extraction of viscera from the thorax alleviates the need for prolonged, aggressive mechanical ventilation with higher inspiratory pressures (50–60 cm H_2O [4.9–5.9 kPa]) needed to achieve tidal volumes of 3 to 5 L and respiratory rates. These manoeuvres do not necessarily improve O_2 exchange as atelectatic lung is difficult to reexpand and pulmonary perfusion may remain poorly distributed. Whereas the incidence of absolute hypoxaemia in horses under anaesthesia for elective procedures is low,[100] Pao_2 values of less than 60 mm Hg (8.0 kPa) may occur in as many as 14% to 25% of horses with colic.[99,162]

As many horses with colic are exhausted and systemically compromised, recovery may be longer than for elective cases. If the horse is lying quietly, fluid administration and cardiovascular support can be continued during the early, lateral phase of recovery. Oxygen should be administered by manually assisting ventilation with a demand valve until spontaneous ventilatory efforts produce good thoracic expansion and are at a normal rate. At this point, O_2 insufflation at 15 L/min should suffice unless the horse was severely hypoxaemic during surgery, in which case the 100% O_2 delivered by continued use of the demand valve may make a difference in the horse's oxygenation and distress. Premature efforts to stand should be discouraged manually and with sedation as needed. The more severely compromised of this population may benefit from assistance in regaining their feet as they are often weak and may continue to be hypovolaemic despite aggressive intraoperative efforts.

Pregnant mares

If possible, elective surgeries on pregnant mares should be postponed until after delivery and, better yet, weaning of

† Noradrenaline (norepinephrine) 1:1000; Abbott Laboratories Ltd., UK.

the foal. When this is not reasonable, the safest period for foetus and mare during a pregnancy is the middle trimester, after most tissue differentiation has taken place and before most of the foetal growth. During early pregnancy, foetal resorption or loss may occur in response to the stress of surgery and anaesthesia but little can be done to prevent this beyond what is basic to good anaesthetic practice—minimise stress and optimise tissue perfusion. Late pregnancy, on the other hand, presents major challenges as the gravid uterus occupies a large portion of the abdomen and the maturing foetus is critically dependent on uterine blood flow. Ventilation and gas exchange are additionally at risk and hypotension is potentially life threatening to the foetus. Monitoring and supporting ventilation and cardiovascular function are essential to a successful outcome.

Third trimester mares that experienced hypoxaemia during exploratory laparotomy for colic are more likely to abort or deliver weak foals that do not survive.[40,41] Exposure to anaesthetic agents is only one factor contributing to foetal loss by a mare stressed by colic and surgery. All anaesthetics do cross the placenta just as they must cross the blood-brain barrier. Restricting anaesthetics with the intent of reducing foetal exposure is likely to be as detrimental to uterine blood flow and foetal stress due to maternal sympathetic stimulation as the anaesthetic agents themselves. Although α_2-agonists increase intrauterine pressure,[163] they have been used extensively to sedate pregnant mares without apparent adverse effects.[164] Maternally administered xylazine and detomidine do significantly decrease foetal heart rate, generally considered an indication of foetal stress, in contrast to acepromazine, which causes an increase.[165,166] In humans, foetal blood levels of diazepam, but not midazolam, are higher than maternal levels and babies from mothers given diazepam are sluggish at birth.[167] Thus, it might be wise to choose midazolam over diazepam for induction when anaesthetising a mare with a live foetus for controlled vaginal delivery or caesarean (Box 4.3). For these mares, using short-acting injectable agents (xylazine, ketamine, ±midazolam) and gas anaesthesia will minimise anaesthetic exposure to the foal. Of the inhalants, sevoflurane is less soluble in blood and therefore will reach the mare's brain, to anaesthetize her, and leave the foal's brain, for its recovery, faster than isoflurane or halothane. The objective of anaesthesia for caesarean section is to have the mare just sufficiently anaesthetised for surgery. In addition to the usual challenge of systemic hypotension due to anaesthesia, the dilated vessels of the pregnant uterus lead to significant haemorrhage on incision. In anticipation, aggressive isotonic fluid administration from the onset of anaesthesia is advisable. Even if the mare is not hypocalcaemic, starting a slow calcium infusion will help cardiac contractility, vascular tone, uterine involution and muscle strength in recovery. Of the inotropes, ephedrine is reputed to specifically improve uterine blood flow while also increasing cardiac output and arterial blood pressure. By comparison, dobutamine and dopamine increase uterine flow secondary to a general increase in cardiac output and tissue perfusion. Once the foal is out of the uterus, anaesthesia of the mare can be managed it would be for any horse undergoing abdominal surgery. Additional analgesics, now no longer a threat to the vigour of the newborn foal, can be given. Cardiovascular support should be tailored to blood loss and cardiovascular status. In reviewing 76 dystocia cases, the mare's blood pressure dropped during foetal delivery of the foal. After delivery, maternal $Paco_2$ decreased and Pao_2 increased. In that same group of mares, there were three horses with hind limb fractures in recovery. The combination of an older, only pasture fit mare, surgical pain, maternal instincts, foetal fluids and blood on the recovery stall floor despite efforts to keep it dry, exhaustion from prolonged labour and perhaps hypocalcaemia is a recipe for trouble in recovery. Sedation and restraint can be inadequate discouragement to premature efforts to stand in these tough, old, veteran broodmares who wake up determined to find their foals. If postoperative analgesics are used, low concentrations would be expected in the milk. The effects of prolonged exposure to oral opioids or non-steroidal anti-inflammatory drugs on the nursing foal are unknown.

Box 4.3. A reasonable anaesthetic protocol for mares during controlled vaginal or caesarean section delivery of a foal

Premedication	0.5 mg/kg xylazine IV
Induction	0.05 mg/kg midazolam IV or guaifenesin to effect (25–50 mg/kg) IV 2.0 mg/kg ketamine IV
Maintenance	
Before delivery	3%–5% sevoflurane or as little as possible Sevoflurane to effect
After delivery	Opioid, ketamine, lidocaine, α_2-agonist by preference and as for any abdominal procedure (see Table 4.3)
Ventilatory support	Mechanical ventilation
Haemodynamic support	≥20 ml/kg/hr balanced electrolyte solution
Before delivery	Ephedrine 0.05 mg/kg IV Dobutamine infusion, 1–5 µg/kg/min Calcium gluconate, 23%, slow infusion 0.25–1 ml/kg
After delivery	Continue rapid fluids and inotropes as needed Add colloid, plasma or blood if significant blood loss
Recovery	Continue fluids if possible Supplement O_2 Sedate (α_2 of preference), restrain and assist

Fractures and distal limb wounds that disrupt support structures

Horses with long bone fractures or distal limb injuries into joints and/or disrupting support structures present in grim pain. The injury often occurs during strenuous exercise; metabolic recovery (rehydration, normalisation of lactate, electrolytes, muscle cell metabolism, etc.) is delayed by the physiological response to tissue damage and pain. Ideally, these horses should be allowed to recover from the acute insult before surgery and anaesthesia. This may not be in the best interest of optimal repair of the bone, joint or tendon, particularly if the overlying skin has been compromised. When possible, a splint, fluids, analgesics and a night in the stall will result in a much better candidate for anaesthesia, surgery and recovery from both. Nonsteroidal anti-inflammatory agents and intramuscular CRI or epidural opioids (see Chapter 6.2) can give these horses enough relief to accommodate their pain without adverse effects. These drugs should then be incorporated in the anaesthetic regimen. Rushing stressed horses to surgery may be part of the reason their mortality rate is the highest of noncolic procedures.[8] Practical anaesthetic choices for horses with distal limb injuries are listed in Box 4.4.

Induction of horses with unstable limbs is gentlest after xylazine sedation followed by ketamine and a BDZ. Supporting the horse in a sling or by the tail and controlling the position of the injured leg while it settles into recumbency will help prevent further injury. Walking the horse to induction well before preanaesthetic sedation will allow it to partially recover from the stress of walking. This, in turn, means lower doses of xylazine will be effective and reduces the risk of α_2-agonist ataxia contributing to fracture fragment displacement. In positioning the horse on the table, muscle groups and nerves should not be sacrificed for surgical site exposure. The inhalant chosen for these horses will be by personal preference. Intraoperatively, arguments could be made in favour of any of them; therefore, behaviour in recovery may be the determining factor. Subjectively, it seems that recoveries from halothane after prolonged procedures (>3 hours) are not necessarily longer than those from the other two inhalants, but they are sloppy, almost rubbery. For most horses, recoveries from sevoflurane seem to be less explosive and more easily modified by sedatives than are those from isoflurane. There is the occasional horse that appears to be angry, almost aggressive on recovery from sevoflurane—an attitude not recognised with halothane or isoflurane. Regardless of the inhalant, these horses are good candidates for balanced anaesthesia with intermittent administration or CRI of opioids, ketamine, lidocaine and/or an α_2-agonist. To reiterate, care must be taken to recognise that drug accumulation, active metabolites and undesirable dysphoria and neuromuscular weakness will adversely impact recovery. As a general rule, consider discontinuing infusions 10 to 30 minutes before moving to recovery and have adequate sedation available to counter residual compulsive activity that may accompany opioid or ketamine administration.

Box 4.4. Possible anaesthetic choices for horses with fractures or disruptive distal limb injuries

Preanaesthetic analgesia	• IM, epidural, CRI or transdermal opioid AND/OR • IM, epidural or CRI detomidine AND • NSAIDs (see chapter on pain management)
Premedication	<0.5 mg/kg xylazine, try to avoid ataxia
Induction	• 0.05–0.08 mg/kg diazepam or midazolam IV • 2.2 mg/kg ketamine IV
Maintenance	• Inhalant of preference: sevoflurane > halothane or isoflurane • Repeated IM or IV bolus or CRI opioid and/or ketamine • CRI lidocaine, α_2-agonist (medetomidine > detomidine > romifidine > xylazine)
Ventilatory support	Mechanical ventilation because of the expected duration
Haemodynamic support	• 10–20 ml/kg/hr isotonic fluids • Dobutamine 1–5 μg/kg/min • Calcium gluconate 23%, 0.5–1.0 ml/kg slowly • Colloids, plasma or blood as appropriate
Recovery	• Discontinue CRI lidocaine and ketamine 20–30 minutes before recovery, slow CRI opioid and α_2-agonist • 2–4 mg acepromazine IV, 15 minutes before end of anaesthesia • Insufflate O_2, warm, quiet and do not rush • Continue IV fluids, catheterise and empty bladder if reasonable • Additional α_2-sedation as needed – 100 mg xylazine IV, beware of ataxia – 5–7 mg romifidine IV – IM before leaving OR if no α_2-agonist CRI for maintenance

Ocular, nasal, sinus and oral procedures

Corneal ulcers, descemetocoels and lacerations with impending global collapse need to be handled with care to avoid actions or drugs that might increase intraocular pressure. Xylazine and acepromazine decrease intraocular pressure unless the horse's head is allowed to drop to a level below its heart and resistance to venous return increases due to gravity.[168,169] Ketamine does increase intracranial and potentially intraocular pressure. Thus, induction with guaifenesin and thiopental is the preferred method if these agents are available. Once the horse is anaesthetised, the globe is in the hands of the surgeons. Intraocular surgery, where an absolutely immobile eye is critical, is most safely done with the addition of a neuromuscular blocking agent. Atracurium‡ (0.2 mg/kg IV) is probably the most commonly used agent for the horse because of its minimal cardiovascular effects, 20- to 30-minute duration of action and spontaneous degradation in addition to hepatic metabolism.[170] When paralysing horses, return of neuromuscular function should be monitored by nerve stimulation. Because of the critical need for normal neuromuscular function in recovery, the acetylcholinesterase inhibitor edrophonium§ (0.5 mg/kg IV) should also be administered before moving to recovery. Ocular manipulation can induce the oculocardiac reflex,[171] and therefore continuous ECG monitoring is recommended. As with any vagally mediated bradycardia, treatment with an anticholinergic (atropine 0.01 mg/kg or glycopyrrolate 0.0025 mg/kg IV) may be necessary if the ventricular rate drops below 20 beats/min and discontinuation of surgical stimulation does not help.

Like ocular procedures, the other common cranial surgeries present the particular challenge of anaesthetizing a horse without access to the head, specifically the ocular signs of anaesthetic depth. Changes in blood pressure, monitored continuously with a catheter in the greater metatarsal artery of the nondependent hind leg, become the most sensitive indicator of anaesthetic depth. Anal tone and reflex response to pinch or poke decrease but, like the ocular reflexes, differ from horse to horse. Having the surgeon or assistant surgeon watch for nystagmus if the horse has not been given atracurium is also helpful. Manipulating the globe, sawing facial bone, deep sinus curettage and hammering teeth are all strong painful stimuli that are usually applied intermittently. As a result, MAP increases during the aggressive surgical stimulation may not truly reflect the anaesthetic plane. Opioids and additional ketamine are commonly used to establish a more stable anaesthetic base. Nasal and sinus procedures are often abruptly terminated if haemorrhage interferes with visualization and threatens patient safety. Rapid debridement, packing and closure can make planning a controlled move to recovery difficult and can be complicated by discovering the horse is not sufficiently anaesthetised for transport when the drapes are removed. This combination of events does justify a pause before going to recovery to continue more energetic fluid administration, stabilise anaesthetic depth and give an analgesic for recovery.

Recoveries from anaesthesia for ocular surgery have been reported to require more attempts to stand and be of poorer overall quality.[172] The role of pain and/or disorientation due to sudden monocular vision in the rough recoveries remains to be determined. Pain may be an important factor as tooth repulsion and other sinus flap surgeries are frequently followed by poor recoveries. The recent use of larger doses of intramuscular opioids seems to have improved recovery quality. Better intraoperative analgesia or use of anaesthetics that may modulate neuropathic pain or hyperalgesia such as CRI ketamine or lidocaine may prove even better at producing postoperative analgesia and less desperate recoveries.

4.3 Total intravenous anaesthesia

TIVA is usually reserved for short, intrahospital procedures, such as cerebrospinal fluid tap, castration, joint lavage, invasive hoof debridement or inferior check desmotomy, that usually take less than 1 hour and often only 5 to 15 minutes. A "simple" cast change can take a deceptively long period of time. For very short procedures such as cerebrospinal fluid taps, xylazine (1.1 mg/kg IV), or another α_2-agonist, and ketamine (2.2 mg/kg IV) will suffice with most horses. The occasional horse will not go down, will go down and get right back up or will go down but clearly not be sufficiently anaesthetised. α_2/Ketamine anaesthesia can be improved with acepromazine (approximately 0.2 mg/kg IM) approximately 20 minutes before induction, a small dose of butorphanol (approximately 0.01 mg/kg IV) with the α_2-agonist and/or diazepam or midazolam (approximately 0.04 mg/kg IV) with the ketamine.[173] The latter two drugs may adversely effect recovery, so large doses should not be given. Detomidine (0.01–0.02 mg/kg IV) or romifidine (0.08–0.12 mg/kg IV) are both longer acting than xylazine but may or may not necessarily prolong the anaesthetic period.[174–176] Additional anaesthesia time can be achieved with supplemental boluses of xylazine and ketamine at one-third to one-half the original dose.[177]

Longer (30–60 minutes) TIVA is best created with combinations of guaifenesin, ketamine and an α_2-agonist. There are numerous formulas and advocates of each. It is important to recognise that the anaesthesia is being provided by the ketamine, and α_2-agonist as guaifenesin, although it may act on the brainstem to reduce awareness, is primarily a muscle relaxant acting on the spinal cord. An easy formula for guaifenesin/ ketamine/xylazine (GKX) to remember is to add 500 mg xylazine and 1000 mg ketamine to 25 grams of 5% guaifenesin (i.e., 500 ml), as these are essentially the common doses used to induce horses. The most frequent variations on this are to half the dose of xylazine relative to ketamine and guaifenesin (500 mg xylazine, 2000 mg ketamine and 50 grams of 5% or 10%

‡Atracurium besylate; Bedford Laboratories, Bedford, OH, USA.

§Enlon; Baxter Healthcare Corporation, Deerfield, IL, USA.

guaifenesin) or double the dose of guaifenesin to xylazine and ketamine (500 mg xylazine, 1000 mg ketamine and 50 grams of 5% or 10% guaifenesin).[178,179] Detomidine (0.005 or 0.01 mg/ml) or romifidine (0.04–0.08 mg/ml) as the α_2-agonist are also effective.[180–182] All are infused to effect (1–2+ ml/kg/hr). Induction should not be attempted with GK α_2-agonist solutions as it is difficult to safely produce effective blood levels in full-sized, adult horses by infusion. Thus, "loading" doses of α_2-agonist, such as xylazine (0.5–1.1 mg/kg IV), followed by ketamine (2.2 mg/kg, IV) or guaifenesin (approximately 50 mg/kg IV) plus ketamine (1.7–2.2 mg/kg IV), are needed. If the procedure is to be painful (e.g., castration, hoof debridement), a local nerve block will reduce the anaesthetic requirement and shorten recovery. Choosing different α_2-agonists for premedication and the TIVA combination is valid if there is some theoretical or practical advantage, such as intramuscular detomidine to control an unmanageable individual followed by additional intravenous xylazine or detomidine for preinduction sedation and in the TIVA. Also, a conservative dose of opioid, with concern for stereotypic behaviour in recovery, can improve the quality of anaesthetic. While recumbent, the horse should be intubated and on O_2 insufflation if breathing well or by demand valve to assist if needed. Positioning to avoid muscle or nerve injury is as important in these horses as for those on an anaesthesia machine (Figure 4.15). If a longer procedure is undertaken on TIVA, efforts should be made to put the horse on a pad. Recovery from this formulation of GKX is usually smooth but takes about as long as the period of anaesthesia. As every horse responds to and metabolizes the drugs differently, 50 to 100 mg xylazine may be useful in recovery to discourage premature, compulsive, ketamine-driven efforts to stand.

An application of TIVA is for moving "down" horses safely. Most of these horses have neurological (West Nile virus, protozoal myelopathy, spinal fracture) or neuromuscular disease (botulism, tetanus). The primary objective is to calm them and slow their flailing legs. It is often convenient to draw a cerebrospinal fluid sample and take radiographs while the horse is unconscious. Although thiopental is cerebroprotective and does not increase intracranial pressure, neither may be critical for these particular horses. Thiopental (2.5–3.0 grams) can be added to guaifenesin (25 g, 5%) and used effectively by infusion but, if the anaesthetist is not familiar with this combination, creating a safe level of anaesthesia is more difficult than with α_2-agonist/ketamine (± muscle relaxant) combinations. Ketamine-induced increases in intracranial pressure may be minor compared to those created by gravity in a horse hoisted by its legs or increases in $Paco_2$ due to hypoventilation. Therefore, perhaps more important than the choice of TIVA is careful handling of the patient with respect to its central nervous system and ventilatory assistance through an endotracheal tube and demand valve. Regardless of the maintenance technique, an induction dose of the primary anaesthetic (ketamine or thiopental) after premedication with an α_2-agonist should be given to achieve unconsciousness. Most of these horses have been sedated for transport and may not need any or only a small dose of α_2-agonist before induction. If the task at hand is merely to reposition a recumbent horse on a mat or waterbed, a single small dose of xylazine/ketamine (or thiopental) will suffice, particularly if the horse is on phenobarbital. As these horses are not expected to get up, including a small dose of BDZ (0.02 mg/kg IV) and further reducing the xylazine (0.3 mg/kg IV) and ketamine (1 mg/kg IV) can be sufficient for a simple rolling to the alternate lateral recumbency. During moving and once repositioned, respiratory effort (rate and thoracic expansion) and pulse rate and quality should be monitored until the horse returns to its preanaesthesia level of consciousness.

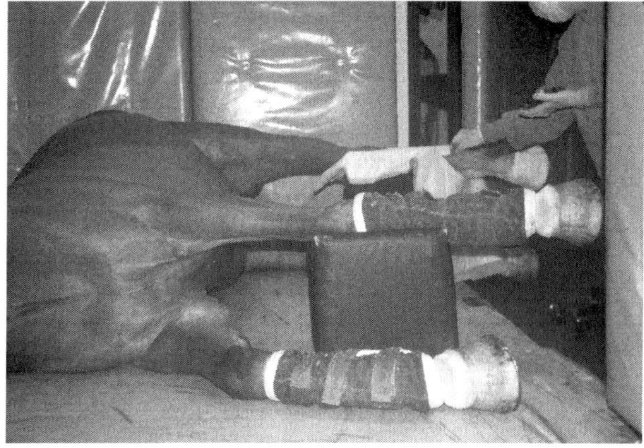

Figure 4.15 Positioning during lateral recumbency under total intravenous anaesthesia. ©Lydia L. Donaldson, 2007.

4.4 Standing surgery sedation and anaesthesia (see Chapter 6.1)

In-hospital standing surgical procedures tend to be involved and take more than 1 hour to complete. They include such procedures as rectovaginal reconstructions, laparoscopies, thoroscopies, cystoscopies, perineal urethrotomies, perineal melanoma resection, uterine polyp excision and any number of upper airway procedures. The foundation sedative for any standing chemical restraint is an α_2-agonist. Logically, for longer duration procedures, the choice would be a longer duration of action drug. Thus, detomidine and, to a lesser extent, romifidine are each a common starting point. Depending on the temperament of the horse, a little intramuscular acepromazine (0.02–0.03 mg/kg) can contribute an underlying calm. Personal preference will determine if repeated doses of detomidine (10–15 μg/kg IV) or CRI (6–15 μg/kg loading dose, 0.1–0.6 μg/kg/min)[183,184] is used. In either case, including butorphanol (0.01–0.02 mg/kg IV) with the first dose of α_2-agonist will add analgesia and sedation. If the horse demonstrates a change in sedation at approximately 1 hour, more butorphanol at this or a lower dose may settle it down. If the procedure is expected to take 1 hour or longer, CRI butorphanol (0.2–0.4 μg/kg/min)[185,186] may help create a stable level of sedation and analgesia. The advantage to CRI detomidine is the rate can be adjusted to produce the desired sedation without unacceptable ataxia. Keep in mind that the α_2-agonists inhibit the release of antidiuretic hormone and these horses will urinate. If the surgery is to be more than 1 hour, passing a catheter will limit the horse's awkward efforts to posture to urinate.

Surgeries caudal to L6 benefit from caudal epidural anaesthesia. Traditionally, single doses of local anaesthetics have been used. Lidocaine and mepivacaine (0.22 mg/kg diluted to 7–10 ml) produce analgesia and muscle relaxation for 60 to 90 minutes. Adding 0.17 mg/kg xylazine will extend the anaesthesia to 3 to 5 hours.[187] It seems that a fair number of horses develop hind limb ataxia with these conventional doses and lower doses (1–1.5 ml 20 mg/ml [2%] xylazine + 8–12 ml 0.5% lidocaine/horse) have proved effective when given through an epidural catheter advanced craniad several centimetres (M. Tomasic, personal communication). Alternately, bupivicaine** (0.06 mg/kg) can be used for longer-duration surgeries (4–5 hours) and immediate postoperative analgesia. Little attention has been paid to the postoperative management of perineal surgeries. It would seem logical to place an epidural catheter preoperatively, perhaps administer epidural morphine (0.1–0.2 mg/kg) several hours before surgery as its peak effect is delayed (approximately 6 hours), use the epidural catheter for regional anaesthesia with local anaesthetic with or without xylazine and have the postoperative pain controlled by the morphine and/or xylazine if the horse is rubbing its tail or straining and potentially disrupting the surgical repair.

4.5 Postanaesthetic morbidity

Finally, postanaesthetic mortality has been reported (approximately 1.6%; range, 0.12%–7.9% depending on the population). Morbidity is a much softer endpoint, and most public communications have been cases reports or anecdotal. The combined results of several studies of nonfatal postanaesthetic lameness (i.e., nonlethal myopathy or neuropathy) suggest an incidence that ranged from 0.6% to 6.4% where the latter defined lameness not attributable to the surgery on exiting the recovery as indication of myopathy.[12,13,27,32,188] The incidence of pneumonia or pleuropneumonia after the stress of shipping to a hospital and anaesthesia with or without surgery is unknown. The hypoventilation, hypotension, decreased cardiac contractility and hypoxaemia compromise tissue perfusion and put all tissues at greater risk of hypoxia. On rare occasions, horses have recovered from inhalant anaesthesia with neurological deficits suggestive of cerebral ischaemia. Subjectively, most commonly this seems to have been blindness. A single case of blindness on recovery that resolved in 24 hours was reported in a retrospective study of complications associated with 1314 general anaesthetics.[27] My experience includes a horse who recovered blind and with a head tilt that lasted a few days, one with minor (head twitching, trembling for 1–2 minutes) seizure activity for several hours postrecovery and one mare treated for dystocia that had grand mal seizures as she emerged from inhalant anaesthesia, never stood and was ultimately euthanised.

Recently, attention has been paid to postanaesthetic colic after nonabdominal surgical procedures. Postoperative ileus has been recognised as a life-threatening complication to emergency exploratory laparotomy with increased risk associated with preoperative physical status, lesions of the small intestine and duration but not type of surgery.[189–191] Increased sympathetic nervous activity due to stress or pain, changes in feeding and nearly all the analgesics and anaesthetics used in equine anaesthesia modify gastrointestinal motility in some way.[192–194] Even standing sedation with an α_2-agonist, with or without butorphanol, delays gastric emptying and decreases intestinal motility,[194–197] and it is common practice to withhold food for at least 1 hour, particularly after prolonged standing procedures. The incidence of postanaesthetic abdominal discomfort after nonabdominal surgery has been reported to be 2.8% to 6.0%.[198–201] Efforts to identify risk factors have produced conflicting results, but morphine (but not butorphanol) remains suspect, as does orthopaedic surgery, emergency procedures and not withholding food preoperatively.[197–199] The use of the anticholinergic agents atropine and glycopyrrolate is discouraged in equine anaesthesia because of their inhibitory effects on gastrointestinal motility.[202,203] Atropine is primarily administered in life-threatening situations such as profound sinus or AV bradycardia or cardiac arrest. However, glycopyrrolate is given fairly often to manage persistent bradycardia accompanied by poor arterial blood pressure.[87] In my experience, glycopyrrolate was probably responsible for horses developing oesophageal obstructions following return from recovery despite being muzzled for 1 hour. Muzzling for 2 hours postoperatively seems to have been preventative. In a brief, in-hospital review of 100 horses given glycopyrrolate intraoperatively, 1 horse with a large colon impaction was identified. As this is well below the incidence of postanaesthetic colic reported, it would seem that glycopyrrolate can safely be considered just another potential contributor to anaesthesia-associated gastrointestinal dysfunction.

Equine anaesthesia is a physiological, pharmacological and physical challenge rewarded by the patients' successful return to their feet in recovery and to a normal life after return to their owners.

** Marcaine; AstraZeneca Pharmaceuticals LP, Wilmington, DE, USA.

References

1. Johnston GM, Taylor PM, Homes MA, Wood JLN: Confidential enquiry of perioperative equine fatalities (CEPEF-1): preliminary results. Equine Vet J 27:193-200, 1995
2. Mee AM, Cripps PJ, Jones RS: A retrospective study of mortality associated with general anaesthesia in horses: elective procedures. Vet Rec 142:275-276, 1998
3. Lindsay WA, Pascoe PJ, McDonell WN, Burgess MLF: Effect of protective padding on forelimb intracompartmental muscle pressures in anesthetized horses. Am J Vet Res 46:688-691, 1985
4. White NA, Suarez M: Change in triceps muscle intracompartmental pressure with repositioning and padding of the lowermost thoracic limb of the horse. Am J Vet Res 47:2257-2260, 1986
5. Taylor PM, Young SS: The effect of limb position on venous and compartmental pressure in the forelimb of ponies. J Assoc Vet Anaesth 17:35-37, 1990
6. Klein LV, Wilson DV: An unusual cause of increasing airway pressure during anesthesia. Vet Surg 18:239-241, 1989
7. Bidwell LA, Bramlage LR, Rood WA: Fatality rates associated with equine general anesthesia. Proc Am Assoc Equine Pract 50:492-493, 2004
8. Johnston GM, Eastment JK, Wood JLN, Taylor PM: The confidential enquiry into perioperative equine fatalities (CEPEF): mortality results of Phases 1 and 2. Vet Anaesth Analg 29:159-170, 2002
9. Cribb PH: The effects of prolonged hypotensive isoflurane anesthesia in horses—post-anesthetic myopathy [abstract]. Proc Am Assoc Vet Anesth 1987
10. Grandy JL, Steffey EP, Hodgson DS, Woliner MJ: Arterial hypotension and the development of postanesthetic myopathy in halothane-anesthetized horses. Am J Vet Res 48:192-197, 1987
11. Lindsay WA, Robinson GM, Brunson DB, Majors LJ: Induction of equine postanesthetic myositis after halothane-induced hypotension. Am J Vet Res 50:404-410, 1989
12. Duke T, Filzek U, Read MR, Read EK, Ferguson JG: Clinical observations surrounding an increased incidence of postanesthetic myopathy in halothane-anesthetized horses. Vet Anaesth Analg 33:122-127, 2006
13. Richey MT, Holland MS, McGrath CJ, Dodman NH, Marshall DB, Court MH, Norman WM, Seeler DC: Equine post-anesthetic lameness: a retrospective study. Vet Surg 19: 392-397, 1990
14. Moens VY, Gootjes P, Lagerweij E, vanDijk P: Uberwachung de saurestoffsattigung von pferden in halthannnarkose durch pulsoximetrie am setum masale. Berl Munch Tierarzt Wschr 104:357-360, 1991
15. Whatney GCG, Norman WM, Schumacher JP, Beck E: Accuracy of reflectance pulse oximeter in anesthetized horses. Am J Vet Res 54:497-501, 1993
16. Matthews NS, Hartsfield SM, Sanders EA, Light GS, Slater MS: Evaluation of pulse oximetry in horses surgically treated for colic. Equine Vet J 26:114-116, 1994
17. Chaffin MK, Matthews NS, Cohen ND, Carter GK: Evaluation of pulse oximetry in anaesthetized foals using multiple combinations of transducer type and transducer attachment site. Equine Vet J 28:437-445, 1996
18. Koenig J, McDonell W, Valverde A: Accuracy of pulse oximetry and capnography in healthy and compromised horses during spontaneous and controlled ventilation. Can J Vet Res 67:169-174, 2003
19. Moens Y, DeMoor A: Use of infra-red carbon dioxide analysis during general anaesthesia in the horse. Equine Vet J 13:229-234, 1981
20. Cribb PH: Capnographic monitoring during anesthesia with controlled ventilation in the horse. Vet Surg 17:48-52, 1988
21. Neto FJ, Luna SPL, Massone F, Thomassian A, Vargas JLR, Junior JRS, D'Ultra Vaz BB, Crocci AJ: The effect of changing the mode of ventilation on the arterial-to-end-tidal CO_2 difference and physiological dead space in laterally and dorsally recumbent horses during halothane anesthesia. Vet Surg 29:200-205, 2000
22. Hopkins PM: Malignant hyperthermia: advances in clinical management and diagnosis. Br J Anaesth 85:118-128, 2000
23. Klein L, Ailes N, Fackelman GE, Kellon E, Rosenberg H: Postanesthetic equine myopathy suggestive of malignant hyperthermia, a case report. Vet Surg 18:479-482, 1989
24. Aleman M, Riehl J, Aldridge BM, LeCouteur RA, Stott JL, Pessah IN: Association of a mutation in the ryanodine receptor 1 gene with equine malignant hyperthermia. Muscle Nerve 30:356-365, 2004
25. Aleman MR, Williams DC, Brosnan RJ, LeCouteur RA, Imai A, Steffey EP: Suspected malignant hyperthermia in a horse anesthetized with halothane. J Vet Intern Med 19:363-366, 2005
26. Tevik A: The role of anesthesia in surgical mortality in horses. Nord Vet Med 35:175-179, 1983
27. Young SS, Taylor PM: Factors influencing the outcome of equine anaesthesia: a review of 1,314 cases. Equine Vet J 25:147-151, 1993
28. Hodgson DS, Dunlop CI: General anesthesia for horses with specific problems. Vet Clin N Am: Equine Pract 6:625-650, 1990
29. Clarke KW, Hall LW: A survey of anaesthesia in small animal practice; AVA/BSAVA report. J Assoc Vet Anaesth 17:4-10, 1990
30. Dyson DH, Maxie MG, Schnurr D: Morbidity and mortality associated with anesthetic management in small animal veterinary practice in Ontario. J Am Anim Hosp Assoc 34:325, 1998
31. Gaynor JS, Dunlop CI, Wagner AE, Wertz EM, Golden AE, Demme WC: Complications and mortality associated with anesthesia in dogs and cats. J Am Anim Hosp Assoc 35:13-17, 1999
32. Johnston GM, Eastment JK, Taylor PM, Wood JLN: Is Isoflurane safer than halothane in equine anaesthesia? Results from a prospective multicenter randomized controlled trial. Equine Vet J 36:64-71, 2004
33. Richardson DW, Kohn CW: Uroperitoneum in the foal. J Am Vet Med Assoc 182:267-271, 1983
34. Whitton DL, Trim CM: Use of dopamine hydrochloride during general anesthesia in the treatment of advanced atrioventricular heart block in four foals. J Am Vet Med Assoc 187:1357-1361, 1985
35. Gasthuys F, Steenhaut M, Van Huffel X, Hoefkens M, Picavet T-M, Deprez P, De Moor A: Perioperative cardiac

and respiratory arrest in three foals with rupture of the urinary bladder. Vlaams Dierg Tijd 56:199-213, 1987

36. Donaldson LL: A retrospective comparison of general anesthesia for geriatric and young horses. Proceedings World Cong Vet Anesth 8:134, 2003
37. Juzwiak JS, Slone DE, Santschi EM, Moll HD: Ceasarean section in 19 mares: results and postoperative fertility. Vet Surg 19:50-52, 1990
38. Freeman DE, Hungerford LL, Schaeffer D, Lock TF, Sertich PL, Baker GJ, Vaala WE, Johnston JK: Caesarean section and other methods for assisted delivery: comparison of effects on mare mortality and complications. Equine Vet J 31:203-207, 1999
39. Byron CR, Embertson RM, Bernard WV, Hance SR, Bramlage LR, Hopper SA: Equine Vet J 35:82-85, 2002
40. Santschi EM, Slone DE, Gronwall R, Juzwiak JS, Moll HD: Types of colic and frequency of postcolic abortion in pregnant mares: 105 cases (1984-1988). J Am Vet Med 199:374-377, 1991
41. Boening KJ, Leendertse IP: Review of 115 cases of colic in the pregnant mare. Equine Vet J 25:518-521, 1993
42. Kotani N, Lin C-Y, Wang J-S, Gurley JM, Tolin FP, Michelassi F, Lin H-S, Sandberg WS, Roisen MF: Loss of alveolar macrophages during anesthesia and operation in humans. Anesth Analg 81:1255-1262, 1995
43. Raphael JH, Selwyn DA, Mottram SD, Langton JA, O'Callaghan C: Effects of 3 MAC of halothane, enflurane and isoflurane on cilia beat frequency of human nasal epithelium *in vitro*. Brit J Anaesth 76:116-121, 1996
44. Larsen G, Hoff G, Wilhelm W, Buchinger H, Wanner GA, Bauer M: Effect of intravenous anesthetics on spontaneous and endotoxin-stimulated cytokine response in cultured human blood. Anesthesiology 89:1218-1227, 1998
45. Nyman G, Funkquist B, Kvart C, Frostell C, Tokics L, Strandberg A, Lundquist H, Lundh B, Brismar B, Hedenstierna G: Atelectasis causes gas exchange impairment in the anaesthetized horse. Equine Vet J 22:317-324, 1990
46. Funakoshi T, Ishibe Y, Okazaki N, Miura K, Liu R, Nagai S, Minami Y: Effect of re-expansion after short-period lung collapse on pulmonary capillary permeability and pro-inflammatory cytokine gene expression in isolated rabbit lung. Brit J Anaesth 92:558-563, 2004
47. Raphel CF, Beech J: Pleuritis secondary to pneumonia or lung abscessation in 90 horses. J Am Vet Med Assoc 181:808-810, 1982
48. Matthews NS, Lindsay SL: Effect of low-dose butorphanol on halothane minimum alveolar concentration in ponies. Equine Vet J 22:325-327, 1990
49. Doherty TJ, Geiser DR, Rohrbach BW: Effect of acepromazine and butorphanol on halothane minimum alveolar concentration in ponies. Equine Vet J 29:374-376, 1997
50. Steffey EP, Eisele JH, Baggot JD: Interactions of morphine and isoflurane in horses. Am J Vet Res 64:166-174, 2003
51. Holland M, Snyder JR, Steffey EP, Heath RB: Laryngotracheal injury associated with nasotracheal intubation in the horse. J Am Vet Med Assoc 189:1447-1450, 1986
52. Heath RB, Steffey EP, Thurmon JC, Wertz EM, Meager DM, Hyyppa T, Van Slyke GL: Laryngotracheal lesions following routine orotracheal intubation in the horse. Equine Vet J 21:434-437, 1989
53. Touzot-Jourde G, Stedman NL, Trim CM: The effects of two endotracheal tube cuff inflation pressures on liquid aspiration and tracheal wall damage in horses. Vet Anaesth Analg 32:23-29, 2005
54. Steffey EP, Howland D: Comparison of the circulatory and respiratory effects of isoflurane and halothane anesthesia in horses. Am J Vet Res 40:821-825, 1980
55. Aida H, Mizuno Y, Hobo S, Yoshida K, Fuginaga T: Cardiovascular and pulmonary effects of sevoflurane anesthesia in horses. Vet Surg 25:164-170, 1996
56. Grosenbaugh DA, Muir WW: Cardiorespiratory effects of sevoflurane, isoflurane, and halothane anesthesia in horses. Am J Vet Res 59:101-106, 1998
57. Steffey EP, Mama KR, Galey FD, Puschner B, Woliner MJ: Effects of sevoflurane dose and mode of ventilation on cardiopulmonary function and blood biochemical variables in horses. Am J Vet Res 66:606-614, 2005
58. Lemke KA, Tranquilli WJ: Anesthetics, arrhythmias, and myocardial sensitization to epinephrine. J Am Vet Med Assoc 205:1679-1684
59. Hikasa Y, Okabe C, Takase K, Ogasawara S: Ventricular arrhythmogenic dose of adrenaline during sevoflurane, isoflurane, and halothane anaesthesia either with or without ketamine or thiopentone in cats. Res Vet Sci 60:134-137, 1996
60. Gaynor JS, Bednarski RM, Muir WW: Effect of xylazine on the arrhythmogenic dose of epinephrine in thiamylal/halothane-anesthetized horses. Am J Vet Res 53:2350-2354, 1992
61. Gaynor JS, Bednarski RM, Muir WW: Effect of hypercapnia on the arrhythmogenic dose of epinephrine in horses anesthetized with guaifenesin, thiamylal sodium, and halothane. Am J Vet Res 54:315-321, 1993
62. Matthews NS, Hartsfield SM: Arrhythmogenic dose of epinephrine in isoflurane- or sevoflurane-anesthetized horses. J Equine Vet Sci 24:110-114, 2004
63. Harvey RC, Gleed RD, Matthews NS, Tyner CL, Short CE: Isoflurane anesthesia for equine colic surgery, comparison with halothane anesthesia. Vet Surg 16:184-188, 1987
64. Raisis AL, Young LE, Blissitt KJ, Brearley JC, Meire HB, Taylor PM, Lekeux P: A comparison of the haemodynamic effects of isoflurane and halothane anaesthesia in horses. Equine Vet J 32:318-326, 2000
65. Yamanaka T, Oku K, Koyama H, Mizuno Y: Time-related changes of the cardiovascular system during maintenance anesthesia with sevoflurane and isoflurane in horses. J Vet Med Sci 63:527-532, 2001
66. Driessen B, Nann L, Benton R, Boston R: Differences in need for hemodynamic support in horses anesthetized with sevoflurane as compared to isoflurane. Vet Anaesth Analg 33:356-367, 2006
67. Donaldson LL, Dunlop GS, Holland MS, Burton BA: The recovery of horses from inhalant anesthesia: a comparison of halothane and isoflurane. Vet Surg 29:92-101, 2000
68. Steffey EP, Howland D, Giri S, Eger EI: Enflurane, halothane, and isoflurane potency in horses. Am J Vet Res 38:1037-1039, 1977
69. Aida H, Mizuno Y, Hobo S, Yoshida K, Fujinaga T: Determination of the minimum alveolar concentration (MAC) and physical response to sevoflurane inhalation in horses. J Vet Med Sci 56:1161-1165, 1994
70. Read MR, Read E, Duke T, Wilson DG: Cardiopulmonary effects of induction and recovery characteristics of isoflurane and sevoflurane in foals. J Am Vet Med Assoc 221:393-398, 2002

71. Matthews NS, Hartsfield SM, Mercer D, Beleau MH, MacKenthun A: Recovery from sevoflurane anesthesia in horses: comparison to isoflurane and effect of postmedication with xylazine. Vet Surg 27:480-485, 1998
72. Matthews NS, Miller SM, Hartsfield SM, Slater MR: Comparison of recoveries from halothane vs isoflurane anesthesia in horses. J Am Vet Med Assoc 210:559-563, 1992
73. Tendillo FJ, Mascias A, Santos M, Lopez-Sanroman J, De Rossi R, San Roman F, Gomez de Segura IA: Anesthetic potency of desflurane in the horse: determination of the minimum alveolar concentration. Vet Surg 26:354-357, 1997
74. Steffey EP, Woliner MJ, Puschner B, Galey FD: Effects of desflurane and mode of ventilation on cardiovascular and respiratory functions and clinicopathologic variables in horses. Am J Vet Res 66:669-677, 2005
75. Santos M, Lopex-Sanroman J, Garcia-Iturralde P, Fuente M, Tendillo FJ: Cardiopulmonary effects of desflurane in horses. Vet Anaesth Analg 32:355-359, 2005
76. Pelletier H, Leith DE: Hypoxia does not contribute to high pulmonary artery pressure in exercising horses. Equine Exercise Physiol 3:30-36, 1991
77. Wilson DV, Rondenay Y, Shance PU: The cardiopulmonary effects of severe blood loss in anesthetized horses. Vet Anaesth Analg 30:81-87, 2003
78. Donaldson LL: Retrospective assessment of dobutamine therapy for hypotension in anesthetized horses. Vet Surg 17:53-57, 1988
79. Swanson CR, Muir WW, Bednarski RM, Skarda RT, Hubbell JAE: Hemodynamic response in halothane-anesthetized horses given infusions of dopamine or dobutamine. Am J Vet Res 46:365-370, 1985
80. Trim CM, Moore JN, White NA: Cardiopulmonary effects of dopamine hydrochloride in anaesthetized horses. Equine Vet J 17:41-44, 1985
81. Young LE, Blissitt KJ, Clutton RE, Molony V: Haemodynamic effects of a sixty minute infusion of dopamine hydrochloride in horses anaesthetized with halothane. Equine Vet J 30:310-316, 1998
82. Lee Y-HL, Clarke KW, Alibhai HIK, Song D: Effects of dopamine, dobutamine, dopexamine, phenylephrine, and saline solution on intramuscular blood flow and other cardiopulmonary variables in halothane-anaesthetized ponies. Am J Vet Res 59:1463-1472, 1998
83. Grandy JL, Hodgson DS, Dunlop CI, Chapman PL, Heath RB: Cardiopulmonary effects of ephedrine in halothane anesthetized horses. J Vet Pharmacol Ther 12:389-396, 1989
84. Gasthuys F, De Moor A, Parmentier D: Cardiovascular effects of low dose calcium chloride infusions during halothane anaesthesia in dorsally recumbent ventilated ponies. J Vet Med Assoc 38:728-736, 1991
85. Grubb TL, Benson GJ, Foreman JH, Constable PD, Thurmon JC, Olson WO, Tranquilli WJ, Davis LE: Hemodynamic effects of ionized calcium in horses anesthetized with halothane or isoflurane. Am J Vet Res 60:1430-1435, 1999
86. Hardy J, Bednarski RM, Biller DS: Effect of phenylephrine on hemodynamics and splenic dimensions in horses. Am J Vet Res 55:1570-1578, 1994
87. Dyson DH, Pascoe PJ, McDonell WN: Effects of intravenously administered glycopyrrolate in anesthetized horses. Can Vet J 40:29-32, 1999
88. Hale GJ, Chambers JP: Bradycardia and asystole following attempted arterial cannulation in a horse under general anesthesia. J Assoc Vet Anaesth 16:10-11, 1989
89. McGoldrick TME, Bowen IM, Clarke KW: Sudden cardiac arrest in an anaesthetized horse associated with low venous oxygen tensions. Vet Rec 142:610-611, 1998
90. Hubbell JAE, Muir WW, Gaynor JS: Cardiovascular effects of thoracic compression in horses subjected to euthanasia. Equine Vet J 25:282-284, 1993
91. Hubbell JAE, Muir WW, Bednarski RM: Atrial fibrillation associated with anesthesia in a Standardbred gelding. Vet Surg 15:450-452, 1986
92. Yamashita K, Satoh M, Umikawa A, Tsuda A, Yajima Y, Tsubakishita S, Seno T, Katoh S, Izumisawa Y, Kontani T: Combiantion of continuous intravenous infusion using a mixture of guaifenesin-ketamine-medetomidine and sevoflurane anesthesia in horses. J Vet Med Sci 62:229-235, 2000
93. Bettschart-Wolfensberger R, Jaggin-Schmucker N, Lendl C, Bettschart RQ, Clarke KW: Minimal alveolar concentration of desflurane in combination with an infusion of medetomidine for the anaesthesia of ponies. Vet Rec 148:264-267, 2001
94. Spadavecchia C, Stucki F, Moens Y, Schatzmann U: Anaesthesia in horses using halothane and intravenous ketamine-guaifenesin: a clinical study. Vet Anaesth Analg 29:20-28, 2002
95. Dzikiti TB, Hellebrekers LJ, van Dijk: Effects of intravenous lidocaine on isoflurane concentration, physiological parameters, metabolic parameters and stress-related hormones in horse undergoing surgery. J Vet Med A Physiol Pathol Clin Med 50:190-195, 2003
96. Kushiro T, Yamashita K, Umar MA, Maehara S, Wakaiki S, Abe R, Seno T, Tsuzuki K, Izumizawa Y, Muir WW: Anesthetic and cardiovascular effects of balanced anesthesia using constant rate infusion of midazolam-ketamine-medetomidine with inhalation of oxygen-sevoflurane (MKM-OS anesthesia) in horses. J Vet Med Sci 67:379-384, 2005
97. Clark L, Clutton RE, Blissitt KJ, Chase-Topping ME: Effects of peri-operative morphine administration during halothane anaesthesia in horses. Vet Anaesth Analg 32:10-15, 2005
98. Valverde A, Gunkel C, Doherty TJ, Giguere S, Pollak AS: Effect of a constant rate infusion of lidocaine on the quality of recovery from sevoflurane or isoflurane general anaesthesia in horses. Equine Vet J 37:559-564, 2005
99. Whitehair KJ, Willits NH: Predictors of arterial oxygen tension in anesthetized horses: 1,610 cases (1992-1994). J Am Vet Med Assoc 215:978-981, 1999
100. Day TK, Gaynor JS, Muir WW, Bednarski RM, Mason DE: Blood gas values during intermittent positive pressure ventilation and spontaneous ventilation in 160 anesthetized horses positioned in lateral or dorsal recumbency. Vet Surg 24:266-276, 1995
101. Moens Y, Lagerweij E, Gootjes P, Poortman J: Distribution of inspired gas to each lung in the anaesthetized horse and influence of body shape. Equine Vet J 27:110-116, 1995
102. Nyman G, Hedenstierna G: Ventilation-perfusion relationships in the anaesthetized horse. Equine Vet J 21:274-281, 1989

103. Dobson A, Gleed RD, Meyer RE, Stewart BJ: Changes in blood flow distribution in equine lungs induced by anaesthesia. Quart J Exp Physiol 70:283-297, 1985
104. Gleed RD, Dobson A: Improvement in arterial oxygen tension with change in posture in anaesthetized horses. Res Vet Sci 44:255-259, 1988
105. Swanson CR, Muir WW: Dobutamine-induced augmentation of cardiac output does not enhance respiratory gas exchange in anesthetized recumbent healthy horses. Am J Vet Res 47:1573-1576, 1986
106. Swanson CR, Muir WW: Hemodynamic and respiratory responses in halothane-anesthetized horses exposed to positive end-expiratory pressure alone and with dobutamine. Am J Vet Res 49:539-542, 1988
107. Wilson DV, Soma LR: Cardiopulmonary effects of positive end-expiratory pressure in anesthetized, mechanically ventilated ponies. Am J Vet Res 51:734-739, 1990
108. Wilson DV, McCGeely AM: Positive end-expiratory pressure during colic surgery in horses: 74 cases (1986-1988). J Am Vet Med Assoc 199:917-921, 1991
109. Wettstein D, Moens Y, Jaeggin-Schmucker N, Bohm SH, Rothen HU, Mosing M, Kastner SB, Schatzmann U: Effects of an alveolar recruitment manoeuvre on cardiovascular and respiratory parameters during total intravenous anesthesia in ponies. Am J Vet Res 67:152-159, 2006
110. Iff I, Moens Y, Levionnois O: An alveolar recruitment maneuver prevents deterioration of gas exchange in ponies undergoing laparoscopic castration in head-down tilt. Proceedings World Cong Vet Anesth 9:148, 2005
111. Robertson SA, Bailey JE: Aerosolized salbutamol (albuterol) improves Pao_2 in hypoxaemic anaesthetized horses—a prospective clinical trial in 81 horses. Vet Anaesth Analg 29:212-218, 2002
112. Trim CM, Wan PY: Hypoxaemia during anaesthesia in seven horses with colic. J Assoc Vet Anaesth 17:45-49, 1990
113. Santos M, Fuente M, Garcia-Iturralde P, Herran R, Lopez-Sanroman K, Tendillo FJ: Effects of alpha-2 adrenoceptor agonists during recovery from isoflurane anaesthesia in horses. Equine Vet J 35:170-175, 2003
114. Bienrt A, Bartmann CP, Von Oppen T, Poppe C, Schiemann B, Deegen E: Recovery phase of horses after inhalant anaesthesia with isoflurane and postanaesthetic sedation with romifidine or xylazine. Dtsch Tierarstl Wschr 110:244-248, 2003
115. Taylor PM: Effect of postoperative pethidine on the anaesthetic recovery period in the horse. Equine Vet J 18:70-72, 1986
116. Love EJ, Lane JG, Murison PJ: Morphine administration in horses anaesthetized for upper respiratory tract surgery. Vet Anaesth Analg 33:179-188, 2006
117. Mama KR, Wagner AW, Steffey EP, Hellyer PW: Use of xylazine and ketamine or propofol to modulate recovery in horses following sevoflurane. Proceedings World Cong Vet Anesth, 2003
118. Steffey EP, Mama KR, Brosnan RJ, Imai A: Use of propofol to modify equine recovery characteristics after 4 hours of isoflurane or desflurane anesthesia. Proceedings World Cong Vet Anesth 8, 2003
119. Waterman AE, Jones RS, Richards DLS: Use of a demand valve for postoperative administration of oxygen to horses. Equine Vet J 14:290-292, 1982
120. Mason DE, Muir WW, Wade A: Arterial blood gas tensions in the horse during recovery from anesthesia. J Am Vet Med Assoc 190:989-993, 1987
121. McMurphy RM, Cribb PH: Alleviation of postanesthetic hypoxemia in the horse. Can Vet J 30:37-41, 1989
122. Watney GCG, Watkins SB, Hall LW: Effects of a demand valve on pulmonary ventilation in spontaneously breathing, anaesthetized horses. Vet Rec 117:358-362, 1985
123. Gallivan GJ, McDonell WN, Forrest JB: Comparative pulmonary mechanics in the horse and the cow. Res Vet Sci 46:322-340, 1989
124. Tomasic M, Mann LS, Soma LR: Effects of sedation, anesthesia, and endotracheal intubation on respiratory mechanics in adult horses. Am J Vet Res 58:641-646, 1997
125. Lukasik VM, Gleed RD, Scarlett JM, Ludders JW, Moon PF, Ballenstedt JL, Sturmer AT: Intranasal phenylephrine reduces post anaesthetic upper airway obstruction in horses. Equine Vet J 29:236-238, 1997
126. Thomas SJ, Corbett WT, Meyer RE: Risk factors and comparative prevalence of rates of equine postanesthetic respiratory obstruction at NCSU. Vet Surg 16:324, 1989
127. Ludders JW, Erb HN, Gleed RD, Moon PF: Case-control analysis for determining possible causes of airway complications during anesthetic recovery in horses. Proc Am College Vet Anesth 2000
128. Kollias-Baker CA, Pipers FS, Heard D, Seeherman H: Pulmonary edema associated with transient airway obstruction in three horses. J Am Vet Med Assoc 202:1116-1118, 1993
129. Ball MA, Trim CM: Post anaesthetic pulmonary oedema in two horses. Equine Vet Educ 8:13-16, 1996
130. Tute AS, Wilkins PA, Gleed RD, Credille KM, Murphy DJ, Ducharme NG: Negative pressure pulmonary edema as a post-anesthetic complication associated with upper airway obstruction in a horse. Vet Surg 25:519-523, 1996
131. Sullivan EK, Klein LV, Richardson DW, Ross MW, Orsini JA, Nunamaker DM: Use of a pool-raft system for recovery of horses from general anesthesia: 393 horses (1984-2000). J Am Vet Med Assoc 221:1014-1018, 2002
132. Tidwell SA, Schneider RK, Ragle CA, Weil AB, Richter MC: Use of a hydro-pool system to recovery horses after general anesthesia: 60 cases. Vet Surg 31:455-461, 2002
133. Ray-Miller WM, Hodgson DS, McMurphy RM, Chapman PL: Comparison of recoveries from anesthesia of horses placed on a rapidly inflating-deflating air pillow or the floor of a padded stall. J Am Vet Med Assoc 229:711-716, 2006
134. Taylor EL, Galuppo LD, Steffey EP, Scarlett CC, Madigan JE: Use of the Anderson sling suspension system for recovery of horses from general anesthesia. Vet Surg 34:559-564, 2005
135. Driessen B: Assisted recovery in horses awakening from general anesthesia, in Steffey EP (ed). Recent Advances in Anesthetic Management of Large Domestic Animals, International Veterinary Information Services, Ithaca, NY (www.ivis.org): 2005
136. Natalini CC, Robinson EP: Evaluation of the analgesic effects of epidurally administered morphine, alfentanil, butorphanol, tramadol, and U50488H in horses. Am J Vet Res 61:1579-1586, 2000
137. Doherty TJ, Geiser DR, Rohrbach BW: Effect of high volume epidural morphine, ketamine and butorphanol on halo-

thane minimum alveolar concentration in ponies. Equine Vet J 29:370-373, 1997
138. Steffey EP, Pascoe PJ: Detomidine reduces isoflurane anesthetic requirement (MAC) in horses. Vet Anaesth Analg 29:223-227, 2002
139. Sammarco JL, Conzemius MG, Perkowski SZ, Weinstein MJ, Gregor TP, Smith GK: Postoperative analgesia for stifle surgery: a comparison of intra-articular bupivacaine, morphine, or saline. Vet Surg 25:59-69, 1996
140. Raikallio M, Taylor PM, Johnson CB, Tulamo R-M, Ruprah M: The disposition and local effects of intra-articular morphine in normal ponies. J Assoc Vet Anaesth 23:23-26, 1996
141. Bauer JE, Asquith RL, Kivipelto J: Serum biochemical indicators of liver function in neonatal foals. Am J Vet Res 50:2037-2041, 1989
142. Norman WM, Court MH, Greenblatt DJ: Age-related changes in the pharmacokinetic disposition of diazepam in foals. Am J Vet Res 58:878-880, 1997
143. Matsui K, Sugano A, Masuyama I, Amada A, Kano Y: Alterations in the heart rate of thoroughbred horse, pony and Holstein cow through pre- and post-natal stages. Jpn J Vet Sci 46:505-510, 1984
144. Tovar P, Escabias MI, Santisteban R: Evolution of the ECG from Spanish bred foals during the post natal stage. Res Vet Sci 46:358-362, 1989
145. Dunlop CI, Hodgson DS, Grandy JL, Chapman PL, Heath RB: The MAC of isoflurane in foals. Proc Am Coll Vet Anesth, 1988
146. Adams JG, Trim CM: Plasma Glucose concentrations in anesthetized foals. Equine Pract 12:25-29, 1990
147. Matthews NS, Chaffin MK, Erickson SW, Overhulse WA: Propofol anesthesia for non-surgical procedures of neonatal foals. Equine Pract 17:15-20, 1995
148. Donaldson LL, Dunlop GS, Cooper WL: A comparison of propofol with ketamine after xylazine and butorphanol as field anesthesia for young foals. Proceedings Am College Vet Anesth, 1998
149. Flaherty D, Reid J, Welsh E, Montiero AM, Lerche P, Nolan A: A pharmacodynamic study of propofol or propofol and ketamine infusions in ponies undergoing surgery. Res Vet Sci 62:179-184, 1997
150. Ohta M, Oku K, Mukai K, Akiyama K, Mizuno Y: Propofol-ketamine anesthesia for internal fixation of fractures in racehorses. J Vet Med Sci 66:1433-1436, 2004
151. Dyson DH, Pascoe PJ: Influence of preinduction methoxamine, lactated Ringer solution, or hypertonic saline solution infusion or postinduction dobutamine infusion on anesthetic-induced hypotension in horses. Am J Vet Res 51:17-21, 1990
152. Hallowell GD, Corley KTT: Preoperative administration of hydroxyethyl starch or hypertonic saline to horses with colic. J Vet Intern Med 20:980-986, 2006
153. Bertone JJ, Gossett KA, Shoemaker KE, Bertone AL, Schneiter HL: Effect of hypertonic vs isotonic saline solution on responses to sublethal *Escherichia coli* endotoxemia in horses. Am J Vet Res 51:999-1007, 1990
154. MacFarlane D: Hetastarch: a synthetic colloid with potential in equine patients. Compendium 21:867-877, 1999
155. Jones PA, Bain FT, Byars TD, David JB, Boston RC: Effect of hydroxyethyl starch infusion on colloid oncotic pressure in hypoproteinemic horses. J Am Vet Med Assoc 218:1130-1135, 2001
156. Kreimeier U, Frey L, Dentz J, Herbel T, Messmer K: Hypertonic saline dextran resuscitation during the initial phase of acute endotoxemia: effect on regional blood flow. Crit Care Med 19:801-809, 1991
157. Moon PF, Snyder JR, Haskins SC, Perron PR, Kramer GC: Effects of a highly concentrated hypertonic saline-dextran volume expander on cardiopulmonary function in anesthetized normovolemic horses. Am J Vet Res 52:1611-1618, 1991
158. Jonas J, Heimann A, Strecker U, Kempski O: Hypertonic/hyperoncotic resuscitation after intestinal superior mesenteric artery occlusion: early effects on circulation and intestinal reperfusion. Shock 14:24-29, 2000
159. Pantaleon LG, Furr MO, McKenzie HC, Donaldson L: Cardiovascular and pulmonary effects of hetastarch plus hypertonic saline solutions during experimental endotoxemia in anesthetized horses. J Vet Intern Med 20:1422-1438, 2006
160. Song S-K, Karl IE, Ackerman JJH, Hotchkiss RS: Increased intracellular Ca^{++}: a critical link in the pathophysiology of sepsis. Proc Natl Acad Sci USA 90:3933-3937, 1993
161. Carlstedt R, Eriksson Mats, Kiiski R, Larsson A, Lind L: Hypocalcemia during porcine endotoxemic shock: effects of calcium administration. Crit Care Med 28:2909-2914, 2000
162. Hubbell JAW, Muir WW, Casey MF: Retrospective study of horses with low arterial oxygen tensions. Vet Surg 15:460, 1986
163. Schatzmann U, Josseck H, Stauffer J-L, Goossens L: Effects of α_2-agonists on intrauterine pressure and sedation in horses: comparison between detomidine, romifidine and xylazine. J Vet Med A 41:523-529, 1994
164. Luukkanen L, Katila T, Koshkinen E: Some effects of multiple administrations of detomidine during the last trimester of equine pregnancy. Equine Vet J 29:400-403, 1997
165. McGladdery AJ, Cottrill CM, Rossdale PD: Effects upon the fetus of sedative drugs administered to the mare [abstract]. Proceedings Int Conf Vet Perinatol 2:14, 1990
166. Smith LJ, Schott: Xylazine-induced fetal bradycardia. Proceedings Int Conf Vet Perinatol 2:36, 1990
167. McElhatton PR: The effects of benzodiazepine use during pregnancy and lactation. Reprod Toxicol 8:461-475, 1994
168. McClure JR, Gelatt KN, Gum GG, Manning JP: The effect of parenteral acepromazine and xylazine on intraocular pressure in the horse. Vet Med 71:1727-1730, 1976
169. Van der Woerdt A, Gilger BC, Wilkie DA, Strauch SM: Effect of auriculopalpebral nerve block and intravenous administration of xylazine on intraocular pressure and corneal thickness in horses. Am J Vet Res 56:155-158, 1995
170. Hildebrand SV, Holland M, Copland VS, Daunt D, Brock N: Clinical use of the neuromuscular blocking agents atracurium and pancuronium for equine anesthesia. J Am Vet Med Assoc 195:212-219
171. Short CE, Rebhun WC: Complications caused by the oculocardiac reflex during anesthesia in a foal. J Am Vet Med Assoc 176:630-631, 1980
172. Parviainen AKJ, Trim CM: Complications associated with anaesthesia for ocular surgery: a retrospective study 1989-1996. Equine Vet J 32:555-559, 2000

173. Marntell S, Nyman G: Effects of additional premedication on romifidine and ketamine anaesthesia in horses. Acta Vet Scand 37:315-325, 1996
174. Wan PY, Trim CM, Mueller POE: Xylazine-ketamine and detomidine-tiletamine-zolazepam anesthesia in horses. Vet Surg 21:312-318, 1992
175. Matthews NS, Miller SM, Slater MR, Hartsfield SM, Short CE: A comparison of xylazine-ketamine and detomidine-ketamine anaesthesia in horses. J Vet Anaesth 20:68-72, 1993
176. Kerr CL, McDonell WN, Young SS: A comparison of romifidine and xylazine when used with diazepam/ketamine for short duration anesthesia in the horse. Can Vet J 37:601-609, 1996
177. McCarty JE, Trim CM, Ferguson D: Prolongation of anesthesia with xylazine, ketamine and guaifenesin in horses: 64 cases (1986-1989)
178. Young LE, Bartram DH, Diamond MJ, Gregg AS, Jones RS: Clinical evaluation of an infusion of xylazine, guaifenesin and ketamine for maintenance of anaesthesia in horses. Equine Vet J 25:115-119, 1993
179. Muir WW, Lerche P, Robertson JT, Hubbell JAE, Beard W, Miller T, Badgley B, Bothwell V: Comparison of four drug combinations for total intravenous anesthesia of horses undergoing surgical removal of an abdominal testis. J Am Vet Med Assoc 217:869-873, 2000
180. Taylor PM, Luna SPL, White KL, Bloomfield M, Fowden AL: Intravenous anaesthesia using detomidine, ketamine and guaiphenesin for laparotomy in pregnant pony mares. Vet Anaesth Analg 28:119-125, 2001
181. Thurmon JC, Ko JCH, Lin HC, Olsen WA: Guaifenesin-ketamine-detomidine anesthesia for castration of ponies. J Equine Vet Sci 17:262-266, 1997
182. McMurphy RM, Young LE, Marlin DJ, Walsh K: Comparison of the cardiopulmonary effects of anesthesia maintained by continuous infusion of romifidine, guaifenesin, and ketamine with anesthesia maintained by inhalation of halothane in horses. Am J Vet Res 63:1655-1661, 2002
183. Hainisch EK: Sedation by continuous intravenous detomidine drip for standing surgical procedures. Equine Vet Ed 13:51-52, 2001
184. Wilson DV, Bohart GV, Evans AT, Robertson S, Rondenay Y: Retrospective analysis of detomidine infusion for standing chemical restraint in 51 horses. Vet Anaesth Analg 29:54-57, 2002
185. Sellon DC, Monroe VL, Roberts MC, Papich MG: Pharmacokinetics and adverse effects of butorphanol administered by single intravenous injection or continuous intravenous infusion in horses. Am J Vet Res 62:183-189, 2001
186. Sellon DC, Roberts MC, Blikslager AT, Ulibarri C, Papich MG: Effects of continuous rate intravenous infusion of butorphanol on physiologic and outcome variables in horses after celiotomy. J Vet Intern Med 18:555-563, 2004
187. Grubb TL, Riebold TW, Huber MJ: Comparison of lidocaine, xylazine, and xylazine/lidocaine for caudal epidural analgesia in horses. J Am Vet Med Assoc 201:1187-1190, 1992
188. Franci P, Leece EA, Brearly JC: Post anaesthetic myopathy/neuropathy in horses undergoing magnetic resonance imaging compared to horses undergoing surgery. Equine Vet J 38:497-501, 2006
189. Blikslager AT, Bowman KF, Levine JF, Bristol DG, Roberts MC: Evaluation of factors associated with postoperative ileus in horses: 31 cases (1990-1992). J Am Vet Med Assoc 205:1748-1752
190. Roussel AJ, Cohen ND, Hooper RN, Rakestraw PC: Risk factors associated with the development of postoperative ileus in horses. J Am Vet Med Assoc 219:72-78, 2001
191. Cohen ND, Lester GD, Sanchez LC, Merritt AM, Roussel AJ: Evaluation of risk factors associated with the development of postoperative ileus in horses. J Am Vet Med Assoc 225:1070-1078, 2004
192. Roberts MC, Argenzio A: Effects of amitraz, several opiate derivatives and anticholinergic agents on intestinal transit in ponies. Equine Vet J 18:256-260, 1986
193. Lester GD, Bolton JR, Cullen LK, Thurgate SM: Effects of general anesthesia on myoelectric activity of the intestine in horses. Am J Vet Res 53:1553-1557, 1992
194. Doherty TJ, Andrews FM, Provenza MK, Frazier DL: The effect of sedation on gastric emptying of a liquid marker in ponies. Vet Surg 28:375-379, 1999
195. Merritt Am, Burrow JA, Hartless CS: Effect of xylazine, detomidine, and a combination of xylazine and butorphanol on equine duodenal motility. Am J Vet Res 59:619-123, 1998
196. Freeman SL, England GCW: Effect of romifidine on gastrointestinal motility, assessed by transrectal ultrasonography. Equine Vet J 33:570-576, 2001
197. Sutton DGM, Preston T, Christley RM, Cohen ND, Love S, Roussel AJ: The effects of xylazine, detomidine, acepromazine and butorphanol on equine solid phase gastric emptying rate. Equine Vet J 34:486-492, 2002
198. Mircica E, Clutton RE, Kyles KW, Blissitt KJ: Problems associated with perioperative morphine in horses: a retrospective case analysis. Vet Anaesth Analg 30:147-155, 2003
199. Senior JM, Pinchbeck GL, Dugdale AHA, Clegg PD: Retrospective study of the risk factors and prevalence of colic in horses after orthopedic surgery. Vet Rec 155:321-325, 2004
200. Andersen MS, Clark L, Dyson SJ, Newton JR: Risk factors for colic in horses after general anaesthesia for MRI or non-abdominal surgery: absence of evidence of effect from peri-anaesthetic morphine. Equine Vet J 38:368-374, 2006
201. Senior JM, Pinchbeck GL, Allister R, Dugdale AHA, Clark L, Clutton RE, Coumbe K, Dyson S, Clegg PD: Post anaesthetic colic in horses: a preventable complication? Equine Vet J 38:479-484, 2006
202. Ducharme NG, Fubini SL: Gastrointestinal complications associated with the use of atropine in horses. J Am Vet Med Assoc 182:229-231, 1983
203. Singh S, McDonell WN, Young SS, Dyson DH: Cardiopulmonary and gastrointestinal motility effects of xylazine/ketamine-induced anesthesia in horses previously treated with glycopyrrolate. Am J Vet Res 57:1762-1770, 1996
204. Doherty TJ, Frazier DL: Effect of intravenous lidocaine on halothane minimum alveolar concentration in ponies. Equine Vet J 30:300-303, 1998
205. Muir WW, Sams R: Effects of ketamine infusion on halothane minimal alveolar concentration in horses. Am J Vet Res 53:1802-1806, 1992

5

Nutritional management of the hospitalised horse

Meri Stratton-Phelps

5.1 The adult horse
5.2 Nutritional management of the hospitalised foal

Critical care nutrition is an integral part of the medical management of the hospitalised adult horse and neonatal foal. Early intervention with either enteral nutrition or parenteral nutrition (PN) is the key to a successful recovery from infection or following surgery. A delay in therapy can lead to protein-calorie malnutrition, immune system impairment, delayed wound healing and a prolonged recovery period and hospitalisation. Nutritional therapy is designed to blunt the effects of malnutrition in the critically ill equine (Box 5.1). This chapter provides the clinician with the information required to perform a basic nutrition consult, starting with the evaluation of the hospitalised horse or foal and ending with the formulation and administration of either enteral or parenteral diets.

5.1 The adult horse

Patient evaluation

A four-step approach is used to evaluate the adult horse before a nutrition plan is developed. Guidelines on the assessment of the equine neonate are provided in Chapter 5.2. Firstly, the horse's clinical condition should be evaluated to determine whether enteral nutrition or PN is appropriate for the patient. Secondly, the horse's body weight should be measured and a body condition score (BCS) should be assigned to the patient. Thirdly, the horse's nutritional history should be reviewed with the owner, referring veterinarian or attending clinician to determine the nutrient intake of the horse prior to initiating therapy. Finally, the horse's serum biochemistry profile should be evaluated to identify metabolic complications in the patient that can be managed with supplemental nutrition. Each of these assessments is discussed separately in the following section.

Box 5.1. Goals of nutrition therapy in the hospitalised equine

1. Slow or eliminate weight loss and protein catabolism
2. Provide sufficient nutrients to enhance wound healing and optimise immune system function
3. In animals that can tolerate enteral feeding, promote gastrointestinal tract barrier function
4. Decrease the complications from sepsis and secondary infections
5. Decrease the time of hospitalisation
6. Decrease recovery time so the horse can return to the former level of work or athletic activity

1. Assessing the horse's clinical condition

The clinical evaluation of the hospitalised horse begins with a thorough physical examination and an examination of the oral cavity. Presenting complaints of anorexia should be distinguished from dysphagia and mechanical disorders of the mouth and gastrointestinal tract. Horses with severe malnutrition may present with clinical signs of nutrient deficiencies that include weight loss, poor muscle condition, muscle weakness and anaemia. The chronicity of the disease and the diet history of the horse provide clues to the type of nutrient deficiency so appropriate diagnostic tests can be selected. Common nutrient deficiencies in the anorectic horse are discussed in detail in the following Nutrient Requirements section of this chapter.

Therapeutic diets are designed to meet the specific nutrient needs of equine patients. Supplemental dietary protein is beneficial for horses with protein-calorie malnutrition if renal and hepatic function is not compromised. Obese equine patients are predisposed to derangements in lipid metabolism including hypertriglyceridaemia, hyperlipaemia and hyperlipidaemia. Any horse that is maintained in

Box 5.2. Equation for estimate of body weight using chest girth and body length

$$\text{Body weight (kg)} = \frac{[\text{chest girth (cm)}]^2 \times \text{length (cm)}}{11877}$$

an NPO status should be treated with supplemental nutrition until they are able to resume food consumption.

The horse's medical condition dictates the form of supplemental nutrition. Assisted enteral feeding (AEF) with a liquid diet, commonly referred to as enteral nutrition, is the treatment of choice for horses that have progressive gastrointestinal motility and that can tolerate placement of a nasogastric tube. PN is usually reserved for horses that cannot tolerate enteral nutrition due to ileus, persistent gastric reflux or a disease condition that prohibits placement of a nasogastric tube. An explanation of how to select the appropriate diet for a critically ill horse is provided later in this chapter.

2. Assessing the horse's body weight and body condition score

The horse's body weight is used in the calculation of both energy and protein requirements and is an essential component in the nutritional management of the equine patient. Changes in the total mass of the patient can be documented with regular body weight measurements. Body weight varies with the hydration status of the horse and with the volume of intestinal tract ingesta. The BCS system helps the clinician to categorise the horse based on the endogenous stores of fat and protein. The horse's body weight and condition scores are complementary measurements that should be monitored throughout the time the horse is hospitalised.

Body weight is most accurately measured using a calibrated scale. Hospitalised horses should be weighed daily. If a scale is not available or if the horse cannot be moved from a stall to a scale every day, then the body weight can be estimated with an equine weight tape. Weight tape measurements are most accurate when a horse has a BCS between 4 and 6. If a weight tape will not fit around the girth of the horse or if the horse has a BCS between 1 and 3, a body weight estimate is made using measurements of the length and girth of the horse.[1,2] Length is measured from the tuber ischium to the point of the shoulder and girth is measured at the withers, behind the elbows at the end of expiration. The equation is given in Box 5.2. Miniature horses should be weighed on a small-animal clinic scale. If a scale is not available, then the equation in Box 5.3 can be used to estimate the body weight of the Miniature horse.[3]

The BCS system enables the clinician to assign a subjective score based on the horse's general muscle condition and the distribution of fat over certain areas of the body (Box 5.4).[4] A score of 1 represents emaciation, and a score of 9 is described as obese. In the horse, the most reliable anatomic sites for BCS assessment include the gluteal area (with an evaluation of the ease of visibility of the tuber coxae, tuber ischii and tail head), the back and the neck. Fat overlying the withers, shoulders and ribs should also be assessed.

Scores between 4 to 6 are considered ideal. Horses in this BCS range have endogenous stores of fat and protein and can tolerate partial to complete anorexia for 48 to 72 hours without severe metabolic complications. Horses with a BCS of 1 to 3 are often affected by PCM. Without early intervention with supplemental nutrition, these horses have difficulty recovering from surgery, sepsis and infectious diseases. Horses with a BCS between 7 to 9 are obese and often suffer complications from hypertriglyceridaemia when they are anorectic. Recommended dietary therapy for horses with different BCSs is discussed in the Nutrient Requirements section.

3. Reviewing the horse's nutritional history

The horse's nutritional history provides essential information about the nutrition of the patient before hospitalisation. When the horse is first evaluated, a complete nutritional history should be obtained from the horse owner. Information should be provided about the type and amount of feed that is normally consumed by the horse, the frequency of feeding, past evidence of dysphagia or quidding and the horse's average water consumption. If a horse has been partially anorectic before presentation, the current and previous diet history should be reviewed. Descriptions that use terms including "flakes of hay" or "scoops of grain" are too vague to permit an accurate estimation of the horse's feed and nutrient intake. The weight of a flake of hay, the number of flakes that are fed and the weight of the grain in the scoop should be obtained, if at all possible. If the horse typically leaves hay or grain behind, the owner should measure the feed remnants and report this information in the history. Owners should provide information on everything that is fed to their horse, including all dietary supplements, salt or trace mineral blocks and treats. The nutritional history should be reviewed to ensure that the diet does not

Box 5.3. Equation for estimate of body weight in Miniature horses using chest girth and body length

$$\text{Body weight (kg)} = \frac{(3.7 \times \text{chest girth in cm}) + (2 \times \text{length in cm}) - 348.5}{2.2}$$

Box 5.4. Description of individual equine body condition scores

Score		Description
1	Poor	Animal extremely emaciated; spinous processes, ribs, tailhead, tuber coxae, and ischii projecting prominently; bone structure of withers, shoulders, and neck easily noticeable; no fatty tissue can be felt
2	Very Thin	Animal emaciated; slight fat covering over base of spinous processes; transverse processes of lumbar vertebrae feel rounded; spinous processes, ribs, tailhead, tuber coxae and ischii prominent; withers, shoulders, and neck structure faintly discernable
3	Thin	Fat buildup about halfway on spinous processes; transverse processes cannot be felt; slight fat cover over ribs; spinous processes and ribs easily discernable; tailhead prominent, but individual vertebrae cannot be identified visually; tuber coxae appear rounded but easily discernable; tuber ischii not distinguishable; withers, shoulders, and neck accentuated
4	Moderately Thin	Slight ridge along back; faint outline of ribs discernable; tailhead prominence depends on conformation, fat can be felt around it; tuber coxae not discernable; withers, shoulders, and neck not obviously thin
5	Moderate	Back is flat (no crease or ridge); ribs not visually distinguishable but easily felt; fat around tailhead beginning to feel spongy; withers appear rounded over spinous processes; shoulders and neck blend smoothly into body
6	Moderately Fleshy	May have slight crease down back; fat over ribs spongy; fat around tailhead soft; fat beginning to be deposited along the side of withers, behind shoulders, and along the sides of the neck
7	Fleshy	May have crease down back; individual ribs can be felt, but noticeable filling between ribs with fat; fat around tailhead soft; fat deposited along withers, behind shoulders, and along neck
8	Fat	Crease down back; difficult to feel ribs; fat around tailhead very soft; area along withers filled with fat; area behind shoulder filled with fat; noticeable thickening of neck; fat deposited along inner thighs
9	Extremely Fat	Obvious crease down back; patchy fat appearing over ribs; bulging fat around tailhead, along withers, behind shoulders, and along neck; fat along inner thighs may rub together; flank filled with fat

Description of equine body condition scores from Table 1-7, Nutrient Requirements of Horses, revised ed 6, Washington, DC, National Academies Press, 2007, p 21.

provide an excess of any nutrients. Most herbal ingredients have not been tested for either safety or efficacy in the equine species, and inclusion of herbal substances could pose a health risk to some horses if fed in excessive amounts or if fed for a prolonged period of time.

During hospitalisation, the type and amount of feed offered to the horse and the amount of feed refused should be documented in a journal. A feed scale should be used to accurately measure feed intake. Daily energy and protein intake can be calculated and compared to requirements. A sample Hospital Feeding Chart is provided in Box 5.5. Close monitoring of the feed consumption of a hospitalised horse allows a clinician to determine the appropriate time to initiate nutritional therapy (Box 5.6).

The basic nutrient content of feeds in the local region can be listed in a feed chart and referenced to calculate the horse's daily intake. Forage analysis provides the most accurate information about the nutrient content of hay and can be performed on hospital hay if sufficiently large shipments are purchased. In the United States, forage analysis can be performed by Equi-analytical Laboratories (www.equi-analytical.com). Regional forage laboratories can provide the service in the United Kingdom, Australia and Europe. If feed cannot be analysed, the nutrient content of forage and grain can be estimated using feed tables in the Nutrient Requirement Council publications or from a forage analysis database. The guaranteed analysis statement on equine commercial feeds and diet supplements includes the concentration of select nutrients. The energy density of the feed can be obtained from the manufacturer. The nutrient content of some common equine feeds is provided in Table 5.1.

4. Evaluating the horse's biochemical profile

The therapeutic diet is designed to match the metabolic profile of the horse at the time the diet is administered. The serum biochemistry profile provides important information about the nutritional status of the equine patient, especially as it relates to lipid and glucose metabolism, and the horse's electrolyte levels.

Many hospitalised horses are septic and have an increased energy requirement due to their altered metabolic state. Proinflammatory cytokines including interleukin (IL)-1, tumor necrosis factor (TNF)-α and IL-6 alter metabolism by enhancing glucose production by the liver, stimulating proteolysis of skeletal muscle, promoting lipolysis and inducing anorexia.[5] The combination of an increase in energy expenditure and a decrease in food intake promotes a metabolic state of catabolism. Essential energy requirements are then met by an increase in lipolysis, protein

Box 5.5. Equine hospital feeding chart

Horse Name __________________ Case Number __________________ Clinician __________________

Diagnosis __________________ Date of Hospitalisation _____________ Date __________________

Horse Body Weight (kg) __________________ Body Condition Score __________________

Daily Nutrient Requirements

a) Resting Energy Requirement
   DE_{Rest} (Mcal) = 0.975 + 0.021 (_____kg) = _____________ Mcal

b) Maintenance Energy Requirement
   DE_{Maint} (Mcal) = 0.0333 × (_____kg) = _____________ Mcal

c) Daily Protein Requirement
   Crude Protein (grams) = 1.26 × (kg) = _____________ grams

Feeding Time	Type of Feed Offered	Volume of Feed Offered (kg, g, lb)	Volume of Feed Consumed (grams) A	Energy in Feed (Mcal/g) B	Protein in Feed (grams) C	Energy Consumed (Mcal) A + B	Protein Consumed (grams) A + C
			Total Energy Consumed				
			Total Protein Consumed				

Energy Deficit _________ Protein Deficit _________

1 Megacalorie (Mcal) = 1000 kilocalories (kcal)
1 kilogram (kg) = 2.2 pounds (lb)
1 pound (lb) = 0.454 kilogram (kg) = 454 grams (g)
1 milligram/kilogram (mg/kg) = 1 part per million (ppm)

To Calculate Protein Content:

$$10\%\ \text{protein} = \frac{10\ \text{grams protein}}{100\ \text{grams feed}} = 0.1\ \text{gram of protein per gram of feed}$$

Box 5.6. Goals of nutrition therapy in the hospitalised equine

Nutrient support should be started when either:

1. The horse's energy intake decreases below 75% of the daily stall resting digestible energy (DE_{Rest}) caloric requirement:

   [DE_{Rest} (Mcal/day) = 0.975 + 0.021 (body weight (kg))]

   AND/OR WHEN

2. The horse's protein intake decreases below 75% of the daily maintenance crude protein requirement:

   [$\text{Crude Protein}_{Maintenance}$ (grams/day) = 1.26 × BW (in kg)]

Energy and protein requirements are listed in Tables 5.2, 5.3, and 5.4.

Table 5.1. Estimated Nutrient Composition of Common Equine Feeds (as Fed)

Feed	kcal/g	Protein (%)	Fat (%)	Calcium (%)	Phosphorus (%)	Magnesium (%)	Potassium (%)
Alfalfa hay*	2.0	15.5	1.8	1.1	0.22	0.25	1.42
Oat hay†	1.8	7.8	2.1	0.32	0.20	0.15	1.64
Timothy hay‡	1.8	8.6	2.3	0.43	0.20	0.12	1.61
Bermudagrass hay†	1.9	9.8	1.7	0.47	0.19	0.19	1.58
Orchardgrass hay§	1.9	11.4	2.6	0.24	0.30	0.10	2.59
Equine Senior**	2.7	14.0	4.0	0.60	0.40	0.37	1.48
Omolene 100**	3.4	10.0	4.5	0.60	0.45	0.23	0.70
Rice bran†	2.8	13.3	14.6	0.61	1.66	0.67	1.31
Wheat bran†	3.0	15.7	1.4	0.14	1.02	0.39	1.11
Beet pulp†	2.4	8.7	1.3	0.87	0.08	0.20	0.71

*Equine NRC, 1989 Feed Composition Table; hay, full bloom, sun cured.
†Dairy One Forage Laboratory Database (May 2000–April 2006).
‡Equine NRC, 1989 Feed Composition Table; hay, mid bloom, sun cured.
§Equine NRC, 1989 Feed Composition Table; hay, early bloom, sun cured.
**Manufacturer Guaranteed Analysis, Purina Mills, St. Louis, MO, USA.

catabolism and an increase in gluconeogenesis. A common metabolic effect of sepsis is hyperglycemia due to insulin intolerance. Animals that are affected by endotoxin may have increased concentrations of serum triglycerides (TG) and may be intolerant of nutritional therapy with high fat solutions due to a reduced activity of lipoprotein lipase.

Markers of protein metabolism in the hospitalised horse
Most horses experience some degree of protein malnutrition before nutritional therapy is started. Protein malnutrition is recognised by a decrease in muscle condition and a reduction in BCS. Mild protein malnutrition is difficult to diagnose with routine biochemical tests, and muscle wasting is often identified in the epaxial and gluteal muscles before the serum urea nitrogen (SUN) and serum albumin decrease below reference concentrations. Severe protein malnutrition is recognised by a decrease in SUN and a low serum albumin concentration. Disease processes that result in a low SUN or serum albumin may occur concurrently with protein malnutrition but can be identified by ancillary diagnostic tests.

The concentration of plasma essential and nonessential amino acids may be useful diagnostic tests to diagnose mild protein malnutrition in the future. Urinary 3-methylhistidine also shows promise as a diagnostic test for protein malnutrition. This amino acid is produced when actin and myosin are degraded. Because 3-methylhistidine cannot be reincorporated into protein, it is excreted into the urine.[6] Although this sampling method has not been widely used in the equine species, results from other species suggest that the test can provide an indication of the protein catabolic state of the horse.

Markers of glucose metabolism in the hospitalised horse
Adult horses maintain their blood glucose within a normal range of 4.16 to 6.39 mmol/L (75–115 mg/dl) during periods of short- and long-term food deprivation. When an animal is septic, proinflammatory cytokines promote hepatic gluconeogenesis and insulin resistance in peripheral tissues. A dysregulation of glucose metabolism should be considered in horses that have abnormally high blood glucose concentrations or in horses that fail to regulate their blood glucose once they have been treated with appropriate nutritional therapy. Horses with equine metabolic syndrome, or other endocrine diseases that alter the regulation of blood glucose and insulin, should be treated with supplemental nutrition that contains a relatively low concentration of dextrose or glucose. Nutritional recommendations for horses with an elevated blood glucose concentration are provided in the section on nutrient requirements.

Markers of lipid metabolism in the hospitalised horse
Nonesterified fatty acids (NEFAs) rise (>100 μmol/L) within 8 hours of feed deprivation, and serum TG begin to increase to >0.62 mmol/L (55 mg/dl) after 36 hours of feed withholding in healthy horses.[7] With feed deprivation beyond 36 hours, serum TG frequently rises as part of the normal physiological response to feed deprivation. When a healthy horse is re-fed, serum concentrations of NEFA and TG gradually decline over 24 to 48 hours and usually return to prefasting levels once the horse consumes enough energy to meet their requirements.

More significant changes occur in the lipid profile of a horse that has been protein-calorie malnourished for greater than 48 hours. In these horses, the concentration of serum TG can reach pathological levels above 5.65 mmol/L (500 mg/dl), resulting in hyperlipaemia. Some horses have severe elevations in their serum TG concentration without concurrent grossly visible lipaemia.[8] In other horses, the prolonged elevation in serum TG concentration will occur concurrently with hepatic lipidosis, a disease that requires aggressive dietary therapy to prevent permanent hepatocyte damage. Ponies, donkeys, Miniature horses and some overweight horses (BCS 7–9) may be at an increased risk of developing hypertriglyceridaemia when they are malnourished. Serum TG should be measured in hospitalised horses before supplemental nutrition is started and throughout the time that the horse is treated. The clinical significance of an increase in serum TG varies between horses, and it is up to the clinician to select the best diet to treat each equine patient. The use of lipid and other energy substrates in parenteral and enteral diets is discussed in the section on nutrient requirements.

Excessive oxidation of fatty acids by the liver may result in the formation of acetoacetate and β-hydroxybutyrate. The concentration of ketone bodies can easily be measured in the urine. Unlike ruminants, horses do not appear to develop severe ketosis following a period of food deprivation, so measurement of urine ketones is a less sensitive indicator of nutritional status than other biochemical measurements.[9]

Prolonged malnutrition and the re-feeding syndrome

The re-feeding syndrome should be suspected in a horse with prolonged protein-calorie malnutrition that develops hypophosphataemia, hypokalaemia and hypomagnesaemia after a period of rapid re-feeding. Rapid re-feeding stimulates glycolysis, and results in an abrupt shift of phosphorus, potassium and magnesium out of the plasma and into cells. In humans, severe electrolyte derangements lead to cardiac, haematological, respiratory and neurological disorders, and results in death in extreme cases. Although the syndrome has been best described in humans, horses show similar electrolyte abnormalities during the re-feeding period. Chronically starved horses re-fed with alfalfa hay, oat hay or a mix of oat hay and Equine Senior (Purina Mills) over 10 days developed hypophosphataemia, a decreased 2,3-DPG and low normal total magnesium (ionised magnesium not measured).[10] Complications from the re-feeding syndrome can be avoided by closely monitoring the serum concentration of macrominerals and by gradually reintroducing the horse to either enteral nutrition or PN. Treatment of electrolyte abnormalities includes oral and/or parenteral mineral supplementation. Patient management is discussed in more detail in the Nutrient Requirements section.

Electrolyte imbalances associated with anorexia, malnutrition and gastrointestinal disease

Serum electrolytes may be altered by the primary clinical disease or by the nutritional status of the horse. During short-term malnutrition, endogenous macromineral stores are mobilised to maintain serum electrolyte concentrations. Prolonged malnutrition often results in whole-body macromineral depletion and clinical signs of mineral deficiencies. Hypokalaemia is a common complication associated with decreased feed intake and may occur alone or in conjunction with other mineral derangements. Because the majority of potassium in the body is obtained from the diet, horses that have partial or complete anorexia can rapidly develop hypokalaemia.[11] Clinical signs associated with hypokalaemia include weakness, fatigue and decreased feed and water intake.[12]

Total body mineral deficiencies often are not recognised by plasma analysis. In the case of calcium and magnesium, the ionised fraction provides a more accurate estimate of available calcium and magnesium. Both hypocalcaemia and hypomagnesaemia have been documented in adult horses with gastrointestinal disease and horses suffering from sepsis. Clinical signs of calcium deficiency in the horse include increased muscle tone, muscle fasciculations, synchronous diaphragmatic flutter, tachycardia, cardiac dysrhythmias and dysphagia. Horses with hypomagnesaemia may develop muscle tremors, cardiac dysrhythmias, ataxia and sweating, and in severe cases, the horse may collapse. Calcium and magnesium are especially important in horses with gastrointestinal disease. In one study of horses with surgical colic, 35% of adult horses had an ionised magnesium below the reference range, and 86% had an ionised calcium below the reference range prior to colic surgery.[13] In this same population of horses, those with postoperative ileus had lower serum ionised magnesium at 3 and 7 days after the surgery compared to horses that did not develop ileus. Plasma phosphorus, glucose and insulin were not measured in these horses, and the use of therapeutic diets in the postoperative period was not discussed by the authors. Horses with enterocolitis frequently suffer from a low serum concentration of ionised calcium and magnesium.[14] Parenteral supplementation with calcium and magnesium is indicated when the serum concentration is below normal. Recommendations for mineral supplementation in intravenous fluids are presented in Chapter 6.5 and in this chapter in the section on nutrient requirements.

Trace mineral and vitamin analysis

Unless a horse is affected by severe malnutrition, clinical signs of trace mineral and vitamin deficiencies usually are not recognised. Although B-vitamin production by gastrointestinal bacteria usually meets requirements in horses with short-term anorexia, horses with gastrointestinal disease are at risk of developing deficiencies. Thiamine deficiency is recognised by ataxia, anorexia, muscle fasciculations, muscle tremors and stiffness.[15] Clinical signs of other B-vitamin deficiencies are not well described. During the initial period of hospitalisation, serum concentrations of trace minerals and vitamins are rarely measured. To ensure adequate intake, trace nutrients should be added to parenteral and enteral diets. Supplementation recommendations are provided in the enteral nutrition and PN sections.

Initiating treatment with therapeutic nutrition

Equine patients with an ideal BCS (4–6) may be able to tolerate short-term anorexia better than horses that are either overconditioned (BCS 7–9) or underconditioned (BCS 1–3). Horses that present with a 1 to 3 BCS at the start of their hospitalisation have minimal reserves of fat and protein to use during a period of anorexia and require earlier intervention with nutritional support compared with horses that present with a BCS between 4 and 6. Overweight horses with a BCS of 7 to 9 should also be managed with supplemental nutrition soon after they develop partial or complete anorexia to prevent complications from hypertriglyceridaemia, hyperlipaemia and hepatic lipidosis (Box 5.7). If a hospitalised horse has lost more than 5% of its body weight since admission (23 kg or 50 lb for a 450-kg [1000-lb] adult horse), or if the horse has dropped in BCS by 1 or more, dietary therapy should be administered.

Because protein-calorie malnutrition is detrimental to immune system function, tissue healing, recovery from systemic disease or following surgery, the daily voluntary energy and protein intake of the hospitalised horse also influence the decision to supplement a horse with either enteral nutrition or PN (Box 5.6). Treatment with any energy or protein source will blunt the severity of protein-calorie malnutrition and will decrease systemic complications associated with anorexia. Supplemental nutrition can be administered to provide part or all of the horse's daily digestible resting energy requirements (DE_{Rest}). The energy requirements of hospitalised horses are discussed later.

Supplemental nutrition should be initiated within the first 24 to 48 hours of hospitalisation to blunt the development of protein-calorie malnutrition. A decision tree for supplemental nutrition is provided in Box 5.8. The horse's diet history, clinical examination and biochemical values are used to determine the nutrient profile of the diet formulation.

Box 5.7. Guidelines for initiating diet therapy based on body condition score

Horses with a BCS between 4 and 6 should receive nutritional supplementation if they consume <75% of their resting digestible energy requirement (DE_{Rest}) for longer than 48 hours.

Horses with a BCS between 1 and 3 should receive nutritional supplementation if they consume <75% of their DE_{Rest} for 24–36 hours.

- In these horses, the DE_{Rest} should be calculated using an average of the current and ideal body weight of the horse.

Horses with a BCS between 7 and 9 should receive nutritional supplementation if they consume <75% if their DE_{Rest} for 24–36 hours.

- In these horses, the DE_{Rest} should be calculated using an average of the current and ideal body weight of the horse.

Early nutrition options: Cafeteria feeding and dextrose-supplemented fluids

During the first 24 to 36 hours of hospitalisation or in the early postoperative period, clinicians can begin treating their patients using a "cafeteria feeding" method and by administering fluids supplemented with dextrose.

Cafeteria feeding

Cafeteria feeding is the common method of offering a wide variety of highly palatable feeds to an anorectic horse. The selection of feeds should include products that have a high concentration of structural carbohydrates such as fresh grass (if available), small amounts of hay and complete pelleted feeds that contain at least 10% dry matter (DM) fibre. Horses should not be offered feeds that contain a high concentration of nonstructural carbohydrates like grain supplements or individual grains like corn, oats or barley. A more complete discussion of dietary carbohydrates and their use in equine therapeutic diets is provided in the nutrient requirements section. A mollased sweet feed may be palatable to some horses, and 114 to 228 grams (g) (½–1 cup) can be added as a top dressing to entice a horse to consume a fibre-based feed. All feeds should be weighed before they are offered. Any feed that has not been consumed after 2 hours should be removed and weighed before it is discarded. Fresh feed should be offered every 4 to 6 hours to maintain the palatability of the feed. The Hospital Feeding Chart (Box 5.5) can be used to track the horse's daily nutrient intake. The goal of cafeteria feeding is to stimulate the horse's appetite and encourage the horse to return to a forage-based diet. Some horses will respond by consuming enough energy and protein to meet their requirements and will not require additional dietary therapy. Other horses will remain anorectic and will become protein-calorie malnourished as their hospitalisation continues. If a horse is offered palatable feeds but consumes less than 75% of its DE_{Rest} in 36 to 48 hours, the horse should be treated with either enteral nutrition or PN.

Intravenous dextrose

Intravenous dextrose or glucose is administered to provide an anorectic horse with supplemental energy. Although this treatment does not provide the horse with a source of protein, the supplemental energy will blunt the catabolism

Box 5.8 Guidelines for Nutritional Management of the Hospitalised Horse

A. Obtain a diet history for the patient prior to hospitalisation
B. Monitor feed intake during hospitalisation (Box 5.5)
C. Calculate energy and protein intake during hospitalisation
D. Calculate the digestible energy requirements (DER) for the horse at rest using the horse's body weight: **DE_{Rest} (Mcal/day) = 0.975 + 0.021 ($BW_{(kg)}$)**
If the horse has a BCS of 1-3 or 7-9, calculate the DER using an average of the horse's current and ideal body weight
E. Decide if the patient requires supplemental nutrition

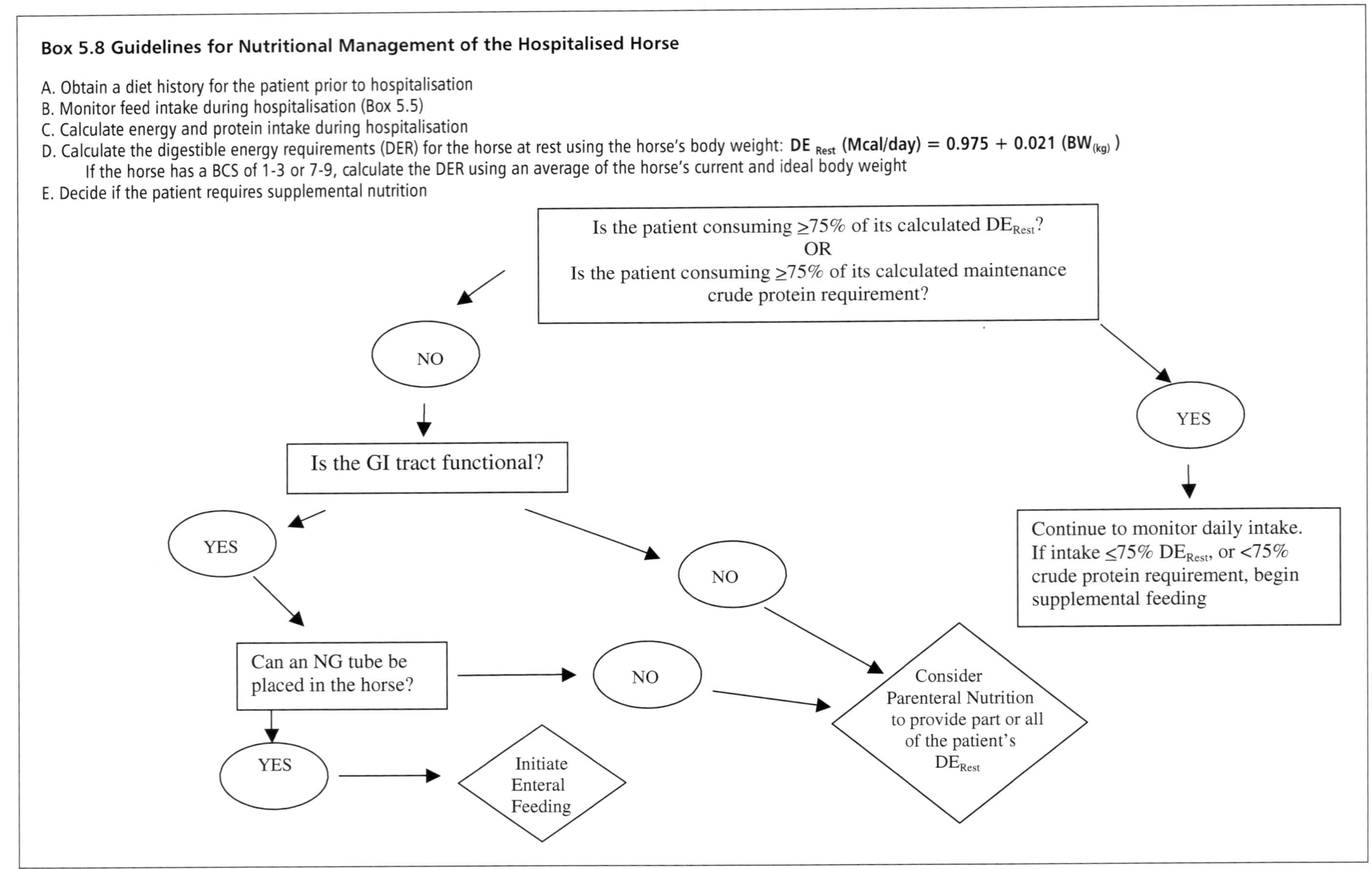

of endogenous lipid and protein stores. Dextrose or glucose is added to make a final solution with a concentration that ranges from 2.5% to 10% and an osmolarity that ranges from 126 to 505 mOsm/L. A 5% dextrose solution approaches the theoretical maximal rate of dextrose oxidation for a horse (extrapolated from the maximal oxidation rate in humans, which is estimated to be approximately 25 kcal/kg/day).[16] When the fluids are infused as a constant rate infusion (CRI), the patient's renal threshold of glucose (10 mmol/L or 180 mg/dl for adult horses; 12 mmol/L or 216 mg/dl for foals) usually is not exceeded. To avoid complications from hyperglycaemia and hyperosmolarity, adult horses are rarely treated with solutions that contain greater than 10% dextrose or glucose.

The energy provided in dextrose or glucose-supplemented fluids (1.7 kcal/ml for 50% dextrose; 1.9 kcal/ml for 50% glucose) should be calculated and recorded. A 450-kg horse, treated with fluids supplemented with 2.5% dextrose, will receive 2295 kcal (close to 23% of the patient's DE_{Rest}) if the fluids are infused at a rate of 60 ml/kg/day (27.0 L/day). If a 2.5% solution of glucose is administered, the horse will receive 2565 kcal from the glucose (close to 25% of the patient's DE_{Rest}). When a 5% dextrose solution is used, a 450-kg horse treated with 120 ml/kg/day (54 L/day) of fluids will receive 9180 kcal. Dextrose-supplemented fluids can be administered as the sole source of nutrition for 24 to 48 hours. During treatment with dextrose-supplemented fluids, the horse should be monitored for hyperglycaemia and glucosuria. Horses that have complications with glucose and insulin regulation may be able to tolerate therapy with a 2.5% solution of dextrose. If the horse is intolerant of the therapy and the horse does not voluntarily consume enough feed to meet greater than 75% of their DE_{Rest} and/or greater than 75% of their maintenance protein requirement, treatment with either enteral nutrition or PN should be initiated (Box 5.6).

Nutrient requirements

Water

Adult horses require 60 ml fluid/kg/day to maintain hydration, and most horses will have their fluid requirements met with intravenous therapy. Horses requiring diuresis or patients suffering from dehydration may be treated with up to 3 times their maintenance requirements. Both enteral and parenteral nutritional therapy provide additional water to the horse. In order to avoid complications from excessive hydration, the fluid infused with the diet must be added to the horse's total daily fluid intake. Water in an enteral diet comes from the fluid used to soak and blend the diet and the water that is infused as a nasogastric tube flush. In some enteral diets, the extra water can exceed 20 L/day.[17] In a parenteral solution of protein, dextrose and lipid, approximately 50% of the total solution volume can be water. Fluid added to a partial parenteral solution should also be tabulated into the horse's daily water intake. Approximately 18% of the fluid volume of a protein, lipid and glucose/water admixture may be metabolised to water.[18] Although the contribution of water from the metabolism of macronutrients is usually not added to the fluid balance of adult horses, this source of water may be significant in equine patients that are at risk of volume overload. Excessive administration of water or fluid in a supplemental diet should be avoided in horses that have hypoalbuminaemia or renal disease or horses that are at risk of developing either peripheral or pulmonary oedema. The intravenous fluid therapy plan of the hospitalised horse may need to be revised to a lower volume to prevent complications from excessive fluid therapy.

Energy

The cornerstone for developing a therapeutic nutrition plan for a hospitalised horse begins with a calculation of the horse's daily resting energy requirement (RER). A scale should be used to measure the weight of the horse; however, an estimation of the horse's body weight can be obtained from a weight tape or from allometric measurements of body length and chest circumference when a scale is not available (Boxes 5.2 and 5.3).

The energy requirement of an adult horse recovering from surgery or from a systemic disease has not been determined using either indirect calorimetry or other measures of cellular metabolism. When therapy is initiated, the horse should be treated with a formulation that will meet their RER. If excess calories are administered at the start of the diet program, the horse may be predisposed to metabolic complications associated with hyperglycaemia and hyperlipaemia. The closest approximation of the RER in the horse is the digestible energy requirement for an adult horse at rest [DE_{Rest} (Mcal/day) = 0.975 + 0.021 (BW in kg)].[19] This DE_{Rest} equation is valid for horses that weigh 125 to 856 kg.[19] (Table 5.2) The true body weight of the horse should be used for the calculation if the horse has a 4 to 6 BCS. The RER for horses that are either underconditioned (BCS 1–3) or overconditioned (BCS 7–9) should be estimated by using an average of the actual and ideal body weight in the DE_{Rest} equation.

If the horse fails to maintain their weight or BCS during treatment at their RER, then additional calories can be added to the formulation. Data from critically ill humans shows that patients with severe trauma, sepsis, and severe head injuries may require up to 1.5 times the RER to meet the metabolic requirements of trauma or disease.[20] Hospitalised horses may also require calories in excess of the calculated DE_{Rest} value. If necessary, supplemental calories can be added to the therapeutic diet to meet and even exceed the horse's energy requirement at a physiological state of maintenance [DE_{Maint} (Mcal/day) = 0.0333 × BW (in kg)][21] (Table 5.2). This DE_{Maint} equation can be used for adult horses that weigh between 200 to 900 kg. Energy requirements for adult horses at DE_{Rest} and DE_{Maint} are listed in Table 5.2. The RER for Miniature horses that weigh less than 125 kg can be estimated from the DE_{Rest}

Table 5.2. Daily Energy and Protein Requirements for Adult Horses Calculated Using the Stall Resting (DE_{Rest}) and Maintenance (DE_{Maint}) Energy Equations[19,21]

Horse Weight (kg)	DE_{Rest} (Mcal/day)[1]	DE_{Maint} (Mcal/day)[2]	Protein (grams/day)[3]
200	5.2	6.7	252
225	5.7	7.5	284
250	6.2	8.3	315
275	6.8	9.2	347
300	7.3	10.0	378
325	7.8	10.8	410
350	8.3	11.7	441
375	8.9	12.5	473
400	9.4	13.3	504
425	9.9	14.2	536
450	10.4	15.0	567
475	11.0	15.8	599
500	11.5	16.7	630
525	12.0	17.5	662
550	12.5	18.3	693
575	13.1	19.1	725
600	13.6	20.0	756
625	14.1	20.8	788
650	14.6	21.6	819
675	15.2	22.5	851
700	15.7	23.3	882
725	16.2	24.1	914
750	16.7	25.0	945
775	17.3	25.8	977
800	17.8	26.6	1,008

[1] DE_{Rest} (Mcal/day) = 0.975 + 0.021 (BW in kg) For horses that weigh 125–856 kg
[2] DE_{Maint} (Mcal/day) = 0.0333 × (BW in kg) For horses that weigh 200–900 kg
[3] Crude Protein (grams/day) = 1.26 × (BW in kg)

Table 5.3. Digestible Energy Requirements (Mcal/day) for Horses In Different Physiologic Conditions[21]

	Mature Body Weight				
	200 kg DE_{Maint}	400 kg DE_{Maint}	500 kg DE_{Maint}	600 kg DE_{Maint}	900 kg DE_{Maint}
Pregnant Mares					
<5 months (feed at maintenance)	6.7	13.3	16.7	20.0	30.0
7 months	7.2	14.3	17.9	21.5	32.2
9 months	7.7	15.4	19.2	23.1	34.6
10 months	8.1	16.2	20.2	24.2	36.4
11 months	8.6	17.1	21.4	25.7	38.5
Lactating Mares					
1 month	12.7	25.4	31.7	38.1	54.4
3 months	12.2	24.5	30.6	36.7	52.4
6 months	10.9	21.8	27.2	32.7	46.3
Growing Horses					
4 months	5.3	10.6	13.3	15.9	23.9
6 months	6.2	12.4	15.5	18.6	28.0
12 months	7.5	15.0	18.8	22.5	33.8
18 months	7.7	15.4	19.2	23.1	34.6
24 months	7.5	15.0	18.7	22.4	33.7

equation. The metabolic energy equation [132 (body weight [kg])$^{0.75}$] provides a calculation of energy in kilocalories (kcal) and likely overestimates the RER but can be used as a guideline for calculating the DE_{Maint} requirement for adult horses that weigh less than 200 kg.

Additional energy is required for horses that are growing and for mares that are either pregnant or lactating. When these animals are treated with a therapeutic diet, their daily energy requirement should be determined using the energy values in Table 5.3. Additional energy values are listed in the *National Research Council Nutrient Requirements of Horses*, sixth revised edition.[21]

Dietary energy is provided in carbohydrates, lipids and protein. The volume of each macronutrient can be varied in a therapeutic diet to meet the requirements of an individual horse.

Protein

Protein is an essential ingredient in the therapeutic diet of a hospitalised horse. Partial and complete anorexia rapidly lead to protein malnutrition and a negative nitrogen balance. Protein catabolism is also stimulated by the release of proinflammatory cytokines. During the time the horse is anorectic, supplemental energy and protein help to blunt the loss of endogenous protein to preserve the lean tissue mass of the horse.

The amount of protein that is included in a therapeutic equine diet should meet the daily protein requirement of the horse (crude protein [g] = BW [in kg] × 1.26).[21] The protein requirements for adult horses at maintenance are listed in Table 5.2. Protein requirements of malnourished horses may be increased from the calculated maintenance value, and horses with a BCS of 1 to 3 should have their protein requirements calculated using their ideal body weight. If a horse is partially or completely anorectic and has a low serum albumin concentration, protein supplementation, with up to 1.5 times the maintenance requirement, is indicated. Additional dietary protein is required during demanding physiological states such as growth, pregnancy and lactation (Table 5.4). Equations used to derive these values are listed in the 2007 *Nutrient Requirements of Horses* publication.[21]

Enteral diets contain protein in the feed ingredients. Protein digestibility varies with the quality of forage, and only high-quality digestible feeds should be chosen for an enteral formulation. Commercial equine complete pelleted feeds usually contain a digestible form of protein and are suitable for use in a liquid enteral diet. Powdered protein supplements including soy, whey and casein typically have

Table 5.4. Protein Requirements (grams/day) of Horses In Different Physiologic Conditions[21]

	Mature Body Weight				
	200 kg Grams	400 kg Grams	500 kg Grams	600 kg Grams	900 kg Grams
Pregnant Mares					
<5 months (feed at maintenance)	252	504	630	756	1134
7 months	291	583	729	874	1311
9 months	319	637	797	956	1434
10 months	336	673	841	1009	1514
11 months	357	714	893	1072	1607
Lactating Mares					
1 month	614	1228	1535	1842	2763
3 months	587	1174	1468	1761	2642
6 months	506	1012	1265	1518	2277
Growing Horses					
4 months	268	535	669	803	1204
6 months	270	541	676	811	1217
12 months	338	677	846	1015	1522
18 months	320	639	799	959	1438
24 months	308	616	770	924	1386

a high digestibility (50%–90%) and are ideal ingredients for equine enteral diets. The essential and nonessential amino acids in parenteral formulations have a high bioavailability and are well tolerated by most horses. Details about protein use in enteral and parenteral diets are presented in the following sections.

The therapeutic diet should provide enough calories from carbohydrates and lipid so that a portion of the dietary protein can be used for protein synthesis. A simple way to assess the calorie and protein content of the formulation is to calculate the calorie-to-nitrogen ratio of the diet. In the example in Box 5.9, all dietary calories (from nonprotein and from protein sources) are included in the calculation of the calorie-to-nitrogen ratio.

The ideal calorie-to-nitrogen ratio for adult horses is extrapolated from data calculated for critically ill humans where the ideal ratio is 120 to 150 : 1 for healthy individuals and 80 to 90 : 1 for acutely ill patients.[16] Horses with systemic inflammatory diseases or severe protein loss or horses recovering from surgery often benefit from a therapeutic enteral or parenteral diet that has a calorie-to-nitrogen ratio between 80 and 100. Horses with hepatic or renal disease should be treated with a diet that has a higher calorie-to-nitrogen ratio.

The amount of protein (in grams) in relationship to the calorie content of the diet (100 kcal) is another way to describe the protein content of the diet. Most equine diets contain approximately 4 g of protein for every 100 kcal of digestible energy. Therapeutic diets for adult horses can be formulated with protein concentrations that are as high as 6 g of protein per 100 kcal, if the horse can tolerate the supplemental protein.

Nutritionists continue to debate if the protein content of a parenteral solution should be included in the total energy calculation for the formulation or if the calories should only be calculated from the dextrose and lipid solutions. Although research has not been performed in horses, an extrapolation of the protein oxidation and synthesis balance evaluations during PN administration in humans suggests that enough protein is oxidised from a PN solution that the protein component of the solution should be included in the total energy calculation of the solution.[18] In horses, the parenteral diet can be formulated using only nonprotein-calories to meet the DE_{Rest} of the animal. The additional contribution of calories from the protein solution will be relatively small compared to the total calories in the parenteral solution. Because some of the protein will be oxidised for energy, the excess energy contribution from the protein will not be detrimental to the horse.

Box 5.9. Calculation of the calorie-to-nitrogen ratio

For a 450-kg adult horse:

DE_{Rest} = 10.4 Mcal (10,400 kcal)
Protein = 567 grams

There is 1 gram of nitrogen in 6.25 grams of protein; 567 grams/6.25 = 91 grams of nitrogen

Calorie : nitrogen ratio = 10,400 : 91 = 114 : 1

Contraindications for protein supplementation

Horses diagnosed with renal or hepatic disease should not be treated with supplemental protein. Instead, the therapeutic diet for horses with renal or hepatic disease should be formulated to meet the patient's protein requirements. Protein restriction beyond maintenance requirements results in catabolism of endogenous protein that is detrimental to the horse. During treatment, it is important to monitor the serum biochemistry profile of the horse to ensure that they are not developing signs of renal or hepatic disease. In some cases, the original enteral or parenteral formulation may need to be altered to adjust the protein concentration to a tolerable level for the patient.

Future trends in amino acid supplementation

Glutamine

Glutamine is a nonessential amino acid that may be conditionally essential in some species during certain disease states. Enteral feeding studies in humans and animals have documented improved immune cell function, decreased bacterial translocation across the gastrointestinal tract and reduced mortality in glutamine-treated groups.[22] Glutamine is a preferred energy source for enterocytes and may be a beneficial nutrient supplement in critically ill horses. Currently, glutamine has not yet been defined as a conditionally essential amino acid in the equine species.

Glutamine supplementation in parenteral formulations is limited because glutamine is not stable in solution. Glutamine supplementation in enteral diets appears to be safe; however, appropriate dose ranges for oral glutamine supplementation have not yet been established in horses. One human study has documented safety at a supplementation rate of 0.5 g glutamine/kg/day.[23] Increased plasma glutamine concentrations were measured following treatment of healthy adult horses with a glutamine dosage of 60 mg/kg body weight.[24] If the human dose was administered to a 450-kg horse, the patient would be treated with 225 g glutamine/day. Treatment with the dose used in the equine study equates to 30 g glutamine/day. Because safety studies with glutamine have not been performed in horses, the glutamine dose of 0.5 g glutamine/kg/day should not be exceeded. Supplemental glutamine should be included in the horse's daily total protein intake. If protein restriction is an important factor of the nutritional management of an equine case, glutamine supplementation should be restricted or avoided completely.

Branched chain amino acids

Branched chain amino acids (BCAA) are oxidised in skeletal muscle in response to starvation, sepsis and physiological stress. Treatment of hospitalised patients with BCAA is proposed to decrease proteolysis in muscle, to provide an amino group for glutamine synthesis and to provide an energy substrate for organs during periods of decreased glucose utilisation.[25] Despite the proposed benefits of BCAA treatment, supplementation of human parenteral formulations with leucine, isoleucine or valine has failed to show a consistent beneficial effect in improving nitrogen metabolism in many groups of human patients.[18] Amino acid solutions supplemented with BCAA appear to be beneficial in human patients with hepatic disease and hepatic encephalopathy who cannot tolerate enteral nutrition or standard parenteral amino acid solutions.[25] Specialised commercial amino acid formulations that contain supplemental BCAA are available for purchase from McGaw (HepatAmine 8%, FreAmine HBC 6.9%) and Abbott (Aminosyn-HBC 7%).[16] These commercial amino acid mixtures have not yet been formally tested in horses. Although the safety of supplemental BCAA in equine parenteral formulations cannot be guaranteed, these formulations may be beneficial in horses that are septic and in horses suffering from hepatic disease. If a BCAA-supplemented amino acid is selected for use, the parenteral formulation calculation worksheets (provided in Boxes 5.15 and 5.16) will need to be adjusted to the correct protein concentration of the amino acid solution.

Use of supplemental BCAA in enteral formulations has not been evaluated in horses; however, oral supplementation with BCAA in horses with hepatic failure may be beneficial. Currently, BCAA supplementation of human enteral formulations has questionable efficacy in improving serum concentrations of BCAA.[26] Due to the lack of data to demonstrate the efficacious use of enteral diet BCAA supplementation, the therapy should not exceed 30 g of leucine, 20 g of isoleucine and 20 g of valine divided into two or three treatments per day.[27]

Lipid

Lipids are a safe component of equine enteral nutrition and PN and should be included whenever the horse can tolerate the ingredient. Lipids provide a higher concentration of energy (9 kcal/g gross energy) compared to either protein or carbohydrate, and dietary lipid is required for the intestinal absorption of fat-soluble vitamins. Linoleic acid, an omega-6 fatty acid, is required in the equine diet at a concentration of 0.5% of the dietary dry matter. Fats in the omega-3 series, including linolenic acid, are also important nutrients, even though a dietary intake has not yet been defined for the horse. During a short period of anorexia, an essential fatty acid deficiency is unlikely to cause health complications in a hospitalised horse. Fatty acid requirements are rarely calculated when a therapeutic diet is formulated for an equine patient. However, if lipids are used in a parenteral formulation or if the horse is treated with a liquid enteral diet that contains forage, canola oil or corn oil, the horse should consume enough linoleic acid to meet their daily requirement. Only fresh feeds that are free of rancidity should be offered to a hospitalised horse.

Because horses rely on endogenous stores of lipid as a primary energy source during short-term anorexia, therapeutic diets that contain lipid are readily utilised by most horses. The benefit of adding lipid to an enteral diet is that the energy density of the diet can be greatly increased without also increasing the volume of the diet. Canola oil (225 ml [1 cup]) contains 1980 kcal of digestible energy, almost one-fifth of the total resting energy required by a 450-kg horse. Although dietary fat delays gastric emptying in some species, this effect may not occur in horses.[28] When lipid is added to a parenteral formulation, the energy density of the solution can be increased without raising the osmolarity of the solution. Inclusion of lipid in parenteral solutions decreases the catabolism of endogenous fat in rats and improves nitrogen balance in dogs when compared to animals that were treated with PN solutions that contained only glucose.[29] Additional information about the specific use of lipid in enteral and parenteral formulations is presented in the following sections on enteral nutrition and PN.

Use of dietary lipid for horses with hypertriglyceridaemia
When a hospitalised horse has a serum TG concentration less than 2.26 mmol/L (200 mg/dl), enteral and parenteral diets can be formulated with a moderate concentration of lipid. Most horses with a serum TG concentration below 2.26 mmol/L (200 mg/dl) will tolerate a liquid enteral diet that contains up to 20% of the total calories as lipid and a parenteral formulation that contains up to 40% of the nonprotein calories as lipid. Colic or diarrhoea may develop in horses that cannot tolerate lipid supplementation in their enteral diet. If the horse's serum TG concentration is between 2.26 and 5.65 mmol/L (200–500 mg/dl), dietary fat should be limited to 10% of the total calories in a liquid enteral formulation and 20% of the nonprotein calories in a parenteral solution. Once treatment with the supplemental diet is initiated, many horses respond with a decrease in their serum TG concentration. When this occurs, the lipid concentration in enteral and parenteral reformulations can be gradually increased. During treatment with a therapeutic diet, the horse's serum TG should be monitored every 24 or 48 hours to ensure that the TG do not continue to increase. The lipid content of the therapeutic diet can be adjusted to meet the horse's changing metabolic profile.

Contraindications for lipid supplementation
An equine patient with hypertriglyceridaemia (TG > 5.65 mmol/L [500 mg/dl]), hyperlipaemia or hepatic lipidosis should not have supplemental lipid added to their therapeutic diet until the TG concentration falls below 5.65 mmol/L (500 mg/dl) or until the hepatic lipidosis has resolved. Horses with hepatic lipidosis that will tolerate enteral nutrition can be treated with a complete feed diet containing 4% DM fat or less, a concentration that is only slightly higher than the fat concentration measured in forages. Another option for fat restriction in an enterally fed horse is to formulate a diet using only low-fat ingredients such as alfalfa meal and whey or casein. Diet formulation is discussed in greater detail in the enteral nutrition section. In healthy feed-deprived ponies, hypertriglyceridaemia was reversed following treatment with a fat-free liquid enteral diet.[30] Administration of a PN solution without lipid is indicated for horses that have hyperlipaemia or hepatic lipidosis. A recent study documented the successful management of hyperlipaemia in three ponies and one donkey following treatment with a partial parenteral nutrition (PPN) solution that contained dextrose and amino acids.[31]

Future trends in lipid supplementation
Lipids from the omega-3 series are being evaluated as supplements in human parenteral formulations. Preliminary work suggests that an inflammatory response may be reduced following parenteral treatment with omega-3 fats; however, studies have not yet been performed in horses, and at this time, parenteral supplementation is not recommended for horses. Enteral diets can be supplemented with omega-3 fatty acids (flaxseed, flax oil, fish oil), but the beneficial effects of omega-3 fatty acids may not be achieved during the short duration of time that the diet is administered.

Medium-chain triglycerides, or MCT, are currently being evaluated as an alternative therapy to long-chain TG in parenteral lipid formulations. Clinical studies with parenteral MCT formulations in humans have demonstrated that MCT are oxidised at a higher rate, that MCT may reduce elevations in liver enzymes and that MCT may provide a protein-sparing effect when compared to long-chain TG.[16] New commercial parenteral lipid formulations of TG made with both long- and medium-chain TG (structured TG) are being tested and appear to show promise in managing critically ill patients compared to traditional long-chain fatty acid supplementation. Although structured TG formulations are not readily available for purchase, they may provide an alternative to traditional parenteral lipid formulations in the future.

Use of oral MCT in equine diets has only been evaluated in one study, by Hallebeek et al.,[32] who documented a significant increase in plasma triacylglycerol and very low density lipoproteins in MCT-treated horses compared to soybean oil–treated horses. The lipids were added to the hay and concentrate–based diets of healthy horses.[32] Until more research is available to document the efficacy of MCT supplementation in enteral diets, the use of MCT in hospitalised horses should be approached with caution.

Carbohydrates

The equine gastrointestinal tract is designed to digest a diet with a high percentage of structural fibre. In addition to the absorption of nonstructural carbohydrates in the small intestine, a large proportion of the daily energy requirement of a horse is met by volatile fatty acids that are produced and absorbed in the caecum and colon following bacterial fermentation of structural carbohydrates. This description of the hindgut fermentation of the horse is overly simplistic; however, for the purpose of this discussion, the term *nonstructural carbohydrate* includes hydrolysable carbohydrates (monosaccharides and disaccharides, some oligosaccharides and starches), and the term *structural carbohydrate* includes insoluble fibre (hemicellulose, cellulose and lignin).

Although an ideal nutrition supplement for an anorectic horse would mimic a typical equine diet that is high in structural carbohydrate, the logistics of diet administration and the general health of the animal may preclude administration of a more natural diet. If the horse can be treated with an enteral diet, either fibre or fibre-free formulations can be administered. Enteral diet formulations that contain grain or feeds with a high concentration of soluble carbohydrates should always be avoided.

Parenteral formulations provide carbohydrates to the horse in the form of dextrose or glucose. A parenteral solution for a horse with a normal blood glucose concentration can include up to 60% of the nonprotein calories as dextrose or glucose. Horses suffering from glucose intolerance should be treated with a PN solution that contains less than 30% of the total nonprotein calories from dextrose. Recent studies in hospitalised humans have documented a decrease in morbidity and mortality in critically ill patients managed with strict regulation of their blood glucose. The trend in veterinary medicine is to manage equine patients in a similar manner. This requires frequent measurements of blood glucose during treatment with PN and solution reformulation if the horse develops persistent hyperglycaemia. Horses that require PN cannot initially be treated with dietary fibre. Because the health of the intestinal villi is supported by the delivery of nutrients directly to the enterocytes, horses treated with PN should be treated with enteral nutrients as soon as possible. A complete discussion about the use of carbohydrates in enteral and parenteral diets is provided in the following sections on enteral nutrition and PN.

Minerals and vitamins

The requirements for macrominerals and microminerals and for fat- and water-soluble vitamins during different disease states are not defined for adult horses. When an enteral or a parenteral diet is formulated, the clinician should evaluate the chronicity of the disease, the severity of malnourishment and the primary disesase condition to determine an appropriate plan for vitamin and mineral supplementation.

If a hospitalised horse is treated with a liquid enteral formulation, the patient's daily electrolyte and mineral requirements often will be met if a complete feed is used and the patient is fed to meet its maintenance energy requirements. Supplemental electrolytes or bicarbonate can be added to an enteral formulation to improve the electrolyte and acid-base balance in an equine patient. Minerals can be added to a parenteral formulation either by using an amino acid solution that contains electrolytes or by adding electrolytes and trace minerals to the formulation. It is often easiest to add electrolyte supplements to the intravenous fluids. This allows for an efficient alteration of the electrolyte therapy without discarding an entire batch of the parenteral solution. Regardless of the route of electrolyte supplementation, consistent monitoring of the horse's serum electrolytes and appropriate electrolyte therapy are important. The maintenance electrolyte requirements for adult horses can be used as a guideline for supplementation of therapeutic diets (Box 5.10).

Trace mineral supplementation is usually reserved for horses that are treated with PN or horses suffering from chronic malnutrition. Most commercial equine complete feeds and enteral diet ingredients contain trace minerals. Supplemental minerals can also be added to an enteral diet. Guidelines for trace mineral supplementation in parenteral formulations are extrapolated from the procedures that are followed by human and small animal nutritionists. Specific recommendations will be made in the sections on enteral nutrition and PN.

Box 5.10. Macromineral requirements for adult horses at a physiologic state of maintenance[12,21]

1. Calcium (grams/day) = 0.04 (BW in kg)
2. Phosphorus (grams/day) = 0.028 (BW in kg)
3. Magnesium (grams/day) = 0.015 (BW in kg)
4. Potassium (grams/day) = 0.05 (BW in kg)

Fat-soluble vitamins are stored in the liver and in lipid-containing cells of the body. Deficiencies of vitamins A, D, E and K are rare in adult horses with short-term anorexia (<7 days). Horses that have experienced prolonged anorexia or that have been fed poor-quality forage without vitamin supplementation may suffer from a deficiency of vitamin A, D or E. Vitamin K is absorbed from dietary sources and is also produced by bacteria in the gastrointestinal tract. Horses with prolonged gastrointestinal disease resulting in a loss of normal gastrointestinal flora may benefit from supplemental dietary vitamin K, especially if the horse demonstrates evidence of increased susceptibility to hemorrhage. Oral vitamin E supplementation with 2000 to 4000 IU for every 224 ml (1 cup) of oil is recommended when oil is added to an enteral diet at concentrations that exceed 113 ml ($\frac{1}{2}$cup)/day. Enteral diets can be supplemented with as much as 10 IU vitamin E/kg body weight/day.[21] Vitamin E can be added in powdered or liquid form. The selected oral vitamin E supplement should not contain selenium. Enteral diets that contain a commercial complete feed product should provide an adult horse with their maintenance vitamin requirements if the diet is fed to meet the maintenance energy requirement of the horse. A vitamin and mineral supplement should be added to enteral diets that do not contain complete feeds. The label daily dosing instructions should be followed for commercial oral vitamin and mineral products. Horses that have abnormalities in lipid absorption in the small intestine may not absorb fat-soluble vitamins. These horses should be treated with a parenteral product if they have intestinal malabsorption or if they remain anorectic for longer than 7 days. Lipid-soluble vitamin products are available for intramuscular injection; however, their use has been associated with complications from myositis and is not recommended. Parenteral formulations can be supplemented with multivitamin products that contain lipid-soluble vitamins.

The B series of vitamins function as essential cofactors in cellular metabolism. Deficiencies of B vitamins have not been reported in healthy horses because these vitamins are normally produced in the gastrointestinal tract. Most B vitamins have a storage time of a few weeks, except for B_{12}, which has a storage time in the liver of at least a few months.

Although current studies do not demonstrate a requirement for B-vitamin supplementation in critically ill horses, equine patients that have had a disruption of the resident flora of the gastrointestinal tract due to colic surgery or colitis or horses that have had an ileal resection or an ileal bypass may benefit from B-vitamin supplementation. Multivitamin products can be added to either enteral or parenteral formulations to ensure adequate B-vitamin intake. Frequently, a B-vitamin supplement is the only vitamin product added to a parenteral diet. The recommended dose is 1 to 2 ml of B-complex vitamins/L of parenteral solution. Adverse effects associated with B-vitamin toxicity have not been described in horses and are unlikely to occur unless a horse is chronically oversupplemented.

Specific vitamin and mineral requirements for healthy adult horses can be found in the *NRC Nutrient Requirements of Horses*, 6th edition, and should be used as a guideline when formulating critical care diets.[21]

Selecting the form of supplemental nutrition

Enteral versus parenteral therapy

Nutritional therapy should be started when a hospitalised horse cannot voluntarily consume greater than 75% of their DE_{Rest} or greater than 75% of their maintenance protein requirement (Table 5.2). The choice between enteral or parenteral therapy depends on the clinical condition of the horse, the resources available for diet preparation and administration at the hospital and the financial restraints of the case (Boxes 5.8 and 5.11).

Assisted enteral feeding

AEF with a liquid enteral formulation is the preferred method of dietary treatment. Enteral nutrition provides nutrients directly to the enterocytes and helps to maintain the protective barrier in the gastrointestinal tract.[33] Studies in laboratory animal species and clinical trials in humans have repeatedly demonstrated decreased complications from sepsis, and improved clinical outcomes in subjects treated with enteral diets compared to groups treated with isocaloric and isonitrogenous parenteral diets.

AEF is the treatment of choice in horses that have progressive gastrointestinal motility, that can tolerate placement of a feeding tube and that can be treated while standing or in sternal recumbency. Horses suffering from neurological disease that are unable to maintain their head in an upright position, horses at risk of aspiration and horses that have severe respiratory disease are not good candidates for AEF.

Equine enteral formulations can be divided into solutions that contain nonstructural carbohydrates (fibre-free) and solutions that contain a moderate (10%–20% DM) concentration of structural carbohydrates (fibre). Horses present a challenge during enteral diet therapy because they frequently develop self-limiting diarrhoea when either low-fibre or fibre-free enteral diets are administered.[17,34,35] One study that evaluated the effects of the human enteral formulation Osmolyte HN in adult horses with systemic disease reported diarrhoea in three of six dysphagic horses fed sufficient Osmolyte HN to meet their maintenance energy requirements.[34] In contrast to this report, other studies that have assessed liquid enteral diet treatment in horses have reported successful dietary management without diarrhoea. A Miniature horse with hyperlipaemia was treated with a fibre-free human enteral diet and did not develop diarrhoea.[36] Hallebeek and Beynen[30] fed one healthy pony a fat- and fibre-free liquid enteral diet for 5 days and did not report any complication from diarrhoea. In the same study, healthy ponies that were fasted for either 8 or 9 days did not develop diarrhoea after 2 to 3 days of treatment with the same fat- and fibre-free enteral diet.

A balanced liquid enteral formulation can be infused as the sole source of nutrition to an adult horse from 2 to beyond 30 days. Liquid enteral diets are almost always infused through a nasogastric tube; however, gastro-oesophageal tubes can be placed in horses that require long-term therapy or in horses that cannot be treated with

Box 5.11. Indications for enteral or parenteral nutritional therapy in the adult horse

Treatment with Assisted Enteral Feeding (AEF)

- Horses that can tolerate a nasogastric tube, that do not have persistent gastric reflux, and that do not require complete feed restriction as part of their medical management
- Horses can be treated with AEF in an equine hospital or in a field setting.
- Minimal equipment and expense are associated with AEF.
- Diarrhoea is the most frequent complication of AEF but can be reduced by using a diet that contains structural fibre.

Treatment with Parenteral Nutrition

- Horses that have ileus, gastrointestinal obstruction or intractable diarrhoea or horses that require complete feed restriction as part of their medical management
- Horses that have nasal, pharyngeal or oesophageal disease, or animals that cannot tolerate a nasogastric tube
- Horses that cannot maintain their head in an upright position, and horses that are at risk of recumbency or aspiration
- Horses that can be treated in a hospitalised setting. A fluid pump is desired. Sterile administration of PN is essential. Frequent monitoring of serum electrolytes and blood glucose is important.
- Treatment can be successful when a portion of the stall resting energy requirement and protein requirement is administered.

a nasogastric tube. Percutaneous gastrostomy tube and jejunostomy tube feeding is not feasible in horses at this time. Equine enteral formulations are relatively inexpensive, with costs as low as US$10.00/day (£6/day; €8/day) for diet ingredients. Equipment requirements are limited to a nasogastric tube and an infusion pump or bag for gravity flow administration. Although AEF is easily administered to hospitalised horses, it can also be used to treat a horse in a field setting.

Some hospitalised patients cannot be fed with a liquid enteral diet. In these patients, therapeutic nutrition is administered using a parenteral formulation. The current evidence supporting the use of PN in adult horses is sparse, but in patients that cannot tolerate enteral feeding, PN is the best option for dietary therapy.

Parenteral nutrition

Equine patients that benefit from treatment from PN include horses managed with prolonged feed restriction, horses with ileus or obstructive gastrointestinal disease, horses with severe diarrhoea, horses with nasal, pharyngeal or oesophageal disease, patients that are recumbent and horses that have severe neurological or respiratory disease. Parenteral nutrition can be administered as the sole source of nutrition, or it can be used in conjunction with enteral feeding to provide nutritional support to a patient that cannot tolerate greater than 50% of the DE_{Rest} with enteral feeding. The high cost of PN for an adult horse (US$300–$400/day if administered at a rate to provide 100% DE_{Rest} [€350–450; £200–300]) usually prohibits use for long (7–10 day) periods of time. From a metabolic and nutritional perspective, equine patients can be maintained on PN for longer than 7 days. Less expensive formulations can be made if solutions provide only 50% to 75% of a patient's stall RER. Provision of even a portion of the patient's daily resting energy and maintenance protein requirements for a few days using PN will help prevent protein-calorie malnutrition.

Practical limitations to PN use include the need for use of a dedicated catheter port and intravenous fluid line and the ability to infuse the PN solution as a CRI. In order to assess the metabolic response to re-feeding with a PN solution, serum biochemical values should be closely monitored. Because complications could arise with PN infusion and because the PN infusion rate or solution may require frequent alteration to meet the changing metabolic profile of an equine patient, horses that are treated with PN are almost always managed in a hospital facility.

Only a few studies have evaluated the efficacy of PN in adult horses. An experimental study performed on four healthy adult horses demonstrated both safety and efficacy of a PN formulation infused in feed-deprived horses for 10 days.[37] The tested PN formulation contained a caloric distribution of 8.5% calories from amino acids, 50.5% calories from glucose and 41% calories from lipid.[37] Two of the horses had glucosuria during the 10 days of therapy, and another two horses had glucosuria during the first 6 to 7 days of the study, suggesting that the concentration of glucose in the PN solution was too high. A wide variation in the energy, protein and lipid contents of PN formulations was described in an 8-year retrospective study of PN therapy in a university hospital.[38] In this population of horses, hyperglycaemia was the most common complication. Treatment consisted of reducing the rate of PN infusion, and insulin therapy if the horse failed to respond to the decreased rate of infusion. The concentration of lipid in the PN solution, as a percent of nonprotein energy, ranged from 8% to 54%. Although serum TG concentration was not reported in the study, the authors did not list hypertriglyceridaemia as a complication from the PN infusion.[38] In another study, the clinical and biochemical effect of PN was compared to feed restriction in adult horses in the immediate period following colic surgery.[39] Horses treated with PN had lower serum concentrations of TG, urea, bilirubin and albumin but higher concentrations of serum glucose and insulin. The same researchers published a second study and concluded that horses treated with PN following resection and anastomosis surgery of the small intestine did not demonstrate a significant clinical improvement compared to horses that were starved.[40]

Nutrition options: Enteral nutrition

A variety of diets can be used in an equine liquid enteral formulation. These include human enteral products, commercial equine complete pelleted feeds or pelleted hay and specially designed equine enteral diet recipes. Recently, an increased number of commercial products have been marketed as equine enteral diets, but their safety and efficacy have not been tested at the time of publication. The nutrient content and ingredient formulations of any equine enteral diet should be closely evaluated by the clinician or by an equine nutritionist before one of these products is selected for use. The choice of a particular type of enteral diet depends on the availability of the diet ingredients, the size of the tube that can be used in the horse and whether or not the horse requires fibre in the diet. An enteral diet formulation worksheet is provided in Box 5.12.

Fibre in enteral diets

The need for structural carbohydrates (fibre) in equine liquid enteral diets is currently being evaluated. Enteral diets that do not contain structural fibre can be administered through a very small diameter (18 F) nasogastric tube. Once structural fibre is added to the enteral formulation, the viscosity of the formulation increases, and a larger-diameter nasogastric tube is required. Although the forage-based diet of the horse typically contains 30% to 60% structural carbohydrates, horses have been successfully treated with fibre-free enteral diets as the sole source of nutrition for a short period of time.[30,34,36]

Diarrhoea is the most common adverse effect of feeding a fibre-free enteral diet to a horse. Eliminating fibre from

Box 5.12. Enteral nutritional formulation worksheet

Patient Information

1. Initial body weight (kg) ____ kg
2. Stall resting energy requirement: DE_{Rest} (kcal/day) = 975 + 21 (BW in kg) ____ kcal
3. Maintenance energy requirement: DE_{Maint} (kcal/day) = 33.3 × (BW in kg) ____ kcal
4. Protein requirements: Crude protein (mg/day) = 1260 × (BW in kg) ____ mg
5. Fluid requirements for maintenance: 60 ml/kg/day ____ ml
6. Total kcal required/day (estimate between **2** and **3** calculated above) ____ kcal
7. Select a product for use using the tables provided in the chapter

Example

For a 450-kg horse

1. Initial body weight (kg) 450 kg
2. Stall resting energy requirement: DE_{Rest} (kcal/day) = 975 + 21 (BW in kg) 10,425 kcal
3. Maintenance energy requirement: DE_{Maint} (kcal/day) = 33.3 × (BW in kg) 14,985 kcal
4. Protein requirements: Crude protein (mg/day) = 1260 × (BW in kg) 567,000 mg
5. Fluid requirements for maintenance: 60 ml/kg/day 27,000 ml
6. Total kcal required/day (estimate between **2** and **3** calculated above) 12,000 kcal

Providing enough energy

If it is decided to use only alfalfa pellets as the energy source, with an energy density of 2156 kcal/kg:

12,000 kcal × 1 kg/2156 kcal = 5.57 kg of alfalfa pellets will be required each day

Providing enough protein

If the horse is fed 5.57 kg of alfalfa pellets, assuming a protein content of 16.7% (16.7 g protein/100 g diet):

Then in each 5.57 kg of diet, a total of 930 g of protein will be provided, well in excess of the 567 g (567,000 mg) required by the horse.

How to feed

In a hospital setting, it is desirable to feed at least 4 times each day:

5.57 kg/4 = 1.39 kg alfalfa pellets/feeding

If all fluids will be provided with enteral nutritional, then 27 L/4 = 6.75 L/feeding. A total of 5 L can be mixed with the pellets, and the remaining 1.75 L can be used for the tube flush.

Electrolytes, vitamins and minerals can be supplemented in the diet to achieve a proper balance of nutrients.

an equine enteral diet may increase the transit time of nutrients through the small intestine, resulting in protein, fat and carbohydrate malabsorption. Fibre-free enteral diets contain nonstructural carbohydrates such as dextrose, glucose and maltodextrin instead of cellulose and hemicellulose. Nonstructural carbohydrates are highly digestible and are normally absorbed in the small intestine. If an excessive concentration of nonstructural carbohydrates is fed, the transport capacity of the small intestine is overwhelmed and the carbohydrates pass into the large intestine, where they serve as substrates for the intestsial microflora. Delivery of macronutrient substrates to caecal and colonic bacteria affect the balance of resident flora. Excessive proliferation of bacterial species such as *Streptococcus bovis* and overgrowth of pathogenic bacteria including *Salmonella* spp. and *Clostridium difficile* may lead to serious complications, including diarrhoea and laminitis. When structural carbohydrates are included in the enteral diet, the fibre provides a substrate for cellulolytic intestinal bacteria. The structural fibre may help to restore the normal balance of intestinal bacteria and should provide the horse with a source of energy from volatile fatty acid production.

Due to the risks associated with gastrointestinal complications, fibre-free enteral diets are not recommended for horses with colitis and/or laminitis, and they may be contraindicated in horses at risk of developing diarrhoea from antibiotic therapy or recent colic surgery. If only a small-diameter nasogastric tube can be placed in a horse with laminitis or colitis or in a horse at risk of developing diarrhoea, every effort should be made to include as much fibre in the diet as possible. Some liquid human formulations (Promote With Fiber) contain fibre. Specialised enteral diet recipes can also be formulated that contain fibre but still have a low viscosity.

Enteral diet formulations

Human formulations

Vital HN and Osmolyte HN* are two human formulations that have been administered to adult horses, and they have

*Ross Laboratories, Columbus, OH, USA.

Table 5.5. Human Liquid Enteral Products*

Product	Caloric Density (kcal/ml)	Osmolarity (mOsm/L)	% Calories Protein	% Calories Fat	% Calories Carbohydrate	Carbohydrate source
Osmolyte	1.06	252	14.0	29.0	57.0	Corn maltodextrin
Osmolite 1 Cal	1.06	252	16.7	29.0	54.3	Corn maltodextrin
Osmolite 1.2 Cal	1.20	295	18.5	29.0	52.5	Corn maltodextrin
Vital HN	1.00	386	16.7	9.5	73.8	Corn maltodextrin, sucrose
Promote	1.00	285	25.0	23.0	52.0	Corn maltodextrin, sucrose
Promote With Fiber	1.00	315	25.0	25.0	50.0	Corn maltodextrin, sucrose, oat fibre, soy fibre

*Ross Nutrition, Abbott Laboratories, North Chicago, IL, USA.

been evaluated in the scientific literature.[34,36] Although the original Osmolyte HN formulation is no longer available, three new Osmolyte solutions are produced by Ross Laboratories. Since the time that the Ross enteral formulations were first evaluated in horses, this company's enteral product line has been expanded to include many different formulations for human patients, some of which contain fibre. A partial nutrient profile of some of the products that could be used in horses is included in Table 5.5. Additional enteral product information can be obtained directly from Ross Laboratories.

Most human enteral formulations contain approximately 1 kcal/ml and 4.1 to 4.2 g of protein/100 kcal. (Table 5.5) All of the human formulations can be administered at room temperature by gravity flow through an 18 Fr or larger nasogastric tube. Based on the energy density of the human formulations, almost 10.5 L is required to meet the DE_{Rest} of 10.4 Mcal for a 450-kg horse. The protein content (approximately 440 g) in 10.5 L of Osmolyte or Vital HN will not meet the 567 g of protein that is required for a 450-kg horse. Supplemental protein (casein, lactalbumin, whey, soy) can be added in a powdered form to a human enteral product to ensure that the diet meets the protein requirements of a hospitalised horse. If a human enteral formulation is selected for a horse that has hypertriglyceridaemia, hyperlipaemia or hepatic lipidosis, a low-fat formulation such as Vital HN (<10% of the total calories from fat) is recommended.

Equine patients that are at risk of developing laminitis or diarrhoea are not good candidates for treatment with a human enteral diet due to the high concentration of soluble carbohydrates in the products. If a human formulation is used in horses that have, or that may develop, diarrhoea, a formulation with fibre, such as Promote With Fiber, should be used. Finely ground fibre sources including alfalfa meal, rice bran or wheat bran may decrease complications from diarrhoea and can be added to the human product. These ingredients will increase the viscosity of the human formulations and may eliminate the option of gravity flow infusion of the diet if a small-diameter (18 F) nasogastric tube is selected for the infusion.

Commercial equine enteral diets and pelleted feeds

Complete pelleted feeds contain 14% to 25% crude fibre (DM) and between 2.6 and 3.1 Mcal/kg of diet (Table 5.6). Between 3.4 and 6.0 kg (7.5–13.2 lb) of diet is required per day to meet the 10.4 Mcal DE_{Rest} of a 450-kg horse. This same volume of feed may not meet the horse's protein requirement. If additional protein is needed, powdered soy, casein, whey or lactalbumin should be added to the diet to ensure adequate protein intake. When a commercial complete pelleted feed is used as an enteral diet and the diet is fed to meet the horse's maintenance energy requirements, the vitamin and mineral requirements of the horse should also be met with the diet.

Hay pellets can be blended into a liquid enteral diet. The nutrient content and quality of pelleted forages vary with the type of hay (Table 5.6). Often, the pellets do not contain sufficient vitamins and minerals to meet a horse's daily requirements. A commercial vitamin and mineral supplement can be added to the diet to ensure adequate nutrient intake. The label directions on the supplement should be followed. Products that contain herbal ingredients should be avoided.

Equine enteral diet recipes

Fibre and fibre-free enteral diets can be formulated if a commercial diet is not available or if a special formulation is required to meet the nutritional needs of the horse. One enteral diet recipe, often called the "Naylor Diet", has been previously published.[17] This formulation provides 12.2 Mcal DE and requires a daily volume of 900 g dextrose, 900 g casein, 2000 g dehydrated alfalfa meal, 21 L of water and 230 g of a mineral mixture (sodium chloride [NaCl], 10 g; sodium bicarbonate [$NaHCO_3^-$], 15 g; potassium chloride [KCl], 75 g; potassium phosphate [dibasic anhydrous, K_2HPO_4], 60 g; calcium chloride [$CaCl_2 \cdot 2H_2O$], 45 g; magnesium oxide [MgO], 25 g).[17] The fat and fibre content in this recipe (2% crude fat, DM; 12% crude fibre, DM) is similar to the concentration in commercial complete feeds; however, this recipe provides additional protein (33% crude protein, DM) which may be

Table 5.6. Commercial and Pelleted Equine Feeds Suitable for Use in a Liquid Enteral Diet

Feed	Digestible Energy (kcal/kg)	Crude Protein (%)	Crude Fat (%)	Crude Fibre (%)
Equine Senior*[a]	2695	14.0	4.0	13.0
Senior†[a]	3124	14.0	7.0	16.0
Senior‡[a]	3146	13.0	4.0	14.0
Senior§[a]	2341	14.0	4.0	20.0
Senior**[a]	3401	14.0	10.0	17.0
Complete Advantage*[a]	3080	12.0	3.75	12.5
Alfalfa Pellets[b]	2156	16.7	2.3	21.5
Timothy Hay Pellets[b]	1760	8.5	2.4	31.5
Oat Hay Pellets[b]	1760	8.6	2.2	29.1

[a] As fed, manufacturer analysis.
[b] As fed, estimated values.
* Purina Mills, St. Louis, MO, USA.
† Seminole Feed, Ocala, FL, USA.
‡ TDI Horse Feeds, Lewis Center, OH, USA.
§ LMF Feeds, Inc., Weiser, ID, USA.
** Triple Crown Nutrition, Wayzata, MN, USA.

beneficial for horses suffering from protein malnutrition or excessive protein loss. The fibre content of this diet may be low enough to infuse into a small-diameter nasogastric tube.

An ingredient-based enteral diet can also be created by a clinician using fibre, protein and energy ingredients that are available in the local region (Table 5.7). A vitamin and mineral supplement can be added to the solution to balance the diet, or the mineral mixture in the preceding paragraph can be used. The consistency of the formulation should be adjusted to ensure that the formulation can be delivered through the nasogastric tube that has been selected for diet administration. Once all ingredients have been combined with water, the final solution can be blended to decrease the viscosity of the solution. The clinician should formulate the diet with a goal to add 50% to 75% of the ingredients as fibre. Diets with high concentrations of oil (>560 ml/day, $2\frac{1}{2}$ cups/day) and dextrose (>1500 g) should be avoided to decrease the likelihood of digestive and metabolic complications.

Nutrition supplements in liquid enteral diets

Oil

The volume of blended feed required to meet the energy and protein requirements of some horses will be too great to be administered over a 24-hour period, even when the feedings are administered 6 times each day. If the horse can tolerate fat supplementation in the diet, oil can be added to the enteral formulation to increase the energy density of the diet. Canola oil (224 ml [1 cup]) contains 1980 kcal, almost one-fifth of the total resting energy required by a 450-kg horse (Table 5.7). Canola, soy, flax and corn oil are all equine enteral diet supplement options. Corn oil contains the highest concentration of omega-6 essential fatty acids in comparison to the other oils and may not be the best oil supplement for horses with systemic inflammation. In contrast, flax oil contains the highest concentration of omega-3 fatty acids of the listed oils. If a horse will be treated with an enteral diet for 7 or more days, dietary supplementation with omega-3 fatty acids may decrease the horse's systemic inflammatory response. Omega-3 fatty acids should be supplemented with caution in horses that have abnormal clotting profiles. To provide antioxidant protection when oil is added to the enteral formulation, vitamin E should be added to the diet at a concentration of 2000 to 4000 IU/224 ml (1 cup) of oil.

If the horse's serum TG is less than 2.26 mmol/L (200 mg/dl), up to 224 ml (1 cup) of oil can be added to an enteral diet each day. Horses with a serum TG between 2.26 and 5.65 mmol/L (200–500 mg/dl) should not be supplemented with more than 112 ml (½ cup) of oil per day. Oil should not be added to the diet of horses with hypertriglyceridaemia (>5.65 mmol/L [500 mg/dl]) or horses that have been diagnosed with hepatic lipidosis. Supplemental dietary oil should be introduced slowly over a 2- to 3-day period.

Protein

Casein, lactalbumin, whey and soy protein are highly digestible sources of protein that can be added to an enteral diet to ensure that the diet meets the protein requirement of the equine patient. The approximate protein and energy content of these protein sources is listed in Table 5.7. Glutamine and BCAA supplementation in enteral diets is discussed in the Nutrient Requirements section.

Table 5.7. Estimated Nutrient Content of Equine Enteral Diet Ingredients

Ingredient	Digestible Energy (kcal/kg)	Crude Protein (%)	Crude Fat (%)	Crude Fibre (%)
Fibre Source				
Alfalfa meal[a]	2156	16.7	2.30	21.5
Wheat bran[a]	2955	15.9	4.1	7.5
Rice bran[a]	2765	13.2	14.7	6.2
Protein Source				
Casein (as sodium caseinate)*	3595	91.0	2.5	1.0
Soy†	3278	63.6	0.46	5.5
ProMod‡ (whey protein)	5606	>71.0	<19.0	<10.0
Energy Source				
Canola oil or corn oil†	1980 kcal/224 ml	0	100	0
50% Dextrose	1.7 kcal/ml	0	0	0
50% Glucose	1.9 kcal/ml	0	0	0

[a] Estimated value, as fed.
*American Casein Company, Burlington, NJ, USA.
†USDA National Nutrient Database for Standard Reference, as fed values (http://www.nal.usda.gov/fnic/foodcomp/search/).
‡Manufacturer Data, Ross Products, Abbott Laboratories, North Chicago, IL, USA.

Feeds to avoid in an enteral diet

Concentrate feeds, grains and commercial supplement feeds are energy-dense products that usually contain high concentrations of nonstructural carbohydrates. In critically ill horses, these feeds may induce complications including diarrhoea, pathogenic bacterial overgrowth and laminitis. The use of these ingredients in equine enteral diets is contraindicated.

Choice and use of indwelling nasogastric tubes

Indwelling nasogastric tubes appear to be relatively safe in adult horses, especially in patients that require treatment 4 to 6 times daily (Figure 5.1). The risk of reflux oesophagitis appears to be relatively uncommon in horses due to the relative alkalinity of gastric secretions compared to other species.[41] Conflicting reports have been published regarding the effect of nasogastric tubes on gastric emptying in horses. One research group determined that placement of a small diameter (1.0-cm inner diameter, 1.6-cm outer diameter) nasogastric tube for 18 hours did not delay the gastric emptying rate of liquids in healthy adult horses.[42] A second group documented a significant delay in gastric emptying of liquids from the stomach in a study in which nasogastric tubes with an outer diameter of 1.6 cm were maintained in adult horses for 72 hours.[43] Treated horses in this study did not have significant gastric ulceration in comparison to the control group of horses; however, treatment horses did have endoscopic evidence of nasal and pharyngeal hyperaemia and ulceration.[43]

The fibre content of the enteral diet dictates the size of the nasogastric tube that is used for infusion. The tube with the smallest internal diameter should be selected to decrease pharyngeal and oesophageal irritation. Fibre-free diets can be administered through an 18 Fr, 250-cm feeding tube†. Diets that contain fibre should be infused through a tube that has an inner diameter of at least 0.65 cm. Silicon tubes are preferred because they are less likely to cause mucosal trauma; however, polyurethane tubes are also suitable. Gravity flow infusion can be used to administer a fibre-free liquid enteral diet and is an ideal method of infusion

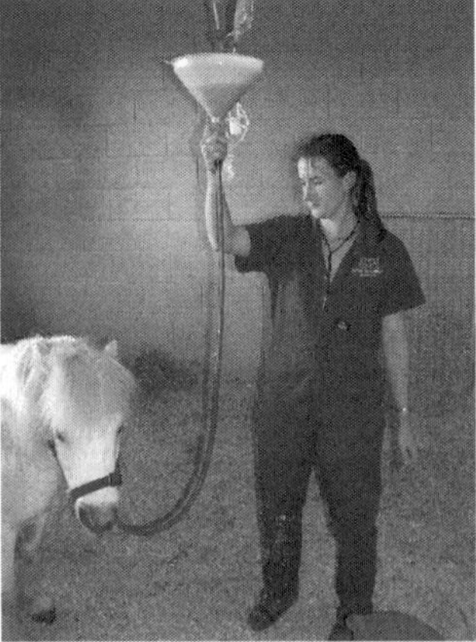

Figure 5.1 Enteral feeding via a large bore nasogastric tube in a pony with hyperlipaemia. ©Kevin Corley 2004.

†NG18100; MILA International, Inc., Florence, KY, USA.

because bolus feeding of large volumes of the diet can be avoided. A bolus feeding method using an infusion pump is usually required to administer an enteral formulation that contains fibre.

Most nasogastric tubes can remain in place for up to 8 days without gastric complications in most horses. When a horse is closely supervised in a hospital setting, the nasogastric tube should remain in place; however, the tube should be removed between feedings if the horse is not monitored. Rigid stomach tubes and large-diameter tubes (>1.9-cm inner diameter) can be used for diet administration. Large-diameter tubes should only be used if smaller tubes are not available because they may cause increased discomfort, may predispose the horse to pharyngeal and oesophageal complications and may not be suitable for indwelling, long-term use. Field practitioners should use any available nasogastric tube to infuse the diet and should remove the tube after the diet has been administered.

Regardless of the size of nasogastric tube that is selected, the enteral diet solution should be tested using the pump and tube to ensure that the solution can be administered without clogging the equipment before the tube is placed in the patient. Additional water can be added to the diet to reduce the viscosity of the enteral solution; however, the volume of diet that can be safely infused may be limited if too much water is added to the solution.

Oesophagostomy tube placement and contraindications

If AEF is required for a prolonged period of time (>21 days) or if a nasogastric tube cannot be used in the horse because of sinus trauma or disease, pharyngeal disorders or proximal oesophageal disease, an oesophagostomy tube should be placed to facilitate enteral feeding (Figure 5.2). Horses that require long-term nutrition support will need to be provided with a complete diet that is balanced in all nutrients including vitamins and trace minerals. A nutritionist can be consulted for complicated cases.

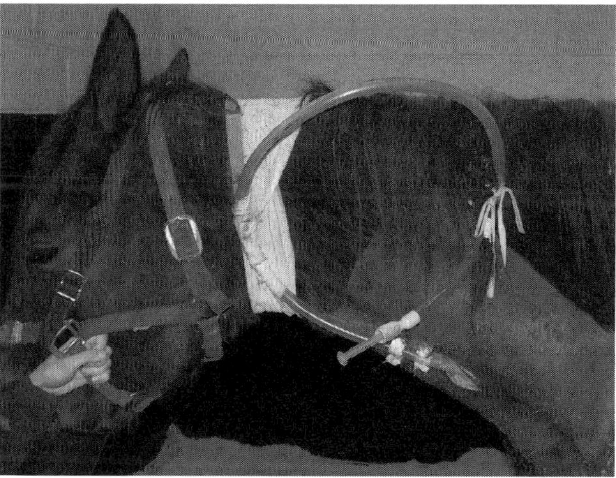

Figure 5.2 An oesophagostomy tube in a Thoroughbred mare. The mare had severe proximal oesophageal necrosis, following an obstruction of 48 hours' duration. The oesophagostomy tube was placed 10 days prior to this photograph. ©Kevin Corley 2007.

The following description of the oesophagostomy procedure is taken from *Equine Surgery*, written by Dr. John Stick.[44] Other descriptions of the procedure and the post-surgical complications associated with an oesophagostomy have been previously published.[45–47] The recommended surgical approach is at the ventrolateral aspect of the mid-cervical oesophagus. The procedure can be performed while the horse is standing, following the infusion of a local anaesthetic, or can be performed while the horse is in right lateral or dorsal recumbency. Passage of a nasogastric tube prior to the procedure aids in identification of the oesophagus during the surgery. Following surgical preparation of the site, a 5-cm (2-inch) incision is made ventral to the left jugular vein. The sternocephalicus and brachiocephalicus muscles are separated; then, the deep cervical fascia is incised. Once the oesophagus is exposed, a 3-cm longitudinal sharp incision is made until the nasogastric tube is identified. The original nasogastric tube is removed, and the feeding tube (14–24-mm outer diameter; ½–1-inch outer diameter) is placed into the oesophagus and passed into the stomach. If the tube does not pass easily, the muscle layer of the oesophagus may not be incised adequately to allow passage of the tube of the chosen diameter. The tube should pass easily through both the elastic inner layer and the inelastic outer muscle layer of the oesophagus. Once the tube is inserted, sutures can be placed around the mucosa to seal the tissue around the tube. The tube should be securely attached to the skin near the entry site with butterfly tape bandages. Elastic tape should then be used to secure the tube to the neck. The tube should remain in place for at least 7 to 10 days to permit a stoma to form with granulation tissue around the surgical site. If the tube is placed around an area with an oesophageal rupture or perforation, the tube should remain in place for a longer period of time. Following removal of the tube, the stoma should heal by second intention. Because of the risk of infection following the oesophagostomy and tube placement, antimicrobial treatment with broad-spectrum therapy is recommended until a stoma forms at the surgery site.[44]

Reported complications following an oesophagostomy in the horse include traction diverticulum at the oesophagostomy site, formation of permanent oesophageal fistulas, possible left laryngeal hemiplegia, dehiscence of the surgical site, formation of fistulas into the thorax and mediastinitis secondary to dissecting infection.[45–47] These serious complications preclude the frequent use of oesophagostomy tubes in equine practice.

The diameter of the oesophagostomy tube and the clinical condition of the horse will dictate the type of liquid enteral diet that is selected. Because horses with oesophagostomy tubes usually require assisted enteral feeding for more than 7 days, fibre should be included in the enteral diet.

Enteral nutrition preparation and administration

Diet preparation

Pelleted diets must be dissolved before nutrition is administered. This can be done either by grinding the pellets before water is added or by processing the pellets in a blender after they have been soaked in warm water. If a large volume of enteral feeding is going to be performed, purchase of a heavy-duty blender like the Vita Mix Blender Super 5000* is recommended. Variable quantities of water will be required to blend each pelleted feed properly. Pellets that contain beet pulp require more water for dissolution than alfalfa-based pellets. The total volume of water that is added to blend the enteral diet should be recorded as part of the horse's daily fluid intake and subtracted from the daily fluid requirement of the horse to ensure that the patient is not overhydrated.

Nutrition administration

When the nutrition is first administered, the equine patient should be treated with 25% to 30% of the total daily volume of diet to avoid metabolic and gastrointestinal complications that can develop with rapid re-feeding (Box 5.13). The monitoring guidelines in Box 5.14 should be followed when enteral nutrition is introduced to an adult horse.

Enteral feedings should be divided into at least 2 treatments each day. In a hospital setting, 4 to 6 daily treatments are preferred. No more than 6 L of fluid should be infused per feeding when the diet is started in an adult horse that weighs greater than 400 kg. This fluid volume includes both the diet formulation and the water infused as a tube flush. A comparatively smaller volume of fluid should be infused in an adult pony or Miniature horse. Draft breeds may tolerate infusion of volumes that exceed 6 L. After the horse has been adapted to the diet for a few days, as much as 8 L can be infused during each feeding in a horse that weighs greater than 400 kg if the horse tolerates the increased fluid volume.

The nasogastric tube should be checked to ensure that the distal end of the tube is in the stomach. Before the diet is infused, the quantity of residual gastric fluid should be removed and measured. If less than 2 L of residual fluid is removed from the stomach, the enteral diet can be infused. If more than 2 L of fluid is removed, the horse should not be fed, and instead should be rechecked for gastric fluid in 1 hour. Horses that have normal gastrointestinal motility will not have greater than 1 to 2 L of residual gastric fluid even if they are fed every 6 hours. If the horse has persistent gastric reflux in volumes that exceed 2 L every 2 hours for more than 12 hours, an alternate method of diet therapy should be initiated.

Box 5.13. Infusion protocol for a liquid enteral diet

Feed 25%–30% of the total volume on days 1–2

Feed 30%–60% of the total volume on days 2–3

Feed 60%–100% of the total volume on days 3–4

Nutrition should be administered slowly to prevent the solution from refluxing around the tube. During manual infusion, the enteral solution should be stirred constantly to prevent the more dense diet ingredients from settling to the bottom of the bucket. If nutrition is administered using a gravity flow method, the infusion can be delivered over 30 to 60 minutes. Diets administered by gravity flow should be frequently monitored to ensure that the diet is flowing at a constant rate.

Once the entire volume of the diet has been administered, 1 to 2 L of water should be infused to flush the tube. After the flush water has been administered, a small amount of air should be pushed through the tube to confirm that the tube is clear of feed debris. The tip of the tube should then be held at the level of the horse's nares. If the stomach is too distended, fluid will flow back out through the tube. Excess fluid should be removed from the stomach before the tube is closed. Before the tip of the tube is closed with a syringe case, a small amount of air should again be pushed through the tube to clear any residual feed from the end of the tube.

If the nasogastric tube remains in place between feedings, the tube should be secured to a leather halter and the horse should wear a muzzle between feedings to prevent removal of the nasogastric tube. A nylon muzzle† is well tolerated, easy to clean, and causes minimal trauma to the face if the horse rubs the muzzle.

Tubes that become blocked should be treated with a gentle water lavage to clear the tube. If this fails to relieve the blockage, 20 to 30 ml of carbonated water can be instilled into the tube, and left in the tube for up to 1 hour to disintegrate the blockage. If the carbonated water fails to dissolve the tube debris, the tube should be removed so it can be properly cleaned, and replaced before the next feeding.

Monitoring guidelines

A complete physical examination should be performed on the horse each day. Elevations in the horse's TPR values beyond the upper normal range are abnormal and require prompt evaluation to identify the etiology of the clinical abnormalities. The examination also includes a measurement of the horse's body weight and an assessment of the horse's BCS. If the horse is in a positive fluid and energy balance, the patent's weight and BCS should remain stable during AEF. Although a small amount of mucoid nasal

*Vita-Mix Corporation, Cleveland, OH, USA.

†Best Friend Grazing Muzzle; Best Friend Equine Supply, Inc., Fairfield Glade, TN, USA.

Box 5.14. Suggested monitoring guidelines during assisted enteral feeding (AEF) and parenteral nutrition (PN)

1. Full physical examination, including temperature, pulse and respiration, every 4–6 hours at the start of therapy; every 6–12 hours once the patient is stable, and the diet has been administered for 48 hours.
2. Body weight every 24 hours with a scale. If a scale is not available, a weight tape should be used.
3. Body condition score (BCS), every 24 hours.
4. Blood glucose every 6–12 hours at the start of therapy; every 8–24 hours once the blood glucose concentration has stabilised during the full nutritional infusion rate.
5. Triglycerides every 24 hours until the patient's serum triglyceride concentration has normalised during the full infusion rate.
6. Electrolytes: Potassium, sodium and chloride, at least every 24 hours; phosphorus, ionised magnesium and ionised calcium, at least once at the start of administration then once every 24 hours until the values have stabilised during the full nutritional infusion rate.
7. Bicarbonate or total CO_2 every 24 hours until stable.
8. Packed cell volume (PCV) and total solid (TS) concentration every 12–24 hours during nutritional therapy.
9. Urine glucose and urine ketones every 8–24 hours during nutritional therapy.
10. Nasogastric tube placement, before each feeding (if using assisted enteral feeding).
11. Intravenous catheter site, at least twice daily (if using parenteral nutrition).

discharge is expected with prolonged nasogastric tube placement, purulent nasal discharge, respiratory stridor, tachypnoea and coughing are abnormal and should be evaluated. Loose faeces and diarrhoea may develop during enteral diet treatment. Diarrhoea is not a reason to stop AEF unless the patient becomes dehydrated, develops colic or develops ileus in association with the enteral feeding. Whenever an equine patient develops diarrhoea during hospitalisation or during treatment with AEF, faecal samples should be evaluated for the presence of pathogenic bacteria. Diarrhoea may also be a sign that the horse cannot tolerate the fat content of the enteral diet. If this is the suspected cause of the diarrhoea, fat supplementation should be discontinued, and the enteral diet should be reformulated to a solution with a lower concentration of fat.

Horses treated with AEF should have daily measurements made of their packed cell volume (PCV), total solids (TS), blood glucose, serum electrolytes and ionised calcium and magnesium. A biochemical panel, including a serum TG measurement, should also be routinely evaluated. Horses that are malnourished before AEF is started are at greater risk of developing complications associated with rapid re-feeding and may require both intravenous and oral electrolyte supplementation.[10] Horses with chronic protein-calorie malnutrition may benefit from an even slower return to re-feeding.[10]

The total volume of water that is added to the diet and used as a flush should be measured and recorded daily. The maintenance fluid requirements (60 ml/kg body weight/day) of a horse can be met during AEF if the horse is fed at least 4 times daily. Complications from overhydration are unlikely. If they occur, the volume of water added to the enteral diet should be reduced. Monitoring guidelines are given in Box 5.14.

Complications associated with assisted enteral feeding

Complications from AEF are rare. Most complications can be avoided if the horse is slowly introduced to the liquid enteral diet and if the horse's condition is closely monitored during the period of diet supplementation. Horses treated with AEF may develop ileus, colic, diarrhoea, oesophageal trauma, laryngeal oedema, aspiration pneumonia or laminitis. Most of these complications are severe enough to warrant immediate cessation of the enteral diet. Horses that will not tolerate or that cannot be treated with AEF should be treated with PN. If complications from ileus or gastric reflux arise during administration of the enteral diet, the volume and frequency of feeding should be reduced until the horse is able to tolerate the feedings. Additional guidelines have been discussed in the diet administration section.

Diarrhoea is one of the most frequent complications of feeding a horse with a liquid enteral diet. If this complication arises in an equine patient, the clinician should assess the problem in a routine manner. Faeces should be submitted for routine bacterial analysis (*Salmonella* spp., *Clostridium difficile, Clostridium perfringens*) according to the hospital protocol. If the lipid concentration of the diet is too high, the enteral diet should be reformulated and administered to determine if the horse can tolerate the lower fat diet. Other strategies to resolve the diarrhoea include increasing the structural fibre in the diet, decreasing the volume infused at each feeding and increasing the frequency of the feedings. Addition of probiotic compounds that contain *Lactobacillus* spp, or *Saccharomyces boulardii*, to a liquid enteral diet may offer some benefit in reducing complications from diarrhoea.[48] Although the efficacy of most probiotic compounds have not been tested in horses, they are relatively safe and inexpensive and can be added to the therapy of enterally fed horses with mild diarrhoea.

In rare cases, horses can develop ulcers and perforations of the pharyngeal and/or oesophageal tissues.[49] If a horse develops bilateral nasal discharge, or signs of discomfort following nasogastric tube placement, an endoscopic examination of the pharynx and oesophagus should be performed to ensure that the mucosal tissues are intact. If oesophageal or pharyngeal ulcers or perforations are identified, the tube should be removed, and the patient should be treated with broad-spectrum antibiotics. Nutritional therapy with PN should be considered in these horses because feed (with the exception of fresh grass) should not be offered in large quantities until the ulcer or perforation has healed.

Gastric ulcers do not appear to be common complications in equine patients that are treated with liquid enteral diets for a short period (7–10 days) of time. If desired, prophylactic treatment with omeprazole (1.1–2.2 mg/kg every 24 hours) may be used in equine patients to aid in the prevention of gastric ulcers.

Return to voluntary feeding

During the time that a liquid enteral diet is administered, the horse should be offered small amounts of fresh feed to stimulate their appetite. If a horse is being treated with a complete feed, the pelleted form can be offered during the transition period back to voluntary feeding. A variety of forages including fresh grass, grass hay, oat hay and alfalfa leaves should also be offered. Supplemental feeds that have a high concentration of nonstructural carbohydrates should be avoided during the re-feeding period. The horse's voluntary total energy and protein intake should be measured and recorded using the Hospital Feeding Chart (Box 5.5). Once the horse is able to consume at least 75% of its DE_{Rest}, the horse can be weaned off from the enteral diet over a 2- to 3-day period of time.

Nutrition options: parenteral nutrition

Formulating a parenteral solution

Parenteral nutrition solutions can be formulated to meet either part or all of the horse's energy and protein requirements. If only a portion of the horse's energy and protein requirements are met with the formulation, the solution is called a *partial parenteral nutrition* (PPN) formulation. More commonly, the PN solution will meet the horse's resting energy and maintenance protein requirements. The term *total parenteral nutrition* (TPN) is not used in this chapter; instead the term is reserved for human formulations that are designed to meet all of the nutrient requirements of a human patient for months to years of administration. Equine PN formulations are rarely formulated to meet all of the nutrient requirements of the horse. In this chapter, the term *parenteral nutrition*, or *PN*, is used to describe a formulation that includes a total nutrient admixture of amino acids, dextrose and, in most cases, lipids in a volume sufficient to meet the horse's DE_{Rest} and maintenance protein requirements. Vitamin and mineral supplements are often added to the PN formulation.

Premixed commercial amino acid and dextrose admixtures provide a convenient option for PPN therapy in adult horses and can be purchased (Table 5.8). These formulations contain a range of amino acid (2.75%–5.0%) and dextrose (5%–25%) concentrations. Some solutions also contain electrolytes. The caloric density (0.17–0.85 kcal/ml) and osmolarity (525–1900 mOsm/L) of the formulations vary widely. Products with a high osmolarity are not suitable for infusion through a small-diameter peripheral vein (cephalic, lateral thoracic).

Total nutrient admixture parenteral formulations can be designed to meet the energy and protein requirements of a hospitalised horse. The solution is made from a mixture of amino acids, dextrose and usually lipid and can be supplemented with B vitamins, electrolytes and trace minerals. Guidelines for selecting the PN ingredients are presented in the following section. A PPN template is shown in Box 5.15. A total nutrient admixture PN formulation template and example is shown in Box 5.16 and Box 5.17, respectively. A nutritionist can be consulted in the formulation of a PN solution for a horse with a complex metabolic condition.

Parenteral solutions: ingredients

Protein

Protein is added to PPN and PN formulations to provide a source of essential and nonessential amino acids to the horse. Commercial amino acid solutions used in equine PN formulations usually contain 8.5% to 15% amino acids, have an energy density of 0.34 to 0.6 kcal/ml, have a pH range between 5.3 and 7.0 and have an osmolarity of 785 to 1160 mOsm/L (Table 5.9). Three percent amino acid solutions are also available. The PPN template (Box 5.15) assumes either a 10% or 15% amino acid solution is used. The total nutrient admixture PN formulation template and example (Boxes 5.16 and 5.17) assume a 10% amino acid solution is used. Adjustments to the protein, energy and osmolarity of the formulation should be made if a different amino acid concentration is used in the PN recipe. Some companies produce amino acid solutions with supplemental amino acids designed to treat human patients with renal or hepatic disease. At this time, the amino acid requirements of horses with renal and hepatic disease have not been defined, and these human formulations should be used with caution in adult horses. Commercially available dextrose–amino acid solutions or complete glucose–amino acid–lipid formulations are also available (Table 5.8).

Amino acid formulas are available both with and without supplemental electrolytes (sodium, potassium, magnesium, chloride, phosphate). Equine patients with severe electrolyte deficiencies should be treated with a solution that contains electrolytes. Recommendations for electrolyte and mineral supplementation are provided below.

Table 5.8. Parenteral Nutrition Commercial Mixtures

Macronutrient Additives	Manufacturer	Amino Acids (g/ml)	Soybean Oil (%)	Safflower Oil (%)	pH	Osmolarity (mOsmol/ml)	kcal/ml	mEq/ml
Clinimix 4.25/5	Baxter*	0.0425			6.0	0.675	0.170	
Clinimix 5.0/15	Baxter*	0.0510			6.0	1.255	0.510	
Clinimix E 4.25/5	Baxter*	0.100			6.5	0.998	0.400	
Sodium								0.035
Potassium								0.030
Magnesium								0.005
Calcium								0.0045
Chloride								0.039
Phosphate								0.015
Kabiven 14 N/2000 kcal (Central)	Fresenius-Kabi†	0.033	3.9		5.6	1.060	1.67	
Sodium								0.08
Potassium								0.06
Magnesium								0.02
Calcium								0.01
Chloride								0.116
Phosphate								0.05

*Baxter Healthcare Corporation, Deerfield, IL, USA.
†Fresenius-Kabi, Bad Homburg, Germany.

Box 5.15. Partial parenteral nutrition (PPN) worksheet

Patient Information

1. Initial body weight (kg) ______ kg
2. Stall resting energy requirement: DE_{Rest} (kcal/day) = 975 + 21 (BW in kg) ______ kcal
3. Maintenance energy requirement: DE_{Maint} (kcal/day) = 33.3 × (BW in kg) ______ kcal
4. Protein requirements: Crude protein (mg/day) = 1260 × (BW in kg) ______ mg
5. Fluid requirements for maintenance: 60 ml/kg/day ______ ml

Parenteral Nutrition Formulation

6. Total kcal to be provided by the PPN solution
   Estimate between 50% and 75% of the DE_{Rest} of the patient ______ kcal
7. Calculate the volume of 5% dextrose or glucose required to meet the energy requirements (from **6**)
   5% dextrose contains 170 kcal/L; 5% glucose contains 190 kcal/L
   kcal (from **6**) × 1 L/170 kcal ______ L
8. Compare the volume of 5% dextrose (from **7**) with the fluid requirement of the patient (from **5**)
   If **5** > **7**, there should not be a complication with overhydration. Additional 5% dextrose may be administered.
   If **7** > **5**, either elect to treat the patient with the increased volume of intravenous fluids
   OR
   Increase the dextrose concentration to provide sufficient calories
   OR
   Add lipid to the solution to increase the energy density of the solution
9. Calculate the volume of 10% amino acids required to meet protein requirement (from **4**)
   Protein (mg) divided by 100 mg/ml of 10% amino acid solution ______ ml
   OR
10. Calculate the volume of 15% amino acids required to meet protein requirement (from **4**)
    Protein (mg) divided by 150 mg/ml of 15% amino acid solution ______ ml
11. Calculate the kcal contained in calculated volume of 10% amino acid solution (from **9**)
    0.4 kcal/ml of 10% AA solution × ml of AA solution ______ kcal
    OR
12. Calculate the kcal contained in calculated volume of 15% amino acid solution (from **10**)
    0.6 kcal/ml of 15% AA solution × ml of AA solution ______ kcal

The energy contribution from protein is NOT included in the calculation for a PPN solution, because the resting energy requirement of the patient is not being met with the dextrose or glucose. This is calculated as a guideline. Some portion of the protein will be oxidised.
The amino acid solution can be added to a solution of 5% dextrose or glucose. The dextrose or glucose (50%) and amino acid solutions can be added to a partially drained bag of polyionic fluids. Sterile water can be added to a dextrose or glucose and amino acid admixture to decrease the osmolarity of the solution.
Calculate the osmolarity of the solution using the guidelines given for PN solutions. A solution of 5% dextrose has an osmolarity of 253 mOsm/L.

Box 5.16. Total nutrient admixture parenteral nutrition worksheet

Patient Information

1. Initial body weight (kg) _____ kg
2. Stall resting energy requirement: DE_{Rest} (kcal/day) = 975 + 21 (BW in kg) _____ kcal
3. Maintenance energy requirement: DE_{Maint} (kcal/day) = 33.3 × (BW in kg) _____ kcal
4. Protein requirements: Crude protein (mg/day) = 1260 × (BW in kg) _____ mg
5. Fluid requirements for maintenance: 60 ml/kg/day _____ ml

Parenteral Nutrition Formulation

6. Total kcal required/day (estimate between **2** and **3** calculated above; use **2** when initiating therapy) _____ kcal
7. Calculate volume of 10% amino acids required to meet protein requirement (from **4**)
   Protein (mg) divided by 100 mg/ml of 10% amino acid solution _____ ml
8. kcal contained in calculated volume of 10% amino acid solution (from **7**)
   0.4 kcal/ml of 10% AA solution × ml of AA solution _____ kcal
9. Total kcal required/day (from **6**) minus total kcal provided by AA (from **8**) _____ kcal

- *The caloric contribution from protein can be omitted from the following calculations, if desired*

10. Determine amount of lipid required to meet 20–70% of the remaining energy requirements
    20% Intralipid contains 2 kcal/ml
    If providing 50% of remaining energy requirements with 20% Intralipid:
    (kcal (from **9**) × 0.5) × 1 ml/2 kcal _____ ml
11. Calculate remaining energy requirements to be provided by 50% dextrose/glucose
    [kcal (from **9**) – kcal (from lipid)] × 1 ml/1.7 kcal (1.9 kcal for glucose) _____ ml
12. Add 1–2 ml of B vitamin complex/L PN solution _____ ml
13. Add up to 5 ml of trace minerals/day _____ ml
14. Determine the total volume of the PN solution (**7 – 10 – 11 – 12 – 13**) _____ ml
15. Determine the energy density of the PN solution [**6** (kcal)/**14** (ml)] _____ kcal/ml
16. Determine the rate of PN infusion for a 24-hour period: ml (from **14**)/24 _____ ml/hour
17. Calculate the calorie:nitrogen ratio for the PN solution
    kcal from protein, lipid and dextrose (from **6**)/(total g of protein)/6.25 _____
18. Calculate osmolarity of the solution

10% Amino acid	_____	ml (from **7**) × 0.998 mOsm/ml	= _____	mOsm
20% Lipid	_____	ml (from **10**) × 0.300 mOsm/ml	= _____	mOsm
50% dextrose	_____	ml (from **11**) × 2.550 mOsm/ml	= _____	mOsm
+_____	+_________			
Total ml	Total mOsm			

PN solution mOsm/L = Total mOsm/Total ml × 1000 ml/L _____ mOsm/L

Dextrose and glucose

Dextrose, a simple carbohydrate, has a nitrogen-sparing effect and provides a source of energy in PN solutions (3.4 kcal gross energy/g of dextrose; 1.7 kcal/ml for 50% dextrose; 1.9 kcal/ml for 50% glucose) (Table 5.9). Although 50% dextrose (U.S.) and 50% glucose (Europe and Australia) are the most common concentrations available at large animal hospitals, dextrose concentrations up to 70% can be purchased. The addition of dextrose/glucose in either PPN or PN solutions is limited by the horse's ability to metabolise the dextrose/glucose. The maximal rate of dextrose oxidation in humans is estimated to be approximately 25 kcal/kg/day.[17] A more complete discussion of dextrose therapy in the horse is provided in the section on nutrient requirements.

The calorie distribution between lipid and dextrose in a parenteral formulation depends on the metabolic profile of the hospitalised horse. A parenteral diet for a horse with a normal blood glucose concentration can include up to 60% of the nonprotein calories as dextrose or glucose. Horses suffering from glucose intolerance should be treated with a PN solution that contains less than 30% of the total non-protein calories from dextrose. These guidelines allow for a wide range of PN solution formulations to be developed for an individual horse.

Lipid

Lipid is the third macronutrient component in the PN formulation, but frequently this ingredient is omitted from equine PPN solutions. If the goal of a PN formulation is to attempt to match the horse's metabolic profile at the time of infusion, then a PN solution that contains lipid should be well utilised by the anorectic equine patient that is relying on endogenous lipid metabolism as their primary source of energy.

Box 5.17. Total parenteral nutrition worksheet example

Patient Information

1. Initial body weight (kg)	500 kg
2. Stall resting energy requirement: DE_{Rest} (kcal/day) = 975 + 21 (BW in kg)	11,475 kcal
3. Maintenance energy requirement: DE_{Maint} (kcal/day) = 33.3 × (BW in kg)	16,650 kcal
4. Protein requirements: Crude protein (mg/day) = 1260 × (BW in kg)	630,000 mg
5. Fluid requirements for maintenance: 60 ml/kg/day	30,000 ml

Parenteral Nutrition Formulation

6. Total kcal required/day (estimate between **2** and **3** calculated above; use **2** when initiating therapy)	12,000 kcal
7. Calculate volume of 10% amino acids required to meet protein requirement (from **4**) Protein (mg) divided by 100 mg/ml of 10% amino acid solution	6300 ml
8. kcal contained in calculated volume of 10% amino acid solution (from **7**) 0.4 kcal/ml of 10% AA solution × ml of AA solution	2520 kcal
9. Total kcal required/day (from **6**) minus total kcal provided by AA (from **8**)	9480 kcal

- *The caloric contribution from protein can be omitted from the following calculations, if desired*

10. Determine amount of lipid required to meet 20–70% of the remaining energy requirements 20% Intralipid contains 2 kcal/ml If providing 53% of remaining energy requirements with 20% Intralipid: [kcal (from **9**) × 0.53] × 1 ml/2 kcal	2500 ml
11. Calculate remaining energy requirements to be provided by 50% dextrose/glucose (kcal (from **9**) – kcal (from lipid)) × 1ml/1.7 kcal (1.9kcal for glucose) 2635 ml	
12. Add 1–2 ml of B vitamin complex/L PN solution	12 ml
13. Add up to 5 ml of trace minerals/day	2 ml
14. Determine the total volume of the PN solution (**7 – 10 – 11 – 12 – 13**)	11,449 ml
15. Determine the energy density of the PN solution [**6** (kcal)/**14** (ml)]	1.05 kcal/ml
16. Determine the rate of PN infusion for a 24-hour period: ml (from **14**)/24	477 ml/hour
17. Calculate the calorie:nitrogen ratio for the PN solution kcal from protein, lipid and dextrose (from **6**)/(total g of protein)/6.25	119

18. Calculate osmolarity of the solution

10% Amino acid	6300 ml (from **7**) × 0.998 mOsm/ml	= 6287 mOsm
20% Lipid	2500 ml (from **10**) × 0.300 mOsm/ml	= 750 mOsm
50% dextrose	2635 ml (from **11**) × 2.550 mOsm/ml	= 6719 mOsm
	+11,435 Total ml	+13,756 Total mOsm

PN solution mOsm/L = Total mOsm/Total ml × 1000 ml/L 1203 mOsm/L

Solutions of lipid in 10%, 20% or 30% concentrations are produced. These formulations are composed primarily of soybean oil, safflower oil or a combination of the two and include the essential fatty acid linoleic acid. Lipid is the most energy dense ingredient in the PN solution (1.1 kcal/ml for 10% Intralipid, 2 kcal/ml for 20% Intralipid) and is iso-osmolar (330 mOsm/L for 20% Intralipid) (Table 5.9). The pH of the lipid solution (pH 8.0 for 20% Intralipid) is also closer to a physiological pH than either the amino acid or dextrose solutions. Lipid is especially useful as an alternate energy source in horses that cannot tolerate a moderate concentration of dextrose in the PN solution.

Two arguments are frequently made against the addition of lipid to PN formulations. The first is that lipids increase the total cost of the PN formulation. Any time PN therapy is chosen, a financial commitment is made by the owner. The additional cost of adding lipid to the final solution will not be great enough to make the formulation cost prohibitive. The second argument against using lipid is that the lipid content of a PN solution is thought to predispose horses to develop hypertriglyceridaemia. Although horses with hepatic lipidosis should be treated with a lipid-free PN formulation, most horses will tolerate PN solutions that contain at least 40% to 50% of the energy from lipid.[37,38] The serum TG concentration of a hospitalised horse is often elevated before diet therapy is started. It is important to regularly monitor the horse's TG concentration during treatment with PN. Once an anorectic horse is treated with energy and protein with a PN solution, their serum TG concentration often decreases even when the PN formulation contains a moderate (30%–60%) concentra-

Table 5.9. Parenteral Nutrition Ingredients

Macronutrient Additives	Manufacturer	Amino Acids (g/ml)	Soybean Oil (%)	Safflower Oil (%)	pH	Osmolarity (mOsmol/ml)	kcal/ ml	mEq/ml
8.5% Travasol with electrolytes	Baxter*	0.085			6.0	1.144	0.313	
Sodium								0.07
Potassium								0.06
Magnesium								0.01
Chloride								0.07
Phosphate								0.06
8.5% Travasol without electrolytes	Baxter*	0.085			6.0	1.144	0.313	
Sodium								0.01
Phosphate								0.02
10% Travasol without electrolytes	Baxter*	0.100			6.5	0.998	0.400	
Chloride								0.04
8.5% FreAmine III without electrolytes	B. Braun†	0.085			6.5	0.810	0.313	
Sodium								0.01
Phosphate								0.02
10% FreAmine III without electrolytes	B. Braun†	0.100			6.5		0.400	
Sodium								0.01
Phosphate								0.02
Vamin 18 Electrolyte Free	Fresenius-Kabi‡	0.114			5.6		0.460	
Intrafusin 22	Fresenius-Kabi‡	0.152				1.400	0.600	
Intralipid 20%	Baxter		20		8	0.260	2.0	
Liposyn III 20%	Abbott§		10	10	8.3	0.258	2.0	
Dextrose, 50%						2.526	1.7	
Glucose 50%						2.780	1.9	

*Baxter Healthcare Corporation, Deerfield, IL, USA.
†B. Braun Medical Inc. Irvine, CA, USA.
‡Fresenius-Kabi, Bad Homburg, Germany.
§Abbott Laboratories, North Chicago, IL, USA.

tion of nonprotein calories from lipid. Once the hypertriglyceridaemia resolves, additional lipid can be added to the PN formulation of some horses. Frequent monitoring of serum TG enables the clinician to determine the appropriate time to either add or restrict dietary lipid.

A hospitalised horse with a serum TG concentration of less than 2.26 mmol/L (<200 mg/dl) can be treated with up to 40% of the nonprotein calories as lipid in a PN solution. If the serum TG concentration is between 2.26 and 5.65 mmol/L (200–500 mg/dl), lipid should be restricted to no more than 20% of the nonprotein calories in a parenteral solution. A hospitalised horse that has severe lipaemia with serum TG in excess of 5.65 mmol/L (500 mg/dl) or that has hepatic lipidosis either should be treated with a restricted lipid PN solution (<10% calories) or should be treated with a solution that does not contain lipid. A dextrose and amino acid PPN solution appears to be effective in resolving hepatic lipidosis as reported by Durham et al.,[31] who documented resolution of hyperlipaemia in three ponies and one donkey following treatment with a PPN formulation that contained 50% dextrose and 15% amino acids.

Minerals and vitamins

Electrolyte supplementation for a patient receiving PN can be managed in two different ways. The first is to provide electrolytes in the PN solution with an amino acid solution that contains electrolytes (Na, K, Mg, Cl, P) or through the addition of electrolytes directly to the PN solution (KCl, NaCl). The second method is to add the macrominerals (Na, K, Ca, Mg, Cl, P) to the horse's intravenous fluids. The benefit of intravenous fluid supplementation is that the horse's electrolyte therapy can be rapidly changed without wasting the costly PN formulation. A combination of these two supplementation plans can be chosen for patients that have severe electrolyte deficiencies and in patients affected by the re-feeding syndrome. Regardless of the form of mineral supplementation that is used, the equine patient should be closely monitored to ensure that they remain in a state of mineral balance. Monitoring guidelines are provided at the end of this section and in Box 5.14.

Most horses benefit from B-vitamin supplementation in PN to facilitate cellular metabolism during a period when intestinal production of B vitamins is likely reduced. Addition of 1 to 2 ml of B-complex vitamins/L of parenteral solution will provide supplementation without excessive therapy.[18] Supplementation of trace minerals and fat-soluble vitamins is recommended if the equine patient is in a state of severe malnutrition at the time of initiation of the PN therapy or if the PN therapy will be administered for longer than 3 days (Box 5.18). In small animals, the current recommendation is to add 1 ml of a parenteral trace mineral supplement for each 100 kcal of the solution.[29] Because the normal gastrointestinal regulation of trace mineral absorption is bypassed during parenteral infusion, toxicity could develop following excess supplementation.[50] In order to avoid oversupplementation of trace minerals, the daily volume of trace minerals should not exceed 5 ml for a horse that weighs greater than 400 kg. This concentration should be proportionately decreased for smaller horses.

Vitamins, especially lipid-soluble vitamins, vary in their stability when exposed to the plastic admixture bag, IV tubing, and light. Vitamin A, as retinol, and vitamin K are the most light-sensitive lipid-soluble vitamins. Riboflavin and pyridoxine are the most light-sensitive B vitamins. If these light-sensitive vitamins are added to a PN solution, the admixture bag and fluid tubing should be shielded from direct light. Fluorescent light does not appear to disrupt the vitamin structure. Thiamine is unstable when exposed to sulfite compounds that are included in amino acid solutions. If thiamine is added to a PN solution, it should only be added once the amino acid solution, dextrose and lipid have been mixed together. Because many B-vitamin preparations contain thiamine, the B-vitamin preparation should only be added once the macronutrient components of the PN have been mixed.

Osmolarity

If the PN solution is administered in the jugular vein, the final osmolarity of the solution should be less than 1200 mOsm/L. If a smaller-diameter vessel is used for administration, the osmolarity should be even lower, preferably between 600 and 900 mOsm/L. Strategies to lower the osmolarity of a solution include (1) using an amino acid solution without electrolytes, (2) adding or increasing the volume of polyionic fluid in the solution, (3) decreasing the volume of 50% dextrose, (4) using a lower concentration of dextrose or (5) by increasing the concentration of lipid in the formulation. If a polyionic solution is administered through the same port as a PN solution, the osmolarity of the solution reaching the vascular endothelium can be decreased. Use of a single-port catheter for PN infusion is not advised, due to potential complications that can develop from contamination of the PN solution or from the potential increased risk of septic thrombophlebitis. A complete discussion of catheters and PN infusion protocols is presented in the following section.

Calculation of the osmolarity of the solution can be made by calculating the contribution of each individual ingredient to the total osmolarity (Box 5.16).

Fluid requirements

Most PN solutions contain at least 50% free water that will be distributed throughout the intracellular and extracellular fluid space. The volume of fluid administered through the PN solution must be calculated into the patient's daily fluid requirements to ensure that the horse is not treated with an excessive volume of fluid.

Formulating the parenteral nutrition for the hospitalised horse

Specific nutrient requirements are provided in the previous requirements section. After the horse's requirements are calculated, Table 5.9 provides a list of different PN solution

Box 5.18. Examples of vitamin and mineral supplements suitable for parenteral nutrition

M.V.I. Adult (Multi-Vitamin Infusion) Mayne Pharma, Inc., Paramus, NJ, USA

Dose per 10 ml: Fat-soluble vitamins [A, 1 mg; E, 10 mg; D, 5 mcg; K 150 mcg]

Water-soluble vitamins [ascorbic acid (C), 200 mg; thiamine, 6 mg; riboflavin, 3.6 mg; niacinamide, 40 mg; pyridoxine, 6 mg; dexpanthenol, 15 mg; biotin, 60 mcg; Folic acid, 600 mcg; cyanocobalamin (B_{12}), 5 mcg]

Multitrace-5 Concentrate American Regent, Inc., Shirley, NY, USA

Dose per 1 ml: Zinc, 5 mg; copper, 1 mg; manganese, 0.5 mg; chromium, 10 mcg; selenium, 60 mcg

Vitamin B Complex Butler Animal Health Supply, Dublin, OH, USA

Cernevit, Baxter Healthcare, Thetford, Norfolk, UK

ingredients and can be used as a guide when formulating a solution.

Compounding the parenteral solution

Commercial compounding options

Commercial companies can be used to prepare PPN or PN formulations. The willingness of a company to provide compounding services to a veterinary hospital depends on the volume of the solution that is required and the frequency that the services are requested. It is best to make logistic arrangements with a compounding service before the solution is required so the PN formulation can be ordered and delivered without complication. Human hospitals and veterinary teaching hospitals may be able to provide compounding services if the veterinary clinic does not wish to purchase the PN components. The commercial compounding pharmacy Central Admixture Pharmacy Services (CAPS)‡ provides human and veterinary compounding services at 19 different locations throughout the United States, allowing for a particular formulation to be ordered and delivered directly to a veterinary hospital. Because some CAPS facilities only work with clinics on a volume basis, this company should be contacted to determine if their service would be available for equine PN formulations. Home PN compounding pharmacies located close to an equine hospital provide another option for PN formulation services.

In-house veterinary clinic compounding

Partial parenteral nutrition formulations

If compounding is done at the veterinary clinic, different methods can be used to either formulate a PPN or a total nutrient admixture PN solution. When a PPN solution is compounded, the formula can be mixed in a solution of polyionic fluids. Exact volume measurements are essential when compounding a solution. The first step is to drain the correct volume of fluid from the bag of polyionic fluids. Once the fluid has been drained, the dextrose, amino acids and lipids (if used) can then be added to the bag. The lipid solution should always be added last to decrease complications from lipid separation in the mixture. An alternate method of formulating a PPN solution is to add an amino acid solution to a bag of 5% dextrose. Sterile water can be added to admixture bags, carboys or sterile glass jars to dilute a PPN solution. Prior to any dilutions, the osmolarity of the final solution should be calculated to ensure that the solution can be administered without causing damage to the vascular endothelium (see guidelines for the optimal osmolarity of a solution earlier).

Total nutrient admixture parenteral nutrition formulations

Selecting a container for the solution

A large volume of fluid is used to formulate a total nutrient admixture for an adult horse, precluding the addition of the dextrose, amino acid and lipid solutions to any other fluids. A variety of PN admixture bags are available for purchase and are recommended for compounding. Because these bags are designed for one-time use, the sterility of the admixture bag is guaranteed. Admixture bags designed for human PN formulations are available that contain two compartments separated by a divider, which allows the dextrose and amino acid solutions to be added into one compartment, and the lipid component to be added into another compartment. Just prior to use, the separator is removed, and the admixture is combined. This type of mixing design is best for patients in which the PN admixture will be made but not immediately used because the product can be stored for at least a week at room temperature (25° C). These compartmentalised admixture bags are available in 1-, 2-, 3- and 4-L volume sizes and are produced by Baxter Healthcare (Deerfield, IL, USA) and by B. Braun Medical Inc. (Irvine, CA, USA). All-in-one admixture bags are also available and are ideal for compounding PN solutions that will be used within 48 hours after the PN solution has been prepared. All-in-one admixture bags§** are available in 2-, 3- and 4-L volume sizes. Sterile glass bottles provide another option for administration; however, the use of large glass vials in a clinic setting is not ideal unless the total solution volume is less than 4 L. Glass bottles are usually reserved for neonatal ICU patients. A sterile carboy can be used for the PN solution. Because carboys are reused, this type of container is the least desirable option and should only be used in an emergency.

Preparing the formulation

Parenteral solutions are relatively easy to compound, but the preparation must be performed in a sterile environment to reduce the risk of contamination. A laminar flow hood should be used, but if one is not available the solution can be mixed in a clean room with minimal traffic, such as a surgical instrument preparation area. Instructions for PN compounding are presented in Box 5.19.

Compounding should be done using a gravity flow method with a closed-circuit tubing apparatus. Many different PN bag products and containers are available and were discussed in the previous section. Once the admixture bag or container has been selected, all of the PN ingredients and equipment required for transferring the solutions should be organised. If only a portion of a solution will be used, the bottle or bag should be marked so the proper infusion volume can be easily determined. Any partially used macronutrient solution should be discarded if it cannot be mixed immediately into a new PN solution. In order to reduce wastage, two PN formulations can be made

‡CAPS: 1-800-853-6498; www.capspharmacy.com.

§Freka Mix + 6; Fresenius-Kabi AG, Bad Homburg, Germany

**Vitalmix, Churchill Medical Systems, Inc., Horsham, PA, USA.

Box 5.19. Instructions for compounding a parenteral nutrition solution

1. Compound the solution in a laminar flow hood, if available. Use a clean room in the hospital if a hood is not available.
2. Organize all ingredients that will be added to the formulation.
   a. If only part of a bottle or bag will be used, place a mark on the bottle or bag to signify the volume that should be infused.
3. Clean the preparation area well, using alcohol as a final preparation on the counter.
4. Wear a gown, mask and sterile gloves when compounding the PN solution.
5. Wipe off all injection sites and infusion ports with alcohol before connecting the infusion lines.
6. Use a new transfer set for each PN ingredient.
7. Add the dextrose and amino acid solution to the compounding bag or container.
8. Add the lipid solution ***AFTER*** the dextrose and amino acid solutions have been mixed together.
9. Gently swirl the solution to mix the ingredients.
10. Add any vitamin or mineral supplements to the solution ***AFTER*** the macronutrients (dextrose, amino acid, lipid) have been added.
    a. Ensure that there are no incompatibilities with the supplemental additives.
11. The PN formulation can be stored in the refrigerator for 24 hours, followed by 24 hours of storage at room temperature.

in one day. The formulation volume can also be adjusted to maximise the use of the complete volume of the lipid and amino acid solutions (available in 250- and 500-ml volumes).

It is easiest to set up a compounding system so each of the macronutrient solutions can be hung to facilitate gravity flow infusion into the admixture bag (Figure 5.3). All of the specialised PN admixture bags come with a set of transfer lines. One line is used for each PN component (amino acid, dextrose, lipid). If the PN is mixed into a fluid bag, sterile glass container or sterile carboy, separate IV infusion lines should be used for each PN component.

The individual who is preparing the PN solution should wear sterile gloves, gown and mask and should ensure that strict sterile technique is followed at all times during the PN preparation. Before any macronutrient solution is added to the admixture bag or compounding container, the top of the bottle or bag containing the macronutrient solution should be swabbed with alcohol. The dextrose or glucose can be added first, followed by the amino acid solution. Following the addition of each PN ingredient, the ingredient transfer line is clamped, disconnected and discarded. If an admixture set is used, then following the addition of all macronutrients, the end of the transfer line

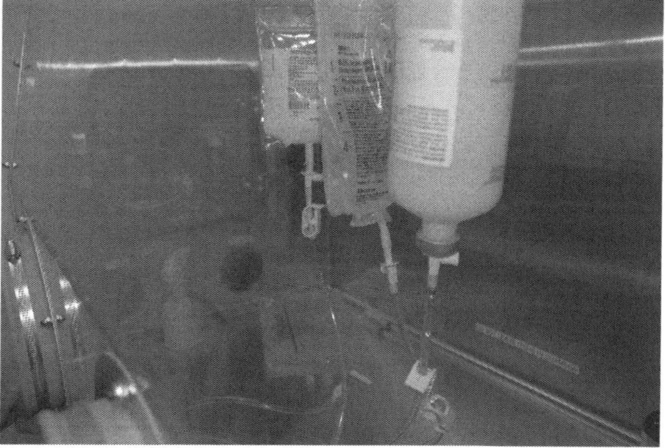

Figure 5.3 Preparation for parenteral nutrition compounding in a laminar flow hood. The dextrose, amino acid and lipid ingredients are connected to the admixture bag using separate transfer lines in a gravity-flow system. The lipid will be added to the mixture last. ©Meri Stratton-Phelps 2007.

that is attached to the admixture bag should be sealed with the sterile cap that is provided with the set. The admixture bag system enables simple, sterile mixing of each of the three PN ingredients. Transfer of solutions using sterile syringes is **not recommended** but can be performed if necessary.

The most important rule about compounding a PN solution is to ***add the lipids last***. If the lipids are added before the dextrose, then the low pH of the dextrose may disrupt the lipid solution, causing it to precipitate or separate in the solution. Slow gradual mixing of the lipid solution will also prevent separation. Any compounded PN solution that has separated should not be used.

Adding supplements to the PN mixture

Vitamin and mineral supplements should be added to a PN solution once all macronutrient ingredients have been mixed together. Multivitamin products (M.V.I. Adult, aai-Pharma, Wilmington, NC) can be added to PN admixtures to provide both lipid and water soluble vitamins. In some formulations only B vitamins are added to the solution. Minerals can be added to PN solutions, as long as drug incompatibilities do not exist (Box 5.20). Multivitamin and trace mineral products for parenteral solutions are designed for one-time use (Box 5.18). Clinicians should follow the dilution instructions that are included with each multivitamin and mineral product to ensure that concentrated solutions are not administered. If PN solutions are frequently used at an equine hospital, a bottle of B vitamins can be reserved for PN use only to help preserve the sterility of the bottle contents. Any opened bottle of B vitamins should be discarded from use in a parenteral formulation if it has been open for more than 30 days.

The top of all supplement bottles should be wiped with alcohol before the contents are withdrawn for use in a PN solution. The injection port on the PN admixture bag should also be wiped with alcohol prior to infusion of any supplemental ingredients. Vitamins and mineral supplements should be injected into the compounded PN solution using the injection port on the PN bag or should be added to a carboy or sterile glass container prior to infusion. Additives should never be added directly to the lipid component of the solution. Once any vitamin or mineral compound has been added to the PN formulation, the solution should be mixed gently.

Many drugs are incompatible with dextrose and amino acids and with total nutrient admixtures (Box 5.20). In order to prevent complications from administration of incompatible pharmaceutical agents, no additional substances should be added to the PN admixture except for the approved multivitamin, B-vitamin, and trace mineral supplements. Vitamin and trace mineral supplements may have their own unique drug interactions, and each product should be evaluated before it is used in a PN formulation.

Administration of the parenteral solution

Parenteral nutrition solutions, either with or without a lipid additive, should be stable when refrigerated at 2° to 8° C for 24 hours but should be used within 24 hours once the solution has been brought to room temperature (25° C). The increased osmolarity and decreased pH of amino acid and dextrose solutions may decrease bacterial growth in solutions that do not include lipid.

To ensure sterility, clinicians should attempt to change the PN solution and infusion lines every 24 hours. Adult horses often require 3 to 5 admixture bags a day, whereas most foal PN formulations can be compounded in one admixture bag. Each time a new bag is started, a new set of infusion lines should be used. Sterile technique should always be followed when working with PN formulations and infusion lines. In order to decrease bacterial contamination, sterile gloves should be worn when the infusion line is being assembled. The PN infusion line should never be broken. If the horse needs to be moved during the time of PN infusion, the PN should remain connected and should be moved with the horse.

Intravenous catheters

Parenteral formulations are almost always infused into a peripheral vein in adult horses. The jugular vein is the most common site for catheterization; however, vascular access can be established in other vessels including the lateral thoracic vein, cephalic vein and medial saphenous vein. The large diameter of the jugular vein allows for infusion of a PN solution that has an increased osmolarity (up to 1200 mOsm/L). Infusion of a PN solution into smaller-diameter vessels requires a formulation with a lower osmolarity (600–900 mOsm/L). Placement of jugular catheters in foals may result in a catheter that is a central line, instead of a peripheral catheter.

PN solutions serve as an excellent medium for bacterial growth, and there is a high risk of sepsis if sterility is not maintained during PN infusion. A separate catheter port should always be used for PN infusion. Blood should never be drawn from a port that will later be used for PN admin-

Box 5.20. Drugs incompatible with parenteral nutrition solutions[16,18]

Drugs that are incompatible with dextrose and amino acid mixtures

Acyclovir	Cyclosporine	**Mannitol**	**Penicillin G**
Amphotericin	Cytarabine	Methotrexate	**Phenytoin**
Ampicillin	Doxorubicin	**Metoclopramide**	**Potassium phosphate**
Cefazolin	Fluorouracil	Metronidazole (with NaHCO3)	**Midazolam**
Promethazine	Cephradine	**Furosemide**	
Sodium bicarbonate	Ciprofloxacin	Ganciclovir	Minocycline
Sodium phosphate	Cisplatin	**Immune globulin**	Mitoxantrone

Drugs that are incompatible with parenteral total nutrient admixture

Acyclovir	**Erythromycin**	Iron dextran	Nalbuphine
Amphotericin	Fluorouracil	Levorphanol	Ondansetron
Cyclosporine	Ganciclovir	Lorazepam	Pentobarbital
Dopamine	Haloperidol	**Magnesium sulfate**	**Phenobarbital**
Doxorubicin	**Heparin**	**Midazolam**	**Phenytoin**
Doxycycline	Hydrochloric Acid	Minocycline	**Potassium phosphate**
Droperidol	Hydromorphone	**Morphine**	**Sodium phosphate**

Drugs indicated in bold are those most commonly used in equine medicine.

istration. A multiple–site infusion port can be attached to a single-lumen catheter if multilumen catheters are not available. Use of this type of infusion arrangement for PN is not recommended due to the increased risk of sepsis and bacterial contamination. Although it is not ideal, this method of infusion may be the sole option for some practices. If a multiport catheter or multiple–infusion port attachment is not available, then a separate intravenous catheter can be placed in another vein for PN administration. Caution should be used if both jugular veins are catheterised in an equine patient due to the complications that can arise from thrombophlebitis.

Double- or triple-lumen, over-the-wire polyurethane catheters are the preferred catheter for PN administration (Figure 5.4). If the catheter site remains healthy, these over-the-wire catheters can be maintained for up to 30 to 60 days. Prior to placing a catheter, the site should be surgically prepared. The entire procedure of catheter insertion should be performed using sterile technique, including securing the catheter with sterile suture. If a double- or triple-lumen catheter is placed in a patient at the time of initial presentation and if PN treatment is an option in the future, a heparin lock should be placed in a port that is taped off and reserved for future PN use. The volume of heparin required for the heparin lock can be found on the catheter package.

When PN solutions are administered through a dedicated port of a multilumen catheter, few complications should occur due to incompatible drug interactions. ***Clinicians should check for potential drug interactions with PN solutions if they elect to use a y-port for PN administration.*** A list of drugs that are incompatible with PN solutions is provided in Box 5.20. Drugs commonly used in equine practice are identified in bold type. A pharmacist should be consulted if there is a question about drug compatibility. If there is a concern about possible drug incompatibility with the PN, the drug should not be administered during the PN infusion. Instead, the PN should be stopped temporarily and the catheter should be thoroughly flushed with saline before the drug therapy is administered. Use of a multiple-lumen catheter should reduce the risk of complications from drug incompatibilities.

Instructions for administration of the parenteral solution

Parenteral solutions are administered at a constant rate of infusion (Box 5.21). Although it is not absolutely required for PN administration, an infusion pump should be used to ensure an accurate delivery rate for the PN. When therapy is started, the PN solution should be infused at 25% to 30% of the total infusion rate. This rate should be maintained for the first 6 to 8 hours. If the horse tolerates the PN and does not develop hyperglycaemia or electrolyte abnormalities, then the rate can be gradually increased to 100% of the total infusion rate over the next 18 to 24 hours. The infusion rate increase may need to be slowed for horses

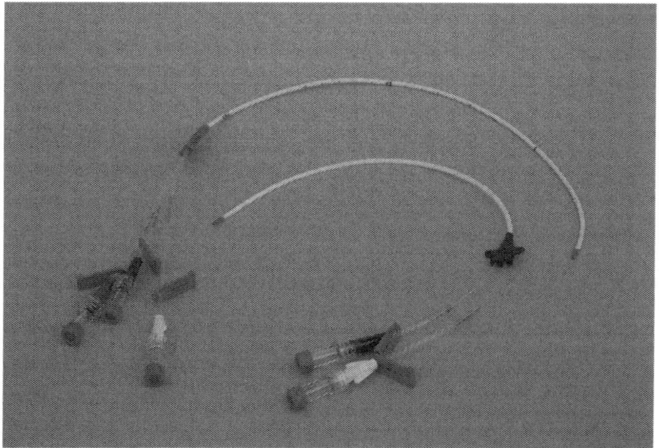

Figure 5.4 Double- and triple-lumen catheters recommended for use during treatment with parenteral nutrition. The white port can be reserved for parenteral nutrition infusion. ©Meri Stratton-Phelps 2007.

Box 5.21. Instructions for parenteral nutrition infusion

1. Begin infusion at 25%–30% of the DE rate that has been calculated for the patient.
2. Infuse the PN for 6–8 hours at the initial rate, then check the blood glucose concentration of the patient. If the glucose concentration is between 4.4 and 8.3 mmol/L (80–150 mg/dl), then the rate of infusion can be increased gradually by 2–4 ml/hr to 100% of the rate over the next 24–36 hours.
3. The patient's packed cell volume, plasma total solids concentration, blood glucose and serum electrolytes should be checked following the first 24 hours of PN infusion to ensure that the patient has not developed marked changes in these values. If fluid, glucose or electrolyte derangements have occurred as the PN is initiated, the clinician can modify the patient's fluid treatment plan to the abnormalities.
4. If the horse develops hyperglycaemia, glucosuria, or hypertriglyceridaemia (elevated from the horse's pretreatment concentrations), during the course of PN therapy, the rate of PN administration should be reduced by 25% for 4–6 hours before the blood glucose and serum triglyceride concentration is rechecked. Cessation of the PN infusion for 15 minutes prior to sampling the patient's serum may be indicated to allow the lipids from the PN solution to be cleared from the peripheral blood. If hyperglycaemia or hypertriglyceridaemia persist after the PN infusion rate has been decreased by 25%, the PN solution should be reformulated to reduce the concentration of dextrose or lipid. If the patient requires PN treatment, but develops persistent hyperglycaemia, and is not a candidate for a high lipid infusion, then insulin therapy can be used to regulate the concentration of blood glucose.

with hyperglycaemia or hypertriglyceridaemia. Once the maintenance rate of PN infusions is reached, the solution must be administered at a constant rate. This requires that the horse is hospitalised, confined to a stall and monitored closely throughout the treatment period. The PN line should never be disconnected, unless the PN bag is being changed.

Patient monitoring

A complete daily physical examination, including a measurement of body weight and BCS, should be performed on horses that are treated with PN. If the horse cannot be weighed, a weight tape can be used. The goal of PN is to prevent the horse from losing additional weight and lean tissue mass. It is unlikely that a hospitalised horse will gain weight or lean tissue mass during treatment with PN; however, some patients may show a modest gain in body weight of 5 to 10 kg. Maintenance of body weight and BCS should be viewed as a treatment success.

The temperature (T), pulse rate (P), respiratory rate (R) (TPR), hydration status and mucous membrane color of the horse should also be evaluated at least every 8 hours during PN therapy. Elevations in the horse's TPR values beyond the upper normal range are abnormal and require prompt evaluation to identify the etiology of the clinical abnormalities. The horse should be closely monitored for signs of peripheral oedema (including ventral or limb oedema) and pulmonary oedema. This is especially important if the horse has an increase in respiratory rate or effort or if the horse develops a soft cough and serous nasal discharge following initiation of the PN therapy. The faecal production of horses treated with PN is expected to drop. Any horse that develops diarrhoea requires a routine evaluation for pathogenic bacteria. Consumption of a forage-based diet is usually required before the gastrointestinal microbial population returns to the normal balance of bacteria. Horses treated with PN are not expected to develop laminitis. The catheter site of PN treated horses should be observed at least every 8 hours. Although the risk of thrombophlebitis is reduced when strict sterile techniques are followed during PN compounding and infusion, thrombophlebitis can still develop in rare cases. Management of this complication is described in Chapter 7.2.

Biochemical monitoring during PN therapy includes measuring the horse's PCV and TS at least every 12 hours, until the values have stabilised. During the first 2 to 3 days of therapy, serum electrolytes and blood glucose should be measured at least every 12 hours. Adjustments can be made to either the PN solution or to the intravenous fluids to manage the patient's electrolyte imbalances. Management of hyperglycaemia is discussed below. The horse's serum TG concentration should be measured every 24 hours until the TG concentration has stabilised below 1.13 mmol/L (100 mg/dl). Strategies to manage hypertriglyceridaemia in a horse treated with PN are described later. Specific guidelines for patient monitoring are listed in Box 5.14.

Fluid therapy during PN infusion

Horses treated with PN may require a reduction in the rate of infusion of their maintenance fluids to prevent overhydration. If the intravenous fluids are supplemented with dextrose or glucose prior to PN therapy, the dextrose or glucose supplementation should be discontinued gradually as the rate of PN infusion is increased.

Complications associated with PN therapy

If sterile compounding procedures are followed, and if the dextrose and lipid content of the PN formula is adjusted as the horse's metabolic condition changes, complications from PN therapy should be minimised. Management strategies for specific complications are discussed below.

Excess fluid administration

If the horse develops signs of fluid overload, such as pulmonary oedema, peripheral oedema or respiratory distress, the maintenance fluid therapy plan for the horse should be revised to a lower fluid administration rate. In rare cases, the volume or rate of administration of the PN infusion may need to be decreased to ensure the patient is not overhydrated.

Electrolyte deficiencies

Common electrolyte deficiencies in anorectic horses are described in the section on nutrient requirements. Electrolyte abnormalities and changes in the acid-base balance of the equine patient are best treated by adding an appropriate supplement to the horse's intravenous fluids. This enables the clinician to meet the changing electrolyte and acid-base profile of the patient without discarding an incorrectly supplemented PN solution. The contribution of electrolytes in the amino acid solution should be included in the electrolyte treatment plan. Horses with severe electrolyte deficiencies should have electrolyte supplements added to the PN solution. Electrolytes and their administration are described in Chapter 6.5. Potential drug interactions must be evaluated before supplements are added to the PN solution (Box 5.20).

Hyperglycaemia

Hyperglycaemia and glucosuria should be avoided during PN therapy. The first step to treat hyperglycaemia (blood glucose >10 mmol/L [>180 mg/dl]) is to decrease the rate of the PN infusion by half. The horse's blood glucose should be checked again in 8 to 12 hours. If the horse has persistent hyperglycaemia, the PN solution should be reformulated to reduce the volume of dextrose or glucose by 30% to 70%, depending on the original formulation. The calorie deficit in the PN solution can be replaced by lipid if the horse has a serum TG less than 2.26 mmol/L (<200 mg/dl) and if the horse can tolerate an increased concentration of lipid. If lipid supplementation is not an option, the PN can be administered as a PPN solution that contains less energy than the DE_{Rest}. The horse's protein requirements can still be met if the PPN solution is adjusted to have an osmolarity less than 1200 mOsm/L.

Horses that cannot tolerate a parenteral solution with a reduced concentration of dextrose/glucose should be treated with a constant rate infusion of regular insulin, titrated to effect from a starting rate of 0.01 IU (unit)/kg/hr. An alternative, which is less reliable to stabilise blood glucose concentrations, is intermittent treatment with protamine zinc insulin (0.1–0.3 IU/kg every 12 hours). The blood glucose concentration of horses treated with insulin must be monitored very closely to ensure that the horse does not become hypoglycaemic. Adjustments in the insulin dose or adjustments in the dextrose/glucose concentration in the PPN or PN should be made to maintain a normal blood glucose concentration.

Hypertriglyceridaemia

Hypertriglyceridaemia should be assessed in relation to the patient's concentration of serum TG before the PN therapy is initiated. The trend in TG concentration is as important as the actual serum concentration. It is not uncommon for anorectic horses to have an elevated serum TG at the start of PN therapy. If the diet therapy is effective, the TG should begin to decrease within 24 hours after initiating treatment. If the concentration of TG in the horse's serum remains elevated (>2.26 mmol/L [>200 mg/dl]) or if it increases after 48 hours of therapy, the PN should be reformulated by reducing the lipid concentration by 50%. Heparin therapy (40 IU/kg every 12 hours) may be beneficial in improving the clearance of serum TG and can be used in horses with persistent hypertriglyceridaemia.

Prior to reformulating the PN solution, the horse's serum TG concentration should be confirmed. Because the concentration of lipids infused in the PN solution can increase the serum TG concentration, the PN infusion should be stopped for 15 to 20 minutes before the blood sample is obtained to allow the liver and peripheral tissues to clear the infused TG. This blood sampling protocol provides a more accurate assessment horse's ability to mobilise fatty acids.

Infections

During treatment with PN, the catheter site must be closely monitored for any signs of infection including swelling, erythema, discharge or pain. If any of these signs are noted and the patient still requires treatment with PN, an alternate infusion site must be chosen. The old PN solution should be discarded, but a culture of the old solution can be taken to determine if the PN solution was contaminated. When changing between the old and new PN bags, the PN should not be discontinued for more than 30 minutes if the horse is receiving the full rate of infusion.

Management of the original catheter site involves removing the catheter in a sterile manner and submitting the tip of the catheter for aerobic and anaerobic bacterial culture and antibiotic sensitivity testing. Treatment of thrombophlebitis is described in Chapter 7.2.

Return to voluntary feeding

Enteral feeding should begin as soon as the horse can tolerate oral nutrition. During the re-feeding period, the horse can be fed cafeteria-style, or it can be treated with a liquid enteral diet to facilitate a return to voluntary food consumption. Once a horse is able to voluntarily consume 75% of their DE_{Rest} or once the horse can tolerate infusion of enough of a liquid enteral diet to meet 75% of their DE_{Rest}, the PN therapy can be discontinued. The rate of PN infusion should be decreased as gradually as it was increased, and the PN can be completely discontinued once the horse is receiving 25% to 30% of the total daily infusion volume. If the infusion is stopped too rapidly, the horse could develop complications from hypoglycaemia. During the transition period, the clinical and biochemical status of the horse should be monitored following the guidelines presented in Box 5.14 to ensure that the horse is transitioned to oral feeding without complications.

References

1. Carroll CL, Huntington PJ: Body condition scoring and weight estimation of horses. Equine Vet J 20:41-45, 1988
2. Reavell DG: Measuring and estimating the weight of horses with tapes, formulae and by visual assessment. Equine Vet Educ December:188-193, 1999
3. Kentucky Equine Research, Inc.: Feeding the miniature horse. Available at http://www.ker.com/library/EQUINEWS/index.html?try = Cookie.
4. Henneke DR, Potter GD, Kreider JL, et al.: Relationship between condition score, physical measurements and body fat percentage in mares. Equine Vet J 15:371-372, 1983
5. Brodsky IG: Hormone, cytokine, and nutrient interactions, in Shils ME, Olson JA, Shike M, Ross AC (eds): Modern Nutrition in Health and Disease, ed 9. Philadelphia, Lippincott Williams and Wilkins, 1999, pp 699-724
6. McNurlan MA, Garlick PJ: Protein synthesis and degradation, in Stipanuk MH (ed): Biochemical and Physiologic Aspects of Human Nutrition. Philadelphia, W.B. Saunders, 2000, pp 211-232
7. Frank N, Sojka JE, Latour MA: Effect of withholding feed on concentration and composition of plasma very low density lipoprotein and serum nonesterified fatty acids in horses. Am J Vet Res 63:1018-1021, 2002
8. Dunkel B, McKenzie HC 3rd: Severe hypertriglyceridaemia in clinically ill horses: diagnosis, treatment and outcome. Equine Vet J 6:590-595, 2003
9. Naylor JM, Kronfeld DS, Acland H: Hyperlipemia in horses: effects of undernutrition and disease. Am J Vet Res 41:899-905, 1980
10. Witham CL, Stull CL: Metabolic responses of chronically starved horses to refeeding with three isoenergetic diets. J Am Vet Med Assoc 212:691-696, 1998
11. Carlson GP: Fluid, electrolyte, and acid-base balance, in Kaneko JJ, Harvey JW, Bruss ML (eds): Clinical Biochemistry

of Domestic Animals, ed 5. San Diego, Academic Press, 1997, pp 485-516
12. Lewis LD: Minerals for horses, in Equine Clinical Nutrition: Feeding and Care. Baltimore, Williams and Wilkins, 1995, pp 25-60
13. Garcia-Lopez JM, Provost PJ, Rush JE, et al.: Prevalence and prognostic importance of hypomagnesemia and hypocalcemia in horses that have colic surgery. Am J Vet Res 62:7-11, 2001
14. Toribio RE, Kohn CW, Chew DJ, et al.: Comparison of serum parathyroid hormone and ionised calcium and magnesium concentrations and fractional urinary clearance of calcium and phosphorus in healthy horses and horses with enterocolitis. Am J Vet Res 62:938-947, 2001
15. Lewis LD: Vitamins for horses, in Equine Clinical Nutrition: Feeding and Care. Baltimore, Williams and Wilkins, 1995, pp 61-89
16. Mirtallo JM: Parenteral formulas, in Rombeau JL, Rolandelli RH (eds): Clinical Nutrition: Parenteral Nutrition, ed 3. Philadelphia, W.B. Saunders, 2001, pp 118-139
17. Naylor JM, Freeman DE, Kronfeld DS: Alimentation of hypophagic horses. Comp Cont Educ Pract Vet 6:S93-S99, 1984
18. Shils ME, Brown RO: Parenteral nutrition, in Shils ME, Olson JA, Shike M, Ross AC (eds): Modern Nutrition in Health and Disease, ed 9. Philadelphia, Lippincott Williams and Wilkins, 1999, pp 1657-1688
19. Nutrient Requirements of Horses, ed 5. Washington, DC, National Academy Press, 1989, pp 2-48
20. Souba WW, Wilmore D: Diet and nutrition in the care of the patient with surgery, trauma and sepsis, in Shils ME, Olson JA, Shike M, Ross AC (eds): Modern Nutrition in Health and Disease, ed 9. Philadelphia, Lippincott Williams and Wilkins, 1999, pp 1589-1618
21. Nutrient Requirements of Horses, ed 6. Washington, DC, The National Academies Press, 2007, pp 3-127, 294-303
22. Heyland DK: Immunonutrition, in Rolandelli RH, Bankhead R, Boullata JI, Compher CW (eds): Clinical Nutrition: Enteral and Tube Feeding, ed 4. Philadelphia, Elsevier, 2005, pp 224-242
23. Sacks G: Glutamine supplementation in catabolic patients. Ann Pharmacother 33:348-354, 1999
24. Harris RC, Harris PA, Routledge NB, et al.: Plasma glutamine concentrations in the horse following feeding and oral glutamine supplementation. Equine Vet J Suppl:637-642, 2006
25. Fan ST, Poon RTP: Liver disease and parenteral nutrition, in Rombeau JL, Rolandelli RH (eds): Clinical Nutrition: Parenteral Nutrition, ed 3. Philadelphia, W.B. Saunders, 2001, pp 392-406
26. Charney P, Russell M: Enteral formulations, in Rolandelli RH, Bankhead R, Boullata JI, Compher CW (eds): Clinical Nutrition: Enteral and Tube Feeding, ed 4. Philadelphia, Elsevier, 2005, pp 216-223
27. Gulick BA, Knight HD, Rogers QR: Use of plasma amino acid patterns in liver disease of the horse. California Vet July:21-23, 1979
28. Lorenzo-Figueras M, Preston T, Ott EA, et al.: Meal-induced gastric relaxation and emptying in horses after ingestion of high-fat versus high-carbohydrate diets. Am J Vet Res 66:897-906, 2005
29. Remillard Rl, Armstrong PJ, Davenport DJ: Assisted feeding in hospitalised patients: Enteral and parenteral nutrition, in Hand MS, Thatcher CD, Remillard RJ, Roudebush P (eds): Small Animal Clinical Nutrition, ed 4. Marceline, Walsworth Publishing Co., 2000, pp 351-399
30. Hallebeek JM, Beynen AC: A preliminary report on a fat-free diet formula for nasogastric enteral administration as treatment for hyperlipaemia in ponies. Vet Q 23:201-205, 2001
31. Durham AE: Clinical application of parenteral nutrition in the treatment of five ponies and one donkey with hyperlipaemia. Vet Rec 158:159-164, 2006
32. Hallebeek JM, Beynen AC: Effect of dietary medium chain triacylglycerols on plasma triacylglycerol levels in horses. Arch Tierernahr 54:159-71, 2001
33. Magnotti LJ, Deitch EA: Mechanisms and significance of gut barrier function and failure, in Rolandelli RH, Bankhead R, Boullata JI, Compher CW (eds): Clinical Nutrition: Enteral and Tube Feeding, ed 4. Philadelphia, Elsevier, 2005, pp 23-31
34. Sweeney RW, Hansen TO: Use of a liquid diet as the sole source of nutrition in six dysphagic horses and as a dietary supplement in seven hypophagic horses. J Am Vet Met Assoc 197:1030-1032, 1990
35. Buechner-Maxwell VA, Elvinger F, Thatcher CD, et al.: Physiological response of normal adult horses to a low-residue liquid diet. J Equine Vet Sci 23:310-317, 2003
36. Golenz MR, Knight DA, Yvorchuk-St. Jean KE: Use of a human enteral feeding preparation for treatment of hyperlipemia and nutritional support during healing of an esophageal laceration in a miniature horse. J Am Vet Met Assoc 200:951-953, 1992
37. Hansen TO, White NA II, Kemp DT: Total parenteral nutrition in four healthy adult horses. Am J Vet Res 49:122-124, 1988
38. Lopes MAF, White NA II: Parenteral nutrition for horses with gastrointestinal disease: a retrospective study of 79 cases. Equine Vet J 34:250-257, 2002
39. Durham AE, Phillips TJ, Walmsley JP, et al.: Nutritional and clinicopathological effects of post operative parenteral nutrition following small intestinal resection and anastomosis in the mature horse. Equine Vet J 36:390-396, 2004
40. Durham AE, Phillips TJ, Walmsley JP, et al.: Study of the clinical effects of postoperative parenteral nutrition in 15 horses. Vet Rec 153:493-498, 2003
41. Stick JA, Derksen FJ, Scott EA: Equine cervical esophagostomy: complications associated with duration and location of feeding tubes. Am J Vet Res 42:727-732, 1981
42. Lammers TW, Roussel AJ, Boothe DM, et al.: Effect of an indwelling nasogastric tube on gastric emptying rates of liquids in horses. Am J Vet Res 66:642-645, 2005
43. Cruz AM, Li R, Kenney DG, et al.: Effects of indwelling nasogastric intubation on gastric emptying of a liquid marker in horses. Am J Vet Res 67:1100-4, 2006
44. Stick JA: Esophagus, in Auer JA, Stick JA (eds): Equine Surgery, ed 3. St Louis, Saunders Elsevier, 2006, pp 351-373
45. Stick JA, Derksen FJ, Scott EA: Equine cervical esophagostomy: complications associated with duration and location of feeding tubes. Am J Vet Res 42:727-732, 1981

46. Stick JA, Slocombe RF, Derksen FJ, et al.: Esophagostomy in the pony: comparison of surgical techniques and form of feed. Am J Vet Res 44:2123-2132, 1983
47. Freeman DE, Naylor JM, Cervical esophagostomy to permit extraoral feeding of the horse. J Am Vet Med Assoc 172:314-320, 1978
48. Desrochers AM, Dolente BA, Roy MF, et al.: Efficacy of *Saccharomyces boulardii* for treatment of horses with acute enterocolitis. J Am Vet Med Assoc 227:954-959, 2005
49. Hardy J, Stewart RH, Beard WL, et al.: Complications of nasogastric intubation in horses: nine cases (1987-1989). J Am Vet Med Assoc 201:483-486, 1992
50. Gabrielson K, Remillard RL, Huso DL: Zinc toxicity with pancreatic necrosis in parenterally fed piglets. Vet Pathol 33:692-696, 1996

5.2 Nutritional management of the hospitalised foal

This section focuses on nutrition therapy for neonatal foals and foals through weaning age. The nutrient requirements of weaned foals are listed in the previous section on adult equine nutrition. The principles of patient assessment and the goals of providing nutrients with enteral nutrition or parenteral nutrition (PN) are the same for foals as for adult horses. In contrast to adult horses, critically ill foals are often in ***immediate*** need of nutritional support due to their high metabolic requirements and their minimal endogenous stores of energy and protein. Because the nutrient requirements of premature foals, septic neonates and clinically ill nursing foals have not been determined, the energy and protein requirements reported here are based on the estimated daily intake of healthy growing foals. This information is a guideline for the therapeutic management of the neonatal patient. Because the nutrient requirements of individual foals vary with their clinical disease and stage of growth, adjustments should be made in the suggested formulations to properly manage each hospitalised foal.

Patient evaluation and initiation of therapy

The newborn foal, whether term, premature or dysmature, is at a high risk of developing protein-calorie malnutrition within the first few days of life if unable to nurse. Neonatal glycogen stores are depleted within 2 hours of birth, and newborn foals have minimal endogenous stores of lipid to use as an energy substrate. Even more energy is required if the foal develops septicaemia or a specific organ disease (respiratory, renal or hepatic disease, gastrointestinal inflammation). In order to meet these energy requirements, early intervention with supplemental nutrition is especially important in the clinically ill equine neonate. Foals older than 7 days may be able to tolerate anorexia for longer than a neonatal foal, but these foals will also fade quickly without adequate nutrition.

The nutritional history of the neonatal foal provides important information about the duration of time before the foal first nursed, the likelihood that colostrum was consumed during the 6- to 8-hour window of maximal antibody absorption in the gastrointestinal tract and how the foal received the colostrum. The late gestation history of the mare should also be discussed with the owner. If the mare leaked colostrum during her pregnancy or if the foal did not consume enough high-quality colostrum within 8 hours of birth, the foal is at great risk of sepsis and will require treatment with intravenous hyperimmune plasma. In some cases, owners will tube feed or syringe feed their foals before a veterinarian examines the foal. Any foal with a history of syringe feeding is at risk of aspiration pneumonia and requires a thorough examination of the respiratory tract. Neonatal foals require a constant supply of milk to maintain their blood glucose. Foals that have not nursed in 12 to 24 hours are deprived both of colostrum and energy and should be managed with dextrose- or glucose-supplemented fluids or enteral nutrition within the first 3 hours after presentation. These foals will also require much more immediate fluid therapy (see Chapter 6.5). Foals that are at least 2 days of age often have had a seemingly normal birth and have nursed adequately. The clinical effects of sepsis can be insidious in onset, and a foal that was bright and alert one day could be obtunded and unwilling or unable to nurse within 12 to 24 hours. Often these foals are evaluated following a period of anorexia and already are affected by protein-calorie malnutrition. The bottom line in the nutritional management of foals is to begin dietary supplementation once the foal has been stabilised.

After reviewing the foal's nutritional history with the owner, the energy intake of the foal should be estimated. In some cases, the foal has not been nursing, protein-calorie malnutrition is apparent, and the need for supplemental nutrition is obvious. The assessment of a nursing foal's nutrient intake and need for dietary therapy can be challenging. Following hospitalisation, one of the easiest measurements of adequate nutrition is to measure the sequential body weight of the foal. This should be done on a scale, because body weight tapes have not been validated for neonatal or young foals. Healthy foals are expected to gain an average of 1.4 to 1.6 kg per day during the first 1 to 2 weeks of life (Table 5.10).

Although the body condition scoring (BCS) system has not been validated for foals, it can be adapted to the equine neonate to monitor the foal for a loss or gain of muscle mass. A rapid loss in a foal's BCS is seen during periods of illness and anorexia. A poor BCS is an overt sign of protein-calorie malnutrition and indicates the need to provide additional nutrients to the foal. Supplemental nutrition should be considered for nursing foals that either fail to gain weight or that lose weight during hospitalisation.

The goal of nutritional management of the neonatal foal is similar to that of the adult horse. Stabilisation of the patient requires supplemental nutrition to meet the resting

Table 5.10. Average Daily Weight Gain for Healthy Foals*

Age	kg/day	lb/day
0–1 month	1.5	3.4
1–2 months	1.35	3.0
2–3 months	1.2	2.6
3–4 months	1.05	2.3
4–5 months	0.9	2.0
5–6 months	0.8	1.8

*Weight gain values estimated for Arabian, Quarter Horse, and Thoroughbred breeds. From Growing horse feeding and care, in Lewis L (ed): Equine Clinical Nutrition, pp 334–349.

energy requirements (RER) of the foal. When the foal is only fed to meet the estimated RER, it will not receive sufficient nutrients to grow, and may not be adequately supplemented to mount an effective immune response or to optimise tissue regeneration. Provision of excess calories to a foal that cannot metabolise the nutrients should be avoided because it can lead to a hypermetabolic state where the foal becomes resistant to insulin and develops persistent hyperglycaemia. Following resolution of the systemic disease, additional dietary calories can be provided to ensure that the foal can meet all of their nutrient requirements, including that for growth.

Glucose- or dextrose-supplemented fluid is often the first type of nutrition support that a foal receives upon admission to a hospital. Anorectic neonates or foals suffering from perinatal asphyxia syndrome often present before they have consumed colostrum or milk. Without this vital caloric intake, these neonates are unable to maintain their blood glucose in a normal range. In some cases, compromised foals will readily respond to the bolus of supplemented fluids and will begin to nurse normally. In most cases, however, critically ill foals are unable to nurse and require immediate treatment with supplemental nutrition.

Foals that require supplemental nutrition can be classified into three different categories: (1) the healthy neonate that cannot ingest enough milk due to reasons associated with the dam (death, illness, inadequate milk production or foal rejection), (2) the anorecic sick neonate or older foal that has a weak to normal suckle reflex but cannot voluntarily or safely consume enough calories to meet its requirements and (3) the critically ill foal that is unable to nurse or to tolerate enteral nutrition due to respiratory, gastrointestinal or neurological complications. In all cases, the clinician must ensure that the foal has absorbed enough colostral antibodies to achieve a serum IgG concentration above 8 g/L (800 mg/dl). Severe sepsis in the equine neonate may necessitate supplemental treatment with hyperimmune plasma. Nutritional therapy is always used in conjunction with appropriate medical management.

Nutrient requirements

Energy

The energy requirements of the neonatal foal have not been studied in great detail. Although the composition of mare's milk changes throughout lactation, the energy and protein content of mare's milk at the start of lactation can be used as a guideline to determine the nutrient requirements of the neonatal foal. A healthy neonatal foal will consume approximately 25% of its body weight in milk daily (12.5 L/day for a 50-kg foal) during the first week of life. Mare's milk has an energy density of approximately 480 kcal/L as fed (AF), which equates to a daily consumption of approximately 6000 kcal/day and an estimated energy requirement of 120 kcal/kg body weight (BW) per day during the first week of life.[1] This energy intake is far greater than the mean RER of 44.36 kcal/kg BW measured using indirect calorimetry in nine foals (three healthy, six clinically ill).[2] Using this RER value, a 50-kg foal would require 2218 kcal/day to maintain its body weight in a thermoneutral environment, following the absorption of a meal.

The large discrepancy in energy values complicates the design of a nutrition plan for the hospitalised neonatal foal. Most hospitalised foals will be housed in a temperature-controlled setting, eliminating environmental factors from the energy requirement. Many hospitalised neonates are recumbent and do not require supplemental energy because they are physically inactive. The energy requirements for foals that are agitated due to colic or neurological complications such as seizures are not known. In order to avoid complications from oversupplementation and hypermetabolism, a conservative approach to the diet should be used by targeting the initial therapy at 45 to 50 kcal/kg/day. This amount of energy will be consumed when the foal is fed to meet approximately 10% of their body weight in mare's milk or a high-quality equine milk replacer. Both enteral and parenteral therapy should be designed to meet this range of energy intake. Because minimal research has documented the energy requirements of a critically ill equine neonate, it is prudent to begin nutritional supplementation to meet the foal's RER. If the foal tolerates the diet, then, as the disease process resolves, the caloric density of the supplement should be gradually increased to match the intake of a healthy age-matched foal.

Protein

At the start of lactation, mare's milk contains approximately 2.7% protein (AF) (27 g protein/L).[1] A healthy 50-kg foal that consumes 12.5 L of milk will consume 338 g of protein/day, or 6.8 g/kg BW. This value is over 2 times greater than the concentration of protein (2–3 g/kg BW/day) that has been traditionally recommended for the supplemental diet of neonatal foals. These lower protein requirements are extrapolated from human infant requirements and may not be appropriate for neonatal foals. Although the actual protein requirement of the clinically ill equine neonate is not known, the nutritional plan should be effective in preventing protein malnutrition. When nutritional therapy is initiated, the foal should be treated at a rate between 2 and 5 g protein/kg BW/day. Hypoproteinaemic foals and foals that have a continual loss of protein may require supplemental dietary protein. If a foal tolerates the initial rate of protein infusion, the protein concentration can gradually be increased towards 6.5 g protein/kg BW/day. Excess protein is contraindicated in foals with renal disease and severe hepatic disease, and these foals should be started on a diet formulation that contains 2 to 3 g protein/kg BW/day.

Lipid

Mare's milk contains a lower concentration of fat (1.8% [AF]) compared to cow's milk (3.5% [AF]) in the first 4 weeks of lactation.[1] References for neonatal nutrition recipes recommend treatment of foals with 1 to 3 g lipid/kg BW/day, which equates to 50 to 150 g lipid/day for a 50-kg foal.[3] If a healthy 50-kg foal consumes 12.5 L of mare's milk, it would ingest 4.5 g lipid/kg BW/day. Most commercial foal milk replacers contain a similar concentration of fat as mare's milk. When enteral therapy is started, the daily volume is usually low enough that foals do not experience complications with the high fat content. Foals treated with PN should be started on a formulation with a concentration between 1 and 2 g fat/kg BW. Many foals will adapt to the parenteral solution and can tolerate a higher fat concentration in subsequent formulations. Fat provides a concentrated source of calories in a low volume of solution. The concentration of fat in a parenteral solution should be limited to 60% of the total calories to prevent complications from hypertriglyceridaemia.

Minerals and vitamins

The mineral and vitamin requirements of neonatal foals are not known, but they can be estimated using the nutrient profile of mare's milk. Hospitalised neonates and nursing foals that are fed using mare's milk or a commercial foal milk replacer should receive a proper balance of minerals and vitamins once the milk consumption rate is between 20% and 25% of the foal's body weight. Parenteral diets can be supplemented with 1 ml of B vitamins per litre and a total of 1 ml of trace minerals every day. Care must be taken to not oversupplement the parenteral fluid with vitamins or trace minerals. Foals with mineral or vitamin deficiencies or foals that have electrolyte imbalances may require supplemental nutrients in their enteral diet and in their maintenance fluids or, in some cases, injectable vitamins and minerals (vitamin E and selenium) may be necessary.

Selecting the form of supplemental nutrition

Enteral versus parenteral therapy

The choice between enteral nutrition or PN depends on the competency of the foal's gastrointestinal tract and respiratory tract and on the foal's neurological condition. Most foals will tolerate treatment with part to all of their daily energy requirements administered as an enteral diet. The small population of hospitalised alert foals that have a strong suckle response can either nurse from the mare or, if the foal is an orphan, be taught to drink from a bucket. Most hospitalised foals are treated with an enteral diet infused through a nasogastric tube. In general, enteral nutrition is the preferred method of nutritional therapy because nutrients are supplied directly to the enterocytes resulting in improved mucosal barrier function and improved local immune function in comparison to PN. The suckle response should be assessed in all neonatal patients before a feeding plan is developed. Foals with a poor suckle response should not be permitted to nurse and should be treated with supplemental nutrition until their suckle response is strong and fully developed. Enteral nutrition is appropriate for all foals that have a healthy gastrointestinal tract.

Foals suffering from gastrointestinal disease (diarrhoea, ileus, enterocolitis, meconium impaction, gastric ulcers) may show a worsening of their clinical disease or may become colicky if they are fed milk or milk replacer at a volume equal to 10% body weight (100 ml/kg/day). These neonatal patients may tolerate a decreased volume of milk; however, in some foals it is preferable to deliver all nutrition via the parenteral route, despite apparent tolerance of the enteral diet. This includes severely affected (recumbent) foals with septicaemia and perinatal asphyxia syndrome. Experience suggests that the hypoxic–ischaemic damage to the gastrointestinal tract in these foals precludes effective uptake of enteral nutrition. Furthermore, it appears that gastrointestinal pathology can be prolonged by early enteral nutrition, resulting in persistent diarrhoea. In foals that present with severe colitis, complete enteral rest for 6 to 72 hours can result in rapid resolution of symptoms. Nutritional support in these foals in supplied by PN (initially intravenous glucose or dextrose). We have found hospital bills to be lower when using early PN in these classes of foals, because of the quicker resolution of disease and earlier hospital discharge.

Obtunded foals, foals that are ventilated and foals showing seizure activity should receive the majority of their nutrients from PN in order to decrease the risk of milk aspiration during enteral feeding. PN can, and in most cases should, be administered in conjunction with enteral nutrition to improve enterocyte integrity and to facilitate the foal's transition to voluntary enteral feeding. Many foals that will not tolerate partial enteral nutrition (>5% of body weight) will tolerate a small volume of mare's milk or milk replacer (10–30 ml) infused into the stomach every 2 to 3 hours once any residual gastric fluid has been removed.

Nutrition options: enteral nutrition

The enteral nutrition options for equine neonates and young foals include mare's milk, commercial equine milk

Table 5.11. Nutrient content of milk and selected milk replacers

	Mare's Milk First Month of Lactation	Goat's Milk	Cow's Milk 2% Fat	Mare's Match*	Foal Lac†	Mare's Milk Plus‡
Total solids (dry matter) (%)	10.7	12.97	10.79			
Crude protein (%)	25	27	31	24	21	21
Crude fat (%)	17	32	18	16	15	14
Crude fibre (%)	0	0	0	0.05	0.04	0.15
Calcium (%)	1.1	1.03	1.13	1.0	0.84	0.7 (min), 1.1 (max)
Phosphorus (%)	0.7	0.85	0.88	0.69	0.69	0.65
Copper (ppm)	4	3.55	0.74	14.9	22.75	35
Zinc (ppm)	23	23.13	36.14	50.24	73.75	110

Modified from Lewis L: Growing Horse Feeding and Care, in. Equine Clinical Nutrition, and the USDA Nutrient Database (http://www.nal.usda.gov/fnic/foodcomp/search/).
*Land O'Lakes, Black River Falls, WI, USA.
†Pet-Ag, Inc., Hampshire, IL, USA.
‡Buckeye Nutrition, Dalton, OH, USA.

replacers and either goat's milk or cow's milk. Multispecies milk replacer products (ProNurse*) can be used for a short period of time but do not provide the balance of nutrients required by growing foals. Human enteral products do not match the nutrient profile of mare's milk and should not be fed for more than 1 to 2 days. Nurse mares can be an excellent source of nutrition for orphan foals, but in a hospital setting, they are usually not immediately available.

Mare's milk is the ideal supplemental feed for critically ill foals, and it provides the foal with all essential nutrients required for growth through about 2 months of age (Table 5.11). When a mare and foal pair is hospitalised, the mare should be milked every 2 to 3 hours to provide milk for the foal and to help the mare maintain her lactation. It is important to follow clean procedures while milking the mare to prevent mastitis. Gloves should be worn by the milker, and debris should be cleaned from the teat. Commercially available milkers† decrease hand contact with the mare and are recommended in busy neonatal units. The volume of milk obtained at each milking should be recorded. Before the milk is offered to the foal, it should be strained to remove any debris. Often, a hospitalised mare will not produce enough milk to meet the daily requirements of the foal. Mares can be treated with domperidone (1.1 mg/kg PO every 24 hours) to improve their milk production. If milk production is still inadequate for the foal, the mare's milk should be mixed with a commercial foal milk replacer, with goat's milk or with cow's milk to ensure that the foal receives enough nutrients. If the mare has maintained her lactation during the foal's hospitalisation, the foal may need to be taught how to nurse from the mare once their illness has resolved. Nursing activity by the foal is likely to increase the yield of milk in a mare that has been hand-milked.

A variety of high-quality commercial foal milk replacers are available for purchase. These products are formulated with highly digestible protein and fat sources and contain a vitamin and mineral profile that closely matches mare's milk (Table 5.11). Supplemental nutrients are not required when these products are used, unless the foal has been diagnosed with a specific nutrient deficiency. Often, critically ill hospitalised foals become functional orphans during a prolonged hospitalisation. In many cases, these foals are managed with a milk replacer product both during hospitalisation and following discharge until they are weaned. Many milk replacer products are available in both a powder and a pellet form, allowing for an easy transition to a dry diet as the foal ages. Although weight gain in foals fed commercial milk replacers is often less than breed-matched mare-fed foals during the first 1 to 2 months of life, growth rates appear to equalize as the milk replacer fed foals reach 4 to 6 months of age.[1] Milk replacers should be reconstituted before each meal but can be refrigerated in between meals to facilitate management of the feedings. The products should be reconstituted according to the label instructions to ensure that the milk solid concentration of the milk replacer matches the milk solid content of mare's milk. However, with some products, mixing according to the manufacturer's instructions can lead to constipation in hospitalised foals. Adding three-quarters of the recommended amount of powder (and therefore making the milk more dilute) for the first week of supplementation can help prevent this. Improper mixing of milk powder and water can lead to hypernatraemia, diarrhoea and constipation. If any electrolyte abnormalities or gastrointestinal disturbances develop during treatment with a milk replacer, the mixing and feeding protocol should be reviewed.

* Purina Mills, LLC, St. Louis, MO, USA.
† Udderly-EZ Milker for Equine, Ellendale, MN, USA.

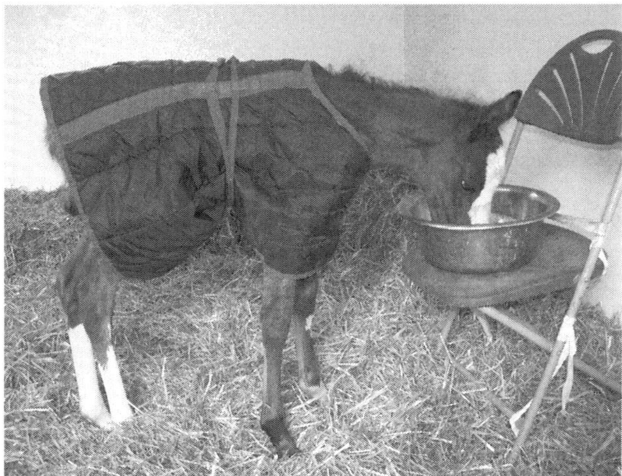

Figure 5.5 Feeding a foal by providing milk in a bowl. This is much less time consuming than bottle feeding, and greatly reduces the risk of aspiration pneumonia. ©Kevin Corley 2006.

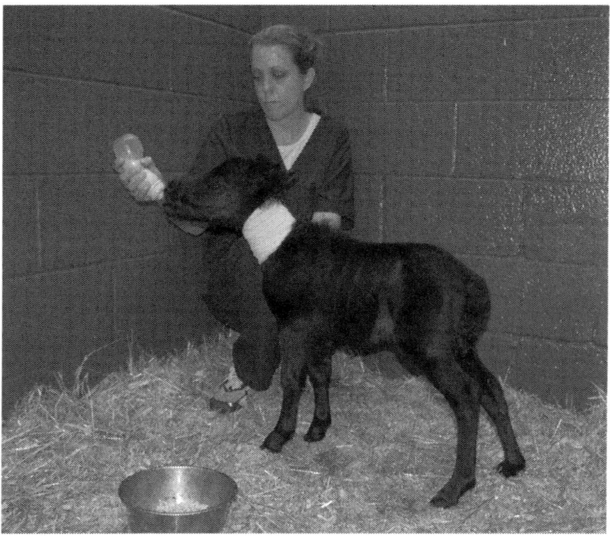

Figure 5.6 Bottle-feeding a foal. There is a risk of aspiration pneumonia with this technique, and it should never be used unless the foal has a very strong suck response. ©Meri Stratton-Phelps 2007.

Milk from goats and cows can be fed to foals, but both can result in gastrointestinal complications due to their higher fat and lower lactose concentrations compared to mare's milk. Goat's milk has a higher energy density than mare's milk (0.69 kcal/g [AF] versus 0.48 kcal/g [AF]), whilst low-fat (2% fat) cow's milk is closer in energy to mare's milk (0.50 kcal/g [AF]). Foals appear to tolerate goat's milk without any alteration of the milk but may develop constipation if they consume a pure diet of goat's milk. When cow's milk is fed to a foal, 2% fat milk should be used, and dextrose should be added to the milk at a concentration of 20 g dextrose (or glucose) per litre of milk. Sucrose (table sugar), honey and corn syrup should not be added to a foal milk substitute because the digestive tract enzymes sucrase and maltase have a low activity in foals. Both goat's milk and cow's milk should be pasteurised (70° C or 170° F for 15 minutes) before they are fed.

Bucket or pan feeding

Bucket or pan feeding is the method of choice for orphan foals and foals that require long-term nutritional support (Figure 5.5). During bucket feeding, if a foal wants to drink, it needs to actively ingest and swallow the milk. This action reduces the chance of aspiration. This method of feeding is efficient and requires minimal time from the caretaker, and it also decreases the behavioural problems that can develop in bottle-fed orphan foals.

Foals must be taught to drink from a bucket. Initially, this procedure can be time consuming, but most foals will learn to drink from a bucket within 2 to 3 days. Foals should be offered milk when they are hungry to facilitate the learning process. Once the foal has a strong suckle response, the trainer should cover their finger in milk, and then have the foal suckle their finger. The pan or bucket is then slowly raised to meet the foal's mouth so the milk is ingested as the foal suckles. The foal's head should never be forced into a bucket. The foal will soon learn to drink the milk without being stimulated to nurse on the trainer's finger. This procedure should be repeated until the foal is able to drink on its own.

The bucket or pan should have a large flat bottom so the foal does not catch its head in a deep bucket. A separate bucket with a measured amount of water should also be provided for the foal. Some foals will consume an excessive amount of water, even if they are fed enough milk to meet their energy requirements. Excessive water consumption can lead to hyponatraemia in some foals. If a foal appears to be drinking too much water, then the foal's packed cell volume (PCV), total protein and serum sodium should be evaluated. The PCV should be compared to earlier measurements in the same foal. It should be borne in mind that foals recovering from critical illness frequently have PCVs in the range of 22 to 30, prior to any possible excessive water consumption. If hyponatraemia or haemodilution develops, controlled water restriction may be necessary.

Bottle feeding

Bottle-feeding should be done with caution in any foal. Only foals that have a strong suckle response should be fed with a bottle (Figure 5.6). The trachea should be auscultated for evidence of aspiration when a bottle is initially introduced to a foal. Foals that have a weak suckle response can easily aspirate if fed from a bottle when their head is in an extended position. If a bottle is used, it should be held so the foal's head remains in a flexed position. The nipple should be selected so it is small enough to force the foal to create suction before the milk is released from the bottle. Infant or lamb nipples are an appropriate size for most young foals. Large nipples used for calves or nipples that leak should not be used.

Enteral feeding for the healthy orphan foal or clinically stable equine neonate

Healthy neonatal foals with normal gastrointestinal tract motility can initially be fed to meet 10% of body weight each day (Table 5.12). If the foal has a normal suckle response, the milk can be offered in a pan or bowl or, possibly, in a bottle. A healthy neonatal foal will nurse for 1 to 2 minutes' duration 3 to 7 times each hour. In the hospital setting, the frequency of offering milk should depend on the age of the foal and the adaptation of the foal to intermittent feeding. A high frequency of feeding allows smaller volumes of milk to be offered, lessening gastric distension and potential complications from colic. Foals less than 48 hours of age should be fed hourly, delivering up to 10% of their body weight in the first 24 hours and up to 20% in the second 24 hours. If the foal continues to tolerate this rate of infusion, the frequency of feeding can be decreased to every 2 hours for the next 3 to 5 days of life, with the volume of each meal accordingly increased to deliver 20% of its body weight over 24 hours. In the second week of life, the foal may be fed every 4 hours. Decreasing the frequency of feeding, and therefore increasing the amount of milk at each feed, should be done at times when the foal can be observed for 30 to 60 minutes after the change. Orphan foals 2 weeks of age or older that are clinically healthy can be fed at a rate between 15% to 20% of their body weight divided into 3 to 6 feedings per day using a commercial foal milk replacer if a nurse mare or mare's milk is not available. As the foal ages, the frequency of feeding can be reduced to 2 to 4 times per day.

Any changes in the diet formulation should be made over 3 to 5 days to decrease the risk of gastrointestinal complications. If the foal develops diarrhoea, ileus or signs of colic, a complete physical examination and ancillary diagnostic tests should be performed to determine the cause of the problem. If the illness appears to be related to the diet, then the frequency of feeding and the volume of each meal should be reduced. If the nutritional requirements of the foal cannot be met with this reduced feeding, supplemental PN should be considered. The suckle response should be monitored throughout the time that the foal is hospitalised. If the foal's health declines, if the foal's suckle response is weak or if the foal cannot voluntarily consume 10% of its body weight in milk, supplemental feeding through a nasogastric tube should be started.

The body weight and height of orphan foals should be monitored every 2 to 4 weeks using a scale or a weight tape. The average daily gain of healthy foals is listed in Table 5.10. An excessive rate of growth can occur even when a foal is managed with a commercial milk product, and routine measurements of body weight and height should be made to ensure that the foal's growth is appropriate.

Enteral feeding for the clinically ill foal

Almost all foals that have signs of clinical illness are managed with supplemental nutrition offered through a nasogastric tube at some point during their hospitalisation. In many cases, septic neonates may appear bright and alert on initial examination, but their condition can rapidly deteriorate to a point where they are unable to maintain their caloric intake. Nasogastric tube placement at presentation provides the clinician the option of enteral therapy and also the ability to assess the foal for residual gastric fluid during hospitalisation. Foal feeding tubes‡ should be used if available. These tubes have a small diameter that allows the foal to nurse around the tube as their condition improves. Foal nasogastric tubes can remain in place for weeks without traumatising the pharyngeal, oesophageal or gastric mucosa. A stallion catheter§ can be used for short-term feeding but is not recommended for use beyond 2 to 3 days. Nasogastric tube placement in the foal is described in Chapter 2.5. It is important to ensure that the tip of the tube is located in the stomach once the tube has been placed. Larger feeding tubes, like a stallion catheter, can be placed with the distal tip in the oesophagus to prevent potential complications from oesophagitis due to gastric reflux. Reflux oesophagitis does not appear to be clinically significant in foals that are managed with small diameter foal feeding tubes. Lateral and ventrodorsal radiographs are useful to document placement of the distal

‡12Fr × 108-cm Nasogastric Feeding Tube (NG1243); MILA International Inc., Florence, KY, USA;

§Portex Horse Catheter; Portex Ltd, Kent, UK.

Table 5.12. Volume of milk *per day* (ml) for foals of varying ages

Weight of foal (kg)	5% (50 ml/kg BW)	10% (100 ml/kg BW)	15% (150 ml/kg BW)	20% (200 ml/kg BW)
10	500	1000	1500	2000
20	1000	2000	3000	4000
30	1500	3000	4500	6000
40	2000	4000	6000	8000
50	2500	5000	7500	10000
60	3000	6000	9000	12000
70	3500	7000	10500	14000

end of the tube. If these are unavailable, it is acceptable to confirm correct placement into the oesophagus with an endoscope. However, this does not give any information regarding the position of the tip of the tube (or if it is kinked). Syringe feeding places foals at great risk of aspiration pneumonia, and is never a suitable method of providing nutrients to a foal.

Volume to feed

When the enteral diet is started, the foal should be fed 5% of its body weight in milk or milk replacer divided into hourly feeds. Even though the foal will not receive all of its nutrient requirements when fed to equal 5% of its body weight, it is always prudent to begin feeding the foal using a low volume. On presentation, a foal may appear to have normal gastrointestinal motility, but, following 6 to 12 hours of milk infusion, signs of ileus, gastric distension or colic may develop. Although it is tempting to be aggressive with enteral feeding, overfeeding during the first 24 hours of treatment should be avoided. In foals less than 48 hours old, milk should be offered at least every hour. In older foals, it should be offered every 1 to 2 hours initially. Although feeding through a constant rate of infusion (CRI) may reduce gastrointestinal complications in human infants, it is often difficult to safely maintain and monitor a critically ill foal that is being fed with a CRI. If the foal tolerates infusion of 5% of its body weight in milk, on the second day of hospitalization the volume of milk offered to the foal can be increased to 7.5% to 10% of body weight. The volume of milk can continue to slowly be increased until the foal is consuming 20% of its body weight in milk each day.

Feeding protocol

Before any milk is infused, proper placement of the tube must be ensured. Occasionally the nasogastric tube migrates out of the stomach, which can lead to milk infusion into the oesophagus and an increased risk of aspiration. In order to lower the risk of aspiration, the foal should be standing or placed in sternal recumbency during the feeding. The procedure should begin by using gentle suction to remove the residual gastric fluid. If the volume is greater than 20 ml in a 50-kg foal, or proportionately less in a smaller foal, the feeding should be delayed for an hour. If the gastric residual fluid is still greater than 20 ml after waiting an hour, then intravenous nutrition should be considered. If less than 20 ml is obtained, the nasogastric tube should be flushed with 10 to 20 ml of warm water, and then freshly mixed warm milk (or milk replacer) should be administered to the foal. Feeding via gravity flow using a commercially available enteral feeding bag** is a convenient method of feeding through a foal feeding tube. As an alternative, a clean 1-L fluid bag and administration line can be used. Alternatively, a gravity flow system can be used by attaching the barrel of 60-ml catheter-tip syringe to the end of the catheter (this works well for a stallion catheter tube). The milk is poured into the syringe barrel during the feeding (Figure 5.7). Gentle pressure may be required to initiate the flow of milk through a stallion catheter. Milk should never be forced through the nasogastric tube. After the foal has been fed, the nasogastric tube should be flushed with 20 to 30 ml of warm water before it is capped. All feeding equipment should be cleaned thoroughly after use. Hospitalised foals should have their own feeding equipment. The daily volume of milk and flush water should be measured, and recorded as part of the foal's daily fluid intake. Adjustments in the intravenous fluid therapy of the foal may be required to take into account the volume of fluid delivered enterally.

Neonatal foals with normal gastrointestinal tract motility should be able to tolerate milk infused at a rate of 10% to 20% of body weight in milk per day, divided into 8 to 12 feedings per day. Foals should be encouraged to nurse from their dam, as soon as they develop a strong suckle response. Nasogastric tube feeding should continue until the foal develops a strong suckle response and is able to repeatedly nurse from the mare, pan or bottle without aspirating milk. When the foal first attempts to nurse from the mare, the trachea should be auscultated. If fluid is auscultated, the foal should not be allowed to nurse. If the trachea is clear of fluid, the foal can be allowed to nurse under supervision while the volume of infused milk is gradually reduced. The foal should gain weight and maintain their BCS before the nasogastric tube is removed.

Foals that are not able to tolerate infusion of 10% of their body weight for more than 2 days or foals that experience weight loss and a loss of BCS because they cannot tolerate more than 100 ml/kg BW/day should be treated with PN.

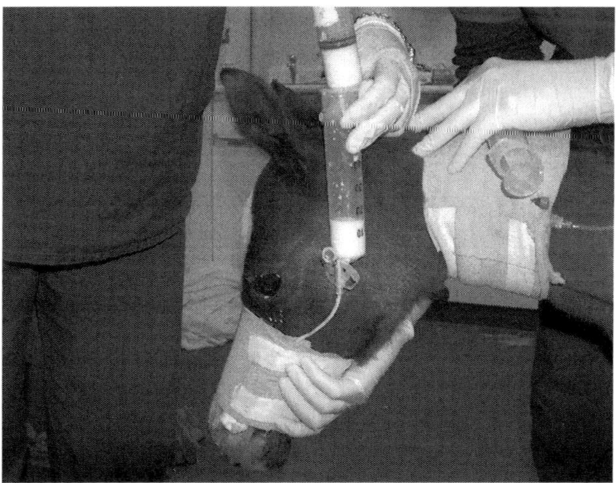

Figure 5.7 Feeding a foal through an indwelling nasogastric tube. A syringe barrel is used as a funnel, to feed the foal by gravity. ©Kevin Corley 2006.

** Flexiflo Gravity Feeding Set, Ross Products, Abbott Laboratories, IL, USA; Enteral Feeding Bag; Plasco Engineered Products, Columbus, MS, USA.

A weekly feeding protocol and daily feeding instructions are given in Boxes 5.22 and 5.23.

Monitoring

Any new change in the foal's condition should be assessed quickly and thoroughly. Because the condition of a neonatal foal can change rapidly, frequent physical examinations and biochemical assessments are necessary to manage and treat new complications.

Foals treated with enteral nutrition should be closely observed for any signs of colic, abdominal distension and ileus. A simple way to monitor the foal's abdominal size is to measure around the area of greatest diameter using a string or umbilical tape. Increased distension is an indication to further evaluate the foal by palpation, abdominal ultrasound and abdominal radiographs, before the foal is offered another meal. Septic neonates can become obtunded rapidly and may not show signs of colic during the early stages of ileus.

The volume and character of the foal's faeces should be recorded daily. It is normal for a foal to pass a small volume (½ cup [125 ml]) of pasty faeces every 24 hours. Persistent watery diarrhoea is not a normal response to enteral feeding. Foals with unresolved diarrhoea should be evaluated with a physical examination and appropriate diagnostic tests. It is also important to monitor the foal's urine output at least every 4 to 6 hours. Any decline in urine output may represent dehydration, hypovolaemia, haemodynamic derangements or, less commonly, renal or postrenal disease.

The hydration status of the foal should be assessed 4 to 6 times each day. If the foal appears underhydrated or overhydrated, has an increasing blood lactate concentration, has a decreasing blood pressure or a decreasing urine

Box 5.22. Weekly feeding plan for hospitalised neonatal foals

Hospital Enteral Feeding Plan

Foal Name: _______ Foal Age: _______ Foal Weight: _______ Weight at Presentation: _______

Day 1

A) Foal weight _______ × 5% = _______ (volume of milk to feed over 24 hours)
B) Number of feedings/day = 24
C) Volume of milk at each feeding = A/B _______

Day 2

A) Foal weight _______ × 7.5% = _______ (volume of milk to feed over 24 hours)
B) Number of feedings/day = 24
C) Volume of milk at each feeding = A/B _______

Day 3

A) Foal weight _______ × 10% = _______ (volume of milk to feed over 24 hours)
B) Number of feedings/day = 18–12
C) Volume of milk at each feeding = A/B _______

Day 4

A) Foal weight _______ × 12.5% = _______ (volume of milk to feed over 24 hours)
B) Number of feedings/day = 18–12
C) Volume of milk at each feeding = A/B _______

Day 5

A) Foal weight _______ × 15% = _______ (volume of milk to feed over 24 hours)
B) Number of feedings/day = 18–12
C) Volume of milk at each feeding = A/B _______

Day 6

A) Foal weight _______ × 17.5% = _______ (volume of milk to feed over 24 hours)
B) Number of feedings/day = 12
C) Volume of milk at each feeding = A/B _______

Day 7

A) Foal weight _______ × 20% = _______ (volume of milk to feed over 24 hours)
B) Number of feedings/day = 12
C) Volume of milk at each feeding = A/B _______

Is the foal gaining weight appropriately? If weight gain is not noted once the foal is consuming 15%–20% of their body weight, consider increasing the foal's daily energy intake.

Box 5.23. Feeding plan for hospitalised neonatal foals

Hospitalised Foal Enteral Feeding Chart

Foal Name: ______________ Patient Number: _______ Day of Hospitalization: _______

Feeding	Time	Gastric Residual (ml) =	Flush water (ml) =	Milk (ml) =
Feeding 1	Time _______	Gastric Residual (ml) = _______	Flush water (ml) = _______	Milk (ml) = _______
Feeding 2	Time _______	Gastric Residual (ml) = _______	Flush water (ml) = _______	Milk (ml) = _______
Feeding 3	Time _______	Gastric Residual (ml) = _______	Flush water (ml) = _______	Milk (ml) = _______
Feeding 4	Time _______	Gastric Residual (ml) = _______	Flush water (ml) = _______	Milk (ml) = _______
Feeding 5	Time _______	Gastric Residual (ml) = _______	Flush water (ml) = _______	Milk (ml) = _______
Feeding 6	Time _______	Gastric Residual (ml) = _______	Flush water (ml) = _______	Milk (ml) = _______
Feeding 7	Time _______	Gastric Residual (ml) = _______	Flush water (ml) = _______	Milk (ml) = _______
Feeding 8	Time _______	Gastric Residual (ml) = _______	Flush water (ml) = _______	Milk (ml) = _______
Feeding 9	Time _______	Gastric Residual (ml) = _______	Flush water (ml) = _______	Milk (ml) = _______
Feeding 10	Time _______	Gastric Residual (ml) = _______	Flush water (ml) = _______	Milk (ml) = _______
Feeding 11	Time _______	Gastric Residual (ml) = _______	Flush water (ml) = _______	Milk (ml) = _______
Feeding 12	Time _______	Gastric Residual (ml) = _______	Flush water (ml) = _______	Milk (ml) = _______

Total Gastric Fluid (ml) = _______ Total Flush water (ml) = _______ Total Milk (ml) = _______

*If gastric residual is >20 ml, skip the feeding, and check the residual gastric fluid in 1 hour. If the volume is still >20 ml, consider parenteral nutrition.

output, develops respiratory crackles, develops a sudden gain in weight or develops peripheral oedema, the total fluid plan and feeding plan for the foal should be examined and revised. The volume of milk and flush water administered to the foal should be included in the maintenance fluid plan for the neonatal patient. Many septic neonates are hypoalbuminaemic and may require supplemental therapy with colloids (or possibly hyperimmune plasma) to maintain their oncotic pressure.

A complete blood count and serum biochemistry panel should be performed as often as necessary to document changes in the foal's condition. Frequent assessments of the foal's serum electrolytes and blood glucose help to determine the appropriate fluid supplementation. Hyperglycaemia and hypertriglyceridaemia are not common in enterally fed foals, but their serum should be monitored for any evidence of glucose or lipid intolerance. Management of this problem involves decreasing the volume of milk infused at each feeding for 12 to 24 hours, until the blood values return to normal.

Complications

The most common complication of enteral nutrition in a neonatal foal is intolerance of the feeding. This usually occurs during the first 1 to 2 days of therapy. Often, the foal has been fed too great a volume of milk, resulting in the development of colic and, in some cases, diarrhoea and enterocolitis. Foals with perinatal asphyxia syndrome may be intolerant of any volume of milk due to persistent gastrointestinal ileus. These foals should be managed with PN, and only a small volume (10–30 ml/feeding) of milk should be infused to directly nourish the enterocytes. Some clinicians prefer to give glutamine (0.4 g/kg/day, divided into 12–24 daily doses) in 10 to 20 ml of water, rather than any milk to these foals. Glutamine, an amino acid, functions as a precursor and regulator of protein synthesis and, as such, supports rapidly proliferating cells, including enterocytes.[4] Intolerance of milk fed at 10% of the foal's body weight is an indication that the foal requires PN.

Overhydration can develop if the total fluid therapy plan for the foal is not managed properly. Usually this problem can be corrected by reducing the rate of infusion of maintenance fluids. If the milk volume must be reduced, then calories can be provided through PN.

Diarrhoea often occurs in neonatal foals after a few days of enteral feeding. This complication should be evaluated by reviewing the diet and the mixing protocol if a milk replacer is being fed. This complication can lead to prolonged hospitalisation in some neonates and may be a reason for avoiding early enteral nutrition in foals with severe perinatal asphyxia syndrome or septicaemia. A diagnostic workup may be indicated if the foal develops signs of septicaemia or enterocolitis. Faecal tests for rotavirus, *Salmonella* spp., *Clostridium perfringens* and *Clostridium difficile* are indicated if the foal develops severe diarrhoea or signs of septicaemia.

Aspiration pneumonia following improper nasogastric tube management is a complication that can be avoided. Radiographs with 2 views of the thorax can confirm placement of the nasogastric tube before the foal is fed. Although the tube can often be palpated in the oesophagus, small flexible foal nasogastric tubes can retroflex and lodge in the oesophagus. Active foals frequently pull their nasogastric tubes during hospitalisation. It is important to remind the nursing staff to notify the clinician if this has occurred. Well-intentioned students and staff may try to replace the tube but if they are unsuccessful, additional feedings could lead to milk aspiration. If aspiration pneumonia is suspected in a patient due to an elevated respiratory rate, an unexplained fever or the sudden decline of a patient, the respiratory tract should be examined, and proper placement of the nasogastric tube should be confirmed.

Nutrition options: parenteral nutrition

PN can be a lifesaving treatment for foals that are unable to tolerate enteral nutrition (Figure 5.8). The general principles of PN therapy in neonatal or young foals are the same as in adult horses, and the clinician is encouraged to review the previous discussion of PN in this chapter.

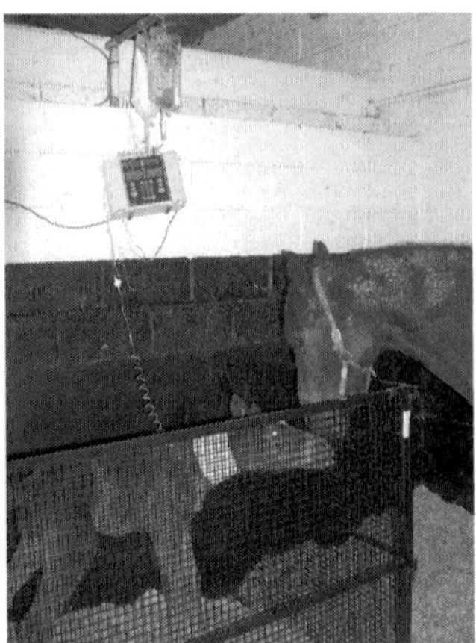

Figure 5.8 Parenteral nutrition in a foal. An electronic infusion pump is used to regulate the flow of the parenteral nutrition and fluids. ©Kevin Corley 2007.

Formulations

The PN solution is formulated to meet the foal's resting energy and maintenance protein requirements. Vitamins and trace minerals are usually added to the formulation to prevent deficiencies of these essential nutrients. Starting formulations should provide approximately 45 to 50 kcal/kg BW, 3 to 5 g protein/kg BW and 1 to 3 g lipid/kg BW/day. The ideal PN formulation will have a total calorie-to-nitrogen ratio of 80 to 100. Foals that have acute renal failure or severe hepatic disease should be treated with the lower concentration of protein (3 g/day). Foals that require more than 5 days of PN therapy may benefit from a higher concentration of energy (75–100 kcal/kg BW) and protein (6–6.5 g/kg/day). Significant changes in the composition of the PN formulation need to be made gradually over 12 to 24 hours so the foal can adapt to the new nutrient profile of the solution. Parenteral solution compounding instructions are provided in the adult equine section of this chapter. A PN worksheet for foals is given in Box 5.24.

The foal PN example in Box 5.24 (525 ml 50% dextrose, 1500 ml 10% amino acid, 500 ml 20% lipid) is designed to provide 5.3/3/2 g/kg/day of dextrose, amino acid and lipid, respectively. This formula will provide approximately 50 kcal/kg/day at a calorie-to-nitrogen ratio of 104 : 1 and an osmolarity of 1141 mOsmol/L. A typical formulation used in Europe is given in Box 5.25. Once the full flow rate is achieved, additional caloric density can be achieved by increasing the proportion of lipid emulsion. Dextrose or glucose calories are usually limited to prevent complications from hyperglycaemia.

Newly marketed commercial amino acid and dextrose admixtures may make parenteral supplementation easier in the future. Both Baxter Healthcare and B. Braun formulate products that contain a preselected volume of amino acids and protein in 1- and 2-L bags. The ingredients are mixed prior to use. The energy density of the solutions can be increased by adding lipid to the solution. The nutrient composition of three products* are listed in the Parenteral Nutrition Ingredients chart in Tables 5.8 and 5.9.

Infusion protocol

Most PN formulations are hyperosmolar and need to be infused through a central venous catheter. If a peripheral catheter is used, the osmolarity of the solution should not exceed 700 mOsmol/L. Co-infusing crystalloid fluids through the same line can achieve this. Multilumen catheters are preferred for administration of PN. The jugular

* CLINIMIX; Baxter Healthcare Corporation, Deerfield, IL, USA.

Box 5.24: Parenteral nutrition worksheet for foals

Patient Information		**Example**
1. Foal Weight (kg)	________	50 kg
2. Estimated Resting Energy Requirement (45-50 kcal/kg/day)	________	
Ex: 50 kcal/kg/day × 50 kg		2,500 kcal
3. Estimated Protein Requirement (2-5 grams/kg/day)	________	
Ex: 3 g/kg/day × 50 kg		150 grams
4. Maintenance fluid requirements (4-5 ml/kg/hour)	________	4,800 ml
Parenteral Nutrition Formulation		
5. Protein Required		
Protein (g) divided by 0.1 g/ml of 10% amino acid solution	________	
Ex: 150 g / 0.1 g/ml		1,500 ml
6. Caloric contribution of 10% amino acid solution (0.40 kcal/ml)	________	
Ex: 0.40 kcal/ml × 1,500 ml of amino acid solution		600 kcal
7. Total calories remaining		
Calories from 2 – calories from 6	________	
Ex: 2,500 kcal – 600 kcal		1,900 kcal
8. Percent of remaining calories from lipid (20-60%)		
Ex: 53% 0.53 × 1,900		1,007 kcal
9. Amount of lipid solution to meet the calories calculated in 8	________	
Ex: 1,007 kcal × 1 ml/2 kcal (20% lipid solution)		500 ml
10. Percent of remaining calories from dextrose	________	
Ex: 47% 0.47 × 1,900		893 kcal
11. Amount of 50% dextrose to meet the calories calculated in 10	________	
Ex: 893 kcal × 1 ml/1.7 kcal		525 ml
12. Add 1-2 ml of B complex vitamins per liter of solution	________	2 ml
13. Add 1 ml of trace minerals per day	________	1 ml
14. Volume of final solution (5+9+11+12+13)	________	
Ex: 1,500 ml + 500 ml + 525 ml + 2 ml + 1 ml		2,528 ml
15. Energy Density (kcal/ml)	________	
Ex: 2,500 kcal/2,528 ml		0.99 kcal/ml
16. Determine the rate of infusion over 24 hours (ml from 14/24)	________	
Ex: 2,528 ml/24 hours		105 ml/hr

Final Solution:	**Energy Contribution:**
1,500 ml 10% amino acid	600 kcal
500 ml 20% lipid	1,007 kcal
525 ml 50% dextrose	893 kcal
2 ml B vitamins	
1 ml trace minerals	

Ratio of Nutrients: 5.3/3/2 g/kg/day of dextrose/amino acid/lipid

Ratio of calories to nitrogen:

150 grams of protein contains 24 grams of nitrogen (1 gram of nitrogen in 6.25 grams of protein)

2,500 kcal (from 2) : 24 grams nitrogen = 104

Remaining Daily Fluid Requirements:

4,800 ml required – (2,528 ml PN × 0.50 free water) = 3,536 ml

vein is commonly selected as the site for placement of a multiple-lumen catheter. It is often easiest to place a multiple lumen catheter in a neonate on initial presentation and to preserve one port for later PN use using a heparin lock. This protocol eliminates the need for a new catheter or placement of a second catheter later during the foal's hospitalisation. Multiple-lumen catheters (double and triple lumen, 5Fr–7Fr, 13–20 cm polyurethane) are available from several manufacturers† and are long enough to permit infusion of the PN into the cranial vena cava in many foals (Figure 5.4). Placing a jugular catheter is described in Chapter 2.6. If jugular catheter placement is not possible, a peripheral catheter can be placed in the cephalic, saphenous or lateral thoracic vein. Multiple-lumen catheters (double and triple lumen, 4F, 8–13 cm polyurethane) suitable for use in Miniature horse foals are also available§.

§Arrow International Inc., Reading, PA, USA; MILA International, Florence, KY, USA.

Box 5.25. Example of a parenteral nutrition formula used in Europe

Glucose 50%*:	1500 ml
Amino acids 15%†:	1000 ml
Lipids 20%‡:	500 ml
3 L Ethyl-vinyl-acetate mixing bag§	
Energy from glucose =	1900 kcal
Energy from amino acids =	600 kcal
Energy from lipids =	1000 kcal

% Nonprotein calories from glucose = 74%
% Nonprotein calories from lipids = 26%

Final infusion rate = 1.266 × body weight in kg

This infusion rate provides 45 kcal/kg/day

*50% Glucose intravenous infusion; Baxter Healthcare, Thetford, Norfolk, UK.
†Intrafusin 22; Fresenius-Kabi AG, Bad Homburg, Germany.
‡Intralipid 20%; Fresenius-Kabi AG, Bad Homburg, Germany.
§Freka Mix + 6; Fresenius-Kabi AG, Bad Homburg, Germany.

The PN should be started at 25% of the final desired infusion rate and must be administered using a constant rate of infusion. It is highly desirable to use an electronic infusion pump, to ensure that the rate of delivery is constant and uninterrupted. If the foal tolerates the infusion, then the rate should be gradually increased by 1 to 2 ml/hr until the foal is at 60% to 70% of the final infusion rate. The foal's physical parameters, serum electrolytes and blood glucose values should be rechecked at this time. If the foal tolerates the infusion, then the rate can be increased by 1 to 2 ml/hr until the maintenance rate is infused. It often takes 24 to 36 hours to achieve the full infusion rate; however, complications from hyperglycaemia are minimized when this protocol is followed. The gradual rate increase also allows the clinician to adjust the formulation according to the foal's response to therapy. If the foal cannot tolerate the lipid or dextrose/glucose content of the PN solution, the rate of infusion should be reduced by one-third. Some clinicians prefer to infuse insulin (starting at 0.01 IU/kg/hr) and achieve their nutritional aims, rather than reduce or reformulate the PN. If an insulin infusion is started, blood glucose concentrations need to be closely monitored (every 1–2 hours initially). The PN solution can be reformulated with a lower concentration of either lipid or dextrose/glucose, if necessary. The energy and protein content of the PN can be increased if the foal tolerates the infusion but experiences a persistent loss of weight or muscle condition. The foal should be maintained at the full infusion rate for 1 to 2 days before the calorie or protein content of the PN is increased. The goal of PN therapy is to maintain the foal's body weight and body condition. Growth is not an expected outcome.

Throughout the time that a foal is treated with PN, it should also be treated with a small volume of mare's milk, milk replacer or a glutamine solution administered through a nasogastric tube every 2 to 4 hours. Residual gastric fluid should be removed before a 10- to 30-ml amount of milk or solution is infused. As the foal begins to tolerate the milk, the volume should be slowly increased by 10 to 20 ml per feeding. Once the foal can tolerate 5% of its body weight (50 ml/kg/day) enterally fed in milk, the PN can be gradually decreased by 1 to 2 ml/hr. The PN can be discontinued once the infusion rate has reached 30% of maintenance.

Monitoring

Foals treated with PN should be monitored using the same criteria listed in Box 5.15 for adult horses. This includes a daily inspection of the catheter site and fluid lines, daily body weight and BCS assessment and measurement of the foal's daily urine and faecal output. Urine glucose should be monitored whenever possible. A physical examination should be performed at least every 4 to 6 hours. A complete blood count and serum biochemistry panel should be evaluated frequently until the foal's condition has stabilised. The foal's blood glucose concentration should be monitored at least every 4 to 6 hours and the electrolyte profile and acid-base balance should be monitored frequently during the time that the foal is in critical condition. As the foal's condition improves, and their electrolyte and glucose levels normalise, the frequency of blood work assessments can be reduced.

Fluid balance is especially important in foals. The foal's maintenance fluid therapy should be adjusted when the foal is receiving parenteral supplementation to ensure that the total infusion does not exceed the current goals of therapy. There is some debate about the appropriate maintenance rate for foals, but a generally accepted rate is 4 to 5 ml/kg/hr (Chapter 6.5). Parenteral solutions usually contain at least 50% free water, which should be calculated into the foal's daily requirements.

Electrolytes are usually not included in commercial amino acid solutions. Unless minerals are added to the PN solution, the formulation is not an adequate source of minerals for the foal. Complications with hypophosphataemia, hypocalcaemia, hypomagnesaemia and hypokalaemia are occasionally encountered and require supplemental therapy. Because most foals require treatment with intravenous crystalloid fluid during PN therapy, supplementation of the maintenance fluid with electrolytes is recommended. The compatibility of electrolyte supplements and pharmacological agents should be confirmed before any additions are made to the PN solution. A list of incompatible additives is available in the adult equine nutrition section (Box 5.21). Sodium bicarbonate is not compatible with nutrient admixtures and, in rare instances when it is required, must be administered in a separate fluid line through a multilumen catheter or into a separate catheter.

Complications

Management strategies for foals that develop complications from electrolyte abnormalities, and infections during

Table 5.13. Guidelines for infusing regular insulin in neonatal foals (SI units)

<u>**Insulin protocol for foals**</u>

0.2 IU (unit) per kg BW normal human insulin in 50 ml 0.9% NaCl (10 IU [units] for 50-kg foal)

Starting rate 2 ml/hr—use syringe driver

Blood glucose concentration	Change in blood glucose in last hour	Instructions to change insulin
>13 mmol/L	Increased or no change	INCREASE by 4 ml/hr
	Decreased by <1 mmol/L	INCREASE by 3 ml/hr
	Decreased by >1 mmol/L and <4 mmol/L	INCREASE by 2 ml/hr
	Decreased by >4 mmol/L	No change
11–13 mmol/L	Increased or no change	INCREASE by 3 ml/hr
	Decreased by <1 mmol/L	INCREASE by 2 ml/hr
	Decreased by >1 mmol/L and <3 mmol/L	INCREASE by 1 ml/hr
	Decreased by >3 mmol/L	No change
9.5–11 mmol/L	Increased or no change	INCREASE by 2 ml/hr
	Decreased by <1.5 mmol/L	INCREASE by 1 ml/hr
	Decreased by >1.5 mmol/L	No change
8.3–9.5 mmol/L	Increased	INCREASE by 1 ml/hr
	No change	INCREASE by 0.5 ml/hr
	Decreased by <0.5 mmol/L	INCREASE by 0.5 ml/hr
	Decreased by >0.5 mmol/L	No change
4.4–8.3 mmol/L	Increased by >1.5 mmol/L	INCREASE by 0.5 ml/hr
	Increased by less than 1.5 mmol/L or decreased by less than 1.5 mmol/L	No change
	Decreased by >1.5 mmol/L	DECREASE by 0.5 ml/hr
3.5–4.4 mmol/L	Increased by >1.5 mmol/L	INCREASE by 0.5 ml/hr
	Increased by less than 1.5 mmol/L	No change
	No change	DECREASE by 0.2 ml/hr
	Decreased by <0.5 mmol/L	DECREASE by 0.5 ml/hr
	Decreased by >0.5 mmol/L	DECREASE by 1 ml/hr
2.5–3.5 mmol/L	Increased by >1.2 mmol/L	INCREASE by 0.2 ml/hr
	Increased by less than 1.2 mmol/L	No change
	No change	DECREASE by 0.3 ml/hr
	Decreased by <0.4 mmol/L	DECREASE by 0.6 ml/hr
	Decreased by >0.4 mmol/L	DECREASE by 1.2 ml/hr
2–2.5 mmol/L	Increased	No change
	No change	DECREASE by 0.5 ml/hr
	Decreased by <0.3 mmol/L	DECREASE by 1 ml/hr
	Decreased by >0.3 mmol/L	DECREASE by 2 ml/hr
<2 mmol/L	**CALL SENIOR CLINICIAN IMMEDIATELY**	

This is intended as a guide only, and has been found to perform LESS WELL than an experienced clinician.

PN infusion are similar to the protocols in adult horses. The clinician is referred to the adult equine section in the earlier part of this chapter for guidelines on the care of these problems.

Hyperglycaemia (blood glucose >8.3 mmol/L; 150 mg/dl) and hypertriglyceridaemia (serum TG >2.5 mmol/L; 220 mg/dl) are the two most common complications of PN infusion in hospitalised foals. Concurrent dextrose supplementation in maintenance fluids is usually unnecessary, and could contribute to the hyperglycaemia. The first step in managing these problems is to decrease the rate of PN infusion by 30%. Some clinicians prefer to infuse insulin and achieve their nutritional aims, rather than reduce the PN infusion rate. The blood glucose should be rechecked in at least 4 to 6 hours and the serum TG should be rechecked in 12 to 18 hours to evaluate the foal's response to therapy. If the hyperglycaemia and hypertriglyceridaemia are not resolved, the PN should be reformulated with a lower concentration of dextrose/glucose, lipid or both. The concentration of lipid should be reduced to 2 g/kg BW in foals that have a serum TG above 2.5 mmol/L (220 mg/dl). Lipid should be excluded from PN solutions if the foal has hyperlipaemia (serum TG >5.65 mmol/L; 500 mg/dl). Foals that remain hyperglycaemic after the PN has been reformulated should be treated with regular insulin‡ as a CRI to achieve glycaemic control. A CRI of insulin allows it to be titrated to blood glucose concentration, with much finer control than intermittent insulin injections. The starting dosage rate is 0.01 IU/kg/hr, and this should be adjusted carefully to maintain glucose in a narrow range (Tables 5.13 and 5.14). If it is

‡Actrapid; Novo Nordisk A/S, Bagsværd, Denmark; Humulin R; Eli-Lilly, Indianapolis, IN, USA.

Table 5.14. Guidelines for infusing regular insulin in neonatal foals (Non–SI units)

Insulin protocol for foals
0.2 IU (unit) per kg BW normal human insulin in 50 ml 0.9% NaCl (10 IU [units] for 50-kg foal)
Starting rate 2 ml/hr—use syringe driver

Blood glucose concentration	Change in blood glucose in last hour	Instructions to change insulin
>234 mg/dl	Increased or no change	INCREASE by 4 ml/hr
	Decreased by <18 mg/dl	INCREASE by 3 ml/hr
	Decreased by >18 mg/dl and <72 mg/dl	INCREASE by 2 ml/hr
	Decreased by >72 mg/dl	No change
200–234 mg/dl	Increased or no change	INCREASE by 3 ml/hr
	Decreased by <18 mg/dl	INCREASE by 2 ml/hr
	Decreased by >18 mg/dl and <54 mg/dl	INCREASE by 1 ml/hr
	Decreased by >54 mg/dl	No change
172–200 mg/dl	Increased or no change	INCREASE by 2 ml/hr
	Decreased by <27 mg/dl	INCREASE by 1 ml/hr
	Decreased by > 27 mg/dl	No change
151–171 mg/dl	Increased	INCREASE by 1 ml/hr
	No change	INCREASE by 0.5 ml/hr
	Decreased by <9 mg/dl	INCREASE by 0.5 ml/hr
	Decreased by >9 mg/dl	No change
80–150 mg/dl	Increased by >27 mg/dl	INCREASE by 0.5 ml/hr
	Increased by less than 27 mg/dl or decreased by less than 27 mg/dl	No change
	Decreased by >27 mg/dl	DECREASE by 0.5 ml/hr
64–79 mg/dl	Increased by >27 mg/dl	INCREASE by 0.5 ml/hr
	Increased by less than 27 mg/dl	No change
	No change	DECREASE by 0.2 ml/hr
	Decreased by <9 mg/dl	DECREASE by 0.5 ml/hr
	Decreased by >9 mg/dl	DECREASE by 1 ml/hr
46–63 mg/dl	Increased by >22 mg/dl	INCREASE by 0.2 ml/hr
	Increased by less than 22 mg/dl	No change
	No change	DECREASE by 0.3 ml/hr
	Decreased by <7 mg/dl	DECREASE by 0.6 ml/hr
	Decreased by >7 mg/dl	DECREASE by 1.2 ml/hr
36–45 mg/dl	Increased	No change
	No change	DECREASE by 0.5 ml/hr
	Decreased by <5.5 mg/dl	DECREASE by 1 ml/hr
	Decreased by >5.5 mg/dl	DECREASE by 2 ml/hr
<36 mg/dl	**CALL SENIOR CLINICIAN IMMEDIATELY**	

This is intended as a guide only, and has been found to perform LESS WELL than an experienced clinician.

not possible to administer a CRI, it is possible to administer intermittent insulin (0.1–0.5 IU regular insulin SQ every 12 hours). In either case, care must be taken not to allow inadvertent interruptions to the PN whilst on insulin therapy, as this may cause blood glucose to fall precipitously. Blood glucose must be monitored very frequently when using insulin therapy (hourly in the initial stages). In the case of very low blood glucose (<2 mmol/L; <36 mg/dl), small boluses (30–50 ml) of 50% glucose or dextrose should be administered, and the blood glucose monitored, until it is stable in the normal range.

Foals that develop fluid overload may require alterations in the volume of crystalloid fluid therapy, and in extreme cases, the PN may need to be reformulated with a higher energy density and a lower total volume.

Conclusion

Supplemental nutrition either with enteral or parenteral therapy should be administered to all equine patients at risk of energy or protein malnutrition. The nutritional history and the clinical condition of the equine patient dictate the type of nutritional therapy that is administered. Although PN is expensive and requires close monitoring during infusion, it is a lifesaving option for many adult horses and foals. Guidelines for diet formulation, administration and patient monitoring are provided throughout this chapter. As the patient responds to therapy, a gradual return to voluntary feed or milk intake is possible in adult horses and foals, respectively. Nutritional therapy prevents protein-calorie malnutrition and is expected to improve the outcome of medical treatment by enhancing immune system function and tissue repair and by decreasing the duration of hospitalisation.

References

1. Lewis LD: Growing horse feeding and care, in Equine Clinical Nutrition: Feeding and Care. Baltimore, Williams and Wilkins, 1995, pp 334-349
2. Paradis MR: Caloric needs of the sick foal—determined by the use of indirect calorimetry. Neonatal Septicemia Workshop, Talloires, France, October 2001
3. Hansen TO: Nutritional support: parenteral feeding, in Koterba AM, Drummond WH, Kosch PC (eds): Equine Clinical Neonatology. Baltimore, Williams and Wilkins, 1990, pp 747-762
4. Dunkel BM, Wilkins PA: Nutrition and the critically ill horse. Vet Clin North Am Equine Pract 20:107-126, 2004

6

Common treatments

6.1 Standing sedation
6.2 Pain management in the hospitalised horse
6.3 Antimicrobial therapy
6.4 Aerosolised antimicrobials
6.5 Fluid therapy

6.1 Standing sedation

Lydia Donaldson

Introduction

Hospitalised horses may need sedation for a variety of reasons and under a variety of circumstances. The most common is short-term sedation to perform a specific procedure. Typically, this might be to encourage a horse to stand still for radiographs or to tolerate such procedures as endoscopy, lumbosacral cerebrospinal fluid aspiration, thoracocentesis, renal biopsy or placement of a subpalpebral lavage system. Thoroscopy and laparoscopy require longer-duration, but still finite, sedation. These situations may only differ from those of the outpatient or farm visit in that the horse may be fundamentally less healthy and the environment and presedation conditions more controlled. The most challenging hospitalised horse is the one in need of behavioural modification to become more accepting of its condition. This may be the horse that does not tolerate confinement, the horse with a cast that insists on stall walking, the horse resentful of life in a sling or the horse unable to overcome its instinctive fear (and pain?) of recumbency. This section reviews the drugs appropriate for sedation of the hospitalised horse and suggests particular circumstances where each agent or class of agents might be applicable. Drugs and doses are listed in Table 6.1.

Tranquilisers, sedatives and hypnotics

α_2-Agonists

The α_2-adrenergic agonists are the mainstays of equine sedation. They include xylazine*, romifidine†, detomidine‡ and medetomidine§ in order of increasing α_2-adrenergic receptor specificity. Only the first three are marketed for use in horses, whereas the potent, specific medetomidine is available for use in small animals. Also, a component of the anaesthetic management of people and currently being explored in horses is dexmedetomidine**. The sedation produced by α_2-agonists is characterised by a lowered head, droopy lips and eyelids, decreased response to auditory, visual and tactile stimulation and reluctance to move.[1] Equisedative intravenous doses are estimated to be 1.1 mg/kg xylazine, 80 μg/kg romifidine, 20 μg/kg detomidine, 7.5 μg/kg medetomidine and 3.0 μg/kg dexmedetomidine.[2–4] Although described as "equisedative", the quality and duration of sedation vary among the agents, with xylazine being the shortest acting and romifidine the least profound.[2,5] Low doses of α_2-agonists are anxiolytic, a feature that allows 1 to 2 μg/kg of detomidine IV to convince a 500-kg racing-fit thoroughbred to trot nicely for lameness evaluation. Analgesia is a component of α_2-sedation, although that of romifidine may be less.[5,6] These agents do produce a characteristic head-to-tail, top-to-bottom gradient of hyposensitivity that results in the head being the easiest body part to work on and the hind foot the most difficult. Response to visceral pain and deep palpation is attenuated better than response to light touch, which may elicit a rapid kick.[7–9]

The price for such good sedation and analgesia is a host of side effects that generally are of little consequence to the healthy horse but may further compromise the critically ill. Of practical importance for someone trying to work around an α_2-sedated horse is the dose-dependent ataxia. Romifidine causes less ataxia than xylazine and detomidine[5] while medetomidine, at an intravenous dose of 10 μg/kg may cause some horses to go down.[10] The cardiovascular effects of α_2-agonists have potential repercussions on peripheral perfusion. The administration of α_2-agonists results in an initial vasoconstriction and increase in arterial blood pres-

* Rompun; Bayer Animal Health, Newbury, Berkshire, UK; Chanazine 10%, Chanelle Animal Health, Liverpool, UK.
† Sedivet; Boehringer Ingelheim, Bracknell, Berkshire, UK.
‡ Domosedan; Pfizer, Sandwich, Kent, UK.
§ Domitor, Pfizer, Sandwich, Kent, UK.

** Precedex; Abbott Laboratories, Abbott Park, IL, USA.

Table 6.1. Common equine sedatives used for standing chemical restraint or behavioural modification (doses are given in mg/kg)

	IV	IM	Sublingual/oral	Constant rate infusion rate
	(Approximate duration of action in minutes)			Loading dose; infusion rate
α_2-Agonists				
Xylazine	0.2–1.1 (15–40)	0.5–2.2 (40–90)	ND	1.0 mg/kg; 12 μg/kg/min
Detomidine	0.004–0.02 (40–90)	0.02–0.05 (90–150)	Sublingual: 0.04–0.08 (90–180)	0.006–0.015 mg/kg; 0.1–0.6 μg/kg/min
Romifidine	0.05–0.12 (40–60)	0.1–0.2 (80–120)	Sublingual not effective at 0.12	ND
Medetomidine	0.004–0.01 (30–50)	0.01–0.02 (60–120)	ND	0.005 mg/kg; 0.06 μg/kg/min
Phenothiazines				
Acepromazine	0.02–0.06 (90–180)	0.03–0.1 (180–360)	0.1–0.5 (240–360)	ND
Fluphenazine	ND	25 mg/horse (4–6 weeks)	ND	ND
Perphenazine	ND	ND	0.375 SID	ND
Benzodazepines				
Diazepam	0.02–0.1 (50–70)	0.1–0.2 (ND)	ND	ND
Midazolam	0.02–0.1 (45–60)	0.1–0.2 (ND)	ND	ND
Opioids				
Butorphanol	0.01–0.04 (45–60)	0.04–0.2 (120–240)	ND	0.018 mg/kg; 0.38 μg/kg/min
Morphine	0.02–0.2 (60–90)	0.2–0.6 (120–180)	ND	ND
Pethidine (Meperidine)	(0.2–0.4) may release histamine	0.4–2.0 (60–90)	ND	ND
Buprenorphine	0.004–0.010 (60–90)	ND	ND	ND
Hypnotics				
Choral hydrate <12% solution	10–50 (60–180)	Caustic	20–60 (240–360)	ND
Pentobarbital	1–2 (30–60)	Caustic	ND	ND
Phenobarbital	1–10 (360–720)	Caustic	11 SID	ND
Reserpine	1.0–2.0 mg/horse, (every 48 hr)	1.0–2.5 mg/horse (≈21 days)	1.04–4.0 mg/horse SID	ND

ND, no data available or not applicable; SID, once daily.
See text for references.

sure that is accompanied by an often pronounced bradycardia and second-degree atrioventricular block. This is followed by hypotension and continued lower than baseline cardiac output that persists beyond the clinically evident sedation.[1] Although the ultimate reduction in cardiac output (40–50%) and blood pressure (≈20%) is comparable for the five drugs for which it has been reported in the horse (xylazine, detomidine, romifidine, medetomidine and dexmedetomidine), it and the atrioventricular block are of shorter duration after xylazine, medetomidine and dexmedetomidine than after romifidine and detomidine.[2,5,11] A consequence of reduced cardiac output is decreased tissue perfusion resulting in a decrease in mixed venous partial pressure of oxygen.[4,11] Intravenous xylazine has been shown to decrease caecal[12,13] and digital blood flow[14] in awake horses. This hypoperfusion may be driven by reduced cardiac performance but regional vascular smooth muscle also contains α_2-receptors that mediate vasoconstriction. Thus, an increase in jejunal vascular resistance has been reported in isolated equine jejunal segments.[15] Within the equine veterinary community, sudden collapse and death have been anecdotally recognised following intravenous xylazine, detomidine and romifidine. Collapse is usually due to severe bradycardia but the mechanism of death in these cases is unknown. Presumably, it is cardiac in origin as xylazine has been shown to enhance the arrhythmogenicity of inhalant anaesthetics[16] and is associated with an increased risk of anaesthesia-related death in horses.[17] Respiratory rates generally decrease after administration of an α_2-agonist, but the occasional horse will become tachypnoeic.[18] In either case and for all four of the available agents, the partial pressure of oxygen in arterial blood decreases 10 to 20% and some horses may become truly hypoxaemic (<60 mm Hg). Again, anecdotally, some of the horses that have an increased respiratory rate after being given an α_2-agonist have been noted to sweat more profusely than is typical of α_2 sedation. Thermoregulation is altered by activation of α_2-adrenoceptors. Rats[19] and foals[20] given xylazine become hypothermic. Detomidine, however, may cause a delayed rise in rectal temperature in rats[19] and horses.[21] There is some suggestion that "puffers" and horses that become hypoxaemic or febrile may have underlying conditions that predispose them to these responses. Hypothalamic α_2-adrenceptors presumably mediate this response and are also the likely explanation for inhibition of antidiuretic hormone release and the dose-dependent diuresis that is a feature of α_2-sedation in the horse.[22–24] Hyperglycaemia may contribute to the diuresis, but the elevated blood glucose concentrations do not always reach glomerular threshold and glycosuria is not a consistent finding.[22,24] α_2-Adrenoceptor activation modulates the stress response in the horse: decreasing circulation catecholamines, cortisol, free fatty acids and insulin.[25–27] Another organ system well populated with α_2-adrenoceptors is the gastrointestinal tract. Liquid and solid phase gastric emptying are delayed.[28,29] Xylazine, detomidine and romifidine have all been shown to decrease duodenal, ileal, caecal and colonic motor activity.[30–33] This may partially explain the pain relief provided by xylazine and detomidine in colicky horses.[34] In summary, there may be instances when the superior sedation induced by α_2-agonists is too costly to a patient's overall well-being and avoiding them, or minimising peak blood concentrations, is wise. One means of reducing peak concentrations and many side effects is to administer the drugs intramuscularly,[35,36] in the case of detomidine sublingually[37] or by constant rate infusion.[18,38,39] Another approach is to combine them with other sedatives or analgesics.

Phenothiazines

The other major family of tranquilisers used in horses is the phenothiazines. Acepromazine†† is the most popular, but descriptions of chlorpromazine‡‡, promazine§§, propionylpromazine*** and the longer-acting agents, fluphenazine†††, perphenazine‡‡‡ and pipothiazine§§§, can be found in the literature of the past two decades.[40–43] Typically, sedation produced by acepromazine given intravenously, intramuscularly or orally is less profound and of longer duration than that of xylazine.[44–46] Repetitive operant behaviour[47] and random movement[48] are slowed. Head position is lowered, reaction to tactile stimulation and apparent awareness of the environment are decreased, but reaction to noise is retained.[48] Sedation is accompanied by dose-dependent penile relaxation.[46,47] A consistent side effect is systemic hypotension, which may be of longer duration than the apparent sedation.[43,45,48,49] The α_1-adrenergic receptor block on arterial smooth muscle responsible for the drop in blood pressure also occurs on the smooth muscle of the venous capacitance vessels and the splenic capsule. Thus, venous return, cardiac output and packed cell volume decrease, whereas plasma volume and total plasma protein concentration remain unchanged. Heart rate may increase or decrease.[47,49,50] Large colon[51] and digital vessels dilate,[14] allowing greater regional blood flow as long as blood volume, blood pressure and cardiac output are adequate. The α_1-adrenergic block is comparable in magnitude but of longer duration following chlorpromazine and promazine than acepromazine.[43] Similar haemodynamic changes have also been reported after the intravenous administration of a combination of propionylpromazine and promethazine to ponies.[42] The shorter duration of action, in addition to greater potency and a lower incidence of paradoxical excitement described with propionylpromazine and chlorpromazine,[43,52] has made acepromazine the preferred phenothiazine. Phenothiazines variously block dopaminergic, α-adrenergic, serotonergic, muscarinic and histaminergic receptors in the central and peripheral nervous systems. A clinically relevant consequence is loss of thermoregulation, which, combined with peripheral vasodilatation allowing greater heat loss, can lead to a decrease in body temperature, particularly in foals.[20,49] Respiratory drive is obtunded.[53] Liquid-, but not solid-, phase gastric emptying is delayed[28,29] and small intestinal myoelectrical activity is decreased[54] by acepromazine. The long-acting phenothiazines have less α-adrenergic but greater dopaminergic blocking activity and cause less hypotension, but stereotypic behaviour and dyskenesia may occur at therapeutic doses.[55] Excitability and hyperaesthesia have been reported following oral perphenazine[56] and muscle spasms and restlessness after intramuscular fluphenazine[41,57] and pipothiazine.[40]

A majority of the undesirable side effects seen with the administration of either the α_2-agonists or acepromazine are dose dependent.[1,47,49] Reducing the doses of acepromazine and xylazine each by 50% and administering them together intravenously attenuated the cardiopulmonary depression yet produced better or comparable sedation to that of the higher doses of either alone.[45] Combining either with an agent with minimal or complementary side effects would be a reasonable approach to optimal sedation.

Opioids

Opioids, when given intravenously to pain-free horses, have been reported to have no significant cardiopulmonary effects[58] or increase heart rate, blood pressure and cardiac output.[59–61] Given to nonpainful horses, morphine****, pethidine (meperidine)††††, oxymorphone‡‡‡‡, methadone§§§§, hydromorphone*****, butorphanol†††††,

†† ACP Injection 10 mg/ml; Novartis Animal Health, Litlington, Herts, UK; PromAce; Fort Dodge Animal Health, Fort Dodge, IA, USA; AceMav; MAVLAB PTY LTD, Slacks Creek, Qld, Australia.

‡‡ Thorazine; SmithKline Beecham, Pittsburgh, PA, USA.

§§ Sparine; Wyeth Laboratories, Philadelphia, PA, USA.

*** Tranvet; Diamond Laboratories, Des Moines, IA, USA.

††† Modecate; Bristol-Myers Squibb Pharmaceuticals, Leopardstown, Dublin, Ireland.

‡‡‡ Trilafon; Schering-Plough, Kenilworth, NJ, USA.

§§§ Piportal Depot, sanofi-aventis, Paris, France.

**** Morphine Sulphate Injection; Antigen Pharmaceuticals, Dublin 4, Ireland.

†††† Pethidine Injection 50 mg/ml; Arnolds Veterinary Products, Shrewsbury, Shropshire, UK; Demerol, Abbott Laboratories, Abbott Park, IL, USA; Pethidine Injection, Parnell Laboratories, Alexandria, NSW, Australia.

‡‡‡‡ Numorphan; DuPont Pharma, Wilmington, DE, USA.

§§§§ Dolophine; Roxane Laboratories, Columbus, OH, USA.

***** Dilaudid; Abbott Laboratories, Abbott Park, IL, USA.

††††† Torbugesic; Fort Dodge Animal Health, Fort Dodge, IA, USA.

pentazocine‡‡‡‡‡, buprenorphine§§§§§, fentanyl****** and alfentanil†††††† have all been shown to produce dysphoria characterised by stereotypic locomotor activity and ataxia.[58–60,62,63] Respiratory rate is increased after the administration of opioids to horses but arterial P_{CO_2} and P_{O_2} are not significantly changed.[58,59,61] Although liquid-phase gastric emptying was delayed by the intravenous administration of larger doses (0.05 mg/kg) of butorphanol than typically used in chemical restraint[28] (0.01–2 mg/kg), gastroduodenal motility and pelvic flexure myoelectric and mechanical activity were minimally affected.[64,65] Likewise, jejunal vascular resistance and metabolism were unchanged by butorphanol given to anaesthetised ponies.[66] In a toxicity study, repeated doses of 1.0 mg/kg intravenous butorphanol over 48 hours decreased auscultable borborygmi in two horses, one of which developed an impaction.[67] Morphine, but not butorphanol, pethidine (meperidine) or oxymorphone prolonged intestinal transit of proethylene glycol.[68] Pethidine (meperidine), morphine and fentanyl inhibited jejunal and colonic motor activity.[54,69]

The contribution that opioids make to the sedation and analgesia created with α_2-agonists and/or tranquilisation with acepromazine is more than additive.[7,8,70–71] Fortunately, administering an α_2-agonist or acepromazine with an opioid reduces the dysphoria to head pressing, occasional head and facial twitching or somnolence.[9,72,73] Depending on the specific opioid and neurolept chosen, their doses and the routes and times of administration, the cardiopulmonary side effects of each are modulated.[7,9,70,72,74] When combined with α_2-agonists, opioids tend to attenuate the late decrease in systemic arterial blood pressure, modify the decrease in cardiac output, but may prolong the duration of atrioventricular block. Generally, mild to moderate decreases in respiratory rates and arterial partial pressure of oxygen with increases in arterial partial pressure of carbon dioxide have been reported.[7,70,72,74] The addition of butorphanol to detomidine or xylazine further slowed solid-phase gastric emptying[29] or duodenal motor activity,[75] respectively. Butorphanol with xylazine prolonged the decrease in caecal motor activity compared to xylazine alone but did not worsen the decrease in caecal blood flow.[30]

Other sedatives, tranquilisers and hypnotics

There is also a scattering of sedatives, tranquilisers or hypnotics that have been used to modify equine behaviour and have potential value in calming the unhappy hospitalised horse. The least marginal of these are the benzodiazepines: diazepam‡‡‡‡‡‡ and midazolam§§§§§§. Given alone to healthy horses, moderate doses of diazepam cause a brief phase of dysphoria and muscle weakness that is rapidly followed by a return to apparently normal mentation and compensated posture. The residual sedation is subtle and the horse appears to be less concerned about its painful or distressing experience. In contrast, foals less than 2 to 3 weeks of age are clearly sedated, become recumbent and tolerate minimally painful manipulations.[20] Used in combination with an α_2-agonist, diazepam balances the sedation much in the way acepromazine does. At clinically conservative doses, diazepam has minimal cardiovascular or pulmonary effects, whereas larger doses cause mild hypotension, a more evident anxiolysis and ataxia and recumbency is possible.[76] As in other species, diazepam stimulates appetite in horses.[77] Midazolam has been shown to delay gastric emptying and gastrointestinal transit time in mice dose dependently,[78] but the gastrointestinal effects of benzodiazepines have not been investigated in the horse. Both the intravenous and intramuscular pharmacokinetics and pharmacodynamics of diazepam vary considerably across individual horses.[76,79] Midazolam differs from diazepam in that it is slightly more potent, water soluble and shorter acting. These characteristics make its pharmacokinetics are more predicable. The haemodynamic and respiratory effects of midazolam have not been studied in the horse. However, in people, hypotension, decreased cardiac output and tachycardia are more common than with diazepam. Mild respiratory depression is similar for the two drugs.[80]

Chloral hydrate******* is a traditional and sometimes useful sedative/hypnotic.[81,82] When given at doses intended for standing sedation, chloral hydrate has little effect on cardiovascular or respiratory function although heart rate may increase.[83,84] As the dose is increased, there is potential for bradycardia, dysrhythmias, decreased gastrointestinal motility and recumbency.[81,83,84] Dosing is slowly to effect as there is considerable individual variation in response. Slight overdose results in ataxia and recumbency. Successful, profound hypnosis is achievable in the presence of marked distress when α_2-agonists, acepromazine and opioids fail. The onset and duration of sedation are dependent on dose and concomitant sedatives or analgesics. Given alone, a low dose of chloral hydrate can produce light sedation for approximately an hour.[85] Given with α_2-agonists and morphine to control unmanageable

‡‡‡‡‡ Talwin; Sanofi-Aventis, Paris, France.

§§§§§ Vetergesic; Alstoe Animal Health, Sherrif Hutton, Yorks., UK; Buprenex, Reckitt Benckiser, Slough, Berks, UK.

****** Sublimaze; Akorn Inc, Buffalo Grove, IL, USA.

†††††† Alfenta; Akorn Inc, Buffalo Grove, IL, USA.

‡‡‡‡‡‡ Valium; Roche Laboratories, Basel. Switzerland; Diazemuls; Dumex Ltd, Whiddon Valley, Barnstaple, EX32 8NS, UK; Diazepam Injection; Parnell Laboratories, Alexandria, NSW, Australia.

§§§§§§ Midazolam Injection; Antigen Pharmaceuticals, Dublin 4, Ireland.

******* Chloral hydrate crystals; available from a variety of suppliers of generic brand pharmaceuticals.

abdominal pain, redosing may be needed at 4 to 6 hours.[82] The sedation created by chloral hydrate is similar in character to that of the benzodiazepines as the horses appear more distracted, with a distant expression on their faces, than sleepy. Choral hydrate is irritating to tissues, even to the gastric mucosa, and should be given as a dilute solution (<12%), through an intravenous catheter or by stomach tube, and not intramuscularly.

The other hypnotics to possibly resort to when all else fails are the barbiturates. Historically, pentobarbital††††††† has been used at sedative doses.[86] In some extreme circumstances, for example, when seizures are a component of the presentation, pentobarbital might be a useful addition to restraint efforts.[57] Phenobarbital§§§§§§§ is a choice for long-term control of seizures and doses may be adjusted, or other sedatives or opioids added, to achieve a degree of additional, titratable sedation.[84] Overdose of barbiturates results in hypotension, myocardial and respiratory depression and, consequently, decrease in tissue perfusion and ultimately death. The therapeutic index is smaller than any of the other agents discussed here.

Reserpine******** blocks the uptake of catecholamines into storage vesicles in nerve terminals. This results in the depletion of the neurotransmitters norepinephrine, serotonin and dopamine, imbalances in central neurotransmission and decreased spontaneous motor activity and response to stimulation (sedation/depression). Concomitantly, autonomic balance is disrupted and bradycardia, hypotension, loss of appetite and thirst and increased gastrointestinal motility occur.[87,88] Today, reserpine is most commonly used for long-term taming of nervous horses. Although dose related, onset is delayed (hours), even after intravenous administration and duration of action is prolonged (days). Ptosis, depression, reduced activity and diarrhoea are the clinical hallmarks of reserpine. Colic and dehydration are concerns.[88] A case of reserpine toxicity in a horse given 12.5 mg IV presented with depression, muscle fasciculations, bradycardia, miosis, paraphimosis, flatulence and episodic abdominal pain that gradually recovered over several days.[89]

Clinical applications

Musculoskeletal conditions

Horses are hospitalised for a wide variety of problems. With the exception of fractures and some myopathies, the least compromising to life are the musculoskeletal diseases. While in residence, orthopaedic cases may need sedation for preoperative or postoperative diagnostic tests such as radiography or ultrasonography. The restraint requirements are of short duration and tolerant of minor breeches of immobility. The exception to this is the case of standing, distal limb magnetic resonance imaging (MRI), where the entire scan may take an hour and any motion during an individual scan sequence will interfere with the image. Another use for sedation is daily wound management. Debridement and lavage of painful, difficult-to-access sites, such as a hind limb tendon sheath or fistulous poll, is needed. Certainly for the average radiographic set of the average, worried horse, xylazine (150–200 mg) is likely to prove sufficient. If the target is the hind leg of a less than cooperative individual, adding butorphanol (5 mg) usually does the trick. If a slightly longer duration is required, combining xylazine (150–200 mg) and detomidine (2.5 mg) or romifidine (50 mg) with or without butorphanol (2.5–5 mg) depending on the extremity and horse's temperament works well. The advantage to using xylazine with detomidine and not just detomidine is that the onset of xylazine is more rapid. This results in an earlier and longer overall peak effect. Simply giving larger doses of xylazine would be more likely to cause ataxia. On the other hand, intramuscular (10–15 mg) or constant rate infusion detomidine will give even longer-duration, more-consistent sedation for standing MRI. Adding IM acepromazine (15 mg) or IV or IM butorphanol (5–10 mg), again depending on which limb and the overall attitude of the horse, could be the little touch of stability needed to achieve reliable immobilisation. For the painful wound, slightly larger doses of xylazine or xylazine plus detomidine with butorphanol (5–10 mg) or possibly morphine (60–100 mg) if the horse is extremely sensitive to wound contact should work. In all cases, the horses should be monitored after returning to their stalls as postsedation choke may occur.

The other category of orthopaedic cases that might benefit from sedation are those unable to accept the stall confinement prescribed for their injury. These horses may be managed with daily or as needed intramuscular acepromazine (20 mg q8–12 hours). In some instances, the slightly more determined sedation of a combination of intramuscular acepromazine and detomidine (10 mg) or romifidine (50 mg) could be used to condition the horse to its new circumstance. As the potential side effects of long-term use of α_2-agonist, particularly with respect to gastrointestinal motility, are unknown, the plan would be to wean the horse of this element of the combination within a day or two. If the recuperation period is expected to be long (weeks), use of one of the long duration of action phenothiazines might be indicated. Likewise, reserpine has been used in such horses. Either choice should be used with care. The side effects of overdoses of fluphenazine are dramatic and an orthopaedic repair could be disrupted or additional damage incurred. Careful dosing to effect (10–15 mg IM; evaluate over several days before 5–10 mg)

††††††† Nembutal; Ovation Pharmaceuticals Inc., Deerfield, IL, USA; Nembutal; Merial Australia PTY, Parramatta NSW, Australia. Nonsterile pentobarbital preparations designed for euthanasia are not suitable for sedation.

§§§§§§§ Epiphen; Vetoquinol UK Ltd, Great Slade, Buckingham, UK; Phenomav; MAVLAB PTY LTD, Slacks Creek, Qld, Australia.

******** Generic reserpine is available in the United States; NV Rakelin Injection; Nature Vet PTY, Glenorie, NSW, Australia.

should avoid this. Effective doses of reserpine (1–2 mg IV, IM, PO) can cause major, persistent disruptions of physiological homeostasis that could debilitate an already stressed individual. Although there are no published reports of the use of a benzodiazepine to manage stall-bound horses, diazepam has been used illegally in performance horses.[90] Diazepam or midazolam may, in fact, be useful given intramuscularly (50 mg).

Horses suffering exertional myopathy have traditionally been managed with acepromazine and supportive care because of both its anxiolytic and vasodilating properties.[91] Nonsteroidal anti-inflammatory agents are also routinely used, but adding an opioid to obtund the pain of muscle spasm and inflammation could help. Theoretically, α_2-agonists might be used for sedation and analgesia but the therapeutic objective to optimise muscle and renal blood flow might be compromised. Inherited muscle diseases such as hyperkalaemic periodic paralysis and polysaccharide storage myopathy are often triggered by exercise or stress.[92,93] Transport to the hospital and hospitalisation may be sufficiently stressful to precipitate an episode. For elective hospitalisations, these horses should be prepared medically and with diet adjustments as appropriate. In the short term, if the required hospital care precipitates myopathic episodes, low-dose intramuscular acepromazine during the hospital stay may control anxiety.

Conditions of the head and neck

The other population of relatively healthy, hospitalised horses that are likely to require sedation consists of the "head cases". These are horses with an upper respiratory, sinus, tooth or eye condition or injury in which a specific objective of sedation is to have the head where it can be worked on, not 10 feet in the air. The α_2-agonists are particularly good at lowering a horse's head. However, noise, sudden movement or light changes will, unpredictably, override this even when large doses are administered. Adding butorphanol will generally contribute the necessary additional sedation and analgesia to permit manipulation of a sinus flap or dental plug. During endoscopic evaluation of upper airway function, xylazine has been shown to distort pharyngeal mechanics.[94,95] If opioids are added to the sedation for ocular procedures, the facial and head twitching may not be completely masked by the concurrent α_2-agonist. This may make working on the globe precarious and examination of intraocular structures frustrating. However, since often the advantage gained by adding an opioid is critical to the horse tolerating the procedure at all, the opioid tick can be minimised for a short procedure, such as a subpalpebral injection, by adding physical restraint with a twitch. Systemically administered sedatives will not render the eye anaesthetic and therefore topical anaesthetic and regional nerve blocks (see Chapter 1.48) are necessary to anaesthetise the cornea and periocular tissues or to paralyse the eyelids. With regard to the eye itself, both α_2-agonists and opioids cause mydriasis[19,21]; therefore, pupillary size and light response should be evaluated before sedation when possible. Many equine ophthalmological cases include some form of corneal injury such that intraocular pressure becomes a concern when sedating a horse for evaluation and treatment. Both acepromazine and xylazine decrease intraocular pressure[96,97]; however, the head-down position assumed by a well-sedated horse may increase intraocular pressure by impeding venous outflow.

Neurological disease

Horses hospitalised with neurological disease are usually the severely affected cases. Those with lesser deficits are more often presented as outpatients for gait abnormalities or loss of athletic performance. Hospitalised neurological cases may be sedated for two reasons: for acquisition of cerebrospinal fluid (CSF) during diagnostic evaluation or to manage the animal's distress related to its inability to ambulate normally. The concerns related to CSF aspiration from a neurologically compromised horse are restraint without additional ataxia and impact on intracranial pressure. Often, these horses are apprehensive, vulnerable and in a strange environment being handled by strange people. Typically, the apprehensive, excited horse requires larger doses to achieve reasonable sedation. Unfortunately, a slightly greater dose than necessary may create excessive sedation and ataxia. Thus, careful dosing using combinations of drugs is most likely to be successful. The veterinary lore that phenothiazines lower the seizure threshold stems from their use in experimental models of epilepsy[98] but has been difficult to confirm in clinical situations. No effort has been made to do so in horses. Adding acepromazine (5 mg IV) certainly allows for the use of lower doses of xylazine (100–150 mg) and together they produce a more stable, quieter horse for longer than would be achieved with a higher dose of xylazine alone. Adding a drop (3 mg) of butorphanol would deepen the sedation. Local anaesthetic infiltration is necessary to prevent painful stimulation with needle insertion. Whether the tendency of romifidine to create less ataxia would be of advantage in this situation has not been reported.

Central neurological disease in the horse is more often infectious than neoplastic and therefore marked increases in intracranial pressure are not a common component of its pathophysiology. However, until that diagnosis is made, the potential for increased intracranial pressure being compounded by agents used for standing chemical restraint should be kept in the back of the clinician's mind. Lumbosacral aspiration of CSF could precipitate pressure shifts and brain stem herniation. Sedation that reduces blood pressure and cardiac output will decrease cerebral perfusion. Elevation of arterial carbon dioxide due to sedation-induced hypoventilation causes cerebral vasodilation that increases intracranial pressure. As with intraocular pressure, gravity and the head-down position increase intracranial pressure by adversely affecting venous outflow from the intracranial compartment.[100] Lumbosacral CSF pressure decreased when horses were allowed to stand in the classic α_2-agonist head-down position after xylazine[99]. Thus, paying attention to the sedated horse's head position is important, not only for successful CSF aspiration from the lumbosacral space but also for optimal intracranial haemodynamics.

The other call for sedation in neurologically abnormal horses is to minimise the distress of their losing the ability to flee, the instinctive response of this prey species to any perceived threat. Most horses that are able to remain standing adapt or at least mask their fear. However, it is rare for a conscious horse to accept recumbency from which it cannot rise and neurologically recumbent horses may fight persistently to be sternal or stand. In such cases, where return to function is expected to take days, not hours, sedation with longer-acting agents, intramuscular administrations or constant rate infusions are the logical approach. Dosing intervals and drug half-lives that allow a glimpse of the less-sedated individual to assess the progression of the disease are also advantageous. Recumbent horses are also often painful from trauma inflicted during their struggles or from myopathy. Adding an opioid will enhance the sedation and provide some analgesia. Concerns to keep in mind include elevated intracranial pressure that may be raised due to position and to hypoventilation secondary to recumbency and sedation. Fluid and electrolyte balance may be challenged by long-term α_2-agonist mediated diuresis and natiuresis.[22–24,101] As has been discussed, most of the drugs mentioned in this chapter have been shown to alter gastrointestinal motility in the normal horse. Combined with recumbency and inability to eat, gastrointestinal stasis, gas distension and/or impaction are potential complications. Although acepromazine might not be an optimal choice in cases of intracranial disease, its use intramuscularly at a moderate dose (10–20 mg) would complement intramuscular (20 mg) or constant rate infusion detomidine (0.5 μg/kg/min, adjusted to effect), with or without butorphanol (20 mg IM or 0.38 μg/kg/min IV),[102] allowing lower doses or rates to create a happier horse. If the cardiovascular side effects of medetomidine are truly less pronounced and its tendency to produce recumbency real,[10,18] its administration by constant rate infusion (0.06 μg/kg/min) might be an interesting choice of α_2-agonist for these horses.[18] The benzodiazepines and barbiturates should be considered as components of the sedative management when, but not necessarily only when, seizures are a component of the signalment. Phenobarbital pharmacokinetics have been studied in the horse and it has been used effectively to control seizures. Depending on the individual case, phenobarbital alone may be sufficient to reduce purposeful struggling. The depth of hypnosis may be fine-tuned to create a quiet but responsive horse, if lower phenobarbital doses are combined with low doses of other agents. Intramuscular diazepam might be complementary. In theory, midazolam would be a better choice because of its more predictable absorption from the muscle and shorter, more-consistent half-life but there is little in the literature on the use of midazolam as a sedative in horses. The additional muscle relaxation with little cardiovascular or respiratory effects of the benzodiazepines could be advantageous during the early phase of recumbency. An indication for adding chloral hydrate to the cocktail would be when combinations of the more commonly available sedatives do not control the horse or do so only for short durations.[82,103]

Respiratory conditions

Horses hospitalised with pneumonia or pleuritis may need sedation for bronchoscopy, lung biopsy, thoracocentesis, drain placement or thoroscopy. The first four of these are relatively short-duration procedures with varying degrees of painful invasion. Sedation for all would best include some degree of cough suppression: moderate in the case of bronchoscopy and complete, if possible, for the other procedures. Once again, the α_2-agonists with or without an opioid are the most reasonable choice. For longer procedures, premedication with intramuscular acepromazine permits a degree of baseline sedation that allows lower doses of detomidine or romifidine or rates of detomidine infusion. Infiltration of local anaesthetic provides anaesthesia at sites of thoracic wall entry. Generally, the α_2-agonists cause nonsignificant decreases in arterial oxygenation in normal horses[1,3,4] and thus may aggravate disease-associated hypoxaemia. This can usually be managed by insufflating oxygen to augment fractional inspired oxygen. Horses with chronic obstructive pulmonary disease that are hospitalised are usually too sick to require sedation. It is best to avoid sedation for pulmonary function testing of less severely affected horses, if possible, as several of the α_2-agonists and opioids, alone and in combination, have been shown to alter respiratory mechanics.[61,104,105]

Cardiac conditions

Atrial fibrillation, congestive heart failure or pericardial tamponade are the cardiac diseases for which a horse might be hospitalised. Most are not likely to require sedation. In the latter two instances, the horses may be distressed but relief of the cause using supportive measures such as oxygen and medication or pericardiocentesis are definitive therapies. Should such horses need sedation, choices that encourage forward arterial flow and maintain venous return without affecting contractility or electrical activity would be ideal. Of course, no such drug exists. Diazepam may be the closest as it is less of an arterial and venous dilator than midazolam and acepromazine in healthy animals. The α_2-agonists would be the worst choice as they increase afterload and are arrhythmogenic. In addition, detomidine has been shown to significantly alter cardiac dimensions and function as determined by echocardiography.[106] However, the subtle quality and undetermined duration of benzodiazepine sedation might not suffice.

Opioids would be helpful if the excitement phase that is accompanied by an increase in heart rate and blood pressure could be controlled. The conservative approach, should sedation be absolutely necessary, would be small doses of a combination of agents (perhaps 15 mg diazepam, 100 mg xylazine and 3 mg butorphanol, with oxygen insufflation) to settle the horse enough for thoracic radiographs, full cardiac evaluation or pericardiocentesis. Horses in atrial fibrillation may be moderately fit athletes and unruly. Their myocardial contractility is usually normal. The concern is that the sedatives most likely to control them, α_2-agonists, slow atrioventricular conduction and ventricular rate could drop to potentially dangerous levels. If given in conjunction with an anti-muscarinic, the risk is of excessive atrioventricular conduction and ventricular tachycardia and dysrhythmias. The degrees to which the various α_2-agonists slow sinus spontaneous activity and atrioventricular conduction are similar. Xylazine may be the safest in that the period of bradycardia, in most horses, is short. Having an antimuscarinic on hand and monitoring the heart rate after xylazine may be the most expedient method of dealing with the horse in atrial fibrillation that will not stand still. Theoretically, an α_2-antagonist (yohimbine, tolazoline or atipamazole) could be administered should the ventricular rate become life threateningly slow.

Gastrointestinal disorders

Horses hospitalised with gastrointestinal disease most commonly suffer from choke, acute abdominal disease, requiring medical or surgical management, or colitis. Acepromazine, detomidine and xylazine with butorphanol decreased spontaneous oesophageal mechanical activity.[107] In addition, the head-down posture assumed by horses sedated with α_2-agonists make these agents ideal for working in the oesophagus whether to relieve an obstruction or evaluate postobstruction damage and healing. For horses with colic, sedation may be needed during the diagnostic phase of the disease but, ultimately, providing analgesia becomes a primary objective and sedation secondary or even a side effect. Because the α_2-agonists are so effective at controlling the painful colicky horse, it is easy to forget that they have been shown to decrease gastrointestinal motility and blood flow in normal horses.[12,13,15,31–33] To the extent that they have been studied in the horse, the inhibitory effects of acepromazine and the opioids on gastrointestinal activity may be less pronounced.[13,28,29,54,69] Chloral hydrate in combination with morphine has been used to sedate colicky horses when xylazine or detomidine were only transiently effective.[82] Relatively large doses of diazepam (50 mg IM) have been helpful in these difficult to manage colics as well. Horses with colic, colitis or peritonitis may be in an acute systemic inflammatory state, one characteristic of which is depression. These horses will be tachycardic, hypertensive or hypotensive, tachypnoeic but numb to all but their abdominal pain. Interestingly, there is some indication that α_2-adrenoreceptors may mediate the gastrointestinal inhibitory effects of endotoxin.[108,109] The tenesmus accompanying colitis is not responsive to systemic sedatives, leaving little indication for sedation in the management of these cases unless for a short-duration diagnostic procedure.

Hepatic and urogenital conditions

Hepatic or renal disease, cystic calculi, pregnancy or postparturient metritis may hospitalise a horse. Frequently, pregnancy is coincidental to the primary indication for hospitalisation. Sedation may be required for hepatic or renal biopsy. Hepatic metabolism and renal excretion are the ultimate elimination routes of all the drugs included in this discussion. Subclinical hepatic disease has been cited as the possible cause for an unusually long duration of analgesia following intravenous detomidine.[110] Should standing chemical restraint be needed for hepatic or renal ultrasound and biopsy, assuming the horse is well hydrated, acepromazine, the α_2-agonists or opioids can be used judiciously. Logical choices would be shorter acting combinations to reduce peak dose, thereby limiting adverse effects such as reduced blood flow that might further compromise the unhealthy tissue. The manipulation of the bladder, urethra or uterus in a standing, detomidine-sedated horse has been anecdotally associated with sudden collapse and death. The mechanism of this acute death is unknown but may be a viscerovagal reflex or, in the case of a uterus distended with air for surgical removal of polyps, air embolisation.

Pregnant and nursing mares pose a multifaceted consideration for sedation: there is the mare, her uterus and her foetus or her milk and her foal. Elevated levels of circulating progesterone and endogenous opioids in pregnant women have a calming effect that reduces sedative and anaesthetic drug requirement. Clinically, this is hard to appreciate in mares, and dosing is based on experience and need. Many professional broodmares, in fact, are not handled extensively and therefore require slightly larger than average doses. Despite the fact that xylazine, detomidine and romifidine increase uterine tone in nonpregnant mares,[111] these drugs have been used extensively and repeatedly in pregnant mares without apparent problems.[112,113] In the third trimester of pregnancy, intramuscular detomidine decreased myometrial electrical activity.[114] In the normal postparturient uterus, detomidine enhances the myotonic activity of oxytocin.[115] Generally, if a drug can cross the blood-brain barrier, it will cross the placenta and will appear in the milk as similar molecular characteristics are determinants of diffusion across these barriers. Thus, it is not surprising that detomidine administered to the third-trimester mare has been found to decrease foetal activity, heart rate and aortic blood flow. Xylazine decreases foetal heart rate and acepromazine increases foetal heart rate without changing aortic flow.[113,116,117] Milk concentrations of sedatives have not been studied in the mare, nor has sedation in suckling foals been reported after administration of sedatives or anaesthetics to lactating mares, but these are concerns in milk-producing species and human neonates.[118–120] Many sedative drugs also alter hormonal secretion in mares. The greater antidopaminergic activity of longer-acting phenothiazines has been shown to increase serum prolactin levels, protect against fescue toxicity and hasten spring ovulation.[121,122] Xylazine has been shown to increase luteinizing hormone and follicle-stimulating hormone pulsatile secretion.[123] Thus, the prolonged or repeated exposure of open broodmares to sedation may influence their ovulation pattern.

Neonatal foals

Sedating the hospitalised neonatal foal is considerably different from sedating the 1- or 6-month-old foal, whose responses rapidly approach those of the adult. Except in the most robust neonate or more painful procedures, diazepam or midazolam (≈0.1 mg/kg IV) with or without butorphanol (≈0.04 mg/kg IV) will produce a recumbent, easily restrained patient for short procedures (15–30 minutes). Using local anaesthetic infiltration provides regional or local anaesthesia as needed. The pharmacokinetics of diazepam in 4-day-old foals showed a smaller volume of distribution and clearance compared to foals older than 21 days, further illustrating the differences between neonatal and older equines.[124] Resistant neonates and older foals sedate well with α_2-agonists, but hypothermia, bradycardia, hypotension and unpredictable depth of sedation are real concerns.[125–128] Given equivalent mg/kg doses of xylazine, some foals will continue to fight restraint and manipulation, whereas others, ostensibly as healthy, will become recumbent and less responsive to stimulation for longer than expected. Progressive hypothermia will compound this, and it is wise to keep these foals warm and consider reversing the α_2-agonist when the need for restraint is satisfied. The less-effective sedation, longer duration of action and potential for hypothermia of acepromazine make it the least useful sedative for young foals.

In conclusion, the hospitalised horse presents many of the same challenges to sedation as those encountered in the field. On the other hand, these horses are often receiving a potpourri of medications and drug interactions will change sedative pharmacokinetics.[129] As a general population, hospitalised horses are less healthy, making it more important to take into consideration the side effects of the drugs chosen for standing chemical restraint. Combinations using smaller doses of several agents are a method of reducing side effects without sacrificing, and often improving, effectiveness.

References

1. England GCW, Clarke KW: Alpha$_2$ adrenergic agonists in the horse—a review. Br Vet J 152:641-657, 1996
2. England GCW, Clarke KW, Goossens L: A comparison of the sedative effects of the α_2-adrenoceptor agonists (romifidine, detomidine and xylazine) in the horse. J Vet Pharmacol Ther 15:194-201, 1992
3. Yamashita K, Tsubakishita S, Futaoka S, Ueda K, Hamaguchi H, Seno T, Katoh S, Izumisawa Y, Kotani T, Muir WW: Cardiovascular effects of medetomidine, detomidine and xylazine in horses. J Vet Med Sci 62:1025-1032, 2000
4. Bettschart-Wolfensberger R, Freeman SL, Bowen IM, Aliabadi FS, Weller R, Huhtinen M, Clarke KW: Cardiopulmonary effects and pharmacokinetics of i.v. dexmedetomidine in ponies. Equine Vet J 37:60-64, 2005
5. Hamm D, Turchi P, Joechle W: Sedative and analgesic effects of detomidine and romifidine in horses. Vet Rec 136:324-327, 1995
6. Moens Y, Lanz F, Doherty MG, Schatzmann U: A comparison of the antinociceptive effects of xylazine, detomidine and romifidine on experimental pain in horses. Vet Anaes Analg 30:183-190, 2003
7. Clarke KW, Paton BS: Combined use of detomidine with opiates in the horse. Equine Vet J 20:331-334, 1988
8. Clarke KW, England CW, Goosens L: Sedative and cardiovascular effects of romifidine, alone and in combination with butorphanol, in the horse. J Vet Anaesth 18:25-29, 1991
9. Klein LV, Baetjer C: Preliminary report: xylazine-morphine sedation in horses. Vet Anesth 2:2-6, 1974
10. Bryant CE, England CGW, Clarke KW: Comparison of the sedative effects of medetomidine and xylazine in horses. Vet Rec 129:421-423, 1991
11. Freeman SL, Bowen IM, Bettschart-Wolfensberger R, Alibhai HIK, England CGW: Cardiovascular effects of romifidine in the standing horse. Res Vet Sci 72:123-129, 2002
12. Clarke ES, Thompson SA, Becht JL, Moore JN: Effects of xylazine on cecal mechanical activity and cecal blood flow in healthy horses. Am J Vet Res 49:720-723, 1988
13. Rutkowski JA, Eades SC, Moore JN: Effects of xylazine butorphanol on cecal arterial blood flow, cecal mechanical activity, and systemic hemodynamics in horses. Am J Vet Res 52:1153-1158, 1991
14. Hunt RJ, Brandon CI, McCann ME: Effects of acetylpromazine, xylazine, and vertical load on digital arterial blood flow in horses. Am J Vet Res 55:375-378, 1994
15. Stick JA, Chou CC, Derksen FJ, Arden WA: Effects of xylazine on equine intestinal vascular resistance, motility, compliance, and oxygen consumption. Am J Vet Res 48:198-203, 1987
16. Gaynor JS, Bednarski RM, Muir WW: Effect of xylazine on the arrhythmogenic dose of epinephrine in thiamylal/halothane-anesthetised horses. Am J Vet Res 53:2350-2354, 1992
17. Johnston GM, Taylor PM, Holmes MA, Wood JLN: Confidential Enquiry of Perioperative Equine Fatalities (CEPEF I): preliminary results. Equine Vet J 27:193-200, 1995
18. Bettschart-Wolfensberger R, Clarke KW, Vainio O, Aliabadi FS, Demuth D: Pharmacokinetics of medetomidine in ponies and elaboration of a medetomidine infusion regime which provides a constant level of sedation. Res Vet Sci 67:41-46, 1999

19. Virtanen R, MacDonald E: Comparison of the effects of detomidine and xylazine on some α_2-adrenoceptor-mediated responses in the central and peripheral nervous systems. Eur J Pharmacol 115:277-284, 1985
20. Robertson SA: Sedation and general anaesthesia of the foal. Equine Vet Educ 9:37-44, 1997
21. Kamerling SG, Cravens WMT, Bagwell CA: Dose-related effects of detomidine on autonomic responses in the horse. J Auton Pharmacol 8:241-249, 1988
22. Thurmon JC, Steffey EP, Zinkl JG, Woliner M, Howland D: Xylazine causes transient dose-related hyperglycemia and increased urine volumes in mares. Am J Vet Res 45:224-227, 1984
23. Gasthuys F, Terpstra P, van den Hende C, de Moor A: Hyperglycaemia and diuresis during sedation with detomidine in the horse. J Vet Med A 34:641-648, 1987
24. Gasthuys F, Martens A, Goosens L, de Moor A: A quantitative and qualitative study of the diuretic effects of romifidine in the horse. J Assoc Vet Anaesth 23:6-10, 1996
25. Greene SA, Thurmon JC, Tranquilli WJ, Benson GJ: Effect of yohimbine on xylazine-induced hypoinsulinemia and hyperglycemia in mares. Am J Vet Res 48:676-678, 1987
26. Raekallio M, Leino A, Vainio O, Scheinin M: Sympathoadrenal activity and the clinical sedative effect of detomidine in horses. Equine Vet J suppl 11:66-68, 1992
27. Carroll GL, Matthews NS, Hartsfield SM, Slater MR, Champney TH, Erickson SW: The effect of detomidine and its antagonism with tolazoline on stress-related hormones, metabolites, physiologic responses, and behavior in awake ponies. Vet Surg 26:69-77, 1997
28. Doherty TJ, Andrews FM, Provenza MK, Frazier DL: The effect of sedation on gastric emptying of a liquid marker in ponies. Vet Surg 28:375-379, 1999
29. Sutton DGM, Preston T, Christley RM, Cohen ND, Love S, Roussel AJ: The effects of xylazine, detomidine, acepromazine and butorphanol on equine solid phase gastric emptying rate. Equine Vet J 34:486-492, 2002
30. Rutkowski JQ, Eades SC, Moore JN: Effects of xylazine butorphanol on cecal arterial blood flow, cecal mechanical activity, and systemic hemodynamics in horses. Am J Vet Res 52:1153-1158, 1991
31. Lester GD, Merritt AM, Neuwirth L, Vetro-Widenhouse T, Steible C, Rice B: Effect of α_2-adrenergic, cholinergic, and non-steroidal anti-inflammatory drugs on myoelectric activity of ileum, cecum, and right ventral colon and on cecal emptying of radiolabeled markers in clinically normal ponies. Am J Vet Res 59:320-327, 1998
32. Merritt AM, Burrow JA, Hartless CS: Effect of xylazine, detomidine, and a combination of xylazine and butorphanol on equine duodenal motility. Am J Vet Res 59:619-623, 1998
33. Freeman SL, England GCW: Effect of romifidine on gastrointestinal motility, assessed by transrectal ultrasonography. Equine Vet J 33:570-576, 2001
34. Roger T, Ruckebusch Y: Colonic α_2-adrenoceptor-mediated responses in the pony. J Vet Pharmacol Ther 10:310-318, 1987
35. Wagner AE, Muir WW, Hinchcliff KW: Cardiovascular effects of xylazine and detomidine in horses. Am J Vet Res 52:651-657, 1991
36. Freeman SL, England GCW: Comparison of sedative effects of romifidine following intravenous, intramuscular, and sublingual administration to horses. Am J Vet Res 60:954-959, 1999
37. Malone JH, Clarke KW: A comparison of the efficacy of detomidine by sublingual and intramuscular administration in ponies. J Vet Anaesth 20:73-77, 1993
38. Kollias-Baker CA, Court MH, Williams LL: Influence of yohimbine and tolazoline on the cardiovascular, respiratory, and sedative effects of xylazine in the horse. J Vet Pharmacol Ther 16:350-358, 1993
39. Wilson DV, Bohart GV, Evans AT, Robertson S, Rondenay Y: Retrospective analysis of detomidine infusion for standing chemical restraint in 51 horses. Vet Anaes Analg 29:54-57, 2002
40. McCrindle CME, Ebedes H, Swan GE: The use of long-acting neuroleptics, perphenazine enanthoate and pipothiazine palmitate in two horses. J South Afr Vet Assoc 60:208-209, 1989
41. Brewer BD, Hines MT, Stewart JT: Fluphenazine induced Parkinson-like syndrome in a horse. Equine Vet J 22:136-137, 1990
42. Gasthuys G, de Moor A, Parmentier D: Haemodynamic changes during sedation in ponies. Vet Res Commun 14:309-327, 1990
43. Hood DM: Alpha-adrenergic blocking effects of phenothiazine tranquilisers. Assoc Equine Sports Med Proc 13:37-39, 1994/1995
44. Kerr DD, Jones EW, Holbert D, Huggins K: Comparison of the effects of xylazine and acetylpromazine maleate in the horse. Am J Vet Res 33:777-784, 1972
45. Muir WW, Skarda RT, Sheehan W: Hemodynamic and respiratory effects of a xylazine-acetylpromazine drug combination in horses. Am J Vet Res 40:1518-1522, 1979
46. Hashem A, Keller H: Disposition, bioavailability and clinical efficacy of orally administered acepromazine in the horse. J Vet Pharmacol Ther 16:359-368, 1993
47. Ballard S, Shults T, Kownacki AA, Blake JW, Tobin T: The pharmacokinetics, pharmacological responses and behavioral effects of acepromazine in the horse. J Vet Pharmacol Ther 5:21-31, 1982
48. Marroum PJ, Well AI, Aeschbacher G, Curry SH: Pharmacokinetics and pharmacodynamics of acepromazine in horses. Am J Vet Res 55:1428-1433, 1994
49. Parry BW, Anderson GA, Gay CC: Hypotension in the horse induced by acepromazine maleate. Aust Vet J 59:148-152, 1982
50. Parry BW, Anderson GA: Influence of acepromazine maleate on the equine haematocrit. J Vet Pharmacol Ther 6:121-126, 1983
51. Sedrish SA, Venugopalan CS, Holmes EP, Koch CE, Moore RM: In vitro response of large colon arterial and venous rings to vasodilating drugs in horses. Am J Vet Res 60:204-210, 1999
52. Hall LW: The effect of chlorpromazine on the cardiovascular system of the conscious horse. Vet Rec 72:85-87, 1960
53. Muir WW, Hamlin RL: Effects of acetylpromazine on ventilatory variables in the horse. Am J Vet Res 36:1439-1442, 1975

54. Davies JV, Gerring EL: Effect of spasmolytic analgesic drugs on the motility patterns of the equine small intestine. Res Vet Sci 34:334-339, 1983
55. Rang HP, Dale MM, Ritter JM, Gardener P (eds): Neuroleptic Drugs in Pharmacology. London, Churchill Livingstone, Inc, 1995, pp 562-575
56. Loch W, Worthy K, Ireland F: The effect of phenothiazine on plasma prolactin levels in non-pregnant mares. Equine Vet J 22:30-32, 1990
57. Kauffman VG, Soma L, Divers TH, Perkons SZ: Extrapyramidal side effects caused by fluphenazine decanoate in a horse. J. Am Vet Med Assoc 195:1128-1130, 1989
58. Robertson JT, Muir WW, Sams R: Cardiopulmonary effects of butorphanol tartrate in horses. Am J Vet Res 42:41-44, 1981
59. Muir WW, Skarda RT. Sheehan WC: Cardiopulmonary effects of narcotic agonists and a partial agonist in horses. Am J Vet Res 39:1632-1635, 1978
60. Kamerling SG, DeQuick DJ, Weckman TJ, Tobin T: Dose-related effects of fentanyl on autonomic and behavioral responses in performance horses. Gen Pharmacol 16:253-238, 1985
61. Szoke MO, Blais D, Cuvelliez SG, Lavoie J-P: Effects of buprenorphine on cardiovascular and pulmonary function in clinically normal horses and horses with chronic obstructive pulmonary disease. Am J Vet Res 59:1287-1291, 1998
62. Combie J, Dougherty J, Nugen E, Tobin T: The pharmacology of narcotic analgesics in the horse. IV. Dose and time response relationships for behavioral responses to morphine, meperidine, pentazocine, anileridine, methadone, and hydromorphone. J Equine Med Surg 3:377-385, 1979
63. Pascoe PJ, Black WD, Claxton JM, Sanson RE: The pharmacokinetics and locomotor activity of alfentanil in the horse. J Vet Pharmacol Ther 14:317-325, 1991
64. Sojka JE, Adams SB, Lamar CH, Eller LL: Effect of butorphanol, pentazocine, meperidine, or metoclopramide on intestinal motility in female ponies. Am J Vet Res 49:527-529, 1988
65. Merritt AM, Campbell-Thompson ML, Lowrey S: Effect of butorphanol on equine antroduodenal motility. Equine Vet J Suppl 7:21-23, 1989
66. Stick JA, Loeffler BS, Arden WA, Ching-Chung C: Effects of butorphanol tartrate on arterial pressure, jejunal blood flow, vascular resistance, O_2 extraction, and O_2 uptake in halothane-anesthetised ponies. Am J Vet Res 50:1202-1206, 1989
67. Orsini JA: Butorphanol tartrate: pharmacology and clinical indications. Comp Cont Educ 10:849-854, 1988
68. Roberts MC, Argenzio A: Effects of amitraz, several opiate derivatives and anticholinergic agents on intestinal transit in ponies. Equine Vet J 18:256-260, 1986
69. Roger T, Bardon T, Ruckebusch Y: Colonic motor responses in the pony: relevance of colonic stimulation by opiate antagonists. Am J Vet Res 46:31-35, 1985
70. Robertson JT, Muir WW: A new analgesic drug combination in the horse. Am J Vet Res 44:1667-1669, 1983
71. Nilsfors L, Kvart C, Kallings P, Carlsten J: Cardiorespiratory and sedative effects of a combination of acepromazine, xylazine and methadone in the horse. Equine Vet J 19:364-367, 1987
72. Nolan AM, Hall LW: Combined use of sedatives and opiates in horses. Vet Rec 114:63-67, 1984
73. Harkins JD, Queiroz-Neto A, Mundy GD, West D, Tobin T: Development and characterization of an equine behaviour chamber and the effects of amitraz and detomidine on spontaneous locomotor activity. J Vet Pharmacol Ther 20:396-401, 1997
74. Muir WW, Skarda RT, Sheehan WC: Hemodynamic and respiratory effects of xylazine-morphine sulphate in horses. Am J Vet Res 40:1417-1420, 1979
75. Merritt AM, Burrow JA, Hartless CS: Effect of xylazine, detomidine, and a combination of xylazine and butorphanol on equine duodenal motility. Am J Vet Res 59:619-623, 1998
76. Muir WW, Sams RA, Huffman RH, Noonan JS: Pharmacodynamic and pharmacokinetic properties of diazepam in horses. Am J Vet Res 43:1756-1762, 1982
77. Brown RF, Houpt KA, Schryver HF: Stimulation of food intake in horses by diazepam and promazine. Pharmacol Biochem Behav 5:495-497, 1976
78. Inada T, Asai T, Yamada M, Shingu K: Propofol and midazolam inhibit gastric emptying and gastrointestinal transit in mice. Anesth Analg 99:1102-1106, 2004
79. Marland A, Sarkar P, Leavitt R: The urinary elimination profiles of diazepam and its metabolites, nordiazepam, temazepam, and oxazepam, in the equine after a 10-mg intramuscular dose. J Analyt Toxicol 23:29-34, 1999
80. Reves JG, Fragen RJ, Vinik HR, Greenblatt DJ: Midazolam: pharmacology and uses. Anesthesiology 62:310-324, 1985
81. Gross JB, Hoff HE: Vagal activity and cardiac arrest in chloral hydrate narcosis. Cardiovasc. Res Center Bull 6:85-98, 1968
82. Ball MA, Peek S: Chloral hydrate: a sedative not to be forgotten. Equine Pract 18:24-27, 1996
83. Gabel AA, Hamlin R, Smith CR: Effects of promazine and chloral hydrate on the cardiovascular system of the horse. Am J Vet Res 25:1151-1158, 1964
84. Muir WW: Standing chemical restraint in horses: tranquilisers, sedatives, and analgesics, in Muir WW, Hubbell JAE (eds.): Equine Anaesthesia: Monitoring and Emergency Therapy. Baltimore, Mosby Year Book, 1991, pp 247-280
85. Fraser AC: Restraint in the horse. Vet Rec 80:56-64, 1967
86. Jones RS: A review of tranquilization and sedation in large animals. Vet Rec 90:613-617, 1972
87. Earl AE: Reserpine (Serpasil) in veterinary practice. J Am Vet Med Assoc 129:227-233, 1956
88. Tobin T: A review of the pharmacology of reserpine in the horse. J Equine Med Surg 2:433-438, 1978
89. Lloyd KCK, Tulleners E: Reserpine toxicosis in a horse. J Am Vet Med Assoc 186:980-981, 1985
90. Ray RS, Sams RA, Huffman R: Detection, identification and quantification of reserpine and diazepam. Proc Equine Pharmacol Symp 2:209-215, 1978
91. Beech J: Treating and preventing chronic intermittent rhabdomyolysis. Vet Med 89:458-461, 1994
92. Meyer TS, Fedde MR, Cox JH, Erickson HH: Hyperkalemic periodic paralysis in horses: a review. Equine Vet J 31:362-367, 1999
93. Firshman AM, Valberg SJ, Bender JB, Finno CJ: Epidemiologic characteristics and management of polysaccharide

storage myopathy in quarter horses. Am J Vet Res 64:1319-1327, 2003

94. Valdes-Vazquez MA, Aguilera-Tejero E, Mayer-Valor R: Effect of xylazine during endoscopic evaluation of functional upper respiratory disorders in horses. J Equine Vet Sci 13:84-86, 1993
95. Duggan VE, MacAllister CG, Davis MS: Xylazine-induced attenuation of dorsal displacement of the soft palate associated with epiglottic dysfunction in a horse. J. Am Vet Med Assoc 221:399-402, 2002
96. McClure JR, Gelatt KN, Manning JP: The effect of parenteral acepromazine and xylazine on intraocular pressure in the horse. Vet Med Sm Anim Clin 71:1727-1730, 1976
97. van der Woerdt A, Gilger BC, Wilkie DA, Staruch SM: Effect of auriculopalpebral nerve block and intravenous administration of xylazine on intraocular pressure and corneal thickness in horses. Am J Vet Res 56:155-158, 1995
98. Redman HC, Wilson GL, Hogan JE: Effect of chlorpromazine combined with intermittent light stimulation on the electroencephalogram and clinical response of the beagle dog. Am J Vet Res 34:929-936, 1973
99. Moore RM, Trim CM: Effect of xylazine on cerebrospinal fluid pressure in conscious horses. Am J Vet Res 53:1558-1562, 1992
100. Brosnan RJ, Steffey EP, LeCouteur RA, Imai A, Farver TB, Kortz GD: Effects of body position on intracranial and cerebral perfusion pressures in isoflurane-anesthetised horses. J Appl Physiol 92:2542-2546, 2002
101. Nunez E, Steffey EP, Ocampo L, Rodriguez A, Garcia AA: Effects of α_2-adrenergic receptor agonists of urine production in horses deprived of food and water. Am J Vet Res 65:1342-1346, 2004
102. Sellon DC, Monroe VL, Roberts MC, Papich MG: Pharmacokinetics and adverse effects of butorphanol administered by single intravenous injection or continuous intravenous infusion in horses. Am J Vet Res 62:183-189, 2001
103. Davis EG, McCue M, Rush BR: Treatment and supportive care of recumbent horses. Compendium 26:216-226, 2004
104. Lavoie JP, Phan ST, Blais D: Effects of a combination of detomidine and butorphanol on respiratory function in horses with or without chronic obstructive pulmonary disease. Am J Vet Res 57:705-709, 1996
105. Lavoie JP, Pascoe JR, Kurpershoek CJ: Effect of head and neck position on respiratory mechanics in horses sedated with xylazine. Am J Vet Res 53:1652-1657, 1992
106. Patteson MW, Gibbs C, Wotton PR, Cripps PJ: Effects of sedation with detomidine hydrochloride on echocardiographic measurements of cardiac dimensions and indices of cardiac function in horses. Equine Vet J suppl 19:33-37, 1995
107. Wooldridge AA, Eades SC, Hosgood GL, Moore RM: Effects of treatment with oxytocin, xylazine-butorphanol, guaifenesin, acepromazine, and detomidine on esophageal manometric pressure in conscious horses. Am J Vet Res 63:1738-1744, 2002
108. Eades SC, Moore JN: Blockade of endotoxin-induced cecal hypoperfusion and ileus with an α_2 antagonist in horses. Am J Vet Res 54:586-590, 1993
109. Meisler SD, Doherty TJ, Andrews FM, Osborne D, Frazier DL: Yohimbine ameliorates the effects of endotoxin on gastric emptying on the liquid marker acetaminophen in horses. Can J Vet Res 64:208-211, 2000
110. Chambers JP, Waterman AE, Livingston A, Goodship AE: Prolonged action of detomidine in thoroughbred horses with abnormal liver function. J Assoc Vet Anaesth 23:27-28, 1996
111. Schatzman U, Josseck H, Stauffer J-L, Goossens L: Effects of α_2-agonists on intrauterine pressure and sedation in horses: comparison between detomidine, romifidine and xylazine. J Vet Med A 41:523-529, 1994
112. Katila T, Oijala M: The effect of detomidine (Domosedan) on the maintenance of equine pregnancy and foetal development: ten cases. Equine Vet J 20:323-326, 1988
113. Luukkanen L, Katila T, Koskeine E: Some effects of multiple administrations of detomidine during the last trimester of equine pregnancy. Equine Vet J 29:400-403, 1997
114. Jedruch J, Gajewski Z, Kuussaari J: The effect of detomidine hydrochloride on the electrical activity of uterus in pregnant mares. Acta Vet Scand 30:307-311, 1989
115. von Reitzenstein M, Callahan MA, Hansen PJ, LeBlanc MM: Aberrations in uterine contractile patterns in mares with delayed uterine clearance after administration of detomidine and oxytocin. Theriogenology 58:887-898, 2002
116. McGladdery AJ, Cottrill CM, Rossdale PD: Effects upon the fetus of sedative drugs administered to the mare. Proc Int Conf Vet Perinatol 2:14, 1990
117. Smith LJ, Schott HC: Xylazine-induced fetal bradycardia. Proc Int Conf Vet Perinat 2:36, 1990
118. Salonen JS, Vahe-Vahe T, Vaino O, Vakkuri O: Single-dose pharmacokinetics of detomidine in the horse and cow. J Vet Pharmacol Ther 12:65-72, 1989
119. Court MH, Dodman MH, Levine HD, Richey MT, Lee JW, Hustead DR: Pharmacokinetics and milk residues of butorphanol in dairy cows after single intravenous administration. J Vet Pharmacol Ther 15:28-35, 1992
120. Borgatta L, Jenny RW, Gruss L, Ong C, Barad D: Clinical significance of methohexital, meperidine, and diazepam in breast milk. J Clin Pharmacol 37:186-193, 1997
121. Bennett-Wimbush K, Loch WE, Plata-Madrid H, Evans T: The effects of perphenazine and bromocriptine on follicular dynamics and endocrine profiles in anestruous pony mares. Theriogenology 49:717-733, 1998
122. Ryan PL, Bennett-Wimbush K, Vaala WE, Bagnell CA: Systemic relaxin in pregnant pony mares grazed on endophyte-infected fescue: effects of fluphenazine treatment. Theriogenology 56:471-483, 2001
123. Fitzgerald BP, Mellbye LB: Effect of administration of an α_2-adrenogeric agonist, xylazine, on pulsatile gondadotrophin secretion in anoestrous horse mares. J Reprod Fertil 84:693-700, 1988
124. Norman WM, Court MH, Greenblatt DJ: Age-related changes in the pharmacokinetic disposition of diazepam in foals. Am J Vet Res 58:878-880, 1997
125. Oijala M, Katila T: Detomidine (Domosedan) in foals: sedative and analgesic effects. Equine Vet J 20:327-329, 1988
126. Carter SW, Robertson SA, Steel CJ, Jourdenais DA: Cardiopulmonary effects of xylazine sedation in the foal. Equine Vet J 22:384-388, 1990
127. Robertson SA, Carter SW, Donovan M, Steele C: Effects of intravenous xylazine hydrochloride on blood glucose,

plasma insulin and rectal temperature in neonatal foals. Equine Vet J 22:43-47, 1990

128. Naylor JM, Garven E, Faser L: A comparison of romifidine and xylazine in foals: the effects on sedation and analgesia. Equine Vet Educ 9:329-334, 1997
129. Burrows GE, MacAllister CG, Tripp P, Black J: Interactions between chloramphenicol, acepromazine, phenylbutazone, rifampin and thiamylal in the horse. Equine Vet J 21:34-38, 1989

6.2 Pain management in the hospitalised horse

Lydia Donaldson

Introduction

In approaching the painful horse, there are a number of factors to consider. There is the type of pain: What tissue(s) or organs are involved? What is the cause or pathology? Is the pain acute or chronic? How long do you expect the painful condition to take to resolve? How debilitating is this pain for this horse? There is the choice of analgesic: What is available? Is an NSAID indicated to reduce inflammation and directly contribute to analgesia? Would the horse also benefit from a degree of sedation or anxiolysis? Are there contraindications for use of any agents due to the primary or concurrent disease(s)? Are there other side effects that this horse might not tolerate well? Is a combination of analgesics likely to be more effective than a single drug? And there is the choice of route of administration: Which is practical for hospital staffing? Which will give optimal, continual pain relief? Or, if appropriate, which will readily permit windows through which glimpses of the horse's true pain level can allow assessment of the progression of healing or pathology? Which will cause the fewest side effects?

The most obviously painful horses are the horses with colic that can barely remain standing and horses with septic synovial structures that wave the affected limb in the air. There are other pains that may be easier to overlook as merely part of the presenting pathology. A blepharospastic eye is painful. Itching a postoperative site indicates discomfort (i.e., pain). Poor appetite and reduced activity may be more than signs of gastrointestinal dysfunction or secondary to fever and malaise. Physiological variables such as heart rate and respiratory rate plus careful observation of a horse's behaviour are used to subjectively, but reasonably accurately, assess degrees of discomfort.[1–5] Importantly, reevaluation of pain is critical not only to monitor the progress of the pathology but also to gauge the effectiveness of pain control. This chapter will discuss the various types of painful horse, choices of analgesics and routes of administration. The doses for systemically and epidurally administered analgesics are shown in Tables 6.2 and 6.3, respectively. For reference, the reader is directed to the in-depth review of pain mechanisms and therapies in the recent veterinary literature.[6]

The overall objective in equine pain management is to diminish pain perception and distress without altering normal physiological homeostasis, mental acuity or jeop-

Table 6.2. Systemic analgesics used in the horse

	IV (mg/kg)	**CRI**	**IM** (mg/kg)	**Other** (mg/kg)
NSAIDs		Dosing interval		
Carpofen	0.5–1.1 SID	—	0.7 SID	PO: 0.7–1.3 SID
Flunixin	0.25–1.1 SID	—	1.1 SID	PO: 1.1 SID
Ketoprofen	2.2 SID	—	2.2 SID	
Meloxicam	0.6 SID	—	0.6 SID	
Phenylbutazone	2.2–4.4 BID	—	Irritant	PO: 4.4 BID <8.8/day
α_2-Agonists		(Approximate duration of effect)		
Xylazine	0.2–1.1 (15–60)	1.0 mg/kg; 12 μg/kg/min	0.5–2.2 (90–240)	
Detomidine	0.004–0.02 (30–90)	6–15 μg/kg; 0.1–0.6 μg/kg/min	0.02–0.05 (50–120)	Sublingual: 0.04–0.08 (60–120)
Opioids				
Butorphanol	0.01–0.1 (30–120)	17.8 μg/kg; 0.38 μg/kg/min	0.04–0.2 (60–240)	
Buprenorphine	0.003–0.006 (≤480)	—	0.01–0.04 (≤480)	
Pethidine (Meperidine)	0.2–0.4 (30)	—	0.5–2.0 (90)	
Methadone	0.12 (60)	—	—	
Morphine	0.02–0.2 (30–90)	—	0.2–0.6 (60–180)	
Oxymorphone	0.005–0.03 (45–60)	—	0.02–0.05 (90–120)	
Fentanyl	0.01–0.04 (15–30)	—	0.22 (30–60)	Transdermal: 2 × 100 μg/hours patches/500 kg (48–72)
Lidocaine	—	1.3–3 mg/kg; 30–50 μg/kg/min	—	
Ketamine	0.2–0.80 (15)	0.5–1 mg/kg; 6.7–13.3 μg/kg/min	1.0–2.0 (30–60)	

NSAIDs, nonsteroidal anti-inflammatory drugs; SID, once daily.

Table 6.3. Analgesics that can be administered in the caudal epidural space in the horse

	Dose (mg/kg)	**Onset*** (minutes)	**Duration*** (minutes)	**Volume‡** (ml)	**References**
Local anaesthetics					
Lidocaine	0.22–0.45	5–20	30–180	8–10	73, 76, 77, 86, 89
Mepivacaine	0.35	21	81	3–5	75
Bupivacaine	0.06	6.0 ± 2.6	320 ± 30	4	78
Ropivacaine	0.08–0.1	5–15	150–230	8–9	79, 80
α_2-Agonists					
Xylazine	0.17–0.35	15–30	165–210	6–10	73, 74, 76, 77, 94
Detomidine	0.06	10–20	120–180	8–10	74, 84
Opioids					
Alfentanil	0.02	20¶	120¶	20	83
Butorphanol	0.05–0.08	Not different from controls		20–70	66, 83,132
Hydromorphone	0.04	30	280	20	155
Pethidine (Meperidine)	0.6–0.8	5–15	240–300	4–5	78, 90
Methadone	0.1	15	300	20	86
Morphine	0.1–0.2	180–300	600–1200	20	83
Tramadol	1.0	20	390	20	83
Ketamine	0.5–2.0	5–10	90	10–70	132, 148, 149
Combinations					
Lidocaine and xylazine	0.22 and 0.17	5.3 ± 1.3	329.8 ± 6.2	6	77
Lidocaine and butorphanol	0.25 and 0.04	<30	150 ± 21	8	89
Morphine and detomidine	0.2 and 0.03	15–30	360–1820	8–20	87, 88
Ropivacaine and fentanyl	0.08 and 0.10	5.67 ± 0.72	217 ± 6.1	10–11	80

*Perineal analgesia.
‡Diluted with 0.9% saline as needed to achieve desired volume.
¶Pain threshold increased but not significantly different from controls.

ardising the healing process. The drugs in our pharmacopoeia with which this is attempted all have potential adverse effects that are generally dose dependent. Of these, α_2-adrenergic agonists cause bradycardia, hypotension, decreases in cardiac output, gastrointestinal motility and intestinal and digital blood flow, diuresis, hyperglycaemia, increased uterine tone, excessive sedation and ataxia.[7–13] Opioids cause excitement, tachycardia, hypertension, dysphoria, compulsive ambulation, decrease propulsive gastrointestinal motility and pruritis.[14–17] Local anaesthetics, administered regionally or locally, cause motor paralysis and complete anaesthesia. Signs of toxicity in the horse include muscle fasciculations, ataxia, bradycardia and seizures.[18] Nonsteroidal anti-inflammatory agents (NSAIDs) potentially cause gastrointestinal ulceration, renal hypoperfusion and thrombosis.[19–21] Ketamine* causes trembling, excitement, tachycardia, hypertension, respiratory depression and recumbency with loss of awareness.[22] Likewise, routes of administration have expected characteristics. Intravenous (IV) bolus is appropriate for immediate, short-term (<1 hour) pain control. Intramuscular (IM) administration results in slower onset, lower peak blood and tissue levels and longer duration of action. Local tissue effects (irritation, vasoconstriction) may limit IM use. Constant rate infusion (CRI) allows dose adjustment to effect but is labour intensive and relatively more expensive. Infusion rates are calculated from pharmacokinetic data of a drug in the species. This information is not available for many drugs in horses. In addition, the pharmacokinetics of a drug are likely to be different in systemically ill, stressed and neonatal or aged horses and therefore pharmacokinetic data determined in young, healthy horses can only serve as guidelines. Most CRI protocols for horses are extrapolated from other species and modified by experience. Intra-articular or synovial analgesics (local anaesthetics, NSAIDs, opioids) have potential but may be more appropriate preemptively as efficacy may be limited by local tissue damage and inflammation. Caudal epidural analgesia (α_2-agonists, opioids, local anaesthetics, ketamine, NSAIDs) targets receptors in the neuronal cell membrane in either the spinal roots or dorsal horn of the spinal cord. Therefore, onset and duration of action depend on diffusion from the epidural space to the site of action and affinity for that site. There is also drug- and dose-dependent systemic absorption. Transdermal absorption (fentanyl†, lignocaine (lidocaine)‡, buprenorphine§) is

* Ketaset; Fort Dodge Animal Health, Fort Dodge, IA, USA.

† Duragesic; Janssen Pharmaceutica, Beerse, Belgium.
‡ Lidoderm; Endo Pharmaceuticals, Chadds Ford, PA, USA.
§ Transtec, Napp Pharmaceuticals, Cambridge, UK.

influenced by skin thickness, preparation and blood flow. Careful combination of two or more analgesics and routes of administration is directed at improved nociceptive control with fewer side effects.[23]

Visceral pain

Abdominal visceral nociception to mechanical, chemical and thermal stimulation, including ischaemia and inflammation, is transmitted through the sympathetic splanchnic nerves and posterior mesenteric plexus to caudal thoracic (T6-T7 to L1) and lumbar (L2-L5) dorsal horn sensory neurons, respectively. Sensory receptors of primary afferent vagal and pelvic nerve (S2-S5) fibres respond to mechanical and chemical stimulation.[24] The sensory branch of the central autonomic network is closely integrated with the enteric nervous system.[25] The parietal peritoneum's sensory innervation is somatic and segmentally distributed. The significance of this anatomical distribution is that modulation of distal colonic, rectal and bladder pain is amenable to caudal epidural analgesic administration. Some relief from peritonitis might also be achieved by this route. However, organs (reproductive, all intestines but the very distal colon, stomach, liver, kidney, pancreas) innervated by sympathetic sensory fibres would require spinally administered analgesics to reach the midlumbar or caudal thoracic dorsal roots and horn neurons and vagally mediated discomfort can only be influenced by systemic analgesic administration.

Analgesia of the colic patient

In the United States, probably 99.9% of acutely colicky horses are given flunixin** for its contribution to analgesia, anti-inflammatory activity and action to ameliorate endotoxaemia.[26–28] In the United Kingdom, a recent survey found dipyrone/hycoscine†† to be the first-choice treatment for mild colic, and flunixin or other NSAIDs to be reserved for more serious pain.[29] Using a standardised caecal distension model to create gastrointestinal pain, dipyrone/hycoscine (0.3 mg/kg IV) proved as effective as butorphanol‡‡ at reducing behaviour indicative of pain.[30] Reports of the clinical efficacy of flunixin and ketoprofen§§ for relief of colic pain have been published,[31,32] although in an experimental model of visceral pain, flunixin (2 mg/kg IM) did not raise the threshold to caecal distension.[33]

More dramatically painful colics or those that do not respond to NSAIDs are most commonly given xylazine*** or detomidine††† IV. All but the most severe will respond: stop pawing, agitating, buckling and stand sedated for at least some period of time. In the caecal distension model of visceral pain, xylazine (1.1 mg/kg IV or 2.2 mg/kg IM) provided better and longer-lasting analgesia than morphine‡‡‡ (0.66 mg/kg IM), pethidine (meperidine) §§§ (1.0 mg/kg IV or 4.4 mg/kg IM), fentanyl**** (0.22 mg/kg IM), oxymorphone†††† (0.033 mg/kg IM), methadone‡‡‡‡ (0.22 mg/kg IM), butorphanol (0.2 mg/kg IV or IM), pentazocine§§§§ (0.99 mg/kg IV or 2.2 mg/kg IM) or flunixin (2.2 mg/kg IM).[33–35] Detomidine-induced (0.020 mg/kg IV) pain relief from caecal distension lasted approximately twice as long as that of xylazine (1.1 mg/kg IV).[36] A multicentre, blinded clinical trial of analgesia for 152 horses with acute abdominal pain found detomidine (0.02 mg/kg IV) superior to xylazine (0.5 mg/kg IV), which was in turn better than flunixin (1.0 mg/kg IV) and butorphanol (0.1 mg/kg IV).[31] The α_2-agonists are so effective that concerns for their negative actions on the cardiovascular, respiratory and gastrointestinal systems are nearly forgotten in the clinical setting. Fortunately, these side effects are dose dependent. They can be reduced by decreasing the α_2-agonist dose while simultaneously administering an opioid and thus taking advantage of the synergism between α_2-agonists and opioids.[35] In the caecal distension model, butorphanol provided better and longer-duration analgesia than the other opioids tested.[33,34] The adverse effects of butorphanol on the gastrointestinal tract may also not be as profound as for the α-agonists, morphine and pethidine (meperidine).[17,37] Butorphanol (0.1 mg/kg IV and 0.2 mg/kg IM) proved less potent a visceral analgesic than xylazine and detomidine[31,33] and, as reported for other opioids,[35] considerable individual variability has been noted.[31] Neither of two doses (0.022 or 0.044 mg/kg IV) of butorphanol lowered the minimum alveolar concentration of halothane in anaesthetised horses.[38] However, a higher dose (0.2 mg/kg IV) did raise the pain threshold to caecal distension for 30 minutes,[39] and a dose of 0.11 mg/kg IV was effective in a clinical trial.[40] The use of opioids as the sole analgesic is limited by the side effects of dyspho-

** Banamine; Fort Dodge Animal Health, Fort Dodge, IA, USA; Finadyne; Schering-Plough Animal Health, Harefield, Middlesex, UK.

†† Buscopan Compositum; Boehringer Ingelheim Limited, Bracknell, Berkshire, UK.

‡‡ Torbugesic; Fort Dodge Animal Health, Fort Dodge, IA, USA.

§§ Ketofen injectable; Fort Dodge Animal Health, Fort Dodge, IA, USA; UK: Merial, Harlow, Essex; Australia: Merial PTY, Parramatta NSW, Australia.

*** Rompun; Bayer Animal Health, Newbury, Berkshire, UK; Chanazine 10%; Chanelle Animal Health, Liverpool, UK.

††† Domosedan; Pfizer, Sandwich, Kent, UK.

‡‡‡ Morphine sulphate injection; Antigen Pharmaceuticals, Dublin 4, Ireland.

§§§ Pethidine injection 50 mg/ml; Arnolds Veterinary Products, Shrewsbury, Shropshire, UK; Demerol; Abbott Laboratories, Abbott Park, IL, USA; Pethidine Injection; Parnell Laboratories, Alexandria, NSW, Australia.

**** Sublimaze; Akorn Inc, Buffalo Grove, IL, USA.

†††† Numorphan; DuPont Pharma, Wilmington, DE, USA.

‡‡‡‡ Dolophine; Roxane Laboratories, Columbus, OH, USA.

§§§§ Talwin; Sanofi-Aventis, Paris, France.

ria and compulsive locomotion. In nonpainful horses, the dose at which stereotypic behaviour is first seen is similar to that of analgesia, although there is some variability among the different drugs. In painful horses, the threshold for excitement is raised.[41] In the presence of caecal distension, mild sedation, shivering and restlessness were reported at various times in some, but not all horses, after 0.2 mg/kg IV or IM butorphanol.[33,34]

The challenge of providing analgesia becomes infinitely more complex when the persistently painful horse is denied surgical relief, appears not to have a surgical lesion or returns from surgery with unrelieved pain. The objective now is relatively long-term modulation of gastrointestinal pain. Giving an α_2-agonist with an opioid by IV bolus with the hope that the colic will resolve with rehydration and interruption of the pain/distress cycle is occasionally successful. On the other hand, IM or CRI can be titrated to more consistent control of pain over time with fewer side effects. Intramuscular xylazine given at twice the IV dose (2.2 mg/kg IM versus 1.1 mg/kg IV) had a comparable peak effect and almost 4 times the duration (60 minutes versus >240 minutes) in reducing the pain response to caecal distension.[33,34] At these large doses in pain-free horses, the cardiovascular depression was not significantly different in magnitude but lasted more than twice as long (≈45 versus 105 minutes) after IM administration.[7] However, in the presence of caecal distension, xylazine caused no significant changes in heart rate by either route, transient hypertension at 5 minutes after IV and hypotension for 90 minutes after IM administration.[33,34] Similar results have been reported for IV and IM detomidine.[7,36] Comparative data for opioids are only available for butorphanol. Administered at 0.1 or 0.2 mg/kg dose IV[30,34] or 0.2 mg/kg IM,[33] the relative change in pain threshold to caecal distension was similar, particularly in relationship to the response to xylazine. The duration of the IM dose was more than 240 minutes, and that after IV administration, 50 minutes. In the presence of caecal distension, both IV and IM butorphanol caused a brief increase in heart rate, but only IV administration was accompanied by an increase in mean arterial blood pressure.[33,34] Thus, using the caecal distension model, IM administration of xylazine and butorphanol increased the duration of analgesia and modified the cardiovascular response when compared to IV administration.

Constant rate infusions

CRIs of α_2-agonists have been described for standing chemical restraint and analgesia in the horse. The use of xylazine was described in an experimental protocol.[42] Detomidine, with and without an opioid, and medetomidine***** for longer-duration protocols, have also been described.[43–46] CRIs of butorphanol have been used for analgesia after colic surgery.[4,47] Profound sedation, bradycardia with second-degree atrioventricular block and no change in mean arterial blood pressure were reported during CRI xylazine at 12 µg/kg/min after a loading dose of 1.1 mg/kg IV.[42] This suggests that, if CRI xylazine were to be used clinically, a smaller loading dose and lower infusion rate would be less compromising. There are no reports of its use clinically. Detomidine, on the other hand, has become popular for chemical restraint because the infusion rate can be titrated to optimise sedation and analgesia while minimising ataxia, thereby improving conditions for standing surgery.[44] Infusion rates high enough to produce marked sedation and ataxia cause bradycardia, hypertension, pulmonary hypertension and decreased cardiac output.[48] Administering IV butorphanol (0.02–0.1 mg/kg) or buprenorphine††††† (6 µg/kg) with the loading dose of detomidine (6–15 µg/kg IV) followed by CRI of detomidine at 0.1–0.6 µg/kg/min results in a moderate bradycardia but little change in mean arterial blood pressure.[44,45,48] Medetomidine, a more specific and potent α_2-agonist, produced stable sedation and only a physiologically acceptable decrease in mean arterial blood pressure (lowest recorded value, 102.4 mm Hg) during the infusion phase (0.058 µg/kg/min). Heart rate, cardiac index and $Pa\text{O}_2$ were decreased from baseline only in the 20 minutes immediately after the loading dose of 5 µg/kg IV.[46] Controlled studies of the analgesic properties of medetomidine have not been reported. A loading dose of butorphanol (17.85 µg/kg IV) followed by an infusion (0.38 µg/kg/min) resulted in heart rates and behaviour in horses that did not differ from those of horses given saline. Gastrointestinal motility was decreased as assessed by auscultation, polyethylene glycol 3500 transit and faecal production but recovered shortly after discontinuation of the infusion.[47] Administered for the first 24 hours after colic surgery butorphanol infusion (0.22 µg/kg/min) improved general behaviour indicative of comfort, delayed faecal output and reduced weight loss, duration of hospitalisation and total treatment cost.[4] Neither the loading dose and higher infusion rate used in healthy horses nor the lower infusion rate used in postoperative colics caused any of the typical opioid side effects of dysphoria or locomotion. Combining CRI butorphanol with CRI detomidine has been recommended for standing chemical restraint where detomidine alone is insufficient.[49]

The administration of a combination of α_2-agonist and opioid to a persistently painful colic may be restricted by the inhibitory action of both these classes of drug have on gastrointestinal motility.[8–10,17,37] Acute death has been anecdotally associated with the use of all the α_2-agonists, and general anaesthetic mortality is increased when an α_2-agonist is used.[50] The abdominal pain of some horses may

***** Domitor; Pfizer, Sandwich, Kent, UK.

††††† Vetergesic; Alstoe Animal Health, Sherrif Hutton, Yorks, UK; Buprenex; Reckitt Benckiser, Slough, Berks, UK.

respond to just CRI butorphanol and flunixin with the occasional IV or IM α_2-agonist supplementation. Alternately, CRI lignocaine (lidocaine)‡‡‡‡‡ has been shown to have antinociceptive activity in that it reduced halothane minimum alveolar concentration in ponies,[51] end-tidal isoflurane requirement for surgery[52] and the electroencephalographic response to castration.[53] In humans and laboratory animals, intravenous lignocaine (lidocaine) decreased neuronal and reflex responses to colorectal distension,[54] decreased postoperative pain after abdominal surgery[55,56] and decreased the duration of postoperative ileus.[55,57] Although lignocaine had no effect on equine pyloric or jejunal smooth muscle activity *in vitro*, it did increase jejunal activity.[58] In a survey of prokinetic drug use in postcolic surgery horses, CRI lignocaine was the most common choice at a loading dose of 1.3 mg/kg followed by 0.05 mg/kg/min infusion.[59] This dosing regimen caused no significant changes in heart rate, mean arterial blood pressure or respiratory rate in a group of healthy horses.[60] A comparable dosing regimen (2 mg/kg loading dose, 50 μg/kg/min CRI), however, showed no increase in pain threshold to duodenal or small colon distension.[61] Intraoperative (0.65 mg/kg then 0.025 mg/kg/min) plus 24-hour postoperative (1.3 mg/kg then 0.05 mg/kg/min) CRI lignocaine resulted in less postoperative small intestinal distension but no significant improvement in reflux, gastrointestinal sounds, faecal production or outcome compared to saline-treated controls.[62] Clinical signs of toxicity, muscle fasciculations, sedation and ataxia, but no changes in heart rate, arterial blood pressure or respiratory rate, were seen at a venous blood concentration of 3.24 ± 0.74 μg/ml 11.4 ± 5.52 minutes after a loading dose of 1.5 mg/kg followed by 0.3 mg/kg/min infusion.[18] Because, in the horse, steady-state volume of distribution and clearance of lignocaine are decreased by sevoflurane anaesthesia,[60] it would be expected that other conditions that decrease cardiac output and hepatic blood flow also affect lignocaine pharmacokinetics. Therefore, sick or stressed horses treated with CRI lignocaine should be carefully observed for signs of toxicity as well as efficacy.

Acupuncture

An additional approach to acute abdominal pain is acupuncture. Practitioners of traditional Chinese medicine attest to successful modulation of colic pain, but few controlled studies have been done.[63] Electrical stimulation of a single gastrointestinal acupuncture point on the bladder meridian prior to balloon distension of the proximal duodenum failed to decrease the frequency of behavioural indicators of abdominal pain (pawing, shifting, neck stretching, kicking at abdomen, looking at flank).[64] However, most treatments stimulate an array of acupuncture points,[63,65] and therefore this may not have been an adequate test. Using five acupoints, electroacupuncture did increase the threshold of response to colorectal distension.[66] In rats, dorsal horn neuronal response to colorectal distension was attenuated by the manual stimulation of the contralateral stomach 36 acupuncture point.[67]

In summary, there is solid evidence that the α_2-agonists are effective analgesics for gastrointestinal pain in the horse. The evidence supporting opioids, systemic lignocaine and acupuncture is less absolute but sufficient to justify their inclusion in combination therapy designed to reduce the dose and adverse effects of the α_2-agonists without compromising pain control. Finally, and often as a last resort, the hypnotics, diazepam§§§§§ and midazolam****** (0.1 mg/kg IM) or chloral hydrate†††††† (20 mg/kg IV or PO),[68,69] have been successful in removing the horse from its abdominal pain. These drugs are not intrinsically analgesic, but their ability to modify the cognitive or emotive response to pain creates clinically apparent relief, allowing the horse to stand or lie quietly.

Other causes of abdominal visceral pain

Colitis that results is tenesmus and potentially rectal prolapse, urethral obstruction and uterine or ovarian pain in the mare are other causes of abdominal pain for the horse. Clinically, the pain induced by the first two conditions appears to be moderate discomfort in that most of the horses fidget and strain rather than paw, pace and roll. They also have a relatively short expected duration as colitis either resolves or is fatal within a few days and urethral obstruction requires removal of the urolith and a finite period of postprocedural analgesia.

Epidural analgesia and anaesthesia for visceral pain

The majority of the afferent and efferent innervation of the rectum, urethra and bladder is sacral (S2-S5). Therefore the discomfort of colitis or urethritis and tenesmus are manageable with caudal epidural analgesics (α_2-agonists, opioids) and/or anaesthesia (local anaesthetics) without undue concern for skeletal motor paralysis. Frequently, a single epidural dose will break the sequence of pain and straining while sufficient healing can occur and further dosing is not needed. Local anaesthetics produce the most profound anaesthesia but will also block sensory and motor fibres to the hind legs if dosed excessively. Cranial spread of epidural injectate is influenced by total volume, speed of injection and drug and patient characteristics.[70] Bupiva-

‡‡‡‡‡ Xylocaine; AstraZeneca Pharmaceuticals LP, Wilmington, DE, USA.

§§§§§ Valium; Roche Laboratories, Basel. Switzerland; Diazemuls; Dumex Ltd, Whiddon Valley, Barnstaple, UK; diazepam injection; Parnell Laboratories, Alexandria, NSW, Australia.

****** Midazolam injection; Antigen Pharmaceuticals, Dublin, Ireland.

†††††† Chloral hydrate crystals. Available from a variety of suppliers of generic brand pharmaceuticals.

caine‡‡‡‡‡‡ and ropivacaine§§§§§§, amides approximately 4 times more potent than lignocaine, have a wider differential of sensory to motor block and a longer duration of action.[71] Less-concentrated solutions of local anaesthetic also tend to selectively block sensory fibres but larger volumes may result in excessive cranial spread. The opioids and α_2-agonists modulate nociceptive input to the neurons in the dorsal horn of the spinal cord, although xylazine also decreases axonal conduction and may cause significant ataxia.[72–74] Generally, local anaesthetics have the most rapid onset (5–20 minutes), α_2-agonists are nearly as rapid (10–30 minutes) and opioids, depending on their lipid solubility, are the slowest (30–180 minutes). Administered epidurally at the first coccygeal intervertebral space, standard doses of 2% lidocaine and mepivacaine******* (0.20–0.35 mg/kg) provide 30–120 minutes of perineal anaesthesia[73,75–77]; 0.5% bupivacaine (0.06 mg/kg), 320 minutes[78]; and 0.5% ropicavaine (0.08 mg/kg), 180 to 320 minutes.[97,80] The perineal analgesia produced by caudal epidural xylazine (0.17 mg/kg) may last 240 minutes; detomidine (0.03–0.06 mg/kg), 180 minutes; morphine (0.1–0.2 mg/kg), up to 32 hours; pethidine (meperidine) (0.8 mg/kg), 5 hours; methadone (0.1 mg/kg), 5 hours; and tramadol††††††† (1 mg/kg), 8 hours.[73,76,77,81–86] Combinations tend to result in an onset consistent with the most rapid component and a duration consistent with the longest acting. The caudal epidural use of combinations of lidocaine and xylazine,[77] morphine and detomidine,[87,88] butorphanol and lidocaine[89] and ropivacaine and fentanyl[80] have shown synergism in horses. Despite textbook recommendations of the use of caudal epidural anaesthesia to manage rectal prolapse, urethral surgery and bladder manipulation, most experimental studies have only tested somatic (cutaneous and superficial muscle) analgesia. Tramadol (1 mg/kg), morphine (0.1 mg/kg) and methadone (0.1 m/kg) at volumes of 20 ml increased the threshold to cutaneous stimulation from the tail to midthorax,[83,86] which suggests visceral afferent sympathetic neurotransmission would also be altered. On the other hand, the analgesia provided by pethidine (meperidine) (0.8 mg/kg, 4–5 ml) only reached the dermatomes innervated by sacral and coccygeal spinal segments.[90] Cutaneous perineal, vaginal and urethral analgesia were achieved with 0.25 mg/kg lignocaine (lidocaine), with or without 0.04 mg/kg butorphanol[89] and 0.196 ± 0.034 mg/kg mepivacaine.[75] Horses have been treated successfully with epidural lignocaine, xylazine or morphine and detomidine for urethral, rectal and rectovaginal lesions, and one horse with nephritis responded to epidural morphine.[81,91] The caveat for epidural management of abdominal pain is that local anaesthetics, alone or in combination with other analgesics, block motor as well as sensory fibre conduction and can result in hindlimb paralysis.[73,75,78,86,92] Therefore, they should be used conservatively for pelvic visceral pain only. Opioids, which may cause mild ataxia and altered gait but not recumbency,[86,90] may be given in doses and volumes expected to reach the dorsal horn of thoracic spinal segments to alleviate visceral pain to structures innervated by the cranial and caudal mesenteric plexus.

Transection of the ovarian pedicle during ovariectomy, tension on the ovarian or uterine mesentery either from a large ovarian tumour, mesenteric haematoma or uterine torsion and uterine wall haematomas appear to be very painful in that the mare will exhibit typical signs of severe colic. The pain can be unresponsive to systemic butorphanol or morphine and only partially controlled by α_2-agonists. The addition of CRI lidocaine and/or caudal epidural analgesics may help. Segmental subarachnoid anaesthesia to localised spinal regions has been described[93] but is not commonly attempted.

Thoracic visceral pain

Causes of thoracic visceral and pleural pain are less commonly encountered in horses and their treatment is confounded by concerns for respiratory depression, which is a side effect of both α_2-agonists[42,46,48] and opioids.[15,16] The sensory innervation of the thoracic viscera is vagal and sympathetic, and that of the parietal pleura, somatic.[24] Thus, a high opioid epidural might offer some pain relief with less chance of further compromise to respiratory function.

Ocular pain

The most common cranial visceral pain encountered in equine practice is that due to corneal injury or inflammation, anterior uveitis or major trauma requiring enucleation. As with other inflammatory conditions, NSAIDs are important in reducing peripheral sensitisation of nerve endings.[6,94] Subconjunctival flunixin has been shown to decrease prostacyclin production in the aqueous humour of the normal equine eye.[95] The recognition of peripheral opioid receptors and their role in nociception has lead to their local administrations.[6,96] In dogs, the topical treatment of experimentally created corneal ulcers with 1% morphine solution reduced blepharospasm and corneal hypersensitivity but not miosis. The healing of the corneal wound was not affected by morphine.[97] Postenucleation pain is expressed by a head tilt and subdued demeanour without noticeable loss of appetite that usually lasts only 24 hours. There are no reports of efforts to attenuate this discomfort, but it might be a pain that could be alleviated

‡‡‡‡‡‡ Marcaine; AstraZeneca Pharmaceuticals LP, Wilmington, DE, USA.

§§§§§§ Naropin; AstraZeneca Pharmaceuticals LP, Wilmington, DE, USA.

******* Intra-Epicaine; Arnolds Veterinary Products, Shrewsbury, Shropshire, UK; Carbocaine; Pharmacia, Bridgewater, NJ, USA; Vetacaine; Troy Laboratories PTY, Smithfield, NSW, Australia.

††††††† Zydol, Searle Pharmaceutical, High Wycombe, Bucks, UK.

by the administration of a long-acting opioid such as buprenorphine (0.02 mg/kg IM) or the preoperative application of transdermal fentanyl (2 × 100 μg/hr [10 mg] patches/500-kg horse).

Somatic pain

Elective orthopaedic cases, whether a simple chip removal or major bone cyst debridement, can benefit from preemptive pain management. Easiest and proved effective in other species is the preoperative use of NSAIDs[98–100] in horses.[1,101] By blocking cyclooxygenase activation in response to surgical tissue trauma, peripheral sensitisation is reduced and, subsequently, postoperative pain should be less. In equine inflammatory joint models, phenylbutazone‡‡‡‡‡‡‡, flunixin, ketoprofen, eltenac§§§§§§§, meloxicam******** and carprofen†††††††† have all proved effective at reducing indicators of inflammation and lameness.[26,101–104]

Postoperative pain equates to postoperative stress, increased sympathetic drive and metabolic demand leading to prolonged recovery and delayed healing.[105,106] In people, preoperative or postoperative epidural or intra-articular bupivacaine and morphine reduced postoperative pain.[107–110] Comparable advantages have been demonstrated in dogs subjected to stifle surgery.[111–113] Preoperatively administered epidural morphine and detomidine resulted in lower mean postoperative lameness scores of horses subjected to bilateral stifle arthroscopy compared to saline-treated controls.[88] There have been no reports of intra-articular opioid use in horses despite the demonstration of opioid receptors in equine carpal and stifle synovial membranes[114] and that morphine (15 mg in 5 ml saline) was not more irritating than saline in the tarsocural joint of ponies.[115,116]

Emergency orthopaedic surgery cases cannot benefit from preemptive analgesia but including preoperative pain management in their anaesthetic protocol will produce a more stable anaesthetic period and, carried into recovery, a safer return to standing. The most painful acute injury seems to be limb fractures as these horses present tachycardic, tachypnoeic, trembling, sweating, and ostensibly focusing on enduring the pain. However, distal limb wounds, septic joints or tendon sheaths, disrupted suspensory apparatus and hoof injuries most often present three-legged lame. Stabilising the limb and providing supportive treatment for pain and distress are immediate goals. An NSAID should help reduce the inflammatory component of the pain. Judicious use of intramuscular opioids, with or without a low dose of α_2-agonist, and intravenous fluids will provide immediate pain relief without pronounced sedation or ataxia and cardiovascular support, respectively. Closed fractures that can be splinted effectively benefit from a night in a stall to allow the horse to adjust and reestablish homeostasis before surgical repair. During this period, an appropriate regimen of systemic, transdermal or epidural opioids can be established for that horse to be maintained through surgery, recovery and postoperative recuperation.

For obvious reasons, controlled studies of the analgesic properties of drugs have used models of cutaneous stimulation or reversible joint inflammation and not of bone or ligament tissue injury. Coronary band heat stimulus response threshold was raised by morphine (0.66 mg/kg IM) less than by xylazine (2.2 mg/kg IM) but more than butorphanol (0.2 mg/kg IM).[33] In that study and similar heat stimulus tests, flunixin (2.2 mg/kg IM or 1.1 mg/kg IV) and phenylbutazone (7.3 mg/kg IV)[117] failed to provide analgesia but the avoidance response threshold was increased by carprofen (0.7 mg/kg IV).[118] Detomidine dose-dependently,[119] and at an equisedative dose (0.02 mg/kg IV), increased the threshold of response to heat, electrical shock or mechanical pressure more than did either xylazine (1.1 mg/kg IV) or romifidine‡‡‡‡‡‡‡‡ (0.08 mg/kg IV).[120,121] Adding butorphanol (0.025 mg/kg IV) or methadone (0.1 mg/kg IV) to detomidine (0.01 mg/kg IV) contributed additional analgesia in response to electrical and mechanical somatic pain.[122] When combined with xylazine (1.1 mg/kg IV), butorphanol (0.1 mg/kg IV) contributed to analgesia in response to a flank skin incision,[123] but neither butorphanol (0.04 mg/kg IV), morphine (0.75 mg/kg IV) nor nalbuphine§§§§§§§§ (0.75 mg/kg IV) changed the response to electrical stimulation of an upper canine tooth compared to xylazine alone.[124] Fentanyl, a potent μ-opioid receptor agonist, also raises the pain threshold, but a single IV bolus of 0.01 mg/kg IV provided only 30 to 40 minutes of relief and stimulated locomotion.[117] Sustained release of fentanyl from a transdermal patch resulted in theoretically analgesic blood levels in 1 to 4 hours[125,126] that were maintained over 8 to 9 days by application of new patches at 48- to 72-hour intervals.[125] Used in combination with phenylbutazone or flunixin on clinically painful horses, subjective pain, but not lameness, scores improved after transdermal fentanyl application without apparent adverse effects.[5] Buprenorphine and lignocaine (lidocaine) are also available as transdermal patches, but no work has been published regarding their application to horses.

‡‡‡‡‡‡‡ Equipalazone; Arnolds Veterinary Products, Shrewsbury, Shropshire, UK; EquiBute; Fort Dodge Animal Health, Fort Dodge, IA, USA.

§§§§§§§ Telzenac; Schering-Plough, Kenilworth, NJ, USA.

******** Metacam; Boehringer Ingelheim, Ingelheim, Germany.

†††††††† Rimadyl; Pfizer, New York, NY, USA; Zenecarp, Pfizer, Sandwich, Kent, UK.

‡‡‡‡‡‡‡‡ Sedivet; Boehringer Ingelheim, Bracknell, Berkshire, UK.

§§§§§§§§ Nubain; Endo Pharmaceuticals, Chadds Ford, PA, USA.

Epidural analgesia for somatic pain

The nociceptive activity of epidurally administered opioids, α_2-agonists, ketamine and NSAIDs is attributed to a similar mechanism albeit involving different specific actions and receptor types.[6,94] As discussed earlier, perineal somatic pain, as tested by pin prick or electrical stimulation, is attenuated by epidural opioids, α_2-agonists or combinations of these with each other or small doses of local anaesthetic. Larger doses and/or larger volumes of injectate result in more cranial distribution of sensory block. In addition, placement of an epidural catheter enables repeated dosing as needed with a low incidence of catheter-related complications.[91,127] The long duration of action (8–32 hours) of epidural morphine (0.1–0.2 mg/kg) makes it extremely useful for the long-term management of any caudal, and some more cranial, pain (Figure 6.1, A and B). The successful control of severe pain due to amputation following fetlock joint luxation and first phalanx fracture with epidural morphine (0.1 mg/kg in 30 ml saline) every 6 to 8 hours for 5 days has been reported.[128] In a review of the use of epidural catheters for pain management in horses, 60% of the horses, 96% of them successfully, were treated with morphine alone (0.04–0.26 mg/kg in 0.9% NaCl to a volume of 10–100 ml) for a variety of orthopaedic problems including a scapular fracture.[91] Side effects of morphine epidural administration potentially include decreased gastrointestinal motility, urinary retention, respiratory depression and pruritis. Of these, only pruritis has been reported in the horse.[129] Excessive dosing results in systemic levels sufficient to cause the typical equine opioid locomotor response. More rapid onset of analgesia has been achieved by adding detomidine (0.03 mg/kg) to morphine[87] at the cost of systemic α_2-adrenergic side effects including sedation, ataxia and bradycardia.[74,85,87,88] For long-term pain management, repeated 2- to 3-hour periods of sedation following detomidine/morphine epidural treatment may not be optimal to patient well-being. Aedation and bradycardia are not features of epidural xylazine, suggesting that it is not absorbed systemically as rapidly as detomidine. The side effects of excessive epidural xylazine are decreased hind limb proprioception and weakness and decreased tail and anal tone attributable to a local anaesthetic–like action on neuronal conduction.[72–74] Neither the clinical nor experimental use of opioid-xylazine combinations has been reported. Combining epidural opioids and local anaesthetics has demonstrated a synergism that permitted reduced doses of both fewer side effects and improved analgesia in humans and rats.[130,131] The only reports of such combinations in horses have compared the combination with the local anaesthetic alone at the same or only a slightly reduced dose[80,89] and found improved somatic analgesia with the addition of opioids that have elsewhere shown little epidural efficacy in horses (fentanyl and butorphanol).[83,132] Cerebrospinal fluid or plasma concentration of β-endorphins increased after multiple-point electroacupuncture that also raised the threshold of response to cutaneous heat stimulus[133] or improved lameness created by applied sole pressure,[134] respectively.

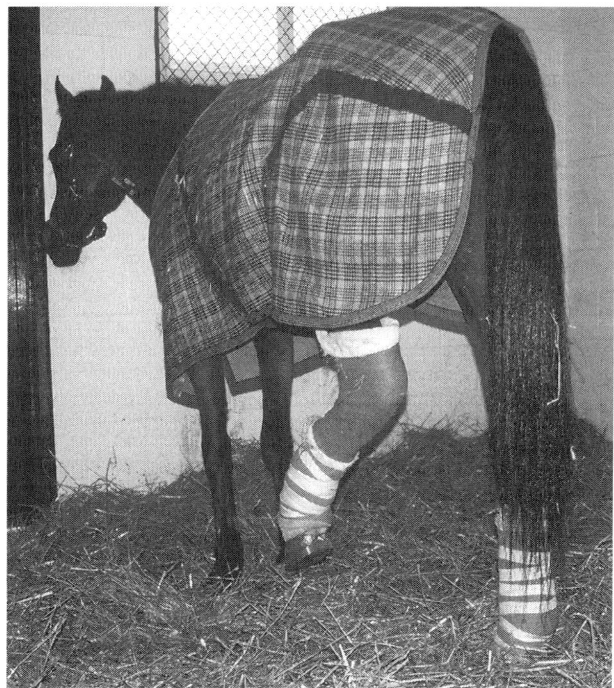

A

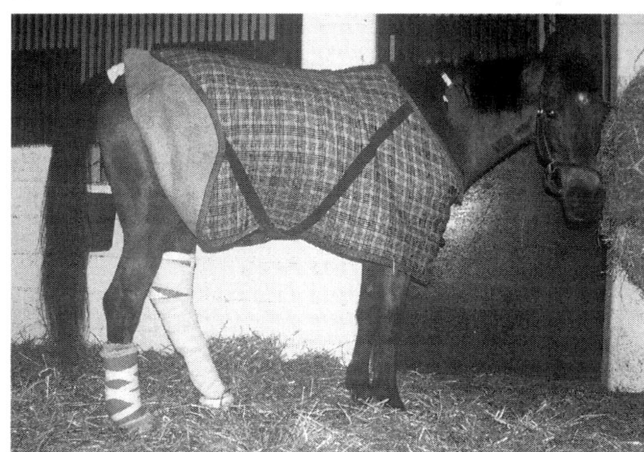

B

Figures 6.1A-B Preepidural and 12-hour postepidural morphine in a horse with a septic tarsal sheath. Note he is standing facing the back of the stall before the morphine and not only is he partially weight bearing with the effective leg (A), but he is in the front of the stall eating after treatment (B). ©Lydia Donaldson 2006.

Secondary hyperalgesia or "wind up"

CRI lignocaine (lidocaine) has been shown to be an effective analgesic for a thermal stimulus applied to the withers of normal horses.[61] Based on research models of pain and use in human patients, systemically administered lignocaine has at least two applications: to reduce acute postoperative pain[55,56] and to modulate secondary hyperalgesia, allodynia and neuropathic pain.[135–137] One of the proposed mechanisms is modulation of synaptic transmission by neurons in the dorsal horn of the spinal cord.[138] Hyperalgesia, allodynia and neuropathic pain are difficult to identify in horses, but severe, longer-duration pain is not. Laminitis may be the classic example, but whether it is associated with "wind up" and hypersensitivity syndromes has yet to be investigated. The sequence of acute injury inducing severe pain followed by chronic, often debilitating pain is reminiscent of the posttraumatic chronic pain syndromes described in people.[94,139] Complex regional pain syndrome or reflex sympathetic dystrophy, a neuropathic syndrome recognised in people, has been a label thrown at laminitis.[140] Traditionally, NSAIDs have been the mainstay of pain management in chronically laminitic horses and have been proved efficacious in a controlled study,[141] but the possibility that aggressive early interruption of nociceptive input to the central nervous system could affect the later chronic phase is intriguing. To this end, systemic lignocaine (lidocaine) has demonstrated some efficacy for reducing hyperalgesia, allodynia and neuropathic pain.[135–137,142] Early administration of systemic lignocaine in severe trauma or acute laminitis may modify the long-term outcome. Ketamine, systemically or epidurally, successfully controls acute postoperative pain and hyperalgesia in human[142,143] and small animal patients[144–146] and chronic pain in people.[147] Subanaesthetic doses of ketamine might be an additional approach to blocking acute laminitic "wind up". In horses, peri-incisional hyperalgesia was reduced by the preemptive epidural administration of ketamine (1 mg/kg in ≈8 ml saline).[148] A level of surgical analgesia of the tail, perineum and proximal hind leg was achieved within 10 to 15 minutes and lasting 30 to 80 minutes after 0.5, 1.0 or 2.0 mg/kg of epidural ketamine in approximately 8 ml saline. Side effects included mild sedation and ataxia.[149] In anaesthetised ponies, epidural ketamine (0.8 and 1.2 mg/kg diluted to a volume of 0.15 ml/kg) decreased halothane minimum alveolar concentration by approximately 15%.[132] Subanaesthetic ketamine CRI (0.006–0.012 mg/kg/min) has been reported to reduce the apparent discomfort in horses with somatic pain (septic joints, burns) but not colic. Ataxia and exaggerated responses to noise were noted at doses greater than 0.027 mg/kg/min.[150]

Newer concepts in pain management have not been investigated for use in horses. Prostaglandins facilitate nociceptive neurotransmission in the dorsal horn of the spinal cord, and the epidural administration of NSAIDs has inhibited nociceptive responses to acute and chronic stimuli in some models.[151] Gabapentin*********, an anticonvulsant, has been shown to decrease postoperative and neuropathic pain in animal models and human patients[152] and to synergistically increase the analgesia of morphine.[153,154] For the average horse owner, treatment with gabapentin is likely prohibitively expensive but it, or similar agents, may become feasible to include as an equine analgesic in the future.

In conclusion, α_2-agonists are the most profound analgesics for both visceral and somatic pain in the horse. Because of their diverse and compromising side effects, combining them with NSAIDs, opioids, local anaesthetics and ketamine in various modalities can affect better control of pain with less impact on behavior and physiological function.

********* Neurontin; Pfizer, New York, NY, USA.

References

1. Raekallio M, Taylor PM, Bennett RC: Preliminary investigations of pain and analgesia assessment in horses administered phenylbutazone or placebo after arthroscopic surgery. Vet Surg 26:150-155, 1997
2. Anil SS, Anil L, Deen J: Challenges of pain assessment in domestic animals. J Am Vet Med Assoc 220:313-319, 2002
3. Price J, Catriona S, Welsh EM, Waran NK: Preliminary evaluation of a behaviour-based system for assessment of post-operative pain in horses following arthroscopic surgery. Vet Anaesth Analg 30:124-137, 2003
4. Sellon DC, Roberts MC, Blikslager AT, Ulibarri C, Papich MG: Effects of continuous rate intravenous infusion of butorphanol on physiologic and outcome variables in horses after celiotomy. J Vet Intern Med 18:555-563, 2004
5. Thomasy SM, Slovis N, Maxwell LK, Kollias-Baker C: Transdermal fentanyl combined with nonsteroidal anti-inflammatory drugs for analgesia in horses. J Vet Intern Med 18:550-554, 2004
6. Muir WW, Woolf CJ: Mechanism of pain and their therapeutic implications. J Am Vet Med Assoc 219:1346-1355, 2001
7. Wagner AE, Muir WW, Hinchcliff KW: Cardiovascular effects of xylazine and detomidine in horses. Am J Vet Res 52:651-657, 1991
8. Stick JA, Chou CC, Derksen FJ, Arden WA: Effects of xylazine on equine intestinal vascular resistance, motility, compliance, and oxygen consumption. Am J Vet Res 48:198-203, 1987
9. Clark ES, Thompson SA, Becht JL, Moore JN: Effects of xylazine on cecal mechanical activity and cecal blood flow in healthy horses. Am J Vet Res 49:720-723, 1988
10. Merritt AM, Burrow JA, Hartless CS: Effect of xylazine, detomidine, and a combination of xylazine and butorphanol on equine duodenal motility. Am J Vet Res 59:619-623, 1998
11. Hunt RJ, Brandon CI, McCann ME: Effects of acetylpromazine, xylazine, and vertical load on digital arterial blood flow in horses. Am J Vet Res 55:375-378, 1994
12. Thurmon JC, Steffey EP, Zinkl JG, Woliner M, Howland D: Xylazine causes transient dose-related hyperglycemia and increased urine volumes in mares. Am J Vet Res 45:224-227
13. Schatzmann U, Josseck H, Stauffer J-L, Goossens L: Effects of α_2-agonists on intrauterine pressure and sedation in horses: comparison between detomidine, romifidine and xylazine. J Vet Med A 41:523-529, 1994

14. Kamerling SG, DeQuick DJ, Weckman TJ, Tobin T: Dose-related effects of fentanyl on autonomic and behavioral responses in performance horses. Gen Pharamcol 16:253-258, 1985
15. Robertson JT, Muir WW, Sams R: Cardiopulmonary effects of butorphanol tartrate in horses. Am J Vet Res 42:41-44, 1981
16. Muir WW, Skarda RT, Sheehan WC: Cardiopulmonary effects of narcotic agonists and a partial agonist in horses. Am J Vet Res 39:1632-1635, 1978
17. Roberts MC, Argenzio A: Effects of amitraz, several opiate derivatives and anticholinergic agents on intestinal transit in ponies. Equine Vet J 18:256-260, 1986
18. Meyer GA, Lin HC, Hanson RR, Hayes TL: Effects of intravenous lidocaine overdose on cardiac electrical activity and blood pressure in the horse. Equine Vet J 33:434-437, 2001
19. McAllister CG, Morgan SJ, Borne AT, Pollet RA: Comparison of adverse effects of phenylbutazone, flunixin meglumine, and ketoprofen in horses. J Am Vet Med Assoc 202:71-77, 1993
20. McKellar QA, Bogan JA, von Fellenberg R-L, Ludwig B, Cawley GD: Pharmacokinetic, biochemical and tolerance studies on carprofen in the horse. Equine Vet J 23:280-282, 1991
21. Blikslager AT: Cyclo-oxygenase-2 inhibitors in equine practice. Compendium 21:548-550, 1999
22. Matthews NS, Fielding CL, Swinebroad E: How to use a ketamine constant rate infusion in horses for analgesia. Am Assoc Equine Pract Proc 50:227-228, 2004
23. Kehlet H, Dahl JB: The value of "multimodal" or "balanced analgesia" in postoperative pain treatment. Anesth Analg 77:1048-1056, 1993
24. Dyce KM, Sack WO, Wensing CJG: Textbook of Veterinary Anatomy, ed 3. Philadelphia, WB Saunders, 2002
25. Goyal RK, Hirano I: The enteric nervous system. N Engl J Med 334:1106-1115, 1996
26. Johnson CB, Taylor PM, Young SS, Brearley JC: Postoperative analgesia using phenylbutazone, flunixin or carprofen in horse. Vet Rec 133:336-338, 1993
27. Semrad SD, Hardee GE, Hardee MM, Moore JN: Low dose flunixin meglumine: effects on eicosanoid production and clinical signs induced by experimental endotoxaemia in horses. Equine Vet J 19:201-206, 1987
28. Bryant CE, Farnfield BA, Janicke HJ: Evaluation of the ability of carprofen and flunixin meglumine to inhibit activation of nuclear factor kappa B. Am J Vet Res 64:211-215, 2003
29. Price J, Marques JM, Welsh EM, Waran NK: Pilot epidemiological study of attitudes towards pain in horses. Vet Rec 151:570-575, 2002
30. Boatwright CE, Fubini SL, Grohn YT, Goosens L: A comparison of N-butylscopolammonium bromide and butorphanol tartrate for analgesia using a balloon model of abdominal pain in ponies. Can J Vet Res 60:65-68, 1996
31. Jochle W, Moore JN, Brown J, Baker GJ, Lowe JE, Fubini S, Reeves MJ, Watkins JP, White NA: Comparison of detomidine, butorphanol, flunixin meglumine and xylazine in clinical cases of equine colic. Equine Vet J Suppl 7:111-116, 1989
32. Longo F, Autefage A, Bayle R, Keister M, Van Gool F: Efficacy of a non-steroidal anti-inflammatory, ketofen 10% (Ketoprofen) in the treatment of colic in horse. Equine Vet Sci 12:311-315, 1992
33. Kalpravidh M, Lumb WV, Wright M, Heath RB: Effects of butorphanol, flunixin, levorphanol, morphine, and xylazine in ponies. Am J Vet Res 45:217-223, 1984
34. Muir WW, Robertson JT: Visceral analgesia: effects of xylazine, butorphanol, meperidine, and pentazocine in horses. Am J Vet Res 46:2081-2084, 1985
35. Pippi NL, Lumb WV: Objective tests of analgesic drugs in ponies. Am J Vet Res 40:1082-1086, 1979
36. Lowe JE, Hilfiger J: Analgesic and sedative effects of detomidine compared to xylazine in a colic model using I.V. and I.M. routes of administration. Acta Vet Scand 82:85-95, 1986
37. Stick JA, Loeffler BS, Arden WA, Chou C-C: Effects of butorphanol tartrate on arterial pressure, jejunal blood flow, vascular resistance, O_2 extraction, and O_2 uptake in halothane-anesthetized horses. Am J Vet Res 50:1202-1206, 1989
38. Matthews NS, Lindsay SL: Effect of low-dose butorphanol on halothane minimum alveolar concentration in ponies. Equine Vet J 22:325-327, 1990
39. Kalpravidh M, Lumb WV, Wright M, Heath RB: Analgesic effects of butorphanol in horses: dose-response studies. Am J Vet Res 45:211-216, 1984
40. Gingerich DA, Rourke JE, Chatfield RC, Strom PW: Butorphanol tartrate: a new analgesic to relieve the pain of equine colic. Vet Med 80:72-77, 1985
41. Kamerling S, Wood T, DeQuick D, Weckman TJ, Tai C, Blake JW, Tobin T: Narcotic analgesics, their detection and pain measurement in the horse: a review. Equine Vet J 21:4-12, 1989
42. Kollias-Baker CA, Court MH, Williams LL: Influence of yohimbine and tolazoline on the cardiovascular, respiratory, and sedative effects of xylazine in the horse. J Vet Pharmacol Ther 16:350-358, 1993
43. Hainisch EK: Sedation by continuous intravenous detomidine drip for standing surgical procedures. Equine Vet Ed 13:43-44, 2001
44. Wilson DV, Bohart GV, Evans ET, Robertson S, Rondenay Y: Retrospective analysis of detomidine infusion for standing chemical restraint in 51 horses. Vet Anaesth Analg 29:54-57, 2002
45. van Dijk P, Lankveld DPK, Rijkenhuizen ABM, Jonker FH: Hormonal, metabolic and physiological effects of laparoscopic surgery using a detomidine-buprenorphine combination in standing horses. Vet Anaesth Analg 30:72-80, 2003
46. Bettschart-Wolfensberger R, Bettschart RW, Vaino O, Marlin D, Clarke KW: Cardiopulmonary effects of a two hour medetomidine infusion and its antagonism by atipamazole in horses and ponies. J Vet Anaes 26:8-12, 1999
47. Sellon DC, Monroe VL, Roberts MC, Papich MG: Pharmacokinetics and adverse effects of butorphanol administered by single intravenous injection or continuous intravenous infusion in horses. Am J Vet Res 62:183-189, 2001
48. Daunt DA, Dunlop CI, Chapman PL, Shafer SL, Ruskoaho H, Vakkuri O, Hodgson DS, Tyler LM, Maze M: Cardiopulmonary and behavioral response to computer-driven infusion of detomidine in standing horses. Am J Vet Res 54:2075-2082, 1993

49. Goodrich LR, Clark-Price S, Ludders J: How to attain effective and consistent sedation for standing procedures in the horse using constant rate infusion. Am Assoc Equine Pract Proc 50:229-232, 2004
50. Johnston GM, Taylor PM, Holmes MA, Wood JLN: Confidential enquiry of perioperative equine fatalities (CEPEF-1): preliminary results. Equine Vet J 27:193-200, 1995
51. Doherty RJ, Fazier DL: Effect of intravenous lidocaine on halothane minimum alveolar concentration in ponies. Equine Vet J 30:300-303, 1998
52. Dzikiti TB, Hellebrekers LJ, van Dijk P: Effects of intravenous lidocaine on isoflurane concentration, physiological parameters, metabolic parameters and stress-related hormones in horses undergoing surgery. J Vet Med A Physiol Pathol Clin Med 50:190-195, 2003
53. Murrell JC, White KL, Johnson CB, Taylor PM, Waterman-Pearson AE. Spontaneous EEG changes in the equine surgical patient: the effect of an intravenous infusion of lidocaine [abstract]. Proc World Cong Vet Anesth 7:114-115, 2000
54. Ness TJ: Intravenous lidocaine inhibits visceral nociceptive reflexes and spinal neurons in the rat. Anesthesia 92:1685-1691, 2000
55. Groudine SB, Fisher HAG, Kaufman RP, Patel MK, Wilkins LJ, Mehta SA, Lumb PD: Intravenous lidocaine speeds the return of bowel function, decreases postoperative pain, and shortens hospital stay in patients undergoing radical retropubic prostatectomy. Anesth Analg 86:235-239, 1998
56. Koppert W, Weigand M, Neumann F, Sittl, Schuettler J, Schmelz M, Hering W: Perioperative intravenous lidocaine has preventive effects on postoperative pain and morphine consumption after major abdominal surgery. Anesth Analg 98:1050-1055, 2004
57. Rimback G, Cassuto J, Tollesson P-O: Treatment of postoperative paralytic ileus by intravenous infusion. Anesth Analg 70:414-419, 1990
58. Nieto JE, Rakestraw PC, Snyder JR, Vatistas NJ: In vitro effects of erythromycin, lidocaine, and metoclopramide on smooth muscle from the pyloric antrum, proximal portion of the duodenum, and middle portion of the jejunum of horse. Am J Vet Res 61:413-419, 2000
59. Van Hoogmoed LLM, Nieto JE, Snyder JR, Harmon FA: Survey of prokinetic use in horses with gastrointestinal injury. Vet Surg 33:279-285, 2004
60. Feary DJ, Mama KR, Wagner AE, Thomasy S: Influence of general anesthesia on pharmocokinetics of intravenous lidocaine infusion in horses. Am J Vet Res 66:574-580, 2005
61. Robertson SA, Sanchez LC, Merritt AM, Doherty TJ: Effects of systemic lidocaine on visceral and somatic nociception in conscious horses. Equine Vet J 37:122-127, 2005
62. Brianceau P, Chevalier H, Karas A, Court MH, Bassage L, Kirker-Head C, Provost P, Paradis MR: Intravenous lidocaine and small-intestinal size, abdominal fluid, and outcome after colic surgery in horses. J Vet Intern Med 16:736-741, 2002
63. Dill SG: Acupuncture for gastrointestinal disorders. Probl Vet Med 4:144-154, 1992
64. Merritt AM, Xie H, Lester GD, Burrow JA, Lorenzo-Figueras M, Mahfoud Z: Evaluation of a method to experimentally induce colic in horses and the effects of acupuncture applied at the Guan-yuan-shu (similar to BL-21) acupoint. Am J Vet Res 63:1006-1011, 2002
65. Feng K-R: A method of electro-acupuncture treatment for equine intestinal impaction. Am J Chin Med 9:174-180, 1981
66. Skarda RT, Muir WW: Comparison of electroacupuncture and butorphanol on respiratory and cardiovascular effects and rectal pain threshold after controlled rectal distension in mares. Am J Vet Res 64:137-144, 2003
67. Rong P-J, Zhu B, Huang Q-F, Gao X-Y, Ben H, Li Y-H: Acupuncture inhibition on neuronal activity of spinal dorsal horn induced by noxious colorectal distension in rat. World J Gastroenterol 11:1011-1017, 2005
68. Ball MA, Peek S: Chloral Hydrate: a sedative not to be forgotten. Equine Pract 18:24-27, 1996
69. Zimmel DN: How to manage pain and dehydration in horses with colic. Am Assoc Equine Pract 49:127-131, 2003
70. Hendrickson DA, Southwood LL, Lopez MJ, Johnson R, Kruse-Elliott KT: Cranial migration of different volumes of new-methylene blue after caudal epidural injection in the horse. Equine Pract 20:12-14, 1998
71. Butterworth JF: Local anesthetics and regional anesthesia, in Hemmings HC, Hopkins PM (eds): Foundations of Anesthesia Basic and Clinical Sciences. Philadelphia, Mosby, 2000, pp 293-304
72. Aziz MA, Martin RJ: α_2-Agonist and local anaesthetic properties of xylazine. Zbl Vet Med A 25:181-188, 1978
73. LeBlanc PH, Caron JP, Patterson JS, Brown M, Matta MA. Epidural injection of xylazine for perineal analgesia in horse. J Am Vet Med Asocc. 193:1405-1408, 1988
74. Skarda RT, Muir WW: Comparison of antinociceptive, cardiovascular, and respiratory effects, head ptosis, and position of pelvic limbs in mares after caudal epidural administration of xylazine and detomidine hydrochloride solution. Am J Vet Res 57:1338-1345, 1996
75. Skarda RT, Muir WW: Continuous caudal epidural and subarachnoid anesthesia in mares: a comparative study. Am J Vet Res 44:2290-2298, 1983
76. Fikes LW, Lin HC, Thurmon JC: A preliminary comparison of lidocaine and xylazine as epidural analgesics in ponies. Vet Surg 18:85-86, 1989
77. Grubb TL, Riebold TW, Huber MJ: Comparison of lidocaine, xylazine, and xylazine/Lidocaine for caudal epidural analgesia in horses. J Am Vet Med Assoc 201:1187-1190, 1992
78. DeRossi R, Sampaio BFB, Varela JV, Junqueira AL: Perineal analgesia and hemodynamic effects of the epidural administration of meperidine or hyperbaric bupivicaine in conscious horses. Can Vet J 45:42-47, 2004
79. Skarda RT, Muir WW: Analgesic, hemodynamic and respiratory effects of caudal epidurally administered ropivacaine hydrochloride in mares. Vet Anaesth Analg 28:61-74, 2001
80. Ganidagli S, Cetin H, Biricik HS, Cimtay I: Comparison of ropivacaine with a combination of ropivacaine and fentanyl for the caudal epidural anaesthesia of mares. Vet Rec 154:329-332, 2004
81. LeBlanc PH, Caron JP: Clinical use of epidural xylazine in the horse. Equine Vet J 22:180-181, 1990

82. LeBlanc PH, Eberhart SW: Cardiopulmonary effects of epidurally administered xylazine in the horse. Equine Vet J 22:389-391, 1990
83. Natalini CC, Robinson EP: Evaluation of the analgesic effects of epidurally administered morphine, alfentanil, butorphanol, tramadol, and U50488H in horses. Am J Vet Res 61:1579-1586, 2000
84. Skarda RT, Muir WW: Caudal analgesia induced by epidural or subarachnoid administration of detomidine hydrochloride solution in mares. Am J Vet Res 55:670-680, 1994
85. Skarda RT, Muir WW: Analgesic, hemodynamic, and respiratory effects of caudal epidurally administered xylazine hydrochloride solution in mares. Am J Vet Res 57:193-200, 1996
86. Olbrich VH, Mosing M: A comparison of the analgesic effects of caudal epidural methadone and lidocaine in the horse. Vet Anaesth Analg 30:156-164, 2003
87. Sysel AM, Pleasant RS, Jacobson JD, Moll HD, Modransky PD, Warnick LD, Sponenberg DP, Eyre P: Efficacy of an epidural combination of morphine and detomidine in alleviating experimentally induced hindlimb lameness in horses. Vet Surg 25:511-518, 1996
88. Goodrich LR, Nixon AJ, Fubini SL, Ducharme NG, Fortier LA, Warnick LD, Ludders JW: Epidural morphine and detomidine decreases postoperative hindlimb lameness in horses after bilateral stifle arthroscopy. Vet Surg 31:232-239, 2002
89. Csik-Salmon J, Blais D, Vaillancourt D, Garon O, Bisaillon A: Utilisation du mélange lidocaine-butorphanol en anesthesia epidurale caudale chez la jument. Can J Vet Res 60:288-295, 1996
90. Skarda RT, Muir WW: Analgesic, hemodynamic, and respiratory effects induced by caudal epidural administration of meperidine hydrochloride in mares. Am J Vet Res 62:1001-1007, 2001
91. Martin CA, Kerr CL, Pearce SG, Landsdowne JL, Boure LP: Outcome of epidural catheterization for delivery of analgesics in horses: 43 cases (1998-2001). J Am Vet Med Assoc 222:1394-1398, 2003
92. Chopin JB, Wright JD: Complications after the use of a combination of lignocaine and xylazine for epidural anaesthesia in a mare. Aust Vet J 72:354-355, 1995
93. Skarda RT, Muir WW: Segmental thoracolumbar spinal (subarachnoid) analgesia in conscious horses. Am J Vet Res 43:2121-2127, 1983
94. Mannion RJ. Woolf CJ: Pain mechanisms and management: a central perspective. Clin J Pain 16:S144-S156, 2000
95. Cooley PL, Milvae R, Riis RC, Laratta LJ: Effect of flunixin meglumine on prostacyclin accumulation in the equine eye. Am J Vet Res 45:1383-1385, 1984
96. Stein C: The control of pain in peripheral tissue by opioids. N Engl J Med 332:1685-1690, 1995
97. Stiles J, Honda CN, Krohne AG, Kazacos EA: Effect of topical administration of 1% morphine sulphate solution on signs of pain and corneal wound healing in dogs. Am J Vet Res 64:813-818, 2003
98. Lascelles BDX, Cripps PJ, Jones A, Waterman-Pearson AE: Efficacy and kinetics of carprofen, administered preoperatively or postoperatively, for the prevention of pain in dogs undergoing ovariohysterectomy. Vet Surg 27:568-582, 1998
99. Lemke KA, Runyon CL, Horney BS: Effects of preoperative administration of ketoprofen on anesthetic requirements and signs of postoperative pain in dogs undergoing elective ovariohysterectomy. J Am Vet Med Assoc 221:1268-1275, 2002
100. Grisneaux E, Pibarot P, Dupuis J, Blais D: Comparison of ketoprofen and carprofen administered prior to orthopedic surgery for control of postoperative pain in dogs. J Am Vet Med Assoc 215:1105-1110, 1999
101. Owens JG, Kamerling SG, Stanton SR, Keowen ML, Prescott-Matthews JS: Effects of pretreatment with ketoprofem and phenylbutazone on experimentally induced synovitis in horses. Am J Vet Res 57:866-874, 1996
102. Hamm D, Turchi P, Johnson JC, Lockwood PW, Thompson KC, Katz T: Determination of an effective dose of eltenac and its comparison with that of flunixin meglumine in horses after experimentally induced carpitis. Am J Vet Res 58:298-302, 1997
103. Armstrong S, Lees P: Effects of R and S enantiomers and a racemic mixture of carprofen on the production and release of proteoglycan and prostaglandin E_2 from equine chondrocytes and cartilage explants. Am J Vet Res 60:98-104, 1999
104. Toutain P-L, Cester CC: Pharmacokinetic-pharmacodynamic relationships and dose response to meloxicam in horses with induced arthritis in the right carpal joint. Am J Vet Res 65:1533-1541, 2004
105. Woolf CJ, Chong M-S: Preemptive analgesia- treating postoperative pain by preventing the establishment of central sensitization. Anesth Analg 77:362-379, 1993
106. Shafford HL, Lascelles BDX, Hellyer PW: Preemptive analgesia: managing pain before it begins. Vet Med 96:478-492, 2001
107. Reuben SS, Sklar J, El-Mansouri M: The preemptive analgesic effect of intraarticular bupivicaine and morphine after ambulatory arthroscopic knee surgery. Anesth Analg 92:923-926, 2001
108. Jaureguito JW, Wilcox JF, Cohn SJ, Thisted RA, Reider B: A comparison of intraarticular morphine and bupivicaine for pain control after outpatient knee arthroscopy. Am J Sports Med 23:350-353, 1995
109. Allen GC, St. Amand MA, Lui ACP, Johnson DH, Lindsay MP: Postarthroscopy analgesia with intraarticular bupivicaine/morphine. Anesthesia 79:475-480, 1992
110. Dalsgaard J, Felsby S, Juelsgaard P, Froekjaer J: Low-dose intra-articular morphine analgesia in day case knee arthroscopy: a randomized double-blinded prospective study. Pain 56:151-154, 1994
111. Day TK, Pepper WT, Tobias TA, Flynn MJ, Clarke KM: Comparison of intra-articular and epidural morphine for analgesia following stifle arthrotomy in dogs. Vet Surg 24:522-530, 1995
112. Sammarco JL, Conzemius MG, Perkowski AZ, Weinstein MJ, Gregor TP, Smith GK: Postoperative analgesia for stifle surgery: a comparison of intra-articular bupivacaine, morphine or saline. Vet Surg 25:59-69, 1996
113. Troncy E, Junot S, Keroack S, Sammut V, Pibarot P, Genevois J-P, Cuvelliez S: Results of preemptive epidural administration of morphine with or without bupivacaine in dogs and cats undergoing surgery: 265 cases (1997-1999). J Am Vet Med Assoc 221:666-672, 2002

114. Sheehy JG, Hellyer PW, Sammonds GE, Mama KR, Powers BE, Hendrickson DA, Magnusson KR: Evaluation of opioid receptors in synovial membranes of horses. Am J Vet Res 62:1408-1412, 2001
115. Raekallio M, Taylor PM, Johnson CB, Tulamo R-M, Ruprah M: The disposition and local effects of intra-articular morphine in normal ponies. J Assoc Vet Anaesth 23:23-26, 1996
116. Tulamo R-M, Raekallio M, Taylor P, Johnson CB, Salonen M: Intra-articular morphine and saline injections induce release of large molecular weight proteoglycans into equine synovial fluid. J Vet Med Assoc 43:147-153, 1996
117. Kamerling SG, DeQuick DJ, Weckman TJ, Sprinkle FP, Tobin T: Differential effects of phenylbutazone and local anesthetics on nociception in the equine. Eur J Pharmacol 107:35-41, 1985
118. Schatzmann U, Gugelmann M, von Cranach J, Ludwig BM, Rehm WF: Pharmacodynamic evaluation of the peripheral pain inhibition by carprofen and flunixin in the horse. Schweiz Arch Tierheilk 132:497-504, 1990
119. Kamerling SG, Cravens WMT, Bagwell CA: Objective assessment of detomidine-induced analgesia and sedation in the horse. Eur J Pharmacol 151:1-8, 1988
120. Hamm D, Turchi P, Jochle W: Sedative and analgesic effects of detomidine and romifidine in horses. Vet Rec 136:324-327, 1995
121. Moens Y, Lanz F, Doherr MG, Schatzmann U: A comparison of the antinociceptive effects of xylazine, detomidine and romifidine on experimental pain in horses. Vet Anaesth Analg 30:183-190, 2003
122. Schatzmann U, Armbuster S, Stucki F, Busato A, Kohler I: Analgesic effect of butorphanol and levomethadone in detomidine sedated horses. J Vet Med Assoc 48:337-342, 2001
123. Robertson JT, Muir WW: A new analgesic drug combination in the horse. Am J Vet Res 44:1667-1669, 1983
124. Brunson DB, Mayors LJ: Comparative analgesia of xylazine, xylazine/ morphine, xylazine/butorphanol, and xylazine/ nalbuphine in the horse, using dental dolorimetry. Am J Vet Res 48:1087-1091, 1987
125. Maxwell LK, Thomasy SM, Slovis N, Kollias-Baker C: Pharmacokinetics of fentanyl following intravenous and transdermal administration in horses. Equine Vet J 35:484-490, 2003
126. Matthews NA, Peck KE, Mealey KL: Transdermal fentanyl: absorption and plasma levels in horses. Proc Int Cong Vet Anaesth 6:116, 1997
127. Sysel AM, Pleasant RS, Jacobson JD, Moll HD, Modransky PD, Warnick LD, Sponenberg DP, Eyre P: Systemic and local effects associated with long-term epidural catheterization and morphine-detomidine administration in horse. Vet Surg 26:144-149, 1997
128. Valverde A, Little CB, Dyson DH, Motter CH: Use of epidural morphine to relieve pain in a horse. Can Vet J 31:211-212, 1990
129. Haitjema H, Gibson KT: Severe pruritis associated with epidural morphine and detomidine. Aust Vet J 79:248-250, 2001
130. Maves TJ, Gebhart GF: Antinociceptive synergy between intrathecal morphine and lidocaine during visceral and somatic nociception in the rat. Anesthesia 76:91-99, 1992
131. de Leon-Casasola OA, Lema MJ: Postoperative epidural opioid analgesia: what are the choices. Anesth Analg 83:867-875, 1996
132. Doherty TJ, Geiser DR, Rohrbach BW: Effect of high volume epidural morphine, ketamine and butorphanol on halothane minimum alveolar concentration in ponies. Equine Vet J 29:370-373, 1997
133. Skarda RT, Tejwani GA, Muir WW: Cutaneous analgesia, hemodynamic and respiratory effects, and β-endorphin concentration in spinal fluid and plasma of horses after acupuncture and electroacupuncture. Am J Vet Res 63:1435-1442, 2002
134. Xie H, Ott EA, Colahan P: Influence of acupuncture on experimental lameness in horses. Am Assoc Equine Pract Proc 47:347-357, 2001
135. Araujo AM, Sinnott CJ, Strichartz GR: Multiple phases of relief from experimental mechanical allodynia by systemic lidocaine: response to early and late infusions. Pain 103:21-29, 2003
136. Dirks J, Fabricius P, Petersen KL, Rowbotham MC, Dahl JB: The effect of systemic lidocaine on pain and secondary hyperalgesia associated with the heat/capsaicin sensitization model in healthy volunteers. Anesth Analg 91:967-972, 2000
137. Ferrante FM, Paggioli J, Cherukuri S, Arthur GR: The analgesic response to intravenous lidocaine in the treatment of neuropathic pain. Anesth Analg 82:91-97, 1996
138. Nagy I, Woolf CJ: Lignocaine selectively reduces C fibre-evoked neuronal activity in rat spinal cord in vitro by decreasing N-methyl-D-aspartate and neurokinin receptor-mediated post-synaptic depolarizations; implications for the development of novel centrally acting analgesics. Pain 64:59-70, 1996
139. Dworkin RH: An overview of neuropathic pain: syndromes, symptoms, signs, and several mechanisms. Clin J Pain 18:343-349, 2002
140. Ahern TJ: Reflex sympathetic dystrophy syndrome (RSDS), complex regional pain syndrome type-1 (CRPS-1), neuropathic pain: an equine perspective. J Equine Vet Sci 16:463-468
141. Owens JG, Kamerling SG, Stanton SR, Keowen ML: Effects of ketoprofen and phenylbutazone on chronic hoof pain and lameness in the horse. Equine Vet J 27:296-300, 1995
142. Gottrup H, Hansen PL, Arendt-Nielsen L, Jensen TS: Differential effects of systemically administered ketamine and lidocaine on dynamic and static hyperalgesia induced by intradermal capsaicin in humans. Br J Anaesth 84:155-162, 2000
143. Schmid RL, Sandler AN, Katz J: Use and efficacy of low-dose ketamine in the management of acute postoperative pain: a review of current techniques and outcomes. Pain 82:111-125, 1999
144. Duque JC, Valadao CAA, Farias A, De Almeida RM, Oleskovicz N: Pre-emptive epidural ketamine or S(+)-ketamine in post-incisional pain in dogs: a comparative study. Vet Surg 33:361-367, 2004
145. Wagner AE, Walton JA, Hellyer PW, Gaynor JS, Mama KR: Use of low doses of ketamine administered by constant rate infusion as an adjunct for postoperative analgesia in dogs. J Am Vet Med Assoc 221:72-75, 2002

146. Hamilton SM, Johnston SA, Broadstone RV: Evaluation of analgesia provided by the administration of epidural ketamine in dogs with a chemically induced synovitis. Vet Anaesth Analg 32:30-39, 2005
147. Hocking G, Cousins MJ: Ketamine in chronic pain management: an evidence-based review. Anesth Analg 97:1730-1739, 2003
148. Redua MA, Valadao CAA, Duque JA, Balestrero LT: The pre-emptive effect of epidural ketamine on wound sensitivity in horses tested by using von Frey filaments. Vet Anaesth Analg 29:200-206, 2002
149. de Segura IAG, de Rossi R, Santos M, San-Roman JL, Tendillo FJ: Epidural injection of ketamine for perineal analgesia in the horse. Vet Surg 27:384-391, 1998
150. Matthews NS, Fielding CL, Swinebroad E: How to use a ketamine constant rate infusion in horses for analgesia. Am Assoc Equine Pract Proc 50:227-228, 2004
151. Vanegas H, Schaible H-G: Prostaglandins and cycloxygenases in the spinal cord. Progr Neurobiol 64:327-363, 2001
152. Mellegers MA, Furlan AD, Mailis A: Gabapentin for neuropathic pain: systematic review of controlled and uncontrolled literature. Clin J Pain 17:284-295, 2001
153. Eckhardt K, Ammon S, Hofmann U, Riebe A, Gugeler J, Mikus G: Gabapentin enhances the analgesic effect of morphine in healthy volunteers. Anesth Analg 91:185-191, 2000
154. Gilron I, Bailey JM, Tu D, Holder RR, Weaver DF, Houlden RL: Morphine, gabapentin, or their combination for neuropathic pain. N Engl J Med 352:1324-1334, 2005

6.3 Antimicrobial therapy

Steeve Giguère

Antimicrobial chemotherapy has played a vital role in the treatment of equine infectious diseases. Since the discovery of penicillin in the 1920s, hundreds of antimicrobial agents have been developed and dozens of these are currently used in human medicine. The arsenal of antimicrobial agents available to the equine clinician is limited, however. Few antimicrobial drugs are licensed for administration to horses and extralabel use is often necessary. Many drugs used in people are not appropriate for use in horses because of poor oral bioavailability, cost, lack of species-specific pharmacokinetic data or development of serious side effects such as enterocolitis.

In choosing the appropriate antimicrobial agent, the equine clinician must consider (1) the likely identity of the infecting microorganism(s), (2) their typical *in vitro* susceptibility patterns or the clinical response in equine patients infected with the same pathogens, (3) the nature and site of the infectious disease process, (4) the pharmacokinetic characteristics of the chosen antimicrobial agent in horses such as bioavailability, tissue distribution and rate of elimination, (5) the pharmacodynamic properties of the antimicrobial agent selected, (6) its safety in horses and (7) the cost of therapy. This chapter provides an overview of current concepts that guide rational antimicrobial therapy in horses and reviews available equine-specific information for antimicrobial agents commonly used in horses.

Antibacterial drugs

Bacterial infections of horses

Because the identity and *in vitro* susceptibility of an infecting microorganism are rarely known when therapy is begun, initial therapy is usually empirical and is based on knowledge of the agents likely to be present and their historical susceptibility. In some cases, the most likely etiologic agent can be highly suspected simply based on the clinical presentation and the horse's history. For example, abscessation of the submandibular and retropharyngeal lymph nodes is most likely caused by *Steptococcus equi* subspecies *equi* (*S. equi*). Lower respiratory tract infection in adult horses is most commonly associated with *S. equi* subspecies *zooepidemicus* (*S. zooepidemicus*), followed by nonenteric Gram-negative bacteria such as *Pasteurella* spp.

On the other hand, pleuropneumonia in an adult horse may be caused by any one or combinations of a number of bacteria and thus requires bacteriological culture of a tracheobronchial aspirate and pleural fluid to determine the etiologic agent(s). Similarly, peritonitis, urinary tract infections, musculoskeletal infections, cellulitis and mastitis may be caused by a variety of bacteria, and initial therapy with broad-spectrum antimicrobial agents is recommended (Table 6.4). The selection of the antimicrobial agent and route of administration will depend on the severity of the disease and the site of infection. A combination of gentamicin for Gram-negative coverage and penicillin for Gram-positive and anaerobic coverage is commonly used as initial broad-spectrum therapy for severe bacterial infections. Enrofloxacin can be used as a substitute to gentamicin in adult horses, whereas ampicillin or cefazolin can replace penicillin. Addition of metronidazole is recommended for disease processes where *Bacteroides fragilis* is commonly isolated such as pleuropneumonia and peritonitis.

Bacterial septicaemia is the leading cause of morbidity and mortality in neonatal foals. Many of the diseases involving the neonatal foal are the sequelae of septicaemia. These diseases include pneumonia, peritonitis, meningitis, osteomyelitis, septic arthritis and omphalophlebitis. Gram-negative bacteria account for 70% to 95% of the microorganisms isolated from cultures of blood samples in equine neonates, with *Escherichia coli* being by far the most common isolate.[1,2] Other Enterobacteriaceae (*Klebsiella* spp., *Salmonella* spp. and *Enterobacter* spp.) and nonenteric Gram-negative rods (*Pasteurella* spp. and *Actinobacillus* spp.) are also commonly isolated. Gram-positive cocci (β-haemolytic streptococci, *Enterococcus* spp. and *Staphylococcus* spp.) account for approximately 15% of isolates in our hospital. Treatment protocols for equine neonates must include antimicrobials with a high level of activity against enteric Gram-negative bacteria while providing adequate coverage against Gram-positive microorganisms. Bactericidal agents

Table 6.4. Suggested choices of antimicrobial agents for selected bacterial infections of horses

Diseases	First choice	Alternative antimicrobials
Foals		
Neonatal infections*	Ampicillin-amikacin	Penicillin-amikacin; ampicillin-gentamicin; penicillin-gentamicin; third- or fourth-generation cephalosporin
Bronchopneumonia (older foals)	Ceftiofur	Penicillin ± gentamicin
Lung/abdominal abscesses	Macrolide† and rifampin	Chloramphenicol-rifampin; doxycycline-rifampin
Adult horses		
Mild bronchopneumonia	Penicillin	Ceftiofur; cefquinome; TMS
Severe pneumonia/pleuropneumonia	Penicillin‡-gentamicin-metronidazole	Penicillin‡-enrofloxacin-metronidazole
Peritonitis	Penicillin‡-gentamicin-metronidazole	Penicillin‡-enrofloxacin-metronidazole
Abdominal abscess	Penicillin-rifampin	TMS-rifampin
Septic arthritis/osteomyelitis	Cefazolin-gentamicin	Penicillin-gentamicin; cefazolin-enrofloxacin; penicillin-enrofloxacin
Cellulitis	Cefazolin-enrofloxacin	Penicillin-enrofloxacin; cefazolin-gentamicin; penicillin-gentamicin
Urinary tract infections	TMS	Ceftiofur; penicillin-enrofloxacin
Mastitis	Penicillin	TMS; ceftiofur

TMS, trimethoprim-sulphonamide.
*Bacteraemia, umbilical infections, septic arthritis, osteomyelitis, and pneumonia (<3–4 weeks of age).
†Erythromycin, clarithromycin, or azithromycin.
‡Cefazolin or ampicilin could replace penicillin.

are preferred because neonatal foals have a naive immune system and their defence mechanisms against bacterial pathogens are often compromised. The combination of an aminoglycoside (amikacin or gentamicin) with either penicillin or ampicillin is often initiated until culture results are available. Such combination provides adequate coverage against approximately 90% of bacterial isolates recovered from blood cultures at the University of Florida. Amikacin, although more expensive, is preferred to gentamicin because of its lower frequency of resistance amongst Enterobacteriaceae.[1,3] Similarly, ampicillin is preferred to penicillin because of its higher activity against enterococci. In situations when an aminoglycosides should not be used such as renal failure, adequate coverage is provided by a third- or fourth-generation cephalosporin such as cefotaxime or cefepime (in Europe, cefquinome), respectively.

In all situations, therapy should be adjusted based on initial clinical response, adverse reactions and results of culture and susceptibility testing. Therapeutic failure may occur when the disease process does not have a bacterial aetiology, when there is a change in the bacterial population at the site of infection or when the pathogens have become resistant to the chosen antimicrobial agent. In addition, therapeutic failure may occur when the microenvironment at the site of infection is not conducive to antimicrobial activity or when there is poor diffusion of the drug at the site of infection. The rate and extent of penetration of a drug into most sites outside the vascular space are determined by the drug's concentration in plasma, molecular charge and size, extent of plasma protein binding, and blood flow.[4] In other tissues such as the central nervous system, the eye and the prostate, a lipid membrane provides a barrier to drug diffusion.[4] There is also a similar barrier between blood and the bronchial epithelium, restricting penetration of some drugs into bronchial secretions and epithelial lining fluid of the lower airways.[5] Drug diffusion into lung tissue, however, is not restricted by such a lipid membrane. Lipophilic drugs such as macrolides, fluoroquinolones, tetracyclines, rifampin, trimethoprim and chloramphenicol are more likely to diffuse across lipid membranes and reach therapeutic concentrations in these tissues. These drugs are also more likely to accumulate within cells and represent an advantage for the treatment of susceptible intracellular bacterial pathogens. Thus, the goal of antimicrobial therapy is to select an antibiotic that, in addition to exhibiting good antimicrobial activity against the infecting microorganism, will achieve therapeutic concentrations in the infected area.

Bacterial susceptibility

Not all bacteria isolated from a specimen should be subjected to susceptibility testing. Bacteria that are typically considered to be contaminants or part of the normal microflora should not be tested. When the offending bacteria are identified, selection of an antimicrobial agent is often simplified because some common equine pathogens have predictable *in vitro* susceptibility profiles. For example, β-haemolytic streptococci, *Pasteurella* spp. and most anaerobes with the exception of *Bacteroides fragilis* are susceptible to penicillins or aminopenicillins. In contrast, Enterobacteraceae, *Pseudomonas* spp., *Enterococcus* spp. and *Staphylococcus* spp. have unpredictable susceptibility. *In vitro* susceptibility testing is particularly important for these bacterial species. Suggested first-line antimicrobial agent and alternative choices for common equine bacterial pathogens are presented in Table 6.5. Tables 6.6 and 6.7

Table 6.5. Suggested choices of antimicrobial agents for common bacterial pathogens of horses

Microorganisms	Antimicrobial of choice	Alternative antimicrobials
Gram positives		
β-Haemolytic streptococci*	Penicillin	Ceftiofur; cefquinome; ampicillin; macrolide; rifampin; chloramphenicol
Staphylococcus spp.	Cefazolin	TMS; enrofloxacin; amikacin; rifampin; chloramphenicol
Enterococcus spp.	Ampicillin ± gentamicin	Penicillin; chloramphenicol
Rhodococcus equi	Macrolide† and rifampin	Chloramphenicol-rifampin; doxycycline-rifampin
Corynebacterium pseudotuberculosis	Penicillin	TMS; rifampin
Nocardia spp.	TMS	Amikacin
Clostridium difficile	Metronidazole	
Gram-positive anaerobes	Penicillin	Metronidazole; chloramphenicol
Gram negatives		
Pasteurella-Actinobacillus spp.	TMS	Ceftiofur; gentamicin
Actinobacillus equuli	Ceftiofur	Gentamicin; amikacin
Bordetella bronchiseptica	Gentamicin; amikacin	TMS; oxytetracycline
Escherichia coli	Amikacin	Gentamicin; enrofloxacin; cefquinome; cefotaxime; cefepime
Klebsiella spp.	Amikacin	Gentamicin; enrofloxacin; cefotaxime; cefepime
Enterobacter spp.	Amikacin	Enrofloxacin; cefepime
Pseudomonas spp.	Amikacin	Ticarcillin; piperacillin; cefepime;
Salmonella spp.	Enrofloxacin	Amikacin; cefepime
Gram-negative anaerobes	Metronidazole	Chloramphenicol; penicillin (not for *B. fragilis*)
Obligate intracellular pathogens		
Lawsonia intracellularis	Erythromycin-rifampin	Doxycycline; chloramphenicol
Anaplasma phagocytophylum	Oxytetracycline	Doxycycline; rifampin; chloramphenicol
Neorickettsia risticii	Oxytetracycline	Erythromycin-rifampin; doxycycline
Spirochetes		
Borrelia burgdorferi	Oxytetracycline	Doxycycline; third-generation cephalosporin
Leptospira spp.	Oxytetracycline	Ampicillin; doxycycline; penicillin

TMS, trimethoprim-sulphonamide.
* *Streptococcus equi* subspecies *equi*, *S. equi* subspecies *zooepidemicus*, and *S. dysgalactiea* subspecies *equisimilis*.
† Erythromycin, clarithromycin, or azithromycin.

provide *in vitro* susceptibilities of common aerobic bacterial pathogens to a variety of antimicrobial agents.

In vitro susceptibility tests

Common methods of performing *in vitro* antimicrobial susceptibility tests in laboratories include disk diffusion (also known as Kirby Bauer test), broth dilution and a concentration gradient test (E test). The decision on which test method to use is based on cost, ease of use and flexibility to meet the needs of the laboratory. They all assess inhibition of growth rather than killing of the bacterium as the endpoint. To provide valid results, *in vitro* susceptibility tests must be performed following standardised procedures.

Interpretation of susceptibility tests and correlation with clinical outcomes

Disk diffusion provides qualitative data, whereas broth dilutions methods and the E test generate a minimal inhibitory concentration (MIC) in μg/ml. The results generated by *in vitro* susceptibility tests, whether they are determined by disk diffusion or dilution methodologies, are usually presented to the clinician by designating the pathogen as susceptible, intermediate or resistant. These designations are determined by comparing the microorganism's MIC (or zone of inhibition) to breakpoints established by the Clinical and Laboratory Standards Institute (CLSI; formerly known as NCCLS). Some countries have their own committee to establish methods of susceptibility, and interpretive criteria for those tests may not be exactly the same as those of the CLSI. Bacteria with an MIC less than or equal to to a given breakpoint are considered susceptible. Susceptibility implies that, at the recommended dosage, the antimicrobial agent should reach serum or tissue concentrations sufficient to inhibit the bacterium's growth *in vivo*. Bacteria with an MIC greater than or equal to to a given breakpoint are considered resistant because these concentrations cannot be achieved at the recommended dosage. Intermediate breakpoints are those zones of inhibition or MIC that fall between susceptible and resistant breakpoints. This intermediate category represents a buffer zone that prevents methodological imprecision to classify a resistant isolate as being susceptible, or vice versa. This category may also represent susceptible microorganisms for antimicrobial agents with low toxicity that allows the drug to be administered at higher than recommended doses. It may also represent susceptibility when the infection occurs at a body site where the drug is concentrated

Table 6.6. In vitro antimicrobial susceptibility of selected Gram-positive aerobic bacterial isolates from horses*

Microorganisms (n)	Antimicrobial†									
	GM	AMI	AZM	CLR	E	CHL	TMS	TE	RIF	P
Staphylococcus aureus (43)	70	86	70	86	70	100	95	78	89	41
Other staphylococci (48)	91	100	76	73	76	97	85	71	97	30
Rhodococcus equi (99)	100	100	93	96	89	96	98	94	86	—
Streptococcus equi subsp. *equi* 45)	29	0	—	—	100	100	76	95	96	100
S.equi subsp. *zooepidemicus* (192)	19	0	—	—	99	100	62	43	98	100
S. dysgalaxiae subsp. equisimilis (34)	18	0	—	—	95	94	60	62	94	100
Enterococcus spp. (38)	—	—	—	—	52	83	68	63	60	77

GM, gentamicin; AMI, amikacin; AZM, azithromycin; CLR, clarithromycin; E, erythromycin; CHL, chloramphenicol; TMS, trimethoprim-sulphonamide; TE, tetracycline; RIF, rifampin; P, penicillin; AM, ampicillin; A/S, ampicillin/sulbactam; OX, oxacillin; TIM, ticarcillin-clavulanic acid (Timentin); CFZ, cefazolin; CFT, cefotaxime; XNL, ceftiofur; CPE, cefepime; IMP, imipenem; ENR, enrofloxacin; CIP, ciprofloxacin; MXF, moxifloxacin; VAN, vancomycin.

—, Not tested or testing not warranted.

*Data from the Clinical Microbiology Laboratory, University of Florida (2003–2005).

†Percent of susceptible isolates (number of susceptible isolates/number of isolates tested × 100).

‡In vivo, ceftiofur is rapidly metabolised to desfuroylceftiofur. Desfuroylceftiofur is as effective as ceftiofur against most bacterial pathogens, but most coagulase-positive *Staphylococcus* spp. are resistant. Therefore, despite *in vitro* susceptibility, ceftiofur is not the ideal choice for the treatment of staphylococcal infections.

Table 6.7. In vitro antimicrobial susceptibility of Gram-negative aerobic bacterial isolates from horses*

Microorganisms (n)	Antimicrobials†																	
	GM	AMI	CHL	TMS	TE	AM	A/S	PI	TIM	CFZ	CAX	CAZ	CFT	XNL	CPE	IMP	ENR	CIP
Escherichia coli (127)	62	90	72	43	51	51	53	52	73	70	79	76	87	69	97	100	82	83
Klebsiella pneumoniae (52)	88	96	94	79	96	6	83	67	88	90	96	96	98	69	98	100	88	100
Enterobacter cloacae (32)	40	83	41	40	57	3	17	40	43	10	63	70	53	34	80	100	78	80
Salmonella enterica (224)	65	99	64	87	62	65	65	65	68	—	78	75	88	64	98	100	100	100
Pseudomonas aeruginosa (48)	70	97	—	—	—	—	—	97	94	—	15	94	15	6	91	97	65	97
Pasteurella spp. (40)	94	94	100	91	100	100	100	100	100	94	100	100	100	95	100	100	100	100
Actinobacillus spp. (31)	100	87	100	93	90	95	100	100	100	100	100	100	100	97	100	100	100	100

GM, gentamicin; AMI, amikacin; CHL, chloramphenicol; TMS, trimethoprim-sulphonamide; TE, tetracycline; AM, ampicillin; A/S, ampicillin/sulbactam; PI, piperacillin; TIM, ticarcillin-clavulanic acid (Timentin); CFZ, cefazolin; CAX, ceftriaxone; CAZ, ceftazidime; CFT, cefotaxime; XNL, ceftiofur; CPE, cefepime; IMP, imipenem; ENR, enrofloxacin; CIP, ciprofloxacin.

*Data from the Clinical Microbiology Laboratory, University of Florida (2003–2005).

†Percent of susceptible isolates (number of susceptible isolates/number of isolates tested × 100).

—, Not tested or testing not warranted.

such as the urinary tract for drugs achieving high concentrations in the urine such as β-lactams, fluoroquinolones and trimethoprim-sulphonamide combinations. The generation of these interpretive criteria involves analysis of three types of data: (1) the distribution of *in vitro* susceptibility results for the bacterial population for which a given antimicrobial is being marketed, (2) the pharmacokinetic parameters of the test agent in the target animal species and, when available, (3) the results of clinical trials. Breakpoints generated from the CLSI for selected antimicrobial agents are presented in Table 6.8.

Many studies, mainly in human medicine, have documented the value of *in vitro* susceptibility testing in predicting efficacy of antimicrobial therapy. In a recent review of the literature, 11 of 12 trials showed a significantly higher response rate in human patients treated with antimicrobial agents to which the offending pathogen was susceptible than in those treated with antimicrobial agents to which the pathogen was resistant.[6] When multiple reports of the correlation of therapeutic outcome with *in vitro* susceptibility were examined, it was consistently found that infections due to susceptible isolates respond to appropriate therapy approximately 90% of the time, whereas infections that are due to resistant isolates respond to therapy about 60% of the time.[6]

Several factors may compromise the ability of *in vitro* susceptibility results to predict clinical efficacy. Very few CLSI breakpoints are generated based on equine-specific

Table 6.6. *Continued*

AM	A/S	OX	TIM	CFZ	CFT	XNL	CPE	IMP	ENR	CIP	MXF	VAN
41	68	68	79	68	68	67‡	68	68	79	81	100	97
30	65	65	—	65	65	85‡	65	65	94	97	100	100
—	—	—	—	—	—	—	—	91	73	100	100	100
100	—	—	100	100	100	96	—	—	84	—	—	100
100	—	—	100	100	100	98	—	—	69	—	—	100
100	—	—	100	100	100	100	—	—	76	—	—	100
83	—	—	—	—	—	34	—	—	53	80	—	95

Table 6.8. Interpretive standards for *in vitro* susceptibility testing of selected antimicrobial agents used in horses*

Antimicrobial agents and microorganisms	MIC breakpoint for susceptibility (μg/ml)
Penicillins	
Penicillin G	
Staphylococci, streptococci	≤0.12
Enterococci	≤8
Ampicillin	
Staphylococci, streptococci	≤0.25
Enterococci, Enterobacteriaceae	≤8
Oxacillin	≤2
Ticarcillin	
P. aeruginosa	≤64
Other Gram-negative bacilli	≤16
Cephalosporins	
Ceftiofur	≤2
Cefpodoxime	≤2
Cefazolin, cephalotin, cefotaxime, cefepime, ceftriaxone	≤8
Cefoperazone	≤16
Other β-lactams	
Imipenem	≤4
Aminoglycosides	
Amikacin	≤16
Gentamicin	≤4
Macrolides	
Erythromycin	≤0.5
Streptococci	≤0.25
Azithromycin, clarithromycin	≤2
Streptococci	≤0.25
Fluoroquinolones	
Enrofloxacin, difloxacin	≤0.5
Ciprofloxacin, orbifloxacin	≤1
Others	
Chloramphenicol	≤8
Streptococci	≤4
Rifampin	≤1
Tetracycline, doxycycline	≤4
Trimethoprim-sulfonamide	≤2/38
Vancomycin	≤4
Streptococci	≤1

*Concentrations based on CLSI breakpoints. Interpretations are valid only when the appropriate methodologies are followed.

data. Most breakpoints are generated from studies using isolates, pharmacokinetic data and clinical trials in humans. For example, the CLSI breakpoint for susceptibility to doxycycline is 4 μg/ml or less based on pharmacokinetic and clinical efficacy data generated in humans (Table 6.8). Administration of oral doxycyline to an adult horse at the recommended dose of 10 mg/kg results in peak serum concentrations of 0.42 ± 0.05 μg/ml.[7] Similar concentrations are achieved in synovial and peritoneal fluids. A pathogen isolated from synovial fluid of a horse with an MIC of 4 μg/ml would be reported as susceptible even though such concentrations are far from being achievable in horses. Based on pharmacokinetic data in horses, a breakpoint of less than or equal to 0.25 μg/ml would be more appropriate for susceptibility.[7,8] Thus the lack of equine-specific interpretation criteria is one of the factors that may explain discrepancies between *in vitro* susceptibility and clinical response. In that regard, MIC, rather than qualitative susceptibility data, may help the clinician in determining if an antimicrobial agent is an appropriate choice by considering the achievable serum and tissue concentrations of the drug in horses, as well as the pharmacodynamic parameters associated with outcome of infection (see later).

Other factors that may compromise the ability of *in vitro* susceptibility results to predict clinical efficacy include poor drug delivery at the site of infection or when the microenvironment at the site of infection is not conductive to antimicrobial activity. For example, gentamicin is inactivated by purulent material and requires an oxidative transport system to penetrate the bacterial membrane. Therefore, a given microorganism may be susceptible to gentamicin *in vitro* but the drug may be ineffective *in vivo* for the treatment of a large abscess.

Pharmacokinetic-pharmacodynamic optimisation of doses

Determination of the appropriate dose and dosing interval of an antimicrobial agent requires knowledge and integration of both its pharmacokinetics and pharmacodynamic properties. The pharmacokinetic properties of a drug describe its disposition within the body and include the process of drug absorption, distribution, metabolism and excretion. On the other hand, pharmacodynamic properties of a drug address the relationship between drug concentration and antimicrobial activity. Drug pharmacokinetic features, such as serum concentrations over time and area under the serum concentration-time curve (AUC), when integrated with MIC values, can predict the probability of bacterial eradication and clinical success. These pharmacokinetic and pharmacodynamic relationships also are important in preventing the selection and spread of resistant strains.

The most significant factor determining the efficacy of β-lactams, trimethoprim-sulphonamide combinations and bacteriostatic agents such as macrolides, tetracyclines and chloramphenicol is the length of time that serum concentrations exceed the MIC of the pathogen.[9] Increasing the concentration of the drug several-fold above the MIC does not significantly increase the rate of microbial killing. Rather, it is the length of time that bacteria are exposed to concentrations of these drugs above the MIC that dictates their rate of killing. Optimal dosing of such antimicrobial agents involves frequent administration. Other antimicrobial agents such as the aminoglycosides, fluoroquinolones and metronidazole exert concentration-dependent killing characteristics. Their rate of killing increases as the drug concentration increases above the MIC for the pathogen, and it is not necessary or even beneficial to maintain drug levels above the MIC between doses. Thus, optimal dosing of concentration dependant drugs involves administration of high doses with long dosing intervals. Some drugs exert characteristics of both time- and concentration-dependent activity. The best predictor of efficacy for these drugs is the 24-hour AUC/MIC ratio. Glycopeptides, rifampin and, to some extent, fluoroquinolones fall within this category.[10]

Antimicrobial agent–associated enterocolitis

The large bowel of the horse makes this species particularly susceptible to antimicrobial-induced enterocolitis secondary to disruption of the normal colonic microflora and overgrowth of pathogenic microorganisms such as *Clostridium* spp., including *C. difficile*. In a historical cohort study using a total of 784 horses, 27 horses developed diarrhoea, for an incidence of 3.4%.[11]

The onset of acute and sometimes fatal diarrhoea in the horse has been anecdotally associated with the use of almost every oral or parenteral antimicrobial agent. However, orally administered antimicrobials with low bioavailability and good activity against anaerobes are most likely to induce diarrhoea. For this reason, oral β-lactam antimicrobials should be used with caution in the horse. Antimicrobials that are partially excreted in the bile after parenteral administration should also be used with caution. Certain antibiotics such as lincomycin and clindamycin are associated with well-recognised enterocolitis syndromes and their use must be avoided in horses.[12,13] Other antibiotics such as oral trimethoprim-sulphonamide combinations, macrolides, ciprofloxacin, moxifloxacin, chloramphenicol, rifampin and metronidazole, as well as parenteral oxytetracycline and cephalosporins, have been occasionally linked to enterocolitis in horses. In one study, administration of oxytetracycline to horses has been associated with the proliferation of *Clostridium perfringens* type A and possible toxin production.[11]

Anecdotally, some antibiotics are known to induce diarrhoea in some parts of the world while used extensively without evidence of such side effect in others. This marked geographic variation in the incidence of antibiotic-induced diarrhoea likely results from differences in colonic microflora. Foals seem less susceptible to antibiotic-induced enterocolitis than do adult horses.

Antibacterial agents used in horses

This section provides an overview of selected relevant information regarding commonly used antimicrobial drug classes in horses. Complete generic information such as mechanisms of action, mechanisms of bacterial resistance, drug interactions and side effects for each class of antimicrobial agent can be found elsewhere.[14] Suggested antimicrobial drug dosages in horses are presented in the Appendix, Table 19.1.

β-Lactams

Benzyl penicillin G

The antimicrobial spectrum of penicillin G includes streptococci, enterococci and approximately 40% to 50% of staphylococci. Most isolates of *Actinobacillus* spp. and *Pasteurella* spp. from horses are also susceptible. Gram-positive anaerobes and many Gram-negative anaerobes including *Bacteroides* spp. (but not *B. fragilis*) are susceptible to penicillin.

The polar nature of penicillin G gives it a volume of distribution similar to the extracellular fluid volume and results in poor tissue penetration. Penicillins are excreted by active renal tubular secretion resulting in high concentrations of active drug in urine.[15] Sodium or potassium salts of penicillin G have a short elimination half-life of less than 1 hour.[16] Because β-lactams do not exert a prolonged postantibiotic effect, frequent dosing is necessary. Intramuscular administration of penicillin G with procaine results in a much longer elimination half-life but peak serum concentrations are low.[16] This limits the antimicrobial spectrum and drug penetration at sites of infection. Procaine has been detected in urine for up to 425 hours after administration of multiple doses of procaine penicillin G.[17] The bioavailability of penicillin administered intragastrically to horses is less than 10%.[18–20]

Penicillin G is generally well tolerated in horses. Many horses develop muscle soreness during prolonged therapy with IM procaine penicillin. Reactions characterised by excitement, seizure activity and rarely death have been observed during or shortly after IM injection of procaine penicillin G.[21] These reactions likely represent accidental IV administration of procaine penicillin G because similar clinical signs can be reproduced by IV administration of low doses of procaine.[22,23] Horses are at least 20-fold more susceptible than humans to the central stimulant effects of procaine.[23] Intravenous administration of sodium or potassium penicillin results in transient hypotension.[24] Reactions to IV potassium penicillin characterised by head shaking, teeth grinding, salivation, mild colic and/or passage of soft faeces have been described, particularly when administration is rapid.[25] IV administration of potassium penicillin G has been shown to stimulate defaecation and myoelectric activity of the caecum and pelvic flexure in horses.[26]

Aminobenzyl penicillins

Ampicillin, amoxicillin and the related esters bacampicillin, talampicillin, and pivampicillin have been studied in horses. Their *in vitro* spectrum of activity against Gram-positive microorganisms and anaerobes is similar to that of penicillin G. They are more active than penicillin G against some Gram-negative bacteria. Nevertheless, the progressive increase in plasmid-mediated resistance that includes β-lactamase production by Gram-negative bacteria has reduced the activity of aminobenzyl penicillins to the point where they only show a slight advantage over penicillin. The spectrum of activity of these drugs can be improved by combining them to a β-lactamase inhibitor such as clavulanic acid, sulbactam or tazobactam.

The elimination half-life of Na ampicillin following IV injection is less than 1 hour, necessitating frequent administration.[27] The trihydrate formulations of ampicillin and amoxicillin are designed for IM injection and provide slow release of the drug but the low serum concentrations achieved limit their spectrum of activity. Ampicillin and amoxicillin are poorly absorbed after oral administration to adult horses with a bioavailability of 2% and 5%, respectively.[28,29] In contrast, oral administration of these drugs to foals result in serum concentrations adequate for the treatment of highly susceptible microorganisms such as β-haemolytic streptococci, *Pasteurella* spp. and non–β–lactamase–producing staphylococci.[30–32]

Bacampicillin, pivampicillin and talampicillin are prodrugs deesterified by the intestinal mucosa to release ampicillin as they are absorbed from the intestinal tract. The oral bioavailability of these drugs in foals and adult horses ranges between 20% and 40%.[33,34] In one study, pivampicillin was effective for the eradication of *S. zooepidemicus* in a soft tissue infection model in ponies.[35] Pivampicillin has also been shown to be safe for prolonged oral administration to hospitalised adult horses. In one study, the incidence of diarrhoea was significantly lower in horses treated with pivampicillin (3%) than in horses treated with trimethoprim-sulphadiazine (7%).[36] Unfortunately, these drugs are unavailable in many countries.

Antistaphylococcal isoxazolyl penicillins

By virtue of their chemical structure, methicillin, cloxacillin, dicloxacillin, nafcillin and oxacillin are resistant to *Staphylococcus aureus* penicillinase. Of these drugs, only oxacillin has been studied in horses.[37] Besides their increased activity against *Staphylococcus* spp., their spectrum of activity against aerobic Gram-positives and *Pasteurella/Actinobacillus* spp. is similar to that of penicillin.[38] Methicillin (oxacillin)-resistant *S. aureus* (MRSA) has emerged as an important zoonotic and veterinary pathogen in some equine veterinary hospitals.[39,40]

Antipseudomonal penicillins

The pharmacokinetics of the antipseudomonal penicillin ticarcillin and piperacillin have been studied in horses.[41–45] These drugs are active against most isolates of *Pseudomonas aeruginosa* and many other Gram-negative bacteria with the notable exception of *Klebsiella* spp., *Salmonella* spp. and *Enterobacter* spp. Ticarcillin is also available in combination with clavulanic acid. However, most *P. aeruginosa* isolates resistant to ticarcillin are also resistant to ticarcillin-clavulanic acid. Nevertheless, coadministration of clavulanic acid considerably improves the spectrum of ticarcillin against Enterobacteriaceae. These drugs are expensive and require high doses with short dosing intervals when administered intravenously. As a result, the major indication for ticarcillin is intrauterine use in mares with endometritis caused by *P. aeruginosa*. Intrauterine administration of ticarcillin results in higher endometrial tissue concentrations than IV administration.[46,47] Addition of clavulanic acid to ticarcillin is of questionable value for intrauterine administration because clavulanate concentrations in endometrial tissue are very low and short lived.[46] An additional indication for ticarcillin-clavulanic acid is the treatment of infections caused by aminoglycoside-resistant Gram-negative bacteria in foals or for the treatment of susceptible bacteria when the use of aminoglycoside is contraindicated because of compromised renal function.

Cephalosporins

Cephalosporins have a wide range on antibacterial activity but show considerable diversity in their antibacterial properties. The cephalosporins are often arbitrarily classified in four generations, according to their order of discovery and antibacterial activity. The first generation cephalosporins were originally introduced for the treatment of β-lactamase–producing *Staphylococcus* spp. Their activity against Gram-negative bacteria is similar to that of extended-spectrum aminobenzyl penicillins. Second generation cephalosporins offer a slightly broader spectrum of activity against Gram-negative bacteria. Third generation cephalosporins offer excellent activity against most Gram-negatives including Enterobacteriaceae, while retaining their activity against equine β-haemolytic streptococci. Their activity against *Pseudomonas* spp. depends on the specific drug, with ceftazidime being the most active. The newest development in the cephalosporin class is the 4th generation drugs. These drugs are active against many Gram-negative bacteria resistant to third-generation cephalosporins and have adequate activity against *Pseudomonas* spp., while retaining activity against many Gram-positive pathogens.

Several first-(cefazolin, cephapirin, cephalotin, cephalexin, cephradine, cefadroxil), second-(cefoxitin), third-(ceftiofur, cefotaxime, ceftriaxone, cefoperazone, cefpodoxime) and fourth-(cefepime, cefquinome) generation cephalosporins have been studied in horses. Most of these drugs have short elimination half-lives and require frequent administration. Although poorly absorbed in adult horses, some first-generation cephalosporins (e.g., cefadroxil and cephradine) have good oral bioavailability in foals.[48,49] In one study, the bioavailability of cefadroxil was 99% in 2-week-old foals and progressively decreased to 14% in 5-month-old foals.[48]

The major indication for the use of third- or fourth-generation cephalosporins, other than ceftiofur, in horses is the treatment of sepsis in neonates with compromised renal function or the treatment of aminoglycoside resistant Gram-negatives. The disposition of orally administered cefpodoxime proxetil was recently investigated in foals and adult horses. Although the peak serum concentrations and AUC were considerably lower than those achieved in humans after administration of the same dose, concentrations sufficient to treat many Gram-negative and Gram-positive bacterial infections were achieved.[50]

In the United States, ceftiofur is the only cephalosporin approved for use in horses. Ceftiofur has a broad antimicrobial spectrum that includes most Gram-positive aerobes, Gram-negative aerobes including most Enterobacteriaceae and many anaerobes including *Clostridium* spp., *Fusobacterium* spp. and some *Bacteroides* spp. (but not *B. fragilis*).[51,52] Resistant bacteria include *Enterococcus* spp., *Pseudomonas* spp. and many *R. equi* isolates. Ceftiofur is rapidly metabolised to an active metabolite, desfuroylceftiofur. Desfuroylceftiofur is as effective as ceftiofur against most bacterial isolates but most coagulase-positive *Staphylococcus* spp. are resistant.[52] Therefore, despite *in vitro* susceptibility, ceftiofur is not an adequate choice for the treatment of staphylococcal infections. Ceftiofur is approved for the treatment of respiratory tract infections caused by β-haemolytic streptococci. Equine β-haemolytic streptococci are highly susceptible to ceftiofur with MIC less than 0.06 μg/ml. Therefore, the label dose of 2.2 to 4.4 mg/kg every 24 hours IM is much lower than that recommended for other third-generation cephalosporins. The MIC of susceptible Enterobacteriaceae is usually in the range of 0.25 to 1.0 μg/ml.[52] As a result, higher doses or more frequent administrations may be necessary to maintain drug concentrations above the MIC of the pathogen for sufficient periods of time. The kinetics of ceftiofur in neonatal foals are better when the drug is administered IM rather than IV. Toxicity studies have shown that horses tolerate doses up to 11 mg/kg per day IM, with pain at the injection site and decrease feed consumption being the most common observed effect at the highest dose.[53] Severe enterocolitis is seen occasionally. Despite a label claim that includes only infection caused by β-haemolytic streptococci, the high susceptibility of this microorganism to penicillin and the low cost of procaine penicillin G make it the treatment of choice in most instances. Third-generation cephalosporins such as ceftiofur are best reserved for the treatment of microorganisms resistant to penicillin G or trimethoprim-sulpha.

In Europe, cefquinome is approved for the treatment of respiratory infections in adult horses, and septicaemia in foals. The drug has good *in vitro* activity against streptococci, *Actinobacillus* spp., *E. coli* and other Enterobacteriacae isolated from horses. *In vitro* activity against *Pseudomonas* spp. and *R. equi* is limited.[54]

Aminoglycosides

The pharmacokinetics of streptomycin, neomycin, kanamycin, gentamicin and amikacin have been investigated in horses. Extensive resistance to neomycin, kanamycin and streptomycin has rendered these drugs much less useful than gentamicin or amikacin, which are consequently the most commonly used aminoglycosides in horses. Amikacin and gentamicin show excellent activity against Gram-negative aerobes. Amikacin has a broader spectrum of activity against Enterobacteriaceae than gentamicin. In contrast, gentamicin is inherently more active against nonenteric Gram-negatives such as *Pasteurella* and *Actinobacillus* spp. than amikacin. Activity against Gram-positive aerobes is generally poor, although many staphylococci are susceptible to amikacin and, to a slightly lesser extent, gentamicin. Obligate anaerobes and facultative anaerobes under anaerobic conditions are resistant to aminoglycosides.

Multiple *in vivo* and *in vitro* studies have shown that the rate of bacterial killing with aminoglycosides increases as the drug concentration increases above the MIC for a given pathogen with optimal C_{max} serum concentration to MIC ratio of approximately 8:1 to 12:1.[55–57] In addition, C_{max}/MIC ratio of at least 10:1 may prevent the emergence of resistant pathogens.[58,59] Unlike β-lactams, aminoglycosides exert a significant postantibiotic effect against susceptible Gram-negative bacteria. The postantibiotic effect is prolonged at higher peak drug concentrations.[60] As a result of their concentration-dependent activity and long postantibiotic effect, once-daily dosage regimens for aminoglycosides are now routinely used in horses and have proved to be effective and relatively safe. Aminoglycosides are not absorbed following oral administration. They can be administered by the IV, IM or SC route. Bioavailability of aminoglycosides administered by IM or SC injection is nearly 100%.[61–63] Aminoglycosides are eliminated by glomerular filtration, resulting in very high concentrations in urine. Concentrations in synovial fluid, peritoneal fluid and tissues are considerably lower than concurrent serum concentrations.[64–69] Intracellular concentrations are very low. Aminoglycosides are distributed throughout the extracellular fluid space, and equine neonates have a considerably higher extracellular fluid volume space than do adult horses. Therefore, foals up to about 4 to 6 weeks of age require much larger doses on a mg/kg basis than do adult horses. There is an age-related maturation in renal function in foals during the first 10 days of life, as indicated by increasing clearance of amikacin.[70,71]

Aminoglycosides are generally well tolerated in horses. The most important side effect is nephrotoxicity, whereas ototoxicity and neuromuscular dysfunctions have not been conclusively demonstrated in horses. The uptake of aminoglycosides by proximal renal tubular cells becomes rapidly saturated. Development of nephrotoxicity depends primarily on sustained exposure of renal tubular cells to the drug rather than on high peak concentrations. Once-daily dosing is theoretically less nephrotoxic than administration of the same total daily dose divided into more frequent administrations, because it allows for longer periods of time with drug concentrations below the putative nephrotoxicity threshold. Nevertheless, nephrotoxicity may occur in horses even with once-daily dosing. Horses with preexisting renal damage, hypovolaemia or, severe systemic illnesses and horses treated concurrently with other nephrotoxic agents such as NSAIDs are at greater risk for the development of renal failure.

All patients receiving aminoglycoside therapy for longer than 5 days should be monitored for evidence of nephrotoxicity. A population pharmacokinetic study in horses showed that creatinine concentration is the best predictor of gentamicin clearance.[72] Serum creatinine concentrations should be monitored every 3 days during treatment, and a 26.5 μmol/L (0.3 mg/dl) or greater increase in creatinine concentrations provides evidence of nephrotoxicity. Serial urinalysis may be a more sensitive method to monitor nephrotoxicity compared to measurement of creatinine concentrations. Mild proteinuria, glucosuria and decreased concentrating ability may occur days before an increase in serum creatinine concentrations. An increase in the ratio of urinary GGT to urinary creatinine concentrations indicates damage to the proximal tubular cells. However, the GGT/creatinine ratio is too sensitive for the clinical monitoring in horses treated with aminoglycosides because it increases considerably in every treated horse and does not indicate the need for withdrawal of aminoglycoside therapy.[73] In a retrospective study of hospitalised equine neonates treated with once-daily amikacin, 2 of 40 foals (5%) developed renal dysfunction as evidenced by an increase in creatinine concentrations of 26.5 μmol/L (0.3 mg/dl) or greater above baseline values during the course of therapy. In another study, 1 of 35 adult horses (2.9%) treated with gentamicin developed evidence of nephrotoxicity.[74] These two studies may represent an underestimation of the true potential for nephrotoxicity as the dose of aminoglycoside was optimised for each animal based on the results of therapeutic drug monitoring (TDM).

TDM is beneficial during aminoglycoside therapy because a wide variation in drug disposition may exist in sick patients, particularly in critically ill neonates. Creatinine concentrations account for only 40% of the variability in the clearance of gentamicin in horses with sepsis.[72] Therefore, monitoring drug concentrations may provide a more sensitive indicator of renal dysfunction as evidenced by decreased clearance and increased trough concentrations. In addition, TDM is helpful to determine if the target C_{max}-to-MIC ratio has been achieved. Aminoglycoside concentrations can easily be measured using fluorescence polarisation immunoassays available on most automated chemistry analysers.

One approach to TDM is to collect a peak drug concentration 0.5 hour after administration along with a trough sample collected immediately prior to the next scheduled dose. However, drug concentrations in the trough sample at 24 hours are often below the limit of quantification of the assay, thereby preventing calculation of pharmacokinetic parameters. The other approach is to obtain two or three samples at 2- to 4-hour intervals to identify the slope of the elimination curve. From the elimination curve, estimates of clearance, volume of distribution and half-life are possible. The use of once-daily amikacin does not necessarily abolish the need for TDM. In one study of once-daily amikacin in hospitalised neonates, optimal peak and trough concentrations were achieved in approximately 88% of the foals treated with a single IV daily dose of 25 mg/kg.[70]

Fluoroquinolones

The pharmacokinetics of several fluoroquinolones have been investigated in horses. Drugs studied include enrofloxacin, ciprofloxacin, norfloxacin, fleroxacin, orbifloxacin, marbofloxacin, danofloxacin and difloxacin.[75–86] With the exception of ciprofloxacin (6%), norfloxacin (9%) and danofloxacin (22%), these drugs have adequate oral bioavailability in horses. The spectrum of activity of these fluoroquinolones includes staphylococci and Gram-negative bacilli such as *Pasteurella* spp., *Actinobacillus* spp. *E. coli*, *Enterobacter* spp., *Klebsiella* spp., *Salmonella* spp. and *Proteus* spp. The drug concentrations needed for activity against some isolates of *Pseudomonas aeruginosa* may require doses higher than those that are typically recommended. The major limitation of these drugs as stand alone therapy for most bacterial infections in horses is their lack of activity against streptococci such as *S. zooepidemicus*, the most common bacterial pathogen of horses. They also lack activity against anaerobic bacteria.

As stated above, fluoroquinolones are generally considered to have concentration-dependent bactericidal activity. Investigators have suggested that AUC/MIC ratios of 100 to 125 or peak/MIC ratios of 8 : 1 to 10 : 1 are required to predict clinical and microbiological success and to limit the development of bacterial resistance.[87,88] Recent evidence suggests that AUC/MIC ratios of 30 to 55 may still be associated with a positive outcome.[89] There is considerable variation in pharmacodynamic calculations, and outcome parameters appear to be quinolone and pathogen specific.[89]

Enrofloxacin has been the most extensively studied fluoroquinolone in horses. After administration, approximately 20% to 25% of the dose is deethylated to ciprofloxacin, which has slightly higher antimicrobial activity than enrofloxacin.[80] Enrofloxacin can be administered to horses by the IV or PO route. Injectable formulations that have been used by the IV route in horses include a 100 mg/ml solution approved for administration to cattle and a 22.7 mg/ml solution for use in dogs. Rapid IV administration to horses may result in ataxia or other neurological signs. Therefore, slow IV administration is recommended. Formulations suitable for oral administration to horses include the tablets for use in small animals and a 32.3 mg/ml poultry formulation.[78,83] In one study, oral administration of the 100 mg/ml bovine solution was highly variable in horses.[78] However, this solution had adequate bioavailability when compounded into a gel.[90] Concentrations of bioactive enrofloxacin and metabolite after long-term oral administration are 5 to 10 times higher in liver, spleen and kidney than in concurrent serum concentrations. Concentrations in brain as well as vitreous and aqueous humour are only 10% to 20% of serum concentrations. Concentrations in most other tissues are similar to those achieved in serum.[91] Concentrations in urine are several 100-fold higher than concurrent serum concentrations.[83]

Prolonged administration of enrofloxacin has been found safe in adult horses even at 4 times the recommended dosage.[92,93] However, administration of enrofloxacin to equine neonates has occasionally resulted in severe arthropathy. In one study, three of four neonatal foals became lame and developed synovial effusion within 4 to 8 days of therapy with oral enrofloxacin at a dose of 10 mg/kg. Gross and histological lesions were present in all four foals and were consistent with quinolone-induced arthropathy.[94] The tibial-tarsal, femoral-tibial and radio-humeral joints were involved.[94] *In vitro* studies have shown that therapeutic concentrations of enrofloxacin do not affect chondrocyte metabolism of adult horses.[95,96] In contrast, *in vitro* cartilage metabolism of equine neonates is affected at therapeutic concentrations.[96] *In vitro* chondrotoxic effects of fluoroquinolones in horses appeared to be the result of irregular integrin signaling and subsequent cellular changes.[97] Therefore, enrofloxacin and other fluoroquinolones are not recommended for use in growing horses unless no other alternatives are available. Problems with tendonitis and tendon ruptures observed in people have not yet been documented conclusively in horses. However, enrofloxacin inhibits cell proliferation, induces morphological changes and decreases proteoglycan synthesis in equine tendon cell cultures.[98] These effects were more pronounced in tendon cells obtained from foals than in adult horses.

The newest generation of fluoroquinolones developed for use in human medicine have a broader spectrum of activity that includes anaerobic bacteria and streptococci. Examples include gatifloxacin, gemifloxacin and moxifloxacin. Of these newer fluoroquinolones, only moxifloxacin has been investigated in horses. Administration at a dosage of 5.8 mg/kg orally at 24-hour intervals to adult horses resulted in therapeutic serum and bronchoalveolar cell concentrations.[99] However, four of six experimental horses studied developed diarrhoea.[99] The routine use of this drug is not recommended until additional safety studies are available.

Macrolides and derivatives

The pharmacokinetics of erythromycin and clarithromycin have been studied in horses.[100–106] Azithromycin, an azalide, has also been studied in foals.[107,108] Azithromycin, clarithromycin and erythromycin show good *in vitro* activity against *R. equi*, β-haemolytic streptococci and *Staphylococcus* spp. They are also active against some anaerobes such as *Bacteroides* spp. (not *B. fragilis*) and *Clostridium* spp. (not *C. difficile*). Of the three, only azithromycin is active against *Pasteurella* spp. and *Salmonella enterica* subspecies *enterica*. Azithromycin, clarithromycin and erythromycin do not show any *in vitro* activity against *E. coli*, *Klebsiella* spp., *Pseudomonas* spp. and *Enterobacter* spp.[38]

Several formulations of erythromycin are commercially available. Although they all show slight differences in bioavailability and elimination, they all result in therapeutic concentrations at recommended dosages. The half-life of azithromycin in foals (15–20 hours) is considerably longer than that of clarithromycin (5.4 hours) or erythromycin (1 hour).[107,108] The longer half-life of azithromycin is attributed to the extensive uptake and subsequent slow release of the drug from tissues. The oral bioavailability of azithromycin (56%) and clarithromycin (57%) in foals having access to hay is considerably higher than that obtained with various erythromycin formulations in foals of the same age despite feed withholding (10–40%).[102–104,106] The bioavailability of erythromycin is decreased by feeding hay.[104] The high lipid solubility of macrolides and derivatives results in excellent penetration and high concentrations in phagocytic cells.[107,108] Administration of azithromycin and clarithromycin to foals results in significantly higher drug concentrations in bronchoalveolar cells and pulmonary epithelial lining fluid compared to those achieved after administration of erythromycin.[109] These properties of the newer-generation macrolides contribute to their lower dosages and longer dosing intervals. Concentrations of clarithromycin in pulmonary epithelial lining fluid and bronchoalveolar cells of foals at steady state are considerably higher than concentrations reported following daily administration of azithromycin to foals.[106,108] However, clarithromycin concentrations at these sites decrease rapidly, whereas the release of azithromycin from cells is much slower, resulting in sustained concentrations of azithromycin in tissues for days following discontinuation of therapy.[109] The terminal half-life of azithromycin in bronchoalveolar cells is 54 hours compared to 6 hours for clarithromycin.[109]

The most common adverse effect of macrolides and derivatives in horses is diarrhoea. Anecdotal evidence suggests that the incidence of diarrhoea is higher in adult horses than in foals. An idiosyncratic reaction characterised by hyperthermia and tachypnoea has also been reported in foals treated with erythromycin during hot weather. In one study, 26 (36%) of 73 foals treated with erythromycin developed diarrhoea, 18 (25%) developed hyperthermia and 11 (15%) developed respiratory distress.[110] Severe enterocolitis has also been reported in mares whose foals are being treated with erythromycin, presumably due to disruption of the mare's normal colonic microflora following ingestion of small amounts of active drug during coprophagia or from contamination of feeders or water buckets with drug present on the foal's muzzle.[111]

The most common indication for the use of macrolides and derivatives in horses is the treatment of *R. equi* infections in foals. For that purpose, these drugs are typically used in combination with rifampin. The MIC at which 90% of *R. equi* isolates were inhibited (MIC_{90}) for azithromycin, clarithromycin and erythromycin were 1.0, 0.12 and ≤0.25 μg/ml, respectively.[38] In a recent retrospective study, clarithromycin-rifampin was found to be superior to both erythromycin-rifampin and azithromycin-rifampin for the treatment of pneumonia caused by *R. equi*.[112] However, the incidence of diarrhoea following administration of clarithromycin was as high as that observed after administration of erythromycin. The incidence of diarrhoea following administration of azithromycin was slightly lower. However, the drug is not as effective as clarithromycin, especially in foals with severe lung lesions.[112] Another indication for the use of macrolides with or without rifampin is the treatment of *Lawsonia intracellularis* infections in foals.[113]

Tetracyclines

The pharmacokinetics of IV and IM oxytetracycline and oral doxycycline have been studied in horses.[8,114–120] Intravenous administration of oxytetracycline is preferred over IM administration because it results in higher and more persistent serum concentrations.[119] A long-acting oxytetracycline–propylene glycol formulation, available in some countries, results in extended release of the drug and a prolonged elimination half-life of approximately 55 hours following IM administration.[121] The clinical use of oxytetracycline in horses has long been controversial because of early anecdotal reports of severe enterocolitis. While oxytetracycline may, like many other antimicrobial agents, cause enterocolitis, the vast majority of treated horses do not exhibit side effects. Nevertheless, the main factor limiting the use of tetracyclines in horses is their limited spectrum against common equine pathogens.

Oxytetracycline is active *in vitro* against most nonenteric Gram-negatives such as *Pasteurella* spp. and *Actinobacillus* spp. and against *Mycoplasma* spp.[38] The drug is also active against approximately 70% of *Staphylococcus* spp.[38] However, at clinically achievable concentrations, oxytetracycline is active against only 50% to 60% of Enterobacteriaceae and β-haemolytic streptococci. Oxytetracycline is the treatment of choice for infections caused by *Borrelia burgdorferi*, *Neoriketsia risticii* and *Anaplasma phagocytophilum* in horses.[122–124] These microorganisms typically have a very low MIC (<0.25 μg/ml).

Another common use for oxytetracycline is the treatment of contracted tendons in foals. In one study, intravenous administration of oxytetracycline at a dose of 44 mg/kg resulted in a decrease in the angle of the metacarpophalangeal joint for approximately 96 hours.[125,126] These effects may be due to oxytetracycline-induced inhibition of collagen gel contraction by myofibroblast through a mechanism mediated by matrix metalloproteinase-1.[127] Administration of these high doses of oxytetracycline to foals with preexisting renal damage or hypovolaemia or to foals unable to nurse sufficiently because of their musculoskeletal problem may result in acute renal failure.[128]

Intravenous administration of doxycycline results in cardiovascular collapse and death in horses, even when slow IV infusions are used.[129] In contrast, oral administration of doxycycline to horses appears safe. However, the usefulness of oral doxycycline in adult horses is limited by the poor oral bioavailability of the drug and resulting low plasma and body fluid concentrations.[7,8,130] In a pilot study in adult horses, feeding considerably decreased oral absorption of doxycycline.[8] On the basis of results of allometric analysis, the oral bioavailability of doxycycline in fasted adult horses is estimated to be only 2.7%.[8] Despite administration at a dose of 10 mg/kg at 12-hour intervals for 5 doses, peak serum concentration was only 0.46 ± 13 μg/ml and trough concentration was 0.23 ± 0.03 μg/ml.[7] Concentrations in synovial and peritoneal fluids were similar to peak serum concentrations, whereas the drug could not be detected in cerebrospinal fluid (CSF).[7] Endometrial tissue concentrations were slightly higher than serum concentrations while concentrations in urine ranged between 75 and 145 μg/ml.[7] Administration at a dose of 20 mg/kg orally twice daily results in higher drug concentrations.[8] However, in one study, this higher dosage regimen resulted in fatal enterocolitis in one of six horses.[8] Therefore, with the exception of urinary tract infections, doxycycline at a dose of 10 mg/kg twice daily or 20 mg/kg once daily would be only appropriate for the treatment of bacterial pathogens with an MIC of 0.25 mg/ml or less.[7,8] These pathogens include *Pasteurella* spp., *Actinobacillus* spp., *Borrelia burgdorferi*, *Neoriketsia risticii* and *Anaplasma phagocyto-*

philum.[131–133] Approximately 50% of staphylococci and β-haemolytic streptococci of equine origin have an MIC of 0.25 μg/ml or less.[38]

The oral bioavailability of doxycycline appears to be better in foals than in adults, allowing a wider range of bacteria to be treated with this drug. In foals between 4 and 8 weeks of age, administration of 10 mg/kg doxycycline by mouth at 12-hour intervals resulted in a peak serum concentration of 4.05 ± 0.83 μg/ml and a trough concentration of 2.67 ± 0.88 μg/ml.[120] These concentrations mean that doxycycline is appropriate for the treatment in foals of bacterial pathogens with an MIC of 3 μg/ml or less. These would include most *Pasteurella* spp., *Actinobacillus* spp., *Staphylococcus* spp., β-haemolytic streptococci, *Rhodococcus equi, Borrelia burgdorferi, Neoriketsia risticii* and *Anaplasma phagocytophilum*.[7,38,132,133] These would also include approximately 50% of *Escherichia coli* and *Klebsiella* spp. isolates.[7,38,134] Oral doxycycline has also been used for the treatment of proliferative enteritis caused by *Lawsonia intracellularis* in foals.[135]

Nitroimidazoles

The pharmacokinetics of metronidazole and tinidazole have been studied in horses. Of the two, metronidazole has been studied and used more extensively. Metronidazole is active against almost all anaerobic bacteria and many protozoa. Susceptible pathogens include Gram-positive anaerobes such as *C. difficile, C. perfringens, Eubacterium* spp. *Peptococcus* spp. and Gram-negative anaerobes including *Bacteroides* spp., *B. fragilis* and *Fusobacterium* spp. These pathogens typically have an MIC of 2 μg/ml or less. Resistance among usually susceptible bacteria is rare but may occur.

The bioavailability of metronidazole following oral administration to adult horses has ranged between 75% and 97%.[136–138] Peak serum concentrations following administration of a dose of 20 mg/kg are 22 ± 8 μg/ml. Bioavailability (30% ± 9%) and peak serum concentrations (9 ± 2 μg/ml) are significantly lower following rectal administration.[137] Nevertheless, intrarectal administration offers an alternative route in horses with gastric reflux, dysphagia or other diseases preventing oral administration. Concentrations in synovial and peritoneal fluids are similar to concurrent serum concentrations, whereas concentrations in CSF and endometrial tissue samples are considerably lower.[136] The drug is concentrated in urine.[136]

A common indication for administration of metronidazole to horses is the treatment of polymicrobial infections that may involve anaerobic bacteria resistant to β-lactams such as pleuropneumonia or peritonitis. Metronidazole is the treatment of choice in horses with enterocolitis caused by *C. difficile* or *C. perfringens*. Metronidazole has also been used for the treatment of idiopatic enterocolitis[139] and, topically, for the treatment of thrush or canker. The incidence of side effects following administration of metronidazole to horses is low. Side effects may include decreased appetite and diarrhoea. In a retrospective study of 200 horses treated with oral metronidazole for various medical illnesses, only 4 (2%) developed anorexia and 2 (1%) developed diarrhoea.[140]

Trimethoprim-sulphonamide combinations

Diaminopyrimidines such as trimethoprim, ormethoprim or pyrimethamine are synergistic with a variety of sulphonamides. The combination of trimethoprim with either sulphadiazine or sulphamethoxazole is commonly used in horses owing to its relatively broad spectrum of activity, good oral bioavailability and low incidence of adverse reactions. Trimethoprim-sulpha (TMS) combinations are active *in vitro* against many Gram-positive bacteria including *Corynebacterium pseudotuberculosis*, streptococci and most *Staphylococcus* spp. They are highly active against *Pasteurella* and *Actinobacillus* spp. However, their activity against Enterobacteriaceae is variable with approximately 50% to 60% of *E. coli* and *Klebsiella* spp. of equine origin being susceptible. TMS is the treatment of choice for *Pneumocyctis carinii* and infection by *Nocardia* spp. in horses. Pyrimethamine in combination with sulphadiazine is commonly used for the treatment of equine protozoal myelitis. *Pseudomonas* spp. and *Mycoplasma* spp. are resistant. TMS is not active against anaerobic bacteria *in vivo*, despite adequate *in vitro* activity. Similarly, recent studies have shown that, in contrast to penicillin, TMS is ineffective in eradicating *S. equi* subspecies *zooepidemicus* in a tissue chamber model of infection.[141,142] This failure of *in vivo* response was observed despite *in vitro* susceptibility of the isolate and high concentrations of TMS in the tissue chamber fluid.[141,142]

TMS can be administered to horses by the IV or oral routes. Oral bioavailability of both trimethoprim and sulphadiazine is approximately 60% to 70%.[143,144] The oral absorption of both drugs is decreased considerably by administration at time of feeding.[143,145] Trimethoprim is absorbed more rapidly than sulphadiazine and has a shorter elimination half-life, resulting in less-than-optimal ratio of the drugs. For this reason, TMS must be administered at least twice daily in horses. Trimethoprim and, to a lesser extent, sulphonamides are well distributed in the body, reaching high concentrations in body fluids, cells and tissues.[146–148] Renal elimination of the drugs results in high concentrations in urine.[148]

The occurrence of diarrhoea following therapy with TMS has ranged between 3% and 7%.[11,36] In most cases, the problem is short-lived once the drug is discontinued.[11] In one study, TMS had minimal effect on the colonic microflora compared to that of oxytetracycline.[147] Rapid IV administration of TMS may result in tremors, excitement, ataxia and, rarely, death. Concurrent use of detomidine with IV TMS should be avoided because this combination has resulted in hypotension, dysrhythmias and death.

Chloramphenicol and florfenicol

The potential for non–dose-related aplastic anaemia in people has led to prohibition of the use of chloramphenicol in food animals in many countries. Albeit extremely rare, a few cases of aplastic anaemia have occurred following contact exposure of the drug in people. Therefore, the use of chloramphenicol in horses should be kept to a minimum. Because of the paucity of antimicrobial agent for oral use in horses, there may be occasional clinical situations when the use of chloramphenicol is justified. Chloramphenicol is active *in vitro* against a wide range of Gram-positive and many Gram-negative bacteria. Susceptible Gram-positive isolates include streptococci, staphylococci and many enterococci. Susceptible Gram-negative isolates include *Pasteurella* spp., and approximately 40% to 80% of Enterobacteraceae. While mycoplasmas often show susceptibility *in vitro*, the outcome of therapy of pulmonary infections caused by this organism is often disappointing. Chloramphenicol is very active against most anaerobes including *B. fragilis*.

Several studies have investigated the pharmacokinetics of chloramphenicol in foals and adult horses.[149–155] The extreme variability of the results between studies complicates general conclusions regarding the pharmacokinetics of the drug and dosage recommendations. The oral bioavailability of chloramphenicol decreases from 40% after administration of a single dose to 20% after administration of multiple doses.[154] The low oral bioavailability of the drug combined with a short elimination half-life of approximately 0.5 to 1 hour results in the necessity for administration of high doses with short dosing intervals. The half-life of chloramphenicol is considerably longer in newborn foals (≈5 hours) and decreases progressively to reach adult values by approximately 7 days of age.[149] Concentrations in synovial and peritoneal fluids are similar to concurrent serum concentrations, whereas concentrations in CSF are lower.[154]

The pharmacokinetics of florfenicol have also been investigated in horses. The bioavailability of the drug is approximately 80% following both IM and oral administration.[156] In one study, all six treated animals developed mild diarrhoea following administration by the IM and by the oral routes.[156] In another study, six horses received florfenicol IM at 48-hour intervals for six treatments.[157] Although no adverse effects were noted, the faecal flora of treated horses were severely altered. There was an increase in the number of *E. coli* and *C. perfringens* and a sharp decrease in the number of streptococci in the faeces of treated horses.[157] The spectrum of activity of florfenicol against equine bacterial pathogens is similar to that of chloramphenicol.[38] The routine use of this drug in horses is not recommended until additional safety studies are available.

Rifamycins

The pharmacokinetics of rifampin in adult horses and foals have been investigated in multiple studies.[11,158–161] Rifampin may be either bactericidal or bacteriostatic depending on the microorganism tested. Resistance to rifampin readily develops particularly if monotherapy is used. As a result, rifampin is typically combined with other antimicrobial agents. Rifampin is mainly active against Gram-positive microorganisms such as *Rhodococcus equi*, β-haemolytic streptococci, *Staphylococcus* spp. and *Corynebacterium pseudotuberculosis*. Rifampin is not active against enteric Gram-negative bacteria. However, rifampin is active against some nonenteric Gram-negatives such as *Actinobacillus* and *Pasteurella* spp.[38] Rifampin is active *in vitro* and *in vivo* against most anaerobes including *B. fragilis*.[162,163] The drug is also active against *Anaplasma phagocytophilum* and *Neoriketsia risticii*.[131,133] Rifampin offers the advantage of oral administration with a bioavailability of approximately 40% to 50%.[158,161,164] Oral absorption is delayed when rifampin is given with feed.[159] At the same oral dose, serum concentrations and AUC are significantly greater in foals that in adult horses as a result of decreased elimination and possibly greater bioavailability in foals.[159] Multiple dosing of rifampin results in lower serum concentrations and decreased half-life because of autoinduction of hepatic enzymes.[165]

Rifampin is lipid soluble and has a high volume of distribution, allowing therapeutic concentrations in most body fluids and tissues, as well as penetration of caseous material. Rifampin is concentrated approximately 2-fold in phagocytic cells and is effective against many intracellular bacteria.[166] The major indications for the use of rifampin in horses are the treatment of *R. equi* infections or internal abscesses caused by *Streptococcus* spp. or *C. pseudotuberculosis*. Another indication for rifampin is the treatment of β-lactamase–producing *Staphylococcus* spp.

Rifampin causes urine and other secretions (tears, saliva, etc.) to turn red-orange but is usually well tolerated when administered orally for long periods of time. Intravenous administration of rifampin may result in severe effects including weakness, unsteadiness, profuse sweating and distress.[159] Although well tolerated by most horses, rifampin may occasionally cause diarrhoea.

Aerosol adminstration of antibacterial agents

(see also Chapter 6.4)

The outcome of respiratory tract infection is more closely associated with antimicrobial drug concentrations within the airways than with concentrations in serum.[167] Aerosol administration of antimicrobial agents can result in high drug concentrations in the respiratory tract while minimising systemic concentrations and their resulting toxicity. Several studies in humans and various animal species have shown that aerosol administration of various antimicrobial agents is effective in the treatment of bacterial infections of the respiratory tract. In some experimental models of pneumonia in mechanically ventilated animals, even poorly ventilated and consolidated areas of the lungs contained higher antimicrobial drug concentrations after aerosol administration than after IV administration.[168] Nevertheless, the administration of antimicrobial agents by inhalation alone may not be sufficient in patients with severe parenchymal involvement or substantial consolidation. In these cases, aerosol therapy may be more appropriate as an adjunct to oral or systemic administration.

Antimicrobial delivery by inhalation is greatly influenced by the product formulation and type of nebuliser. Use of intravenous formulations can lead to exposure to potentially irritant or toxic additives and inappropriate pH or osmolality ranges. In one study, the particle size distribution and particle density of gentamicin sulfate and ceftiofur sodium aerosols were affected by the antimicrobial concentration of the solution.[169] Gentamicin concentrations of 50 mg/ml or ceftiofur concentrations of 25 mg/ml produced the optimal combinations of particle size and aerosol density when using a medical ultrasonic nebuliser.[169]

In healthy horses, aerosolisation of 20 ml of the commercially available IV gentamicin sulfate solution (diluted to 50 mg/ml) using an ultrasonic nebuliser resulted in bronchial lavage fluid concentrations approximately 12 times higher than concentrations achieved by IV administration at a dose of 6.6 mg/kg.[170] In the same study, serum concentrations following aerosol administration were below 1 µg/ml at all times.[170] Once-daily aerosol administration of gentamicin to healthy horses for 7 consecutive days did not result in pulmonary inflammation or drug accumulation in the respiratory tract.[171] Serum concentrations were below 0.8 µg/ml at all times sampled.[171] The major limitation to the use of aerosolised gentamicin in horses is its lack of activity against *S. zooepidemicus*, the most common bacterial pathogen of the equine respiratory tract.

Local therapy for musculoskeletal infections

Infection of the synovial structures or bone of the limbs is a common complication of lacerations and athletic injuries in horses. It is also a common and life-threatening complication of septicaemia in foals. Many commonly used antimicrobials such as β-lactams and aminoglycosides do not diffuse particularly well in tissues. As a result, bone and synovial fluid concentrations after systemic administration are considerably lower than concurrent serum concentrations. In many instances, concentrations at these sites are lower than the CLSI breakpoints for susceptibility and do not permit adequate C_{max}/MIC ratio or T > MIC required for optimal efficacy. Local delivery of antimicrobial agents is an important adjunct to joint lavage, systemic antimicrobial therapy and, when necessary, surgical therapy. Intra-articular (IA) administration of antimicrobial agents is the preferred local delivery method in cases of septic arthritis. Intravenous or intraosseous infusions are useful alternatives in horses with osteomyelitis of the distal limb, when multiple joints are involved or when the drug of choice is too much of an irritant for IA use.

Intra-articular therapy

Intra-articular injection of antimicrobial agents represents an easy and efficient way of achieving high and sustained concentrations at the site of infection in cases of septic arthritis. An ideal antimicrobial agent for IA administration must induce no or only minimal chemical synovitis and be poorly absorbed in the systemic circulation to minimise the risks of systemic toxicity. Intra-articular administration of 150 mg of gentamicin sulfate in a normal joint induces only a mild and transient inflammatory reaction.[172] Peak synovial fluid concentrations of gentamicin following IV administration are approximately 5 µg/ml. Peak concentrations of gentamicin in synovial fluid following IA administration of 150 mg in the antebrachial joint of normal horses are in excess of 1000 µg/ml and mean concentrations 24 hours later remain high at approximately 15 µg/ml.[173] In the same study, concentrations of gentamicin in serum following IA administration were below 1 µg/ml at all times. In an experimental model of *E. coli* infectious arthritis, IA gentamicin was more effective at eradicating *E. coli* from the joint than was IV gentamicin.[174] Buffering gentamicin with sodium bicarbonate is not recommended as it exacerbates synovial inflammation and reduces the antibacterial activity of the drug.[174,175] Continuous infusion of gentamicin is safe and results in persistently high synovial fluid concentrations.[176] Because aminoglycosides are concentration dependent and a single IA injection results in high synovial fluid concentrations for longer than 24 hours, a continuous delivery system may be of little clinical benefit compared to intermittent injections. A delivery system for continuous infusion would be better suited for the IA delivery of time-dependent antimicrobial agents. Amikacin IA has also been shown to prevent infection following inoculation of *S. aureus*.[177] Following IA administration, concentrations of amikacin are lower in inflamed joints compared to normal joints.[178] When 500 mg of amikacin is administered in a normal antebrachiocarpal joint, synovial fluid concentrations are maintained above 4 µg/ml for 72 hours, but when the same dose is administered in an inflamed joint, concentrations remain above 4 µg/ml for only 48 hours.[178]

Ceftiofur administered by the IA route does not result in synovial inflammation as assessed by synovial fluid cytology and histopathology of the synovial membrane and articular cartillage.[179] Ceftiofur concentrations in synovial fluid following IA injection of 150 mg remain above 2 µg/ml for longer than 24 hours. In contrast, synovial fluid concentrations following IV administration remain above 1 µg/ml for only 8 hours.[179]

Intravenous and intraosseous regional limb perfusion

Regional perfusion of an antimicrobial agent to a distal limb is an excellent method for delivering high concentrations at the site of infection while minimizing systemic delivery of the drug. Regional perfusion delivers antimicrobials into the venous system by using either a superficial vein or the medullary cavity of a bone. For both techniques, vasculature proximal to the treatment site is occluded with a tourniquet to restrict venous outflow, and antibiotics are infused into the distal portion of the limb. As the diluted antimicrobial agent enters the venous system, it distends the vasculature which promotes diffusion of the drug into tissues. Both the IV or intraosseous (IO) techniques can be done with the horse standing with nerve block and sedation or under general anaesthesia.[180,181]

In most situations IV is preferred to IO regional perfusion because it results in similar or higher drug concentrations in synovial fluid, bone and tendon sheath, and it is less likely to result in serious complications.[182–184] In addition, most antimicrobial agents with an IV formulation can be used for IV regional perfusion. In contrast, some antimicrobial agents may induce significant inflammation when injected into the medullary cavity. Selection of the optimal site of IV infusion and tourniquet placement depends on the site of infection. The cephalic or saphenous veins are used when infection involves the carpus or tarsus, respectively. The palmar/plantar digital vein may be used for the treatment of septic conditions involving the metacarpal/metatarsal-pharyngeal joint or the interphalangeal joints.[180] A 20-gauge catheter or butterfly needle is typically used in adult horses and a 22-gauge catheter or butterfly needle is used in foals. Proper tourniquet placement (see Chapter 1.53) is the most important aspect of a successful perfusion to minimise loss of the drug into the systemic circulation. There are no data on the optimal dose of antimicrobial agents. In adult horses, doses ranging from 500 mg to 1 g have been used for amikacin and gentamicin.[180,185] In foals, doses ranging from 50 to 250 mg of amikacin or gentamicin are commonly used.[185] Ceftiofur is also commonly used for regional IV perfusion at a dose of 4 mg/kg.[186] Vancomycin (300 mg in adult horses) is also safe for administration by regional limb perfusion.[187,188] However, the use of vancomycin in horses should be limited to the treatment or severe infections caused by microorganisms resistant to all other antimicrobial agents. Enrofloxacin (1.5 mg/kg) may also be used for IV regional limb perfusion.[189] However, its use often results in perivascular oedema and mild cellulitis.[189] Therefore, it should be reserved for the treatment of microorganisms resistant to safer antimicrobial agents. Other antimicrobial agents that have not been studied thoroughly but that have been used for regional limb perfusion with satisfactory clinical outcomes in adult horses include sodium or potassium penicillin (10×10^6 units), ticarcillin-clavulanic acid (1 g) and sodium ampicillin (9 g).[190]

The optimal volume of perfusate is not accurately known. As a general rule, higher volumes result in higher intravascular pressure and greater diffusion into surrounding tissues. Conversely, higher intravascular pressures will increase the likelihood of perfusate leakage under the tourniquet into the systemic circulation. In clinical practice, drugs used in regional IV perfusion are typically diluted in a volume of approximately 60 ml of a balanced electrolyte solution for an adult horse, or 10 ml for a foal.[190] The solution is usually injected by hand over 1 minute. After 30 minutes, the tourniquet and catheter (or butterfly needle) are removed. Complications are rare but may include soft tissue swelling at the site of catheter placement and thrombosis of the port of entry.

Drug concentrations in bone, synovial or tendon sheath fluid, and serum following regional IV perfusion depend on the dose used and tourniquet placement. In one study, regional IV perfusion with 125 mg amikacin in anaesthetised horses resulted in average peak amikacin concentrations in the distal interphalangeal joint of 110 μg/ml.[191] In contrast, another study found that regional IV perfusion with 250 mg amikacin was not sufficient to attain effective tissue concentrations in standing horses.[189] In another study, 500 mg amikacin administered in a similar fashion resulted in peak drug concentrations of 896 μg/ml in the same joint.[183] In all studies, serum amikacin concentrations following removal of the tourniquet were below 4 μg/ml.[183,191]

Regional perfusion by the IV route may be difficult or impossible in animals with severe soft tissue swelling of the distal limb or when venous thrombosis has occurred. The IO route eliminates the need for localisation and catheterisation of a peripheral vein. The IO technique also results in high concentrations of the drug in synovial or tendon sheath fluid, and it has proved more effective than systemic antimicrobial administration in experimentally induced septic arthritis.[181,183,192] An area of the bone lacking overlying muscle, nerves, large blood vessels or tendons is selected. An incision is made through the skin and the periosteum. Several surgical approaches have been used. A simple approach is to drill a 4-mm hole through the cortex into the medullary cavity. This allows tight fitting of a regular IV extension set into the cortical hole. The surgical site can be protected by bandaging between treatments, and the same hole can be used repeatedly for drug delivery. Doses of gentamicin or amikacin ranging between 500 mg and 1 g have been used in a volume of approximately 60 ml.[181–183,192] Potential complications include soft tissue swelling at the site of entry and, rarely, cortical fracture or avascular necrosis of the bone.

Antifungal drugs

With the exception of dermatophytosis, fungal diseases are relatively rare in horses. Fungal diseases are often divided into four categories. Superficial or cutaneous mycosis (dermatophytosis) such as *Trichophyton* spp. and *Microsporum* spp. infect the epidermis, dermis or hair. Subcutaneous fungal infections are much less common. Fungi isolated from affected horses include *Sporothrix schenckii*, *Pythium insidiosum*, *Conidiobolus coronata* and other fungi that cause mycetoma (e.g., *Pseudallescheria boydii*) and phaeohyphomycosis (e.g., *Drechslera spicifera*). These agents are opportunistic invaders of damaged skin surfaces or are introduced by penetration through the skin or mucous membranes. Systemic mycoses are even rarer in horses except in specific geographical areas. The three most important systemic pathogens are *Histoplasma capsulatum*, *Coccidioides immitis* and *Blastomyces dermatidis*. Infection with opportunistic fungi such as *Candida* spp., *Aspergillus* spp., *Mucor* spp., *Cryptococcus neoformans* and *Pneumocyctis carinii* occurs with increasing frequency in horses. Some of these opportunistic fungi may occur as a nosocomial infection in hospitalised patients. Risk factors, common to many hospitalised patients, may include malnutrition, indwelling catheters, immunosuppression and the use of broad-spectrum antibacterial agents.

In vitro antifungal susceptibility tests are similar in design to tests for antibacterial agents. However, antifungal susceptibility testing is not routinely performed in most veterinary clinical microbiology laboratories and requires sending the isolate to a specialised laboratory. This results in a considerable increase in costs and an additional delay in obtaining the results. For this reason, the clinician must be familiar with the fungal agents most likely to be involved in various disease processes in order to initiate appropriate therapy prior to obtaining the results of *in vitro* susceptibility testing. For example, pneumonia caused by *Aspergillus* spp. is a relatively common complication in horses with diseases resulting in loss of integrity of the gastrointestinal tract such as severe colitis or colic.[193,194] Similarly, colonisation of the mouth (thrush) or indwelling catheter sites with *Candida* spp. is not uncommon in neonatal foals treated with broad-spectrum antibacterial agents and may result in systemic infections at various sites including the joints.[195] Table 6.9 provides a summary of various fungi reported to cause disease in horses at selected body systems. In addition, the clinician must be familiar with the spectrum of activity of available antifungal agents (Table 6.10).

Systemic therapy of fungal infections is challenging in horses because of the paucity of pharmacokinetic data, the poor absorption of many drugs commonly used in other species and the high cost of many antifungal agents. As a result, empirical therapy is often based on dosage regimens used in people, measurement of serum levels in selected clinical cases and anecdotal observation of positive clinical response in a few equine patients. Because of the limitations and cost of systemic therapy, local therapy is of primordial importance when the lesions are accessible. When possible, complete surgical excision of the lesions should be performed. In addition, topical, intralesional or regional perfusion of antifungal agents are excellent means of providing high drug concentrations at the site of infection, while minimizing systemic adverse reactions and limiting the cost of therapy. For some diseases, such as *Pythium insidiosum*, immunotherapy has also been shown to be of benefit.[196] In cases of guttural pouch mycosis, surgical arterial occlusion using the balloon catheter technique or transarterial coil is the treatment of choice with little evidence for the necessity for adjunctive medical therapy.[197,198]

Pharmacodynamics of antifungal agents

In vitro and animal models studies have begun to define the pharmacodynamic characteristics of antifungal agents. Analysis of clinical data in humans also suggests that pharmacodynamic targets identified in animal models is predictive of outcome in humans.[199] Polyenes and echinocandins antifungal agents exert a long postantifungal effect and are concentration dependent. The best predictor of efficacy for these drugs is a C_{max}/MIC ratio of 3:1 to 10:1, with high ratios conferring better activity.[199,200] In contrast, flucyto-

Table 6.9. Most common fungal pathogens at selected sites in horses*

Site of infection	Common fungal agents
Skin	*Trichophyton* spp., *Microsporum* spp.
Subcutaneous tissues/cellulitis	*Pythium insidiosum, Sporothrix schenckii, Drechslera spicifera*
Upper airway/pharynx	*Aspergillus* spp., *Conidiobolus coronatus, Pseudallescheria boydii, Cryptococcus neoformans*
Lung	*Aspergillus* spp., *Pneumocyctis carinii, Cryptococcus neoformans, Coccidioides immitis, Histoplasma capsulatum, Blastomyces dermatitidis*
Guttural pouch mycosis	*Aspergillus* spp., *Emericella nidulans*
Bone	*Pythium insidiosum, Coccidioides immitis, Scedosporium prolificans*
Joint	*Candida* spp.
Oral cavity, IV catheter, blood cultures	*Candida* spp.
Placenta	*Aspergillus* spp., *Cryptococcus neoformans*
Endometritis	*Candida* spp.
Keratitis	*Aspergillus* spp., *Fusarium* spp.

*The relative prevalence of many fungi depends on the geographical location.

Table 6.10. Spectrum of activity of antifungal agents

Antifungal	*Aspergillus*	*Candida*	*Blastomyces*	*Cryptococcus*	*Coccidioides*	*Histoplasma*	*Sporothrix*	*Pythium*	*Conidiobolus*	*Pseudo-allescheria*
Amphotericin B	+*	+	+	+*	+*	+	+	–	+	–
Flucytosine	+	+	–	+	–	–	–	–	–	–
Ketoconazole	–	+†	+	+	+	+	+	+	±	+*
Fluconazole	–	+*†	±	+*	+*	+	+	+	±	±
Itraconazole	+*	+†	+*	+	+	+*	+*	–	±	+*
Voriconazole	+	+	+	+	+	+	+	–	–	+
Miconazole	+	+†	+	+	+	–	+	+*	±	+
Caspofungin	+	+	–	–	–	–	–	–	–	–
Iodides	–	–	–	–	–	–	+‡	–	+‡	–

+ Most isolates are susceptible.
– Most isolates are resistant.
± Variable susceptibility or conflicting data.
* Agent(s) of choice in most clinical situations.
† *Candida* species other than *albicans* are more commonly resistant to fluconazole, itraconazole, ketoconazole, and miconazole
‡ Clinical response has been documented despite the lack of *in vitro* susceptibility.

sine has a short postantifungal effect and the best predictor of efficacy is T > MIC.[201] The best predictor of efficacy with the triazoles is an AUC/MIC ratio of 25 : 1.[199]

Antifungal agents used in horses

This section provides an overview of selected information on antifungal agents that have been used in horses. A complete list of available antifungal agents with generic information such as mechanisms of action, drug interactions and side effects can be found elsewhere.[202]

Polyenes

Amphotericin B is a polyene macrolide with broad-spectrum antifungal activity. Amphotericin B was the mainstay of systemic antifungal therapy for many years until the introduction of the azoles. It is still the treatment of choice for life-threatening yeast or dimorphic fungal infections in people. A major advantage of this drug is its fungicidal nature against most pathogenic fungi (Table 6.10). The main limitation of amphotericin B therapy is its high potential for nephrotoxicity. Lipid-based formulations (liposomal, colloidal or lipid complex) of amphotericin B are less nephrotoxic, but they are cost prohibitive for most equine patients.

There is no pharmacokinetic data available for the use of amphotericin B in horses. There are several reports of intralesional or systemic use of amphotericin B in horses.[195,203–207] A wide range of doses and administration protocols have been used for systemic administration. Most reported doses range from 0.3 to 0.9 mg/kg diluted and given IV over 1 hour. In one report, successful treatment of pulmonary cryptococcosis was reported with daily infusions of amphotericin B at 0.5 mg/kg for a month.[208] Natamycin is a polyene antifungal produced by *Streptomyces natalensis*. It is active against a wide variety of fungi. Its main indication is the topical therapy of fungal keratomycosis in horses. In one study, natamycin was active *in vitro* against 95% of fungal isolates from horses with keratomycosis.[209] Nystatin, another polyene, has a limited spectrum of activity and is rarely indicated in horses. The only indication for nystatin would be the topical treatment of *Candida* spp. infections

Azoles

Imidazole (ketoconazole, miconazole, clotrimazole, enilconazole) and triazoles (fluconazole, itraconazole, voriconazole, posaconazole) exert activity against a broad range of fungi (Table 6.10). All are fungistatic, so that prolonged therapy is required, especially in immunosuppressed partients. Triazoles are less toxic than imidazoles because they bind more specifically to fungal cell cytochromes than to mammalian cells cytochromes.

The pharmacokinetics of ketokonazole, fluconazole, itraconazole and voriconazole have been studied in horses. Administration of ketokonazole orally at a dose of 30 mg/kg did not result in detectable serum concentrations.[210] Administration of the same dose in 0.2% HCl resulted in peak serum concentrations of 3.7 mg/ml.[210] The bioavailability was only 23%. The drug was detected at therapeutic concentrations in synovial fluid, peritoneal fluid and endometrial tissue. Low concentrations were measured in the CSF of only one of three horses.[210] Administration of ketokonazole in HCl requires placement of a nasogastric tube to prevent irritation of the nasopharynx.

As opposed to ketokonazole, fluconazole and voriconazole are completely absorbed following oral administration to adult horses.[211,212] Long term oral administration of fluconazole at 24-hour intervals results in adequate concentrations in plasma, CSF, synovial fluid, urine and aqueous humor.[211] Oral or topical administration of voriconazole to adult horses results in therapeutic concentrations in aqueous humour.[213] Itraconazole is also suitable for oral administration to horses. The oral solution is better absorbed than the capsules in horses with bioavailabilities of 65% and 12%, respectively.[214] The absorption of azoles antifungal agents is considerably reduced by administration of gastric acid suppressant.

There are many reports of successful use of various azoles for the treatment of fungal infections in horses. It is difficult to assess the true efficacy of many of these drugs as multiple treatment modalities were often used concurrently. Intranasal miconazole was part of successful multimodal therapy against nasopharyngeal *Pseudallescheria boydii* in a horse.[215] Regional perfusion with miconazole was successful in a pregnant mare with osteomyelitis caused by *Pythium* spp.[216] Topical enilconazole has also been used with apparent success for the treatment of guttural pouch mycosis in horses.[217,218] Enilconazole administered by aerosolisation also resolved *Scopulariopsis* pneumonia in a mare.[219] Oral itraconazole has been used for the treatment of coccidioidomycosis osteomyelitis and mycotic rhinitis in horses.[220,221] Itraconazole (1%)-dimethyl sulfoxide (30%) petrolatum-based ointment has been used successfully for the topical treatment keratomycosis in horses.[222] Topical miconazole is also commonly used for that purpose.

Fluconazole has been used for the treatment of candidiasis in foals.[195] Fluconazole has also been used successfully for the treatment of *Coccidioides immitis* in two horses.[223] In a recent report, oral fluconazole was apparently successful in resolving granulomatous mass caused by *Conidiobolus coronatus* in two mares.[224] Paradoxically, most *C. coronatous* isolates are highly resistant to azoles *in vitro*.[225,226] Systemic therapy with fluconazole and itraconazole appears to be well tolerated in horses.

Systemic iodide therapy

Iodides have been used for many years to treat mycotic infections. Iodides have little, if any, *in vitro* antifungal activity. Their mechanism of action is unknown but may include enhancement of the immune response of the host. Sodium or potassium iodide therapy may be of benefit in horses with infections caused by *Conidiobolus* or *Sporothrix*. Treatment with organic iodide is inexpensive, but toxicity may occur. Iodide toxicosis is evidenced by excessive lacrimation, skin scaling and a dry nonproductive cough. Iodide is not recommended in pregnant mares because excessive iodide in the diet may result in congenital hypothyroidism in foals.

References

1. Marsh PS, Palmer JE: Bacterial isolates from blood and their susceptibility patterns in critically ill foals: 543 cases (1991-1998). J Am Vet Med Assoc 218:1608-1610, 2001
2. Wilson WD, Madigan JE: Comparison of bacteriologic culture of blood and necropsy specimens for determining the cause of foal septicemia: 47 cases (1978-1987). J Am Vet Med Assoc 195:1759-1763, 1989
3. Paradis MR: Update on neonatal septicemia. Vet Clin North Am Equine Pract 10:109-135, 1994
4. Nix DE, Goodwin SD, Peloquin CA, Rotella DL, Schentag JJ: Antibiotic tissue penetration and its relevance: impact of tissue penetration on infection response. Antimicrob Agents Chemother 35:1953-1959, 1991
5. Baldwin DR, Honeybourne D, Wise R: Pulmonary disposition of antimicrobial agents: in vivo observations and clinical relevance. Antimicrob Agents Chemother 36:1176-1180, 1992
6. Rex JH, Pfaller MA: Has antifungal susceptibility testing come of age? Clin Infect Dis 35:982-989, 2002
7. Bryant JE, Brown MP, Gronwall RR, Merritt KA: Study of intragastric administration of doxycycline: pharmacokinetics including body fluid, endometrial and minimum inhibitory concentrations. Equine Vet J 32:233-238, 2000
8. Davis JL, Salmon JH, Papich MG: Pharmacokinetics and tissue distribution of doxycycline after oral administration of single and multiple doses in horses. Am J Vet Res 67:310-316, 2006
9. Andes D, Anon J, Jacobs MR, Craig WA: Application of pharmacokinetics and pharmacodynamics to antimicrobial therapy of respiratory tract infections. Clin Lab Med 24:477-502, 2004
10. Craig WA: Basic pharmacodynamics of antibacterials with clinical applications to the use of beta-lactams, glycopeptides, and linezolid. Infect Dis Clin North Am 17:479-501, 2003
11. Wilson DA, MacFadden KE, Green EM, Crabill M, Frankeny RL, Thorne JG: Case control and historical cohort study of diarrhea associated with administration of trimethoprim-potentiated sulphonamides to horses and ponies. J Vet Intern Med 10:258-264, 1996
12. Staempfli HR, Prescott JF, Brash ML: Lincomycin-induced severe colitis in ponies: association with *Clostridium cadaveris*. Can J Vet Res 56:168-169, 1992
13. Prescott JF, Staempfli HR, Barker IK, Bettoni R, Delaney K: A method for reproducing fatal idiopathic colitis (colitis X) in ponies and isolation of a clostridium as a possible agent. Equine Vet J 20:417-420, 1988
14. Giguère S, Prescott JF, Baggot JD, Walker RD, Dowling PM: Antimicrobial Therapy in Veterinary Medicine, ed 4. Ames, IA, Blackwell, 2006
15. Stover SM, Brown MP, Kelly RH, Farver TB, Knight HD: Aqueous procaine penicillin G in the horse: serum, synovial, peritoneal, and urine concentrations after single-dose intramuscular administration. Am J Vet Res 42:629-631, 1981
16. Love DN, Rose RJ, Martin IC, Bailey M: Serum concentrations of penicillin in the horse after administration of a variety of penicillin preparations. Equine Vet J 15:43-48, 1983
17. Stevenson AJ, Weber MP, Todi F, Young L, Beaumier P, Kacew S: Plasma elimination and urinary excretion of procaine after administration of different products to standardbred mares. Equine Vet J 24:118-124, 1992

18. Horspool LJ, McKellar QA: Disposition of penicillin G sodium following intravenous and oral administration to Equidae. Br Vet J 151:401-412, 1995
19. Baggot JD, Love DN, Love RJ, Raus J, Rose RJ: Oral dosage of penicillin V in adult horses and foals. Equine Vet J 22:290-291, 1990
20. Ducharme NG, Dill SG, Shin SJ, Schwark WS, Ducharme GR, Beilman WW: Phenoxymethyl penicillin in the horse: an alternative to parenteral administration of penicillin. Can J Comp Med 47:436-439, 1983
21. Nielsen IL, Jacobs KA, Huntington PJ, Chapman CB, Lloyd KC: Adverse reaction to procaine penicillin G in horses. Aust Vet J 65:181-185, 1988
22. Chapman CB, Courage P, Nielsen IL, Sitaram BR, Huntington PJ: The role of procaine in adverse reactions to procaine penicillin in horses. Aust Vet J 69:129-133, 1992
23. Tobin T, Blake JW, Sturma L, Arnett S, Truelove J: Pharmacology of procaine in the horse: pharmacokinetics and behavioral effects. Am J Vet Res 38:637-647, 1977
24. Hubbell JA, Muir WW, Robertson JT, Sams RA: Cardiovascular effects of intravenous sodium penicillin, sodium cefazolin, and sodium citrate in awake and anesthetized horses. Vet Surg 16:245-250, 1987
25. Wilson WD: Rational selection of antimicrobials for use in horses. Proc Am Assoc Equine Pract 47:75-93, 2001
26. Roussel AJ, Hooper RN, Cohen ND, Bye AD, Hicks RJ, Schulze JL: Evaluation of the effects of penicillin G potassium and potassium chloride on the motility of the large intestine in horses. Am J Vet Res 64:1360-1363, 2003
27. Horspool LJ, Sarasola P, McKellar QA: Disposition of ampicillin sodium in horses, ponies and donkeys after intravenous administration. Equine Vet J Suppl 59-61, 1992
28. Ensink JM, Vulto AG, Van Miert AS, Tukker JJ, Winkel MB, Fluitman MA: Oral bioavailability and in vitro stability of pivampicillin, bacampicillin, talampicillin, and ampicillin in horses. Am J Vet Res 57:1021-1024, 1996
29. Ensink JM, Klein WR, Mevius DJ, Klarenbeek A, Vulto AG: Bioavailability of oral penicillins in the horse: a comparison of pivampicillin and amoxicillin. J Vet Pharmacol Ther 15:221-230, 1992
30. Baggot JD, Love DN, Stewart J, Raus J: Bioavailability and disposition kinetics of amoxicillin in neonatal foals. Equine Vet J 20:125-127, 1988
31. Love DN, Rose RJ, Martin IC, Bailey M: Serum levels of amoxycillin following its oral administration to thoroughbred foals. Equine Vet J 13:53-55, 1981
32. Brown MP, Gronwall R, Kroll WR, Beal C: Ampicillin trihydrate in foals: serum concentrations and clearance after a single oral dose. Equine Vet J 16:371-373, 1984
33. Ensink JM, Moi A, Vulto AG, Tukker JJ: Bioavailability of pivampicillin and ampicillin trihydrate administered as an oral paste in horses. Vet Q 18(Suppl 2):S117-S120, 1996
34. Ensink JM, Barneveld A, Klein WR, Van Miert AS, Vulto AG: Oral bioavailability of pivampicillin in foals at different ages. Vet Q 16 Suppl 2:S113-S116, 1994
35. Ensink JM, Klein WR, Barneveld A, Vulto AG, Van Miert AS: Clinical efficacy of ampicillin, pivampicillin and procaine penicillin G in a soft tissue infection model in ponies. J Vet Pharmacol Ther 19:445-453, 1996
36. Ensink JM, Klein WR, Barneveld A, Van Miert AS, Vulto AG: Side effects of oral antimicrobial agents in the horse: a comparison of pivampicillin and trimethoprim/sulphadiazine. Vet Rec 138:253-256, 1996
37. Stover SM, Brown MP, Kelly RH, Farver TB: Sodium oxacillin in the horse: serum, synovial fluid, peritoneal fluid, and urine concentrations after single-dose intramuscular administration. Am J Vet Res 42:1826-1828, 1981
38. Jacks S, Giguère S, Nguyen A: In vitro susceptibilities of *Rhodococcus equi* and other common equine pathogens to azithromycin, clarithromycin and 20 other antimicrobials. Antimicrob Agents Chemother 47:1742-1745, 2003
39. Weese JS, Archambault M, Willey BM, et al.: Methicillin-resistant *Staphylococcus aureus* in horses and horse personnel, 2000-2002. Emerg Infect Dis 11:430-435, 2005
40. Seguin JC, Walker RD, Caron JP, et al.: Methicillin-resistant *Staphylococcus aureus* outbreak in a veterinary teaching hospital: potential human-to-animal transmission. J Clin Microbiol 37:1459-1463, 1999
41. Wilson WD, Spensley MS, Baggot JD, Hietala SK, Pryor P: Pharmacokinetics and bioavailability of ticarcillin and clavulanate in foals after intravenous and intramuscular administration. J Vet Pharmacol Ther 14:78-89, 1991
42. Sweeney RW, Beech J, Simmons RD, Soma LR: Pharmacokinetics of ticarcillin and clavulanic acid given in combination to adult horses by intravenous and intramuscular routes. J Vet Pharmacol Ther 11:10310-10318, 1988
43. Sweeney RW, Beech J, Simmons RD: Pharmacokinetics of intravenously and intramuscularly administered ticarcillin and clavulanic acid in foals. Am J Vet Res 49:23-26, 1988
44. Sweeney CR, Soma LR, Beech J, Reef V, Simmons R: Pharmacokinetics of ticarcillin in the horse after intravenous and intramuscular administration. Am J Vet Res 45:1000-1002, 1984
45. el Komy AA: Disposition kinetics and bioavailability of piperacillin and cephapirin in mares. Dtsch Tierarztl Wochenschr 102:244-248, 1995
46. Van Camp SD, Papich MG, Whitacre MD: Administration of ticarcillin in combination with clavulanic acid intravenously and intrauterinely to clinically normal oestrous mares. J Vet Pharmacol Ther 23:373-378, 2000
47. Spensley MS, Baggot JD, Wilson WD, Hietala SK, Mihalyi JE: Pharmacokinetics and endometrial tissue concentrations of ticarcillin given to the horse by intravenous and intrauterine routes. Am J Vet Res 47:2587-2590, 1986
48. Duffee NE, Stang BE, Schaeffer DJ: The pharmacokinetics of cefadroxil over a range of oral doses and animal ages in the foal. J Vet Pharmacol Ther 20:427-433, 1997
49. Henry MM, Morris DD, Lakritz J, Aucoin D: Pharmacokinetics of cephradine in neonatal foals after single oral dosing. Equine Vet J 24:242-243, 1992
50. Carrillo NA, Giguère S, Gronwall RR, Brown MP, Merritt KA, O'Kelley JJ: Disposition of orally administered cefpodoxime proxetil in foals and adult horses and minimum inhibitory concentration of the drug against common bacterial pathogens of horses. Am J Vet Res 66:30-35, 2005
51. Samitz EM, Jang SS, Hirsh DC: In vitro susceptibilities of selected obligate anaerobic bacteria obtained from bovine and equine sources to ceftiofur. J Vet Diagn Invest 8:121-123, 1996
52. Salmon SA, Watts JL, Yancey RJ Jr: In vitro activity of ceftiofur and its primary metabolite, desfuroylceftiofur, against

organisms of veterinary importance. J Vet Diagn Invest 8:332-326, 1996

53. Mahrt CR: Safety of ceftiofur sodium administered intramuscularly in horses. Am J Vet Res 53:2201-2205, 1992
54. Thomas E, Thomas V, Wilhelm C: Antibacterial activity of cefquinome against equine bacterial pathogens. Vet Microbiol 115:140-147, 2006
55. Ebert SC, Craig WA: Pharmacodynamic properties of antibiotics: application to drug monitoring and dosage regimen design. Infect Control Hosp Epidemiol 11:319-326, 1990
56. Jackson GG, Lolans VT, Daikos GL: The inductive role of ionic binding in the bactericidal and postexposure effects of aminoglycoside antibiotics with implications for dosing. J Infect Dis 162:408-413, 1990
57. Deziel-Evans LM, Murphy JE, Job ML: Correlation of pharmacokinetic indices with therapeutic outcome in patients receiving aminoglycosides. Clin Pharm 5:319-324, 1986
58. Moore RD, Lietman PS, Smith CR: Clinical response to aminoglycoside therapy: importance of the ratio of peak concentration to minimal inhibitory concentration. J Infect Dis 155:93-99, 1987
59. Karlowsky JA, Zhanel GG, Davidson RJ, Hoban DJ: Once-daily aminoglycoside dosing assessed by MIC reversion time with *Pseudomonas aeruginosa*. Antimicrob Agents Chemother 38:1165-1168, 1994
60. Godber LM, Walker RD, Stein GE, Hauptman JG, Derksen FJ: Pharmacokinetics, nephrotoxicosis, and in vitro antibacterial activity associated with single versus multiple (three times) daily gentamicin treatments in horses. Am J Vet Res 56:613-618, 1995
61. Magdesian KG, Hogan PM, Cohen ND, Brumbaugh GW, Bernard WV: Pharmacokinetics of a high dose of gentamicin administered intravenously or intramuscularly to horses. J Am Vet Med Assoc 213:1007-1011, 1998
62. Orsini JA, Soma LR, Rourke JE, Park M: Pharmacokinetics of amikacin in the horse following intravenous and intramuscular administration. J Vet Pharmacol Ther 8:194-201, 1985
63. Gilman JM, Davis LE, Neff-Davis CA, Koritz GD, Baker GJ: Plasma concentration of gentamicin after intramuscular or subcutaneous administration to horses. J Vet Pharmacol Ther 10:101-103, 1987
64. Anderson BH, Firth EC, Whittem T: The disposition of gentamicin in equine plasma, synovial fluid and lymph. J Vet Pharmacol Ther 18:124-131, 1995
65. Brown MP, Stover SM, Kelly RH, Farver TB: Gentamicin sulfate in the horse: serum, synovial, peritoneal, and urine concentrations after single dose intramuscular administration. J Vet Pharmacol Ther 5:119-122, 1982
66. Beech J, Kohn C, Leitch M, Weinstein AJ, Gallagher M: Therapeutic use of gentamicin in horses: concentrations in serum, urine, and synovial fluid and evaluation of renal function. Am J Vet Res 38:1085-1087, 1977
67. Haddad NS, Pedersoli WM, Ravis WR, Fazeli MH, Carson RL Jr: Pharmacokinetics of gentamicin at steady-state in ponies: serum, urine, and endometrial concentrations. Am J Vet Res 46:1268-12671, 1985
68. Snyder JR, Pascoe JR, Hietala SK, Holland M, Baggot DJ: Gentamicin tissue concentrations in equine small intestine and large colon. Am J Vet Res 47:1092-1095, 1986
69. Orsini JA, Park MI, Spencer PA: Tissue and serum concentrations of amikacin after intramuscular and intrauterine administration to mares in estrus. Can Vet J 37:157-160, 1996
70. Bucki EP, Giguère S, Macpherson M, Davis R: Pharmacokinetics of once-daily amikacin in healthy foals and therapeutic drug monitoring in hospitalised equine neonates. J Vet Intern Med 18:728-733, 2004
71. Magdesian KG, Wilson WD, Mihalyi J: Pharmacokinetics of a high dose of amikacin administered at extended intervals to neonatal foals. Am J Vet Res 65:473-479, 2004
72. Martin-Jimenez T, Papich MG, Riviere JE: Population pharmacokinetics of gentamicin in horses. Am J Vet Res 59:1589-1598, 1998
73. Rossier Y, Divers TJ, Sweeney RW: Variations in urinary gamma glutamyl transferase/urinary creatinine ratio in horses with or without pleuropneumonia treated with gentamicin. Equine Vet J 27:217-220, 1995
74. Sweeney RW, Divers TJ, Rossier Y: Disposition of gentamicin administered intravenously to horses with sepsis. J Am Vet Med Assoc 200:503-506, 1992
75. Lavy E, Ziv G, Glickman A: Intravenous disposition kinetics, oral and intramuscular bioavailability and urinary excretion of norfloxacin nicotinate in donkeys. J Vet Pharmacol Ther 18:101-107, 1995
76. Park SC, Yun HI: Clinical pharmacokinetics of norfloxacin-glycine acetate after intravenous and intramuscular administration to horses. Res Vet Sci 74:79-83, 2003
77. Rebuelto M, Otero P, Albarellos G, et al.: Pharmacokinetics of fleroxacin in horses. J Vet Pharmacol Ther 23:103-105, 2000
78. Haines GR, Brown MP, Gronwall RR, Merritt KA: Serum concentrations and pharmacokinetics of enrofloxacin after intravenous and intragastric administration to mares. Can J Vet Res 64:171-177, 2000
79. Haines GR, Brown MP, Gronwall RR, Merritt KA, Baltzley LK: Pharmacokinetics of orbifloxacin and its concentration in body fluids and in endometrial tissues of mares. Can J Vet Res 65:181-187, 2001
80. Kaartinen L, Panu S, Pyorala S: Pharmacokinetics of enrofloxacin in horses after single intravenous and intramuscular administration. Equine Vet J 29:378-381, 1997
81. Papich MG, Van Camp SD, Cole JA, Whitacre MD: Pharmacokinetics and endometrial tissue concentrations of enrofloxacin and the metabolite ciprofloxacin after i.v. administration of enrofloxacin to mares. J Vet Pharmacol Ther 25:343-350, 2002
82. Dowling PM, Wilson RC, Tyler JW, Duran SH: Pharmacokinetics of ciprofloxacin in ponies. J Vet Pharmacol Ther 18:7-12, 1995
83. Giguère S, Sweeney RW, Belanger M: Pharmacokinetics of enrofloxacin in adult horses and concentration of the drug in serum, body fluids, and endometrial tissues after repeated intragastrically administered doses. Am J Vet Res 57:1025-1030, 1996
84. Adams AR, Haines GR, Brown MP, Gronwall R, Merritt K: Pharmacokinetics of difloxacin and its concentration in body fluids and endometrial tissues of mares after repeated intragastric administration. Can J Vet Res 69:229-235, 2005

85. Fernandez-Varon E, Ayala I, Marin P, et al.: Pharmacokinetics of danofloxacin in horses after intravenous, intramuscular and intragastric administration. Equine Vet J 38:342-346, 2006
86. Fernandez-Varon E, Carceles CM, Marin P, Martos N, Escudero E, Ayala I: Pharmacokinetics of difloxacin after intravenous, intramuscular, and intragastric administration to horses. Am J Vet Res 67:1076-1081, 2006
87. Drusano GL, Johnson DE, Rosen M, Standiford HC: Pharmacodynamics of a fluoroquinolone antimicrobial agent in a neutropenic rat model of *Pseudomonas sepsis*. Antimicrob Agents Chemother 37:483-490, 1993
88. Forrest A, Nix DE, Ballow CH, Goss TF, Birmingham MC, Schentag JJ: Pharmacodynamics of intravenous ciprofloxacin in seriously ill patients. Antimicrob Agents Chemother 37:1073-1081, 1993
89. Wright DH, Brown GH, Peterson ML, Rotschafer JC: Application of fluoroquinolone pharmacodynamics. J Antimicrob Chemother 46:669-683, 2000
90. Epstein K, Cohen N, Boothe D, Nieuwoudt C, Chandler J: Pharmacokinetics, stability, and retrospective analysis of use of an oral gel formulation of the bovine injectable enrofloxacin in horses. Vet Ther 5:155-167, 2004
91. Giguère S, Belanger M: Concentration of enrofloxacin in equine tissues after long-term oral administration. J Vet Pharmacol Ther 20:402-404, 1997
92. Bertone AL, Tremaine WH, Macoris DG, et al.: Effect of long-term administration of an injectable enrofloxacin solution on physical and musculoskeletal variables in adult horses. J Am Vet Med Assoc 217:1514-1521, 2000
93. Giguère S, Sweeney RW, Habecker PL, Lucas J, Richardson DW: Tolerability of orally administered enrofloxacin in adult horses: a pilot study. J Vet Pharmacol Ther 22:343-347, 1999
94. Vivrette S, Bostian A, Bermingham E, Papich MG: Quinolone induced arthropathy in neonatal foals. Proc Am Assoc Equine Pract 47:376-377, 2001
95. Beluche LA, Bertone AL, Anderson DE, Kohn CW, Weisbrode SE: In vitro dose-dependent effects of enrofloxacin on equine articular cartilage. Am J Vet Res 60:577-582, 1999
96. Davenport CL, Boston RC, Richardson DW: Effects of enrofloxacin and magnesium deficiency on matrix metabolism in equine articular cartilage. Am J Vet Res 62:160-166, 2001
97. Egerbacher M, Edinger J, Tschulenk W: Effects of enrofloxacin and ciprofloxacin hydrochloride on canine and equine chondrocytes in culture. Am J Vet Res 62:704-708, 2001
98. Yoon JH, Brooks RL Jr, Khan A, et al.: The effect of enrofloxacin on cell proliferation and proteoglycans in horse tendon cells. Cell Biol Toxicol 20:41-54, 2004
99. Gardner SY, Davis JL, Jones SL, et al.: Moxifloxacin pharmacokinetics in horses and disposition into phagocytes after oral dosing. J Vet Pharmacol Ther 27:57-60, 2004
100. Ewing PJ, Burrows G, MacAllister C, Clarke C: Comparison of oral erythromycin formulations in the horse using pharmacokinetic profiles. J Vet Pharmacol Ther 17:17-23, 1994
101. Jacks S, Giguère S, Gronwall RR, Brown MP, Merritt KA: Disposition of oral clarithromycin in foals. J Vet Pharmacol Ther 25:359-362, 2002
102. Lakritz J, Wilson WD, Mihalyi JE: Comparison of microbiologic and high-performance liquid chromatography assays to determine plasma concentrations, pharmacokinetics, and bioavailability of erythromycin base in plasma of foals after intravenous or intragastric administration. Am J Vet Res 60:414-419, 1999
103. Lakritz J, Wilson WD, Marsh AE, Mihalyi JE: Pharmacokinetics of erythromycin estolate and erythromycin phosphate after intragastric administration to healthy foals. Am J Vet Res 61:914-919, 2000
104. Lakritz J, Wilson WD, Marsh AE, Mihalyi JE: Effects of prior feeding on pharmacokinetics and estimated bioavailability after oral administration of a single dose of microencapsulated erythromycin base in healthy foals. Am J Vet Res 61:1011-1015, 2000
105. Prescott JF, Hoover DJ, Dohoo IR: Pharmacokinetics of erythromycin in foals and in adult horses. J Vet Pharmacol Ther 6:67-73, 1983
106. Womble AY, Giguère S, Lee EA, Vickroy TW: Pharmacokinetics of clarithromycin and concentrations in body fluids and bronchoalveolar cells of foals. Am J Vet Res 67:1681-1686, 2006
107. Davis JL, Gardner SY, Jones SL, Schwabenton BA, Papich MG: Pharmacokinetics of azithromycin in foals after i.v. and oral dose and disposition into phagocytes. J Vet Pharmacol Ther 25:99-104, 2002
108. Jacks S, Giguère S, Gronwall PR, Brown MP, Merritt KA: Pharmacokinetics of azithromycin and concentration in body fluids and bronchoalveolar cells in foals. Am J Vet Res 62:1870-1875, 2001
109. Suarez-Mier G, Giguère S, Lee EA: Pulmonary disposition of erythromycin, azithromycin, and clarithromycin in foals. J Vet Pharmacol Ther 30:109-115, 2007
110. Stratton-Phelps M, Wilson WD, Gardner IA: Risk of adverse effects in pneumonic foals treated with erythromycin versus other antibiotics: 143 cases (1986-1996). J Am Vet Med Assoc 217:68-73, 2000
111. Baverud V, Franklin A, Gunnarsson A, Gustafsson A, Hellander-Edman A: *Clostridium difficile* associated with acute colitis in mares when their foals are treated with erythromycin and rifampicin for *Rhodococcus equi* pneumonia. Equine Vet J 30:482-488, 1998
112. Giguère S, Jacks S, Roberts GD, Hernandez J, Long MT, Ellis C: Retrospective comparison of azithromycin, clarithromycin, and erythromycin for the treatment of foals with *Rhodococcus equi* pneumonia. J Vet Intern Med 18:568-573, 2004
113. Lavoie JP, Drolet R, Parsons D, et al.: Equine proliferative enteropathy: a cause of weight loss, colic, diarrhoea and hypoproteinaemia in foals on three breeding farms in Canada. Equine Vet J 32:418-425, 2000
114. Papich MG, Wright AK, Petrie L, Korsrud GO: Pharmacokinetics of oxytetracycline administered intravenously to 4 to 5-day-old foals. J Vet Pharmacol Ther 18:375-378, 1995
115. Horspool LJ, McKellar QA: Disposition of oxytetracycline in horses, ponies and donkeys after intravenous administration. Equine Vet J 22:284-285, 1990
116. Larson VL, Stowe CM: Plasma and tissue concentrations of oxytetracycline in the horse after intravenous administration. Am J Vet Res 42:2165-2166, 1981

117. Brown MP, Stover SM, Kelly RH, Farver TB, Knight HD: Oxytetracycline hydrochloride in the horse: serum, synovial, peritoneal and urine concentrations after single dose intravenous administration. J Vet Pharmacol Ther 4:7-10, 1981
118. Pilloud M: Pharmacokinetics, plasma protein binding and dosage of oxytetracycline in cattle and horses. Res Vet Sci 15:224-230, 1973
119. Teske RH, Rollins LD, Condon RJ, Carter GG: Serum oxytetracycline concentrations after intravenous and intramuscular administration in horses. J Am Vet Med Assoc 162:119-120, 1973
120. Womble A, Giguère S, Lee EA: Pharmacokinetics of oral doxycycline and concentrations in body fluids and bronchoalveolar cells of foals. J Vet Pharmacol Ther 30:187-193, 2007
121. Dowling PM, Russell AM: Pharmacokinetics of a long-acting oxytetracycline-polyethylene glycol formulation in horses. J Vet Pharmacol Ther 23:107-110, 2000
122. Palmer JE, Benson CE, Whitlock RH: Effect of treatment with oxytetracycline during the acute stages of experimentally induced equine ehrlichial colitis in ponies. Am J Vet Res 53:2300-2304, 1992
123. Palmer JE, Whitlock RH, Benson CE: Equine ehrlichial colitis: effect of oxytetracycline treatment during the incubation period of *Ehrlichia risticii* infection in ponies. J Am Vet Med Assoc 192:343-345, 1988
124. Chang YF, Ku YW, Chang CF, et al.: Antibiotic treatment of experimentally *Borrelia burgdorferi*-infected ponies. Vet Microbiol 107:285-294, 2005
125. Kasper CA, Clayton HM, Wright AK, Skuba EV, Petrie L: Effects of high doses of oxytetracycline on metacarpophalangeal joint kinematics in neonatal foals. J Am Vet Med Assoc 207:71-73, 1995
126. Madison JB, Garber JL, Rice B, Stumf AJ, Zimmer AE, Ott EA: Effect of oxytetracycline on metacarpophalangeal and distal interphalangeal joint angles in newborn foals. J Am Vet Med Assoc 204:246-249, 1994
127. Arnoczky SP, Lavagnino M, Gardner KL, Tian T, Vaupel ZM, Stick JA: In vitro effects of oxytetracycline on matrix metalloproteinase-1 mRNA expression and on collagen gel contraction by cultured myofibroblasts obtained from the accessory ligament of foals. Am J Vet Res 65:491-496, 2004
128. Vivrette S, Cowgill LD, Pascoe J, Suter C, Becker T: Hemodialysis for treatment of oxytetracycline-induced acute renal failure in a neonatal foal. J Am Vet Med Assoc 203:105-107, 1993
129. Riond JL, Riviere JE, Duckett WM, et al.: Cardiovascular effects and fatalities associated with intravenous administration of doxycycline to horses and ponies. Equine Vet J 24:41-45, 1992
130. Gilmour MA, Clarke CR, MacAllister CG, et al.: Ocular penetration of oral doxycycline in the horse. Vet Ophthalmol 8:331-335, 2005
131. Branger S, Rolain JM, Raoult D: Evaluation of antibiotic susceptibilities of *Ehrlichia canis*, *Ehrlichia chaffeensis*, and *Anaplasma phagocytophilum* by real-time PCR. Antimicrob Agents Chemother 48:4822-4828, 2004
132. Hunfeld KP, Bittner T, Rodel R, Brade V, Cinatl J: New real-time PCR-based method for in vitro susceptibility testing of *Anaplasma phagocytophilum* against antimicrobial agents. Int J Antimicrob Agents 23:563-571, 2004
133. Rikihisa Y, Jiang BM: In vitro susceptibilities of *Ehrlichia risticii* to eight antibiotics. Antimicrob Agents Chemother 32:986-991, 1988
134. Ensink JM, van Klingeren B, Houwers DJ, Klein WR, Vulto AG: In-vitro susceptibility to antimicrobial drugs of bacterial isolates from horses in the Netherlands. Equine Vet J 25:309-313, 1993
135. Sampieri F, Hinchcliff KW, Toribio RE: Tetracycline therapy of *Lawsonia intracellularis* enteropathy in foals. Equine Vet J 38:89-92, 2006
136. Specht TE, Brown MP, Gronwall RR, Rib WJ, Houston AE: Pharmacokinetics of metronidazole and its concentration in body fluids and endometrial tissues of mares. Am J Vet Res 53:1807-1812, 1992
137. Steinman A, Gips M, Lavy E, Sinay I, Soback S: Pharmacokinetics of metronidazole in horses after intravenous, rectal and oral administration. J Vet Pharmacol Ther 23:353-357, 2000
138. Sweeney RW, Sweeney CR, Soma LR, Woodward CB, Charlton CA: Pharmacokinetics of metronidazole given to horses by intravenous and oral routes. Am J Vet Res 47:1726-1729, 1986
139. McGorum BC, Dixon PM, Smith DG: Use of metronidazole in equine acute idiopathic toxaemic colitis. Vet Rec 142:635-638, 1998
140. Sweeney RW, Sweeney CR, Weiher J: Clinical use of metronidazole in horses: 200 cases (1984-1989). J Am Vet Med Assoc 198:1045-1048, 1991
141. Ensink JM, Smit JA, van Duijkeren E: Clinical efficacy of trimethoprim/sulfadiazine and procaine penicillin G in a *Streptococcus equi* subsp. *zooepidemicus* infection model in ponies. J Vet Pharmacol Ther 26:247-252, 2003
142. Ensink JM, Bosch G, van Duijkeren E: Clinical efficacy of prophylactic administration of trimethoprim/sulfadiazine in a *Streptococcus equi* subsp. *zooepidemicus* infection model in ponies. J Vet Pharmacol Ther 28:45-49, 2005
143. van Duijkeren E, Vulto AG, Sloet van Oldruitenborgh-Oosterbaan MM, Kessels BG, Van Miert AS, Breukink HJ: Pharmacokinetics of trimethoprim/sulphachlorpyridazine in horses after oral, nasogastric and intravenous administration. J Vet Pharmacol Ther 18:47-53, 1995
144. van Duijkeren E, Vulto AG, Sloet van Oldruitenborg Oosterbaan MM, et al.: A comparative study of the pharmacokinetics of intravenous and oral trimethoprim/sulfadiazine formulations in the horse. J Vet Pharmacol Ther 17:440-446, 1994
145. Bogan JA, Galbraith A, Baxter P, Ali NM, Marriner SE: Effect of feeding on the fate of orally administered phenylbutazone, trimethoprim and sulphadiazine in the horse. Vet Rec 115:599-600, 1984
146. van Duijkeren E, Ensink JM, Meijer LA: Distribution of orally administered trimethoprim and sulfadiazine into noninfected subcutaneous tissue chambers in adult ponies. J Vet Pharmacol Ther 25:273-277, 2002
147. White G, Prior SD: Comparative effects of oral administration of trimethoprim/sulphadiazine or oxytetracycline on the faecal flora of horses. Vet Rec 111:316-318, 1982
148. Brown MP, Gronwall R, Castro L: Pharmacokinetics and body fluid and endometrial concentrations of trime-

thoprim-sulfamethoxazole in mares. Am J Vet Res 49:918-922, 1988

149. Adamson PJ, Wilson WD, Baggot JD, Hietala SK, Mihalyi JE: Influence of age on the disposition kinetics of chloramphenicol in equine neonates. Am J Vet Res 52:426-431, 1991
150. Brown MP, Kelly RH, Gronwall RR, Stover SM: Chloramphenicol sodium succinate in the horse: serum, synovial, peritoneal, and urine concentrations after single-dose intravenous administration. Am J Vet Res 45:578-580, 1984
151. Brumbaugh GW, Martens RJ, Knight HD, Martin MT: Pharmacokinetics of chloramphenicol in the neonatal horse. J Vet Pharmacol Ther 6:219-227, 1983
152. Buonpane NA, Brown MP, Gronwall R, Stone HW, Miles N: Serum concentrations and pharmacokinetics of chloramphenicol in foals after a single oral dose. Equine Vet J 20:59-61, 1988
153. Davis LE, Neff CA, Baggot JD, Powers TE: Pharmacokinetics of chloramphenicol in domesticated animals. Am J Vet Res 33:2259-2266, 1972
154. Gronwall R, Brown MP, Merritt AM, Stone HW: Body fluid concentrations and pharmacokinetics of chloramphenicol given to mares intravenously or by repeated gavage. Am J Vet Res 47:2591-2595, 1986
155. Varma KJ, Powers TE, Powers JD: Single- and repeat-dose pharmacokinetic studies of chloramphenicol in horses: values and limitations of pharmacokinetic studies in predicting dosage regimens. Am J Vet Res 48:403-406, 1987
156. McKellar QA, Varga KJ: Pharmacokinetics and tolerance of florfenicol in equidae. Equine Vet J 28:209-213, 1996
157. Dowling PM: Florfenicol in horses: pharmacokinetics and tolerance. Proc 19th Annu Vet Med Forum Am Coll Vet Intern Med 19:198-199, 2001
158. Burrows GE, MacAllister CG, Beckstrom DA, Nick JT: Rifampin in the horse: comparison of intravenous, intramuscular, and oral administrations. Am J Vet Res 46:442-446, 1985
159. Burrows GE, MacAllister CG, Ewing P, Stair E, Tripp PW: Rifampin disposition in the horse: effects of age and method of oral administration. J Vet Pharmacol Ther 15:124-132, 1992
160. Castro LA, Brown MP, Gronwall R, Houston AE, Miles N: Pharmacokinetics of rifampin given as a single oral dose in foals. Am J Vet Res 47:2584-2586, 1986
161. Kohn CW, Sams R, Kowalski JJ, Powers J, Wallace S: Pharmacokinetics of single intravenous and single and multiple dose oral administration of rifampin in mares. J Vet Pharmacol Ther 16:119-131, 1993
162. Fu KP, Lasinski ER, Zoganas HC, Kimble EF, Konopka EA: Therapeutic efficacy and pharmacokinetic properties of rifampicin in a *Bacteroides fragilis* intra-abdominal abscess. J Antimicrob Chemother 14:633-640, 1984
163. Bach VT, Thadepalli H: Susceptibility of anaerobic bacteria in vitro to 23 antimicrobial agents. Chemotherapy 26:344-353, 1980
164. Wilson WD, Spensley MS, Baggot JD, Hietala SK: Pharmacokinetics, bioavailability, and in vitro antibacterial activity of rifampin in the horse. Am J Vet Res 49:2041-2046, 1988
165. Burrows GE, MacAllister CG, Ewing P, Stair E, Burrows SL: Rifampin disposition in the horse: effects of repeated dosage of rifampin or phenylbutazone. J Vet Pharmacol Ther 15:305-308, 1992
166. Maurin M, Raoult D: Antibiotic penetration within phagocytic cells, in Raoult D (ed): Antimicrobial Agents and Intracellular Pathogens. Boca Raton, FL, CRC Press, 1993, pp 23-37
167. Valcke Y, Pauwels R, Van der SM: Pharmacokinetics of antibiotics in the lungs. Eur Respir J 3:715-722, 1990
168. Goldstein I, Wallet F, Nicolas-Robin A, Ferrari F, Marquette CH, Rouby JJ: Lung deposition and efficiency of nebulized amikacin during *Escherichia coli* pneumonia in ventilated piglets. Am J Respir Crit Care Med 166:1375-1381, 2002
169. McKenzie HC III: Characterization of antimicrobial aerosols for administration to horses. Vet Ther 4:110-119, 2003
170. McKenzie HC III, Murray MJ: Concentrations of gentamicin in serum and bronchial lavage fluid after intravenous and aerosol administration of gentamicin to horses. Am J Vet Res 61:1185-1190, 2000
171. McKenzie HC III, Murray MJ: Concentrations of gentamicin in serum and bronchial lavage fluid after once-daily aerosol administration to horses for seven days. Am J Vet Res 65:173-178. 2004
172. Stover SM, Pool RR: Effect of intra-articular gentamicin sulfate on normal equine synovial membrane. Am J Vet Res 46:2485-2491, 1985
173. Lloyd KC, Stover SM, Pascoe JR, Baggot JD, Kurpershoek C, Hietala S: Plasma and synovial fluid concentrations of gentamicin in horses after intra-articular administration of buffered and unbuffered gentamicin. Am J Vet Res 49:644-649, 1988
174. Lloyd KC, Stover SM, Pascoe JR, Adams P: Synovial fluid pH, cytologic characteristics, and gentamicin concentration after intra-articular administration of the drug in an experimental model of infectious arthritis in horses. Am J Vet Res 51:1363-1369, 1990
175. Lloyd KC, Stover SM, Pascoe JR, Pool RR, Kurpershoek C: Effect of gentamicin sulfate and sodium bicarbonate on the synovium of clinically normal equine antebrachiocarpal joints. Am J Vet Res 49:650-657, 1988
176. Lescun TB, Ward MP, Adams SB: Gentamicin concentrations in synovial fluid and joint tissues during intravenous administration or continuous intra-articular infusion of the tarsocrural joint of clinically normal horses. Am J Vet Res 67:409-416, 2006
177. Gustafson SB, McIlwraith CW, Jones RL, Dixon-White HE: Further investigations into the potentiation of infection by intra-articular injection of polysulfated glycosaminoglycan and the effect of filtration and intra-articular injection of amikacin. Am J Vet Res 50:2018-2022, 1989
178. Taintor J, Schumacher J, DeGraves F: Comparison of amikacin concentrations in normal and inflamed joints of horses following intra-articular administration. Equine Vet J 38:189-191, 2006
179. Mills ML, Rush BR, St Jean G, et al.: Determination of synovial fluid and serum concentrations, and morphologic effects of intraarticular ceftiofur sodium in horses. Vet Surg 29:398-406, 2000
180. Palmer SE, Hogan PM: How to perform regional limb perfusion in the standing horse. Proc Am Assoc Equine Pract 45:124-127, 1999

181. Mattson S, Boure L, Pearce S, Hurtig M, Burger J, Black W: Intraosseous gentamicin perfusion of the distal metacarpus in standing horses. Vet Surg 33:180-186, 2004
182. Scheuch BC, Van Hoogmoed LM, Wilson WD, et al.: Comparison of intraosseous or intravenous infusion for delivery of amikacin sulfate to the tibiotarsal joint of horses. Am J Vet Res 63:374-380, 2002
183. Butt TD, Bailey JV, Dowling PM, Fretz PB: Comparison of 2 techniques for regional antibiotic delivery to the equine forelimb: intraosseous perfusion vs. intravenous perfusion. Can Vet J 42:617-622, 2001
184. Werner LA, Hardy J, Bertone AL: Bone gentamicin concentration after intra-articular injection or regional intravenous perfusion in the horse. Vet Surg 32:559-565, 2003
185. Santschi EM, Adams SB, Murphey ED: How to perform equine intravenous digital perfusion. Proc Am Assoc Equine Pract 44:198-201, 1998
186. Pille F, De Baere S, Ceelen L, et al.: Synovial fluid and plasma concentrations of ceftiofur after regional intravenous perfusion in the horse. Vet Surg 34:610-617, 2005
187. Rubio-Martinez LM, Lopez-Sanroman J, Cruz AM, Santos M, Andres MS, Roman FS: Evaluation of safety and pharmacokinetics of vancomycin after intravenous regional limb perfusion in horses. Am J Vet Res 66:2107-2113, 2005
188. Rubio-Martinez LM, Lopez-Sanroman J, Cruz AM, Tendillo F, Rioja E, San Roman F: Evaluation of safety and pharmacokinetics of vancomycin after intraosseous regional limb perfusion and comparison of results with those obtained after intravenous regional limb perfusion in horses. Am J Vet Res 67:1701-1707, 2006
189. Parra-Sanchez A, Lugo J, Boothe DM, et al.: Pharmacokinetics and pharmacodynamics of enrofloxacin and a low dose of amikacin administered via regional intravenous limb perfusion in standing horses. Am J Vet Res 67:1687-1695, 2006
190. Rubio-Martinez LM, Cruz AM: Antimicrobial regional limb perfusion in horses. J Am Vet Med Assoc 228:655, 706-712, 2006
191. Murphey ED, Santschi EM, Papich MG: Regional intravenous perfusion of the distal limb of horses with amikacin sulfate. J Vet Pharmacol Ther 22:68-71, 1999
192. Whithair KJ, Bowersock TL, Blevins WE, Fessler JF, White MR, Van Sickle DC: Regional limb perfusion for antibiotic treatment of experimentally induced septic arthritis. Vet Surg 21:367-373, 1992
193. Sweeney CR, Habecker PL: Pulmonary aspergillosis in horses: 29 cases (1974-1997). J Am Vet Med Assoc 214:808-811, 1999
194. Slocombe RF, Slauson DO: Invasive pulmonary aspergillosis of horses: an association with acute enteritis. Vet Pathol 25:277-281, 1988
195. Reilly LK, Palmer JE: Systemic candidiasis in four foals. J Am Vet Med Assoc 205:464-466, 1994
196. Mendoza L, Mandy W, Glass R: An improved *Pythium insidiosum*-vaccine formulation with enhanced immunotherapeutic properties in horses and dogs with pythiosis. Vaccine 21:2797-2804, 2003
197. Leveille R, Hardy J, Robertson JT, et al.: Transarterial coil embolization of the internal and external carotid and maxillary arteries for prevention of hemorrhage from guttural pouch mycosis in horses. Vet Surg 29:389-397, 2000
198. Freeman DE, Ross MW, Donawick WJ, Hamir AN: Occlusion of the external carotid and maxillary arteries in the horse to prevent hemorrhage from guttural pouch mycosis. Vet Surg 18:39-47, 1989
199. Andes D: Clinical utility of antifungal pharmacokinetics and pharmacodynamics. Curr Opin Infect Dis 17:533-540, 2004
200. Andes D, Stamsted T, Conklin R: Pharmacodynamics of amphotericin B in a neutropenic-mouse disseminated-candidiasis model. Antimicrob Agents Chemother 45:922-926, 2001
201. Andes D, van Ogtrop M: In vivo characterization of the pharmacodynamics of flucytosine in a neutropenic murine disseminated candidiasis model. Antimicrob Agents Chemother 44:938-942, 2000
202. Giguère S: Antifungal chemotherapy, in Giguère S, Prescott JF, Baggot JD, Walker RD, Dowling PM (eds): Antimicrobial Therapy in Veterinary Medicine. Ames, IA, Blackwell, 2006, pp 301-322
203. Chaffin MK, Schumacher J, McMullan WC: Cutaneous pythiosis in the horse. Vet Clin North Am Equine Pract 11:91-103, 1995
204. Madison JB, Reid BV, Raskin RE: Amphotericin B treatment of Candida arthritis in two horses. J Am Vet Med Assoc 206:338-341, 1995
205. Zamos DT, Schumacher J, Loy JK: Nasopharyngeal conidiobolomycosis in a horse. J Am Vet Med Assoc 208:100-101, 1996
206. Cornick JL: Diagnosis and treatment of pulmonary histoplasmosis in a horse. Cornell Vet 80:97-103, 1990
207. Ziemer EL, Pappagianis D, Madigan JE, Mansmann RA, Hoffman KD: Coccidioidomycosis in horses: 15 cases (1975-1984). J Am Vet Med Assoc 201:910-916, 1992
208. Begg LM, Hughes KJ, Kessell A, Krockenberger MB, Wigney DI, Malik R: Successful treatment of cryptococcal pneumonia in a pony mare. Aust Vet J 82:686-692, 2004
209. Brooks DE, Andrew SE, Dillavou CL, Ellis G, Kubilis PS: Antimicrobial susceptibility patterns of fungi isolated from horses with ulcerative keratomycosis. Am J Vet Res 59:138-142, 1998
210. Prades M, Brown MP, Gronwall R, Houston AE: Body fluid and endometrial concentrations of ketoconazole in mares after intravenous injection or repeated gavage. Equine Vet J 21:211-214, 1989
211. Latimer FG, Colitz CM, Campbell NB, Papich MG: Pharmacokinetics of fluconazole following intravenous and oral administration and body fluid concentrations of fluconazole following repeated oral dosing in horses. Am J Vet Res 62:1606-1611, 2001
212. Davis JL, Salmon JH, Papich MG: Pharmacokinetics of voriconazole after oral and intravenous administration to horses. Am J Vet Res 67:1070-1075, 2006
213. Clode AB, Davis JL, Salmon J, Michau TM, Gilger BC: Evaluation of concentration of voriconazole in aqueous humor after topical and oral administration in horses. Am J Vet Res 67:296-301, 2006
214. Davis JL, Salmon JH, Papich MG: Pharmacokinetics and tissue distribution of itraconazole after oral and intravenous administration to horses. Am J Vet Res 66:1694-1701, 2005

215. Davis PR, Meyer GA, Hanson RR, Stringfellow JS: *Pseudallescheria boydii* infection of the nasal cavity of a horse. J Am Vet Med Assoc 217:707-709, 2000
216. Worster AA, Lillich JD, Cox JH, Rush BR: Pythiosis with bone lesions in a pregnant mare. J Am Vet Med Assoc 216:1795-1798, 2000
217. Davis EW, Legendre AM: Successful treatment of guttural pouch mycosis with itraconazole and topical enilconazole in a horse. J Vet Intern Med 8:304-305, 1994
218. van Nieuwstadt RA, Kalsbeek HC: Air sac mycosis: topical treatment using enilconazole administered via indwelling catheter. Tijdschr Diergeneeskd 119:3-5, 1994
219. Nappert G, Van Dyck T, Papich M, Chirino-Trejo M: Successful treatment of a fever associated with consistent pulmonary isolation of *Scopulariopsis* sp. in a mare. Equine Vet J 28:421-424, 1996
220. Foley JP, Legendre AM: Treatment of coccidioidomycosis osteomyelitis with itraconazole in a horse. A brief report. J Vet Intern Med 6:333-334, 1992
221. Korenek NL, Legendre AM, Andrews FM, et al.: Treatment of mycotic rhinitis with itraconazole in three horses. J Vet Intern Med 8:224-227, 1994
222. Ball MA, Rebhun WC, Gaarder JE, Patten V: Evaluation of itraconazole-dimethyl sulfoxide ointment for treatment of keratomycosis in nine horses. J Am Vet Med Assoc 211:199-203, 1997
223. Higgins JC, Leith GS, Pappagianis D, Pusterla N: Treatment of *Coccidioides immitis* pneumonia in two horses with fluconazole. Vet Rec 159:349-351, 2006
224. Taintor J, Crowe C, Hancock S, Schumacher J, Livesey L: Treatment of conidiobolomycosis with fluconazole in two pregnant mares. J Vet Intern Med 18:363-364, 2004
225. Guarro J, Aguilar C, Pujol I: In-vitro antifungal susceptibilities of *Basidiobolus* and *Conidiobolus* spp. strains. J Antimicrob Chemother 44:557-560, 1999
226. Yangco BG, Okafor JI, TeStrake D: In vitro susceptibilities of human and wild-type isolates of *Basidiobolus* and *Conidiobolus* species. Antimicrob Agents Chemother 25:413-416, 1984

6.4 Aerosolised antimicrobials

Harold C. McKenzie III

One of the major limitations of systemic antimicrobial therapy for the treatment of lower respiratory infectious disease is the low pulmonary penetration of many antimicrobials, and it has been shown in human patients that the therapeutic outcome of respiratory infections is more closely associated with airway rather than serum antimicrobial concentrations.[1] Aerosol administration of antimicrobials has been demonstrated to achieve high antimicrobial concentrations at the respiratory mucosal surface, while minimising the development of systemic side effects.[2–5] Other potential advantages to delivering medications to the lower respiratory tract by aerosolisation include a decrease in the total dose administered, avoidance of systemic side effects and a rapid onset of action.[6,7] The administration of antimicrobials by aerosolisation does have limitations, however, including potential problems with drug delivery and pulmonary irritation, as well as the expense of the required equipment and the time required for administration.

There is limited mention in the literature of aerosol antimicrobial therapy in foals or adult horses, and concern has been expressed regarding the potential lack of efficacy of this treatment modality.[8,9] There is one report of aerosolised gentamicin used as an adjunct to systemic antimicrobial therapy in a case of bronchopneumonia in a 6-month-old colt.[10] In that report, the addition of aerosol antimicrobial therapy was associated with resolution of mucopurulent nasal discharge within 2 days of initiation of aerosol therapy and normalisation of respiratory sounds after 7 days of aerosol therapy.

While no controlled studies have been performed to assess efficacy of aerosolised antimicrobial therapy in horses, a number of human studies have demonstrated the effectiveness of aerosol antimicrobial administration in preventing the development, or decreasing the severity or duration, of lower respiratory bacterial infections.[2,11–18] Studies in guinea pigs, dogs and calves have demonstrated the effectiveness of aerosolised antimicrobials, as either the primary or an adjunctive therapy in the treatment of bacterial pneumonia.[19–21] The aerosol administration of antimicrobials has been advocated for treatment of lower respiratory infectious disease in adult horses.[22] This treatment modality was reported to have been used in horses with airway infections characterised by the presence of one or more clinical signs of lower respiratory disease but not exhibiting signs of systemic inflammation or involvement of the pulmonary parenchyma. Aerosol administration of gentamicin (2.2 mg/kg once daily) and/or ceftiofur (2.2 mg/kg twice daily) was reported to have been effective in reducing the numbers of bacteria present within the airways and resolving the clinical signs of lower respiratory disease in this subset of equine patients. Parenteral administration of antimicrobials remains the primary treatment for infections with parenchymal and systemic involvement, but aerosol administration of antimicrobials was suggested as an adjunct to parenteral therapy.

The delivery of gentamicin to the lower respiratory tract of adult horses has been compared following intravenous and aerosol administration and with repeated aerosol administration.[3,4] The gentamicin concentrations in the bronchial lavage fluid following aerosol administration were significantly greater than after intravenous administration for at least 8 hours. Because the maximum bronchial lavage fluid gentamicin concentrations after aerosol administration were approximately 12 times greater than those measured following intravenous administration, aerosol administration would appear to achieve sufficiently high airway concentrations of gentamicin to be of clinical benefit.[3] This appears especially true as one study of once-daily (6.6 mg/kg) intravenous gentamicin administration in horses concluded that intravenous gentamicin administration could not be recommended for treatment of airway infections due to the low concentrations achieved within the respiratory secretions.[23] Repeated daily aerosol administration of gentamicin to horses for 7 days was not associated with lower respiratory inflammation, drug accumulation or other adverse effects.[4]

Aerosol theory

The effect of an aerosolised medication is achieved following deposition of the aerosolised particles on the mucosal surface of the respiratory tract. The pattern of deposition of aerosol particles and the efficiency of aerosol delivery are influenced by the characteristics of the aerosol itself, including the size distribution of the aerosol particles and the aerosol density, and these characteristics can vary significantly with different delivery systems and drug formulations.[24,25] The most important characteristic of therapeutic aerosols is the size of the individual particles. The size of the particle determines the degree to which it will be able to penetrate the respiratory tract, as particles of 10-μm diameter or greater are deposited within the nasal passages and nasopharynx, while particles of less than 10 μm diameter are deposited within the lower respiratory tract.[26] Patient-dependent factors are also important in determining aerosol deposition, including both ventilatory parameters and respiratory morphology.[27] The respiratory pattern of the horse has been described as being well suited to inhalation therapy, because the large tidal volume and high flow rate enhance deep pulmonary deposition of aerosols.[28] Deposition of small particles in the lung periphery may also be enhanced by the low respiratory rate of the resting horse, which increases the residence time of particles within the peripheral airways and may enhance deposition due to sedimentation and diffusion.

The presence of pulmonary disease is an important consideration in the administration of therapeutic aerosols, because changes in pulmonary function and mechanics associated with pulmonary disease can impair the delivery of aerosolised medications to the affected region. Inflammation and airway sensitization are commonly associated with pulmonary disease and can cause bronchoconstriction, mucus hypersecretion and mucosal oedema, resulting in variable airway obstruction. Airway obstruction increases particle deposition at the site of obstruction but diverts airflow to nonobstructed airways, resulting in increased delivery of therapeutic particles to the less-affected portions of the lung.[26] The net result is a shift toward more central deposition of drug and decreased peripheral distribution.[29] Administration of an aerosolised bronchodilator to horses with recurrent airway obstruction has been shown to significantly improve pulmonary distribution of a radiolabeled aerosol.[30] Total airway obstruction is generally thought to prevent deposition of aerosol particles in the affected region peripheral to the site of obstruction, and as a result no medication will reach a consolidated region of the lung following aerosol administration.[29] Interestingly, a recent experimental study demonstrated significantly higher antimicrobial concentrations in the consolidated regions of pneumonic lungs following aerosol administration compared to intravenous administration.[31]

Aerosol administration

Aerosol delivery of therapeutic substances presents several challenges. The substance to be delivered must be available in a formulation, liquid or powdered, which can be delivered directly to the respiratory tract as an aerosol, or it must be soluble in a liquid that can be safely aerosolised into the respiratory tract. The therapeutic agent should be nonirritating and nonallergenic and lack local toxicity.[32] The therapeutic substance must be capable of exerting its action on the mucosal surface or of being absorbed into the respiratory mucosa, but if the therapeutic substance has the potential for systemic toxicity, it should be poorly absorbed.[32] The delivery method must be capable of producing particles that are of an appropriate size to deliver the medication to the desired portion of the respiratory tract, and the delivery method should be able to deliver the total dose in a reasonable period of time with reasonable efficiency.

Devices

The generation of therapeutic aerosols is accomplished using several different inhalation drug delivery systems. None of these systems, however, is capable of delivering aerosolised medication with high efficiency, with less than 10% of the original dose being deposited in the lower respiratory tract regardless of delivery system.[33] Antimicrobial aerosols are generated from liquids by nebulisers, either ultrasonic or compressed-gas driven (jet). Nebulisation is considered to be the optimal method of administration when the dose to be delivered exceeds 200 μg[34] and does not require coordination of administration and inhalation, depending only on normal tidal breathing.[25] Nebulisers must be used with a facemask in the conscious animal patient, with attendant aerosol wastage on the face and facemask and in the nasal passages and nasopharynx.[35] Snug-fitting valved facemasks are commercially available for the administration of aerosols to adult horses and foals.* Nebulisers are attached to the facemask using plastic aerosol tubing.

Jet nebulisers are more widely used than ultrasonic nebulisers in human medicine, because they are inexpensive and relatively easy to use. Jet nebulisers are usually limited to reservoir volumes of 3 to 6 ml, however, and the time required to aerosolise this volume of fluid is anywhere from 10 to 15 minutes.[36] This means that the time required to deliver a single dose (10–20 ml) may become excessive with adult horses. Ultrasonic nebulisers are generally capable of producing more aerosol per unit time than jet nebulizers, resulting in shorter treatment times and greater

* Equine Aeromask; Canadian Monaghan Ltd., London, Ontario, Canada.

ease of use.[37] Larger fill volumes (up to 30 ml or more) also allow convenient administration of larger doses. These devices are expensive and fragile, however, limiting their clinical application outside of referral institutions.[35]

Drug formulations for nebulisation

The formulation of a therapeutic nebulisation solution can have a major impact on the aerosol produced and on the patient response to aerosol administration. The concentration of solute is of major importance, because increased solute concentrations result in decreases in aerosol output and in particle size.[38] A recent study of antimicrobial aerosol generation from medical nebulisers determined that the antimicrobial concentration in a nebulisation solution, regardless of the specific antimicrobial, should ideally be 100 mg/ml or less, in a saline solution of 0.23% to 0.45% concentration.[38] Lower antimicrobial concentrations were recommended for ultrasonic nebulisers, with an ideal concentration of approximately 50 mg/ml.[38] The ideal nebulisation solution would also be isotonic and have a neutral pH, to minimize the development of coughing and/or bronchoconstriction.[39] A study that characterised the aerosols produced by an ultrasonic nebuliser using antimicrobial solutions appropriate for therapy of equine lower respiratory bacterial infections found that solutions containing 50 mg/ml gentamicin or 25 mg/ml of ceftiofur yielded the optimal combinations of particle size and aerosol density.[39]

Limitations

There a number of limitations associated with aerosolised antimicrobial administration.[40] Most importantly, severe bacterial infections of the respiratory tract often have a systemic component and therefore require systemic antimicrobial therapy. Also, due to concerns regarding the ability of aerosol administration to deliver adequate amounts of medication to poorly ventilated areas of the lung, the administration of antimicrobials by inhalation alone is not appropriate in cases with substantial consolidation or parenchymal involvement. There is an increasing body of evidence, however, that systemic antimicrobial therapy may be effectively augmented by the concurrent administration of antimicrobials by the inhaled route.

There are several reports of altered pulmonary mechanics in human patients following aerosol administration of antimicrobials, primarily as the result of bronchoconstriction resulting from irritation induced by the antimicrobial compound, the preservatives or carriers present within the solution or the tonicity of the solution itself.[38,41] While the repeated administration of gentamicin aerosol to horses was not associated with any evidence of bronchoconstriction or a pulmonary inflammatory response, pretreatment with an aerosolised β_2-agonist bronchodilator may attenuate any coughing and bronchoconstriction that may be induced by aerosolised antimicrobials.[4,42]

References

1. Valcke Y, Pauwels R, Van der Straeten M: Pharmacokinetics of antibiotics in the lungs. Eur Respir J 3:715-722, 1990
2. Palmer LB, Smaldone GC, Simon SR, et al.: Aerosolized antibiotics in mechanically ventilated patients: delivery and response. Crit Care Med 26:31-39, 1998
3. McKenzie HC 3rd, Murray MJ: Concentrations of gentamicin in serum and bronchial lavage fluid after intravenous and aerosol administration of gentamicin to horses. Am J Vet Res 61:1185-1190, 2000
4. McKenzie HC 3rd, Murray MJ: Concentrations of gentamicin in serum and bronchial lavage fluid after once-daily aerosol administration to horses for seven days. Am J Vet Res 65:173-178, 2004
5. Tonnellier M, Ferrari F, Goldstein I, et al.: Intravenous versus nebulized ceftazidime in ventilated piglets with and without experimental bronchopneumonia: comparative effects of helium and nitrogen. Anesthesiology 102:995-1000, 2005
6. Duvivier DH, Votion D, Vandenput S, et al.: Aerosol therapy in the equine species. Vet J 154:189-202, 1997
7. Lipworth BJ: Pharmacokinetics of inhaled drugs. Br J Clin Pharmacol 42:697-705, 1996
8. Beech J: Therapeutic strategies involving antimicrobial treatment of the lower respiratory tract in large animals. J Am Vet Med Assoc 185:1199-1202, 1984
9. Clarke AF: Practicalities of nebulisation. Equine Vet Educ 3:45-49, 1991
10. Rhodes CH, Genetzky RM: Nebulization therapy in the foal. Iowa State Univ Vet 44:104-108, 1982
11. Burns JL, Van Dalfsen JM, Shawar RM, et al.: Effect of chronic intermittent administration of inhaled tobramycin on respiratory microbial flora in patients with cystic fibrosis. J Infect Dis 179:1190-1196, 1999
12. Hamer DH: Treatment of nosocomial pneumonia and tracheobronchitis caused by multidrug-resistant *Pseudomonas aeruginosa* with aerosolized colistin. Am J Respir Crit Care Med 162:328-330, 2000
13. Lin HC, Cheng HF, Wang CH, et al.: Inhaled gentamicin reduces airway neutrophil activity and mucus secretion in bronchiectasis. Am J Respir Crit Care Med 155:2024-2029, 1997
14. MacLeod DL, Nelson LE, Shawar RM, et al.: Aminoglycoside-resistance mechanisms for cystic fibrosis *Pseudomonas aeruginosa* isolates are unchanged by long-term, intermittent, inhaled tobramycin treatment. J Infect Dis 181:1180-1184, 2000
15. Wiesemann HG, Steinkamp G, Ratjen F, et al.: Placebo-controlled, double-blind, randomized study of aerosolized tobramycin for early treatment of *Pseudomonas aeruginosa* colonization in cystic fibrosis. Pediatr Pulmonol 25:88-92, 1998
16. Drobnic ME, Sune P, Montoro JB, et al.: Inhaled tobramycin in non-cystic fibrosis patients with bronchiectasis and chronic bronchial infection with *Pseudomonas aeruginosa*. Ann Pharmacother 39:39-44, 2005
17. Klepser ME: Role of nebulized antibiotics for the treatment of respiratory infections. Curr Opin Infect Dis 17:109-112, 2004
18. Hodson ME, Gallagher CG, Govan JR: A randomised clinical trial of nebulised tobramycin or colistin in cystic fibrosis. Eur Respir J 20:658-664, 2002

19. Bemis DA, Appel MJG: Aerosol, parenteral, and oral antibiotic treatment of Bordetella bronchiseptica infections in dogs. J Am Vet Med Assoc 170:1082-1086, 1977
20. Makhoul IR, Merzbach D, Lichtig C, et al.: Antibiotic treatment of experimental *Pseudomonas aeruginosa* pneumonia in guinea pigs: comparison of aerosol and systemic administration. J Infect Dis 168:1296-1299, 1993
21. Vermeersch H, Vandenbossche G, Remon JP, et al.: Pharmacokinetics of nebulized sodium ceftiofur in calves. J Vet Pharmacol Ther 19:152-154, 1996
22. Murray MJ: New diagnostic techniques and treatment for lower respiratory disease. Proc 15th Forum Am Coll Vet Intern Med 380-382, 1997
23. Godber LM, Walker RD, Stein GE, et al.: Pharmacokinetics, nephrotoxicosis, and in vitro antibacterial activity associated with single versus multiple (three times) daily gentamicin treatments in horses. Am J Vet Res 56:613-618, 1995
24. Brain JD, Valberg PA: Deposition of aerosol in the respiratory tract. Am Rev Respir Dis 120:1325-1373, 1979
25. Hardy JG, Newman SP, Knoch M: Lung deposition from four nebulizers. Respir Med 87:461-465, 1993
26. Brain JD, Blanchard JD: Mechanisms of particle deposition and clearance, in Moren F, Dolovich MB, Newhouse MT, et al. (eds): Aerosols in Medicine: Principles, Diagnosis and Therapy. London, Elsevier Science, 1993, pp 117-156
27. Martonen T, Yang Y: Deposition mechanics of pharmaceutical particles in human airways, in Hickey AJ (ed): Inhalation Aerosols: Physical and Biological Basis for Therapy. New York, Marcel Dekker, 1996, pp 57-68
28. Rush BR: Aerosolized drug delivery devices, in Robinson NE (ed): Current Therapy in Equine Medicine, ed 5. St Louis, WB Saunders, 2003, pp 436-440
29. Hiller FC: Therapeutic aerosols: an overview from a clinical perspective, in Hickey AJ (ed): Pharmaceutical Inhalation Aerosol Technology. New York, Marcel Dekker, 1992, pp 289-306
30. Rush BR, Hoskinson JJ, Davis EG, et al.: Pulmonary distribution of aerosolized technetium Tc 99m pentetate after administration of a single dose of aerosolized albuterol sulfate in horses with recurrent airway obstruction. Am J Vet Res 60:764-769, 1999
31. Elman M, Goldstein I, Marquette CH, et al.: Influence of lung aeration on pulmonary concentrations of nebulized and intravenous amikacin in ventilated piglets with severe bronchopneumonia. Anesthesiology 97:199-206, 2002
32. Gough PA, Jordan NS: A review of the therapeutic efficacy of aerosolized and endotracheally instilled antibiotics. Pharmacotherapy 2:367-377, 1982
33. Smith SJ, Bernstein JA: Therapeutic uses of lung aerosols, in Hickey AJ (ed): Inhalation Aerosols: Physical and Biological Basis for Therapy. New York, Marcel Dekker, 1996, pp 233-269
34. Atkins PJ, Barker NP, Mathisen D: The design and development of inhalation drug delivery systems, in Hickey AJ (ed): Inhalation Aerosols: Physical and Biological Basis for Therapy. New York, Marcel Dekker, 1996, pp 155-185
35. Votion D, Ghafir Y, Munsters K, et al.: Aerosol deposition in equine lungs following ultrasonic nebulisation versus jet aerosol delivery system. Equine Vet J 29:388-393, 1997
36. Hickey A: Pharmaceutical Inhalation Aerosol Technology. New York, Marcel Dekker, 1992, p 365
37. Faurisson F, Dessanges JF, Grimfeld A, et al.: Nebulizer performance: AFLM study. Respiration 62(Suppl 1):13-18, 1995
38. Weber A, Morlin G, Cohen M, et al.: Effect of nebulizer type and antibiotic concentration on device performance. Pediatr Pulmonol 23:249-260, 1997
39. McKenzie HC: Characterization of antimicrobial aerosols for administration to horses. Vet Ther 4:110-119, 2003
40. O'Riordan T, Faris M: Inhaled antimicrobial therapy. Respir Care Clin N Am 5:617-631, 1999
41. Chua HL, Collis GG, Le Souef PN: Bronchial response to nebulized antibiotics in children with cystic fibrosis. Eur Respir J 3:1114-1116, 1990
42. Harrison KS, Laube BL: Bronchodilator pretreatment improves aerosol deposition uniformity in HIV-positive patients who cough while inhaling aerosolized pentamidine. Chest 106:421-426, 1994

6.5 Fluid therapy

Kevin Corley

Fluid therapy is a relatively simple treatment, which is highly likely to make a significant impact on outcome of many severely ill horses. There are relatively few pitfalls, and, for the most part, these are easily avoided. The keys to successful fluid therapy are given in Box 6.1.

Recognising the need for fluid therapy

Some horses have obvious large fluid losses, such as those with high volume reflux or diarrhoea. However, fluid losses may be insidious or internal, and therefore may not be immediately apparent. It is extremely important to recognise hypovolaemia, because it requires immediate treatment with large volumes of fluid. It is my experience that many clinicians do not administer adequate fluids acutely to hypovolaemic horses, and in many cases it is because they underestimate the severity of the fluid deficits. This is particularly true in the treatment of neonatal foals, which can be markedly hypovolaemic, with minimal clinical signs.

Clinical Signs of hypovolaemia and dehydration

Even though they may coexist in the same horse, hypovolaemia and dehydration are important to distinguish,

Box 6.1. Approach to fluid therapy in the horse

1. Recognise the need for fluid therapy.
2. Select the appropriate route of administration.
3. Select an appropriate fluid delivery system.
4. Select appropriate fluid type to administer.
5. Rapid reversal of hypovolaemia.
6. Match fluid amounts to needs after hypovolaemia reversal.
7. Careful correction of electrolyte imbalances, if present.

because their therapy is different. Hypovolaemia requires emergency intravenous treatment to rapidly restore circulating volume. There is considerable evidence linking markers of hypovolaemia on hospital admission with morbidity and decreased survival in equine colic[1,2] and neonatal foals.[3,4] Dehydration may be treated over a more prolonged period and may be corrected with intravenous, nasogastric or, occasionally, free-choice oral fluid therapy.

Hypovolaemia is defined as a decrease in circulating blood volume. The classic example of hypovolaemia is acute arterial haemorrhage, in which the circulating volume is decreased without a change in the remainder of the extracellular fluid volume. *Dehydration* is defined as a loss of interstitial fluid without a change in the circulating volume. The classic example is moderate sweating during exercise or high ambient temperatures. There are powerful physiological mechanisms protecting the circulating volume during dehydration at the expense of extravascular fluid, and it is only with severe dehydration that animals will also become hypovolaemic. Clinical signs of hypovolaemia and dehydration in the adult horse are given in Box 6.2.

Box 6.2. Clinical signs of hypovolaemia and dehydration in the horse

Hypovolaemia
- Tachycardia
- Decreased pulse pressure
- Reduced jugular fill
- Tachypnoea
- Cold extremities
- Decreased urine output

Dehydration
- Tacky mucous membranes
- Prolonged skin tent
- Sunken eyes

Neonatal foals appear to compensate poorly for hypovolaemia, which makes the consequences not only more severe than in mature horses but also harder to identify. For example, approximately 40% of neonatal foals do not increase their heart rate in response to hypovolaemia.[5] Therefore, foals can be severely hypovolaemic and demonstrate only few or mild clinical signs or even none at all. When clinical signs are present, they are similar to those in adult horses (Box 6.2). If any of these signs is present, hypovolaemia should be strongly suspected. Historical information is also extremely important, and given much more weight than in the adult horse. Neonatal foals (<7 days old) are likely to be hypovolaemic if they have not nursed within the last 4 to 6 hours and may be dehydrated if they have not nursed within the previous 3 hours.

Laboratory signs of hypovolaemia and dehydration

The results of laboratory tests that suggest hypovolaemia or dehydration are given in Tables 6.11 and 6.12.

Packed cell volume and total solids

Packed cell volume (PCV) and plasma total solids are commonly used to assess the circulating volume. Unfortunately, neither test is sensitive or specific. Splenic contraction, in response to stress or exercise, can markedly change the PCV in the horse, making small increases very hard to interpret. Splenic contraction may, in fact, be partially responsible for the very high PCV seen in horses with marked hypovolaemia, such as in severe colitis. Nonexercising horses with a PCV of over 50% are almost always hypovolaemic. Plasma total solids (protein measured by refractometer) or total protein (measured by a chemistry analyzer) concentration also increases with hypovolaemia. However, significant protein loss can occur in gastrointestinal disease (particularly with colitis) resulting in a low or normal protein concentration despite hypovolaemia. Protein loss can also occur with nephropathy, although this is much less common in the horse. Further, hypergammaglobulinaemia (e.g., in cyathostomiasis) can increase the plasma total protein concentration without the presence of

Table 6.11. Laboratory signs of hypovolaemia in the horse (clinical decisions should be based on history, clinical signs, and laboratory data, and certainly not on a single laboratory value in isolation)

Hypovolaemia	Value above which hypovolaemia should be suspected (adults)	Normal range (adults)	Value above which hypovolaemia should be suspected (foals)	Normal range (foals)
Lactate (blood or plasma)	>2.0 mmol/L	0.2–0.7 mmol/L	>2.5 mmol/L	2.38 ± 1.03 mmol/L (2 hours old) 1.24 ± 0.33 mmol/L (24 hours old) 1.08 ± 0.27 mmol/L (48 hours old)
Packed cell volume (blood)	>45%	32–42%	>44%*	28–44%
Total solids (plasma)	>75 g/L (7.5 g/dl)	52–72 g/L (5.2–7.2 g/dl)	>80 g/L (8.0 g/dl)	42–78 g/L (4.2–7.8 g/dl)
Creatinine (blood or plasma)	>160 μmol/L (1.8 mg/dl)	80–160 μmol/L (0.9–1.8 mg/dl)	>180 μmol/L (2.0 mg/dl)†	70–180 μmol/L (0.8–2.0 mg/dl)†

*Increased packed cell volume is not common in foals with hypovolaemia.
†Can be very high in newborn foals (<48 hr old) due to *in utero* placental dysfunction, with no hypovolaemia.

Table 6.12. Laboratory signs of dehydration in the horse (clinical decisions should be based on history, clinical signs, and laboratory data, and certainly not on a single laboratory value in isolation)

Dehydration	Value above which dehydration should be suspected (adults)	Normal range (adults)	Value above which dehydration should be suspected (foals)	Normal range (foals)
↑ **Specific Gravity** (urine)	>1.035	1.021–1.035	>1.012	1.008–1.012 (<48 hours old) 1.000–1.008 (>48 hours old)

hypovolaemia. The PCV and plasma total solids are most useful when greatly increased or when used serially to monitor the response to fluid therapy.

Creatinine concentration

Plasma or serum creatinine concentrations are useful to assess hydration status in the absence of renal dysfunction. High normal (130–160 μmol/L; 1.5–1.8 mg/dl) creatinine concentrations can be associated with subclinical hypovolaemia and should be evaluated in light of the history and clinical signs. Creatinine concentrations up to 310 μmol/L (3.5 mg/dl) are common with moderate to severe hypovolaemia, and concentrations as high as 450 μmol/L (5.0 mg/dl) are possible with prolonged hypovolaemia. Even with marked hypovolaemia, the creatinine concentration will not increase by much more than 200 μmol/L (2.3 mg/dl) per day.[6] If the creatinine concentration does not decrease appropriately with fluid therapy, renal dysfunction should be suspected.

In newborn foals, creatinine concentrations reflect placental function and very high concentrations (up to 2200 μmol/L; 25 mg/dl) are possible without either hypovolaemia or renal dysfunction. If placental insufficiency is the cause of the high creatinine concentration, it will decrease rapidly over the first 24 hours of life, and will often have returned to the normal range by 36 to 48 hours of life.[7]

Lactate concentration

Increased blood lactate concentrations (Table 6.11) in the nonexercising horse are sufficient evidence of a metabolic disturbance to initiate fluid therapy. The major cause of increased blood lactate concentrations in the horse is inadequate tissue perfusion, due to hypovolaemia. Endotoxaemia and sepsis can also increase tissue lactate production by inappropriate anaerobic metabolism, despite adequate circulation. Increased blood lactate concentration was associated with worse outcomes in equine colic[2] and referred neonatal foals.[4] Lactate can be measured in the field by hand-held blood gas analysers* or hand-held lactate meters†. The expected lactate concentration can also be calculated by means of equations based on electrolyte and acid-base measurements, although these are not as accurate as direct measurement.[4] An increased circulating lactate should be suspected in a metabolic acidosis (decreased pH, negative base excess) in the absence of hyperchloraemia or hyponatraemia.[8]

* i-STAT; Heska, Fort Collins, CO, USA.

† Accutrend Lactate System; Roche Diagnostics, Basel, Switzerland.

Urine specific gravity

Urine specific gravity is measured with a refractometer and is a useful marker to monitor dehydration. Although urine specific gravity also increases with hypovolaemia, it is often hard to obtain a urine sample, because urine production can be markedly decreased. High urine specific gravities (Table 6.12) indicate probable dehydration and normal renal concentration of urine. Isothenuria (1.008–1.012), after the first 2 days of life, indicates possible renal damage or a recent high fluid load. Urine specific gravity is most useful to monitor the response to fluid therapy because rising or continually high specific gravities in the face of fluid therapy may indicate insufficient fluid is being delivered to the horse.

Neonatal foals normally have very dilute urine (Table 6.12) (Scott, Stoneham and Corley, unpublished data, 2005). Critically ill neonatal foals may also show inappropriately high urine specific gravity for their hydration status. These foals most often respond well to a frusemide (furosemide) continuous rate infusion (0.5–4.2 μg/kg/min). However, because of the propensity of this treatment to worsen hypovolaemia and dehydration, it is vital to be certain that the foal has received adequate fluid therapy before starting the infusion. The infusion can also cause chloride and potassium loss, and this author always monitors these electrolytes and starts a concurrent potassium chloride infusion (not to exceed 0.5 mmol/kg/hr of potassium (taking into account potassium in all fluids being administered)).

Selecting route of administration for fluids

The first decision, once the need for fluid therapy has been established, is the route of administration. When there are signs of hypovolaemia, the only effective route is intravenous. For dehydrated horses, there are really only three viable routes: oral (free choice), intragastric and intravenous. Attempts to use other routes, such as indwelling caecal catheters, have been beset by complications and cannot be recommended.[9]

Table 6.13. Recipes for oral and nasogastric fluids

Solution	Amount of salt per litre (grams)	Approximate amount of salt granules per litre (ml)	Amount of low sodium salt per litre (grams)	Approximate amount of low sodium salt per litre (ml)	Amount of sodium bicarbonate powder per litre (grams)	Approximate amount of sodium bicarbonate powder per litre (ml)
Isotonic sodium-potassium-chloride	0.45	3.75	0.45	3.75	—	—
Slightly hypotonic sodium-potassium-chloride	0.4	3.33	0.4	3.33	—	—
Isotonic sodium chloride	0.9	7.5	—	—	—	—
Slightly hypotonic sodium chloride	0.8	6.6	—	—	—	—
Isotonic sodium bicarbonate	—	—	—	—	12	12
Slightly hypotonic sodium bicarbonate	—	—	—	—	10	10

The approximate amount is given in ml so that the salt can be measured in a syringe barrel, rather than on a weigh scale. Readers should check that the volume in ml given matches the weight for the preparation of sodium chloride or sodium bicarbonate that they are using.

Enteral fluid therapy

Free choice water

Free choice water is the simplest way to provide fluid therapy. It can be effective in replacing mild deficits and in providing fluids for maintenance. Clearly, free choice fluid intake is dependent on the willingness and ability of the patient to imbibe and absorb sufficient fluids. In hypovolaemia, blood is diverted away from the gastrointestinal tract to vital organs such as the heart, brain and muscles. This severely limits the ability to absorb fluids from the intestine. Furthermore, the thirst reaction is often blunted or absent in moderately to severely ill horses. For these reasons, free choice intake can rarely be relied upon to provide sufficient fluid intake during the early stages of hospital care. In horses with continued moderate fluid loss, such as mild to moderate diarrhoea, free choice fluids can be a useful source or adjunct source of fluids. Electrolytes can also be replaced in this way, and some horses will preferentially drink from water buckets containing electrolytes than from those containing plain water. When making water buckets containing electrolytes, it is extremely important not to make the fluids more concentrated than isotonic. Slightly hypotonic fluids are generally more palatable than isotonic fluids. Possible recipes for making free choice or intragastric electrolyte replacement fluids are given in Table 6.13.

Intragastric fluid administration

Intragastric fluid administration, using a nasogastric tube, is an extremely effective way of ensuring adequate fluid intake, when the gastrointestinal tract is able to absorb fluids. It can also be used to hydrate the gastrointestinal contents, as a very effective method of treating primary large-colon impactions. As outlined earlier, hypovolaemia may prevent effective gastrointestinal absorption of fluids, and therefore this route should be avoided in moderately to severely hypovolaemic animals.

Delivery of nasogastric fluids

Nasogastric administration of fluids is achieved through a soft plastic tube, passed along the ventral meatus of the nose, through the nasopharynx and into the oesophagus (see Chapter 1.7). It is important to ascertain that the tube is in the correct position prior to putting any fluid through it. This can be achieved most easily by palpation at the left base of the neck (deep to the jugular furrow), where the tube can be felt as a hard round object within the oesophagus, on the side of the trachea. Repeated administration of nasogastric fluids can be delivered through an indwelling tube. The tube should be plugged with a syringe barrel between administrations to prevent excessive air influx. Continuous enteral fluid therapy can be provided with an enteral feeding tube* connected to a coiled administration set designed for intravenous fluid therapy[10] (Figures 6.2 and 6.3). Tubes and delivery systems used for nasogastric administration of fluids need to be clean but not sterile. However, they should be sterilised after use on a horse with a known or suspected infectious agent, including those with anterior enteritis.

Types of fluid for enteral fluid therapy

It is possible to treat moderately dehydrated horses effectively with enteral replacement solutions.[11,12] Nasogastric fluids do not need to be sterile and can be made up on the farm and are therefore considerably cheaper and easier to transport than intravenous fluids. It is apparently not necessary to add glucose to enteral fluids for horses but, if

* 18 Fr, 100-inch nasogastric feeding tube; MILA International Inc., Florence, KY, USA.

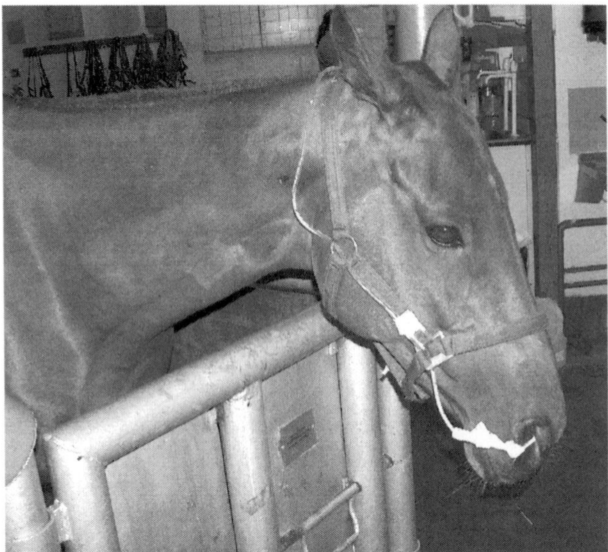

Figure 6.2 An indwelling narrow nasogastric tube placed in a polo pony for constant delivery of intragastric fluids. ©Kevin Corley 2002.

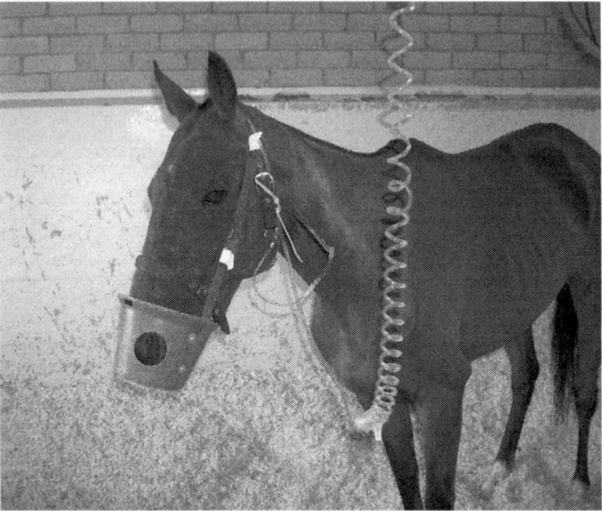

Figure 6.3 The indwelling nasogastric tube shown in Figure 6.2 has been connected to a resterilised intravenous fluid delivery set. Nonsterile fluids are placed in the bags, and a constant rate of intragastric fluids is delivered. ©Kevin Corley 2002.

feasible, electrolytes should be added. Isotonic or hypotonic fluids should be administered.[13]

Oral fluids can be a successful alternative or adjunct to intravenous fluids in many mildly dehydrated horses with large colon impactions.[14,15] Unfortunately, enteral fluids are insufficient for moderately to severely dehydrated horses. Rapid administration of a glucose- and glycine-containing electrolyte solution (8 L/30 min) resulted in incomplete fluid absorption in horses with castor oil–induced diarrhoea.[16] The enteral rehydration solutions available commercially may not be ideal for fluid replacement in horses.[16] Further research is necessary to refine enteral fluid therapy for horses.

The administration of plain water is of minimal benefit to restore plasma volume in horses exercised in hot and humid conditions.[17] However, the administration of an oral rehydration solution or an electrolyte paste together with provision of fresh drinking water may be sufficient to supplement water and electrolytes following vigorous or prolonged exercise in dehydrated horses.[17,18]

Composition, recipes and amounts to give

(see Table 6.13)

A possible isotonic solution consists of 4.9 g/L table salt and 4.9 g/L Lite salt† (potassium chloride and sodium chloride, sold in supermarkets for people on sodium-restrictive diets) to produce final concentrations of 123 mmol/L sodium, 34 mmol/L potassium and 157 mmol/L chloride.[13] This is approximately equal to 15 ml of table salt and 15 ml of Lite salt per 4 L of water. If using sodium chloride alone, no more than 9 g (approximately half a tablespoon or 7.5 ml) should be added per litre. A measured quantity of these fluids should be given via a nasogastric tube. The amount administered at any one time should not exceed 6 to 8-L for a 500-kg horse, with at least 30 minutes allowed to elapse between each administration. Before each dose, the stomach should be refluxed and the administration delayed if more than 2 L of fluid are recovered. Repeated doses of nasogastric fluids overrun the capacity of the small intestine to absorb these fluids. This limits the quantity of ongoing fluid loss that can be replaced with nasogastric fluids (e.g., in colitis) Conversely, however, it provides a method for hydrating colonic material in large colon impactions. The author uses 5 to 6 L of isotonic fluid by nasogastric tube for a 500-kg horse with a primary pelvic flexure impaction, given at 30-minute intervals for 5 times. Some horses will show signs of abdominal pain when large doses of nasogastric fluids are administered, especially if the fluids are cold.

Continuous nasogastric fluids with an indwelling tube have the advantage that they are much less likely to induce abdominal pain. The maximum rate administered should be 20 ml/kg/hr. Often, the narrow bore of the feeding tube and giving set will limit the fluid rate to considerably lower than this, in the region of 5 to 6 L/hr in a 500-kg horse.

For both intermittent and continuous enteral fluids, the rate given is decided based on degree of dehydration, maintenance requirements and ongoing losses (see later).

Intravenous fluid therapy

Intravenous fluid administration is the only suitable route for horses with moderate to severe hypovolaemia. This allows rapid restoration of circulating volume, and therefore return of oxygen delivery to the tissues. Intravenous

† Morton Salt, Chicago, IL, USA.

Table 6.14. Flow rate chart: Drops per second for various flow rates

Bag size/flow time	Flow rate (litres/hr)	STAT Set* (drops/sec)	Straight set, single spike† (drops/sec)	Coil set, single spike‡ (drops/sec)	Six spike set§ (drops/sec)	10 Solution set** (drops/sec)	Mini (60) set** (drops/sec)
5 L/1 hr	5	15	—	—	—	13.8	—
5 L/1.5 hr	3.33	10	—	—	—	9.2	—
5 L/2 hr	2.5	7.5	—	—	—	6.9	—
5 L/3 hr	1.66	5	3.2	—	—	4.6	—
5 L/4 hr	1.25	3.8	2.3	2.5	—	3.5	—
5 L/5 hr	1	3	2.1	2.4	2.9	2.8	—
1 L/1 hr	1	3	2.1	2.4	2.9	2.8	16.7
1 L/1.5 hr	0.75	—	1.5	1.7	2.1	2.1	12.5
1 L/2 hr	0.5	—	1.1	1.1	1.3	1.4	8.3
1 L/3 hr	0.33	—	0.9	0.8	1.2	0.9	5.5
1 L/4 hr	0.25	—	0.7	0.7	1.1	0.7	4.2
1 L/5 hr	0.2	—	0.6	0.5	1.0	—	3.3
1 L/6 hr	0.16	—	0.4	0.4	0.5	—	2.8

*Stat Large Animal IV Set; International WIN, Kennett Square, PA, USA.
†V-LACT-24-200-S-C-EC1; Cook Veterinary Products, Spencer, IN, USA.
‡V-LACT-24-450-S-C-EC2; Cook Veterinary Products, Spencer, IN, USA.
§V-LACT-14-60-6S-C-EA3; Cook Veterinary Products, Spencer, IN, USA.
**Baxter Healthcare Corp; Deerfield, IL, USA.
Adapted from: Corley KTT. Fluid therapy for horses with gastrointestinal diseases. In Smith BP (ed): Large Animal Internal Medicine, ed 3. St. Louis, Mosby, 2002. Used with permission.

fluid therapy is also necessary when the enteral route is unavailable. The classic example is a horse that has gastrointestinal ileus and nasogastric reflux after colic surgery. Other examples include any cause of ileus (botulism, grass sickness, etc., in horses and sepsis and perinatal asphyxia syndrome in foals) and lesions of the oesophagus or stomach that prevent oral fluid delivery or gastric emptying.

Intravenous delivery systems

Delivery of intravenous fluids usually requires placement of a catheter (see Chapters 1.14, 1.15 and 2.6). The exception is in neonatal foals, where 1 to 2 L of fluid can be delivered via a 16-gauge needle, prior to referral.

The choice of catheter and administration set depends on the clinical status of the horse. Large-gauge catheters are essential for rapid reversal of moderate to severe hypovolaemia but have the disadvantage of being more thrombogenic. A 10- or 12-gauge catheter is recommended for severely hypovolaemic adult horses, and a 12- or 14-gauge catheter for moderately hypovolaemic horses. Large-bore short extension sets‡ should be used for 10- and 12-gauge catheters. Sixteen-gauge catheters are sufficient for neonatal foals and moderately hypovolaemic weanlings and Miniature horses. For administration of parenteral nutrition (PN), double-lumen catheters can provide a dedicated line for the PN and avoid the need to interrupt the PN when administering incompatible drugs.

A variety of fluid administration sets are available commercially. Sets that include large-bore tubing and a coil§ are suitable for most situations in adult horses and are recommended. Coils** can also be helpful in neonatal foals, but wide-bore tubing is unnecessary. The flow rate can be estimated by counting the number of drops per second in the drip chamber (Table 6.14) or can be set by using an electronic infusion pump. In all situations, a record should be kept of the time the infusion was started and the desired infusion rate to ensure that the correct volume is being delivered in the appropriate time.

Intravenous fluid types

General principles: Resuscitation, rehydration and maintenance

Hypovolaemia

Hypovolaemia is treated with rapid volume expanders, such as large-volume intravenous crystalloids, colloids or hypertonic saline. Studies in pediatric and adult human sepsis have shown dramatic improvements in outcome with early restoration of volume.[19,20] The author's recom-

‡ET3002 Large animal 7-inch extension set; International WIN Ltd, Kennett Square, PA, USA.

§IV8001S, Coiled Primary I.V. Set; International WIN Ltd, Kennett Square, PA, USA.
**International WIN, Kennett Square, PA, USA.

mendations for fluids and volumes for hypovolaemia are given in the section on rapid reversal of hypovolaemia. However, it should be noted that fluid type used remains a controversial area in both human medicine, where studies have been conflicting or equivocal,[21–30] and in the horse, where there is very little primary evidence from clinical cases.[31]

Dehydration

For treatment of dehydration, fluids that restore the interstitial fluid are required. Crystalloid fluids are ideal for this purpose, as 70% of isotonic intravenous fluids leave the circulation with 30 minutes of infusion.[32] Resuscitation formula polyionic crystalloids are often the most suitable fluids for rehydration, providing that there are no gross electrolyte or acid-base imbalances after reversal of hypovolaemia. Treatment of these disturbances is covered in a later section. The aim of treatment in all cases is to rehydrate the horse completely over 12 to 24 hours.

Maintenance

All horses have a daily fluid requirement to replace losses from metabolic processes, sweat, urination, defaecation, evaporation from the respiratory tract and any lost salivation or lacrimation. The electrolyte losses in these processes are not in proportion to either the fluid content, or the electrolyte composition of plasma. For example, urine is relatively high in potassium and low in sodium and chloride, relative to plasma. Normally this requirement is met by a combination of drinking and the water and electrolyte content of feed. If a horse is deprived of feed, it will normally drink more to match these losses. In horses with reduced water intake, the maintenance requirement must be met by administered nasogastric or intravenous fluids.

Because the electrolyte loss is not in proportion to the concentration in plasma, it follows that fluids used for maintenance therapy should not necessarily have the same proportion of electrolytes as plasma. There are specifically manufactured maintenance fluids available for the human market, which have lower sodium and chloride and higher potassium concentrations than resuscitation formulas. However, these fluids are only currently available in litre bags and are slightly more expensive than resuscitation formulas. Therefore, these fluids are not commonly used in equine medicine. Most adult horses with normal kidney function are able to tolerate the high sodium and chloride infusions when resuscitation fluids are used as maintenance fluids. The low potassium concentration relative to losses means that many of these animals become hypokalaemic. For this reason, many hospitals add potassium chloride (10–20 mmol/L per 5-L bag of resuscitation fluids) to reduce the incidence of hypokalaemia.

Neonatal foals are generally not able to handle the high sodium and chloride loads associated with resuscitation formulas, and these foals may become hypernatraemic and hyperchloraemic.[33] Use of maintenance formula fluids is ideal in these patients. However, if this is not possible, 0.45% sodium chloride/2.5% glucose solutions, with added potassium chloride (added according to administration rate, not to exceed 0.5 mmol/kg/hr potassium infusion), is an alternative.

General principles: Oncotic pressure

The net amount of fluid that leaves the circulation in the capillaries is determined by the difference in oncotic pressure and hydrostatic pressure between the fluid in the capillary and the interstitial space. *Colloidal oncotic pressure* refers to the osmotic pressure exerted by the molecules that do not freely pass from the vascular into the interstitial space. *Hydrostatic pressure* refers to the pressure of the fluid within the capillary, which is generated by the forward flow (pumping action of the heart) and the resistance to flow in the arterioles, capillaries and venules. This drives fluid out of the vessels at the beginning of the capillary bed. The hydrostatic pressure falls as the flow passes through the capillary bed. The oncotic pressure holds water in the circulation and draws fluid back into the circulation at the end of the capillary beds,[34] when it exceeds hydrostatic pressure. The fluid remaining outside the capillaries may be returned to the circulation via the lymphatic system, but, if excessive, will result in tissue oedema.

The number of particles in a solution determines its osmotic pressure. Thus, solutions containing smaller molecules can exert a higher osmotic pressure because saturated solutions will contain more molecules per unit volume. However, small molecules diffuse more easily out of the vascular space. Therefore, the net oncotic pressure exerted by a solution is a balance between the osmotic pressure exerted by that solution and the rate of diffusion of that solution out of the vascular bed. In normal plasma, most of the oncotic pressure gradient (approximately 80%) is produced by albumin. Globulins contribute the remainder of the oncotic pressure, with fibrinogen exerting little effect (<0.01% of total).[35] The normal plasma colloid oncotic pressure of plasma is less in neonatal foals (17–21 mm Hg) than in mature Thoroughbred horses (20–22 mm Hg).[36,37]

Albumin has other important physiological functions. A major function is to bind ions, drugs and hormones and serve as a carrier for fatty acids and other water-insoluble compounds within the plasma.[38] When the plasma concentration of albumin is decreased, the free (or nonbound) fraction of an albumin-binding drug will increase. However, for most drugs, plasma clearance will also increase, resulting in an unchanged free concentration of the drug, and therefore no change in drug activity.[39,40] Albumin also acts as a buffer in acid-base disturbances, and decreased albumin contributes to a metabolic alkalosis.[8]

General principles: Crystalloids

Crystalloid solutions consist of electrolytes in water. Crystalloid solutions may be isotonic, hypertonic or hypotonic. Isotonic solutions have approximately the same osmolality as plasma and thus may be given rapidly, in large volumes or into peripheral veins. Hypertonic solutions act to draw water into the extracellular fluid from the intracellular fluid and represent a method of rapidly reversing hypovolaemia at the expense of tissue hydration. Hypotonic solutions are usually only used to correct plasma hypertonicity. Because true hypotonic solutions (e.g., sterile water) cause erythrolysis,[41] they can only be given slowly via a central vein.[42] For this reason, isotonic solutions containing a metabolisable substrate, such as dextrose and no electrolytes are usually used to correct hypertonicity.

Crystalloid fluids pass rapidly from the circulation to the interstitial fluid. This means that their resuscitation effect may be short-lived and that they can cause oedema. Only 30% of isotonic fluids and 10% of hypotonic fluids remain in the circulation after 30 minutes.[32] The increase in interstitial fluid may actually decrease tissue oxygen uptake in normal animals by increasing the diffusion distance between capillaries and cells.[43] Large volumes of crystalloids also dilute plasma proteins, reducing the colloidal oncotic pressure, and further promoting oedema. However, crystalloids remain the cheapest and, in many circumstances, the best fluids for administration to the horse. All fluid therapy plans involve crystalloid fluids, and these are frequently the only fluids administered.

Homemade or "Carboy" fluids, while considerably cheaper than fluids available commercially, have been associated with producing clinical signs of endotoxaemia in normal horses[44] and a 7-fold increase in the risk of thrombophlebitis[45] (see Chapter 7.2) and thus cannot be recommended.

General principles: Colloids

Colloids are solutions containing large sugar or protein molecules, in addition to the water and electrolytes found in crystalloid solutions. All colloids, except albumin, contain a range of molecule sizes. The larger molecules allow colloid solutions to persist longer in the circulation than crystalloid solutions. The smaller molecules exert osmotic pressure to draw fluid into the circulation in a similar way to hypertonic saline. Solutions with a large number of smaller molecules allow a rapid increase in the circulating volume, greater than the actual volume infused.

Colloids have been recommended for the resuscitation in hypovolaemia and for the treatment of severe hypoproteinaemia in horses.[46] Colloids have two advantages over crystalloids, which makes them attractive for fluid therapy. Firstly, because of their persistence in the circulation, a 3 to 6 times lower volume is required to produce the same resuscitative effect as a crystalloid.[47] This is particularly useful in acute resuscitation of severely hypovolaemic horses or in the field where large amounts of crystalloids may be difficult to transport. Secondly, the administration of colloids can increase colloidal oncotic pressure, in contrast to the administration of large volumes of crystalloids.[37,48]

The molecular weight of a colloid solution is the most important factor in determining its pharmacology. All currently available synthetic colloids are polydisperse (made up of a mixture of molecules of differing molecular weights). Albumin is a monodisperse solution, as all molecules have a molecular weight of 69 kDa. The *weight average molecular weight* refers to the average size of molecule in the solution. As a rule, the higher the average molecular weight, the longer the colloid will persist in the circulation. The chemical nature of the colloid also influences the persistence in the circulation but generally to a lesser degree. The number of molecules in the solution determines the osmotic pressure, which can be considerably greater than plasma (e.g., 342 mm Hg for urea-linked gelatin, compared to approximately 200 mm Hg for plasma). Colloids with a smaller average molecular weight exert a higher osmotic pressure and expand the plasma volume more rapidly, by drawing fluid from the interstitial space into the vasculature and thus increasing the circulating volume in excess of the amount of fluid infused. However, smaller molecular weight colloids are cleared faster from the circulation and may leak more readily into the interstitium.

Leakage of proteins into the interstitium is important in oedema formation. This occurs relatively commonly in critically ill horses (particularly in colitis) and foals (particularly in severe septicaemia and perinatal asphyxia syndrome). Oedema impairs delivery of oxygen to the tissues, as it both compresses capillary beds and increases the diffusion distance between the capillaries, and the cells. Therefore, oedema may contribute significantly to morbidity and mortality. Endotoxin[49] and ischaemia–reperfusion injury[50,51] induce capillary damage, which allows plasma albumin to leak out into the interstitium. This not only reduces the oncotic pressure within the vasculature but also allows the extravasated albumin to exert an osmotic pressure that holds fluid in the interstitial space. Large colloid molecules do not leak as readily, allowing their oncotic pressure to draw fluid back into the vasculature. Larger colloid molecules may also plug the gaps in the capillary endothelium.[52,53] Even in conditions of severe capillary leak, very large molecules are not able to escape the vasculature unless the integrity of the capillary endothelium is totally destroyed.[54]

All of the currently available artificial colloid solutions are removed from the circulation by the reticuloendothelial system resulting in colloid-containing vacuoles, which may persist for years.[55,56] The presence of these vacuoles does not appear to interfere with the function of the reticuloendothelial system.[57] One precaution when using colloids is that the plasma total solids or total protein concentration is no longer a useful guide to plasma oncotic pressure.[58]

In the author's clinical experience, colloids (particularly the hydroxyethyl starch solutions) have a very useful role in rapid reversal of hypovolaemia (Box 6.3) and treatment

Box 6.3. "Shock doses" of fluids for reversal of hypovolaemia in both adult horses and foals

Type of fluid	Shock dose
Balanced electrolyte solutions	60–80 ml/kg
Pentastarch	10–15 ml/kg
Hetastarch	10 ml/kg

of hypoproteinaemia. One small study in horses demonstrated better cardiac outputs during colic surgery when the colloid pentastarch was used to reverse hypovolaemia at admission, compared to hypertonic saline.[31]

Crystalloid fluids

Balanced electrolyte solutions

For most situations, commercial isotonic polyionic crystalloid resuscitation-formula solutions (Normosol-R*, Plasma-lyte 148†, Isolec‡, lactated Ringer's solution§, etc.) are the safest fluids with which to resuscitate hypovolaemic horses. They increase plasma volume without directly causing profound electrolyte disturbances, because they contain approximately the same electrolyte concentrations as plasma. Therefore, balanced polyionic fluids are always a good choice when laboratory information is not available immediately. It also follows that polyionic crystalloid solutions are often not sufficient to correct electrolyte imbalances.

Two classes of polyionic fluids are available—those for resuscitation and those for maintenance. Resuscitation fluids contain electrolyte concentrations similar to plasma. Maintenance fluids (Normosol-M*, Plasma-lyte M†, Plasmalyte-56† etc.) contain higher potassium (15–30 mmol/L) and lower sodium (40–60 mmol/L) and chloride (40–60 mmol/L) concentrations than resuscitation fluids. Currently, maintenance fluids are not available commercially in volumes of greater than one litre. For adult horses, this has led to the practice of adding potassium chloride (at 10–20 mmol/L) to resuscitation formulas so that they can be used as maintenance fluids. Commercial maintenance fluids are a useful treatment option in equine neonates, because these foals have problems handling the high sodium loads found in resuscitation fluids, and may become hypernatraemic if these are used for maintenance.[33]

The different alkalinising agents used (or "bicarbonate substitutes") in resuscitation fluids are clinically relevant. The alkalinising agent in plasma is bicarbonate. Bicarbonate-containing fluids are unstable when stored and may produce profound metabolic alkalosis, which has led to different anions being used to replace bicarbonate in commercial fluids. Lactate (in lactated Ringer's solution and Hartmann's solution) is metabolised in the liver, but this process is slow enough to avoid the rapid changes in plasma pH seen with bicarbonate. It may seem counterintuitive to administer lactate-containing fluids to a horse with lactic acidosis resulting from poor tissue perfusion. However, it appears that in shock there is poor delivery of lactate to the liver by the circulation, rather than any direct impairment of lactate metabolism by the liver. Restoring the circulating volume, even with fluids containing moderate amounts of lactate, is sufficient to allow the liver to clear the circulating lactate.[59] Whereas this is true for haemorrhagic shock, uptake of lactate by the liver may be impaired in severe septicaemia.[60] In endotoxic and septic horses and foals, and those with liver disease, lactated Ringer's solution should be used with caution. Alternative alkalinizing agents to lactate are found in some commercial polyionic fluids (e.g., acetate and gluconate in Normosol-R). The muscles primarily metabolise acetate and a variety of tissues throughout the body metabolise gluconate. Lactated Ringer's solution contains calcium, whereas Normosol-R contains magnesium. Calcium solutions should not be mixed with whole blood; blood and its products should be stored with a compound that chelates calcium ions; similarly, calcium solutions should not be mixed with sodium bicarbonate as they react to produce calcium carbonate. Clearly, calcium solutions are contraindicated in hypercalcaemia. Fluids containing magnesium can therefore be used in more clinical situations than those containing calcium.

Normal saline

Isotonic (0.9%) sodium chloride is used commonly as an intraoperative intravenous replacement fluid in species other than the horse. Isotonic sodium chloride has a higher ratio of chloride to sodium than plasma and therefore reduces the strong ion difference. This results in a mild hyperchloraemic acidosis in normal ponies.[61] This limits its utility as a resuscitation fluid in the horse, as most horses requiring fluid resuscitation are acidotic. Furthermore, there is some evidence that hyperchloraemic acidosis may be harmful. Hyperchloraemic acidosis resulted in hypotension in a rat model of sepsis[62] reduced the glomerular filtration rate by 30% in rats[63] and was found to be proinflammatory *in vitro*.[64] Isotonic sodium chloride should not be used for resuscitation of horses unless indicated by measured electrolyte abnormalities. Sodium chloride solution has been advocated in hyperkalaemia, in order to avoid the potassium-containing polyionic fluids. However, this does not apply to the horse; in the absence of clinical signs of hyperkalaemia and with the exception of horses with hyperkalaemic periodic paralysis or with a ruptured bladder, the hyperkalaemia is likely to reflect acidosis and polyionic fluids are appropriate. Many, but not

* Abbott Laboratories, North Chicago, IL, USA.

† Baxter Healthcare Corporation, Deerfield, IL, USA.

‡ Ivex Division, Dechra Veterinary Products, Shrewsbury, Shropshire, UK.

all, foals with a ruptured bladder have profound electrolyte disturbances (hyponatraemia, hypochloraemia, hyperkalaemia).[65] In these foals, 0.9% to 1.8% sodium chloride solutions are a good choice for resuscitation. Many of these foals require further strategies aimed at reducing plasma potassium concentration.

Sodium bicarbonate

Sodium bicarbonate has been advocated for the correction of metabolic acidosis in horses.[66,67] However, the cause of the acidosis needs to be considered carefully prior to starting treatment. Sodium bicarbonate may be beneficial in acidosis due to hyponatraemia or hyperchloraemia.[8] However, in lactic acidosis, which is far more common in the horse, treatment with sodium bicarbonate is highly controversial.

It is the author's opinion that there are no grounds for administering sodium bicarbonate to cases with lactic acidosis, irrespective of the arterial (or venous) pH. This contradicts previous recommendations that it should be used when the pH decreases below 7.1[66] or 7.2.[67] Treatment of lactic acidosis with sodium bicarbonate is based on four suppositions: low blood pH is directly harmful, sodium bicarbonate is able to increase blood pH when infused intravenously, raising the blood pH with sodium bicarbonate improves patient status and any adverse effects of sodium bicarbonate are outweighed by its benefits.[68] These suppositions are not supported by data available currently in horses, humans and experimental animals:

Metabolic acidosis is reported to result in reduced cardiac contractility, constriction of the peripheral vasculature, inhibition of glycolysis, a decrease in oxygen uptake by haemoglobin in the lungs and central nervous system depression.[69,70] However, the *in vitro* reduction in cardiac contractility with acidosis[71] does not occur or is slight in whole animal models.[72,73] The lactate itself, rather than the pH, caused decreased contractility in a frog heart muscle model of lactic acidosis.[74] Glycolysis is inhibited at low intracellular pH.[75] However, the intracellular environment is protected from extracellular changes in pH. Lowering extracellular pH from 7.4 to 6.9 was not associated with any change in the pH gradient across the mitochondrial membrane in isolated rat hepatocytes and an extracellular pH of 6.6 was not associated with any deleterious effects to the cells.[76] Decreasing pH causes a shift to the right in the hemoglobin-oxygen dissociation curve.[70] Although this leads to decreased oxygen uptake in the lungs, it also results in increased oxygen liberation from haemoglobin in the tissues and the net effect may actually be an increase in tissue oxygen uptake. There is little compelling evidence that a low pH is directly harmful. Indeed, transient acidosis may actually be beneficial as it is associated with delayed cell death in anoxia[76] and decreases infarction size after myocardial ischaemia.[77]

In normal horses, the administration of sodium bicarbonate results in an increase in plasma pH,[78,79] fulfilling the second supposition. Unfortunately, this is not true for the cerebrospinal fluid (CSF). In one study, intravenous administration of sodium bicarbonate to normal horses resulted in a mild decrease in CSF pH, which was still statistically significant 2 hours after the infusion was complete.[78] The blood-brain barrier is not permeable to sodium, and intravenous sodium bicarbonate administration does not change the CSF sodium concentration[78] or the CSF strong ion gap. Therefore, intravenous sodium bicarbonate does not produce alkalization of the CSF. Sodium bicarbonate may also cause a decrease in intracellular pH. Intracellular pH falls in response to extracellular sodium bicarbonate in the brain in normal humans[80] and in isolated lymphocytes[81] and myocardial cells.[82] The observed increase in plasma pH in normal horses may only be short-lived in clinical cases. In ponies treated with a low dose of endotoxin, the plasma pH was increased for less than 30 minutes after sodium bicarbonate administration,[83] whereas in normal horses the plasma pH was increased for at least 3 hours.[78]

Many uncontrolled studies can be found in the literature demonstrating improved haemodynamics following the administration of sodium bicarbonate.[84,85] However, this effect is almost certainly due to increased cardiac preload, because no benefit was documented in studies where an equivalent sodium load is given as a control.[86,87] No other clinical benefits of sodium bicarbonate administration have been documented. In diarrheoic calves, there was no difference in clinical score between the sodium bicarbonate group and the saline controls at the end of infusion, despite a statistically different increase in plasma pH.[88] Some authors argue for the use of sodium bicarbonate in lactic acidosis based on the finding that acidosis results in decreased hepatic uptake of lactate.[89] The theory is that lactate cannot be cleared until pH is corrected, and the low pH results is a vicious circle of increasing lactic acidosis. However, other authors have demonstrated that low pH does not inhibit hepatic lactate metabolism.[90,91] Furthermore, it has been demonstrated that increased extracellular carbon dioxide tension, a feature of bicarbonate administration, does inhibit hepatic lactate metabolism.[92]

It might be acceptable to administer sodium bicarbonate to improve plasma pH based on anecdotal evidence, if it caused no harmful effects. Unfortunately, this is not the case. The production of carbon dioxide and accompanying respiratory acidosis causes a more profound depression in myocardial contractility than metabolic acidosis.[71] Therefore, sodium bicarbonate is totally contraindicated in acidotic horses with normal or increased plasma carbon dioxide tensions, as they have not adequately compensated for the current acidosis and cannot be expected to eliminate the increased carbon dioxide load efficiently. Other potentially harmful effects of sodium bicarbonate include increasing plasma lactate concentration, hypernatremia, hypokalemia and hyperosmolality.[83]

Hypertonic sodium bicarbonate solutions (>1.3%) are not suitable for use in neonatal foals.

Glucose-containing solutions

Five-percent dextrose and 5% glucose solutions (5%G) are used to replace a deficit of pure water (without accompanying electrolyte deficits) and are effectively hypotonic because the dextrose is rapidly metabolised to carbon dioxide and water. They are indicated in cases where fluid loss exceeds electrolyte loss, which can occur in horses with strangulating intestinal lesions[93] and colitis. Hypernatraemia and hyperchloraemia are also relatively common in neonatal foals where resuscitation formulas are used as maintenance fluids.[33] The volume of distribution of 5%G is likely to be larger than that of a balanced electrolyte solution, which could result in a diminished ability to maintain the circulating volume. Horses receiving 5%G should be monitored carefully because rapid administration can lead to hyperglycaemia. If the plasma glucose concentration exceeds the renal threshold (approximately 10 mmol/L [180 mg/dl] in adults; 12.5 mmol/L [225 mg/dl] in foals), osmotic diuresis will result, which can reduce the benefit of the fluid administration. In species other than the horse (humans, pigs and dogs), high concentrations of glucose have been shown to be detrimental in both acute renal and acute cerebral injury.[94–96] The effect in the horse is undocumented. In human surgical (but not medical) critical care patients, preventing hyperglycaemia is associated with lower mortality and morbidity.[97,98]

An alternative to the 5% solutions is a solution of 2.5% glucose or dextrose and 0.45% sodium chloride, which, once the sugar has been metabolised, has an effective osmolality one-half of that of plasma. It is retained better in the circulation (20% after 30 minutes compared with 10% for D_5W)[32] and can be used in the treatment of moderate plasma hypertonicity or when plasma glucose concentration is a concern. It should be noted that a rapid reduction in plasma tonicity has been associated with the development of cerebral oedema, resulting in coma, seizures and death in other species.[99] This has not been documented in the horse.

Five-percent dextrose and 5%G solutions should not be considered a form of parenteral nutrition. One litre of 5% dextrose provides approximately 170 kcal (712 kJ) of energy, and 1 L of 5% glucose provides approximately 190 kcal (796 kJ). In order to provide 11.5 Mcal/day, the caloric requirement of a 500-kg horse standing in a stall,[100] it would be necessary to administer 60 to 70 L per day, which would produce serious electrolyte abnormalities. Similarly, to meet the resting energy requirements of a 50 kg neonatal foal (40–45 kcal/kg/day),[101] 11 to 13 L per day would be required; 50% dextrose and 50% glucose solutions may be preferable for providing energy requirements to the 5% solutions. Each millilitre of 50% dextrose is equivalent to 1.7 kcal (7.1 kJ), and each ml of 50% glucose is equivalent to 1.9 kcal (8 kJ).

Hypertonic saline

Hypertonic saline (2–4 ml/kg of 7%–7.5% sodium chloride) is used as a method of quickly restoring circulating volume in horses with severe endotoxaemia.[102] Administration of 7% sodium chloride results in an increase in the extracellular fluid of 4 to 5 times the infused volume for at least 60 minutes after it is infused.[103] The hypertonic saline draws fluid into the extracellular fluid from the intracellular fluid, principally from muscle and liver cells[103] without providing significant fluid replacement. The administration of hypertonic saline should always be followed by large volumes of isotonic polyionic crystalloids within 2.5 hours of administration. The volume of crystalloid fluids given should be based on the severity of clinical signs of hypovolaemia and dehydration but should be in excess of 5 times the volume of hypertonic saline infused.

Administration of hypertonic saline solution, at a dose rate of 5 ml/kg immediately after experimental endotoxin infusion to horses, attenuated the cardiovascular derangements associated with endotoxaemia more effectively than an equivalent volume of isotonic saline.[102] In horses with naturally occurring colic, hypertonic saline resulted in lower cardiac outputs during surgery than pentastarch, when the fluids were used as alternates for resuscitation at hospital admission.[31] Additional possible benefits of hypertonic saline include reduction the capillary endothelial swelling that may occur as part of the systemic inflammatory response syndrome and therefore improvement of tissue microcirculation and oxygen delivery.[104] Furthermore, in experimental haemorrhagic shock, hypertonic saline reduces neutrophil activation resulting in reduced lung injury.[105]

Hypertonic saline, at a dose of 2 to 4 ml/kg, has clear benefits in treatment of haemorrhagic shock, where the bleeding has been controlled or has stopped.[106] The role in animals that have dehydration as well as hypovolaemia is less clear, because experimental animal evidence shows decreased survival and greater renal dysfunction.[107,108] The author uses hydroxyethyl starch in preference to hypertonic saline for resuscitation of non-haemorrhage hypovolaemia (Box 6.3), except when there are budgetary constraints. In horses with extreme hypovolaemia (severe colitis cases), I use combined hydroxyethyl starch (10 ml/kg) and hypertonic saline (2–4 ml/kg). If used, this combination should be followed up with crystalloid fluids. Combination of a colloid with hypertonic saline has been shown to be beneficial in experimental models.[109,110]

Neonatal foals are at particular risk from rapid changes in plasma osmolality,[99] and therefore the author does not use 7% saline in these patients. However, 1.8% saline may have a role in treatment of foals with a ruptured bladder and 3% saline in slightly older foals with closed head trauma[111] (foals that have "flipped over" backwards).

Colloid fluids

Hydroxyethyl starches

Hydroxyethyl starches are modified polymers of amylopectin. Several different hydroxyethyl starch preparations are marketed around the world. They all consist of a polydisperse solution of starch molecules in which hydroxyethyl groups have been substituted for a number of the glucose subunits. The solutions differ in the number of glucose units substituted and the weight average molecular weight. The greater the number of glucose molecules substituted, the longer is the half-life of the solution *in vivo*. The degree of substitution is usually given as a proportion of substituted residues, which results in a number between 0 and 1, with higher numbers representing greater substitution and hence a longer half-life. The average molecular weight is also important, with lower molecular weight solutions having a greater oncotic pressure but a shorter persistence in the circulation. Ideally lower molecular weight starches would be selected for treatment of hypovolaemia (<200 kDa), and higher molecular weight starches for treatment of hypoproteinaemia (>400 kDa). However, in many countries, only one molecular weight of hydroxylethyl starch is available commercially.

Hydroxyethyl starches are eliminated by renal excretion, extravasation and uptake by the reticuloendothelial system and, for a very small percentage (<1%) of molecules, by biliary excretion.[55,112] Larger molecules are cleaved by serum α-amylase prior to elimination. This cleavage generates smaller molecules, with a higher oncotic pressure, and contributes to a long persistence of increased colloid oncotic pressure in normal animals.[37] Uptake by the reticuloendothelial system can result in the presence of phagocytic cells containing starch granules in the liver, spleen, skin, small intestine, striated muscle and lymph nodes.[56,57] These deposits are dose dependent and decrease with time but may persist for up to 4.5 years following the infusion of hydroxyethyl starch in humans.[56]

Hetastarch

Hetastarch is the only hydroxyethyl starch marketed for resuscitation in the United States. It is available as a 6% solution in isotonic saline* or in an isotonic lactated electrolyte solution†. Hetastarch is a polydisperse solution with a wide range of molecular sizes (10–3000 kDa) and a high average molecular weight (450 kDa) and degree of substitution (0.75). In normal dogs, hetastarch expands the plasma by 140% of the volume infused.[55] The effects on plasma volume in the normal horse are likely to be similar but have not been investigated. Hetastarch is slowly degraded in the circulation and thus has a long half-life. In normal ponies, the increase in colloidal oncotic pressure after a dose of 10 ml/kg lasts longer than 120 hours.[37] However, in hypoproteinemic horses and foals, the clinical effects appear to be shorter, typically lasting 24 to 36 hours.[48]

In normal ponies, a single dose of 20 ml/kg of hetastarch decreased circulating von Willebrand factor, factor VIII coagulant activity and activated partial thromboplastin time and prolonged bleeding times.[37] A dose of 10 ml/kg of hetastarch did not affect haemostasis in normal ponies.[37] However, endotoxaemia may produce coagulation derangements[113] that might render endotoxic horses susceptible to clinically important changes in the clotting profile at this or lower doses. There is no difference in the effect on coagulation between the solution in isotonic saline or in an isotonic lactated electrolyte solution.[114] A study from human medicine suggested that administration of hydroxyethyl starches was associated with a higher incidence of renal failure than administration of gelatins.[115] However, this finding has not been replicated in subsequent studies.[116–118]

Hetastarch may decrease vascular permeability following ischaemia-reperfusion injury,[52,53] which makes it a theoretically attractive solution for administration to horses prior to the surgical correction of strangulating intestinal lesions. This effect on reperfusion injury is not simply a function of high molecular weight; a similar effect could not be demonstrated for a dextran solution with an average molecular weight of 250 kDa.[119] There is evidence that hetastarch reduces neutrophil chemotaxis through the endothelium *in vitro*.[120] Thus, there is a potential for hetastarch to reduce neutrophil-mediated damage in ischaemia-reperfusion, endotoxaemia and other inflammatory tissue insults. However, this effect has not yet been demonstrated *in vivo*.

The rapid increase in circulating volume seen following the administration of hypertonic saline (2–4 ml/kg) and the increase in oncotic pressure and more prolonged effects of hetastarch (up to 10 ml/kg) make this combination appropriate for the resuscitation of extremely hypovolaemic horses, especially those with severe colitis. If used, this combination should be followed up with crystalloid fluids.

Pentastarch

In Europe, several hydroxyethyl starch preparations are available commercially. Pentastarch, one of the more commonly used preparations, has been used clinically in horses[31,121,122] and is approved for use in horses in Switzerland. It is available as a 6% or 10% solution in isotonic sodium chloride. Pentastarch has a smaller average molecular weight than hetastarch (130–200 kDa)**** and thus is expected to produce a greater initial increase in the plasma

* Hespan; B. Braun Medical, Sheffield, UK.

† Hextend; Hospira, Inc., Lake Forest, IL, USA.

**** HAES-Steril (200/0.5); Fresenius Kabi, Bad Homburg, Germany; Voluven (130/0.4); Fresenius Kabi, Bad Homburg, Germany.

volume. The initial increase in plasma volume in human patients is reported as 145% of the volume infused for the 10% solution and 100% of the volume infused for the 6% solution.[123] The degree of substitution (0.5) is less than hetastarch, which is expected to lead to faster degradation by serum amylases.

In human medicine, smaller average molecular weight starches have less profound effects on haemostasis.[124] This may also be the case in horses, although only one dose has been tested. In healthy horses, an 8 ml/kg dose of a 10% pentastarch solution resulted in a slight decrease in the thrombin time 12 hours after administration, which returned to normal after 24 hours. No effect on prothrombin time or partial thromboplastin time was documented.[122] In healthy horses, the initial phase half-life of pentastarch is 5.6 hours and the terminal phase half-life is 122 hours. However, the effects on PCV, plasma total solids and plasma viscosity appear to last only 12 to 24 hours.[122] In naturally occurring horses disease, the clinical effects may be as short as 2 to 3 hours.[31,121] Pentastarch, although available in the United States, is only approved for leukapheresis in human medicine.

For reversal of hypovolaemia, pentastarch is used at a dose of up to 15 ml/kg (Box 6.3). The maximum daily dose to avoid problems with coagulation has not been properly documented in the horse. This author uses 15 ml/kg as a maximum daily dose and has not seen overt problems with coagulation.

Dextrans

Dextrans are polysaccharides composed of linear glucose residues. They are produced from a polysaccharide synthesised by the bacteria *Leuconostoc mesenteroides* grown on sucrose media. Different molecular weight dextrans are produced by acid hydrolysis of the parent molecule. Two dextran solutions are available commercially in the United States: dextran 40 (10% solution in isotonic saline) and dextran 70 (6% solution in isotonic saline). Both of these solutions are polydisperse. The number refers to the weight average molecular weight: 40 kDa and 70 kDa, respectively. Dextran molecules less than 50 to 55 kDa are excreted in the urine.[55] Dextran 40 was reported to cause acute renal failure in 4.7% of human patients.[125] It is not known whether this is a risk in the horse.

Because of the poor persistence in the circulation and the possibility of acute renal failure, the author does not currently use the dextrans.

Gelatins

Gelatins should be considered as a slightly longer lasting version of hypertonic saline, rather than as an alternative to the hydroxyethyl starches. Their main use is therefore in acute resuscitation of severely hypovolaemic horses, at a dose of 2 to 4 ml/kg. Like hypertonic saline, they should be followed up with large volumes (at least 5 times the volume of gelatin infused) of balanced electrolyte solutions.

Gelatins have a low weight average molecular weight (30 kDa for succinylated gelatin†††† and 35 kDa for urea-linked gelatin‡‡‡‡). This molecular weight is below the size that is freely filtered in the glomerulus of the kidney (55 kDa), and therefore gelatins are rapidly eliminated by the kidneys. The small size means that they have a very high osmotic pressure (342 mm Hg), meaning that they draw fluid from the interstitial fluid into the circulation, in a similar manner to hypertonic saline. The small size of the molecules also means that more of this colloid is extravasated than other colloids, leading to greater oedema formation.[126,127] Gelatins are produced by chemical modification of bovine collagen. Despite their bovine origin, the risk of transmission of bovine spongiform encephalopathy by these products is apparently negligible.[128]

The high osmotic pressure of gelatins means that it is possible to cause fluid overload in normal horses. In one study, normal ponies undergoing anaesthesia were given an extremely large dose of urea-linked gelatin (average dose, 48 ml/kg). This caused significant fluid overload and pulmonary oedema.[129] In human patients, allergic reactions are reported to both gelatin preparations, with urea-linked gelatins having the higher incidence at 0.146%.[130] There is no evidence that urea-linked gelatin causes allergic reactions in horses.[129]

Blood, blood components and blood substitutes

Whole blood

Blood transfusion is a potentially life-saving treatment and should be given swiftly when required. However, there is a small risk of transfusion reaction and a smaller risk of transmission of infectious disease, and horses that receive blood transfusions should be monitored carefully. A transfusion should be considered in all horses with a PCV of less than 18% (haemoglobin concentration < 6 g/dl) and is usually imperative in horses with a PCV of less than 12%. Parameters other than the PCV, such as heart rate, blood lactate concentration and venous oxygen tension, should also be considered when deciding whether to transfuse a patient. Blood transfusion is not necessary in mild anaemia (PCV > 24%); human patients with mild anaemia who received blood transfusion therapy have a worse outcome.[131] In septic shock, blood transfusion has been suggested as a method of increasing oxygen delivery to the tissues by increasing the oxygen-carrying capacity of the blood. However, in septic human patients, blood transfusion was associated with an increase in oxygen delivery but not in oxygen uptake,[132] suggesting that the increased supply of oxygen is not available to the tissues. This is supported by work in experimental animals that suggests that tissue oxygen uptake is superior at a PCV of 20% or 30% to that at a PCV of 40%, despite the higher oxygen delivery at the higher PCV.[133] The most likely explanation for this is that

†††† Gelofusine®, B. Braun Medical Ltd, Sheffield, UK.
‡‡‡‡ Haemaccel®, Intervet, Cambridge, UK.

the increasing PCV increases blood viscosity,[134] causing blood sludging and reduced flow through the capillaries. However, the relevance of these findings to the horse, which can tolerate very high PCVs during exercise, is unclear. Horses with haemoperitoneum may present in acute pain and may, occasionally, require transfusion.

In other species, blood transfusion recipients are usually cross-matched with potential donors prior to blood collection. However, the reliability of these tests in the horse is questionable.[135,136] For this reason, the author prefers to select donors negative for the major antigens (Aa and Qa) so that cross-matching is not as necessary.[135] Several laboratories* offer blood-typing for horses. For neonatal isoerythrolysis, washed red cells from the dam are another option. Washing removes the plasma, which contains antierythrocyte antibodies. The red cells are washed by repeatedly separating the cells from the plasma and resuspending them in isotonic saline. Ideally, the separation of the cells from the plasma or saline should be done with a centrifuge or plasmaphoresis machine, but it is acceptable to allow the cells to settle, remove the plasma and then resuspend them. Three washes are usually adequate. The advantage of blood from the dam is that it is guaranteed not to carry the specific antigenic blood group. However, this advantage may be offset by the long time lag in being able to administer blood to the foal, due to the length of the washing process (typically 4–6 hours).

In all cases, the recipient should be monitored very closely for signs of a transfusion reaction during the infusion of the initial 50 ml of blood. Signs of transfusion reactions include pyrexia, tachycardia, tachypnea, sweating, icterus, lying down, frequent defecation, proteinuria and haemoglobinuria.[137] None of these signs are invariably present, but pyrexia and sweating are frequently the most prominent signs. In one study of normal horses given repeated incompatible transfusions, icterus and proteinuria were the only clinical signs that lasted for longer than 24 hours and transfusion reactions did not occur before the sixth incompatible transfusion.[137] In another study, one horse died, apparently of an anaphylactoid reaction, during the second transfusion.[136] Transfusion reactions should be treated with corticosteroids (e.g., dexamethasone 0.05 mg/kg IV or IM once) and stopping the administration of blood or blood products.

Disease transmission is possible with administration of blood or blood products and is a particular concern in areas where equine infectious anaemia is endemic.[138] All donor animals should be tested regularly for this disease.

Whole blood should be collected into bags containing acid-citrate-dextrose†. If possible, the blood should be used immediately, but erythrocytes may remain viable in a refrigerator for as long as 3 to 4 weeks.[135]

The amount of blood needed for transfusion can be calculated using the following equation:

$$\text{Amount of blood (ml)} = \frac{\text{Bodyweight (kg)} \times \left(\text{Desired PCV} - \text{Current PCV}\right) \times Z}{\text{PCV of Donor}}$$

where Z is blood volume of the recipient per kg of body weight (80 ml/kg for adult horses[135]; 150 ml/kg for a 2-day-old foal[139,140]).

Studies of the length of survival of transfused erythrocytes in recipient horses have produced variable results. In adult horses, the half-life of ^{59}Fe-labeled donor erythrocytes was 4 days in three of six horses and less than 24 hours in the other three recipients.[136] This methodology does not permit autologous transfusions as a control. In 2- to 5-day old foals, the mean half-life of ^{50}Cr-labeled donor erythrocytes was 5.5 days compared with 11.7 days for autologous erythrocytes.[141]

Plasma

Plasma has been used extensively in horses with colitis and in neonatal foals for the passive transfer of immunity. Large amounts of plasma are required to treat clinically significant hypoproteinaemia in adult horses, and even so the effects may be short-lived. Six to 8 L is required to increase the plasma total protein concentration by 5 to 10 g/L (0.5–1.0 g/dl).[142] Plasma administration does not have the advantage of the larger molecular weight colloids (e.g., hydroxyethyl starches) of potentially drawing fluid back into the circulation in damaged capillaries, but it may prevent a low plasma oncotic pressure,[142] leading to generalised oedema. Plasma may have a role in replacing antithrombin III, protein C and other cofactors that are depleted during the systemic inflammatory response syndrome (which occurs during endotoxaemia, sepsis, trauma and ischaemia). When used for this purpose, fresh plasma is preferable because plasma that has been frozen for longer than 1 year may no longer contain high concentrations of these proteins.

Plasma may either be purchased commercially or collected from donors. As for whole blood, disease transmission is a possibility with plasma transfusion. This is particularly a concern in areas where equine infectious anaemia is endemic.[138] Imported plasma was thought to be responsible for an outbreak of equine infectious anaemia in Ireland in 2006.

The ideal plasma donor is a young, healthy gelding with a known, entire history that has never been administered a blood product. It is safe to collect 1.6% of the animal's body weight (e.g., 9.5 L for a 600-kg horse), at 3- to 4-week intervals.[143] For blood collection from the donor, a catheter

*Weatherbys Ireland Bloodtyping Laboratory, Irish Equine Centre, Naas, County Kildare, Ireland.

† Plasma collection kit; Arnolds Veterinary Products, Shropshire, UK.

is placed in the jugular vein with the tip pointing towards the head of the animal. Using a 10- or 12-gauge catheter speeds up collection. A collection bag containing anticoagulant* (100 ml acid-citrate-dextrose for each 900 ml whole blood collected[142]) is connected to the catheter and the jugular vein occluded beneath the catheter until the bag is full. Centrifugation and plasmapheresis are the most effective methods of separating the plasma from the cells. It is possible to get reasonable separation of the plasma and cells by sedimentation. The bag should be placed with the administration set uppermost in an ice bucket. There is reasonable separation after 2 hours but the bag should ideally be left for 12 hours, if the circumstances allow.[135] However, if the plasma is being collected for replacement of clotting factors, no more than 6 hours should elapse between collection and administration or freezing, because factors V and VIII are not stable beyond 6 hours.[144] These clotting factors are also depleted if frozen plasma is stored for longer than 1 year. Albumin, globulin and factors II, VII, IX and X are stable for at least 1 year.[144] Horses with colitis[113] and foals with septicaemia[145] are at high risk of coagulopathy, and therefore fresh plasma, collected and administered within 6 hours, is preferred to frozen plasma, if available.

Although classically prescribed for hypoalbuminaemia, the utility of plasma for replacing protein is unclear. Approximately 80% of the colloidal oncotic pressure of plasma is provided by albumin. Because albumin is lost in hypoproteinaemia, it is expected that exogenously administered albumin would also be lost. Large artificial colloid molecules may maintain plasma oncotic pressure more effectively.

Blood substitutes

Stroma-free haemoglobin preparations have been developed in response to the need for safe, infection-free, sustainable sources of blood in human medicine and to eliminate the need for cross-matching. Unfortunately, unmodified free haemoglobin has too high an affinity for oxygen, is rapidly eliminated by the kidneys, causes a substantial increase in oncotic pressure and may cause renal injury. For this reason, research has focused on modified polymers of haemoglobin. Polymerised bovine haemoglobin has already been registered in the United States and Europe for use in dogs‡, where the recommended dose is 10 to 30 ml/kg. Successful use of this product has been reported in a foal with neonatal isoerythrolysis[146] and an early version of the product was used with apparent success in an anaemic Miniature horse[147]—in both cases, a compatible blood donor could not be found. Although not clinically significant in this case, the anaemic mare showed increased pulmonary and systemic pressure, reported side effects in humans,[148] following infusion of the haemoglobin product.[147] More concerning is that, in an experimental trial of ponies with normovolaemic anaemia, one of six ponies experienced an anaphylactic reaction.[149] The main clinical use of polymerised bovine haemoglobin to date has been in the treatment of neonatal isoerythrolysis. There are two ways in which it is used. If used as a "bridge" until a blood transfusion can be prepared, a dose of 10 to 20 ml/kg is recommended.[150] If used as a replacement for a blood transfusion, a dose of 22[146] to 30 ml/kg is recommended.

These products are an exciting development that may have a particular application in equine medicine due to the difficulty of reliable cross-matching for blood transfusion. However, because of reports of anaphylaxis, currently available products do not appear optimal for use in the horse.

Reversal of hypovolaemia

Reversal of hypovolaemia is the most important phase of fluid therapy. Although no specific experiments have been performed in the horse, there is a great deal of evidence from human medicine that early reversal of hypovolaemia dramatically improves outcome.[19,20] The clinical and laboratory signs of hypovolaemia are given in Box 6.2 and Table 6.11. There is no good evidence for choosing between balanced electrolyte solutions and colloids for treatment of hypovolaemia. Therefore, factors such as availability, speed of administration, ease of transport and clinician preference will determine this choice.

The most common concept used to describe treatment of hypovolaemia is the "Shock Dose" (Box 6.3). This describes the maximum dose of fluids to be given acutely, as a bolus, to animals in shock. In practice, one-fourth to one-half of the shock dose is given as a bolus. The animal is then quickly reassessed. If any evidence of continuing hypovolaemia is present, a further one-fourth of the shock dose is then given. This process is then repeated, with the animal being reassessed and given further boluses of one-fourth of the shock dose as necessary, until hypovolaemia has been reversed or a full shock dose has been given. It should be possible to deliver a full shock dose to a foal in 30 to 40 minutes and to an adult horse in 60 to 90 minutes. Delivering fluid this fast requires a large-gauge catheter and a wide-bore delivery system. In the author's practice, wide-bore tubing designed for delivery of fluid during arthroscopy is used for reversal of hypovolaemia in adult horses. Drip sets with inbuilt coils provide a much greater resistance to flow and are reserved for treatment of dehydration and ongoing losses and provision of maintenance needs.

In the neonatal foal, there is an alternative method to the "Shock Dose" method, which is more practical. For this method, give a bolus of 1 L of crystalloids (i.e., approximately 20 ml/kg for a 50-kg foal) and reassess the foal to decide if hypovolaemia has been reversed. Up to three further boluses may be given, reassessing the foal after each. Most obviously hypovolaemic foals require at least two boluses. In foals whose body weight is obviously dif-

*Weatherbys Ireland Bloodtyping Laboratory, Irish Equine Centre, Naas, County Kildare, Ireland.

‡Oxyglobin; Biopure, Cambridge, MA, USA.

ferent from 50 kg, the method needs to be adjusted so that the bolus is approximately 20 ml/kg. In pony foals and very premature Thoroughbred foals, a bolus of 500 ml is usually appropriate. In large draft foals, the first bolus should be 2 L.

Deciding that hypovolaemia has been reversed, and no further fluids are required, is not always straightforward. In adult horses, the clinical signs of hypovolaemia should improve dramatically. Particularly useful to judge is heart rate, jugular fill and urination. Heart rate may not return to the normal range (particularly if other factors, such as pain, are also driving heart rate), but should decrease. Jugular fill may be noticeably quicker. Adult horses will often urinate once sufficient acute fluids have been given. In foals, the clinical signs of hypovolaemia may not have been present. Often there is an improvement in degree of consciousness with administration of fluids. As for adults, foals will often urinate once hypovolaemia has been reversed. There may also be a change in mean arterial blood pressure with fluid administration in foals, and a mean arterial pressure that was reduced and now is consistently above 65 mm Hg probably indicates that sufficient acute fluids have been administered.

It is important to remember that reversal of hypovolaemia represents the beginning of fluid therapy, and not the end. Almost all horses that have been hypovolaemic will also be dehydrated, and this will need to be addressed over the next 12 to 24 hours. Furthermore, these horses may be sufficiently compromised to limit their fluid intake, or increase their losses, resulting in a continued need for fluid therapy.

Uncontrolled haemorrhage

There is one important exception to aggressive fluid therapy for hypovolaemia. This is in the case of uncontrolled haemorrhage (intra-abdominal bleeds etc.).[151,152] Fluid therapy should be given at a rate of 2 to 3 ml/kg/hr until the haemorrhage has been controlled (usually by surgical intervention). Where arterial blood pressure can be measured, therapy should be titrated to a moderate mean arterial pressure (60 mm Hg).

Matching fluid amounts to needs

Following resuscitation, fluid therapy is aimed at reversing dehydration and matching ongoing losses and maintenance requirements. Delivering insufficient fluid is highly likely to be detrimental. The horse will remain or become dehydrated, and will again develop hypovolaemia, resulting in decreased gastrointestinal perfusion, poor wound healing and increased morbidity and mortality. The speed with which the horse will become hypovolaemic depends on how effective the reversal of hypovolaemia has been and the degree of ongoing losses. Delivering too much fluid during this phase generally carries less risk to the horse than delivering too little. For the majority of patients, over administration of fluid will only result increased expense for the client and possible electrolyte losses. In horses with oliguric or anuric renal failure, and with cardiac failure, the consequences of over zealous fluid administration are more severe, and can result in circulatory overload and pulmonary oedema.

Dehydration

Estimating the degree of dehydration and replacing it with fluid is not as straightforward as it sounds. Although tables relating clinical signs to an estimated percentage dehydration have been published,[153] it is unlikely that these are sufficiently accurate to be a useful clinical guide. Evidence from dogs and cats demonstrates that similar tables are not accurate in those species,[154] and clinical experience suggests that the same is true of the tables designed for horses.

This therefore leaves the clinician without a set recipe to treat dehydration, and with a quandary. The key is monitoring. Once the hypovolaemia has been treated, the horse should be examined for clinical and laboratory signs of dehydration (Box 6.2 and Table 6.12). The horse should then be given fluids in excess of the ongoing losses plus the maintenance requirements, until the clinical and laboratory signs of dehydration are no longer present. The aim should be for dehydration to be reversed in 12 to 24 hours. In practical terms, dehydration is usually treated by giving fluids at twice the maintenance rate (see later) with the addition of fluids for ongoing losses. Thus, a dehydrated adult horse will receive 5 ml/kg/hr and ongoing losses, and a foal will receive 9 ml/kg/hr and ongoing losses, until dehydration is reversed. In horses with normal renal function, urine specific gravity is probably the most reliable indicator of when dehydration is reversed. Horses with urine specific gravities below 1.020 and foals with a urine specific gravity of 1.010 or less are unlikely to be dehydrated. Adult horses with normal renal function, frequent urination and a urine specific gravity of 1.012 or below are probably receiving too much fluid. It is important, however, to check the other clinical signs of dehydration, as isosthenuria (urine specific gravity 1.008–1.012) can also occur in horses and foals with renal failure. These horses will usually have increased plasma creatinine concentrations. Horses with polyuric renal failure could become markedly dehydrated or hypovolaemic, if fluid monitoring were based on urine specific gravity alone. Skin tent is a reasonably reliable clinical sign to judge dehydration in adult horses. It is less reliable in neonatal foals and geriatric horses. Tacky mucous membranes are also reasonably reliable method of detecting ongoing dehydration, providing the animal is maintaining its mouth shut most of the time.

Ongoing losses

Excessive fluid losses from horses with acute abdominal disease frequently do not stop when treatment is initiated, and these must be taken into account in the fluid plan. The most dramatic ongoing fluid losses are with severe diarrhoea or nasogastric reflux, which may reach 200 ml/kg/day (100 L/day for a 500-kg horse).[155] Even without such obvious losses, horses may lose significant amounts of fluid through sweating, inadequate intake or, rarely, through polyuric renal failure.

Treatment for ongoing losses is aimed to exactly replace the amount lost to maintain hydration. This is relatively simple when the amount of fluid lost can be measured, as in the case of nasogastric reflux. Reflux is collected in a bucket and measured (Figure 6.4), and the amount collected over a 4- to 12-hour period is compared to the amount of fluid administered. If the fluid lost is in excess of the amounts given, the fluid rates are adjusted both to replace this over the next 12 to 24 hours, and to account for the higher level of ongoing losses than originally estimated. If the excessive losses have resulted in hypovolaemia (on the basis of clinical and laboratory evidence), this must be treated acutely. It is much harder to estimate losses from diarrhoea, sweating and urination. In the case of diarrhoea and urination, it is possible to attempt to either collect the faeces or urine, or to use absorbent bedding and measure the increase in weight. These are almost never done in clinical practice, except in the case of recumbent neonatal foals, for which faeces or urine may be readily collected and weighed on incontinence pads, or urine may be collected with an indwelling Foley catheter and closed collection system (see Figure 2.34). When ongoing losses cannot be collected, they must be estimated. These estimates may be inaccurate and the amount of ongoing loss can dramatically change, and therefore it is important to frequently reassess the adequacy of fluid therapy through clinical examination and relevant laboratory investigations. Horses in which ongoing losses are not adequately replaced will become dehydrated initially and then hypovolaemic. Urine specific gravity and the clinical signs of dehydration are the best methods of ensuring sufficient fluids delivery.

Maintenance

The mean daily water intake (including the water content of feed) of normal resting adult horses is 57 to 64 ml/kg/day at ambient temperatures of 5° to 25° C (41° to 77° F).[156,157] When mares were restricted to 40 ml/kg/day, they demonstrated significant dehydration.[158] The quantity of 60 ml/kg/day is a useful guideline for maintenance rate (2.5 ml/kg/hr) in adult horses. Thus, a 500-kg horse requires approximately 30 L/day for maintenance, in addition to any fluids to replace ongoing losses. The maintenance requirement of neonatal foals is significantly higher and is usually taken to be 4 to 5 ml/kg/hr,[159,160] although some authors use a lower estimate.[161] The fluid intake of nursing foals considerably exceeds this figure.[162,163] It should be emphasised that it is important to take into account the fluid component of all infusions when calculating fluid rates to avoid inadvertent volume overload in neonatal foals receiving a number of intravenous infusions. For both horses and foals with normal enteral function, it is possible to meet maintenance requirements with nasogastric fluids, if this is clinically appropriate.

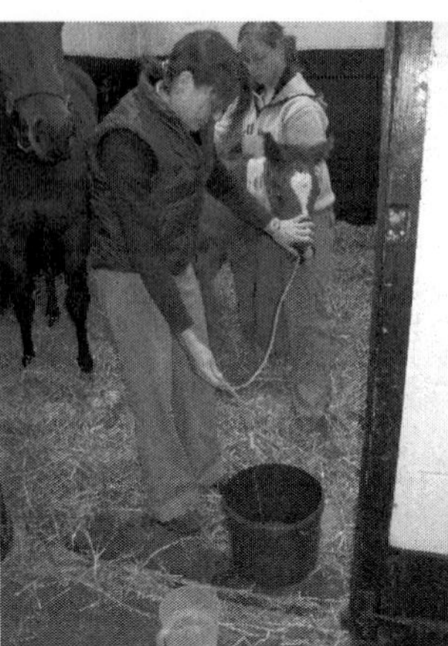

Figure 6.4 Collecting gastric reflux from a foal with colic. The amount of reflux is measured and used to calculate ongoing losses. ©Kevin Corley 2007.

Monitoring of adequacy of fluid delivery is vital even when dehydration has been addressed, and there are no major ongoing losses. The fluid requirements of the animal can change during treatment, and it is important to check that they are matched to requirements. Again, this is best done by monitoring urine specific gravity and for the clinical signs of dehydration.

Correction of electrolyte imbalances

General principles: Acid-base balance

The most common acid-base disturbance in compromised horses is metabolic acidosis, due to lactic acidosis (hypovolaemia, endotoxaemia). Causes of acid-base disturbances are given in Boxes 6.4, 6.5, 6.6 and 6.7.

Acid-base balance is determined by the examination of arterial pH, arterial carbon dioxide tension ($Paco_2$) and the

Box 6.4. Common causes of respiratory acidosis in horses

Respiratory acidosis: ↑Pco_2
(Compensatory response ↑BE)

Reduced gas exchange
- Pneumonia
- Upper airway obstruction
- Neonatal respiratory distress syndrome
- Cardiac arrest

Local causes of hypoventilation
- Fractured ribs and associated pain
- Tetanus
- Botulism

Central causes of hypoventilation
- CNS diseases
- Anaesthetics
- Opiates

Box 6.5. Common causes of respiratory alkalosis in horses

Respiratory alkalosis: ↓P_{CO_2}
(Compensatory response ↓BE)

Tachypnoea

- Excitement, fear, pain, transport
- Gram-negative septicaemia
- Neurological disorders
- Severe anaemia
- Lung disease
- Anaphylaxis
- Intracarotid injection

Box 6.6. Common causes of metabolic acidosis in horses

Metabolic acidosis: ↓ BE
(Compensatory response ↓ P_{CO_2})

Unidentified anion acidosis

- Lactic acidosis
  - Tissue underperfusion
    Hypovolaemic shock
    Septic shock
    Cardiac failure
  - Reduced O_2 uptake in lungs
    Pulmonary conditions
    Right-sided heart failure
  - Strenuous exercise
  - Underexcretion
    Renal failure
  - Cell lysis
    Rhabdomyolysis
  - Intoxications
    Ethylene glycol
- Anion acidosis
  - Phosphate can contribute to acidosis
  - Sulphate can contribute to acidosis
  - Unknown anion
    Sepsis
    Endotoxaemia
  - Other anions
    Ethylene glycol (oxalate, glycolate)

Hyponatraemic acidosis

- Primary sodium loss
  - Diarrhoea
  - Excessive sweating
  - Blood loss
  - High volume pleural drainage
  - Renal tubular acidosis
- Third spacing of sodium
  - Bladder rupture
  - Peritonitis
  - Gut torsion/volvulus

Hyperchloraemic acidosis

- Renal tubular acidosis
- Compensation for respiratory alkalosis

base excess (Table 6.15). The pH gives the overall acid-base balance. It is calculated as the negative log of the hydrogen ion concentration. A decreased pH represents an overall acidosis and an increased pH represents an overall alkalosis. The normal range is approximately 7.35 to 7.48.[8] The arterial carbon dioxide tension gives the respiratory component of the acid-base balance. Base excess gives the metabolic component of the acid-base balance. Base excess is a measure of the required strong acid needed to restore pH to 7.4 at a P_{CO_2} of 40 mm Hg in whole blood. Positive base excess represents a metabolic alkalosis, and a negative base excess, a metabolic acidosis.

Classification of acid-base disturbances is important to effectively direct treatment. They are classified as acidosis or alkalosis, metabolic or respiratory and compensated or uncompensated. The majority of acid base disturbances can be classified by the following three steps (Table 6.15). The first step is to look at the measured pH. If the pH is below 7.40, the primary problem is likely to be an acidosis. If the pH is above 7.40, the primary problem is likely to be an alkalosis. The second step is to look for which of the Pa_{CO_2} or base excess matches the pH. An increased Pa_{CO_2} or negative base excess matches an acidotic pH. A decreased Pa_{CO_2} or positive base excess matches an alkalotic pH. If Pa_{CO_2} matches the pH, the primary problem is respiratory. If the base excess matches the pH, the primary problem is metabolic. If both match the pH, then it is a mixed respiratory and metabolic problem. The third step is to decide if there is compensation. This depends on the direction of whichever of the Pa_{CO_2} or base excess that does not match the pH. If this is within its normal range, there is almost certainly no compensation. If it is in the opposite direction to the primary problem (e.g., a decreased Pa_{CO_2} for a primary metabolic acidosis), it most likely represents compensation. There are a few cases that do not fit this scheme. For example, metabolic acidosis may be primary, due to hypovolaemia, and not compensatory in a horse with colitis and pain-induced tachypnea.

Abnormalities of major electrolytes and their treatment

Horses and foals can have profound changes in the plasma concentrations of the major electrolytes. Understanding the roles of these electrolytes and the prevalence and causes of changes in their concentrations can help prioritise therapy. Electrolyte and acid-base abnormalities are usually corrected after treatment for hypovolaemia, during rehydration therapy. The choice of fluid composition for this phase of therapy is therefore dependent on the plasma electrolyte concentrations. Common causes of

Box 6.7. Common causes of metabolic alkalosis in horses

Metabolic alkalosis: ↑ BE
(Compensatory response ↑P_{CO_2})

Hypochloraemic alkalosis
- High-volume gastric reflux
  - Grass sickness
  - Proximal enteritis
- Exhausted horse syndrome
- Rhabdomyolysis
- Compensation for respiratory acidosis
- Furosemide (frusemide) administration

Hypoproteinaemic alkalosis
- Hypoalbuminaemia
  - Severe enterocolitis
  - Glomerulonephritis
  - Severe parasitism
  - Excessive fluid therapy

Hypernatraemic alkalosis
- Excessive sodium bicarbonate administration

Table 6.15. Scheme for identification of the majority of acid-base disturbances

Disturbance	pH	Pa_{CO_2}	Base excess (BE)
Uncompensated metabolic acidosis	Decreased	Unchanged	Negative
Compensated metabolic acidosis	Decreased	Decreased	Negative
Uncompensated respiratory acidosis	Decreased	Increased	Unchanged
Compensated respiratory acidosis	Decreased	Increased	Positive
Mixed metabolic and respiratory acidosis	Decreased	Increased	Negative
Uncompensated metabolic alkalosis	Increased	Unchanged	Positive
Compensated metabolic alkalosis	Increased	Increased	Positive
Uncompensated respiratory alkalosis	Increased	Decreased	Unchanged
Compensated respiratory alkalosis	Increased	Decreased	Negative
Mixed metabolic and respiratory alkalosis	Increased	Decreased	Positive

Pa_{CO_2}, arterial tension of carbon dioxide.

electrolyte derangements are given in the Appendix (see Chapter 19).

Sodium

Sodium is the major cation in plasma, and sodium and glucose concentrations are the main determinants of plasma osmolality.[93] Changes in plasma osmolality can lead to central nervous system oedema or dehydration,[99,164] because the cerebrospinal fluid equilibrates slowly with the plasma but will change rapidly if osmotic gradients are high. Plasma sodium concentration is mainly controlled by the hormone vasopressin (formerly called antidiuretic hormone).

Treatment of sodium disturbances

The fluid choice for hyponatraemia depends on whether there is concurrent hypochloraemia (Table 6.16). Sodium chloride is the best choice, if the plasma chloride concentration is also low. If the chloride concentration is normal or increased, then sodium bicarbonate should be administered. In adult horses that are not markedly dehydrated[108] with severe hyponatraemia, hypertonic solutions may be indicated (7%–7.5% sodium chloride and 5%–8.4% sodium bicarbonate, respectively). In other species, the rapid correction of sodium deficits has been shown to cause demyelination of the pontine and extra pontine neurons, resulting in severe neurological dysfunction.[164] It has not been established whether or not this is a risk in the horse and therefore it is necessary to follow the guidelines for sodium restoration in other species. These guidelines state that sodium should be corrected at a rate of 1 mmol/L/hr in acute hyponatraemia and at less than 0.5 mmol/L/hr in chronic hyponatraemia, in neither case to exceed 8 mmol/L during the first 24 hours.[165] Sodium can be replaced in oral fluids. Some horses with hyponatraemia will preferentially drink electrolyte-supplemented water. The water should be isotonic or slightly hypotonic (Table 6.13). For concurrent hyponatraemia and hypochloraemia, sodium chloride granules should be added to water. For hyponatraemia without hypochloraemia, sodium bicarbonate should be added to water. Fresh water should always be provided in addition to the electrolyte-supplemented water. These sodium-supplemented solutions may also be delivered by nasogastric tube. In foals, sodium chloride and sodium bicarbonate (1 teaspoon, up to 4 times a day) may be supplemented more empirically by oral syringe. Mixing the sodium salt with yoghurt makes a paste, which foals tend to retain better when given by oral syringe.

Hypernatraemia is corrected with low sodium fluids such as 5% dextrose or 2.5% dextrose and 0.45% sodium chloride should be administered. Again, in other species, it is recommended that hypernatraemia not be corrected too rapidly: Sodium should be lowered by 0.5 mmol/L/hr, not to exceed 12 mmol/L in the first 24 hours.[165]

Potassium

Potassium is primarily an intracellular ion, and thus decreases in whole body potassium may not be detected by plasma measurements.[166] Although erythrocyte potassium content has been used to estimate whole body potassium,[166] its accuracy has not been validated. Moreover, the extracellular potassium concentration (reflected in the plasma) is critical for neuromuscular transmission and thus more

Table 6.16. Fluids of choice for specific metabolic disturbances

Metabolic disturbance	Recommended fluid	Dose
Lactic acidosis	Polyionic crystalloids—resuscitation formulas (Normosol-R, lactated Ringer's solution)	Up to 60–80 ml/kg as a bolus Continuous rate depends on fluid requirements and losses
	Hetastarch	Up to 10 ml/kg as a bolus
	Pentastarch	Up to 15 ml/kg as a bolus
Hyponatraemia		
• With hypochloraemia	Sodium chloride (0.9%–1.8%)	Sodium should be corrected no faster than 1 mmol/L/hr
• without hypochloraemia	Sodium bicarbonate (1.3%–5%)	
Hypernatraemia	5% Glucose (or 5% dextrose)	To lower sodium no faster than 0.5 mmol/L/hr
	2.5% Dextrose/0.45% sodium chloride	
Hypokalaemia	Potassium chloride IV	0.2–0.5 mmol/kg/hr, never to exceed 0.5 mmol/kg/hr
	Potassium chloride PO	0.1–0.2 g/kg per os (divide into 3–4 doses in foals)
Hyperkalaemia		
• With clinical signs or >7 mEq/L	Calcium gluconate 23%	1 ml/kg IV over 10 minutes
	Calcium borogluconate 40%	0.5 ml/kg IV over 10 minutes
	50% Glucose (or dextrose) solution	2 ml/kg IV over 5 minutes
	± insulin (to follow glucose)	Regular insulin—0.1 unit/kg bolus
	Sodium bicarbonate	1–2 mmol/kg IV over 15 minutes
• Without clinical signs	Polyionic crystalloid fluids	
Hypochloraemia	Sodium chloride (0.9%–1.8%)	To effect
Hyperchloraemia		
• With hypernatraemia	5% Glucose (or 5% dextrose)	To lower sodium no faster than 0.5 mmol/L/hr
• Without hypernatraemia	Sodium bicarbonate	1.3–5%, slowly, to effect
Hypocalcaemia	Calcium borogluconate 40%	0.1–0.5 ml/kg over 2–3 hours
	Calcium gluconate 23%	0.2–1.0 ml/kg over 2–3 hours
Hypercalcaemia	Magnesium sulphate	4–16 mg/kg IV as an initial dose
Hypomagnesaemia	Magnesium sulphate	8–32 mg/kg IV over 4–6 hours as an initial dose
Hypermagnesaemia	Calcium borogluconate 40%	125–250 ml IV over 15 minutes
	Calcium gluconate 23%	250–500 ml IV over 15 minutes
Hypophosphataemia	Sodium-potassium-phosphate	0.01–0.03 mmol phosphate/kg/hr (small animal dose)

Always take into account all disturbances present before commencing treatment.

relevant to clinical signs than whole body potassium stores.[167]

Hypokalaemia is very common in critically ill horses maintained on prolonged fluid therapy. In other species, mild to moderate hypokalaemia is a cause of reduced intestinal motility.[165,168] In the horse, clinical experience suggests there is also a relationship between hypokalaemia and ileus. Other clinical signs include muscle weakness, lethargy and inability to concentrate urine.[165] Cardiac conduction abnormalities are rare except in severe hypokalaemia and in preexisting cardiac dysfunction.[168] The effect of potassium on acid-base status is small and need not be considered clinically.[8]

Treatment of potassium disturbances

Treatment of hypokalaemia involves potassium replacement, either intravenously or orally. Rapid administration of intravenous potassium can lead to very high circulating potassium concentrations and cardiac dysrhythmias. Therefore, potassium should be infused at a maximum rate of 0.5 mmol/kg/hr. Potassium chloride is the ideal replacement salt, especially in horses that are concurrently hypochloraemic[168] (including those that are on frusemide therapy). High crystalloid flow rates result in increased urine production and kalliuresis and therefore can make it harder to replace potassium intravenously. Oral supplementation can therefore be more effective, in horses and foals in which this route is available. The dose is 0.1 to 0.2 g/kg, by mouth or nasogastric tube. For foals, this is usually divided into 3 or 4 doses given at intervals of at least 4 hours. Horses that are also hypomagnesaemic may be refractory to potassium replacement therapy, unless the magnesium deficit is simultaneously corrected.[169]

There are several treatment options for hyperkalaemia. In the absence of clinical signs, polyionic fluids should be administered. Possible treatments for symptomatic or severe (>7 mmol/L) hyperkalaemia include 40% calcium gluconate (0.5 ml/kg intravenously over 10 minutes), 50% glucose (or dextrose) solution (2 ml/kg intravenously over

5 minutes) and sodium bicarbonate (1–2 mmol/kg intravenously over 15 minutes).[165] Normal insulin, at 0.1 unit/kg bolus IV, may be given after the glucose and can speed up entry of potassium into the cells. Of these possible treatments, calcium is the quickest at reversing cardiac signs, and glucose with insulin is usually the most effective at reducing circulating potassium concentrations. In foals with hyperkalaemia due to a ruptured bladder, there is often a concurrent hyponatraemia and hypochloraemia.[65] In these foals, 0.9% to 18% sodium chloride solution intravenously, at appropriate doses for the degree of hypovolaemia or dehydration, can be very effective at restoring the electrolyte balance. Peritoneal drainage or lavage is also a useful adjunct at restoring metabolic balance in these foals.

Chloride

Chloride is the major anion in the extracellular fluid. Chloride ions are important in maintaining acid-base balance, renal tubular function and the production of gastric acid.[170] Chloride is an important determinant of metabolic acid-base status.[171] High concentrations of chloride are found in gastric acid and small intestinal secretions, and it is normally absorbed from the upper small intestine.[172] In the kidney, its reabsorption is heavily influenced by both plasma sodium concentration and acid-base balance. Both active and passive chloride transport mechanisms contribute to its reabsorption. Renal reabsorption of chloride is affected by a number of hormones including parathyroid hormone, calcitonin, antidiuretic hormone and angiotensin II.[172] Chloride ion concentration is dependent on whole body water balance. Therefore, plasma chloride concentrations must be interpreted relative to plasma sodium ion concentrations.[8,172]

Treatment of chloride disturbances

Treatment of hypochloraemia can usually be achieved with intravenous 0.9% sodium chloride, which contains more chloride relative to sodium than plasma. In horses with high volume gastric reflux, administration of intravenous histamine$_2$ receptor antagonists (e.g., cimetidine at 6.6 mg/kg IV 4 times daily) reduces gastric hydrochloric acid secretion and may therefore reduce chloride loss. In humans, intravenous hydrochloric acid has been used to treat severe hypochloraemia[173] but carries substantial risks for the patient.[174]

Hyperchloraemia should be treated with 5% dextrose if accompanied by hypernatraemia and with sodium bicarbonate if severe and accompanied by a low or normal plasma sodium concentration.[165]

Calcium

Calcium is involved in excitation and contraction of cardiac muscle and the maintenance of vascular tone. It is a positive inotrope, causing an increase in smooth muscle contractility.[175–177] Other functions of calcium include neuromuscular transmission, enzyme and hormone production and coagulation.[175] It is also involved in cell messaging and receptor coupling.[178] Calcium is primarily extracellular, with 99% being found in bones and teeth. Only 1% is found in the extracellular fluid, of which roughly half of this is protein bound, and approximately 47% ionised in the plasma.[179] Many commonly used analyzers measure total plasma calcium, which is partly dependent on the plasma albumin concentration. The formulas for correcting total calcium for the measured albumin concentration are:

Corrected calcium (mmol/L) = Measured calcium (mmol/L) + 0.02 (40 – albumin [g/L])

Corrected calcium (mg/dl) = Measured calcium (mg/dl) + 0.8 (4 – albumin [g/dl])[180]

Acid-base alterations will affect the protein binding of calcium, with acidosis increasing ionised calcium as it is displaced from protein bound sites by hydrogen ions.[181]

Clinical signs of hypocalcaemia reported in the horse include synchronous diaphragmatic flutter, tetany, muscle spasm and seizures.[182] In horses following colic surgery, decreasing ionised calcium concentrations were correlated with the following changes on the electrocardiogram: increased heart rate, increased QT interval corrected for heart rate, decreased PR interval and decreased QRS interval.[177] Experimentally induced hypocalcaemia (<0.83 mmol/L; 3.52 mg/dl) induced cardiac dysrhythmias in four of seven ponies, which were fatal in two.[183] Hypocalcaemia may be associated with postoperative ileus in the horse,[179,184] but a causal relationship has not been established. The most prominent clinical signs of hypocalcaemia in neonatal foals tend to be ataxia and weakness, rather than synchronous diaphragmatic flutter seen in adult horses.

Hypercalcaemia can cause muscle weakness, depression and seizures due to elevated CSF calcium concentrations.[175] Experimentally induced hypercalcaemia in ponies resulted in ventricular fibrillation or cardiac arrest at ionised calcium concentrations of 4.55 to 10.0 mmol/L (18.2 to 40 mg/dl).[183]

Treatment of calcium disturbances

Whenever possible, the plasma ionised calcium concentration should be measured rather than the total concentration. If total plasma calcium measurements are used to guide therapy, the calcium concentration should be corrected for changes in albumin concentration (see earlier). The level at which intervention is required in the treatment of hypocalcaemia is unknown. Administration of calcium exacerbates endotoxaemia and increases mortality in rodent models.[178,185] While the relevance of these observations to the horse has not been determined, aggressive supplementation of calcium in endotoxaemic horses may be inadvisable. However, the plasma ionised calcium concentration is directly related to myocardial contractility[186]; thus, close attention to the ionised calcium concentration is warranted. Even in endotoxic horses, calcium should probably be supplemented if the ionised calcium concentration is less than 0.9 mmol/L (3.6 mg/dl).

Hypocalcaemia is usually treated with 20%, 23% or 40% calcium gluconate or calcium borogluconate solution administered intravenously. Approximately 0.2 to 1.0 ml/kg of the 20% or 23% solution or 0.1 to 0.5 ml/kg of the 40% solution will be required,[179] but the amount will depend on the ongoing losses and the ionised calcium concentration should be checked frequently during therapy. Calcium solutions are irritating to the veins and should be diluted in crystalloid fluids prior to administration. Calcium solutions should not be mixed with sodium bicarbonate or whole blood. Following calcium supplementation, the plasma calcium concentration should be checked after 4 to 8 hours because ongoing losses and redistribution into cells may result in further hypocalcaemia. Hypocalcaemia can be a sequel to magnesium deficiency, and therefore magnesium should be supplemented in horses with refractory hypocalcaemia.

Treatment for severe hypercalcaemia (ionised calcium concentration of greater than 2.0 mmol/L [8 mg/dl]) should include non–calcium-containing intravenous fluids (sodium chloride or Normosol-R) and intravenous magnesium sulphate (Table 6.16).

Magnesium

Magnesium plays a crucial role in many metabolic and cellular functions in the body, especially those involving adenosine triphosphate (ATP) and the production of energy.[187] It is an important coenzyme for the sodium-potassium ATPase pump.[188] Abnormalities of the normal resting membrane potential can result from interference with the normal function of this pump, causing membrane destabilisation and hyperexcitability. Magnesium is an essential cofactor in many enzymatic reactions in the body.[188] Magnesium also directly competes with calcium for some of its binding sites, allowing greater binding of calcium to enzymes in hypomagnesaemia. One example is phospholipase A_2; increased calcium binding results in greater activity of this enzyme, which leads to the increased formation of eicosanoids, particularly thromboxane A_2,[189] which may play a role in thrombophlebitis.[190]

In the horse, severe hypomagnesaemia can result in ventricular dysrhythmias and also muscle tremors, ataxia, seizures and calcification of elastic tissue.[191] Other clinical manifestations of hypomagnesaemia reported in humans include supraventricular tachycardia, atrial fibrillation, thrombosis, anaemia, decreased muscle strength, increased nephrotoxicity of aminoglycoside drugs, increased pulmonary vascular resistance and sudden death.[188,189,192,193] Hypomagnesaemia can also result in hypokalaemia that is refractory to potassium supplementation in human[169] and equine patients. Magnesium antagonises the effects of calcium at the neuromuscular junction, and signs of hypermagnesaemia include sweating, flaccid paralysis, coma and recumbency due to a blockade of peripheral neuromuscular transmission.[194]

Treatment of magnesium disturbances

Hypomagnesaemia can be treated by intravenous or oral supplementation. Intravenous magnesium sulphate (at 2 mg/kg/min, not to exceed 50 mg/kg) is recommended for the treatment of ventricular dysrhythmias associated with hypomagnesaemia.[195] Higher doses should be avoided because they cause significant muscle weakness; 140 mg/kg of intravenous magnesium sulphate can induce recumbency in normal horses.[194] For the treatment of hypomagnesaemia in the absence of cardiac signs, 8 to 32 mg magnesium sulphate/kg can be used as an initial dose in horses with normal renal function. Oral or nasogastric supplementation with magnesium-lactate-citrate or magnesium oxide is possible but large oral doses of magnesium sulphate should be avoided due to its laxative effects. Treatment of iatrogenic hypermagnesaemia has been reported in horses.[196] The horses were treated with 250 ml of 23% calcium gluconate solution, repeated after 1 hour, and polyionic intravenous fluids to promote diuresis.

Phosphate

Only 1% of total body phosphorus is present in the blood, with the majority of the remainder in the bone.[197] Phosphate (inorganic phosphorus) is the most abundant intracellular anion.[170] Phosphate homeostasis is controlled by parathyroid hormone, calcitonin and vitamin D, involving the intestine, kidneys and bone. Absorption of phosphate from the intestine is affected by calcium, which binds to intraluminal phosphate to form insoluble complexes, thus reducing bioavailability of both ions.[197] Phosphate in the body is important as an enzyme cofactor, a buffer and in the production of ATP for energy. It is an important part of proteins and lipids and is also essential for normal functioning of the coagulation cascade and the immune system.[170]

Clinical signs of hypophosphataemia reported in small animals and humans include haemolysis, skeletal muscle weakness and rhabdomyolysis, leukocyte dysfunction, ventricular dysrhythmias and reduced cardiac output.[198] These clinical signs occur in horses and neonatal foals, but it is often hard to be sure whether they are related to low blood phosphate concentrations. Clinical findings of hyperphosphataemia reported in small animals include diarrhoea, hypocalcaemia, hypernatraemia and an increased propensity to metastatic soft tissue calcification.[198]

Treatment of phosphate disturbances

Treatment of hypophosphataemia has not been reported in the horse, and in humans there is no good evidence for commencing treatment in the absence of clinical signs.[197] Treatment options reported in small animals include intravenous (0.01–0.03 mmol phosphate/kg/hr) and oral (0.5–2 mmol phosphate/kg/day) potassium phosphate or sodium-potassium phosphate.[198] This phosphate dose has been used with apparent clinical success by the author in mature horses. The potential effects of potassium phosphate on the plasma potassium concentration must be considered before commencing treatment. Intravenous glucose-1-phosphate[199] and intravenous sodium phosphate administration has also been reported in humans. The safety of these treatments has not been evaluated in the horse.

Hyperphosphataemia may not require treatment. It appears that increased plasma phosphate concentrations are not directly toxic.[200] The treatment recommended in small animals includes intravenous fluids to correct any acidosis and promote renal phosphorus excretion and dextrose-containing fluids to promote translocation of phosphorus into cells.[198]

Iatrogenic complications of fluid therapy

Fluid overload

Clinical signs of fluid overload are very rare in horses with normal cardiac and renal function. The most important clinical sign of overhydration is pulmonary oedema, manifested by dyspnoea and a pink-white foamy nasal discharge. Treatment for overhydration should include frusemide administered intravenously (0.5–1 mg/kg) and a reduction in the rate of fluid administration. Intranasal oxygen supplementation is indicated where there is significant hypoxaemia (based on clinical examination or arterial blood gas analysis). Further fluid therapy in these horses should be monitored carefully, ideally using central venous pressure measurements (Chapter 1.23).

Fluid overload can be avoided in most cases by careful monitoring of patients during fluid therapy. Utmost caution should be exercised in horses with pronounced pathological jugular fill. Fluid therapy may only be required in these horses after other treatments to reduce cardiac preload, such as frusemide therapy, have been attempted. Any fluid therapy given should be monitored by means of central venous pressure measurements, if possible. Horses with anuric renal failure are even more of a challenge for fluid therapy. Fortunately, this condition is rare in horses. These horses may be hypovolaemic, but overestimating the amount of fluids required acutely will result in rapid fluid overload. Giving these horses more conservative boluses of fluid (5–10 ml/kg) when treating hypovolaemia is probably prudent. All available monitoring, including careful physical examination of the cardiovascular system, should be used to determine whether further fluid is required, after each bolus.

Iatrogenic electrolyte abnormalities

Iatrogenic induction of electrolyte abnormalities is very rare. This usually only occurs with human error, when there has been a mistake calculating doses, reading bottle labels or interpreting laboratory results. Treatment is exactly the same as for naturally occurring electrolyte disturbances and is given in Table 6.16. Avoiding iatrogenic electrolyte disturbances is a question of attention to detail, in most cases. The frequency of measuring electrolytes depends on the degree of disturbance and the speed at which the electrolyte concentration has been changing. Ideally, when there is a large derangement (>20%–25% change from the upper or lower limit of the normal range), electrolytes should be measured at least every 4 hours. The same is true when an electrolyte is changing rapidly (>10% change from the upper or lower limit of the normal range in 4–8 hours). However, financial constraints may limit the frequency of electrolyte monitoring possible. When electrolyte derangements are less marked and fairly stable, they should be measured every 8 to 12 hours until they have normalised. It is much less likely that an electrolyte disturbance will be overcorrected if oral, rather than intravenous, therapy is given. However, it can occur by both routes.

Extravasation of fluids

Catheters may become displaced or may develop leaks, allowing extravasation of fluids. If only fluids (and not drugs) have been administered by the catheter, the problems associated with the extravasation will be relatively short term. Crystalloids will be reabsorbed from the tissue planes fairly quickly. The exact speed depends on the hydration status and plasma oncotic pressure (mainly dictated by the total protein concentration). Colloids may take longer to be reabsorbed. Fluids in the tissue planes will cause discomfort and may obscure the vein (and in the neck, the contralateral jugular vein) for replacement of an intravenous catheter. Certain drugs, such as phenobarbital, will cause tissue inflammation and possible sloughing if extravasated.

Hypothermia and energy loss

Treatment with large quantities of fluids that are below the horse's body temperature can cause hypothermia and energy loss.[201] This may be a particular problem in neonatal foals, which are more prone to hypothermia. The simple remedy is to prewarm fluids before administration to the horse. Large laboratory incubators are suitable for this purpose and may be often be obtained second-hand from hospitals and other medical equipment outlets. Prewarmed fluids will lose their heat as they travel through delivery systems, especially when the ambient temperature is low. The ideal solution is an in-line fluid warming system§, which is available commercially. If this is not available, minimising the length of tubing and maximising the bore of the tubing will reduce heat loss.

Possible exceptions to warming fluids are in the foal with perinatal asphyxia syndrome at admission and in animals after cardiopulmonary resuscitation. I do not warm fluids

§ Bair Hugger 241 Fluid Warming Set, Prairie, MN, USA.

for these horses, based on human medical research demonstrating that hypothermia is beneficial for reduction of neurological injury in these circumstances.[202–205]

Conclusion

Fluid therapy is a routine and life-saving therapy in the equine hospital. Rapid reversal of hypovolaemia is the most important phase to get right, in that it will be the major influence on morbidity and mortality. Throughout all the phases of fluid therapy, frequent monitoring and attention to detail will yield the best outcomes.

References

1. Cohen ND, Lester GD, Sanchez LC, et al.: Evaluation of risk factors associated with development of postoperative ileus in horses. J Am Vet Med Assoc 225:1070-1078, 2004
2. Furr MO, Lessard P, White NA: Development of a colic severity score for predicting the outcome of equine colic. Vet Surg 24:97-101, 1995
3. Furr M, Tinker MK, Edens L: Prognosis for neonatal foals in an intensive care unit. J Vet Int Med 11:183-188, 1997
4. Corley KTT, Donaldson LL, Furr MO: Arterial lactate concentration, hospital survival, sepsis and SIRS in critically ill neonatal foals. Equine Vet J 37:53-59, 2005
5. Corley KTT: Monitoring and treating haemodynamic disturbances in critically ill neonatal foals. Part I, haemodynamic monitoring. Equine Vet Educ 14:270-279, 2002
6. Tennant B, Lowe JE, Tasker JB: Hypercalcemia and hypophosphatemia in ponies following bilateral nephrectomy. Proc Soc Exp Biol Med 167:365-368, 1981
7. Corley KTT, Axon JE, Herron C, et al.: Acute renal failure in critically-ill neonatal foals [abstract]. J Vet Int Med 19:446, 2005
8. Corley KTT, Marr CM: Pathophysiology, assessment and treatment of acid-base disturbances in the horse. Equine Vet Educ 10:255-265, 1998
9. Mealey RH, Carter GK, Roussel AJ, et al.: Indwelling cecal catheters for fluid administration in ponies. J Vet Int Med 9:347-352, 1995
10. Lopes MA, Walker BL, White NA, et al.: Treatments to promote colonic hydration: enteral fluid therapy versus intravenous fluid therapy and magnesium sulphate. Equine Vet J 34:505-509, 2002
11. McGinness SG, Mansmann RA, Breuhaus BA: Nasogastric electrolyte replacement in horses. Compend Contin Educ Pract Vet 18:942-951, 1996
12. Lopes MAF: Physiological aspects, indications and contraindications of enteral fluid therapy. Equine Vet Educ 14:257-262, 2002
13. Sosa León LA, Davie AJ, Hodgson DR, et al.: The effects of tonicity, glucose concentration and temperature of an oral rehydration solution on its absorption and elimination. Equine Vet J Suppl:140-146, 1995
14. Lopes MAF, Moura GS, Filho JD: Treatment of large colon impaction with enteral fluid therapy, in Proceedings of the 45th Annual Conference of the American Association of Equine Practitioners, Albuquerque, NM, pp 99-102
15. Lopes MAF, White NA, Donaldson L, et al.: Effects of enteral and intravenous fluid therapy, magnesium sulfate, and sodium sulfate on colonic contents and feces in horses. Am J Vet Res 65:695-704, 2004
16. Ecke P, Hodgson DR, Rose RJ: Induced diarrhoea in horses. Part 2: response to administration of an oral rehydration solution. Vet J 155:161-170, 1998
17. Marlin DJ, Scott CM, Mills PC, et al.: Rehydration following exercise: effects of administration of water versus an isotonic oral rehydration solution (ORS). Vet J 156:41-49, 1998
18. Sosa León LA, Hodgson DR, Carlson GP, et al.: Effects of concentrated electrolytes administered via a paste on fluid, electrolyte, and acid base balance in horses. Am J Vet Res 59:898-903, 1998
19. Carcillo JA, Davis AL, Zaritsky A: Role of early fluid resuscitation in pediatric septic shock. J Am Med Assoc 266:1242-1245, 1991
20. Rivers E, Nguyen B, Havstad S, et al.: Early goal-directed therapy in the treatment of severe sepsis and septic shock. N Engl J Med 345:1368-1377, 2001
21. Finfer S, Bellomo R, Boyce N, et al.: A comparison of albumin and saline for fluid resuscitation in the intensive care unit. N Engl J Med 350:2247-2256, 2004
22. Choi PT, Yip G, Quinonez LG, et al.: Crystalloids vs. colloids in fluid resuscitation: a systematic review. Crit Care Med 27:200-210, 1999
23. Schierhout G, Roberts I: Fluid resuscitation with colloid or crystalloid solutions in critically ill patients: a systematic review of randomised trials. Br Med J 316:961-964, 1998
24. Shoemaker WC, Schluchter M, Hopkins JA, et al.: Comparison of the relative effectiveness of colloids and crystalloids in emergency resuscitation. Am J Surg 142:73-84, 1981
25. Velanovich V: Crystalloid versus colloid fluid resuscitation: a meta-analysis of mortality. Surgery 105:65-71, 1989
26. Cochrane Injuries Group Albumin Reviewers: Human albumin administration in critically ill patients: systematic review of randomised controlled trials. Br Med J 317:235-240, 1998
27. Vassar MJ, Perry CA, Gannaway WL, et al.: 7.5% Sodium chloride/dextran for resuscitation of trauma patients undergoing helicopter transport. Arch Surg 126:1065-1072, 1991
28. Holcroft JW, Vassar MJ, Perry CA, et al.: Use of a 7.5% NaCl/6% dextran 70 solution in the resuscitation of injured patients in the emergency room. Prog Clin Biol Res 299:331-338, 1989
29. Vassar MJ, Perry CA, Holcroft JW: Prehospital resuscitation of hypotensive trauma patients with 7.5% NaCl versus 7.5% NaCl with added dextran: a controlled trial. J Trauma 34:622-632; discussion, 1993
30. Vassar MJ, Fischer RP, O'Brien PE, et al.: A multicenter trial for resuscitation of injured patients with 7.5% sodium chloride. The effect of added dextran 70. The Multicenter Group for the Study of Hypertonic Saline in Trauma Patients. Arch Surg 128:1003-1011, 1993
31. Hallowell GD, Corley KTT: Preoperative administration of hydroxyethyl starch or hypertonic saline to horses with colic. J Vet Int Med 20:980-986, 2006
32. Spalding HK, Goodwin SR: Fluid and electrolyte disorders in the critically ill. Semin Anesth Perioper Med Pain 18:15-26, 1999

33. Buchanan BR, Sommardahl CS, Rohrbach BW, et al.: Effect of a 24-hour infusion of an isotonic electrolyte replacement fluid on the renal clearance of electrolytes in healthy neonatal foals. J Am Vet Med Assoc 227:1123-1129, 2005
34. Starling EH: On the absorption of fluids from the connective tissue spaces. J Physiol (Lond) 19:312-326, 1896
35. Roberts JS, Bratton SL: Colloid volume expanders. Problems, pitfalls and possibilities. Drugs 55:621-630, 1998
36. Runk DT, Madigan JE, Rahal CJ, et al.: Measurement of plasma colloid osmotic pressure in normal thoroughbred neonatal foals. J Vet Int Med 14:475-478, 2000
37. Jones PA, Tomasic M, Gentry PA: Oncotic, hemodilutional, and hemostatic effects of isotonic saline and hydroxyethyl starch solutions in clinically normal ponies. Am J Vet Res 58:541-548, 1997
38. Weil MH, Tang W: Albumin versus crystalloid solutions for the critically ill and injured. N Engl J Med 32:2154-2155, 2004
39. Tumer N, Scarpace PJ, Lowenthal DT: Geriatric pharmacology: basic and clinical considerations. Annu Rev Pharmacol Toxicol 32:271-302, 1992
40. Toutain PL, Bousquet-Melou A: Free drug fraction vs. free drug concentration: a matter of frequent confusion. J Vet Pharmacol Ther 25:460-463, 2002
41. Krumbhaar EB: Hemolysis due to intravenous injection of distilled water. JAMA 62:992-993, 1914
42. Worthley LI: Hyperosmolar coma treated with intravenous sterile water. A study of three cases. Arch Intern Med 146:945-947, 1986
43. Gow KW, Phang PT, Tebbutt-Speirs SM, et al.: Effect of crystalloid administration on oxygen extraction in endotoxemic pigs. J Appl Physiol 85:1667-1675, 1998
44. Denkhaus M, Van Amstel S: Adverse effects following intravenous fluid therapy in the horse using non-commercial fluids: preliminary findings. J S Afr Vet Assoc 57:105-107, 1986
45. Traub-Dargatz JL, Dargatz DA: A retrospective study of vein thrombosis in horses treated with intravenous fluids in a veterinary teaching hospital. J Vet Int Med 8:264-266, 1994
46. McFarlane D: Hetastarch: A synthetic colloid with potential in equine patients. Compend Contin Educ Pract Vet 21:867-877, 1999
47. Rackow EC, Weil MH, Macneil AR, et al.: Effects of crystalloid and colloid fluids on extravascular lung water in hypoproteinemic dogs. J Appl Physiol 62:2421-2425, 1987
48. Jones PA, Bain FT, Byars TD, et al.: Effect of hydroxyethyl starch infusion on colloid oncotic pressure in hypoproteinemic horses. J Am Vet Med Assoc 218:1130-1135, 2001
49. Mills PC, Ng JC, Seawright AA, et al.: Kinetics, dose response, tachyphylaxis and cross-tachyphylaxis of vascular leakage induced by endotoxin, zymosan-activated plasma and platelet-activating factor in the horse. J Vet Pharmacol Ther 18:204-209, 1995
50. Henninger DD, Snyder JR, Pascoe JR, et al.: Microvascular permeability changes in ischemia/reperfusion injury in the ascending colon of horses. J Am Vet Med Assoc 201:1191-1196, 1992
51. Dabareiner RM, Snyder JR, White NA, et al.: Microvascular permeability and endothelial cell morphology associated with low-flow ischemia/reperfusion injury in the equine jejunum. Am J Vet Res 56:639-648, 1995
52. Zikria BA, King TC, Stanford J, et al.: A biophysical approach to capillary permeability. Surgery 105:625-631, 1989
53. Zikria BA, Subbarao C, Oz MC, et al.: Macromolecules reduce abnormal microvascular permeability in rat limb ischemia-reperfusion injury. Crit Care Med 17:1306-1309, 1989
54. Conhaim RL, Watson KE, Potenza BM, et al.: Pulmonary capillary sieving of hetastarch is not altered by LPS-induced sepsis. J Trauma 46:800-808; discussion 808-810, 1999
55. Thompson WL, Fukushima T, Rutherford RB, et al.: Intravascular persistence, tissue storage, and excretion of hydroxyethyl starch. Surg Gynecol Obstet 131:965-972, 1970
56. Sirtl C, Laubenthal H, Zumtobel V, et al.: Tissue deposits of hydroxyethyl starch (HES): dose-dependent and time-related. Br J Anaesth 82:510-515, 1999
57. Lenz G, Hempel V, Junger H, et al.: Auswirkungen von hydroxyäthylstärke, oxypolygelatine und humanalbumin auf die phagozytosefunktion des retikuloendothelialen systems (RES) gesunder probanden. Anaesthesist 35:423-428, 1986
58. Bumpus SE, Haskins SC, Kass PH: Effect of synthetic colloids on refractometric readings of total solids. J Vet Emerg Crit Care 8:21-26, 1998
59. Lupo MA, Cefalu WT, Pardridge WM: Kinetics of lactate transport into rat liver in vivo. Metabolism 39:374-377, 1990
60. Chrusch C, Bands C, Bose D, et al.: Impaired hepatic extraction and increased splanchnic production contribute to lactic acidosis in canine sepsis. Am J Respir Crit Care Med 161:517-526, 2000
61. Gossett KA, French DD, Cleghorn B, et al.: Effect of acute acidemia on blood biochemical variables in healthy ponies. Am J Vet Res 51:1375-1379, 1990
62. Kellum JA, Song M, Venkataraman R: Effects of hyperchloremic acidosis on arterial pressure and circulating inflammatory molecules in experimental sepsis. Chest 125:243-248, 2004
63. Bullivant EM, Wilcox CS, Welch WJ: Intrarenal vasoconstriction during hyperchloremia: role of thromboxane. Am J Physiol 256:F152-157, 1989
64. Kellum JA, Song M, Li J: Lactic and hydrochloric acids induce different patterns of inflammatory response in LPS-stimulated RAW 264.7 cells. Am J Physiol Regul Integr Comp Physiol 286:R686-692, 2004
65. Dunkel B, Palmer JE, Olson KN, et al.: Uroperitoneum in 32 foals: influence of intravenous fluid therapy, infection, and sepsis. J Vet Intern Med 19:889-893, 2005
66. Divers TJ: Diarrheal diseases—adults, in Orsini JA, Divers TJ (eds): Manual of Equine Emergencies. Philadelphia, WB Saunders, 1998, pp 217-225
67. Johnson PJ: Electrolyte and acid-base disturbances in the horse. Vet Clin N Am: Equine Pract 11:491-514, 1995
68. Forsythe SM, Schmidt GA: Sodium bicarbonate for the treatment of lactic acidosis. Chest 117:260-267, 2000
69. Cohen RD, Woods HF: Disturbances of acid-base homeostasis, in Weatherall DJ, Ledingham JGG, Warrell DA (eds):

Oxford Textbook of Medicine, ed 3. Oxford, Oxford University Press, 1996, pp 1533-1544

70. Smale K, Anderson LS, Butler PJ: An algorithm to describe the oxygen equilibrium curve for the thoroughbred racehorse. Equine Vet J 26:500-502, 1994
71. Poole-Wilson PA, Langer GA: Effect of pH on ionic exchange and function in rat and rabbit myocardium. Am J Physiol 229:570-581, 1975
72. Cooper DJ, Herbertson MJ, Werner HA, et al.: Bicarbonate does not increase left ventricular contractility during L-lactic acidemia in pigs. Am Rev Respir Dis 148:317-322, 1993
73. Downing SE, Talner NS, Gardner TH: Cardiovascular responses to metabolic acidosis. Am J Physiol 208:237-242, 1965
74. Yatani A, Fujino T, Kinoshita K, et al.: Excess lactate modulates ionic currents and tension components in frog atrial muscle. J Mol Cell Cardiol 13:147-161, 1981
75. Halperin ML, Connors HP, Relman AS, et al.: Factors that control the effect of pH on glycolysis in leukocytes. J Biol Chem 244:384-390, 1969
76. Bonventre JV, Cheung JY: Effects of metabolic acidosis on viability of cells exposed to anoxia. Am J Physiol 249:C149-159, 1985
77. Kitakaze M, Takashima S, Funaya H, et al.: Temporary acidosis during reperfusion limits myocardial infarct size in dogs. Am J Physiol 272:H2071-2078, 1997
78. Pedrick TP, Moon PF, Ludders JW, et al.: The effects of equivalent doses of tromethamine or sodium bicarbonate in healthy horses. Vet Surg 27:284-291, 1998
79. Rumbaugh GE, Carlson GP, Harrold D: Clinicopathologic effects of rapid infusion of 5% sodium bicarbonate in 5% dextrose in the horse. J Am Vet Med Assoc 178:267-271, 1981
80. Nakashima K, Yamashita T, Kashiwagi S, et al.: The effect of sodium bicarbonate on CBF and intracellular pH in man: stable Xe-CT and 31P-MRS. Acta Neurol Scand Suppl 166:96-98, 1996
81. Bjerneroth G, Sammeli O, Li Y-C, et al.: Effects of alkaline buffers on cytoplasmic pH in lymphocytes. Crit Care Med 22:1550-1556, 1994
82. Li Y-C, Wiklund L, Bjerneroth G: Influence of alkaline buffers on cytoplasmic pH in myocardial cells exposed to hypoxia. Resuscitation 34:71-77, 1997
83. Gossett KA, French DD, Cleghorn B, et al.: Blood biochemical response to sodium bicarbonate infusion during sublethal endotoxemia in ponies. Am J Vet Res 51:1370-1374, 1990
84. Fanconi S, Burger R, Ghelfi D, et al.: Hemodynamic effects of sodium bicarbonate in critically ill neonates. Intensive Care Med 19:65-69, 1993
85. Vukmir RB, Bircher NG, Radovsky A, et al.: Sodium bicarbonate may improve outcome in dogs with brief or prolonged cardiac arrest. Crit Care Med 23:515-522, 1995
86. Benjamin E, Oropello JM, Abalos AM, et al.: Effects of acid-base correction on hemodynamics, oxygen dynamics, and resuscitability in severe canine haemorrhagic shock. Crit Care Med 22:1616-1623, 1994
87. Graf H, Leach W, Arieff AI: Evidence for a detrimental effect of bicarbonate therapy in hypoxic lactic acidosis. Science 227:754-756, 1985
88. Kasari TR, Naylor JM: Clinical evaluation of sodium bicarbonate, sodium L-lactate, and sodium acetate for the treatment of acidosis in diarrheic calves. J Am Vet Med Assoc 187:392-397, 1985
89. Lloyd MH, Iles RA, Simpson BR, et al.: The effect of simulated metabolic acidosis on intracellular pH and lactate metabolism in the isolated perfused rat liver. Clin Sci Mol Med 45:543-549, 1973
90. Sestoft L, Bartels PD, Folke M: Pathophysiology of metabolic acidosis: effect of low pH on the hepatic uptake of lactate, pyruvate and alanine. Clin Physiol 2:51-58, 1982
91. Sestoft L, Marshall MO: Hepatic lactate uptake is enhanced by low pH at low lactate concentrations in perfused rat liver. Clin Sci 70:19-22, 1986
92. Baron PG, Iles RA, Cohen RD: Effect of varying PCO2 on intracellular pH and lactate consumption in the isolated perfused rat liver. Clin Sci Mol Med 55:175-181, 1978
93. Brownlow MA, Hutchins DR: The concept of osmolality: its use in the evaluation of dehydration in the horse. Equine Vet J 14:106-110, 1982
94. Li PA, Shamloo M, Katsura K, et al.: Critical values for plasma glucose in aggravating ischaemic brain damage: correlation to extracellular pH. Neurobiol Dis 2:97-108, 1995
95. Moursi M, Rising CL, Zelenock GB, et al.: Dextrose administration exacerbates acute renal ischemic damage in anesthetized dogs. Arch Surg 122:790-794, 1987
96. Park WS, Chang YS, Lee M: Effects of hyperglycemia or hypoglycemia on brain cell membrane function and energy metabolism during the immediate reoxygenation-reperfusion period after acute transient global hypoxia-ischemia in the newborn piglet. Brain Res 901:102-108, 2001
97. Van den Berghe G, Wilmer A, Hermans G, et al.: Intensive insulin therapy in the medical ICU. N Engl J Med 354:449-461, 2006
98. Van den Berghe G, Wouters P, Weekers F, et al.: Intensive insulin therapy in critically ill patients. N Engl J Med 345:1359-1367, 2001
99. Adrogue HJ, Madias NE: Hypernatremia. N Engl J Med 342:1493-1499, 2000
100. Ralston SL: Clinical nutrition of adult horses. Vet Clin N Am: Equine Pract 6:339-354, 1990
101. Paradis MR: Caloric needs of the sick foal—determined by the use of indirect calorimetry, presented at the Dorothy R. Havemeyer Neonatal Septicemia Workshop III. Talloires, France, 2001
102. Bertone JJ: Intravenous hypertonic saline solution and endotoxaemia in horses. Proc Am Coll Vet Intern Med 7:476-479, 1989
103. Onarheim H: Fluid shifts following 7% hypertonic saline (2400 mosmol/L) infusion. Shock 3:350-354, 1995
104. Mazzoni MC, Borgström P, Intaglietta M, et al.: Capillary narrowing in hemorrhagic shock is rectified by hyperosmotic saline-dextran reinfusion. Circ Shock 31:407-418, 1990
105. Angle N, Hoyt DB, Coimbra R, et al.: Hypertonic saline resuscitation diminishes lung injury by suppressing neutrophil activation after hemorrhagic shock. Shock 9:164-170, 1998
106. Rocha e Silva M: Hypertonic saline resuscitation. Medicina (B Aires) 58:393-402, 1998

107. Krausz MM, Ravid A, Izhar U, et al.: The effect of heat load and dehydration on hypertonic saline solution treatment of controlled hemorrhagic shock. Surg Gynecol Obstet 177:583-592, 1993
108. Malcolm DS, Friedland M, Moore T, et al.: Hypertonic saline resuscitation detrimentally affects renal function and survival in dehydrated rats. Circ Shock 40:69-74, 1993
109. Constable PD, Gohar HM, Morin DE, et al.: Use of hypertonic saline-dextran solution to resuscitate hypovolemic calves with diarrhea. Am J Vet Res 57:97-104, 1996
110. McKirnan MD, Williams RL, Limjoco U, et al.: Hypertonic saline/dextran versus lactated Ringer's treatment for hemorrhage in dehydrated swine. Circ Shock 44:238-246, 1994
111. Peterson B, Khanna S, Fisher B, et al.: Prolonged hypernatremia controls elevated intracranial pressure in head-injured pediatric patients. Crit Care Med 28:1136-1143, 2000
112. Lenz K, Schimetta W, Polz W, et al.: Intestinal elimination of hydroxyethyl starch? Intensive Care Med 26:733-739, 2000
113. Dolente BA, Wilkins PA, Boston RC: Clinicopathologic evidence of disseminated intravascular coagulation in horses with acute colitis. J Am Vet Med Assoc 220:1034-1038, 2002
114. Dailey SE, Dysart CB, Langan DR, et al.: An in vitro study comparing the effects of Hextend, Hespan, normal saline, and lactated Ringer's solution on thrombelastography and the activated partial thromboplastin time. J Cardiothorac Vasc Anesth 19:358-361, 2005
115. Schortgen F, Lacherade JC, Bruneel F, et al.: Effects of hydroxyethylstarch and gelatin on renal function in severe sepsis: a multicentre randomised study. Lancet 357:911-916, 2001
116. Wiesen P, Canivet JL, Ledoux D, et al.: Effect of hydroxyethylstarch on renal function in cardiac surgery: a large scale retrospective study. Acta Anaesthesiol Belg 56:257-263, 2005
117. Dehne MG, Muhling J, Sablotzki A, et al.: Hydroxyethyl starch (HES) does not directly affect renal function in patients with no prior renal impairment. J Clin Anesth 13:103-111, 2001
118. Sakr Y, Reinhart K, Schiller F, et al.: Effects of hydroxyethyl starch administration on renal function in critically ill patients [abstract]. Crit Care Med 33:A175, 2005
119. Moore RM, Bertone AL, Muir WW: Effect of high-molecular weight dextran macromolecules on low-flow ischemia and reperfusion of the large colon in horses. Am J Vet Res 57:1067-1073, 1996
120. Hofbauer R, Moser D, Hornykewycz S, et al.: Hydroxyethyl starch reduces the chemotaxis of white cells through endothelial cell monolayers. Transfusion 39:289-294, 1999
121. Hermann M, Bretscher R, Thiébaud G, et al.: Erste erfahrungen bei der schockbehandlung des pferdes mit einem plasmaexpander auf stärkebasis. Schweiz Arch Tierheilkd 132:5-12, 1990
122. Meister D, Hermann M, Mathis GA: Kinetics of hydroxyethyl starch in horses. Schweiz Arch Tierheilkd 134:329-339, 1992
123. Anonymous: HAES-steril®. Scientific product information, Bad Homburg, Fresenius AG, 1998, p 100
124. Treib J, Baron JF, Grauer MT, et al.: An international view of hydroxyethyl starches. Intensive Care Med 25:258-268, 1999
125. Biesenbach G, Kaiser W, Zazgornik J: Incidence of acute oligoanuric renal failure in dextran 40 treated patients with acute ischemic stroke stage III or IV. Ren Fail 19:69-75, 1997
126. Allison KP, Gosling P, Jones S, et al.: Randomized trial of hydroxyethyl starch versus gelatine for trauma resuscitation. J Trauma 47:1114-1121, 1999
127. Holbeck S, Bentzer P, Wikstrand C, et al.: Dextran, gelatin, and hydroxyethyl starch do not affect permeability for albumin in cat skeletal muscle. Crit Care Med 29:123-128, 2001
128. Peano S, Reiner G, Carbonatto M, et al.: Determination of the clearance factor for transmissible spongiform encephalopathy agents during the manufacturing process of polygeline. Intensive Care Med 26:608-612, 2000
129. Taylor PM: Endocrine and metabolic responses to plasma volume expansion during halothane anesthesia in ponies. J Vet Pharmacol Ther 21:485-490, 1998
130. Ring J, Messmer K: Incidence and severity of anaphylactoid reactions to colloid volume substitutes. Lancet 1:466-469, 1977
131. Hébert PC, Wells G, Blajchman MA, et al.: A multicenter, randomized, controlled clinical trial of transfusion requirements in critical care. N Engl J Med 340:409-417, 1999
132. Lorente JA, Landin L, De Pablo R, et al.: Effects of blood transfusion on oxygen transport variables in severe sepsis. Crit Care Med 21:1312-1318, 1993
133. Creteur J, Sun Q, Abid O, et al.: Normovolemic hemodilution improves oxygen extraction capabilities in endotoxic shock. J Appl Physiol 91:1701-1707, 2001
134. Stone HO, Thompson HKJ, Schmidt-Nielsen K: Influence of erythrocytes on blood viscosity. Am J Physiol 214:913-918, 1968
135. Durham AE: Blood and plasma transfusion in the horse. Equine Vet Educ 8:8-12, 1996
136. Kallfelz FA, Whitlock RH, Schultz RD: Survival of 59Fe-labeled erythrocytes in cross-transfused equine blood. Am J Vet Res 39:617-620, 1978
137. Hata R, Sonoda M: Clinical and hematological observations on repeated experimental blood transfusions in horses. Exp Rep Equine Hlth Lab 11:133-151, 1974
138. Issel CJ, Adams WVJ, Meek L, et al.: Transmission of equine infectious anemia virus from horses without clinical signs of disease. J Am Vet Med Assoc 180:272-275, 1982
139. Spensley MS, Carlson GP, Harrold D: Plasma, red blood cell, total blood, and extracellular fluid volumes in healthy horse foals during growth. Am J Vet Res 48:1703-1707, 1987
140. Persson SG, Ullberg LE: Blood-volume determination with Evans blue dye in foals. Acta Vet Scand 20:10-15, 1979
141. Smith JE, Dever M, Smith J, et al.: Post-transfusion survival of 50Cr-labeled erythrocytes in neonatal foals. J Vet Int Med 6:183-185, 1992
142. Collatos C: Blood and blood component therapy, in Robinson NE (ed): Current Therapy in Equine Medicine, ed 4. Philadelphia, WB Saunders, 1997, pp 290-292

143. Malikides N, Mollison PJ, Reid SW, et al.: Haematological responses of repeated large volume blood collection in the horse. Res Vet Sci 68:275-278, 2000
144. Cotter SM: Clinical transfusion medicine. Adv Vet Sci Compend Med 36:187-223, 1991
145. Barton MH, Morris DD, Norton N, et al.: Hemostatic and fibrinolytic indices in neonatal foals with presumed septicemia. J Vet Int Med 12:26-35, 1998
146. Perkins GA, Divers TJ: Polymerized hemoglobin therapy in a foal with neonatal isoerythrolysis. J Vet Emerg Crit Care 11:141-146, 2001
147. Maxson AD, Giger U, Sweeney CR, et al.: Use of a bovine hemoglobin preparation in the treatment of cyclic ovarian hemorrhage in a minature horse. J Am Vet Med Assoc 203:1308-1311, 1993
148. Fromm RE: Blood substitutes. Crit Care Med 28:2150-2151, 2000
149. Belgrave RL, Hines MT, Keegan RD, et al.: Effects of a polymerized ultrapurified bovine hemoglobin blood substitute administered to ponies with normovolemic anemia. J Vet Int Med 16:396-403, 2002
150. Giguère S, Polkes AC: Immunologic disorders in neonatal foals. Vet Clin North Am Equine Pract 21:241-272, v, 2005
151. Burris D, Rhee P, Kaufmann C, et al.: Controlled resuscitation for uncontrolled hemorrhagic shock. J Trauma 46:216-223, 1999
152. Soucy DM, Rudé M, Hsia WC, et al.: The effects of varying fluid volume and rate of resuscitation during uncontrolled hemorrhage. J Trauma 46:209-215, 1999
153. Corley KTT: Fluid therapy for horses with gastrointestinal diseases, in Smith BP (ed): Large Animal Internal Medicine, ed 3. St. Louis, Mosby, 2002, pp 682-694
154. Hansen B, DeFrancesco T: Relationship between hydration estimate and body weight change after fluid therapy in critically ill dogs and cats. J Vet Emerg Crit Care 12:235-243, 2002
155. Rose RJ: A physiological approach to fluid and electrolyte therapy in the horse. Equine Vet J 13:7-14, 1981
156. Groenendyk S, English PB, Abetz I: External balance of water and electrolytes in the horse. Equine Vet J 20:189-193, 1988
157. Tasker JB: Fluid and electrolyte studies in the horse. III. Intake and output of water, sodium and potassium in normal horses. Cornell Vet 57:649-657, 1967
158. Houpt KA, Eggleston A, Kunkle K, et al.: Effect of water restriction on equine behaviour and physiology. Equine Vet J 32:341-344, 2000
159. Corley KTT: Fluid therapy, in Bertone JJ, Horspool LL (eds): Equine Clinical Pharmacology. London, WB Saunders, 2004, pp 327-364
160. Spurlock SL, Furr M: Fluid therapy, in Koterba AM, Drummond WH, Kosch PC (eds): Equine Clinical Neonatology. Philadelphia, Lea and Febiger, 1990, pp 671-700
161. Palmer JE: Fluid therapy in the neonate: not your mother's fluid space. Vet Clin North Am Equine Pract 20:63-75, 2004
162. Martin RG, McMeniman NP, Dowsett KF: Milk and water intakes of foals sucking grazing mares. Equine Vet J 24:295-299, 1992
163. Oftedal OT, Hintz HF, Schryver HF: Lactation in the horse: milk composition and intake by foals. J Nutr 113:2096-2106, 1983
164. Adrogue HJ, Madias NE: Hyponatremia. N Engl J Med 342:1581-1589, 2000
165. Schaer M: Disorders of serum potassium, sodium, magnesium and chloride. J Vet Emerg Crit Care 9:209-217, 1999
166. Muylle E, Nuytten J, Van den Hende C, et al.: Determination of red blood cell potassium content in horses with diarrhoea: a practical approach for therapy. Equine Vet J 16:450-452, 1984
167. Rose BD: Clinical Physiology of Acid-Base and Electrolyte Disorders, ed 4. New York, McGraw-Hill, 1994, p 916
168. Gennari FJ: Hypokalemia. N Engl J Med 339:451-458, 1998
169. Hamill-Ruth RJ, McGory R: Magnesium repletion and its effect on potassium homeostasis in critically ill adults: results of a double-blind, randomized, controlled trial. Crit Care Med 24:38-45, 1996
170. Maloney DG, Appadurai IR, Vaughan RS: Anions and the anaesthetist. Anaesthesia 57:140-154, 2002
171. Funk G-C, Doberer D, Heinze G, et al.: Changes of serum chloride and metabolic acid-base status in critical illness. Anaesthesia 59:1111-1115, 2004
172. de Morais HSA: Chloride ion in small animal practice: the forgotten ion. J Vet Emerg Crit Care 2:11-24, 1993
173. Kwun KB, Boucherit T, Wong J, et al.: Treatment of metabolic alkalosis with intravenous infusion of concentrated hydrochloric acid. Am J Surg 146:328-330, 1983
174. Rothe KF, Schimek F: Necrotic skin lesion following therapy of severe metabolic alkalosis. A case report. Acta Anaesthesiol Belg 37:137-139, 1986
175. Grubb TL, Foreman JH, Benson GJ, et al.: Hemodynamic effects of calcium gluconate administered to conscious horses. J Vet Int Med 10:401-404, 1996
176. Gasthuys F, De Moor A, Parmentier D: Cardiovascular effects of low dose calcium chloride infusions during halothane anaesthesia in dorsally recumbent ventilated ponies. J Vet Med A Physiol Pathol Clin Med 38:728-736, 1991
177. Garcia-Lopez JM, Provost PJ, Rush JE, et al.: Prevalence and prognostic importance of hypomagnesemia and hypocalcemia in horses that have colic surgery. Am J Vet Res 62:7-12, 2001
178. Zaloga GP, Sager A, Black KW, et al.: Low dose calcium administration increases mortality during septic peritonitis in rats. Circ Shock 37:226-229, 1992
179. Dart AJ, Snyder JR, Spier SJ, et al.: Ionized calcium concentration in horses with surgically managed gastrointestinal disease: 147 cases (1988-1990). J Am Vet Med Assoc 201:1244-1248, 1992
180. Payne RB, Little AJ, Williams RB, et al.: Interpretation of serum calcium in patients with abnormal serum proteins. Br Med J 4:643-646, 1973
181. Cooper DJ, Walley KR, Dodek PM, et al.: Plasma ionized calcium and blood lactate concentrations are inversely associated in human lactic acidosis. Intensive Care Med 18:286-289, 1992
182. Beyer MJ, Freestone JF, Reimer JM, et al.: Idiopathic hypocalcemia in foals. J Vet Int Med 11:356-360, 1997

183. Glazier DB, Littledike ET, Evans RD: Electrocardiographic changes in induced hypocalcemia and hypercalcemia in horses. J Equine Med Surg 3:489-494, 1979
184. Delesalle C, Dewulf J, Lefebvre RA, et al.: Use of plasma ionized calcium levels and Ca2+ substitution response patterns as prognostic parameters for ileus and survival in colic horses. Vet Q 27:157-172, 2005
185. Malcolm DS, Zaloga GP, Holaday JW: Calcium administration increases the mortality of endotoxic shock in rats. Crit Care Med 17:900-903, 1989
186. Lang RM, Fellner SK, Neumann A, et al.: Left ventricular contractility varies directly with blood ionized calcium. Ann Intern Med 108:524-529, 1988
187. Page S, Salem M, Laughlin MR: Intracellular Mg2+ regulates ADP phosphorylation and adenine nucleotide synthesis in human erythrocytes. Am J Physiol 274:E920-E927, 1998
188. Tso EL, Barish RA: Magnesium: clinical considerations. J Emerg Med 10:735-745, 1992
189. Gunther T: Biochemical bases of the therapeutic actions of magnesium. Magnes Bull 13:46-52, 1992
190. Morris DD: Thrombophlebitis in horses: The contribution of hemostatic dysfunction to pathogenesis. Compend Contin Educ Pract Vet 11:1386-1394, 1989
191. Harrington DD: Pathological features of magnesium deficiency in young horses fed purified rations. Am J Vet Res 35:503-513, 1974
192. Landon RA, Young EA: Role of magnesium in regulation of lung function. J Am Diet Assoc 93:674-677, 1993
193. Salem M, Munoz R, Chernow B: Hypomagnesemia in critical illness. A common and clinically important problem. Crit Care Clin 7:225-252, 1991
194. Bowen JM, Blackmon DM, Heavner JE: Effect of magnesium ions on neuromuscular transmission in the horse, steer, and dog. J Am Vet Med Assoc 157:164-173, 1970
195. Bonagura JD, Reef VB: Disorders of the cardiovascular system, in Reed SM, Bayly WM, Sellon DC (eds): Equine Internal Medicine, ed 2. St. Louis, WB Saunders, 2004, pp 355-459
196. Henninger RW, Horst J: Magnesium toxicosis in two horses. J Am Vet Med Assoc 211:82-85, 1997
197. Bugg NC, Jones JA: Hypophosphataemia. Pathophysiology, effects and management on the intensive care unit. Anaesthesia 53:895-902, 1998
198. Macintire DK: Disorders of potassium, phosphorus, and magnesium in critical illness. Compend Contin Educ Pract Vet 19:41-48, 1997
199. Bollaert PE, Levy B, Nace L, et al.: Hemodynamic and metabolic effects of rapid correction of hypophosphatemia in patients with septic shock. Chest 107:1698-1701, 1995
200. Sutters M, Gaboury CL, Bennett WM: Severe hyperphosphatemia and hypocalcemia: a dilemma in patient management. J Am Soc Nephrol 7:2056-2061, 1996
201. Carlson GP: Energy loss in fluid therapy. N Engl J Med 285:1328-1329, 1971
202. Shankaran S, Laptook AR, Ehrenkranz RA, et al.: Whole-body hypothermia for neonates with hypoxic-ischemic encephalopathy. N Engl J Med 353:1574-1584, 2005
203. Holzer M, Cerchiari E, Martens P, et al.: Mild therapeutic hypothermia to improve the neurologic outcome after cardiac arrest. N Engl J Med 346:549-556, 2002
204. Compagnoni G, Pogliani L, Lista G, et al.: Hypothermia reduces neurological damage in asphyxiated newborn infants. Biol Neonate 82:222-227, 2002
205. Bernard SA, Gray TW, Buist MD, et al.: Treatment of comatose survivors of out-of-hospital cardiac arrest with induced hypothermia. N Engl J Med 346:557-563, 2002

7

Common problems encountered in the hospitalised horse

7.1 Unexplained fever
7.2 Thrombophlebitis
7.3 Inappetence
7.4 Unwillingness to drink
7.5 Hyperlipaemia

7.1 Unexplained fever

Veronica Roberts and Shaun McKane

In adult horses, the normal range of body temperature is 37.5° to 38.5° C (99.5°–101.5° F). In neonatal foals, there is a wider normal range of 37.2° to 38.9° C (99.0°–102.0° F). The body temperature setpoint is subject to diurnal variation of up to 1° C (2° F), lowest in the morning and peaking in the evening. This setpoint is the temperature that homeostasis attempts to maintain, primarily via neuronal control operating through the thermoregulatory centre in the hypothalamus.[1–3]

A variety of disorders may cause increased body temperature. Hyperthermic conditions are those in which the setpoint is unaltered and include exercise-related hyperthermia,[3] heat stroke,[4] malignant hyperthermia,[5,6] anhidrosis,[4,7] central nervous system disorders and reactions to certain toxins or drugs.[8] Hyperthermia has been reported in the foal following administration of erythromycin.[9] True fever occurs when the setpoint is increased and then maintained by the same mechanisms that maintain the normal body temperature. Common causes of fever are not limited to infections and also include immune-mediated, neoplastic and noninfectious causes. The common causes of fever in hospitalised horses are listed in Box 7.1.

Box 7.1. Common causes of fever in the hospitalised horse

Infectious causes
- Wound infection
- Viral respiratory diseases
- Thrombophlebitis
- Peritonitis
- Enterocolitis (e.g., salmonellosis)
- Strangles
- Pleuropneumonia
- Rotavirus (foals)
- Umbilical abscess (foals)
- Septic arthritis (foals)

Noninfectious causes
- Hyperlipaemia
- Hepatic lipidosis
- Chronic active hepatitis
- Occular trauma
- Acute renal failure

Immune-mediated causes
- Purpura haemorrhagica
- Drug reactions
- Urticaria

Neoplastic causes
- Lymphosarcoma
- Metastatic melanoma
- Squamous cell carcinoma

Pathogenesis

The pathogenesis of the febrile response[10,11] is through the release of microbial products (exogenous pyrogens) and several endogenous pyrogens, especially interleukin 1 (IL-1) and tumour necrosis factor α (TNF-α). Both types of pyrogens act on the thermoregulatory centre of the hypothalamus leading to the production of arachidonic acid metabolites, particularly prostaglandin E_2, hence the effectiveness of cyclooxygenase inhibitors and corticosteroids on reducing the febrile response. Multiple feedback mechanisms, via endogenous cryogens, act to prevent extremes that are incompatible with life.

Investigation

In many cases, the cause for the development of fever in the hospitalised horse is evident from history and physical examination. Investigation of fever in the horse postoperatively requires particular consideration of postoperative infection. This includes the skin incision, surgical site, catheter site and respiratory tract. In horses that have undergone abdominal surgery, peritonitis is an important consideration. Infectious diseases are the most common cause of fever (43% of horses in a study of 63 cases)[12] and often easily identified from clinical signs such as nasal discharge, tachypnoea, coughing or diarrhoea. Some inflammatory, immunologic or neoplastic causes of fever can also be easily identified from clinical examination, for example, pemphigus foliaceus.

Taking body temperature twice a day over several days helps to identify a pattern to the fever. Sustained fevers are those where the pyrexia is consistent. Intermittent fevers typically demonstrate diurnal variation, with the period of pyrexia being most common in the evening. These are often associated with infectious causes. If after thorough history, physical examination and haematological and serum biochemical profile the cause is not evident, further investigation is required. Further physical examination should include rectal examination and a more thorough examination of the respiratory system and abdomen in particular.

Remittent fevers are characterised by a state alternating between days of pyrexia followed by days of normal temperature. Differential diagnoses include equine infectious anaemia, equine viral arteritis, equine ehrliciosis, purpura haemorrhagica and autoimmune haemolytic anaemia. Thorough history, clinical examination and clinical pathology are required to differentiate between these causes.

The housing of many horses from varying backgrounds in a hospital affords a great opportunity for the spread of respiratory viruses. Equine rhinovirus is of particular importance because of its rapid spread and ability to produce fever and anorexia. General anaesthesia can result in pulmonary compromise, thus predisposing horses to bacterial bronchopneumonia. Full examination of the respiratory system should include auscultation at rest and during the application of a rebreathing bag, upper and lower respiratory tract endoscopy and tracheal wash. Thoracic radiography and ultrasonography may be included and thoracocentesis may be useful when there is an increase in pleural fluid. Pleuroscopy and biopsy may be useful where neoplasia is suspected.

Postoperative infections of laporotomy incisions are relatively common, especially following intestinal resection or enterotomy. These infections may produce fever prior to the production of significant exudate, so careful examination and ultrasonography of the wound should be undertaken in horses that become pyrexic in the first 10 days following colic surgery. Peritonitis and abdominal abscessation are also common causes of fever, so abdominocentesis should be performed and the fluid cultured and evaluated for protein and cytology. In cases of neoplasia, peritoneal fluid cytology is a specific, but not a sensitive, indicator. Exploratory laparotomy or laparoscopy may be indicated if the horse becomes progressively debilitated and does not respond to therapy.

In cases of fever associated with gastrointestinal protein loss and diarrhoea, faecal worm egg count and faecal culture are indicated. Salmonellosis is an important cause of fever in stressed hospitalised horses, with the recrudescence of infection in carrier animals and the potential for spread to immunocompromised patients. Isolation procedures to prevent the spread of infectious enterocolitis should be instigated where *Salmonella* or *Clostridia* is a possibility. Isolation and biosecurity are discussed in depth in Chapter 3.3.

Thrombophlebitis following catheterisation is another relatively common complication of the hospitalised horse, especially in cases involving marked endotoxaemia. Catheter sites should be examined twice daily for swelling and ultrasonography of the jugular vein should be conducted in the event of fever. Bacterial endocarditis is not as common in the horse as many other species; however, cardiac evaluation including electrocardiography and echocardiography is indicated, where a new murmur, dysrhythmia or persistent tachycardia is identified in the hospitalised horse.

Clinical pathological testing should include haematology, fibrinogen, serum biochemistry and urinalysis. Minimum recommended panels are summarised in Box 7.2. Hyperfibrinogenaemia and hyperglobulinaemia are typical findings of chronic inflammation or infection. As an acute-phase reactant protein, hyperfibrinogenaemia is the first indicator of active inflammatory disease and is more sensitive than leukocytosis or neutrophilia. Fibrinogen normally increases in response to inflammation and then declines as the condition improves. Hyperfibrinogenaemia remains associated with chronic inflammation as long as the disease remains active, but values are not always in direct correlation with disease severity. Serum amyloid A (SAA) is an acute-phase protein that increases rapidly with infection/inflammation, and decreases more rapidly than fibrinogen. SAA is a sensitive marker of infection in the neonatal foal.[14,15] However, in animals with a well-walled off abscess, SAA may be low.[16] Fibrinogen often continues to be increased in these animals.

Causes of hypoproteinaemia are usually from increased consumption or loss into gastrointestinal tract, urine or into a third space (e.g., pleuropneumonia). Blood cultures may be useful; ideally, three to five samples should taken at least 45 minutes apart, when the horse is pyrexic but not receiving antibiotics. Serology for specific pathogens (e.g., equine infectious anaemia, *Streptococcus equi equi*, babesiosis) may be considered but is often of limited value.

Box 7.2. Minimum recommended clinical pathology panels

Haematology
- White blood cells
- Neutrophils
- Bands
- Lymphocytes
- Monocytes
- Eosinophils
- Basophils
- Neutrophil-to-lymphocyte ratio
- PCV
- Erythrocytes
- Haemoglobin
- MCV
- MCH
- MCHC

Biochemistry
- Glucose
- Blood urea nitrogen (BUN)
- Creatinine
- Creatinine phosphokinase (CK)
- Aspartate aminotransferase (AST)
- Inositol dehydrogenase (IDH)
  - previously called sorbitol dehydrogenase (SDH)
- γ-Glutamyl transferase (GGT)
- Alkaline phosphatase (ALP)
- Bilirubin (total)
- Bile acids
- Total protein
- Albumin (Total protein − albumin = globulin)
- Sodium
- Potassium
- Calcium
- Phosphate
- Fibrinogen

Helpful, if available
- Serum amyloid A

Urinalysis

References

1. Dinarello CA: Thermoregulation and the pathogenesis of fever. Infect Dis Clin North Am 10:433-450, 1996
2. Guyton AC, Hall JE: Body temperature, temperature regulation and fever, in Guyton AC, Hall JE (eds): Textbook of Medical Physiology, ed 10. Philadelphia, WB Saunders, 2000, pp 823-833
3. Guthrie AJ, Lund RJ: Thermoregulation: base mechanisms and hyperthermia Vet Clin North Am Equine Pract 14:45-59, 1998
4. Hubert JD, Beadle RE, Norwood G: Equine anhidrosis. Vet Clin North Am Equine Pract 18:355-69, 2002
5. Aleman M, Brosnan RJ, Williams DC, LeCouteur RA, Imai A, Tharp BR, Steffey EP: Malignant hyperthermia in a horse anaesthetised with halothane. J Vet Intern Med 19:363-366, 2005
6. Manley SV, Kelly AB, Hodgson D: Malignant hyperthermia-like reactions in three anaesthetised horses. J Am Vet Med Assoc 183:85-89, 1983
7. Mayhew IG, Ferguson HO: Clinical, clinicopathological, and epidemiological features of anhidrosis in central Florida thoroughbred horses, J Vet Intern Med 1:136-141, 1987
8. Stratton-Phelps M, Wilson WD, Gardner IA: Risk of adverse effects in pneumonic foals treated with erythromycin versus other antibiotics: 143 cases (1986-1996). J Am Vet Med Assoc 217:68-73, 2000
9. Clayman MD, Capaldo RA: Vancomycin allergy presenting as fever of unknown origin. Arch Intern Med 149:1425-1426, 1989
10. Dinarello CA: Infection, fever, and exogenous and endogenous pyrogens: some concepts have changed. J Endotoxin Res 10:201-222, 2004
11. Hines MT: Changes in body temperature, in Reed SM, Bayly WM, Sellon DC: Equine Internal Medicine, ed 2. Philadelphia, WB Saunders, 2004, pp 148-155
12. Mair TS, Taylor FG, Pinsent PJ: Fever of unknown origin in the horse: a review of 63 cases. Equine Vet J 21:260-265, 1989
13. White SA: Alterations in body temperature, in Smith BP (ed): Large Animal Internal Medicine, ed 3. St. Louis, Mosby, 2002
14. Stoneham SJ, Palmer L, Cash R, et al.: Measurement of serum amyloid A in the neonatal foal using a latex agglutination immunoturbidimetric assay: determination of the normal range, variation with age and response to disease. Equine Vet J 33:599-603, 2001
15. Hulten C, Demmers S: Serum amyloid A (SAA) as an aid in the management of infectious disease in the foal: comparison with total leucocyte count, neutrophil count and fibrinogen. Equine Vet J 34:693-698, 2002
16. Jacobsen S, Andersen PH: The acute phase protein serum amyloid A (SAA) as a marker of inflammation in horses. Equine Vet Educ 19:38-46, 2007

7.2 Thrombophlebitis

Harold C. McKenzie III

One of the most common complications in hospitalised equine patients is phlebitis or thrombophlebitis, which is typically associated with venipuncture sites or indwelling intravenous catheters. *Phlebitis* refers to inflammation of the blood vessel wall, while *thrombophlebitis* is characterised by formation of a thrombus on the vessel wall, in combination with vessel wall inflammation. Risk factors for the development of thrombophlebitis include patient factors such as the presence of clinical endotoxaemia (odds ratio [OR] = 18.5), hypoproteinaemia (OR = 4.7), large intestinal disease (OR = 3.6), diarrhoea, postoperative shock and debilitation, as well as exposure factors including the type of intravenous fluid administered and duration of intravenous catheterisation.[1–5] While type of catheter material, catheter length, method of catheter placement and catheter stability are all demonstrated to be related to the incidence of thrombophlebitis in human patients, and would logically be of concern in equine patients, there is inadequate evidence in the equine literature to substantiate their role.[1,3] Additional factors that may be involved in the development of thrombophlebitis are altered function of the coagulation system leading to a hypercoagulable state and the development of the syndrome of disseminated intravascular coagulation (DIC).[1–3,6]

Thrombophlebitis and phlebitis can be present as septic or nonseptic processes; however, the distinction may be difficult to make on clinical grounds as the predominant clinical signs are associated with inflammation regardless of aetiology. These clinical signs most often include pain, heat and swelling or drainage at the affected site, while fever, leukocytosis and hyperfibrinogenaemia may be present, especially if infection is present. Peripheral venous distension will be present if a thrombus is causing complete vascular obstruction. Cases involving both jugular veins may develop profound swelling of the head due to impaired venous drainage, potentially causing respiratory distress and necessitating placement of a tracheotomy.

Diagnosis

Monitoring for thrombophlebitis begins with daily palpation of intravenous catheter sites for heat or swelling (Figure 7.1). In some cases, the first sign of thrombophlebitis is the loss of patency of an intravenous catheter. This is especially true in the case of catheters of sufficient length that the tip of the catheter may not be present in the palpable portion of the catheterised vein, and a thrombus at the tip of the catheter is not detectable. If heat, swelling or catheter dysfunction is detected, then the area should be more thoroughly investigated using ultrasonography to examine the perivascular soft tissues and the vessel wall, as well as to assess whether any thrombus is present within the vascular lumen. Ultrasonographic examination is best performed using a high frequency probe (7.5–10 MHz) with a standoff to allow for detailed examination of the skin and subcutaneous region as well as the affected vessel. Distension of the affected region of the vein facilitates ultrasonographic assessment by increasing the vessel diameter and this can be accomplished by manual compression of the vein below the site. Failure of the vein to distend indicates that the vessel is no longer patent. The ultrasonographic appearance of phlebitis is characterised by thickening of the wall of the affected vessel, while a thrombus is typically characterized by a variably heterogenous area of increased echogenicity within the vessel lumen. The presence of cavitary areas of decreased echogenicity within the thrombus may be indicative of a septic process.[7] Sterile aspiration of cavitary lesions may yield a sample for culture and sensitivity testing,[7] but in the author's experience, it can be associated with clinical deterioration of the condition and is only used in cases poorly responsive to treatment. Septic thromboembolism can occur in association with thrombophlebitis, with vegetative endocarditis being perhaps the most common manifestation, and this should possibility be considered in cases with persistent fever, leukocytosis and/or hyperfibrinogenaemia.

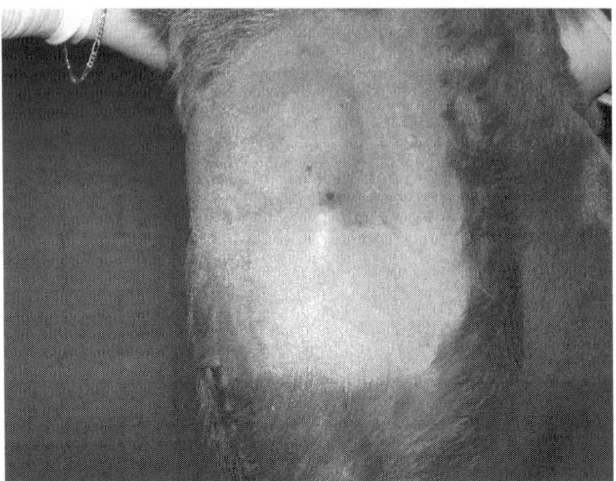

Figure 7.1 Jugular thrombophlebitis in the site of a previous indwelling intravenous catheter in a foal. ©Kevin Corley 2004.

Treatment

Suspicion of thrombophlebitis represents a clear indication for immediate removal of the intravenous catheter, if present. If infection is suspected then the catheter should be removed in a sterile manner and the tip of the catheter collected sterilely for culture and sensitivity testing. If the affected vein is a jugular vein, then one should avoid placing an intravenous catheter in the opposite jugular vein, due to the risk of bilateral jugular vein thrombosis. Treatment of phlebitis and thrombophlebitis relies heavily upon anti-inflammatory therapies, with both systemic nonsteroidals, such as phenylbutazone and flunixin meglumine, and topical anti-inflammatories, such as DMSO, being frequently used. Hot-packing of the affected area with a moist clean towel appears to be clinically beneficial and can be repeated several times daily. Systemic antimicrobial therapy is indicated if infection is suspected, and should ideally consist of drugs capable of penetrating into the thrombus. Staphylococcal infections are common, and it is reasonable to target this organism initially.[1] Highly lipophilic drugs, such as enrofloxacin, chloramphenicol, doxyxcycline and trimethoprim-sulpha, represent reasonable choices for initial therapy. Rifampin has been used by the author as an adjunctive antimicrobial due to its highly lipophilic nature and reported efficacy against staphylococcal organisms.[8,9] Rifampin cannot be used alone due to rapid development of resistance but can be used in combination with any of the listed antimicrobials to provide an enhanced antimicrobial effect.[8] Drainage is indicated if a large fluid pocket is detected ultrasonographically or is palpable just below the skin surface, and often requires only reopening of the catheter insertion site. Severe cases that are not responsive to medical treatment may require surgical resection of the affected segment of the jugular vein. With time, however, many cases will recanalise as the thrombus resolves, and normal venous drainage will be restored.[7]

Prevention

Minimisation of venipuncture in critically ill horses will aid in preventing thrombophlebitis, and sparing of the jugular vein in particular is helpful, as this preserves the jugulars for intravenous catheterisation. The facial venous plexus can be used as an alternative site for collection of blood samples (see Chapter 1.5), and this site appears less susceptible to thrombosis.[1] The use of minimally thrombogenic catheter materials is helpful in prevention, with polyutherane being best.[1] The type of catheter used may be helpful as well, with over-the-wire catheters being less traumatic to place and easier to maintain, especially in critically ill patients. Use of over-the-wire catheters is essential when utilising alternative sites for intravenous catheter placement, such as the lateral thoracic vein and the cephalic vein (see Chapter 1.15). When using Teflon catheters, the duration of catheterisation should be limited to 1 to 2 days, due to the irritant effects of these catheters on the vascular endothelium. The catheter insertion site should be kept clean and dry, and this can be aided by placing the area under a light bandage, but this should only be used in horses likely to lie down or otherwise soil the catheter site, as the bandage can interfere with careful monitoring of the site for heat, swelling, pain and discharge.

References

1. Divers TJ: Prevention and treatment of thrombosis, phlebitis, and laminitis in horses with gastrointestinal diseases. Vet Clin North Am Equine Pract 19:779-790, 2003
2. Dolente BA, Beech J, Lindborg S, et al.: Evaluation of risk factors for development of catheter-associated jugular thrombophlebitis in horses: 50 cases (1993-1998). J Am Vet Med Assoc 227:1134-1141, 2005
3. Lankveld DP, Ensink JM, van Dijk P, et al.: Factors influencing the occurrence of thrombophlebitis after post-surgical long-term intravenous catheterization of colic horses: a study of 38 cases. J Vet Med A Physiol Pathol Clin Med 48:545-552, 2001
4. Mair TS, Smith LJ: Survival and complication rates in 300 horses undergoing surgical treatment of colic. Part 2: short-term complications. Equine Vet J 37:303-309, 2005
5. Traub-Dargatz JL, Dargatz DA: A retrospective study of vein thrombosis in horses treated with intravenous fluids in a veterinary teaching hospital. J Vet Intern Med 8:264-266, 1994
6. Morris DD: Thrombophlebitis in horses: the contribution of hemostatic dysfunction to pathogenesis. Compend Contin Educ Pract Vet 11:1386-1395, 1989
7. Gardner SY, Reef VB, Spencer PA: Ultrasonographic evaluation of horses with thrombophlebitis of the jugular vein: 46 cases (1985-1988). J Am Vet Med Assoc 199:370-373, 1991
8. Clumeck N, Marcelis L, Amiri-Lamraski MH, et al.: Treatment of severe staphylococcal infections with a rifampicin-minocycline association. J Antimicrob Chemother 13(Suppl C):17-22, 1984
9. Lilenbaum W, Veras M, Blum E, et al.: Antimicrobial susceptibility of staphylococci isolated from otitis externa in dogs. Lett Appl Microbiol 31:42-45, 2000

7.3 Inappetence

Bettina Dunkel

Inappetence is a common and particularly frustrating problem in hospitalised horses. The exact cause remains obscure in the majority of these cases. The condition is most likely the result of a combination of unfamiliar environment and feed, systemic effects of the primary disease process, infection, pain, fever and depressed mentation. The inappetant patient is easily identified by close observation and recording of the amount of feed consumed (weighing or measuring the amount of grain/complete feed and hay offered and the amount left in the stall).

Investigation

A thorough clinical and oral examination is necessary to rule out a mechanical inability to prehend, chew and swallow or inappetence due to pain associated with eating. Examples of reduced ability to eat include neurological deficits, dental disease, oral and oesophageal ulcerations or wounds in the oral cavity. Once a mechanical reason is excluded, inappetence is addressed by reducing or excluding any other features potentially contributing to the anorexia of the patient. The history obtained on admission should include the exact type of feed used, the amount and frequency of feeding and any known feed preferences of the individual horse. The information can be recorded on a feed card in front of the stall door, obvious to the personnel feeding, allowing them to mimic the home feeding schedule as closely as possible. Asking owners to provide some of their own feed can also help.

Hyperlipaemia and hyperlipidaemia are important causes of inappetence in hospitalised horses and are discussed in Chapter 7.5. Measurement of serum triglycerides should be part of the workup of inappetence, especially when accompanied by depression and there is a history of a negative energy balance.

The importance of adequate pain control and its effects on feed intake and weight gain have been reported in horses and other animals.[1-4] A constant rate infusion of butorphanol in addition to flunixin meglumine improved behavioural score and decreased weight loss in horses after exploratory celiotomy.[2] Unfortunately, recognition of pain is difficult and subjective, with signs of pain being largely unspecific. Behavioural scores and heart rate may be used clinically as indicators of pain,[5] but often more subtle changes in behaviour remain unnoticed by a person not familiar with the individual horse.[6] Sometimes a trial of different or additional analgesia (see Chapter 6.2) and observation for subsequent changes in behavior and appetite are most revealing.

Anorexia of infection is part of the acute-phase response and is thought to be initially beneficial, while chronic anorexia has devastating effects by compromising host defense and delaying recovery.[7] Although the exact mechanisms have not been fully elucidated, multiple peripherally and centrally produced proinflammatory cytokines play an important role in promoting lack of appetite. Due to the complex and reciprocal nature of the cytokine response involved, blockage of individual cytokines has produced mixed results at best.[7] For the veterinary patient, treatment of the primary disease and nutritional support therefore remain momentarily the best therapeutic approach.

High fever and anorexia frequently occur together. Although a low to moderate fever in itself does not require treatment, it can contribute to decreased feed intake. Antipyretic drugs may encourage appetite in those cases and can be used as needed.

Exercise in form of turn-out in a paddock, frequent hand walks and grazing increases the spirits of some patients remarkably and anecdotally stimulates appetite and gastrointestinal function.

Treatment

Once these possible causes of anorexia have been addressed, there is, unfortunately, little else that can increase the appetite of an anorectic horse. Offering a variety of feeds and different hay types, such as oats, complete feed, a high protein grain, beet pulp, grass and alfalfa hay, may be tried. It is worthwhile to offer feeds repeatedly as some horses change their preference on a daily basis, but success is frequently limited to less-affected patients.

Fresh grass can be an amazing appetite stimulant and is sometimes accepted when any other feed is refused. The caloric content of small amounts of grass is minimal, and additional supplementation is absolutely essential. If the appetite does not improve within 1 to 3 days, depending on the body condition of the horse, enteral or parenteral nutritional support should be instituted (see Chapter 5).

Unwillingness to drink may accompany inappetence and is described in Chapter 7.4.

References

1. Liles JH, Flecknell PA, Roughan J, et al.: Influence of oral buprenorphine, oral naltrexone or morphine on the effects of laparotomy in the rat. Lab Anim 32:149-161, 1998
2. Sellon DC, Roberts MC, Blikslager AT, et al.: Effects of continuous rate intravenous infusion of butorphanol on physiologic and outcome variables in horses after celiotomy. J Vet Intern Med 18:555-563, 2004
3. Zulauf M, Gutzwiller A, Steiner A, et al.: The effect of a pain medication in bloodless castration of male calves on the concentrated feed intake, weight gain and serum cortisol level. Schweiz Arch Tierheilkd 145:283-290, 2003
4. Malavasi LM, Nyman G, Augustsson H, et al.: Effects of epidural morphine and transdermal fentanyl analgesia on physiology and behaviour after abdominal surgery in pigs. Lab Anim 40:16-27, 2006
5. Pritchett L, Ulibarri, C, Roberts, MC, et al.: Identification of potential physiological and behavioral indicators of postoperative pain in horses after exploratory celiotomy. Appl Anim Behav Sci 80:31-43, 2003
6. Ashley FH, Waterman-Pearson AE, Whay HR: Behavioural assessment of pain in horses and donkeys: application to clinical practice and future studies. Equine Vet J 37:565-575, 2005
7. Langhans W: Anorexia of infection: current prospects. Nutrition 16:996-1005, 2000

7.4 Unwillingness to drink

Harold C. McKenzie III

Occasionally, one will encounter patients that are unwilling to consume water while hospitalised. The first distinction to be made is whether this represents a functional inability or a true reluctance to drink. If the horse has demonstrated the ability to normally prehend, masticate and swallow food, then it is unlikely that it is unable to drink. If the horse is unwilling to eat or drink, or if it is unclear whether the horse is capable of ingesting food or water, then further investigation will be required. Manual and visual examination of the oral cavity and tongue will allow for assessment of potential neurological dysfunction, oral ulceration, oral foreign bodies, severe dental abnormalities or musculoskeletal abnormalities such as a mandibular fracture that might interfere with drinking or result in pain associated with drinking. Care should be taken when applying an oral speculum to a horse with any possibility of a mandibular fracture, as this may result in fracture displacement. If no oral abnormalities are identified, then upper respiratory endoscopy is indicated to determine if laryngeal or pharyngeal dysfunction is present that may be associated with dysphagia, or if severe inflammation or foreign bodies are present. Infusing a small amount of water (20–30 ml) through the biopsy channel of the endoscope will allow for the assessment of pharyngeal function, as the animal should respond to this stimulus by swallowing within a few seconds. This swallow response should result in the complete closure of the glottis and the pharyngeal space and clearing of the infused water from the pharynx. If the response is delayed or incomplete, then neurological dysfunction (dysphagia) may be present. Oesophagoscopy is also indicated, in order to rule out oesophageal foreign bodies and oesophageal ulceration.

If the horse is not drinking water while receiving intravenous fluid supplementation, it is likely that the individual is fluid replete and has no need to consume water. However, some individuals may simply be unwilling to drink from containers different from those used in the home farm environment or will not accept the water offered in the hospital environment. These issues can be addressed by requesting that the owner provide the hospital with the horse's accustomed water container and water from the farm. Alternatively, the horse's water can be flavoured to try and improve palatability, using apple juice, other fruit juices, commercially available electrolyte powders or powdered human sports drink mix. A "water buffet" can be set up, with two or three different solutions offered, to increase the likelihood that the horse will select one preferentially. Thirst may also be stimulated by oral dosing of small amounts of table salt (30–60 g NaCl for an adult horse) as a paste every 8 to 24 hours. If voluntary intake is not forthcoming, consideration should be given to placing a small bore (18 Fr × 250 cm) nasogastric feeding tube*, which can remain in place for ongoing fluid delivery, without impairing the horse's ability to eat or to drink if interest returns. Long-term unwillingness to drink is extremely unusual, and if encountered may require that the horse undergo one or more 6- to 12-hour periods of water deprivation to stimulate drinking. This should only be done in patients that are clinically stable and that exhibit no evidence of renal impairment, to avoid the possibility of the development of severe dehydration.

7.5 Hyperlipaemia

Bettina Dunkel

Pathophysiology of hyperlipaemia and hyperlipidaemia

Hyperlipaemia and *hyperlipidaemia* describe an increased amount of lipids in the bloodstream, while *hypertriglyceridaemia* refers to an increased serum concentration of triglycerides. Serum triglycerides are the most commonly routinely measured fraction of lipids in equine medicine, and their serum concentration is used to differentiate milder increases, frequently referred to as hyperlipidaemia, from the more severe, potentially life-threatening hyperlipaemia (serum triglycerides >5.65 mmol/L [500 mg/dl]).[1,2] Increases in triglycerides, free fatty acids (FFAs) and very low density lipoproteins (VLDLs) can be observed in healthy fasting horses and ponies as peripheral fat reserves are mobilised for energy generation.[2–4] Triglycerides stored in adipose tissue are broken down into FFAs and glycerol in a process regulated in part by the insulin responsive enzyme hormone sensitive lipase and are transported via the bloodstream to the liver. In the hepatic tissue, triglycerides are re-esterified and released into the systemic circulation in form of VLDLs to be transported to and utilised by the peripheral tissues. Uptake in the periphery is regulated by the enzyme lipoprotein lipase. If disease or additional stress is superimposed on starvation, the natural response can become uncontrolled, resulting in excessive breakdown of fat and release of VLDLs from the liver.[4]

* NG18100; MILA International, Florence, KY, USA.

Overproduction and defective clearance of VLDLs have both been suggested as potential reasons for the accumulation of lipids in the blood of equids.[3,5] As activities of lipoprotein lipase and hepatic lipase, the enzymes responsible for catabolism of VLDLs, are increased in naturally occurring equine hyperlipaemia, the former is currently the more plausible explanation.[5]

Clinical signs and diagnosis

Clinical signs of hyperlipaemia are unspecific and difficult to differentiate from signs associated with a primary disease process. Inappetence, lethargy and depression are the most commonly reported.[5–8] Opaque discolouration of the plasma is considered the classic sign of hyperlipaemia, and is obvious when present.[8] In severe cases, lipid deposition in liver, kidney and other organs may result in compromised organ function or even hepatic rupture.[7] Diagnosis relies on determination of serum triglyceride concentrations. Hyperlipaemia is diagnosed with a serum triglyceride concentration greater than 5.65 mmol/L (>500 mg/dl). Hyperlipidaemia is a serum triglyceride concentration above the normal range but less than this value. The absence of plasma opacity does not indicate normal triglyceride levels. In horses (as opposed to ponies) in particular, a significant increase in triglycerides may be present without visible changes in the plasma.[9]

Differences between horses, ponies and donkeys

There are large interindividual differences in the magnitude of the response and inherent differences between horses on one hand and ponies, Miniature horses and donkeys on the other.[2–4,6] The latter group is predisposed to the condition and is negatively affected by feed deprivation much more readily than horses.[10] Triglyceride values for fasted healthy horses are lower compared to those of healthy fasted ponies and donkeys.[2,3,11] In ponies and donkeys, severe, sometimes life-threatening hyperlipaemia can occur without an obvious underlying disease process, a condition termed *primary hyperlipaemia*.[7,10–12] Hyperlipaemia during disease is also more common and more dramatic in ponies, Miniature horses and donkeys.[6,10–12] Compared to horses, normal ponies show a mildly impaired glucose tolerance and less sensitivity to insulin following an oral glucose challenge, and a degree of insulin resistance was found in healthy ponies using a glucose clamp technique.[13] The effect is even more pronounced in obese and laminitic ponies and may play a role in the development of hyperlipaemia.[14] A reduction in tissue sensitivity to the glucoregulatory action of insulin during fasting and a positive correlation between plasma insulin and triglyceride concentration in naturally occurring hyperlipaemia has been documented in donkeys.[11,15] Following *in vitro* stimulation of pony adipocytes with norepinephrine, FFAs are released in a linear fashion, an effect not observed in horses, further supporting the hypothesis that differences in fat and glucose metabolism contribute to the observed breed differences.[16] Nevertheless, significant increases in serum triglycerides also occur in horses. The values remain relatively low with simple starvation or following withholding of feed after abdominal surgery but can increase more dramatically with severe systemic diseases.[2,9,17–19] Primary hyperlipaemia has, to the author's knowledge, not been reported in adult horses. The classic opaque plasma may not be evident, and measurement of triglycerides is necessary to accurately identify affected horses.[9] Predisposing factors for development of hypertriglyceridaemia in horses are not known, but azotaemia[2,10] and increased levels of circulating proinflammatory cytokines have been suggested[6,9] as increased triglyceride levels are associated with chronic renal failure and inflammatory conditions in human medicine.[20–22]

Treatment

The most effective treatment is resolution of any underlying disease process and establishment of a positive energy balance. Most patients are inappetant and will not consume sufficient amounts of calories voluntarily. In these cases, enteral or parenteral nutritional support is essential. In horses with mild to moderate hyperlipaemia, a glucose or dextrose infusion at 1 to 2 mg/kg/min (0.15–0.25 ml/kg/hr of a 50% glucose or 50% dextrose solution) providing 5 to 10 kcal/kg/day may be sufficient. Ponies, Miniature horses and donkeys may require more aggressive support, including tube feeding or parenteral nutrition containing amino acids, in addition to glucose or dextrose. Guidelines for enteral and parenteral nutrition are given in Chapter 5. Enteral liquid diets have been used successfully in the treatment of hyperlipaemia in the latter group.[6,23] Insulin and heparin have been suggested as adjacent therapies—insulin for its inhibitory effects on hormone-sensitive lipase and heparin as an activator of peripheral lipoprotein lipase; none of these treatments have been proved to improve outcome above providing a positive energy balance alone. Insulin is useful in horses and ponies with difficulties controlling their blood glucose levels and can be given as injection or as a constant rate infusion.[6,24] Triglyceride levels should be monitored on a daily basis until returned to normal limits to ensure the success of therapy.

References

1. Jeffcott LB, Field JR: Current concepts of hyperlipaemia in horses and ponies. Vet Rec 116:461-466, 1985
2. Naylor JM, Kronfeld DS, Acland H: Hyperlipemia in horses: effects of undernutrition and disease. Am J Vet Res 41:899-905, 1980
3. Bauer JE: Plasma lipids and lipoproteins of fasted ponies. Am J Vet Res 44:379-384, 1983
4. Frank N, Sojka JE, Latour MA: Effect of withholding feed on concentration and composition of plasma very low density lipoprotein and serum nonesterified fatty acids in horses. Am J Vet Res 63:1018-1021, 2002
5. Watson TD, Burns L, Love S, et al.: Plasma lipids, lipoproteins and post-heparin lipases in ponies with hyperlipaemia. Equine Vet J 24:341-346, 1992
6. Moore BR, Abood SK, Hinchcliff KW: Hyperlipemia in 9 miniature horses and miniature donkeys. J Vet Intern Med 8:376-381, 1994
7. Gay CC, Sullivan ND, Wilkinson JS, et al.: Hyperlipaemia in ponies. Aust Vet J 54:459-462, 1978
8. Schotman AJ, Wagenaar G: Hyperlipemia in ponies. Zentralbl Veterinarmed A 16:1-7, 1969
9. Dunkel B, McKenzie HC 3rd: Severe hypertriglyceridaemia in clinically ill horses: diagnosis, treatment and outcome. Equine Vet J 35:590-595, 2003
10. Watson TD, Murphy D, Love S: Equine hyperlipaemia in the United Kingdom: clinical features and blood biochemistry of 18 cases. Vet Rec 131:48-51, 1992
11. Forhead AJ, French J, Ikin P, et al.: Relationship between plasma insulin and triglyceride concentrations in hypertriglyceridaemic donkeys. Res Vet Sci 56:389-392, 1994
12. Mogg TD, Palmer JE: Hyperlipidemia, hyperlipemia, and hepatic lipidosis in American miniature horses: 23 cases (1990-1994). J Am Vet Med Assoc 207:604-607, 1995
13. Rijnen KE, van der Kolk JH: Determination of reference range values indicative of glucose metabolism and insulin resistance by use of glucose clamp techniques in horses and ponies. Am J Vet Res 64:1260-1264, 2003
14. Jeffcott LB, Field JR, McLean JG, et al.: Glucose tolerance and insulin sensitivity in ponies and Standardbred horses. Equine Vet J 18:97-101, 1986
15. Forhead AJ, Dobson H: Plasma glucose and cortisol responses to exogenous insulin in fasted donkeys. Res Vet Sci 62:265-269, 1997
16. Breidenbach A, Fuhrmann H, Deegen E, et al.: Studies on equine lipid metabolism. 2. Lipolytic activities of plasma and tissue lipases in large horses and ponies. Zentralbl Veterinarmed A 46:39-48, 1999
17. Durham AE, Phillips TJ, Walmsley JP, et al.: Nutritional and clinicopathological effects of post operative parenteral nutrition following small intestinal resection and anastomosis in the mature horse. Equine Vet J 36:390-396, 2004
18. Murray M: Hepatic-lipidosis in a post parturient mare. Equine Vet J 17:68-69, 1985
19. Field JR: Hyperlipemia in a quarter horse. Comp Cont Educ pract vet 10:218-221, 1988
20. Vaziri ND: Dyslipidemia of chronic renal failure: the nature, mechanisms, and potential consequences. Am J Physiol Renal Physiol 290:F262-F272, 2006
21. Esteve E, Ricart W, Fernandez-Real JM: Dyslipidemia and inflammation: an evolutionary conserved mechanism. Clin Nutr 24:16-31, 2005
22. Feingold KR, Grunfeld C: Role of cytokines in inducing hyperlipidemia. Diabetes 41 Suppl 2:97-101, 1992
23. Hallebeek JM, Beynen AC: A preliminary report on a fat-free diet formula for nasogastric enteral administration as treatment for hyperlipaemia in ponies. Vet Q 23:201-205, 2001
24. Lopes MA, White NA 2nd: Parenteral nutrition for horses with gastrointestinal disease: a retrospective study of 79 cases. Equine Vet J 34:250-257, 2002

8

Monitoring and treating the coagulation system

8.1 Monitoring the coagulation system
8.2 Management of horses with coagulopathies

8.1 Monitoring the coagulation system

Luis Monreal

Dysfunctions of the coagulation system can become an important complication in hospitalised horses due to the close relationship of this system with inflammation, vascular integrity (endothelium and platelets) and liver function. In addition, the coagulation system can be easily activated by common aggressions such as surgery, trauma, infections or tissue necrosis. Therefore, haemostatic dysfunctions may develop in many hospitalised horses, especially in intensive care patients, and they may significantly contribute to poor outcomes and high mortality rates.

From a clinical standpoint, coagulopathies should be grouped according to two main pathophysiological processes:

- Excessive activation of the coagulation system causing hypercoagulable states
- Deficient activation of the coagulation system causing hypocoagulable states

Coagulopathies caused by an excessive activation of the coagulation system (hypercoagulable state)

Activation of the coagulation system occurs in both physiological and pathological conditions in people and animals. Activation of haemostasis is normally compensated by a proportional increase in the activity of the coagulation inhibitory systems (antithrombin III [AT-III], protein C and the fibrinolytic system).[1,2] When coagulation is activated, the coagulation inhibitors act to avoid fibrin formation, fibrin deposition in the microvasculature and subsequent impairment of the tissue blood supply (compensated hypercoagulation). However, in severe pathological conditions, a marked activation of coagulation may occur without a corresponding inhibitory response, and uncompensated situations may arise causing increased predisposition to thrombosis or excessive thrombus formation.[3–7]

In all these situations, clinical management should be focused on (1) early recognition of patients with identified at-risk diseases, (2) laboratory confirmation of the prothrombotic state and (3) establishment of prophylactic measures to reduce the ongoing excessive activation of coagulation before an uncompensated situation arises.

The haemostatic disorders most often diagnosed in hospitalised horses due to an excessive activation of the coagulation system are:

1. Disseminated intravascular coagulation (DIC)
2. Jugular thrombophlebitis
3. Other thrombotic events

Disseminated intravascular coagulation

DIC is the most frequently diagnosed haemostatic dysfunction in hospitalised horses, and the one most associated with mortality. DIC is characterised by a severe, systemic hypercoagulable state, which can lead to massive fibrin and microthrombi formation and deposition in different tissues.[3,5] This severe prothrombotic situation can be partially controlled by the coagulation inhibitors (AT-III, protein C) and the fibrinolytic system (compensated DIC) or not (uncompensated DIC).[3,5]

Clinical forms of disseminated intravascular coagulation

There are three main clinical forms of DIC. Which one arises depends on the intensity and duration of the prothrombotic stimulus and on the efficacy of the inhibitors.

Compensated/subclinical form of DIC

In this situation, activation of the coagulation system is strong, but the amount of fibrin formed is well controlled by the coagulation inhibitors and the proportional increase in fibrinolytic activity. No clinical signs are observed, but patients show an increased predisposition to thrombosis. In these cases, diagnosis can be reached when specific markers of coagulation (e.g., thrombin—AT-III [TAT] complexes, fibrin monomers) and fibrinolysis (e.g., D-dimers) indicate the existence of a hypercoagulable and a hyperfibrinolytic state.[8–10] In addition, the coagulation profile might reveal mild changes (e.g., prolonged clotting times) consistent with a mild consumption of coagulation factors.[10]

Bleeding form of DIC
In this form, the activation of the coagulation system is stronger and/or prolonged in time. It is most often described in cases of inflammatory gastrointestinal disorders or disseminated neoplasms.[11] The high amounts of fibrin formed and the elongated formation time cause depletion of platelets, coagulation factors and coagulation inhibitors. The severe consumption of coagulation factors promotes a secondary hypocoagulable state, which causes prolonged bleeding or spontaneous haemorrhagic diatheses (Figure 8.1).

In both the compensated and bleeding forms, the coagulation disorder is clinically recognised when bleeding occurs, although it may be erroneously associated with a primary hypocoagulable disorder.

This form of DIC can be confirmed by identification of the primary disease and performance of a clotting profile. The clotting profile will show changes consistent with platelet, coagulation factor and coagulation inhibitor consumption. Mortality can be very high in these cases, because the coagulation disorder is frequently associated with primary diseases difficult to resolve, and because of the profuse bleeding that affected animals may show.

Multiorgan failure form of DIC
When there is an exaggerated activation of the coagulation system in a very short period of time (such as it occurs in cases of gastrointestinal ischaemia), the huge amount of fibrin formed in the microvasculature leads to a severe tissue hypoperfusion and subsequent multiorgan failure syndrome (MOFS), with clinical signs of shock, renal failure, hypoxia, colic, cardiac dysrhythmias, and death.[11–14] MOFS is often underdiagnosed due to the difficulty in identifying these signs as a clinical form of a coagulation disorder.

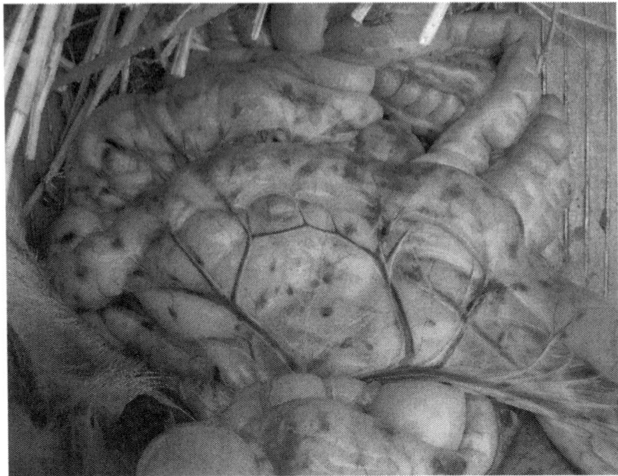

Figure 8.1. Post-mortem of a foal with the bleeding form of disseminated intravascular coagulation (DIC). There are ecchymotic haemorrhages across the gastrointestinal tract. ©Kevin Corley 2004.

In the MOFS form of DIC, laboratory testing easily confirms the marked hypercoagulable state with or without a proportional increase in the fibrinolytic activity. Laboratory abnormalities consistent with MOFS can also be found (e.g., an increase in plasma creatinine and blood urea nitrogen). The rapid and severe development of DIC causes a very high mortality rate. Detection of the preliminary forms in patients at risk is important in order to prevent the development of MOFS.

Patients at risk of disseminated intravascular coagulation
The diagnoses associated with an increased risk of DIC are given in Box 8.1.[4–6,11,12,15–18]

Other clinical situations that have also been identified as causes or predisposing factors for thrombotic disorders in human medicine are some surgical procedures, especially those related to abdominal, traumatic and orthopaedic problems. This has not yet been confirmed in horses.

Coagulation testing profile to diagnose hypercoagulability and disseminated intravascular coagulation
In all forms of DIC, the marked activation of coagulation cascade causes a rapid consumption of platelets, clotting factors and coagulation inhibitors (AT-III, protein C). At the same time, large amounts of fibrin degradation products (FDPs) (D-dimers) are produced as a result of the consequent enhancement in fibrinolytic activity. Therefore, DIC is confirmed in a patient at risk when at least three of the following laboratory abnormalities are present: thrombocytopenia, prolonged clotting times, decreased fibrinogen and coagulation inhibitor activity and increased fibrinolytic products.[11] However, this traditional criterion is not specific enough, as these alterations can also be found in other coagulopathies due to hypocoagulable states (e.g., hepatic disease).[7] To avoid misdiagnoses, new laboratory markers of hypercoagulation have been developed recently, but many of them are not available in emergency settings. A sensitive marker of hypercoagulation and

Box 8.1. Primary diagnoses associated with an increased risk of disseminated intravascular coagulation

- Colic with ischaemic gastrointestinal injury
- Intestinal inflammatory disorder and protein-losing enteropathy
- Endotoxaemia
- Septicaemia and other severe septic disorders
- Disseminated neoplasia (e.g., melanosarcoma, etc.)
- Severe haemolytic disease
- Obstetrical disorder
- Others: trauma, heat stroke, burns, acute renal failure

Box 8.2. Laboratory tests to diagnose disseminated intravascular coagulation

- Platelet count (<100 × 10^9/L; <100,000/μl)
- Clotting times (PT > 15 seconds, aPTT > 65 seconds)
- Plasma D-dimer concentration (>500 ng/ml)
- Concentration of fibrin degradation products (FDPs > 40 μg/ml)
- Fibrinogen concentration (<1.3 g/L; 130 mg/dl)

The most reliable and sensitive parameters are prolonged clotting times, increased D-dimers, and decreased platelet count.

Box 8.3. Results of specialised laboratory tests to diagnose disseminated intravascular coagulation

- Decrease in coagulation inhibitor (antithrombin III, protein C) activities
- Increase in other markers of hypercoagulation, such as thrombin—antithrombin III (TAT) complexes, fibrin monomers, etc. Determination of these constitutes the most sensitive test to confirm the subclinical form of disseminated intravascular coagulation.
- Increase in other markers of fibrinolysis, such as plasmin-antiplasmin (PAP) complexes
- Increase in markers of platelet activation

hyperfibrinolysis that can be easily performed in clinical settings is the determination of plasma D-dimer concentration.[19–21] A definitive diagnosis of DIC can be easily made in any hospital setting by determination of the parameters given in Box 8.2.[1,4,5,7,11,12,22,23] Other sensitive laboratory findings are given in Box 8.3. However, these determinations can only be performed in special laboratory settings.

Clinical considerations

Diagnosis of DIC (subclinical, bleeding or MOFS forms) requires clinicians to be aware of its occurrence in patients at risk and the presence of laboratory findings consistent with a coagulation consumption.[1,5,7] Patients at risk of DIC should be monitored in order to detect animals with preliminary and subclinical forms of DIC. In these patients, prophylactic therapy with LMWH for 3 to 4 days is advised to reduce the likelihood of progression to clinical DIC.[24] It has been demonstrated that most horses with ischaemic colic, septicaemia, endotoxaemia and enteritis have coagulation profiles consistent with marked hypercoagulable states.[10,19–21] In addition, DIC has been confirmed in these animals by post-mortem examination findings, which included presence of fibrin deposits in the endothelia of several tissues.[25] All surgical colic horses should receive thromboprophylaxis for a few days.[24]

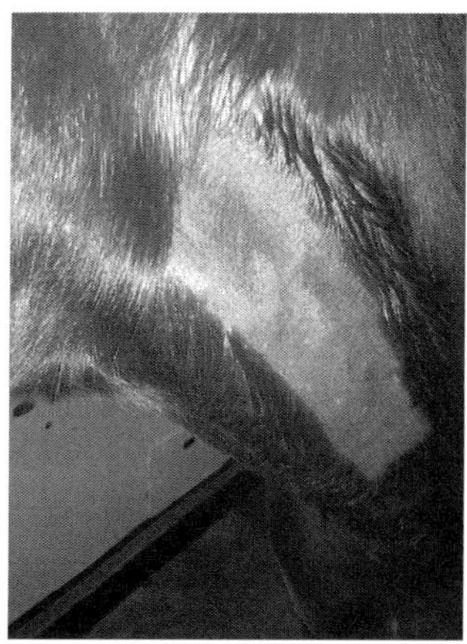

Figure 8.2. Jugular thrombophlebitis in a horse with colitis, secondary to presumed endotoxaemia. ©Kevin Corley 2004.

Box 8.4. Factors reported to be associated with thrombophlebitis

- **Presence of a hypercoagulable state**
  The use of catheters and/or continuous venipuncture for blood sampling in horses with hypercoagulability are the main clinical procedures that induce thrombophlebitis.[27] Patients at risk of excessive activation of the coagulation cascade have a higher incidence of thrombophlebitis.[11,26]

- **Catheter**
  Daily care, material, size and length of the catheter are factors that influence the risk of endothelial damage and subsequent thrombus formation. Polyurethane and silicone catheters are the least thrombogenic.[28,29] On the other hand, long catheters are associated with less complications than are short catheters.

- **Fluids or drugs infused through the catheter**
  Infusion of solutions with nonphysiological pH or osmolality, such as hypertonic solutions, some anaesthetic drugs, etc., predispose to endothelial damage and thrombus formation.[27,29,30]

Jugular thrombophlebitis

Thrombophlebitis is also a frequent problem in hospitalised horses (see Chapter 7.2). This is not only because placement of venous catheters and repeated venipunctures are common in these animals but also because hypercoagulable states may trigger the problem. Thus, horses at risk of DIC (see Box 8.1) are also prone to develop thrombophlebitis[11,26] (Figure 8.2). The factors reported to be associated with thrombophlebitis in horses with a venous catheter are given in Box 8.4.

Clinical considerations

The measures to reduce the incidence of jugular thrombophlebitis are (1) to control the hypercoagulable state with antithrombotics, (2) to minimise venous damage with adequate catheter placement and reduction of venipunctures, (3) to use the less thrombogenic catheter materials, appropriate bores and lengths, (4) to perform special daily catheter care (flushing generously with heparinised saline every 6 hours) and (5) to slowly infuse thrombogenic solutions/drugs in order to decrease their blood concentration at the catheter tip and to minimise endothelial damage. When these clinical measures are taken, the incidence of thrombophlebitis is significantly reduced.

Other reported thrombotic events

Other thrombotic insults have been sporadically diagnosed in neonates or mature horses, but they are rare. These include thrombosis of limb arteries,[31,32] pulmonary thromboembolism following orthopaedic surgery,[33,34] aortoiliac thrombosis,[35,36] congenital deficiency of coagulation inhibitors (protein C)[37] and others.

Coagulopathies caused by a deficient activation of the coagulation system (hypocoagulable state)

These coagulation disorders are characterised by a deficiency in coagulation and a haemorrhagic syndrome, which causes prolonged bleeding following wounds, surgery, venipuncture, or spontaneous bleeding. Hypocoagulable states are less frequently observed in hospitalised horses than hypercoagulable states. However, they are easily detected because prolonged bleeding is commonly viewed as a haemostatic disorder.

The hypocoagulable disorders that can be observed in hospitalised horses are

1. Due to a haemostatic defect
2. Due to a consumption of coagulation factors

Coagulopathies due to an haemostatic defect

Vasculitis

Vasculitis is manifested by petechiation in mucous membranes and subcutaneous oedema.

Vasculitis in these horses is mainly related to an immune-mediated reaction that may appear a few weeks after viral or bacterial respiratory infections (e.g., *Streptococcus equi*, *Rhodococcus equi* infections), although it may also occur with septicaemia, endotoxaemia and equine viral arteritis.[38] The coagulation profile and platelet count are frequently normal or mildly altered in these animals.

Thrombocytopenia

Several diseases may cause a decrease in platelet count ($<100 \times 10^9$/L; 100,000/μl), but clinical signs related to thrombocytopenia, such as petechial and ecchymotic haemorrhages of the mucous membranes, epistaxis, haematuria and other spontaneous bleeding signs, are usually only evident with a severe reduction in platelet count ($<30 \times 10^9$/L; 30,000/μl).[39]

Mild to moderate degrees of thrombocytopenia are mainly caused by hypercoagulation and platelet consumption, but the most severe forms of thrombocytopenia observed in neonates or adult horses (in some cases, platelet count may fall below 10,000/μl) usually result from immune-mediated platelet destruction, secondary to bacterial or viral infections, neoplasia or vasculitis[39,40] (Figure 8.3). Other possible causes of thrombocytopenia have included bone marrow disease, infectious diseases (e.g., equine infectious anaemia) that cause increased platelet destruction and other rare situations.[41,42]

Laboratory diagnosis can be easily achieved when a reduced platelet count is observed and there are no other alterations in the coagulation profile. However, care should be taken when using EDTA anticoagulant, which can cause an *ex vivo* pseudothrombocytopenia and may lead to false diagnoses.[43] Iatrogenic causes of thrombocytopenia are given in Box 8.5.

Vitamin K deficiency

Although uncommon in horses, a hypocoagulable state with a bleeding tendency due to coumarin or warfarin toxicosis or chronic intestinal malabsorption could occur. In these cases, presence of prolonged clotting times (prothrombin time [PT], activated partial thromboplastin time [aPTT]) in patients that are not at risk of DIC supports the diagnosis of vitamin K deficiency.[42]

Hepatopathies

Liver diseases might produce a hypocoagulable state due to decreased production of coagulation factors.[42] However, liver damage must be very severe to cause coagulation failure.

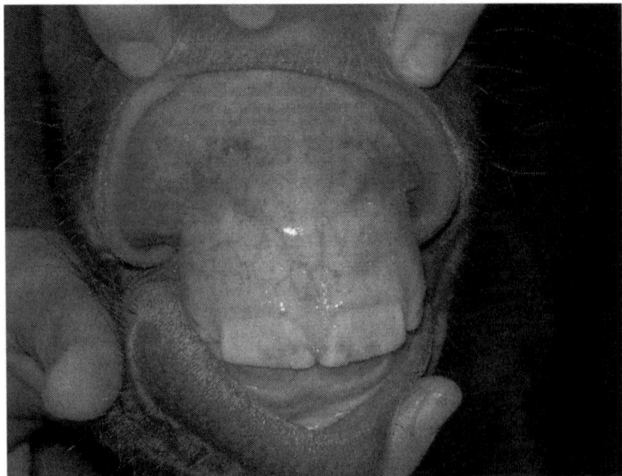

Figure 8.3. Petechial haemorrhages in the oral mucous membranes of a 2-month-old foal that presented with a severe pneumonia (*Streptococcus equi zooepidemicus* and *Pasteurella*) and thrombocytopenia (12×10^9/L; 12,000/μl). This progressed to a decreasing platelet count (8×10^9/L; 8000/μl), anemia (packed cell volume 12%) and spontaneous bleeding. The foal was treated with antibiotics, whole blood transfusion and NSAIDs, and responded well. ©Luis Monreal 2007.

Box 8.5. Iatrogenic causes of thrombocytopenia

- **Administration of high doses of heparin** (therapeutic or higher) or other antithrombotic drugs may increase the risk of haemorrhage. In these cases, a prolonged thrombin time (TT) helps to confirm the diagnosis.
- **Administration of antiplatelet drugs** (e.g., aspirin) to surgical patients may promote a haemorrhagic syndrome. Prolonged template bleeding time or closure times (measured using a platelet function analyser, PFA-100*) are observed in these patients.[44,45]
- **The administration of fibrinolytic drugs** (e.g., t-PA, streptokinase) to reduce fibrin formation and adhesions in joints and abdominal cavity has been recently proposed in horses due to their use in human medicine. No studies have been conducted in horses. However, clinical experience in people confirms that these drugs are not highly effective, and the associated risk of spontaneous bleeding can be very high.

*Dade-Behring (Siemens), Deerfield, IL, USA.

Inherited haemostatic disorders in young animals

Haemophilia A

(factor VIII deficiency) has been reported to occur in young Thoroughbred, Standardbred, Quarter Horse and Arabian males and can be confirmed when an abnormally prolonged aPTT is detected.[46,47]

Other very rare coagulation factor defects or platelet dysfunctions, such as **von Willebrand's disease**, **prekallikrein deficiency**, and others, have been reported in horses.[48–50]

Coagulopathies due to consumption of coagulation factors

After surgically or wound-induced profuse bleeding

The large amount of platelet and coagulation factors consumed after a profuse haemorrhage could lead to a temporary lack of coagulation components and a mild hypocoagulable state, which may cause further impairment in coagulation function and bleeding. Therefore, an impairment of the coagulation system function may be observed after some surgical procedures (e.g., upper respiratory surgeries), which can be confirmed by detecting a coagulation consumption profile (mild thrombocytopenia, prolonged clotting times, increased D-dimer concentration, decreased concentration of several coagulation factors).

Disseminated intravascular coagulation

Although DIC is associated with a hypercoagulable state, it can cause a secondary haemorrhagic syndrome, due to an excessive consumption of coagulation factors. The clinical management of these animals needs to be focused at decreasing the primary hypercoagulable state and at resolving the primary or underlying disease.

Laboratory tests to monitor coagulation system disorders

During the past years, many tests have been developed to improve the assessment of the coagulation system function in people and animals. Some of them have been demonstrated to have improved sensitivity in assessing activation of coagulation, and therefore to diagnose the hypercoagulable states. Others are useful to detect coagulation deficits or bleeding syndromes. Coagulation tests can be grouped by their availability in a clinical setting.

Initial coagulation profile: Useful tests for emergencies

The following are the most reliable and sensitive parameters that can be easily determined in emergency settings and allow a quick assessment of coagulation system function.

Platelet count

Platelet count is useful to detect thrombocytopenias due to consumption (DIC) or destruction/sequestration (e.g., immune mediated).[5] It is very easy to perform, and very reliable to monitor patients with petechiation in mucous membranes and bleeding problems. In patients at risk of DIC, a decreasing platelet count may indicate a hypercoagulable state, which should be confirmed by assessment of other clotting tests (e.g., clotting times and D-dimers as a DIC profile).[4,5,12,18,19]

Mean platelet component

This new platelet parameter determined by current CBC analysers is linearly related with platelet granularity and is reduced when platelets have undergone activation, as demonstrated in humans and small animals. In horses, mean platelet component (MPC) has been assessed, and its value significantly decreases in different conditions consistent with platelet activation.[51]

Clotting times (prothrombin time and activated partial thromboplastin time)

Prolonged clotting times can be observed in cases of marked haemostatic activation (hypercoagulation and DIC), but also in coagulation factor defects (inherited factor deficiencies, vitamin K deficiency, etc).[4,12] These tests are useful to diagnose coagulation disorders, but their specificity is low because they do not allow differentiation between hypercoagulable and hypocoagulable states.[5,7] Other clotting times (such as thrombin time [TT] and activated clotting time [ACT]) have been shown to be less accurate in the study of coagulation disorders.

Fibrinogen concentration

This parameter is commonly used to assess acute inflammatory response in horses. It may be decreased in cases of severe coagulation consumption (e.g., DIC).[4,5]

Fibrin degradation products/D-dimers
Measurement of FDPs using a polyclonal test has been used during many years to confirm an increase in fibrinolytic activity. However, elevated FDPs may result not only from increased fibrinolysis but also from increased fibrin formation.[4,7,19] On the other hand, the development of more sensitive and specific monoclonal tests (D-dimers by semi-quantitative and quantitative techniques) has improved the diagnosis of hypercoagulation, thrombotic disorders and DIC. In addition, these tests have been shown to be good prognostic indicators.[5,52,53] In human medicine, normal D-dimer plasma values confirm the absence of any prothrombotic condition, which means that the test has the highest negative predictive value (close to 100%).[19,54]

In prospective clinical studies, determination of plasma D-dimer concentrations has shown to be very sensitive and effective to detect hypercoagulation associated with gastro-intestinal insults in horses and with septicaemia in neonates.[20,21]

Template bleeding time
This has been used to detect functional platelet defects, especially inherited deficiencies and those induced by drugs.[44,55] However, as platelet inhibitory dysfunctions are rare in horses and the test has shown to have a low reproducibility, it is rarely performed.[56,57]

Closure time
A very simple platelet function analyser (PFA-100*) has recently been marketed to substitute measurement of bleeding time in human and veterinary emergency settings. It easily assesses platelet function *in vitro* by simulating platelet adhesion and aggregation phenomena after a vascular injury, and results are given in terms of closure times.[58]

It has been reported that it is more reliable and sensitive than bleeding time and its results are similar to those obtained by optical aggregometry to detect platelet aggregation dysfunctions (such as thrombocytopenia, thrombopathies and drug-induced platelet inhibition) in people and dogs.[59–62] Recently, its assessment has also been performed in horses.[45]

Markers not routinely available (to study haemostasis in depth)

There are other sensitive and reliable tests that are not easily determined in emergency settings but have been introduced in research studies and can be performed in specialised laboratories. The following are the most commonly reported.

Coagulation inhibitor activities (antithombin III, protein C)
A decrease in these inhibitors is associated with an increased risk of thrombosis and poor prognosis.[63,64] Monitoring their plasma levels is recommended in patients with DIC, because heparin therapy becomes ineffective when AT-III activity drops below 70%.

Markers of coagulation activity (TAT complexes, fibrin monomers, etc)
These markers have been shown to have a very high sensitivity to detect hypercoagulable states, not only in pathological but also in physiological situations (e.g., endurance exercise).[2,4,5,8–10,18]

Markers of fibrinolytic activity (tissue plasminogen activator [t-PA], plasminogen activator inhibitor [PAI], plasmin–[alpha]2-antiplasmin [PAP] complexes, plasminogen, FgDP, etc)
These markers have also been shown to have a very high sensitivity to assess fibrinolytic activity, not only in pathological but also in physiological situations.[8,65,66]

Measurement of coagulation factors
The measurement of specific coagulation proteins may better define an underlying coagulation defect.[67]

Aggregometry
This technique assesses the response of platelets to different agonists (thrombin, collagen, ADP, epinephrine), and it has been mainly used to study defects in platelet function for many years. Platelet activation has also been assessed using this technique. However, it requires the use of platelet-rich plasma, in which manipulation may induce an *ex vivo* activation.

In horses, many studies have been conducted using this technique to assess platelet function in different situations (endotoxaemia, during exercise, after drug administration, etc.).[68–75]

Flow cytometry
This technique is widely used to assess platelet function in human and veterinary medicine because it allows accurate quantification of circulating activated platelets, platelet–platelet aggregates and platelet–leukocyte aggregates. It is also used to study platelet activation processes through detection of platelet membrane glycoproteins and to determine procoagulant activity.[76–78] In fact, this is the technique currently recommended to assess platelet activation in depth.

In horses, it has shown to be very reliable to assess platelet activation during exercise and other clinical situations.[77–83]

Post-mortem detection of fibrin deposits
It has been recently studied that massive fibrin deposits formed in horses with DIC can be histologically detected

* Dade-Behring (Siemens), Deerfield, IL, USA.

in several tissues (lung, kidney, liver) using PTAH staining and immunohistochemistry methods.[25,84]

Other techniques

Other techniques, such as thromboelastography[85] and perfusion studies,[78] have also been proposed to assess the coagulation system. Finally, the upcoming laboratory tests to assess haemostasis in the near future seem to be centred on the measurement of sensitive markers of coagulation and fibrinolysis, as well as markers of endothelial and platelet activation.

Conclusion

Coagulation disorders are a frequent finding in hospitalised horses because excessive activation of the coagulation system occurs in many diseases. Horses in critical care units are especially prone to develop coagulation complications. These coagulopathies are characterised by being difficult to recognise, and they need proper monitoring. On the other hand, coagulopathies due to haemostatic defects that cause spontaneous bleeding may also occur, and these are very easily recognised and diagnosed.

A horse that suddenly shows a bleeding tendency may have a coagulation defect or a consumption coagulopathy secondary to a hypercoagulation state. These two situations should be well differentiated because management and therapy are completely different.

Finally, a very severe clinical form of MOFS should be taken into account in patients at risk of DIC. Clinicians do not commonly associate this form of DIC to a coagulopathy, and it should be diagnosed before fulminant DIC is established.

References

1. Darien BJ: Hypercoagulation: pathophysiology, diagnosis and treatment. Equine Vet Educ 5:37-40, 1993
2. Monreal L, Anglés A, Monreal M, et al.: Changes in haemostasis in endurance horses: detection by highly sensitive ELISA-tests. Equine Vet J Suppl 18:120-123, 1995
3. Schafer AI: The hypercoagulable states. Ann Intern Med 102:814-828, 1985
4. Monreal L, Anglés A, Espada Y, et al.: Hypercoagulation and hypofibrinolysis in horses with colic and DIC. Equine Vet J Suppl 32:19-25, 2000
5. Dallap BL: Coagulopathy in the equine critical care patient. Vet Clin North Am Equine Pract 20:231-251, 2004
6. Zbanyszek M, Procajlo A, Stopyra A, et al.: The coagulation system in horses with colic. Pol J Vet Sci 7:53-58, 2004
7. Smith SA: Update on diagnosis of disseminated intravascular coagulation. Proc ACVIM annual meeting, 2005
8. Asakura H, Jokaji H, Saito M, et al.: Study of the balance between coagulation and fibrinolysis in disseminated intravascular coagulation using molecular markers. Blood Coagul Fibrinol 5:829-832, 1994
9. Wada H, Wakita Y, Nakase T, et al.: Diagnosis of pre-disseminated intravascular coagulation stage with haemostatic molecular markers. Pol J Pharmacol 48:225-228, 1996
10. Feige K, Kastner SB, Dempfle CE, et al.: Changes in coagulation and markers of fibrinolysis in horses undergoing colic surgery. J Vet Med A 50:30-36, 2003
11. Morris DD: Recognition and management of disseminated intravascular coagulation in horses. Vet Clin North Am Equine Pract 4:115-143, 1988
12. Morris DD, Beech J: Disseminated intravascular coagulation in six horses. J Am Vet Med Assoc 183:1067-1072, 1983
13. Divers TJ, Whitlock RH, Byars TD, et al.: Acute renal failure in six horses resulting from haemodynamic causes. Equine Vet J 19:178-184, 1987
14. Guglick MA, MacAllister CG, Ewing PJ, et al.: Thrombosis resulting in rectal perforation in a horse. J Am Vet Med Assoc 209:1125-1127, 1996
15. Johnstone IB, Blackwell TE: Disseminated intravascular coagulation in a horse with postpartum ulcerative colitis and laminitis. Can Vet J 25:195-198, 1984
16. Prasse KW, Topper MJ, Moore JN, et al.: Analysis of haemostasis in horses with colic. J Am Vet Med Assoc 203:685-693, 1993
17. Barton MH, Morris DD, Norton N, et al.: Haemostatic and fibrinolytic indices in neonatal foals with presumed septicaemia. J Vet Intern Med 12:26-35, 1998
18. Dallap BL, Dolente B, Boston R: Coagulation profiles in 27 horses with large colon volvulus. J Vet Emerg Crit Care 13:215-225, 2003
19. Monreal L: D-dimer as a new test for the diagnosis of DIC and thromboembolic disease. J Vet Intern Med 17:757-759, 2003
20. Armengou L, Monreal L, Segura D, et al.: Plasma D-dimer concentration in sick newborn foals. J Vet Intern Med 22: 2008 (in press)
21. Armengou L, Monreal L, Segura D, et al.: Plasma D-dimers in horses with colic. Proc Equine Colic Res Symp, Quebec, Canada, 2005
22. Welch RD, Watkins JP, Taylor TS, et al.: Disseminated intravascular coagulation associated with colic in 23 horses (1984-1989). J Vet Intern Med 6:29-35, 1992
23. Kirby R, Rudloff E: Acquired coagulopathy VI: disseminated intravascular coagulation, in Feldman BF, Zinkl JG, Jain NC (eds): Veterinary hematology. Philadelphia, Lippincott Williams & Wilkins, 2000, pp 581-587
24. Feige K, Schwarzwald CC, Bombeli T: Comparison of unfractioned and low molecular weight heparin for prophylaxis of coagulopathies in 52 horses with colic: a randomised double-blind clinical trial. Equine Vet J 35:506-513, 2003
25. Cotovio M, Monreal L, Navarro M, et al.: Detection of fibrin deposits in tissues from horses with gastrointestinal disorders. J Vet Intern Med 21:308-313, 2007
26. Morris DD: Thrombophlebitis in horses: the contribution of haemostatic dysfunction to pathogenesis. Compend Contin Educ Pract Vet 11:1386-1394, 1989
27. Traub-Dargatz JL, Dargatz DA: A retrospective study of vein thrombosis in horses treated with intravenous fluids in a veterinary teaching hospital. J Vet Intern Med 8:264-266, 1994
28. Spurlock SL, Spurlock GH, Parker G, et al.: Long-term jugular vein catheterization in horses. J Am Vet Med Assoc 196:425-430, 1990
29. Hay CW: Equine intravenous catheterization. Equine Vet Educ 4:319-323, 1992

30. Dickson LR, Badcoe LM, Burbidge H, et al.: Jugular thrombophlebitis resulting from an anaesthetic induction technique in the horse. Equine Vet J 22:177-179, 1990
31. Triplett EA, O'Brien RT, Wilson DG, et al.: Thrombosis of the brachial artery in a foal. J Vet Intern Med 10:330-332, 1996
32. Brianceau P, Divers TJ: Acute thrombosis of limb arteries in horses with sepsis: five cases (1988-1998). Equine Vet J 33:105-109, 2001
33. Jones RS, Payne-Johnson CE, Seymour CJ: Pulmonary microembolism following orthopaedic surgery in a Thoroughbred gelding. Equine Vet J 19:382-384, 1987
34. Carr EA, Carlson GP, Wilson WD, et al.: Acute hemorrhagic pulmonary infarction and necrotizing pneumonia in horses: 21 cases (1967-1993). J Am Vet Med Assoc 210:1774-1778, 1997
35. Edwards GB, Allen WE: Aorto-iliac thrombosis in two horses: clinical course of the disease and use of real-time ultrasonography to confirm diagnosis. Equine Vet J 19:384-391, 1987
36. Barrelet A: Aorto-iliac thrombosis in a breeding stallion and an eventer mare. Equine Vet Educ 5:86-89, 1993
37. Edens LM, Morris DD, Prasse KW, et al.: Hypercoagulable state associated with a deficiency of protein C in a thoroughbred colt. J Vet Intern Med 7:190-193, 1993
38. Sweeney CR, Timoney JF, Newton JR, et al.: *Streptococcus equi* infections in horses: guidelines for treatment, control, and prevention of strangles. J Vet Intern Med 19:123-134, 2005
39. Sellon DC, Levine J, Millikin E, et al.: Thrombocytopenia in horses: 35 cases (1989-1994). J Vet Intern Med 10:127-132, 1996
40. Davis E, Wilkerson MJ: Thrombocytopenia, in Robinson NE (ed): Current Therapy in Equine Medicine, ed 5. Philadelphia, WB Saunders, 2003, pp 349-350
41. Crawford TB, Wardrop KJ, Tornquist SJ, et al.: A primary production deficit in the thrombocytopenia of equine infectious anaemia. J Virol 70:7842-7850, 1996
42. Sellon DC: Disorders of the hematopoietic system, in Reed SM, Bayly WM, Sellon DC (eds): Equine Internal Medicine, ed 2. St. Louis, WB Saunders, 2004, pp 721-768
43. Hinchcliff KW, Kociba GJ, Mitten LA: Diagnosis of EDTA-dependent pseudothrombocytopenia in a horse. J Am Vet Med Assoc 203:1715-1716, 1993
44. Kopp KJ, Moore JN, Byars TD, et al.: Template bleeding time and thromboxane generation in the horse: effects of three non-steroidal anti-inflammatory drugs. Equine Vet J 17:322-324, 1985
45. Segura D, Monreal L, Espada Y, et al.: Assessment of a platelet function analyser in horses: reference range and influence of a platelet aggregation inhibitor. Vet J 170:108-112, 2005
46. Henninger RW: Hemophilia A in two related quarter horse colts. J Am Vet Med Assoc 193:91-94, 1988
47. Littlewood JD, Bevan SA, Corke MJ: Haemophilia A (classic haemophilia, factor VIII deficiency) in a Thoroughbred colt foal. Equine Vet J 23:70-72, 1991
48. Geor RJ, Jackson ML, Lewis KD, et al.: Prekallikrein deficiency in a family of Belgian horses. J Am Vet Med Assoc 197:741-745, 1990
49. Brooks M, Leith GS, Allen AK, et al.: Bleeding disorder (von Willebrand disease) in a quarter horse. J Am Vet Med Assoc 198:114-116, 1991
50. Fry MM, Walker NJ, Blevins GM, et al.: Platelet function defect in a thoroughbred filly. J Vet Intern Med 19:359-362, 2005
51. Segura D, Monreal L, Armengou L, et al.: Mean platelet component as an indicator of platelet activation in foals and adult horses. J Vet Intern Med 21:1076-1082, 2007
52. Sandholm M, Vidovic A, Puotunen-Reinert A, et al.: D-dimer improves the prognostic value of combined clinical and laboratory data in equine gastrointestinal colic. Acta Vet Scand 36:255-272, 1995
53. Stokol T, Brooks MB, Erb HN, et al.: D-dimer concentrations in healthy dogs and dogs with disseminated intravascular coagulation. Am J Vet Res 61:393-398, 2000
54. Bates SM, Kearon C, Crowther M, et al.: A diagnostic strategy involving a quantitative latex D-dimer assay reliably excludes deep venous thrombosis. Ann Intern Med 138:787-794, 2003
55. Monreal L, Villatoro AJ, Monreal M, et al.: Comparison of the effects of low-molecular-weight and unfractioned heparin in horses. Am J Vet Res 56:1281-1285, 1995
56. Rodgers RP, Levin J: Bleeding time: a guide to its diagnostic and clinical utility. Arch Pathol Lab Med 114:1187-1188, 1990
57. Rodgers RP, Levin J: A critical reappraisal of the bleeding time. Semin Thromb Hemost 16:1-20, 1990
58. Kundu SK, Heilmann EJ, Sio R, et al.: Description of an in vitro platelet function analyzer—PFA-100. Semin Thromb Hemost 21 Suppl 2:106-112, 1995
59. Cattaneo M, Lecchi A, Agati B, et al.: Evaluation of platelet function with the PFA-100 system in patients with congenital defects of platelet secretion. Thromb Res 96:213-217, 1999
60. Callan MB, Giger U: Assessment of a point-of-care instrument for identification of primary haemostatic disorders in dogs. Am J Vet Res 62:652-658, 2001
61. Tarnow I, Kristensen AT, Texel H, et al.: Decreased platelet function in Cavalier King Charles Spaniels with mitral valve regurgitation. J Vet Intern Med 17:680-686, 2003
62. Mischke R, Keidel A: Influence of platelet count, acetylsalicylic acid, von Willebrand's disease, coagulopathies, and haematocrit on results obtained using a platelet function analyser in dogs. Vet J 165:43-52, 2003
63. Holland M, Kelly AB, Snyder JR, et al.: Antithrombin III activity in horses with large colon torsion. Am J Vet Res 47:897-900, 1986
64. Darien BJ, Potempa J, Moore JN, et al.: Antithrombin III activity in horses with colic: an analysis of 46 cases. Equine Vet J 23:211-214, 1991
65. Collatos C, Barton MH, Moore JN: Fibrinolytic activity in plasma from horses with gastrointestinal diseases: changes associated with diagnosis, surgery, and outcome. J Vet Intern Med 9:18-23, 1995
66. Collatos C, Barton MH, Prasse KW, et al.: Intravascular and peritoneal coagulation and fibrinolysis in horses with acute gastrointestinal tract diseases. J Am Vet Med Assoc 207:465-470, 1995
67. Topper MJ, Prasse KW: Chromogenic assays for equine coagulation factors VII, VIII:C, IX, and X, and C1-esterase inhibitor. Am J Vet Res 59:538-541, 1998

68. Meyers KM, Lindner C, Grant B: Characterization of the equine platelet aggregation response. Am J Vet Res 40:260-264, 1979
69. Jarvis GE, Evans RJ: Endotoxin-induced platelet aggregation in heparinised equine whole blood in vitro. Res Vet Sci 57:317-24, 1994
70. Jarvis GE, Evans RJ, Heath MF: The role of ADP in endotoxin-induced equine platelet activation. Eur J Pharmacol 315:203-212, 1996
71. Ablett JM, Fairbairn SM, Page CP, et al.: Influence of antigen challenge on platelet responsiveness in horses with chronic obstructive pulmonary disease. Equine Vet J 29:382-386, 1997
72. Heath MF, Evans RJ, Hayes LJ: Dextran-70 inhibits equine platelet aggregation induced by PAF but not by other agonists. Equine Vet J 30:408-411, 1998
73. Weiss DJ, Evanson OA, McClenahan D, et al.: Evaluation of platelet activation and platelet-neutrophil aggregates in ponies with alimentary laminitis. Am J Vet Res 58:1376-1380, 1997
74. Kingston JK, Sampson SN, Beard LA, et al.: The effect of supramaximal exercise on equine platelet function. Equine Vet J Suppl 30:181-183, 1999
75. Bailey SR, Andrews MJ, Elliott J, et al.: Actions and interactions of ADP, 5-HT, histamine and PAF on equine platelets. Res Vet Sci 68:175-180
76. Michelson AD, Barnard MR, Krueger LA, et al.: Evaluation of platelet function by flow cytometry. Methods 21:259-270, 2000
77. Segura D, Monreal L, Perez-Pujol S, et al.: Effects of etamsylate on equine platelets: in vitro and in vivo studies. Vet J 174:325-329, 2007
78. Segura D, Monreal L, Perez-Pujol S, et al.: Assessment of platelet function in horses: ultrastructure, flow cytometry, and perfusion techniques. J Vet Intern Med 20:581-588, 2006
79. Weiss DJ, Evanson OA, McClenahan D, et al.: Evaluation of platelet activation and platelet-neutrophil aggregates in ponies with alimentary laminitis. Am J Vet Res 58:1376-1380, 1997
80. Weiss DJ, Evanson OA: Detection of activated platelets and platelet-leukocyte aggregates in horses. Am J Vet Res 58:823-827, 1997
81. Weiss DJ, Evanson OA, Fagliari JJ, et al.: Evaluation of platelet activation and platelet-neutrophil aggregates in Thoroughbreds undergoing near-maximal treadmill exercise. Am J Vet Res 59:393-396, 1998
82. Kingston JK, Bayly WM, Meyers KM, et al.: Evaluation of binding of fibrinogen and annexin V to equine platelets in response to supramaximal treadmill exercise. Equine Vet J Suppl 34:502-505, 2002
83. Kingston JK, Bayly WM, Sellon DC, et al.: Measurement of the activation of equine platelets by use of fluorescent-labeled annexin V, anti-human fibrinogen antibody, and anti-human thrombospondin antibody. Am J Vet Res 63:513-519, 2002
84. Cotovio M, Monreal L, Navarro M, et al.: Detection of fibrin deposits in horse tissues by immunohistochemistry. J Vet Intern Med 21:1083-1089, 2007
85. Donahue SM, Otto CM: Thromboelastography: a tool for measuring hypercoagulability, hypocoagulability, and fibrinolysis. J Vet Emerg Crit Care 15:9-16, 2005

8.2 Management of horses with coagulopathies

Luis Monreal and Escolástico Aguilera

Horses are infrequently hospitalised because of coagulation disorders. However, coagulopathies are common complications in hospitalised horses. In these patients, a pathological activation of the coagulation mechanism, with a subsequent disseminated intravascular coagulation (DIC), is the most frequent coagulation disorder observed.

This chapter describes (1) the most common treatments for coagulopathies and (2) the clinical management and therapeutic measures to be taken in hospitalised horses that develop clinical signs consistent with a coagulation disorder.

Therapy of coagulation disorders

Haemostatic abnormalities in hospitalised horses are always related to the existence of either hypercoagulable or hypocoagulable states. Therapeutic measures in these animals will therefore be classified into those aimed at treating hypercoagulation and those aimed at resolving hypocoagulable states (Box 8.6).

Hypercoagulation (disseminated intravascular coagulation) therapy

Treatment of hypercoagulable states in equine critical care patients requires early identification of the prothrombotic

Box 8.6. Treatments recommended in hospitalised horses with coagulopathies

Treatments in horses with hypercoagulable states

- Antithrombotic drugs:
  - Heparin
  - Low-molecular-weight heparin (LMWH)
  - Ancillary drugs (antiaggregants, anti–vitamin K, etc)
- Fresh (frozen) plasma
- Other treatments
  - Treatments for the primary (underlying) disease
  - Fluid therapy to reduce the deleterious effects of fibrin deposits

Treatments in horses with hypocoagulable states

- Antihaemorrhagic drugs
  - ε-Aminocaproic acid (EACA) or tranexamic acid
  - Ethamsylate
  - Others
- Blood and blood component therapy
  - Whole blood transfusion
  - Fresh (frozen) plasma transfusion
  - Platelet and platelet-rich plasma
  - Other components
- Vitamin K
- Other treatments

> **Box 8.7. Therapeutic protocol for disseminated intravascular coagulation in a hospitalised patient**
>
> **In subclinical cases**
> - Administration of antithrombotics to avoid progression to severe forms: 50 U/kg dalteparin SQ q24h ***or*** 0.5 mg/kg enoxaparin SQ q24h while clinical signs of endotoxaemia are present
> - Treatment of the underlying disease if possible
> - Monitoring clotting times (PT, aPTT) or plasma D-dimers
>
> **In cases of haemorrhagic diathesis**
> - Administration of fresh (frozen) plasma until bleeding stops: at least 3–10 L may be required in a 450-kg horse
> - Administration of antithrombotics: 50 U/kg dalteparin SQ q24h ***or*** 0.5 mg/kg enoxaparin SQ q24h for 3–5 days
> - Specific treatment of the primary disease if possible
> - Monitoring clotting times or plasma D-dimers
>
> **In cases of multiorgan failure syndrome**
> - Detection of patients at risk at the preliminary stages
> - Administration of fluid therapy (minimum twice maintenance rate), DMSO, Hetastarch, etc, which may also have a mild antiplatelet effect
> - Administration of antithrombotics: 50 U/kg dalteparin SQ q24h ***or*** 0.5 mg/kg enoxaparin SQ q24h for 3–5 days
> - Administration of fresh (frozen) plasma to replace plasma antithrombin III levels if they are very decreased
> - Emergency treatment of the primary problem (e.g., surgical repair)
> - Monitoring clotting times or plasma D-dimers

state in patients at risk, administration of antithrombotic drugs at prophylactic doses, and specific treatment of the primary or underlying disease.[1–4] Treatment of patients which are already in a severe hypercoagulable state and develop haemorrhagic diathesis (bleeding form of DIC) may require the addition of fresh plasma transfusions.[1] Finally, therapy for animals with DIC and subsequent multiorgan failure (MOFS) is difficult and requires antithrombotic drugs, fluid therapy, and other treatments to improve tissue blood supply and to avoid organ failure due to fibrin deposition in capillary vessels (Box 8.7).[1,5,6]

In summary, hypercoagulable states in horses are best managed using the following treatments (see Box 8.6):

- Antithrombotic drugs
- Fresh (frozen) plasma
- Specific treatments to resolve the primary or underlying disease (e.g., antiendotoxic drugs, etc.)

Antithrombotic drugs

The main therapeutic goal when managing hypercoagulation is to reduce the excess of activated thrombin and to avoid further thrombus formation. Antithrombotics are the best drugs to achieve these goals. Among all antithrombotics, heparin has been shown to be the most effective and safe drug to treat all types of hypercoagulation disorders. Heparin has been successfully used to treat mild (compensated) and severe DIC situations.[1,5,7]

Thrombin is the main activator of coagulation, and it is also an important platelet activator in horses. Thus, administration of antithrombin drugs (e.g., heparin) reduces activation of both platelets and coagulation. In contrast, antiaggregant drugs (e.g., aspirin) decrease platelet activation but do not have any effect on fibrin formation.[8,9]

Heparin

Heparin is the most effective drug to control hypercoagulation. It increases the activity of the main coagulation inhibitor (antithrombin-III [AT-III]) by 2000-fold, thereby reducing excess thrombin. However, undesirable effects such as bleeding, thrombocytopenia, individual variability in dose response and dose-dependent erythrocyte agglutination with a subsequent decrease in packed cell volume have been reported in horses.[9–11]

The recommended dose for thrombus prophylaxis is 80 to 100 IU/kg IV or SQ q12h.[9] However, due to the severe erythrocyte agglutination observed when using this dose, lower doses (40–60 IU/kg q8h or q12h) are used.[1]

Low-Molecular-Weight Heparins

Fragmented standard heparin shows an increase in bioavailability, in affinity for AT-III and in thrombin inhibition, while reducing bleeding risks and avoiding erythrocyte agglutination.[3,9,12–14] Because low-molecular-weight heparins (LMWHs) are more effective and safer than unfractioned heparin, they have become the best recommended antithrombotics in hospitalised horses.[9,14]

The dose for thrombus prophylaxis is 50 U/kg for dalteparin, and 0.5 mg/kg for enoxaparin q24h SQ.[13]

In patients at high risk of DIC (horses with surgical colic, with inflammatory gastrointestinal disorders or with severe endotoxaemia), administration of LMWHs for several days helps to normalise the coagulation profile, reduce thrombotic complications and fibrin deposition and improve outcome.[14,15]

Other antithrombotics

Although hypercoagulable states are best managed using heparins, other, less-effective treatments may also be used.

Antiplatelet drugs. Aspirin is one of the best known antiaggregant drugs, and its efficacy in people has been well established. However, because thromboxane is not the main platelet activator in horses, aspirin does not effectively reduce platelet aggregation in equine patients.[9,16,17]

The use of aspirin in horses has also been limited by its short half-life, although recent studies have shown that rectal administration of acetylsalicylic acid improved its pharmacokinetics significantly.[18]

Vitamin K antagonists. Warfarin is widely used in people because it is an effective anticoagulant drug and it can be administered orally. However, its use in horses has been associated with a high risk of bleeding complications and requires close monitoring.[9] Therefore, it is not commonly used in equine patients.

Fibrinolytics. The use of fibrinolytic drugs to control thrombus formation in patients at risk has been proposed but is not well established due to low efficacy and the high risk of associated bleeding complications.

Fresh (frozen) plasma

Fresh (frozen) plasma is used to stop bleeding in severe cases of hypercoagulation, in which the high consumption of coagulation factors may cause haemorrhagic diathesis (bleeding form of DIC). Plasma transfusion should be a very early treatment when there is excessive consumption of coagulation factors and AT-III. If sufficient plasma can be given to restore AT-III concentration, it will ensure adequate function of heparins and will stop haemorrhagic diathesis.[1,3] In these cases, fresh plasma transfusion might be better than fresh-frozen plasma, because it will also replace platelets. Because fresh plasma needs to be collected from blood donors, stored fresh-frozen plasma may be more readily available and can be administered initially to try to stop bleeding in emergency situations.

The volume of plasma required for a horse with bleeding DIC is variable, but plasma should be administered at least until bleeding stops. Thus, as a general rule, a bleeding adult horse may require between 3 and 10 L of fresh plasma.[1,19]

Concentrates of anticoagulant proteins (AT-III and protein C) might be used to reduce the incidence of thrombosis in horses with endotoxaemia. AT-III concentrates have been shown to improve the clinical outcome in people with DIC due to septic shock.[20] However, to our knowledge, these are not marketed for use in horses.

Other treatments

Treatment of the primary underlying disease and its consequences is paramount in cases of hypercoagulation to stop the pathologic stimulation of coagulation and to restore normal physiological haemostasis. Therefore, in cases of endotoxaemia, low doses of flunixin meglumine, polymixin B, should be administered to ameliorate the effects of endotoxin and, hopefully, to improve the patient's outcome. Septic horses should be treated with appropriate antimicrobial drugs. Ischaemic gastrointestinal insults should be surgically repaired.[1,3,4,6,19]

Additionally, adequate fluid therapy (see Chapter 6.5) is essential to improve tissue perfusion in patients prone to develop microthrombi.[6]

Hypocoagulation therapy

True hypocoagulable states in horses are infrequent clinical presentations and they may be related to either congenital (e.g., haemophilia A) or acquired (e.g., warfarin toxicosis) defects in the coagulation system. In some instances, a coagulation defect may cause spontaneous bleeding, but haemorrhages are more often caused by an initial insult (e.g., venipuncture, wound, trauma, etc.) and are then complicated or exacerbated by a subclinical coagulation deficit.

In practice, treatments for hypocoagulation are administered to horses that are bleeding. The most effective therapy to manage these bleeding problems and coagulation deficits in horses are as follows (see Box 8.6)[4,21]:

- Antihaemorrhagic drugs
- Blood and blood component therapy
- Other treatments (e.g., vitamin K)

Antihaemorrhagic drugs

The rationale for use of antihaemorrhagic drugs is to stop haemorrhage. In most instances, this means potentiating coagulation mechanisms, rather than correcting coagulation deficits. The use of antihaemorrhagic drugs in equine medicine is controversial. Although they are widely used to reduce bleeding complications, there are few data supporting their effectiveness. The antihaemorrhagic drugs that are more frequently advocated in horses are given next.

ε-Aminocaproic acid and tranexamic acid

ε-Aminocaproic acid (EACA) is an antifibrinolytic drug that has the ability to irreversibly bind to plasminogen, and thereby to inhibit the conversion of plasminogen to plasmin.[21,22] Consequently, it increases plasma levels of the main plasmin inhibitor (α_2-antiplasmin), as it has been observed in people and clinically normal horses and ponies.[23,24] It has been demonstrated that EACA reduces bleeding in a variety of clinical situations. In fact, it is one of the most used antihaemorrhagic drugs in people, and one of the most recommended in horses.[21]

The recommended dosage is 20 to 40 mg/kg diluted 1:9 in saline and delivered slowly as an intravenous infusion (over 30–60 minutes). The treatment can be repeated every 6 hours if necessary.[21]

Tranexamic acid is a newer related drug that has approximately 8 times the antifibrinolytic activity of EACA. Little published work is available on tranexamic acid in horses, although there are older reports of efficacy.[25] Tranexamic acid is marketed for horses in Australia*, and the manufacturer's recommended dose is 5 to 25 mg/kg IV, IM or SQ.

Ethamsylate

Ethamsylate is a mild antihaemorrhagic drug that has been used in human and veterinary medicine for many years. It

*Vasolamin S 100; Troy Laboratories PTY, Smithfield, NSW, Australia.

has been shown to shorten the bleeding time in experimental animals and to reduce haemorrhage in several clinical situations in people and dogs.[26–28] It appears that ethamsylate improves platelet adhesiveness to other platelets and to leukocytes.[29,30]

In horses, it is used in Europe for exercise-induced pulmonary haemorrhage (EIPH) prophylaxis and to reduce bleeding in some surgical procedures, although its effectiveness in horses has not been documented. However, a mild activation of equine platelets has been recently observed when ethamsylate is used *in vitro* and *in vivo*.[31]

The recommended dosage is 10 to 15 mg/kg IV.

Formaldehyde

Although the mechanism of action of formaldehyde is unknown, its intravenous administration has been advocated as an effective method to stop haemorrhage in horses with profuse bleeding. However, the effectiveness of such treatment is purely anecdotal.[21] When formaldehyde was compared with lactated Ringer's solution in a two-way crossover study, no detectable effect of formaldehyde on haemostatic variables was observed in healthy horses. In addition, higher doses of formaldehyde (0.74%) induced unwanted side effects (muscle fasciculations, tachycardia, tachypnea, restlessness, etc.).[32] Thus, scientific evidence does not support the use of fomaldehyde as an antihaemorrhagic drug.

Blood and blood component therapy

Blood and blood component therapy are important in the management of horses with coagulopathies. The rationale behind the use of blood or blood derived products in these horses is to supply the blood components that are necessary with hypocoagulation disorders.[4] In addition, in bleeding patients, blood and blood component therapy help to maintain haemodynamics and to ensure adequate oxygen transportation.

Whole blood transfusion

The use of whole blood in horses with coagulation disorders is reserved for patients with severe haemorrhages that have lost a substantial amount of red blood cells. In these horses, transfusion of whole blood provides coagulation factors and platelets that are needed to treat the coagulation disorder and to restore a sufficient red cell number for adequate oxygen delivery to the tissues. Before performing this procedure, the benefits of whole blood transfusion should be weighed against the potential risks (posttransfusion reactions), and it is also necessary to take into account the short half-life of transfused erythrocytes (compatible allogenic equine erythrocytes are removed from the bloodstream within 4 days of administration). Thus, whole blood transfusions should be limited to cases where sufficient tissue oxygen delivery cannot be guaranteed, due to a low blood haemoglobin concentration.[33]

Procedures for donor selection, blood collection and transfusion are described in Chapter 6.5.

Fresh (frozen) plasma transfusion

Plasma transfusions are preferred to whole blood in horses with coagulopathies because plasma incorporates all the essential coagulation factors and does not have the potential problems associated with red blood cell transfusion. To prevent red blood cell contamination and ensure sterility, plasma is best collected by apheresis, although sedimentation under gravity during 2 hours is the most common method used in horses.[34,35] However, when using plasma transfusions to treat bleeding disorders, it is important to remember that the time elapsed from plasma collection until its administration to the bleeding patient must be less than 6 hours to avoid deterioration of coagulation factors. Thus, both fresh plasma or fresh-frozen plasma can be used to provide the essential coagulation factors, although the former might be preferred to treat horses with coagulopathies because it also provides platelets. The volume of plasma transfusion may be roughly estimated based on the decrease of plasma protein concentration. As a general rule, to elevate plasma proteins 10 g/L (1 g/dl), transfusion of 1.4 L/100 kg body weight of plasma of normal protein concentration (70 g/L [7 g/dl]) is needed.[35] Therefore, administration of 5 to 10 L of plasma may be the recommended volume in a 450-kg patient with a coagulopathy.

Clinical indications for plasma transfusion include diseases in which coagulation factors are required, which are listed in Box 8.8.

Platelets and platelet-rich plasma

Platelets can be provided as a concentrate or as platelet-rich plasma. The latter is more commonly used in equine medicine. Platelet-rich plasma can be harvested by centrifugation of fresh blood for 3 to 5 minutes at 250g.[36] However, when obtained by apheresis, platelets expire about 4 hours after collection. Therefore, in most clinical situations platelets are transfused together with freshly collected plasma. The survival of transfused platelets averages 3 to 5 days unless a consumptive disorder is present. It is also impor-

Box 8.8. Disease conditions in which plasma transfusions are recommended to replace coagulation factors

- Congenital defects of the coagulation system (e.g., haemophilia A)
- Acquired defects of the coagulation system: these can be related to the ingestion of products that interfere with vitamin K metabolism (dicoumarin derivatives) or to systemic diseases in which there is a deficit in the hepatic synthesis of coagulation factors (liver disease)
- Profuse bleeding secondary to trauma or to a surgical procedure that may cause an excessive consumption of coagulation factors
- Advanced disseminated intravascular coagulation (bleeding form)

tant to remember that the effectiveness of platelet transfusions decreases under certain circumstances (e.g., uraemia or treatment with nonsteroidal anti-inflammatory drugs). Clinical indications for platelet or platelet-rich plasma administration include situations in which a profound thrombocytopenia is detected.[36] The guidelines for platelet transfusions are extrapolated from human medicine. Although the platelet count must decrease below 10×10^9/L (10,000/μl) for spontaneous bleeding to occur, it is recommended to maintain platelet count above 50×10^9/L (50,000/μl) in the bleeding patient. It is also important to consider that the patient may have an abnormal platelet function and thus may show a platelet-derived coagulation problem with normal platelet values. To increase the platelet count by 10×10^9/L (10,000/μl), a 450-kg horse will require approximately 5 to 10 L of fresh plasma with a normal platelet count.

Other components

Cryoprecipitate, which is a combination of fibrinogen, von Willebrand factor, factor VIII, factor IX and fibronectin, could be useful in some specific conditions (e.g., treatment of haemophilia), but it is not readily available in horses.[35,37] In addition, these coagulopathies are very rare in these animals.

Vitamin K

The main uses of exogenous vitamin K in horses are the treatment of coumarin toxicity (warfarin, rodenticide, sweet clover, *Ferula* spp., etc.) and the treatment of a vitamin K deficiency associated with chronic enteropathy.[38] Vitamin K exerts an antihaemorrhagic effect only in patients with a deficiency, by restoring the synthesis of the deficient coagulation factors.

Vitamin K is administered parenterally (IV, IM or SQ) at a dose range of 0.5 to 2.5 mg/kg body weight for 3 to 5 days, or until normalisation of the PT value occurs.

Clinical approach and management of the main coagulation problems detected in hospitalised horses

The approach to the management of coagulation disorders in hospitalised horses can be summarised into four main clinical scenarios:

1. The horse with spontaneous bleeding
2. The horse developing DIC
3. The horse with petechial haemorrhages in mucous membranes
4. The horse with profuse bleeding after a surgical procedure

Clinical approach and management of a hospitalised patient presenting a spontaneous bleeding episode

Bleeding episodes in hospitalised horses can occur spontaneously, but they are more commonly associated to minor trauma (e.g., nasogastric intubation). These bleeding episodes can be due to:

- A marked hypercoagulable state, in which the rapid consumption of coagulation factors has induced a secondary hypocoagulable state (bleeding form of DIC)

or

- A hypocoagulable state due to a haemostatic defect (platelets, coagulation factors, drug induced)

Clinical considerations

First, it is paramount to elucidate whether the patient is in a hypercoagulable or a hypocoagulable state. This would allow differentiation of patients at risk of developing DIC from those showing clinical signs of haemostatic defects.

Once the bleeding problem has been classified as a hypercoagulable or hypocoagulable state, the therapeutic plan can then be selected (see Box 8.6):

- **Antithrombotic therapy** (e.g., LMWH) is recommended in patients with DIC after fresh plasma transfusion, but it is contraindicated in cases with haemostatic defects.
- **Antihaemorrhagic drugs** (e.g., antifibrinolytics) are recommended in horses with hypocoagulation but are contraindicated in DIC cases.

Diagnostic tests

- Platelet count, bleeding time/closure times
- Clotting times (PT, aPTT, TT), fibrinogen
- D-dimers
- Other examinations (i.e., radiology, ultrasonography, etc.) to diagnose the primary problem

In cases of DIC, the coagulation profile will show haemostatic alterations consistent with a consumption coagulopathy (mild thrombocytopenia, prolonged clotting times, increased D-dimers).

In cases of haemostatic defects, results of diagnostic tests might be variable depending on the defect.

In some patients, the coagulation tests will not allow a clear differentiation between DIC and haemostatic defects (in these cases, the history and the presence of clinical signs consistent with diseases that cause DIC are very important).

Therapeutic plan

When the problem is due to a hypercoagulable state (DIC)

1. Fresh (frozen) plasma transfusion
2. Antithrombotics (LMWHs)
3. Try to control the primary problem (gastrointestinal inflammatory disorder, neoplasia, etc.).
4. Monitor plasma D-dimer or clotting times.

When the problem is due to a hypocoagulable state induced by a platelet defect

1. Platelet-rich plasma transfusion
2. Whole blood transfusion in cases of severe bleeding
3. Antihaemorrhagic drugs (EACA, ethamsylate)
4. If possible, treat the primary disease that is causing massive platelet destruction.
5. Monitor platelet count.

When the problem is due to a hypocoagulable state induced by a coagulation defect

1. Fresh (frozen) plasma
2. Consider administration of vitamin K in cases of acquired deficiencies.
3. Monitor clotting times.

Clinical approach and management of a hospitalised horse that is developing DIC

This is a fairly common situation in hospitalised horses. DIC, a pathological activation of the coagulation system, may be triggered by endotoxaemia, sepsis and other conditions such as gastrointestinal disorders. Because these disorders, particularly endotoxaemia, are so common, DIC represents the main coagulopathy in hospitalised horses.

Clinical considerations

From a clinical point of view, it is important to remember that development of DIC can be assessed by changes in the coagulation profile, but from a practical point of view, it is also very important to consider that DIC is better prevented than treated. Thus, in many clinical situations the main objective will be to detect the patients that are at risk of developing DIC and to initiate prophylactic treatment in these patients.

Which patients will be considered at risk of developing DIC?

All horses with severe endotoxaemia. This will include not only gastrointestinal problems (ischaemic and inflammatory disorders) but also some infections (neonatal septicaemia, pleuroneumonia, metritis) and other conditions such as disseminated neoplasia (e.g., melanosarcoma) and severe haemolytic disorders.

Diagnostic tests

In DIC, several (more than three) of the routine coagulation parameters will be abnormal. The coagulation profile will be consistent with consumption of coagulation factors:

- Platelet count: thrombocytopenia ($<100 \times 10^9$/L [100,000/μl])
- Clotting times (PT, aPTT): significantly prolonged
- D-dimers: increased levels
- Fibrinogen: decreased concentration
- AT-III (difficult to measure in emergency settings): decreased activity

Therapeutic plan

Therapeutic plan in a patient that is at high risk of DIC to prevent the development of fulminant forms

1. Antithrombotic agents (LMWHs) for a few days
2. Monitor plasma D-dimer or clotting times.

Therapeutic plan for impending DIC in a patient that is showing deterioration in the coagulation profile

1. Fresh (frozen) plasma
2. Antithrombotics (LMWHs) for a few days
3. Monitor plasma D-dimer or clotting times.

Clinical approach and management of a hospitalised patient with petechial haemorrhages

In the course of being hospitalised, a horse may develop mucous membrane haemorrhages. The most common causes for development of petechial and ecchymotic haemorrhages are:

- Vasculitis that may be associated to immune-mediated diseases
- Marked thrombocytopenia
- Severe platelet dysfunction
- Secondary to a hypercoagulable state, DIC and platelet consumption

Clinical considerations

When a hospitalised horse develops mucous membrane petechiations, there are several questions that should be addressed.

- Does the patient show other clinical signs consistent with vasculitis (e.g., cutaneous oedema), or is there a history of diseases that may predispose to vasculitis (e.g., viral, immune mediated)?
- Is there a history of diseases that may predispose to an immune-mediated thrombocytopenia (e.g., strangles) or to a severe platelet dysfunction (e.g., antiaggregant therapy)?
- Is the patient at risk of DIC? (see earlier)

Diagnostic tests

Emergency diagnostic tests in these patients should include a coagulation profile to determine if there is a hypocoagulation or a hypercoagulation problem:

- Platelet count
- Bleeding time/closure times
- Clotting times (PT, aPTT, TT), fibrinogen
- D-dimers

Other diagnostic examinations (i.e., thoracic radiology, ultrasonography, blood biochemistry, etc.) should be performed to detect a primary problem.

Therapeutic plan

Vasculitis

1. Control the immune-mediated vasculitis (e.g., immunosuppressant therapy) and the primary problem (e.g., antibiotics, etc).
2. If there is thrombocytopenia ($<30 \times 10^9$/L [30,000/μl]), platelet-rich plasma

Due to a hypocoagulable state induced by a severe thrombocytopenia and/or platelet dysfunction (prolonged bleeding time/closure times)

1. Fresh plasma/platelet-rich plasma

Due to a hypocoagulable state induced by a coagulation defect (prolonged clotting times)

1. Fresh (frozen) plasma
2. Consider administration of vitamin K in cases of acquired deficiency.
3. Treat the primary problem.

Due to a hypercoagulable state induced by DIC

1. DIC therapy

Clinical approach and management of a hospitalised patient that bleeds profusely after surgery

Profuse bleeding after surgery can occur in the horse. In these patients, bleeding may be a consequence of poor surgical haemostasis, subclinical coagulation disorders that went unnoticed before the surgery or a combination of both. There are three basic situations:

- Bleeding due to extensive vessel damage or poor surgical technique
- Bleeding due to a consumption coagulopathy caused by haemorrhagic losses, but without underlying hypercoagulable state
- Haemorrhage due to a hypocoagulable state not detected before surgery (e.g., moderate thrombocytopenia, previous administration of an antiaggregant drug, etc.)

Clinical considerations

- In practice, it is very difficult to isolate the effects of poor surgical haemostasis.
- Coagulation profiles are necessary to detect if there is a coagulation defect in addition to poor surgical haemostasis.
- Because antihaemorrhagic drugs need to be avoided in DIC, it is important to differentiate hypocoagulable and hypercoagulable states.

Diagnostic tests

- Platelet count
- Bleeding time/closure times
- Clotting times (PT, aPTT, TT), fibrinogen
- D-dimers

Therapeutic plans

When an extended area is bleeding continuously

1. Improve surgical management if possible.
2. If the patient is not one of those at risk of DIC, use antihaemorrhagic drugs (e.g., 20 g of EACA in 5 L lactated Ringer's solution infused over 30–60 minutes), followed by 10 g more every 6 hours if necessary.

When a coagulopathic consumption is already detected due to continuous bleeding

1. Add whole blood/fresh plasma transfusion.
2. Antihaemorrhagic drugs (e.g., EACA)
3. Monitor platelet count and clotting times.

When a hypocoagulable state is detected

1. Fresh plasma transfusion/platelet-rich plasma
2. Antihaemorrhagic drugs (e.g., EACA)
3. Monitor clotting times.

References

1. Darien BJ: Hypercoagulation: pathophysiology, diagnosis and treatment. Equine Vet Educ 5:37-40, 1993
2. Wada H, Wakita Y, Nakase T, et al.: Outcome of disseminated intravascular coagulation in relation to the score when treatment was begun. Thromb Haemost 74:848-852, 1995
3. Dallap BL: Coagulopathy in the equine critical care patient. Vet Clin North Am Equine Pract 20:231-251, 2004
4. Sellon DC: Disorders of the hematopoietic system, in Reed SM, Bayly WM, Sellon DC (eds): Equine Internal Medicine, ed 2. St. Louis, WB Saunders, 2004, pp 721-768
5. Darien BJ, Williams MA: Possible hypercoagulation in 3 foals with septicemia. Equine Vet Educ 5:19-22, 1993
6. Kirby R, Rudloff E: Acquired coagulopathy. VI: Disseminated intravascular coagulation, in Feldman BF, Zinkl JG, Jain NC (eds): Veterinary Hematology, ed 5. Philadelphia, Lippincott Williams & Wilkins, 2000, pp 581-587
7. Provost PJ, Stick JA, Patterson JS, et al.: Effects of heparin treatment on colonic torsion-associated hemodynamic and plasma eicosanoid changes in anesthetized ponies. Am J Vet Res 52:289-297, 1991
8. Poole AW: Thrombosis in the horse: the role of platelets in its pathogenesis and therapy. Equine Vet Educ 5:99-102, 1993
9. Ruiz de Gopegui R, Monreal L: Anticoagulant and fibrinolytic drugs, in Feldman BF, Zinkl JG, Jain NC (eds): Veterinary Hematology, ed 5. Philadelphia, Lippincott Williams and Wilkins, 2000, pp 588-593
10. Moore JN, Mahaffey EA, Zboran M: Heparin-induced agglutination of erythrocytes in horses. Am J Vet Res 48:68-71, 1987
11. Moore BR, Hinchcliff KW: Heparin: a review of its pharmacology and therapeutic use in horses. J Vet Intern Med 8:26-35, 1994
12. Monreal L, Villatoro AJ, Monreal M, et al.: Comparison of the effects of low-molecular-weight and unfractioned heparin in horses. Am J Vet Res 56:1281-1285, 1995
13. Schwarzwald CC, Feige K, Wunderli-Allenspach H, et al.: Comparison of pharmacokinetic variables for two low-

molecular-weight heparins after subcutaneous administration of a single dose to horses. Am J Vet Res 63:868-873, 2002

14. Feige K, Schwarzwald CC, Bombeli T: Comparison of unfractioned and low molecular weight heparin for prophylaxis of coagulopathies in 52 horses with colic: a randomised double-blind clinical trial. Equine Vet J 35:506-513, 2003
15. Cotovio M, Monreal L, Navarro M, et al.: Detection of fibrin deposits in tissues from horses with severe gastrointestinal disorders. J Vet Intern Med 21:308-313, 2007
16. Cambridge H, Lees P, Hooke RE, et al.: Antithrombotic actions of aspirin in the horse. Equine Vet J 23:123-127, 1991
17. Heath MF, Evans RJ, Poole AW, et al.: The effects of aspirin and paracetamol on the aggregation of equine blood platelets. J Vet Pharmacol Ther 17:374-378, 1994
18. Broome TA, Brown MP, Gronwall RR, et al.: Pharmacokinetics and plasma concentrations of acetylsalicylic acid after intravenous, rectal, and intragastric administration to horses. Can J Vet Res 67:297-302, 2003
19. Zimmel DN: Hemostatic disorders, in Robinson NE (ed): Current Therapy in Equine Medicine, ed 5. Philadelphia, WB Saunders, 2003, pp 351-354
20. Fourrier F, Chopin C, Huart JJ, et al.: Double-blind, placebo-controlled trial of antithrombin III concentrates in septic shock with disseminated intravascular coagulation. Chest 104:882-888, 1993
21. Smith CL: Critical care therapeutics for mature horses, in Robinson NE (ed): Current Therapy in Equine Medicine, ed 5. Philadelphia, WB Saunders, 2003, pp 19-23
22. Xia VW, Steadman RH: Antifibrinolytics in orthotopic liver transplantation: current status and controversies. Liver Transpl 11:10-18, 2005
23. Ray MJ, Hales M, Marsh N: Epsilon-aminocaproic acid promotes the release of alpha2-antiplasmin during and after cardiopulmonary bypass. Blood Coagul Fibrinolysis 12:129-135, 2001
24. Heidmann P, Tornquist SJ, Qu A, et al.: Laboratory measures of hemostasis and fibrinolysis after intravenous administration of epsilon-aminocaproic acid in clinically normal horses and ponies. Am J Vet Res 66:313-318, 2005
25. Balun J, Sutta J, Janda J: [Follow-up study on the hemostatic effect of the Vasolamin preparation in domestic animals]. Vet Med (Praha) 21:119-124, 1976
26. Ment LR, Stewart WB, Duncan CC: Beagle puppy model of intraventricular hemorrhage: ethamsylate studies. Prostaglandins 27:245-256, 1984
27. Chen JY: Ethamsylate in the prevention of periventricular-intraventricular hemorrhage in premature infants. J Formos Med Assoc 92:889-893, 1993
28. Hutton RA, Hales M, Kernoff PB: A study of the effect of ethamsylate (Dicynene) on the bleeding time, von Willebrand factor level and fibrinolysis in patients with von Willebrand's disease. Thromb Haemost 60:506-507, 1997
29. Alvarez-Guerra M, Hernández MR, Escolar G, et al.: The hemostatic agent ethamsylate enhances P-selectin membrane expression in human platelets and cultured endothelial cells. Thromb Res 107:329-335, 2002
30. Hernández MR, Alvarez-Guerra M, Escolar G, et al.: The hemostatic agent ethamsylate promotes platelet/leukocyte aggregate formation in a model of vascular injury. Fundam Clin Pharmacol 18:423-430, 2004
31. Segura D, Monreal L, Perez-Pujol S, et al.: Effects of etamsylate on equine platelets: in vitro and in vivo studies. Vet J 174:325-329, 2007
32. Taylor EL, Sellon DC, Wardrop KJ, et al.: Effects of intravenous administration of formaldehyde on platelet and coagulation variables in healthy horses. Am J Vet Res 61:1191-1196, 2000
33. Durham AE: Blood and plasma transfusion in the horse. Equine Vet Educ 8:8-12, 1996
34. Feige K, Ehrat FB, Kastner SB, et al.: Automated plasmapheresis compared with other plasma collection methods in the horse. J Vet Med A 50:185-189, 2003
35. Porter MB, Green E: Blood and blood component therapy, in Robinson NE (ed): Current Therapy in Equine Medicine, ed 5. Philadelphia, WB Saunders, 2003, pp 355-357
36. Davis E, Wilkerson MJ: Thrombocytopenia, in Robinson NE (ed): Current Therapy in Equine Medicine, ed 5. Philadelphia, WB Saunders, 2003, pp 349-350
37. Morris DD: Blood products in large animal medicine: a comparative account of current and future technology. Equine Vet J 19:272-275, 1987
38. Byars TD, Greene CE, Kemp DT: Antidotal effect of vitamin K1 against warfarin-induced anticoagulation in horses. Am J Vet Res 47:2309-2312, 1986

9

Monitoring and treating the cardiovascular system

9.1 Monitoring the cardiovascular system
9.2 Treating the cardiovascular system

9.1 Monitoring the cardiovascular system

9.1.1 Monitoring the heart

Mary Durando

It is very important to monitor the hospitalised patient's cardiovascular system critically, as the patient is at risk for developing disorders that increase morbidity and mortality, both as a primary problem and secondary to other diseases. For this purpose, both daily physical examinations and other diagnostic aids can be used that will help to determine the involvement of the cardiovascular system in the disease process, the effect of other diseases on the heart, or the progression of disease.

Physical examination

Thorough auscultation is the cornerstone of the cardiac examination and is a key factor in directing the remainder of the examination.[1–5] Knowledge of normal heart sounds, as well as their genesis is essential to the recognition of abnormal heart sounds. A quiet location, free from distractions is ideal to detect subtle murmurs and sounds.[6] If too much activity and/or commotion surrounds the examination area, not only is it difficult for the examiner, but the horse's cardiovascular status will be influenced.

One should always use a systematic approach for the physical examination, as well as for auscultation. The horse should first be observed from a distance for anxiety, discomfort, nostril flair and dyspnoea. The peripheral arteries should be palpated, both to determine pulse quality and character, and to note if pulse deficits are present during auscultation, indicating a dysrhythmia. Pulse character is an indication of the difference between systolic and diastolic blood pressure, and is related to and influenced by cardiac output and systemic vascular resistance. It can help determine the severity of underlying cardiac disease. For instance, in a horse with aortic insufficiency, bounding pulses may indicate more severe regurgitation and left ventricular volume overload, while a horse in circulatory shock or congestive heart failure will likely have rapid, weak pulses that may be an indication of impending cardiovascular deterioration. A tachycardic horse with pulse deficits may have a dysrhythmia such as ventricular tachycardia or atrial fibrillation. Pulse character in extremities helps to determine peripheral perfusion or if local vascular thromboses are present. Peripheral perfusion can also be assessed by temperature of extremities, as these are usually cooler to the touch if systemic circulation is severely decreased.

Jugular venous filling and distension, as well as the presence of jugular pulses, should be assessed. Jugular distension may be present in congestive heart failure or any obstruction to venous return such as a mediastinal mass, large pericardial effusions, or constrictive pericarditis. Jugular pulses are present in cases of severe tricuspid regurgitation and atrioventricular dissociation (most commonly, ventricular tachycardia; uncommonly, third-degree atrioventricular block). Care must be taken to determine that a true jugular pulse exists. This is done by occluding the vein midway up the neck and milking the blood distally towards the heart whilst holding the horse's head up in a natural position. It is abnormal for the vein to then fill with blood. Abnormalities in other peripheral veins should also be noted.

Auscultation

All valve areas on both sides of the thorax should be auscultated. In addition, all valve areas should be palpated for the presence of a precordial thrill. The pulmonic, aortic, and mitral valves are located on the left side.[3,5] The cardiac impulse, or left apical beat, can be palpated as a reference point for the ventricular inlet and the mitral valve. It is located medial to the left elbow in the fifth intercostal space (ICS); deviations from this may indicate displacement or enlargement of the cardiac silhouette. The mitral valve is located in the fifth ICS, between the point of the elbow and the point of the shoulder. In most horses standing relatively squarely, the fifth ICS is just caudal to or under the triceps musculature. The aortic valve is auscultated in the fourth ICS, cranial and dorsal to the mitral valve. The pulmonic valve is cranial to the aortic valve, in the third ICS. To reach the pulmonic valve, the stethoscope must be pushed rather far forward, under the triceps musculature, which many horses object to. Placing the horse's fore limb forward facilitates auscultation.

On the right side, the tricuspid valve is best heard in ICS 3–4.[3,5] Heart sounds on the right are generally less intense than those on the left side. It is helpful to have the leg on the side of the examiner positioned forward to allow easier placement of the stethoscope in the third and fourth ICS, as many times, if the tricuspid valve is difficult to hear it is because the examiner is listening too far caudally.

Heart sounds

In many horses, four heart sounds can normally be appreciated, although not all four sounds may be heard at the same time or in the same location. S_1 corresponds to the onset of systole and is loudest near the apex beat and mitral valve. The intensity of S_1 may vary with a dysrhythmia such as atrial fibrillation or ventricular tachycardia, and may be related to ventricular filling. S_2 (onset of diastole) is usually loudest around the aortic valve, although the pulmonic component of a split S_2 is heard best over the pulmonic valve.[7] S_2 is often split in normal horses, with variability in the order of closure of the pulmonic and aortic valves. Although the order of valve closure may be variable in normal horses, if the pulmonic component becomes noticeably louder than the aortic component, it may indicate pulmonary hypertension. S_3 is associated with rapid ventricular filling and is the most difficult of the heart sounds to hear consistently. It may be loud with left ventricular volume overload such as seen with severe aortic insufficiency in older horses or an extracardiac shunt in foals. S_3 is heard best in the region of the ventricular inlet. S_4 occurs at the end of diastole, after atrial contraction, and is heard in most horses. It is frequently heard alone in horses with second-degree atrioventricular block and is never heard in horses in atrial fibrillation, because of the lack of atrial contraction.

Rate, rhythm, and character of the heart sounds

When evaluating the patient, the heart rate should be assessed first. Normal values for the particular breed, type, and age of the horse should be considered, as well as any change in rate or character over time in the individual. Changes or trends in heart rate over time give very important information regarding the clinical status of the horse. When taking the heart rate, it is important to allow the horse to adjust to the examiner listening, as often excitement will result in an initial heart rate increase. Next, the heart should be evaluated for abnormal rhythm. Any irregularities suspected in rhythm, inconsistencies or variations in intensity of heart sounds, or pulse deficits should be further worked up with electrocardiography. After the rate and rhythm have been determined, auscultation should be performed separately over each valve area for abnormal noises and heart sounds, and the presence of murmurs. Other sounds, such as clicks, knocks, rubs or squeaks, may be present and should be noted. The intensity of the heart sounds should be noted, as deviations from normal may indicate pathological conditions (e.g, a very loud S_3 may indicate ventricular volume overload).[8] However, one should keep in mind that external factors that influence sound transmission, such as obesity, effusions, masses, etc, can also affect heart sounds.

Murmurs

Murmurs are sounds that occur in a normally silent portion of the cardiac cycle and can be physiological ("innocent") or pathological. They are caused by abnormal or turbulent blood flow, or vibrating structures (e.g, valves or chordae tendinae). Abnormal blood flow can be caused by a number of factors, such as high velocity, turbulence, decreased viscosity or anything that influences Reynold's number. Many horses hospitalised in ICUs have problems that alter these factors, causing murmurs even if the heart is not abnormal. The challenge lies in determining whether the murmur is secondary to other abnormalities, and not a problem on its own, or if it indicates primary cardiac disease that should be addressed. Murmurs are described by their timing, duration, intensity, quality, shape and point of maximal intensity (PMI)/radiation to try to help determine their significance. **Timing** refers to relationship to the events of the cardiac cycle (e.g, systolic, diastolic or continuous). A peripheral pulse can be palpated simultaneously if it is difficult to determine systolic versus diastolic timing. **Duration** refers to the length of time within a portion of the cardiac cycle the murmur is audible, and is usually described as holo, pan, early, mid or late systolic or diastolic. **Intensity**, or loudness, of a murmur is graded on a scale of either I to VI or I to V. A general description on a grade I to VI scale is given in Box 9.1.

The **quality** is similar to the pitch, and can be described in terms of soft and blowing, harsh, or musical. Musical murmurs often have an associated vibrating structure and, because they are easy to hear, may sound loud. The **shape**

Box 9.1. Grading of cardiac murmurs

Grade	Description
I	Murmurs can only be heard after careful auscultation in a quiet place and are usually focal.
II	Murmurs are clearly audible, yet soft, and do not typically radiate over a large area.
III	Murmurs are immediately apparent and usually heard over a wider area than grade II murmurs.
IV	Murmurs have a faint, but palpable precordial thrill.
V and VI	Murmurs are progressively louder, and the loudest may be heard with the stethoscope removed from the chest wall. They always have a palpable thrill associated with them.

describes the intensity and pitch of the murmur over the duration of the cycle and is most commonly band-shaped, decrescendo, crescendo or crescendo-decrescendo. It is usually influenced by pressure differences between the chambers. Certain types of murmurs often have a typical shape, such as a decrescendo murmur in diastole, often indicative of aortic regurgitation, or a systolic crescendo murmur that may occur with mitral valve prolapse. **PMI**, the point of maximal intensity, is where the murmur is heard loudest, and the direction it radiates. A detailed description of auscultation technique is available in several texts for the interested reader.[1,3–5] In addition, correlation of murmur descriptions with echocardiographic findings has been described in detail.[9]

Changes in any of these aspects over time should be noted, as well as changes that occur with changes in heart rate. Horses that are admitted with or develop murmurs or abnormal heart sounds while hospitalised should be evaluated echocardiographically to assess their importance. Any changes in intensity, duration or character of a murmur while hospitalised should also be evaluated with echocardiography, even if previously assessed.

Laboratory Investigations

Most laboratory tests cannot specifically diagnose or confirm cardiac disease, with the possible exception of cardiac specific enzymes and proteins. However, laboratory monitoring in horses with known cardiac disease can be very useful and aid in determining the aetiology of certain abnormalities and their correction.

Electrolyte assessment

Electrolyte assessment is particularly useful in cases with dysrhythmias, especially horses hospitalised with gastrointestinal disturbances[10,11] or upper (e.g, renal failure) or lower (e.g, ruptured bladder) urinary tract disease. Disturbances in potassium, calcium and magnesium are commonly associated with dysrhythmias,[12] and until these are corrected, the dysrhythmia is often likely to be refractory to treatment, if severe imbalances exist. There may be multiple concurrent electrolyte derangements, so it is important to address all abnormalities, as correction of one may require simultaneous correction of the others (see Chapter 6.5).

Potassium

Hypokalaemia is often associated with prolongation of the QT interval and ST-segment depression, as well as supraventricular and ventricular tachycardias. Whole body potassium depletion is thought to be a contributing factor to the development of atrial fibrillation (AF) in horses,[13] and hypokalaemia predisposes to digitalis intoxication.[14] Hyperkalaemia slows conduction time, and can shorten ventricular repolarisation. It is classically associated with tall, tented T waves on an electrocardiogram (ECG), but other disturbances such as bradycardia with prolongation of the PR interval or broadening and flattening of the P wave and slowing of conduction leading to atrial standstill commonly occur.[3] Third-degree atrioventricular block may be secondary to hyperkalaemia and can be seen in foals with ruptured bladders[15]; less commonly, premature depolarisations and ventricular tachycardia may be seen. The QRS complex may widen, and ventricular fibrillation or asystole may occur as the concentrations become lethal. Plasma potassium concentrations greater than 6 mmol/L (>6 mEq/L) may be associated with abnormalities of the ECG.

Magnesium

Hypomagnesaemia, rather than hypermagnesaemia, occurs most commonly in sick horses. Although the exact roles magnesium plays in the genesis of cardiac disease are controversial, there is no doubt that it is important in normal cardiovascular function. Magnesium deficiencies typically result in ventricular dysrhythmias (premature depolarisations and tachycardia), although rarely supraventricular dysrhythmias will occur.[12] In people, magnesium also likely plays a role in hypertension and ischaemic myocardial disease. Hypomagnesaemia commonly occurs in horses hospitalised with gastrointestinal lesions[11,16] and may be associated with ventricular dysrhythmias. It is usually seen in conjunction with other electrolyte deficiencies. Hypermagnesaemia is more likely to be iatrogenic, from oversupplementation; this probably occurs less frequently in large animals than in small animals. In a report of two horses with magnesium toxicosis, tachycardia was seen.[17]

Calcium

Hypocalcaemia can occur with several diseases, most notably gastrointestinal diseases,[10,11] but also with exhaustive exercise and in association with lactation. It is usually associated with sinus tachycardia, although ventricular tachycardia and premature depolarisations may be present. Prolonged QT interval and cardiac arrest may also occur. Synchronous diaphragmatic flutter also occurs with hypocalcaemia. Horses may have an abnormal hind limb gait, ataxia, seizures, or flaccid paralysis and recumbency, depending on the severity of the deficiency and the presence of other electrolyte derangements. Hypercalcaemia is most often seen with chronic, severe renal failure but can also be a manifestation of neoplasia. It can cause bradycardia or tachycardia, ectopic depolarisations, prolonged QT interval, cardiac arrest and ventricular fibrillation.

Plasma biochemistry

Biochemical analysis of organ function can help to assess the effects of cardiac disease on other organs, the effects of organ function on the cardiovascular system or the concurrent effects of a particular disease.[3] Indices of renal and hepatic function, fractional excretion of electrolytes and serum albumin concentrations should be measured. Venous blood gas analysis (including bicarbonate, pH and

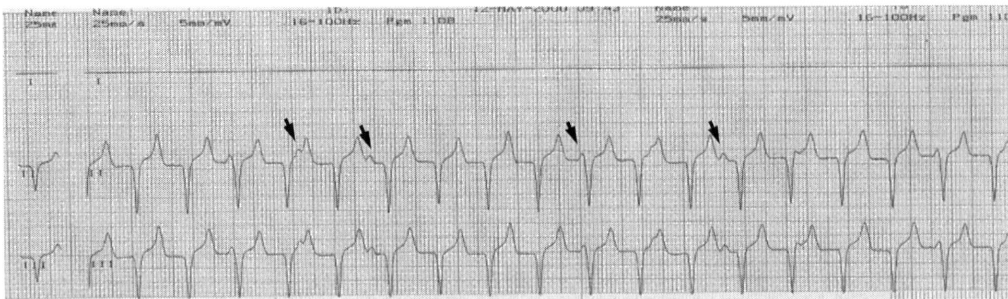

Figure 9.1 Uniform ventricular tachycardia in a horse with oleander toxicity. Note the regularity of the RR interval and the similar morphology of the QRS waves. *Arrowheads* denote some of the P waves that can be seen at varying places buried within the QRS-T complexes, but not associated with the QRS. ©Mary Durando 2006.

base deficit determination), anion gap and lactate concentrations are useful to assess the presence of and effect of low-output cardiac failure on tissue perfusion/oxygenation and oxygen extraction.[18] Assessment of arterial and venous blood gas differences and mixed venous oxygen can give a crude idea of cardiac output, provided pulmonary function is normal.[19] Arterial blood gases can also indicate the presence of venous admixture from a complex congenital cardiac disease or can be used to assess pulmonary function. Severe pulmonary disease, such as seen in horses with severe recurrent airway obstruction in acute crisis or pulmonary thromboembolism, can cause pulmonary vasoconstriction, increased pulmonary vascular resistance, pulmonary hypertension, reduced right heart function and cor pulmonale. Inflammation or infection associated with pulmonary disease may also affect cardiac function (e.g, myocarditis associated with influenza or streptococcal infections). Severe acid-base disorders or evidence of endotoxaemia is noteworthy and may depress myocardial function or cause myocarditis.[20–25] This may occur more often than is realized in strangulating intestinal diseases or severe colitis.

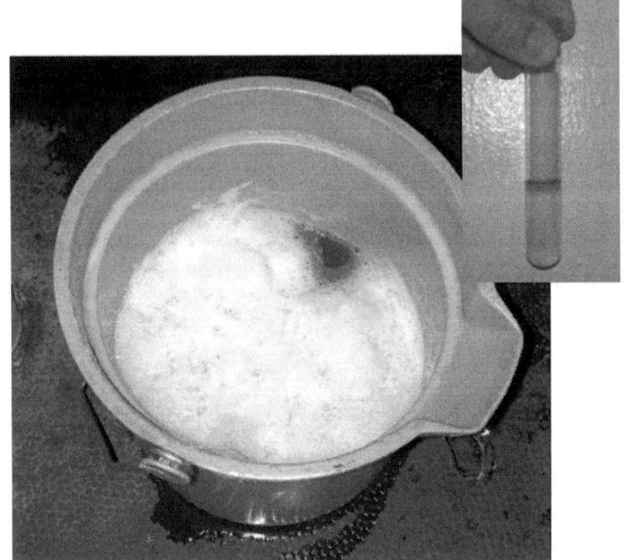

Figure 9.2 Pericardial effusion from a foal with septic pericarditis. Courtesy of Dr. Whitcomb, University of California, Davis, CA. ©Dr. Whitcomb, 2006.

Specific indicators of cardiac disease

Specific indicators of cardiac disease used in veterinary medicine include the cardiac troponins (cTn), the cardiac isoenzyme of creatine kinase (CK-MB) and the cardiac isoenzymes of lactate dehydrogenase (LDH-1, LDH-2). Cardiac troponins (e.g, cTnI and cTnT) are regulatory proteins in the cardiomyocyte and are considered to be much more cardiac specific than the cardiac isoenzymes.[26–34] Circulating concentrations increase with myocardial necrosis and inflammation[35,36] and have been documented to increase in association with myocardial disease and trauma in dogs and horses.[37–40] The cTnI assay has now been validated in horses;[41] however, its sensitivity and specificity for myocardial diseases have yet to be determined in the horse.

Other laboratory tests that help determine an aetiology can be used in suspected cases of toxicoses, such as oleander, ionophore or blister beetle (cantharidin) ingestion. These cases may present with dysrhythmias or myocarditis of varying severity (Figure 9.1), along with disease in multiple other body systems, making diagnosis more challenging without a thorough history. Although a strong index of suspicion is needed, laboratory tests can be helpful for confirmation in some cases. In cases with suspected or confirmed endocarditis, blood culture and antimicrobial sensitivity testing help in the selection of appropriate therapy. Sampling of pericardial effusions for cytological evaluation, Gram stain, culture and sensitivity, and virus isolation and titres help to differentiate septic, inflammatory/idiopathic and neoplastic causes of pericarditis (Figure 9.2). Complete blood count and fibrinogen concentrations can provide supportive data for acute inflammatory etiologies such as bacterial endocarditis and septic pericarditis, and monitoring serum protein concentrations (globulin and albumin) may indicate chronicity of disease.

Electrocardiography

Although many cardiac abnormalities can be diagnosed with careful auscultation, electrocardiography provides essential information for confirming the presence of and accurately diagnosing rhythm disturbances. An appropriate ECG can identify conclusively that a particular dysrhythmia is present, allow changes in rhythm to be appreciated over time, aid in determining the need for treatment and follow response to treatment. The technique for obtaining an ECG is described in Chapter 1.24.

Systems such as continuous 24-hour Holter monitors and radiotelemetry, which allow monitoring of a patient's rhythm from a distance without having to be directly connected to the animal, are extremely useful for hospitalised patients.[42,43] Telemetric electrocardiography allows clinicians to monitor the rhythm continuously, which is of particular importance when converting an abnormal rhythm to normal sinus rhythm or performing invasive procedures such as pericardiocentesis or cardiac catheterisation.[44,45] When performing these procedures, there is a risk of inducing dysrhythmias by inadvertently irritating the myocardium. Therefore, telemetry or some means of directly monitoring the ECG should always be used during these procedures. Because of the risks that antiarrhythmic drugs have to precipitate other unwanted dysrhythmias, it is also important to monitor the effect of any antiarrhythmic treatment on the heart rhythm during and after treatment. For instance, the use of electrocardiography is a valuable aid in monitoring the conversion of atrial fibrillation to sinus rhythm with quinidine (Figure 9.3). Quinidine is a type 1 fast sodium channel blocker, and one of its negative effects is to prolong the width of the QRS.[13] This is an indication of quinidine toxicity; therefore, the width should be monitored before each treatment, and if it increases by more than 25% of the original width, treatment should be discontinued and plasma concentrations obtained.

Many disease processes result in disturbances in cardiac rhythm, even in the absence of underlying cardiac disease, and critical care patients with electrolyte or metabolic disorders, organ failure or endotoaxemia are particularly prone to dysrhythmias. These are most often secondary disorders, and resolve with treatment of the underlying disease; however, conversion may be necessary if the rhythm disturbance worsens. Those critical care patients with known or suspected, or at high risk for the development of, dysrhythmias should be monitored with telemetry. It is used to confirm the presence of or determine the need for conversion of the dysrhythmia, in the event the patient deteriorates. For instance, many patients with gastrointestinal diseases may have intermittent or paroxysmal dysrhythmias[46,47] (Figure 9.4). Although most do not need specific antidysrhythmic treatment, as they disappear once the underlying disease has resolved, they should be monitored to take appropriate action. If the dysrhythmia becomes sustained and causes cardiovascular deterioration it will need to be addressed. Horses with primary myocarditis, congestive heart failure, and other cardiac diseases also commonly develop dysrhythmias[40,48–51] (Figure 9.5). Continuous electrocardiographic monitoring is also useful for foetal monitoring in high-risk pregnancy cases.

Telemetry is the best means to directly evaluate the effects of exercise on rhythm.[3,42] The clinician can assess

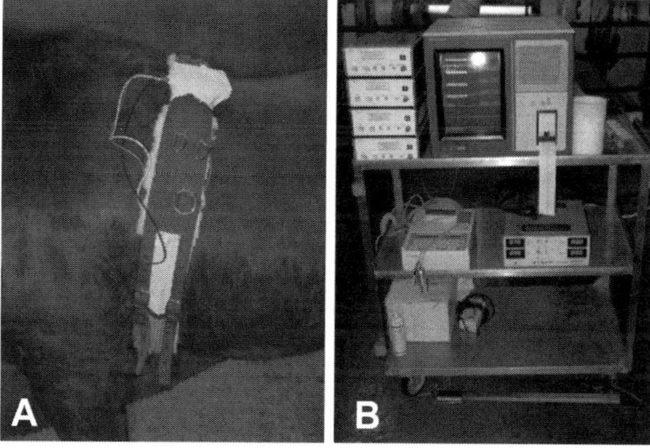

Figure 9.3 Telemetric monitoring of cardiac rhythm in a horse during conversion of atrial fibrillation using quinidine sulphate. (**A**) Horse with leads in a modified base-apex configuration secured in place with a surcingle. The transmitter is taped to the surcingle near the withers for protection. (**B**) Picture of the receiver with four channels on the top shelf. A portable ECG machine and blood pressure monitor are on the middle shelf. ©Mary Durando 2006.

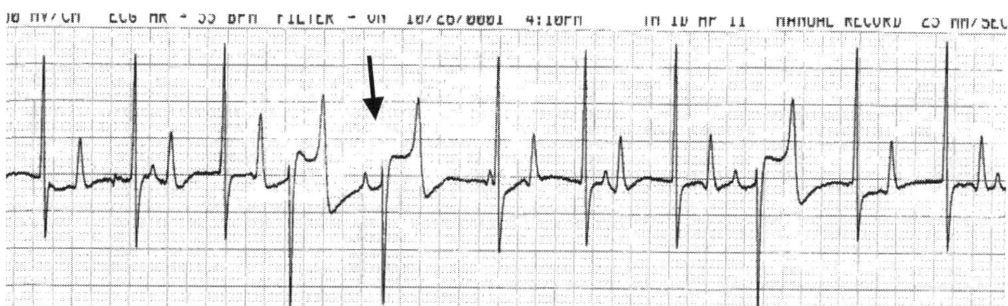

Figure 9.4 Ventricular ectopy in a postsurgical colic horse. Note the different configuration of the QRS complexes, with most of the QRS having no associated P waves. *Arrow* denotes one of the normally conducted sinus depolarisations. Base-apex lead system, paper speed 25 mm/sec. ©Mary Durando 2006.

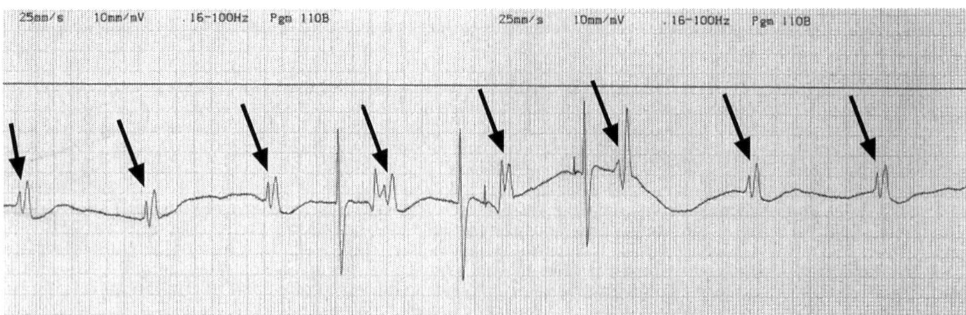

Figure 9.5 Horse with myocarditis that developed third-degree atri-ventricular block. Note the regularity of the PP interval (*arrows*) and the lack of association with the QRS. Long, irregular stretches without a QRS occurred between ventricular escape beats. Base-apex lead system, paper speed 25 mm/sec. ©Mary Durando 2006.

the presence of exercise-induced dysrhythmias and the heart rate response to exercise in horses with dysrhythmias (e.g, atrial fibrillation), to determine the maximal realistic work they are capable of doing or if conversion is needed. While this is not necessary for the critical care patient, it can be useful to perform in horses admitted with a history of collapse.[52]

Continuous 24-hour recordings with a Holter monitor may also be used to describe the horse's rhythm over a longer time.[43,44] Often the telemetry display cannot be continuously observed or printed out for prolonged periods, and the equipment may not have the capability of automatically digitally storing the ECG. Holter monitors are used if a more accurate documentation of the dysrhythmia or the frequency of the dysrhythmia in a 24-hour period is necessary. They are also often utilised to try to determine a cardiac aetiology in a horse with a history of collapse.[52] As these horses often have a normal resting physical and cardiac examination, and only intermittent collapse, it is useful to document the heart rhythm over a longer period of time, in their resting environment and, potentially, under conditions known to precipitate an episode of collapse. Holter recordings are not useful if an ongoing display of the rhythm is needed, such as while converting an abnormal rhythm or during an invasive procedure, as they do not display in real-time, but rather record, either digitally or on a magnetic tape, for future evaluation.

Analysis of an electrocardiographic recording

When evaluating an ECG, it is critical to have a methodical approach. Simplifying the evaluation makes determining the rhythm less overwhelming. The heart rate is calculated first to determine if a severe tachyarrhythmia or bradyarrhythmia is present, as these are the rhythm disturbances most likely to need immediate correction. This can be done by counting the number of beats in a known time (e.g, in a 6-second period and multiplying by 10) or dividing 60 by the RR duration (in seconds). If each small box is 1 mm, the duration of the RR interval can be calculated as long as the paper speed is known (e.g, at a paper speed of 25 mm/sec, 25 small boxes = 1 second, 1 small box = 0.04 second). However, if this method is used, it must be noted if the heart rate was calculated during sinus rhythm or during a dysrhythmia. It is useful to calculate the heart rate occurring during both normal sinus rhythm and during any paroxysms of dysrhythmia such as atrial or ventricular tachycardia, and to calculate both the atrial and ventricular rate. The longer the duration used to calculate the heart rate, the more accurate is the representation of overall heart rate. However, if paroxysms of rapid tachycardia or prolonged asystole occur, this is also very important information, even if the overall heart rate is not significantly abnormal.

Once the heart rate is calculated, the presence and origin of all abnormal complexes should be determined, along with their pattern and frequency of occurrence (e.g, intermittent or sustained). If there is an association with some stimulus, this should be noted. Normal sinus rhythm has a P wave for every QRS, and a QRS for every P wave; any deviations from this indicate dysrhythmias. There should also be a regular RR interval and a regular PP interval. Calipers are extremely useful for determining regularity of intervals and detecting P waves that may be partially buried in T waves or ST segments (Figure 9.6). The appearance of each complex should be observed; all QRS complexes should look similar, and have an appropriate appearance for the lead system used, although there may be some variations in the T waves. Depolarisations are commonly described as supraventricular or ventricular in origin (Figure 9.7). Usually, the configuration of a supraventricular beat has a similar appearance as the QRS of the normally conducted sinus beats, and should be associated with a P wave, although the P wave may be difficult to find, if buried in the preceding T wave. Ventricular depolarisations almost always have a very different appearance to the QRS from normal sinus beats, and the T wave is usually larger than normal, and opposite in orientation to the QRS. No P wave will be associated with the QRS-T, and there is often (though not always) a compensatory pause after the premature depolarisation. If it is difficult to determine the origin, particularly in rapid tachyarrhythmias, more than one lead system may be necessary, and the paper speed can

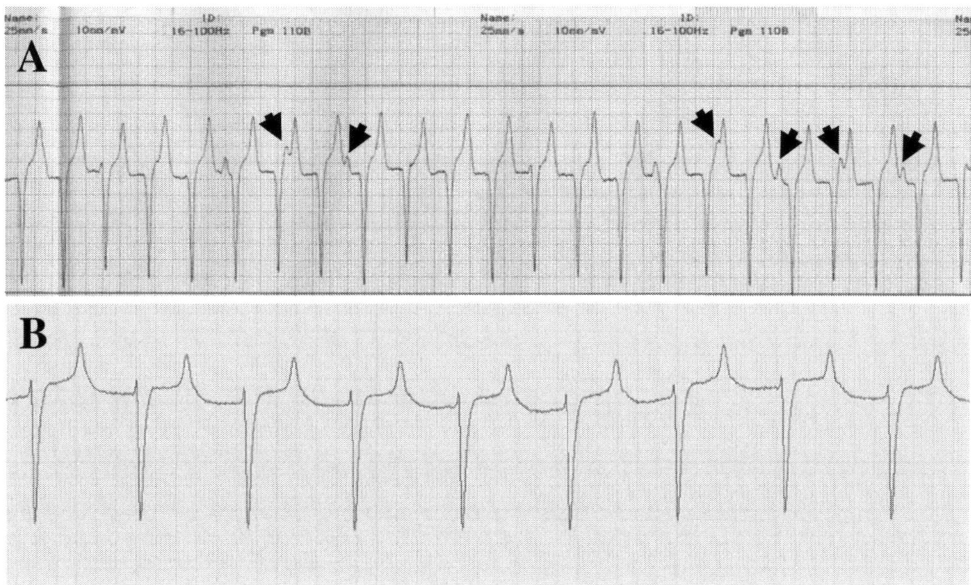

Figure 9.6 (**A**) Uniform ventricular tachycardia. Note the regular RR interval and similar appearance of QRS-T complexes. However, P waves are not associated with QRS complexes, and are found in varying places within the QRS-T complexes. Calipers are extremely useful to help detect the P waves. *Arrowheads* mark some of the P waves. (**B**) Supraventricular tachycardia. The RR interval is regular and the QRS-T complexes have a similar appearance. The QRS morphology is the same as the sinus beats (not shown). P waves are buried in the preceding T waves. Base-apex lead system. ©Mary Durando 2006.

be increased to 50 mm/second to try to better discern the complexes. ECGs should be monitored daily on horses with rhythm disturbances, to record any changes in frequency, pattern or type of dysrhythmia, as this may indicate a change in status of the disease. It is also important to remember to evaluate the effect of the dysrhythmia on the clinical status of the horse, and if this has changed (Figure 9.8). For a detailed description of the appearance of specific dysrhythmias, the reader can consult several publications on this topic.[3,6,44,53–55]

Echocardiography

Echocardiography has tremendously improved the clinician's ability to diagnose cardiac diseases in the horse and has all but eliminated the need for more invasive techniques. The basic technique is described in Chapter 1.25. Although in some cases cardiac catheterisation can add important information, it is rarely needed for diagnoses in clinical cases. Because of the lack of sensitivity of ECGs and radiographs in the evaluation of anatomic and functional abnormalities of the heart, the equine clinician relies almost exclusively on echocardiography. Echocardiography allows evaluation of both normal and abnormal cardiac structure and function, and the effects of training and exercise on the heart.[3] It is also invaluable for monitoring disease progression and/or response to therapy and for formulating a prognosis for future performance and life expectancy. It is important to remember that an orderly, thorough examination should be done, even when reassessing patients, so that unexpected changes or new complications are not overlooked.

Indications for echocardiography

There are many situations when echocardiography is useful to monitor hospitalised patients, or to determine the need for hospitalisation and further treatment. Although the clinical cardiac examination, particularly auscultation, provides the basis for the need for echocardiography, echocardiography (including M-mode and Doppler studies) is required to definitively diagnose the abnormality, classify its severity and determine the need for treatment. Often, serial examinations are needed to assess progression of disease.

Horses quite commonly have murmurs and dysrhythmias; however, most are physiological or not clinically relevant.[56–61] Echocardiography is invaluable to determine whether a murmur has a physiological or a pathological basis, and, in the case of the latter, the severity of the disease process causing it, or whether underlying cardiac disease is associated with an observed dysrhythmia.

Echocardiography is useful in the neonate and adult for diagnosing both congenital (Figure 9.9) and acquired cardiac diseases.[2,9,62–66] Clinical examination findings that should prompt evaluation for congenital cardiac disease in neonates include a persistent ≥grade 3/6 holosystolic murmur, ≥grade 1/6 holodiastolic murmur, ≥grade 1/6 continuous murmur lasting beyond 4 days or cyanosis in the face of oxygen therapy.

Clinical findings often associated with adult cardiac disease are grade >3/6 systolic murmur, ≥3/6 diastolic murmur, tachycardia unexplained by other clinical examination findings or tachycardia >100 beats/min, dysrhythmias other than second-degree atrioventricular block or

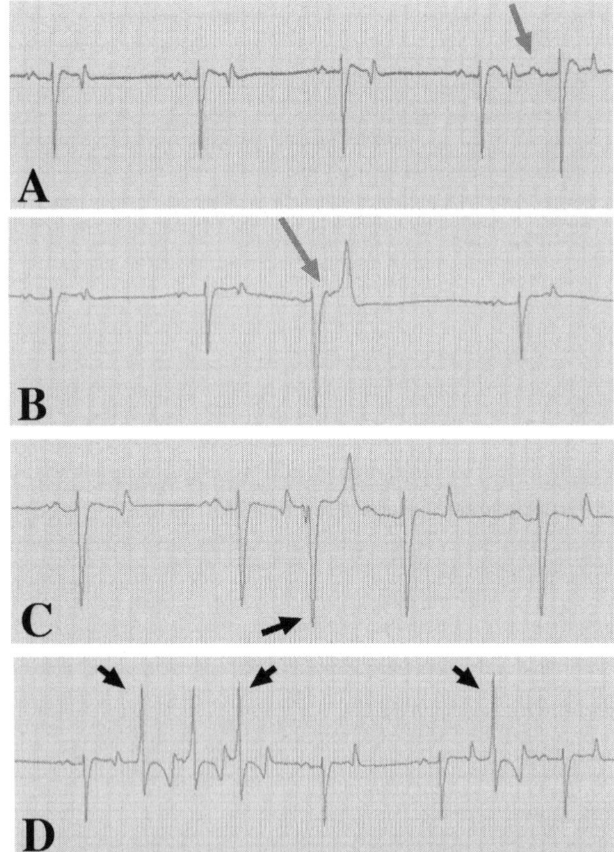

Figure 9.7 (**A**) Supraventricular premature depolarisation. The QRS-T following the early P wave looks similar to the sinus beats. Note the slightly different appearance of the premature P wave (*arrow*), compared with the sinus beats. (**B**) Ventricular premature depolarisation. The premature QRS-T has a different morphology than the sinus beats, and is not associated with a P wave (*arrow*). This ventricular premature beat is followed by a compensatory pause. (**C**) Interpolated ventricular premature depolarisation. The arrow marks the interpolated beat. (**D**) Run of three ventricular premature beats not followed by a compensatory pause. Base-apex lead systems for each figure. ©Mary Durando 2006.

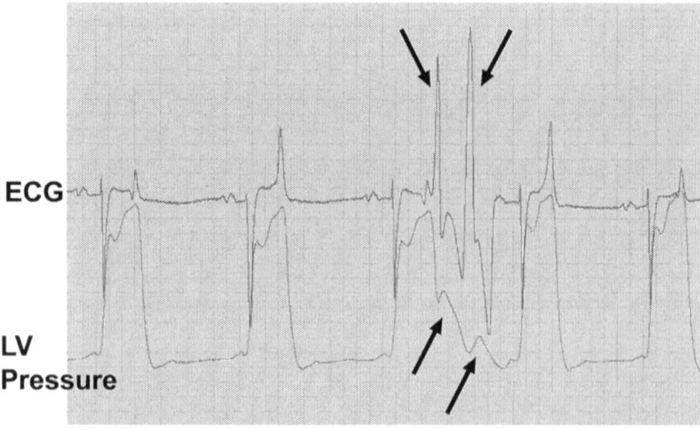

Figure 9.8 Effect of ventricular premature beats on left ventricular (LV) pressures. A base-apex ECG (*top*) and a high-fidelity catheter-tipped transducer in the left ventricle (*bottom*) are shown. A normal LV pressure trace immediately follows each QRS that is conducted normally. *Arrows* point to the premature ventricular depolarisations (VPDs), and their effect on LV pressures. These VPDs would result in a pulse deficit (not enough LV pressure to open the aortic valve), which could contribute to syncopal episodes if frequent. ©Mary Durando 2006.

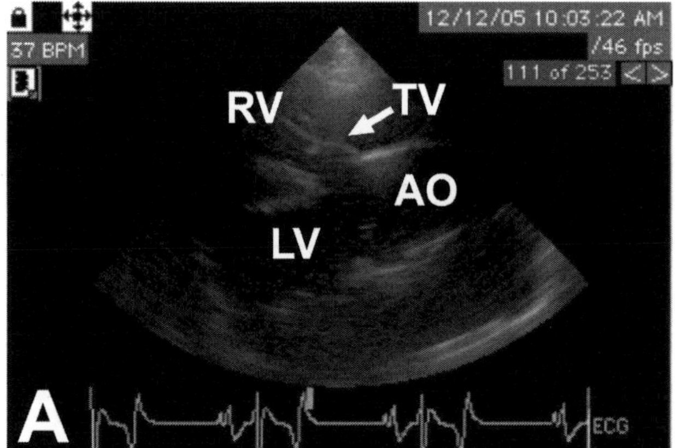

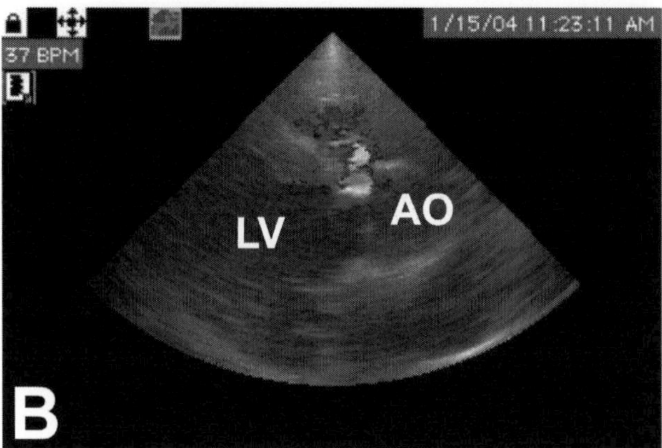

Figure 9.9 An adult Standardbred horse with a ventricular septal defect. (A) Right parasternal long axis view of the left outflow tract showing a membranous septal defect beneath the aortic and tricuspid valves. This is the most common location for a VSD. (B) Colour flow Doppler of the VSD showing turbulent dark flow through the defect. Abbreviations are as follows: AO, aorta; LV, left ventricle; RV, right ventricle; TV, tricuspid valve. Images courtesy of Dr. V. Reef, University of Pennsylvania. ©Dr. V. Reef 2006.

sinus dysrhythmia, pulse deficits, generalised venous distension, pericardial friction rubs or muffled or dull heart sounds. The presence of any of these warrants further evaluation using echocardiography. Changes in the character of a murmur or recent onset of a murmur, cough or dyspnoea, ventral oedema, fever of unknown origin, or unexplained poor performance or exercise intolerance may also signify cardiac disease, although all of the above are also associated with diseases of other body systems. Depending on other clinical examination and diagnostic findings, these clinical signs may also warrant further echocardiographic investigation.

Valvular lesions

Echocardiography is particularly useful in the diagnosis of valvular abnormalities, and is the most sensitive means of diagnosing bacterial endocarditis[67] (Figure 9.10). It can be used to determine which valves are affected and the severity

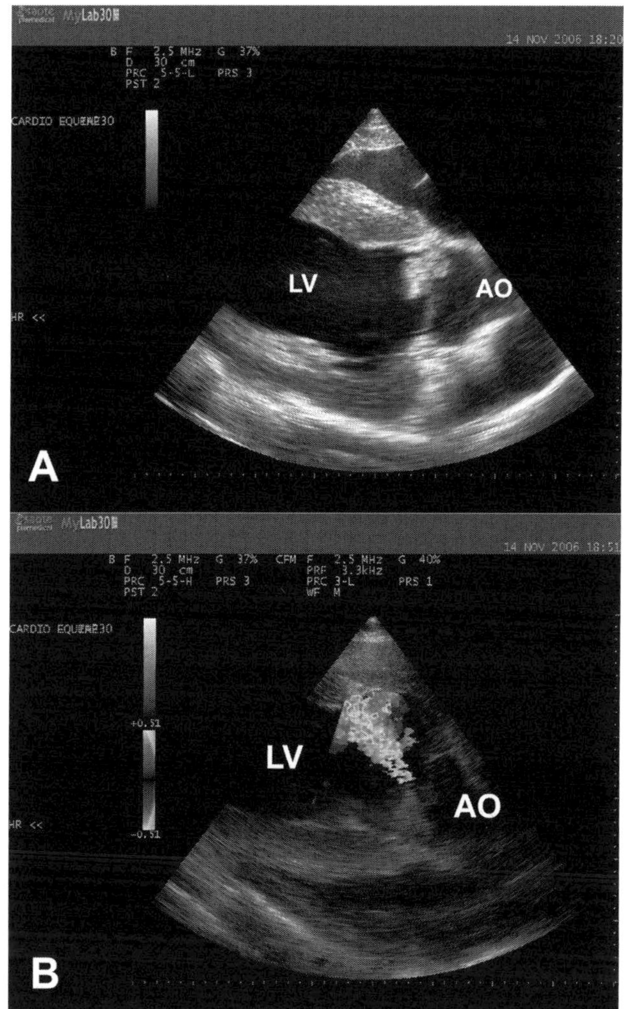

Figure 9.10 Horse with severe bacterial endocarditis. (A) Right parasternal long-axis view of the aortic valve and left outflow tract. Marked thickening of the right coronary cusps is seen. In addition, there is left ventricular hypertrophy secondary to aortic stenosis from the distorted valve. (B) Colour flow Doppler of the aortic valve in a left parasternal long-axis view, showing aortic regurgitation during diastole. Because of the distortion of the aortic valve, both stenosis and regurgitation were present. Abbreviations are as follows: AO, aorta; LV, left ventricle. ©Kevin Corley 2006.

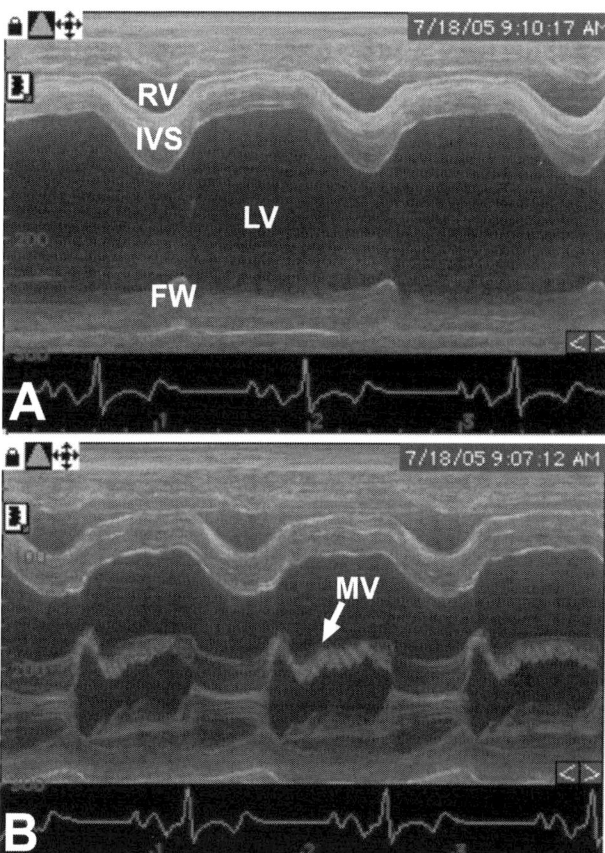

Figure 9.11 Horse with severe aortic insufficiency and left ventricular volume overload. (A) M-mode image of the left ventricle showing an enlarged left ventricle with a reduced fractional shortening (contractility). Note the wavy motion of the septal wall and the compressed appearance to the right ventricle in diastole. (B) M-mode of the mitral valve. The *arrow* points to the high frequency fluttering of the mitral valve in diastole, from the jet of aortic regurgitation. Abbreviations are as follows: RV, right ventricle; LV, left ventricle; IVS, interventricular septum; FW, free wall; MV, mitral valve. Images courtesy of Dr. V. Reef, University of Pennsylvania. ©Dr. V. Reef 2006.

of the structural changes. It can also show if other endocardial surfaces are involved. Echocardiography allows the clinician to monitor the effect of treatment by following the size and appearance of the lesion, and, importantly, the effect on valve structure and function as it resolves. This is important, because even after resolution of the infection the valve may be permanently scarred, with worsening of the regurgitation over time.

Severe aortic and mitral regurgitation, leading to congestive heart failure, also are easily diagnosed with echocardiography.[8,68] Not only can the affected valves be determined, but the effect of the dysfunction on chamber size, valvular competence, and myocardial function should also be evaluated. Aortic insufficiency is one of the most common valvular diseases in older horses, and may be associated with degenerative changes or endocarditis. While it is often a slowly progressive disease that does not significantly impact performance or life expectancy when caused by degenerative valve disease, it can proceed more rapidly to severe disease.[49] As aortic regurgitation becomes more severe, the aortic root and left ventricle become enlarged, and fractional shortening increases above normal. This is the normal compensatory response to volume overload. As the myocardium begins to fail, the fractional shortening will decrease back to normal, and then below normal (Figure 9.11). Other echocardiographic findings related to aortic insufficiency include fluttering of the aortic and mitral valve leaflets (Figure 9.11). Left ventricular enlargement can eventually lead to stretching of the mitral valve annulus, mitral regurgitation, left atrial enlargement and, eventually, pulmonary oedema and hypertension (congestive heart failure). These cases can advance to right heart failure over time, and the horse may be presented with signs of right heart failure (e.g, venous distension and ventral oedema) rather than left heart failure. Because of atrial enlargement, these horses commonly develop atrial fibrillation. Horses with left ventricular enlargement can also have ventricular ectopic depolarisations, which may be related to poor coronary perfusion.

Mitral valve lesions are also common, and it is the valve lesion most often resulting in poor performance or congestive heart failure. Ruptured chordae tendinae of the mitral valve can lead to acute onset respiratory distress. Lesions of the mitral valve are best seen from the left parasternal approach, and often better alignment with blood flow for Doppler studies is achieved from this window. A more accurate measurement of left atrial size and secondary enlargement can be determined from the left parasternal two-chamber view.

Other causes of acute-onset distress that might be encountered in an intensive care setting or emergency basis that are best detected with echocardiography include intact or ruptured aortic aneurysms.[69,70] These may present with clinical signs that can be mistaken for colic, and often these horses have concurrent ventricular tachycardia.

Myocarditis and cardiomyopathies

Echocardiography is also useful to evaluate myocarditis and cardiomyopathies. Frequent dysrhythmias not attributable to other diseases may be due to primary myocarditis. In these cases, one may see abnormalities in myocardial echogenicity, along with focal, regional or global decreases in contractility and wall motion.[51]

Pericardial disease

Pericardial diseases are easily recognised with echocardiography.[3,45,71,72] Echocardiography allows determination of the volume and character of effusion, effect of the effusion on cardiac function, optimal location for pericardiocentesis and depth needed to perform pericardiocentesis and gives the ability to monitor progression of disease and effect of treatment (see Chapter 1.27 and Figure 1.102).

Pericarditis

Pericardiocentesis to obtain fluid samples is used for both diagnostic and therapeutic purposes in horses with pericarditis. The technique is described in Chapter 1.27. Whilst recognition and general assessment of pericarditis and pericardial effusion are best done with echocardiography, evaluation of the recovered fluid can be extremely helpful to determine a specific aetiology and to direct therapy. Pericardiocentesis is essential as a treatment aid in horses with large volumes of pericardial effusion. Should sufficient fluid be present to cause cardiac tamponade, immediate, aggressive drainage is necessary.[3,45,71,73,74]

Clinical signs

Horses with pericarditis may initially appear painful or reluctant to move, depressed and/or anorexic and, dependent on the aetiology, may be febrile or tachypnoeic.[45] These clinical signs are commonly confused with colic or pleuritis. On auscultation, biphasic or triphasic friction rubs, which should not be mistaken for murmurs or pleural friction rubs, may be heard when the volume of effusion is small. As the volume of effusion increases, the friction rubs may disappear and heart sounds will be muffled. If the volume of effusion is large enough, particularly if the onset is rapid, it can result in cardiac tamponade. Clinically, this is seen as tachycardia with muffled heart sounds, generalised venous distension with jugular pulses (Figure 9.12), weak peripheral arterial pulses and ventral/pectoral oedema. Pericardiocentesis should be performed in horses with effusion that results in cardiovascular compromise or has a septic appearance echocardiographically.

Evaluation of the fluid

Horses most commonly develop pericarditis due to bacterial or viral infections, or idiopathic or inflammatory/immune-mediated conditions, although neoplasia and

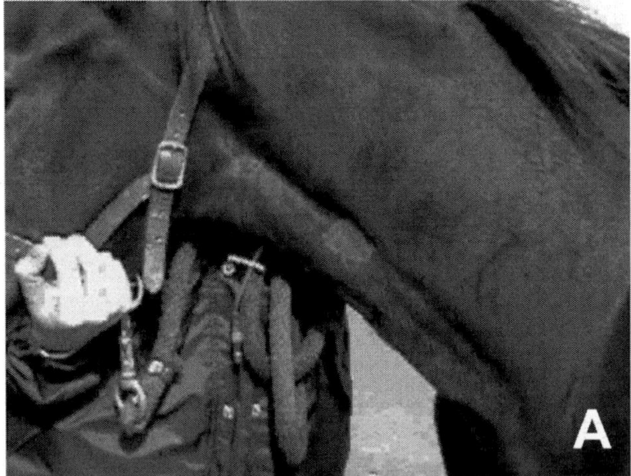

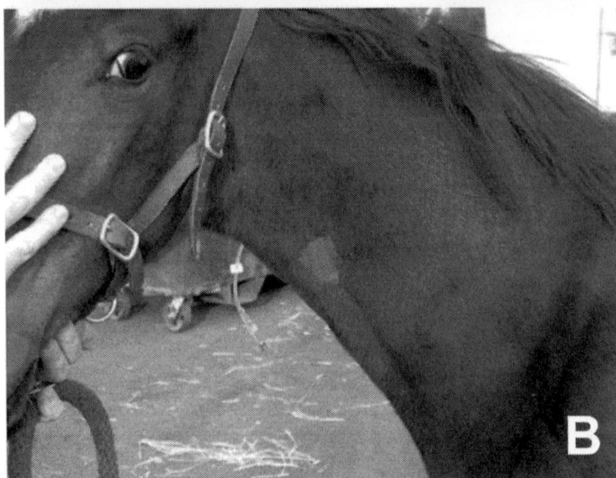

Figure 9.12 Foal with pericardial effusion causing tamponade. **(A)** Note the distended jugular vein before pericardiocentesis and drainage. **(B)** Normal jugular vein postdrainage. Photos courtesy of Dr. Whitcomb, University of California, Davis, CA. ©Dr. Whitcomb, 2006.

trauma can also result in effusion. Evaluation of the fluid is used to help distinguish between causes. Aspirated fluid should be submitted to clinical and microbiological laboratories for the following evaluations: cytology for cell type and morphology, bacterial culture and antimicrobial sensitivity testing, virus isolation and titres, and biochemical analysis of pH, glucose and lactate. If a concurrent pleural effusion is present or pneumonia is suspected, a transtracheal aspirate and/or pleural fluid should also be submitted for similar tests.

Horses with septic pericarditis typically have a neutrophilia with degenerate neutrophils present in the fluid. Bacteria may be seen on cytology or Gram stain and may be cultured from the effusion, although cultures are often negative with septic pericarditis. Culture and cytology of transtracheal and pleural fluid may help confirm a septic cause, if a concurrent pleuropneumonia exists. Inflammatory/immune-mediated causes and idiopathic pericarditis most commonly have a neutrophilia composed primarily of well-preserved neutrophils, although cases with idiopathic effusive pericarditis may have a histiocytic or eosinophilic effusion.[72] The presence of neoplastic cells confirms neoplasia as a cause of pericarditis. A haemorrhagic effusion would most likely be secondary to trauma, although other causes may be possible.

Drainage

The amount and type of effusion present should dictate whether a single sampling of fluid or placement of a large-bore catheter for repeated drainage and lavage is necessary. If a large volume of fluid is present, particularly if fibrinous or echogenic in appearance, if it is accumulating rapidly, or if the horse is exhibiting signs of cardiovascular compromise, a large-bore tube should be placed[45,71] (Figures 9.13 and 9.14). This tube can be used for repeated drainage and lavage of the pericardial sac with instillation of antibiotics,

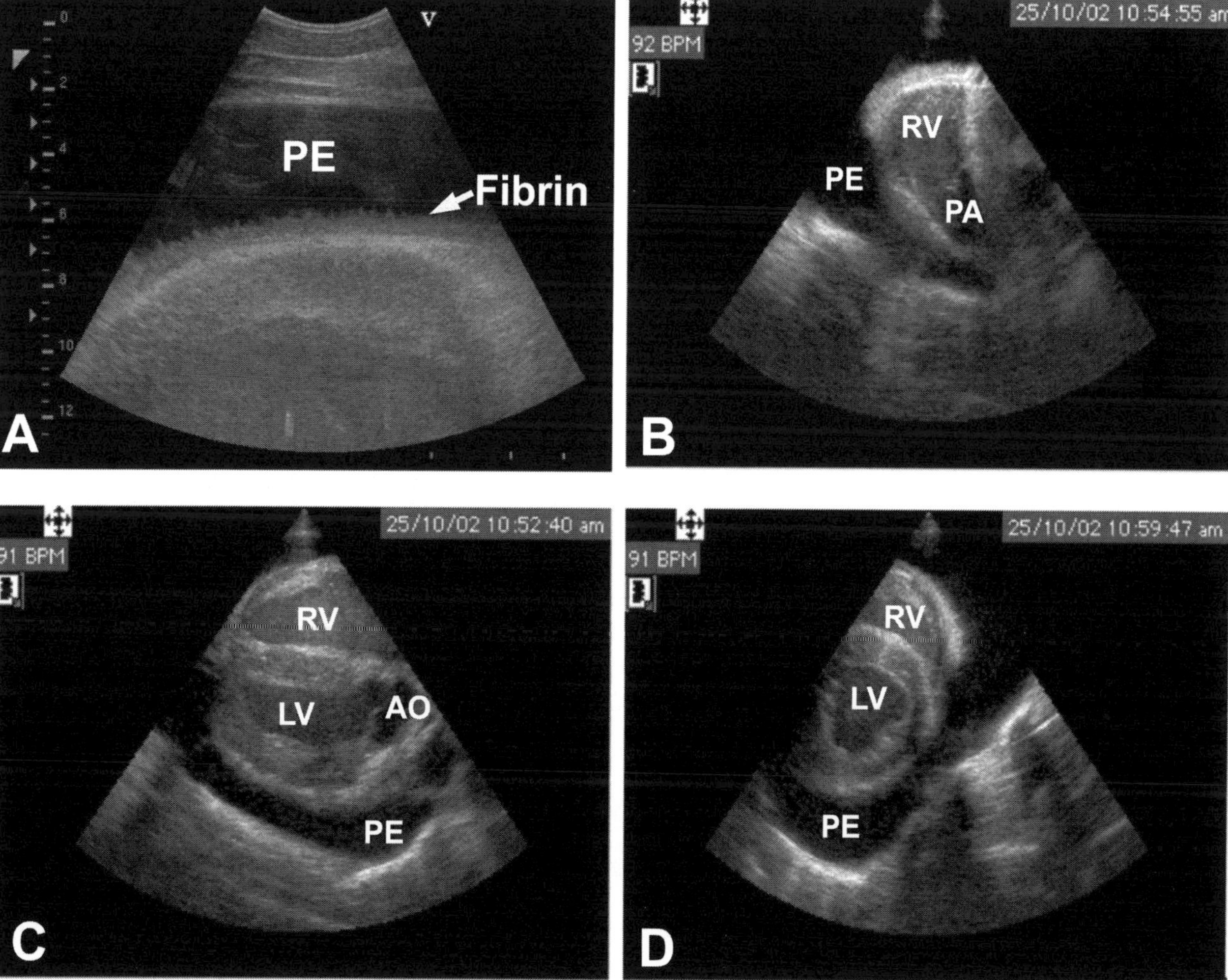

Figure 9.13 Echocardiograms of a foal with pericarditis. (**A**) Note the shaggy appearance of the fibrin lining the endocardial surface. (**B–D**) Right parasternal two-dimensional echocardiograms showing pericardial effusion and decreased right and left ventricular filling. A long-axis view of the right (**B**) and left (**C**) outflow tracts and a short-axis view of the left ventricle (**D**) are shown. Abbreviations: PE, pericardial effusion; RV, right ventricle; PA, pulmonary artery; LV, left ventricle; AO, aorta. Images courtesy of Dr. Whitcomb, University of California, Davis, CA. ©Dr. Whitcomb, 2006.

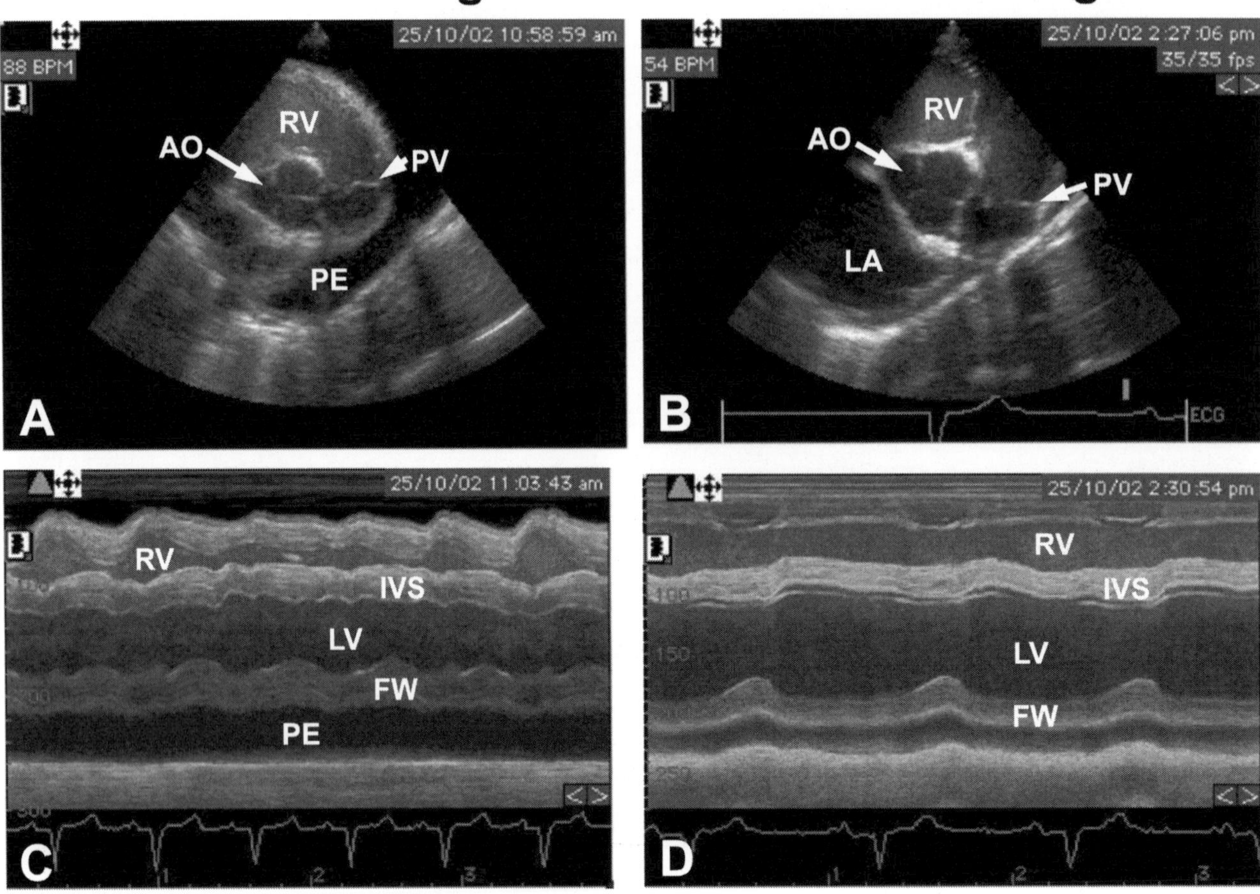

Figure 9.14 Predrainage and postdrainage echocardiograms showing the effect of fluid removal on the heart. Right parasternal short axis view of the aorta (**A**) before (*left*) and (**B**) after (*right*) drainage. Note the improved filling of the right ventricle and larger aortic root and left atrium following removal of fluid. M-mode of the left ventricle (**C**) before (*left*) and (**D**) after (*right*) fluid removal. Left ventricular filling and function have improved and the right ventricle is larger. Heart rate is also significantly slower. Abbreviations are as used earlier. PV, pulmonic valve; LA, left atrium; IVS, interventricular septum; FW, free wall. Images courtesy of Dr. Whitcomb, University of California, Davis, CA. ©Dr. Whitcomb, 2006.

if needed. If an indwelling tube or catheter is placed, it is important to secure it well so that it does not get repositioned and to ensure that it is capped or clamped off completely. After drainage, the pericardial sac can be lavaged with at least 2 L of warmed isotonic fluids, followed by instillation of 1 L of fluids containing antimicrobials (e.g, sodium penicillin, $1–10 \times 10^6$ units or gentamicin). Potassium penicillin should not be used, because of the potential negative effects of potassium on the heart. Ideally, drainage and lavage should be performed every 12 hours. This should be continued until the volume of fluid initially drained is small (i.e, <1 L) over a couple of attempts, at which time the catheter can be removed. The volume of residual fluid should be assessed with echocardiography before removing the catheter, in the event that fibrin has clogged the tube, preventing adequate drainage, or the tube position has shifted. Lavage and instillation of fluids with antibiotics are done to remove fluid, fibrin, inflammatory mediators and bacteria and bacterial products and to prevent fibrin deposition and adhesion formation between the pericardial sac and the epicardium, which could result in a chronic constrictive pericarditis. Installation of antimicrobials in the pericardial fluid results in higher concentrations of antibiotics locally. The horse should also receive broad-spectrum antibiotics systemically if a septic aetiology is suspected or until proved otherwise. Anti-inflammatory doses of corticosteroids may be helpful for a suspected idiopathic pericarditis if sepsis is ruled out.[72,74] Prophylactic antimicrobial therapy can be instituted in these cases. Nonsteroidal anti-inflammatory agents can be administered for anti-inflammatory and analgesic purposes.

If only a small volume of effusion is present and/or drainage is likely only needed once, a smaller over-the-needle catheter system or teat cannula in smaller, thinner horses for sample collection and drainage can be used.

Once the catheter is removed, the horse should continue to receive stall rest and be monitored carefully for signs of reoccurrence of effusion by clinical examination and echocardiography. The horse should also continue to be treated for the underlying aetiology (if it is known).

References

1. Reef VB: Evaluation of the equine cardiovascular system. Vet Clin N Am: Equine Pract 1:275-288, 1985
2. Bonagura JD, Blissitt KJ: Echocardiography. Equine Vet J Suppl:5-17, 1995
3. Bonagura JD, Reef VB: Cardiovascular diseases, in Reed SM, Bayly WM (eds): Equine Internal Medicine. Philadelphia, WB Saunders, 1998, pp 290-370
4. Durando MM, Young LE: Cardiovascular examination and diagnostic techniques, in Robinson NE (ed): Current Therapy in Equine Medicine, ed 5. St. Louis, WB Saunders, 2003, pp 572-585
5. Fregin GF: Cardiovascular sound and cardiac auscultation in the normal horse. Compend Contin Educ Pract Vet 1:S28-S32, 1979
6. McGuirk SM, Muir WW: Diagnosis and treatment of cardiac arrhythmias. Vet Clin N Am: Equine Pract 1:353-370, 1985
7. Welker FH, Muir WW: An investigation of the second heart sound in the normal horse. Equine Vet J 22:403-407, 1990
8. Reef VB, Bain FT, Spencer PA: Severe mitral regurgitation in horses: clinical, echocardiographic and pathological findings. Equine Vet J 30:18-27, 1998
9. Reef VB: Heart murmurs in horses: determining their significance with echocardiography. Equine Vet J Suppl 19:71-80, 1995
10. Dart AJ, Snyder JR, Spier SJ, et al.: Ionized calcium concentration in horses with surgically managed gastrointestinal disease: 147 cases (1988-1990). J Am Vet Med Assoc 201:1244-1248, 1992
11. Garcia-Lopez JM, Provost PJ, Rush JE, et al.: Prevalence and prognostic importance of hypomagnesemia and hypocalcemia in horses that have colic surgery. Am J Vet Res 62:7-12, 2001
12. Chakraborti S, Chakraborti T, Mandal M, et al.: Protective role of magnesium in cardiovascular diseases: a review. Moll Cell Biochem 238:163-179, 2002
13. Reef VB, Reimer JM, Spencer PA: Treatment of atrial fibrillation in horses: new perspectives. J Vet Int Med 9:57-67, 1995
14. Muir WW, McGuirk SM: Pharmacology and pharmacokinetics of drugs used to treat cardiac disease in horses. Vet Clin N Am: Equine Pract 1:335-352, 1985
15. Marr CM: Treatment of cardiac arrhythmias and cardiac failure, in Robinson NE (ed): Current Therapy in Equine Medicine, ed 4. Philadelphia, WB Saunders, 1997, pp 250-255
16. Protopapas K: Studies on metabolic disturbances and other post-operative complications following equine surgery, in Department of Farm Animal and Equine Medicine and Surgery. London, Royal Veterinary College, University of London, 2000, p 298
17. Henninger RW, Horst J: Magnesium toxicosis in two horses. J Am Vet Med Assoc 211:82-85, 1997
18. Divers T: Monitoring tissue oxygenation in the ICU patient. Clin Tech Equine Pract 2:138-144, 2003
19. Wetmore LA, Derksen FJ, Blaze CA, et al.: Mixed venous oxygen tension as an estimate of cardiac output in anesthetized horses. Am J Vet Res 48:971-976, 1987
20. Cohen RI, Huberfeld S, Genovese J, et al.: A comparison between the acute effects of nitric oxide synthase inhibition and fluid resuscitation on myocardial function and metabolism in endotoxemic dogs. J Crit Care 11:27-36, 1996
21. Fish RE, Burns AH, Lang CH, et al.: Myocardial dysfunction in a nonlethal, nonshock model of chronic endotoxemia. Circ Shock 16:241-252, 1985
22. Peng T, Lu X, Lei M, et al.: Inhibition of p38 MAPK decreases myocardial TNF-alpha expression and improves myocardial function and survival in endotoxemia. Cardiovasc Res 59:893-900, 2003
23. Romanosky AJ, Giaimo ME, Shepherd RE, et al.: The effect of in vivo endotoxin on myocardial function in vitro. Circ Shock 19:1-12, 1986
24. Rubin LJ, Keller RS, Parker JL, et al.: Contractile dysfunction of ventricular myocytes isolated from endotoxemic guinea pigs. Shock 2:113-120, 1994
25. Sosa G, Milstein JM, Bennett SH: Escherichia coli endotoxin depresses left ventricular contractility in neonatal lambs. Pediatr Res 35:62-67, 1994
26. Adams JE, Bodor GS, Davila-Roman VG, et al.: Cardiac troponin I. A marker with high specificity for cardiac injury. Circulation 88:101-106, 1993
27. Bennett AE, R.L. B: Discordant results of CK-MB and troponin I measurements: a review of 14 cases. Ann Clin Lab Sci 30:167-173, 2000
28. La Vecchia L, Mezzena G, Zanolla L, et al.: Cardiac troponin I as diagnostic and prognostic marker in severe heart failure. J Heart Lung Transplant 19:644-652, 2000
29. Mair J, Wagner I, Puschendorf B, et al.: Cardiac troponin I to diagnose myocardial injury. Lancet 341:838-839, 1993
30. Mair J, Wagner I, Morass B, et al.: Cardiac troponin I release correlates with myocardial infarction size. Eur J Clin Chem Clin Biochem 33:869-872, 1995
31. Mair J, Genser N, Morandell D, et al.: Cardiac troponin I in the diagnosis of myocardial injury and infarction. Clin Chim Acta 245:19-38, 1996
32. Mair J: Cardiac troponin I and troponin T: are enzymes still relevant as cardiac markers? Clin Chim Acta 257:99-115, 1997
33. O'Brien PJ, Landt Y, Ladenson JH: Differential reactivity of cardiac and skeletal muscle from various species in a cardiac troponin I immunoassay. Clin Chem 43:2333-2338, 1997
34. Voderwinkler KP, Mair J, Puschendorf B, et al.: Cardiac troponin I increases in parallel to cardiac troponin T, creatine kinase and lactate dehydrogenase in effluents from isolated perfused rat hearts after hypoxia-reoxygenation-induced myocardial injury. Clin Chim Acta 251:113-117, 1996
35. Edouard AR, Benoist JF, Cosson C, et al.: Circulating cardiac troponin I in trauma patients without cardiac contusion. Intensive Care Med 24:569-573, 1998
36. Horwich TB, Patel J, MacLellan WR, et al.: Cardiac troponin I is associated with impaired hemodynamics, progressive left ventricular dysfunction, and increased mortality rates in advanced heart failure. Circulation 108:833-838, 2003
37. Oyama MA, Sisson DD: Cardiac troponin-I concentration in dogs with cardiac disease. J Vet Int Med 18:831-839, 2004
38. Schober KE, Kirbach B, Oechtering G: Noninvasive assessment of myocardial cell injury in dogs with suspected cardiac contusion. Eur J Vet Cardiol 1:17-25, 2000
39. Schober KE, Cornand C, Kirbach B, et al.: Serum cardiac troponin I and cardiac troponin T concentrations in dogs

with gastric dilatation-volvulus. J Am Vet Med Assoc 221:381-388, 2002
40. Schwarzwald CC, Hardy J, Buccellato M: High cardiac troponin I serum concentration in a horse with multiform ventricular tachycardia and myocardial necrosis. J Vet Int Med 17:364-368, 2003
41. Rishniw M, Simpson KW: Cloning and sequencing of equine cardiac troponin I and confirmation of its usefulness as a target analyte for commercial troponin I analyzers. J Vet Diagn Invest 17:582-584, 2005
42. Reef VB: Electrocardiography and echocardiography in the exercising horse, in Robinson NE (ed): Current Therapy in Equine Medicine, ed 4. Philadelphia, WB Saunders, 1997, pp 234-239
43. Reef VB: Ambulatory and exercise electrocardiography and post-exercise echocardiography, in Marr CM (ed): Cardiology of the Horse. London, WB Saunders, 1999, pp 150-160
44. Reef VB: Arrhythmias, in Marr CM (ed): Cardiology of the Horse. London, WB Saunders, 1999, pp 179-209
45. Worth LT, Reef VB: Pericarditis in horses: 18 cases (1986-1995). J Am Vet Med Assoc 212:248-253, 1998
46. Cornick JL, Seahorn TL: Cardiac arrhythmias identified in horses with duodenitis/proximal jejunitis: six cases (1985-1988). J Am Vet Med Assoc 197:1054-1059, 1990
47. Rebhun WC: Exopthalmos in horses. Equine Vet Educ 10:63-65, 1998
48. Button C, Scrutchfield WL, Clark RG, et al.: Multiple atrial dysrhythmias in a horse. J Am Vet Med Assoc 177:714-719, 1980
49. Marr CM: Heart failure, in Marr CM (ed): Cardiology of the Horse. London, WB Saunders, 1999, pp 289-311
50. Reimer JM, Reef VB, Sweeney RW: Ventricular arrhythmias in horses: 21 cases (1984-1989). J Am Vet Med Assoc 201:1237-1243, 1992
51. Traub-Dargatz JL, Schlipf JW, Boon J, et al.: Ventricular tachycardia and myocardial dysfunction in a horse. J Am Vet Med Assoc 205:1569-1573, 1994
52. Piercy RJ, Marr CM: Collapse, in Marr CM (ed): Cardiology of the Horse. London, WB Saunders, 1999, pp 268-288
53. Bonagura JD: Diagnosis of cardiac arrhythmias, in Robinson NE (ed): Current Therapy in Equine Medicine (ed 4th). Philadelphia, WB Saunders, 1997, pp 240-250
54. Bowen IM: Cardiac dysrhythmias, in Robinson NE (ed): Current Therapy in Equine Medicine, ed 5. St. Louis, WB Saunders, 2003, pp 602-613
55. Patteson MW: Equine Cardiology. Oxford, Blackwell, 1996, p 254
56. Holmes JR, Alps BJ: The effect of exercise on rhythm irregularities in the horse. Vet Rec 78:672-683, 1966
57. Kriz N, Hodgson D, Rose R: Prevalence and clinical importance of heart murmurs in racehorses. J Am Vet Med Assoc 216:1441-1445, 2000
58. Marr CM, Reef VB: Physiological valvular regurgitation in clinically normal young racehorses: prevalence and two-dimensional colour flow Doppler echocardiographic characteristics. Equine Vet J Suppl 19:56-62, 1995
59. Patteson MW, Cripps PJ: A survey of cardiac auscultatory findings in horses. Equine Vet J 25:409-415, 1993
60. Young LE, Wood JLN: Effect of age and training on murmurs of atrioventricular valvular regurgitation in young thoroughbreds. Equine Vet J 32:195-199, 2000
61. Young LE: Cardiac responses to training in 2-year-old thoroughbreds: an echocardiographic study. Equine Vet J Suppl 30:195-198, 1999
62. Long KJ, Bonagura JD, Darke PG: Standardised imaging technique for guided M-mode and Doppler echocardiography in the horse. Equine Vet J 24:226-235, 1992
63. Marr CM, Reef VB, Reimer JM, et al.: An echocardiographic study of atrial fibrillation in horses: before and after conversion to sinus rhythm. J Vet Int Med 9:336-340, 1995
64. Reef VB: Echocardiographic examination in the horse: the basics. Compend Contin Educ Pract Vet 12:1312-1320, 1990
65. Reef VB: Evaluation of ventricular septal defects in horses using two-dimensional and Doppler echocardiography. Equine Vet J Suppl:86-95, 1995
66. Reef VB: Echocardiographic findings in horses with congenital cardiac disease. Compend Contin Educ Pract Vet 13:109-117, 1991
67. Maxson AD, Reef VB: Bacterial endocarditis in horses: ten cases (1984-1995). Equine Vet J 29:394-399, 1997
68. Reef VB, Spencer P: Echocardiographic evaluation of equine aortic insufficiency. Am J Vet Res 48:904-909, 1987
69. Marr CM, Reef VB, Brazil TJ, et al.: Aorto-cardiac fistulas in seven horses. Vet Radiol Ultrasound 39:22-31, 1998
70. Sleeper MM, Durando MM, Miller M, et al.: Aortic root disease in four horses. J Am Vet Med Assoc 219:491-496, 2001
71. Bernard W, Reef VB, Clark ES, et al.: Pericarditis in horses: six cases (1982-1986). J Am Vet Med Assoc 196:468-471, 1990
72. Freestone JF, Thomas WP, Carlson GP, et al.: Idiopathic effusive pericarditis with tamponade in the horse. Equine Vet J 19:38-42, 1987
73. Reef VB, Gentile DG, Freeman DE: Successful treatment of pericarditis in a horse. J Am Vet Med Assoc 185:94-98, 1984
74. Robinson JA, Marr CM, Reef VB, et al.: Idiopathic, aseptic, effusive, fibrinous, nonconstrictive pericarditis with tamponade in a standardbred filly. J Am Vet Med Assoc 201:1593-1598, 1992

9.1.2 Monitoring tissue perfusion

Kevin Corley

It is not possible to monitor tissue perfusion directly in animals. Cardiovascular measurements such as arterial blood pressure and cardiac output (Chapter 9.1.3) are extremely useful indicators of global cardiovascular disturbances but give no information about perfusion of individual organ beds. Assessments of tissue perfusion should be considered together, rather than individually, to allow a rational treatment plan to be formulated.

Physical examination

The clinical examination is an important part of any assessment of the cardiovascular system. However, it is important to recognise its limitations and to combine observations made on physical examination with all other available data.

Animals with major haemodynamic derangements are almost universally depressed, and most, but not all, are recumbent. Changes in mentation may only be apparent 2 to 3 hours after the onset of cardiovascular shock. Therefore, other parameters should also be monitored in high-risk animals to allow early intervention. Improvements in alertness are often a useful indicator that therapeutic interventions are having a beneficial effect at the organ level.

A high heart rate is the expected physiological response in hypovolaemic shock, septic shock and severe anaemia. In horses with surgical colic lesions, the high heart rate may be a consequence of hypovolaemia, pain or a combination of both. In neonatal foals, however, the heart rate may be within the normal range despite marked hypovolaemia.[1] This failure to mount an appropriate, protective physiological response may explain the high morbidity and mortality for these conditions in foals. Additionally, in foals, very low heart rates (less than 60 bpm) are often associated with hypothermia.[1] In adult horses and foals, persistently abnormal heart rates and dysrhythmias should be further investigated by means of an electrocardiogram (see Chapters 1.24 and 9.1.1).

In the adult horse, the facial artery is usually easily palpated. This artery may be hard to feel in the foal, but the dorsal metatarsal and femoral arterial pulses are easily palpated. The pulse pressure is often reduced in hypotension. In severe hypotension, the pulse may be impalpable. The pulse pressure represents the difference between systolic and diastolic arterial pressure and is independent of their absolute value and that of the mean pressure. Therefore, in hypotensive animals with markedly decreased diastolic pressure but a reasonable stroke volume, the pulse pressure can feel normal.

Traditionally, red mucous membranes with a fast capillary refill time have been associated with peripheral vasodilation accompanied by adequate cardiac output ("hyperdynamic shock"). Pale or blanched mucous membranes are considered indicative of peripheral vasoconstriction or anaemia. Purple mucous membranes with a prolonged capillary refill time have been associated with a low cardiac output or poor peripheral perfusion. Prolonged capillary refill times are an indicator of hypovolaemia. Dry mucous membranes have been reported to indicate dehydration. Whilst these colour changes are reasonably reliable in the adult horse, they have only a weak association with specific haemodynamic derangements in the neonatal foal.

Other parts of the clinical examination may give additional information on the haemodynamic status. Cold extremities are often a feature of cardiovascular shock. Prolonged skin tent is a sign of dehydration, not hypovolaemia. However, hypovolaemia and dehydration are usually associated in critically ill animals (see Chapter 6.5). Increased respiratory rates may be seen with tissue hypoperfusion, as a result of respiratory compensation for metabolic acidosis or impaired gas exchange.

Urine output

Urine output is an extremely useful indicator of end organ perfusion in critically ill foals, except where renal function is compromised by intrinsic renal failure. Although theoretically equally useful in adult horses, limitations to maintaining urinary catheters and collection devices in ambulatory adult horses means that urine output is rarely accurately and continuously measured in adult horses. Placement of a closed urinary collection system in the foal is described in Chapter 2.9, and urinary catheterisation of the adult horse is described in Chapter 1.42. The normal urine output of a 4-day-old foal is 148 ml/kg/day, which is approximately 6 ml/kg/hr.[2]

Glomerular filtration is partially a function of the difference in hydrostatic pressure in the glomerular capillaries and Bowman's capsule. In the normal physiological range, changes in arterial pressure are damped by inherent autoregulatory mechanisms resulting in little change in renal blood flow and glomerular hydrostatic pressure, and therefore glomerular filtration rate and urine output. However, in the failing circulation, renal blood flow is decreased both directly and via neuroendocrine feedback mechanisms, resulting in decreased urine output.[3]

Therapies aimed to improve cardiovascular status that result in decreased urine output are highly unlikely to be beneficial and should be urgently reviewed. Conversely, improved urine output is one of the earliest signs of successful therapy. Decreased urine output may be the first sign of impending hypovolaemia and may occur very early in cardiovascular shock from any cause. It is important to note that many variables other than circulatory status can decrease urine output. Acute renal failure may result in oliguria, anuria or polyuria. Measuring the urine specific gravity can help distinguish haemodynamic (prerenal) renal insufficiency from renal failure. The specific gravity is expected to be close to isotonic (1.010) in renal failure and is usually higher than this with significant dehydration or hypovolaemia.

Other causes of decreased urine output include blocked urinary catheters and defects in bladder wall integrity. Therefore, any investigation of low urine output should include an ultrasonographic examination of the peritoneal space and confirmation of an empty bladder. Hyperglycaemia is relatively common in critically ill animals and may result in an osmotic diuresis when blood glucose is above renal threshold for resorption. This diuresis may result in increased urine outputs except in severe circulatory collapse. If an osmotic diuresis is occurring, glucose will be present in the urine. Some critically ill foals produce small amounts of urine despite apparently adequate haemodynamics. These foals may respond to furosemide (frusemide) therapy. However, because of the potential detrimental effects of furosemide on a failing circulation, it is vital to rule haemodynamic causes of oliguria before its use.

Ascending infection is a risk of urinary catheterisation. This risk needs to be weighed against the benefits of accurate determination of urine output and the avoidance of urine scalding, particularly in recumbent foals. Attempts to reduce the risk of infection with antibacterial impregnated catheters have not been successful in human medicine.[4]

Lactate

Blood lactate concentration is a useful indicator of decreased organ perfusion. Lactate is produced from pyruvate in conditions of low cellular oxygenation, with the production of one molecule of ATP. Decreased supply of oxygen to the tissues therefore results in an increasing lactate concentration. Lactate is metabolised by the liver (50%) and kidneys (20%), and decreased blood flow through these organs decreases lactate clearance.[5] Therefore, the production of lactate is increased and the clearance decreased, in times of inadequate tissue perfusion. However, increased lactate concentrations can occur in pathophysiological states other than decreased tissue perfusion. Lactate has been reported to be increased in sepsis, the systemic inflammatory response syndrome (SIRS), trauma, following seizures and during periods of increased circulating catecholamines.[5–9] Therefore, blood lactate concentrations should always be evaluated in the context of the physical examination and other indicators of tissue perfusion.

Lactate concentrations are associated with hospital survival in neonatal foals and colic patients.[10–13] There are also many studies showing the association of lactate concentration with survival in critically ill human patients.[5,14,15]

Lactate can be measured on whole blood or plasma. Some bench-top critical care analysers measure lactate alongside other parameters, such as blood gas analysis. Inexpensive handheld devices are available that have been validated for the horse[16,17] (Figure 9.15). Because these analysers measure colourimetric changes, they are affected by high packed cell volume.[17] For this reason, it is recommended to measure lactate on plasma samples rather than whole blood for handheld machines that have settings for both whole blood and plasma. In our lab, we collect samples for lactate measurement into lithium heparin (green top) vacutainer tubes and immediately centrifuge the sample for 3 minutes before making the measurement on plasma. We believe that the increase in accuracy justifies the minor delay in obtaining a result.

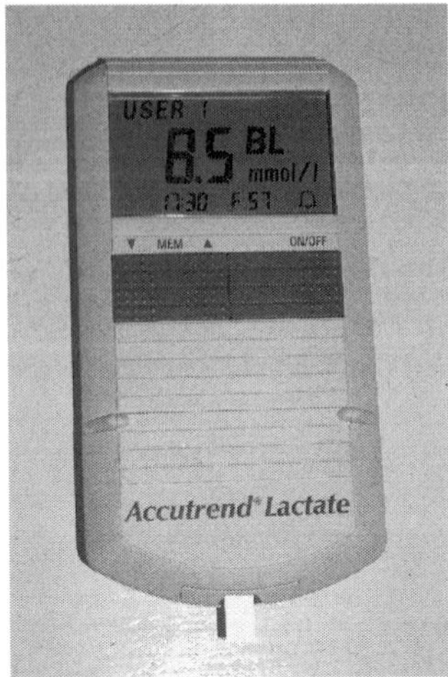

Figure 9.15 Handheld analyser for measurement of lactate. ©Kevin Corley 2006.

Despite the limitations, blood lactate concentrations can be a very useful guide to the adequacy of tissue oxygen delivery and thus help guide haemodynamic therapy. Where hyperlactaemia is due to haemodynamic disturbances, decreasing blood lactate concentrations suggest that tissue perfusion is being improved. Conversely, if blood lactate concentrations increase in response to therapies aimed at improving haemodynamics, these therapies should be urgently reviewed. Unfortunately, decreases in plasma lactate concentration may lag behind improved cardiovascular status[8] and therefore blood lactate concentrations are not the most sensitive measure by which to titrate therapy.

Arterial blood pressure

Arterial blood pressure is the product of cardiac output (flow) and the resistance to flow in the vasculature. Organ perfusion is dependent on blood flow, rather than blood pressure. However, there seems to be a critical threshold for blood pressure below which organ function is compromised. In some organs, such as the kidney, heart and brain, there is autoregulation of blood pressure. This autoregulation results in blood pressure being maintained within narrow limits across a wide range of systemic arterial pressures. The mean blood pressure at which autoregulation fails and flow becomes pressure dependent is unknown in the foal but in other species is approximately 60 mm Hg.[18–20] Based on a comparison of mean arterial blood pressure and blood lactate concentrations in 59 foals, there is circumstantial evidence that tissue perfusion is inadequate below 60 mm Hg in foals.[10] Organ hypoperfusion can quickly result in severe tissue injury, which may be exacerbated when flow is returned (reperfusion injury). For these reasons, blood pressure should be monitored and hypotension appropriately and promptly treated in critically ill animals.

The most accurate way to measure blood pressure is to place an indwelling catheter in an artery (see Chapters 2.8 and 1.20) and directly measure blood pressure (see Chapter 1.22). Noninvasive blood pressure monitoring, via a pressure cuff (see Chapters 1.21 and 2.7), has several advantages over direct pressure monitoring. The first measurement may be taken within 3 minutes of admission of the hospital, measurements require less technical expertise than arterial catheterisation and there is no arterial catheter to maintain. The disadvantages of noninvasive blood pressure measurements are that it only provides intermittent measurements and that it is not as accurate as direct measurements. However, in foals, the accuracy of noninvasive blood pressure measurements is good for diastolic and mean arterial pressure but not for systolic pressure.[21,22]

The Doppler technique is an alternative method of measuring arterial blood pressure noninvasively, but it is reported not to be accurate in adult anaesthetised horses.[23]

Pulse oximetry

Pulse oximetry offers a noninvasive method of monitoring arterial haemoglobin oxygenation saturation. It is based on detection of light emitted by two light-emitting diodes of differing wavelengths that are preferentially absorbed by oxyhaemoglobin and deoxyhaemoglobin, respectively. This allows the percentage saturation of blood passing by the sensor to be calculated. Most pulse oximeters also calculate pulse rate, based on the pulsatile flow within the arteriolar bed. Pulse oximetry probes intended for human fingers can be placed on tongues, ears or lips; reflective probes can be used on the forehead[24]; and rectal probes may also be used. In conscious animals, all probes can be difficult to maintain.

Theoretically, the pulse oximeter gives useful information regarding oxygen delivery to the tissues and the functioning of the cardiopulmonary unit. Decreases in saturation below 90% should warrant investigation of a cause for hypoxaemia or hypoperfusion.[25,26] Pulse oximetry may be particularly useful in mechanically ventilated foals. Although clinically useful to follow trends and warn of arterial desaturation, pulse oximetry in the foal is only moderately accurate and varies with probe site.[24]

References

1. Corley KTT: Monitoring and treating haemodynamic disturbances in critically ill neonatal foals. Part I: haemodynamic monitoring. Equine Vet Educ 14:270-279, 2002
2. Brewer BD, Clement SF, Lotz WS, et al.: A comparison of inulin, para-aminohippuric acid, and endogenous creatinine clearances as measures of renal function in neonatal foals. J Vet Int Med 4:301-305, 1990
3. Vander AJ: Renal blood flow and glomerular filtration, in Vander AJ (ed): Renal Physiology, ed 5. New York, McGraw-Hill, 1995, pp 24-50
4. Riley DK, Classen DC, Stevens LE, et al.: A large randomized clinical trial of a silver-impregnated urinary catheter: lack of efficacy and staphylococcal superinfection. Am J Med 98:349-356, 1995
5. De Backer D: Lactic acidosis. Intensive Care Med 29:699-702, 2003
6. Chrusch C, Bands C, Bose D, et al.: Impaired hepatic extraction and increased splanchnic production contribute to lactic acidosis in canine sepsis. Am J Respir Crit Care Med 161:517-526, 2000
7. Gore DC, Jahoor F, Hibbert JM, et al.: Lactic acidosis during sepsis is related to increased pyruvate production, not deficits in tissue oxygen availability. Ann Surg 224:97-102, 1996
8. James JH, Luchette FA, McCarter FD, et al.: Lactate is an unreliable indicator of tissue hypoxia in injury or sepsis. Lancet 354:505-508, 1999
9. Magdesian KG, Madigan JE: Volume replacement in the neonatal ICU: Colloids and crystalloids. Clin Tech Equine Pract 2:20-30, 2003
10. Corley KTT, Donaldson LL, Furr MO: Arterial lactate concentration, hospital survival, sepsis and SIRS in critically ill neonatal foals. Equine Vet J 37:53-59, 2005
11. Furr MO, Lessard P, White NA: Development of a colic severity score for predicting the outcome of equine colic. Vet Surg 24:97-101, 1995
12. Gossett KA, Cleghorn B, Martin GS, et al.: Correlation between anion gap, blood L lactate concentration and survival in horses. Equine Vet J 19:29-30, 1987
13. Moore JN, Owen RR, Lumsden JH: Clinical evaluation of blood lactate levels in equine colic. Equine Vet J 8:49-54, 1976
14. Smith I, Kumar P, Molloy S, et al.: Base excess and lactate as prognostic indicators for patients admitted to intensive care. Intensive Care Med 27:74-83, 2001
15. Husain FA, Martin MJ, Mullenix PS, et al.: Serum lactate and base deficit as predictors of mortality and morbidity. Am J Surg 185:485-491, 2003
16. Lindner A: Measurement of plasma lactate concentration with Accusport. Equine Vet J 28:403-405, 1996
17. Evans DL, Golland LC: Accuracy of Accusport for measurement of lactate concentrations in equine blood and plasma. Equine Vet J 28:398-402, 1996
18. Hollenberg SM, Ahrens TS, Astiz ME, et al.: Practice parameters for hemodynamic support of sepsis in adult patients in sepsis. Crit Care Med 27:639-660, 1999
19. Johnson PC: Autoregulation of blood flow. Circ Res 59:483-495, 1986
20. Robertson CR, Deen WM, Troy JL, et al.: Dynamics of glomerular ultrafiltration in the rat. 3. Hemodynamics and autoregulation. Am J Physiol 223:1191-1200, 1972
21. Nout YS, Corley KTT, Donaldson LL, et al.: Indirect oscillometric and direct blood pressure measurement in anesthetized and conscious neonatal foals. J Vet Emerg Crit Care 12:75-80, 2002
22. Giguere S, Knowles HA, Jr, Valverde A, et al.: Accuracy of indirect measurement of blood pressure in neonatal foals. J Vet Intern Med 19:571-576, 2005
23. Bailey JE, Dunlop CI, Chapman PL, et al.: Indirect Doppler ultrasonic measurement of arterial blood pressure results in a large measurement error in dorsally recumbent anaesthetised horses. Equine Vet J 26:70-73, 1994
24. Chaffin MK, Matthews NS, Cohen ND, et al.: Evaluation of pulse oximetry in anaesthetised foals using multiple combinations of transducer type and transducer attachment site. Equine Vet J 28:437-445, 1996
25. Daily EK, Schroeder JS: Monitoring of oxygenation, in Daily EK, Schroeder JS (eds): Techniques in Bedside Hemodynamic Monitoring, ed 5. St. Louis, Mosby, 1994, pp 215-240
26. Van de Louw A, Cracco C, Cerf C, et al.: Accuracy of pulse oximetry in the intensive care unit. Intensive Care Med 27:1606-1613, 2001

9.1.3 Cardiac output monitoring

Mary Durando

Although less frequently used than other diagnostic modalities, the measurement of cardiac output (CO) can give valuable information, and help in the management of horses with cardiac disease or cardiovascular/circulatory compromise. The limited use of CO is primarily due to the fact that the most commonly available procedures are rather complicated, are invasive to perform and require equipment not routinely available to practitioners or even all referral hospitals. However, with the development of less-invasive means of measuring cardiac output that have been validated in horses, such as the lithium dilution method, monitoring is becoming more feasible. The technique for measuring cardiac output by the lithium dilution technique is described in Chapter 1.26.

In equine medicine, the haemodynamic status of the patient is commonly estimated using selected physical examination findings such as heart rate, quality or intensity of heart sounds, peripheral pulse quality, mucus membrane colour, capillary refill time (CRT), venous distension and/or filling and temperature of extremities. Diagnostic aids such as direct and indirect blood pressure measurement, central venous pressure (CVP), blood gas analysis, lactate measurement and pulse oximetry supplement clinical examination findings and give valuable information[1] (see Chapter 9.1.2). However, measurement of cardiac output allows direct interpretation of cardiovascular function and the heart's ability to deliver oxygen globally. A direct measurement of cardiac output can greatly enhance understanding of the particular disease process and thus potentially greatly improve patient management. It also allows calculation of a number of other haemodynamic parameters, which give further information about the cardiovascular system (see Chapter 9.1.4).

CO is the product of stroke volume and heart rate and is the basis for adequate tissue perfusion and normal organ function. Although many other controls regulate blood flow to organs, without sufficient cardiac output, these regulations will eventually fail. Blood pressure, which is critical in the determination of adequate organ perfusion, is determined by CO and systemic vascular resistance. Therefore, a decrease in blood pressure could be secondary to either a decrease in systemic vascular resistance or a decrease in cardiac output, and without a direct measurement of CO, the clinician cannot always determine the cause of inadequate tissue perfusion. CO monitoring in situations such as this would help guide the clinician and may decrease unnecessary administration of certain potentially harmful drugs.[2,3] If CO is low, other diagnostics could then be used to try to determine the reason (i.e., inadequate fluid volume or cardiomyopathy). If CO is suspected to be reduced based on clinical parameters such as decreased perfusion of extremities, prolonged CRT, poor peripheral pulse quality and/or tachycardia despite fluid therapy, it would be advantageous to directly record and monitor. For instance, in horses with elevated CVP, measurement of CO may provide insight as to the reason for the elevation. Management of critically ill neonates, hypotensive patients, horses with cardiac disease and horses with significant fluid, acid-base, and electrolyte derangements such as those with colitis or other gastrointestinal diseases, as well as horses under general anesthesia, are just a few of the possible situations in which monitoring CO could be of benefit.[2–4]

In human medicine, measurement of CO with treatment strategies aimed at improving this variable, along with improvement in oxygen delivery and other haemodynamic variables, are thought to be important and have been shown to improve outcome in critically ill patients.[5–7] However, the positive or negative impact of pulmonary artery catheterisation for measuring cardiac output and other variables remains controversial in human medicine.[8–11] Much less has been published regarding the clinical usefulness of monitoring CO in horses, but it has been evaluated and found to yield important adjunctive information for case management of neonatal foals.[3,12] Normal resting values measured in healthy, conscious, adult horses range from 72 to 93 ml/kg/min.[2,4,13] Although the effect of various diseases and the expectations of effect of treatments on CO in horses have not been studied, it has the potential to be helpful in critically ill adult horses and horses with significant cardiac disease.

Normal values for cardiac output are given in the Appendix (see Tables 19.17 and 19.18).

References

1. Divers T: Monitoring tissue oxygenation in the ICU patient. Clin Tech Equine Pract 2:138-144, 2003
2. Blissitt KJ, Young LE, Jones RS, et al.: Measurement of cardiac output in standing horses by Doppler echocardiography and thermodilution. Equine Vet J 29:18-25, 1997
3. Corley KTT: Monitoring and treating haemodynamic disturbances in critically ill neonatal foals. Part II—Assessment and treatment. Equine Vet Educ 14:328-336, 2002
4. Muir WW, Skarda RT, Milne DW: Estimation of cardiac output in the horse by thermodilution techniques. Am J Vet Res 37:697-700, 1976
5. Edwards JD, Brown GC, Nightingale P, et al.: Use of survivors' cardiorespiratory values as therapeutic goals in septic shock. Crit Care Med 17:1098-1103, 1989
6. Mimoz O, Rauss A, Rekik N, et al.: Pulmonary artery catheterization in critically ill patients: a prospective analysis of outcome changes associated with catheter-prompted changes in therapy. Crit Care Med 22:573-579, 1994
7. Steingrub JS, Celoria G, Vickers-Lahti M, et al.: Therapeutic impact of pulmonary artery catheterization in a medical/surgical ICU. Chest 99:1451-1455, 1991
8. Vender JS: Resolved: A pulmonary artery catheter should be used in the management of the critically ill patient. Pro J Cardiothorac Vasc Anesth 12:9-12, 1998

9. Becker K: Resolved: A pulmonary artery catheter should be used in the management of the critically ill patient. Con J Cardiothorac Vasc Anesth 12:13-16, 1998
10. Connors AF, Speroff T, Dawson NV, et al.: The effectiveness of right heart catheterization in the initial care of critically ill patients. J Am Med Assoc 276:889-897, 1996
11. Murdoch SD, Cohen AT, Bellamy MC: Pulmonary artery catheterization and mortality in critically ill patients. Br J Anaesth 85:611-615, 2000
12. Corley KTT: Monitoring and treating haemodynamic disturbances in critically ill neonatal foals. Part I—Haemodynamic monitoring. Equine Vet Educ 14:270-279, 2002
13. Hinchcliff KW, McKeever KH, Muir WW: Hemodynamic effects of atropine, dobutamine, nitroprusside, phenylephrine, and propranolol in conscious horses. J Vet Int Med 5:80-86, 1991

9.1.4 Derived haemodynamic parameters

Kevin Corley

Several haemodynamic variables can be calculated from cardiac output, heart rate, blood pressure and blood gases. These include stroke volume, systemic vascular resistance, oxygen extraction ratio, global oxygen delivery and global oxygen uptake. The calculations are given in the Appendix (see Table 19.19).

Stroke volume

Stroke volume is an indirect indicator of myocardial contractile function and should be interpreted in light of the fluid status and central venous pressure of the animal. A low stroke volume, despite a high central venous pressure or in spite of an adequate fluid challenge is consistent with cardiac failure. A greater than normal stroke volume suggests that hypovolaemia is unlikely.

Systemic vascular resistance

Resistance to flow cannot be directly measured but can be calculated by dividing the blood pressure by the flow. Resistance to flow is dependent on a number of factors, but a major contributor is the state of contraction in the arterioles. During very early systemic inflammatory response syndrome (SIRS), there is increased arteriolar contraction and increased resistance.[1] This stage is rarely recognised clinically. This is followed by marked vasodilation.[2,3]

Systemic vascular resistance (SVR) is calculated by the pressure in the systemic system (difference between arterial blood pressure and central venous pressure) divided by the cardiac output (see Table 19.19). This gives the systemic vascular resistance in Woods units. Conventionally, this figure is multiplied by 80 to convert to SI units (dynes $\times$ sec $\times$ cm^{-5}). Knowledge of the SVR can help distinguish hypotension caused by vasodilation from that caused by low cardiac output.

Global oxygen delivery and oxygen uptake

Global oxygen delivery is a measure of the amount of oxygen delivered from the heart per minute and is an indicator of both cardiovascular and respiratory system function. It only describes the rate at which oxygen is entering the systemic circulation and not its distribution to the various tissues, which varies markedly between individual organs in both normal as well as disease states. Global oxygen delivery is calculated by multiplying the cardiac index by the arterial oxygen content.

Global oxygen uptake is the amount of oxygen removed in the systemic circulation and indicates overall tissue oxygen utilization. It indicates whether organs are able to utilize the delivered oxygen. In normal animals, the oxygen uptake reflects metabolic oxygen requirements and increasing oxygen delivery will not increase oxygen uptake when there is no increase in oxygen demand by the tissue. In diseased animals, treatments that increase oxygen uptake are, in general, likely to be beneficial.

Increasing oxygen delivery will not increase a reduced oxygen uptake in two situations. The first is where there is an effective anatomical shunt. If some organs are adequately perfused, but local vascular constriction or dilation is preventing perfusion of other organs, increasing cardiac output may simply increase flow through the already perfused organs. The second situation is a physiological shunt in sepsis. Biochemical changes to the cells may reduce oxygen uptake in sepsis despite adequate oxygen delivery.[4] In both these cases, central venous oxygen saturation is likely to be over 80%, reflecting the return of oxygenated blood to the venous system. As in the case of global oxygen delivery, individual organs may vary markedly from the global parameter in both normality and disease.

Global oxygen delivery is calculated by multiplying the cardiac index by the difference between arterial and central venous oxygen contents.

Oxygen extraction ratio

Oxygen extraction ratio describes the percent of oxygen delivered that is utilised by the tissues. Its main advantage over the global oxygen delivery and uptake parameters is that it does not require cardiac output measurement. The disadvantage is that it cannot distinguish between the contribution of these two factors to the ratio. A decreasing oxygen extraction ratio may result from decreased oxygen uptake without a change in oxygen delivery or increased oxygen delivery without a change in oxygen uptake. Conversely a high oxygen extraction ratio may represent decreased relative oxygen delivery or increased relative oxygen uptake.

References

1. Lavoie JP, Madigan JE, Cullor JS, et al.: Haemodynamic, pathological, haematological and behavioural changes during endotoxin infusion in equine neonates. Equine Vet J 22:23-29, 1990
2. Corley KTT, McKenzie HC, Amoroso LM, et al.: Initial experience with norepinephrine infusion in hypotensive critically ill foals. J Vet Emerg Crit Care 10:267-276, 2000

3. Corley KTT: Monitoring and treating haemodynamic disturbances in critically ill neonatal foals. Part II: assessment and treatment. Equine Vet Educ 14:328-336, 2002
4. Fink M: Cytopathic hypoxia in sepsis. Acta Anaesthesiol Scand Suppl 110:87-95, 1997

9.2 Treating the cardiovascular system

9.2.1 Treating problems of the heart

Mary Durando

The success of management or treatment of horses with cardiovascular diseases depends greatly on the abnormality present and its severity, the aetiology of the disease and any concurrent problems. While we have improved our ability to monitor and correct many cardiac diseases, we are still limited in management of certain diseases compared with human and small animal medicine. Many drugs used in people are not used in horses because of expense and lack of safety and efficacy studies. Surgical as well as medical treatments used in small animal and human medicine allow the clinician more options. There are additional concerns, such as the expected use of the horse and safety of the rider, that are unique to the management of equine cardiac diseases. Episodes of syncope, collapse or sudden death have the potential to seriously injure a rider and must be taken into consideration when treating certain diseases or giving a prognosis. The majority of the drugs used to manage cardiac disease in horses are either antidysrhythmic drugs or medications used to improve cardiac function and decrease oedema formation. The more commonly used treatments are described below.

Antidysrhythmic therapy

Horses frequently have dysrhythmias; however, the proportion of those requiring treatment is quite low.[1–3] In order to decide upon the appropriate treatment, it is essential to determine the type of dysrhythmia present, as well as the probable aetiology. This will help to determine if specific antidysrhythmic therapy is needed, or if correction of the underlying disease is sufficient. In some cases, both may be necessary. With some dysrhythmias that are not life-threatening or likely to deteriorate, such as persistent atrial fibrillation, effect on performance is also helpful to decide if conversion to sinus rhythm with antidysrhythmic drugs is necessary.

Criteria for determining the necessity for specific treatment include the heart rate, the effect on cardiovascular status (i.e., whether the horse is exhibiting clinical signs of circulatory compromise or collapse) and the likelihood the rhythm disturbance will deteriorate if left untreated.[4–6] Severe, persistent tachydysrhythmias and profound bradydysrhythmias (which are rare in the horse) are the dysrhythmias most likely to need immediate attention. If the rhythm disturbance is urgent, a definitive aetiology may not be determined prior to therapy. However, it is important to try to determine the cause in a timely manner and ascertain severe electrolyte or acid-base disturbances, as some treatments may not be successful in the face of these disturbances and correction of some electrolyte abnormalities may correct the dysrhythmia. Ventricular tachycardia (VT) is the rhythm most likely to need immediate attention in the intensive care setting. Conversion of VT is required if the heart rate is greater than 100 to 120 beats/min at rest (in adults), polymorphic VT or the R-on-T phenomenon is seen (these are more likely to deteriorate into ventricular fibrillation) (Figure 9.16), or the horse is exhibiting clinical signs associated with cardiovascular compromise.[6,7]

Ventricular premature depolarisations (VPDs), even if frequent, may not need specific antidysrhythmic therapy, unless the R-on-T phenomenon exists or they are multiform in origin. In these cases, it is important to try to

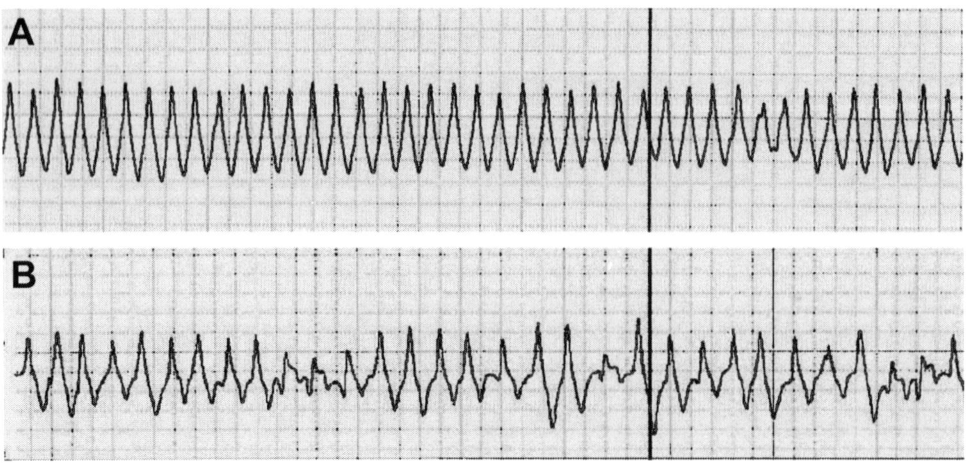

Figure 9.16 Base-apex electrocardiograms from a horse exhibiting different types of ventricular tachycardia. (**A**) Torsades de pointes. Note the wide QRS configuration and how the QRS and T waves twist around the baseline and are difficult to distinguish from one another. (**B**) The torsades de pointes deteriorated into multiform ventricular tachycardia. ©Mary Durando 2006.

determine and correct the underlying cause. If frequent, VPDs can impact performance and an exercise test with telemetric electrocardiography should always be performed to determine if they are abolished or worsened by exercise. If they remain during exercise they should be treated, as not only will they affect ability to perform, they can increase the risk of collapse, and thus harm to the rider. Other tachydysrhythmias such as atrial fibrillation and supraventricular tachycardia are also frequently converted with specific therapy.

Classes of antidysrhythmic drug

Antidysrhythmic drugs can be broadly separated by their class, or mechanism of action.[8] Class I drugs are sodium channel blockers and fall into three major categories: class IA (i.e., quinidine and procainamide), class IB (i.e., lidocaine and mexiletine) and class IC (i.e., propafenone and flecainide). Class II drugs are β-adrenergic blockers, such as propranolol and atenolol. Class III drugs are potassium channel blockers such as amiodarone, and class IV drugs are calcium channel blockers such as verapamil and diltiazem. These drugs have varying effects on conduction velocity, action potential duration, the refractory period and repolarisation. Some drugs may have multiple mechanisms and thus do not fit "neatly" into one class. Other drugs with different mechanisms of action, such as magnesium sulphate and corticosteroids, are also used in the treatment of various dysrhythmias. Additional drugs used for managing cardiovascular diseases, including diuretics, vasodilators and positive inotropes, are discussed later. As always, appropriate supportive care and rest are also imperative for successful treatment. The typical indications for some of the more commonly used specific antidysrhythmic drugs are described and are summarised in Table 9.1.

Ventricular Tachycardia

Ventricular tachycardia is defined as more than three PVDs in succession. As mentioned earlier, it is the most common dysrhythmia likely to need immediate conversion in the hospital setting, as it is more likely to result in hemodynamic compromise and can have a profound effect on cardiac output and organ perfusion. If rapid (>120 beats/

Table 9.1. Antidysrhythmic agents commonly used in horses

Drug	Indications	Dose	Adverse effects
Lidocaine	VT—acute onset, rapid	0.5–1 mg/kg IV; 20–50 μg/kg/min CRI	CNS excitability, seizures
Quinidine gluconate	Supraventricular and ventricular tachyarrhythmias, acute AF	1 mg/kg IV boluses q 5–10 min, total dose ≤12 mg/kg; 10–12 mg/kg CRI over 1–2 hours	Depression, mild gastrointestinal signs, similar to quinidine sulphate
Quinidine sulphate*	AF, supraventricular and ventricular tachyarrhythmias	22 mg/kg via NG tube q 2 hours for ≤5 treatments, converted, toxic or [plasma] >5 μg/ml; then 22 mg/kg q 6 hours until converted, adverse effects	Tachyarrhythmias, negative inotropy, hypotension, colic, diarrhea, laminitis, nasal oedema and stertor, depression, anorexia, hives, paraphimosis, neurologic/ataxia
Procainamide	Supraventricular and ventricular tachyarrhythmias, AF	1 mg/kg/min IV CRI, total dose ≤20 mg/kg; 25–35 mg/kg PO q 8 hours	Similar gastrointestinal disturbances as quinidine
Phenytoin	Digitalis glycoside toxicity, supraventricular and ventricular tachyarrhythmias	20 mg/kg PO q 12 hours 3–4 doses, then 10–15 mg/kg PO q 12 hours	Sedation and drowsiness, excitability at high concentrations
Magnesium sulphate	Torsades de pointes, quinidine-induced ventricular arrhythmias, VT	1–2.5 g/450 kg/min IV CRI, total dose ≤25 gm	
Digoxin*	Supraventricular tachyarrhythmias, CHF	0.0022 mg/kg IV; 0.011 mg/kg PO q 12 hours	Depression, anorexia, colic, dysrhythmias
Propafenone	Supraventricular and ventricular tachyarrhythmias	0.5–1 mg/kg IV over 5–10 min; 2 mg/kg PO q 8 hours	Gastrointestinal, bronchoconstriction in horses with respiratory disease
Propranolol	Rapid, unresponsive SVT or VT	0.03 mg/kg IV	Negative inotrope, bronchoconstriction in horses with severe respiratory disease
Atropine	Advanced second- or third-degree AV block	0.005–0.01 mg/kg IV	Ileus, mydriasis, supraventricular dysrhythmias
Glycopyrrolate	Same as atropine	0.05–0.1 mg/kg IV	Same as atropine
Bretylium	Life-threatening VT, VF	3–5 mg/kg IV, total dose ≤10 mg/kg	Gastrointestinal
Dexamethasone	Suspected inflammatory myocarditis	0.05–0.2 mg/kg IV	Laminitis, immunosuppression

*Best to monitor plasma concentrations during therapy.

AF, atrial flutter; AV, atrioventricular; CHF, congestive heart failure; CNS, central nervous system; CRI, constant rate infusion; SVT, supraventricular tachycardia; VF, ventricular fibrillation; VT, ventricular tachycardia.

min) and left uncorrected, particularly if multiform in origin, it can result in clinical signs of congestive heart failure and collapse. VT often occurs in association with gastrointestinal diseases and primary cardiac diseases.[9–14] While the immediate goal is to correct the rate and rhythm disturbance, discerning the underlying cause and addressing and managing this are also critical. Correction of severe acid-base and electrolyte changes, as well as fluid deficits in horses with gastrointestinal disease, recognition or index of suspicion of toxin exposure such as oleander or monensin, and identification of an underlying cardiac problem such as bacterial endocarditis, ruptured aortic root or myocardial disease are necessary for both acute management and long-term prognosis. If necessary, intranasal O_2 and a diuretic such as furosemide (frusemide) should be administered for pulmonary oedema. While overall treatment may vary depending on the aetiology or additional problems the horse may have, specific antidysrhythmic therapy is discussed here.

Lidocaine (lignocaine)

Lidocaine is a Class IB agent that is most commonly used in acute-onset rapid VT.[8] Lidocaine is thought to suppress dysrhythmias involving depolarised or partially depolarised arrhythmogenic tissue, such as occurs in myocardial ischaemia, but to not affect normally polarised tissue.[15] Advantages of lidocaine are its relative safety if recommended dosages are used, ease of infusion and rapidity of response, availability and cost, and it is often a first-line treatment for these reasons. Clinically significant haemodynamic impairment rarely occurs from lidocaine administration.[16] It has the potential to cause central nervous system excitability with high doses (2 mg/kg)[16] but rarely causes a problem if boluses of 0.5 to 1.0 mg/kg are used. Diazepam can be administered (0.05 mg/kg) if excessive excitability or seizures occur. Lidocaine administration can be repeated every 5 to 10 minutes for multiple doses or, alternatively, can be given as a continuous infusion at a rate of 30 to 50 μg/kg/min. The therapeutic range is 1.5 to 5 μg/ml.[15] Lidocaine affects ventricular myocardium and Purkinjie fibres, with no effect on atrial function. Lidocaine for intravenous injection without epinephrine should always be used for treatment of dysrhythmias.

Quinidine

Quinidine is one of the most commonly used antidysrhythmic agents in the horse.[15] It is a class IA drug that prolongs the action potential duration and effective refractory period of atrial and ventricular muscle.[17,18] It has a vagolytic effect on the heart, which can accelerate conduction through the atrioventricular node, and has α-adrenergic blocking effects, which can cause hypotension.[16] Quinidine is eliminated primarily via hepatic metabolism. It is the drug of choice for treatment of atrial fibrillation (AF) in horses with no underlying cardiac disease[19–21] but is also used successfully to convert horses with a variety of tachyarrhythmias including VT. The intravenous preparation, quinidine gluconate, is used if the dysrhythmia is more severe, needing acute treatment. Quinidine gluconate can be given at a dosage rate of 1 mg/kg boluses repeated every 5 to 10 minutes, up to a total dose of approximately 12 mg/kg; alternatively, this dosage can be given as an infusion over 1 to 2 hours.[17,22] It should not be used in horses that are obviously hypotensive, as it can exacerbate this condition. It should also be used with care in horses receiving digoxin, as they compete for tissue binding sites, resulting in elevated concentrations of digoxin, which has a narrow therapeutic range.[23] Quinidine sulphate, the preparation commonly used for oral administration, can induce many side effects including depression and anorexia, diarrhoea, colic, laminitis, nasal oedema, paraphimosis and hives.[21,24] Depression and mild gastrointestinal abnormalities have been reported with intravenous use of quinidine gluconate.[22]

Procainamide

Procainamide is also a Class 1A drug that has actions similar to quinidine in prolonging the effective refractory period and action potential duration.[8] It does not have the vagolytic and α-adrenergic blocking effects of quinidine,[15] so it is less likely to cause hypotension or an elevated ventricular response in horses with AF. It is used for converting a variety of supraventricular and ventricular tachyarrhythmias and is effective in horses with VT. Procainamide is available in intravenous or oral preparations. It is administered at a dosage rate of 1 mg/kg/min IV infusion, up to a maximum of 20 mg/kg for emergency treatment of tachyarrhythmias.[25] The major metabolite, *N*-acetylprocainamide (NAPA), is excreted by the kidneys, so horses with reduced renal function should have their drug levels monitored, and dosages adjusted accordingly. Therapeutic levels of 4 to 10 μg/ml for procainamide and 10 to 30 μg/ml for procainamide and NAPA combined have been reported.[25] Although there are reported adverse side effects in people, it is a relatively safe drug in horses. The gastrointestinal side effects are not as common as in quinidine, and although it can induce similar conduction disturbances, ventricular tachyarrhythmias do not seem to occur as frequently as with quinidine. Co-administration of procainamide and digoxin does not result in elevated digoxin levels, so would perhaps be safer than quinidine in horses on digoxin that develop ventricular dysrhythmias.

Propafenone

Propafenone is a Class 1C drug that is effective in correcting atrial and ventricular dysrhythmias, including VT.[26] It can be given intravenously, at a dose of 0.5 to 1 mg/kg slowly over 5 to 10 minutes,[26] but the intravenous formulation is not available in many countries. It can also be given orally at a dose of 2 mg/kg every 8 hours for control of less immediately life-threatening dysrhythmias. Because of lack of availability and use in horses, published information regarding efficacy and adverse effects is lacking; however, anecdotally it has been used successfully and seems to be well tolerated.

Phenytoin

Phenytoin has effects of Class 1B drugs and has been available for many years as an anticonvulsant.[27] It is also used for the treatment of atrial and ventricular dysrhythmias, including VT,[28] although it is currently used much less frequently in people than it was in the past. It is particularly useful in dysrhythmias secondary to digitalis glycoside toxicity, one of its primary indications.[27] In recent reports, phenytoin has been used for the successful conversion of a tachyarrhythmia secondary to oleander toxicity in a donkey[29] and VT secondary to foxglove ingestion in a pony.[30] It was also used successfully to correct VT or VPDs in seven horses refractory to other treatments.[31] On the basis of this report, the authors recommend a loading dose of 20 mg/kg orally every 12 hours for 3 or 4 doses and then decreasing to a maintenance dose of 10 to 15 mg/kg every 12 hours. Therapeutic drug levels in this study were 8.8 ± 2.1 µg/ml.[31] Pharmacokinetic studies have been performed in the horse with this drug, and it has been found to have a variable excretion pattern, making prediction of plasma concentrations difficult.[32,33] Phenytoin is generally very well tolerated in people and is inexpensive compared with many newer antidysrhythmic agents, which is a very important consideration in equine medicine. It has not been used in horses extensively for the treatment of dysrhythmias; however, it seems relatively safe and most side effects are related to sedation and drowsiness, although with elevated plasma concentrations excitement can occur. In people, the cardiac benefits are attained at similar serum concentrations as its anticonvulsant effects (10–20 µg/ml); therefore, if overt central nervous system signs such as ataxia and nystagmus are seen, drug concentrations are too high, and further administration of the drug is unlikely to correct the dysrhythmia.

Magnesium sulphate

Magnesium sulphate is used for correction of ventricular dysrhythmias, including VT, in several situations. It is particularly useful in quinidine-induced torsades de pointes, a wide ventricular tachyarrhythmia.[34] The term means "twisting around a point," which is an accurate description of its appearance as the QRS and T waves twist around the baseline (Figure 9.16). It is also especially useful in horses with VT that are hypomagnesaemic, although it may also be successful in normomagnesaemic horses. It has the advantage of minimal adverse effects and is very well tolerated. It does not have the negative inotropic effects of many of the other antidysrhythmic drugs and acts, at least in part, as a physiological calcium channel blocker. The typical dosage is 1 to 2.5 g/450 kg/min up to a total dose of 25 g, and it is usually infused over 10 to 20 minutes.[4,6]

Propranolol

If the horse has not responded to any of the above treatments, propranolol, at 0.03 mg/kg IV, can be tried.[16,18] Propranolol may control the ventricular response rate, to slow the heart rate, but is not often successful in converting horses in VT. Because propranolol acts primarily through β-adrenergic blockade, its effects depend on the underlying sympathetic tone.[35] Propranolol should be used with caution in horses clinically affected with recurrent airway obstruction or severe respiratory disease, as it could exacerbate bronchoconstriction.[16] Use of other nonspecific β-blockers such as atenolol or sotalol have not been reported in the horse. Esmolol is an ultra-short-acting, selective β_1-adrenergic receptor antagonist that would have similar antidysrhythmic effects as propranolol but would not have deleterious side effects seen with β_2-blockade.[15] Although anecdotally it is safe and effective to use, there are no reports in the literature of its use in horses.

Bretylium tosylate

If the horse is in ventricular fibrillation or life-threatening VT that has not responded to the previous agents, bretylium tosylate can be tried as a last resort. The recommended dose is 3 to 5 mg/kg IV, up to a total dose of 10 mg/kg. However, once an adult horse is in ventricular fibrillation, it is unlikely that medical therapy will be successful.

General guidelines for treating ventricular tachycardia

When treating VT, if the horse has not responded to one antidysrhythmic agent, treatment should be attempted with a different drug; it is emphasised that it may be necessary to use several before conversion occurs. It is also important to remember that any antidysrhythmic drug has the potential to be prodysrhythmic; thus all horses should be monitored closely during treatment with continuous electrocardiography and drug administration stopped if problems are encountered. Additional supportive care may be necessary, including intranasal oxygen, intravenous fluid therapy and, as mentioned previously, correction of any electrolyte and acid-base abnormalities. Diuretics should be administered if concurrent congestive heart failure and/or pulmonary oedema is present. Horses that are extremely agitated may need antianxiety agents such as diazepam.

Ventricular ectopic depolarisations

Ventricular ectopic beats are those that originate from the ventricle, rather than going through the normal conduction pathway. Normal horses can have occasional premature depolarisations in a 24-hour period[3,36,37]; however, if they are numerous, occur in runs, are multiform in configuration indicating origination from multiple sites in the ventricle or persist during exercise, they are abnormal. Usually, VPDs do not need specific antidysrhythmic therapy as they do not typically cause cardiovascular compromise in a resting horse; however, the underlying cause should be determined and corrected. This will often result in correction of the dysrhythmia. If no other underlying disease is found, and an inflammatory cause is suspected (e.g., myocarditis), they may resolve with corticosteroid treatment and rest. Standard treatment with antiinflammatory doses of dexamethasone is usually used.[38] Active infection should be ruled out before initiation of steroid therapy. This must be accompanied by adequate rest. If the VPDs are numerous, are multiform and/or remain during exercise, despite resolution of the primary disease process or rest and a course of corticosteroids, antidysrhythmic therapy may be necessary. Although antidysrhythmics may correct the dysrhythmia, they are likely to return on cessation of treatment, if the primary disease process is not eliminated. Many of the same agents used to control VT are used to abolish frequent VPDs, although the oral preparations can be used because these dysrhythmias are not immediately life threatening.

Procainamide
Procainamide can be administered orally and is often effective in abolishing or decreasing VPDs. It is given at a dosage of 25to 35 mg/kg every 8 hours.[25] When using it orally, the extended release form should not be used. The oral formulation of procainamide can be expensive and is not always available.

Propafenone
Oral propafenone (2 mg/kg every 8 hours) may correct ventricular dysrhythmias,[6] although there is minimal literature describing its use in horses.

Quinidine sulphate
Quinidine sulphate can be administered to correct ventricular dysrhythmias. For a more detailed protocol, and adverse effects, see the next section, on treatment of supraventricular tachydysrhythmias.

Supraventricular tachydysrhythmias
Supraventricular tachydysrhythmias are rhythm disturbances originating above the ventricle and include atrial fibrillation, atrial flutter, supraventricular or atrial tachycardia, and supraventricular premature depolarisations.

Atrial fibrillation
Atrial fibrillation (AF) is the supraventricular dysrhythmia most often requiring specific treatment, primarily because of its effect on performance.[19–21,24] It is not a dysrhythmia that requires emergency treatment, and, in fact, treatment should wait at least 1 to 2 days after onset, because the horse may self-convert. It is often associated with no underlying cardiac disease, although it commonly develops in horses with congestive heart failure (CHF) and enlarged atria. The prognosis for successful conversion is very good if no underlying cardiac disease is present and the horse has not been in AF long.[19,20,24,38] If the horse is in CHF, treatment should be directed at improving cardiac performance and decreasing pulmonary oedema rather than correcting the AF.

Supraventricular tachycardia
Supraventicular tachycardias (SVTs) can be associated with both primary cardiac disease and diseases in other body systems. They can also be seen following the resolution of AF with medical therapy. Usually, correction of any underlying disease if noncardiac in origin, or adequate rest and corticosteroids, will correct the SVT; however, if it persists or is very rapid, specific antidysrhythmic therapy may be needed.

Supraventricular premature depolarisation
Supraventricular premature depolarisations (SVPDs) seldom require specific therapy. Occasional SVPDs are present in many normal horses and should disappear with exercise. If the SVPDs are numerous, they indicate some type of pathology and can be secondary to either cardiac abnormalities or disease in another body system. Usually, correction of the underlying problem corrects the dysrhythmia.

Quinidine
Quinidine gluconate can be used in horses with acute-onset (<1 month duration) AF but is less effective in more chronic cases.[22] The same dosing protocol as described under ventricular tachycardia can be used.

Quinidine sulphate is the oral preparation used in most other situations and still seems to be the most effective medical treatment of AF in horses. It is used at a dosage of 22 mg/kg given orally via nasogastric tube every 2 hours for 1 day.[16,17] This regimen is based on the pharmacokinetics of the drug, with the goal of reaching and maintaining therapeutic plasma concentrations. The longer plasma levels remain in the therapeutic range, the greater is the likelihood of efficacy. This protocol is continued until the horse converts to sinus rhythm, has a negative reaction to the drug or has had four or five treatments. At this time, if the horse has not converted, plasma concentrations of quinidine should be measured, as most horses will have reached therapeutic concentrations by this time, and continued treatment every 2 hours may result in toxic levels.[16,17,21] Treatment frequency should then be decreased to every 6 hours (the mean half-life of the drug in horses) to maintain therapeutic levels. This protocol can be continued until the horse converts to normal sinus rhythm or has a negative response to treatment or the owner wishes to discontinue treatment. It is less common for horses to have difficulty with the treatments once the frequency has been decreased to every 6 hours, but they certainly can, so the horse should continue to be monitored continuously throughout the treatment period.

Because of the possibility of negative cardiovascular effects, horses receiving quinidine should always be monitored closely.[19,20,24] An intravenous catheter should always be placed before treatment begins, for rapid venous access. In emergency situations, prompt treatment of a potentially life-threatening dysrhythmia is paramount, and in the face of a rapid tachydysrhythmia and hypotension, catheter placement becomes a more challenging procedure. Cardiovascular drugs that may be needed to correct an emergency should be nearby, with dosages calculated beforehand. The horse should have continuous telemetry to monitor for the development of tachyarrhythmias, allowing correction in a timely manner. Quinidine can cause both atrial and ventricular tachyarrhythmias, so it is important to evaluate the ECG carefully, to determine the type of dysrhythmia induced. Table 9.2 gives recommended treatments for quinidine-induced dysrhythmias. A base-apex electrocardiogram should be performed before each dose, to measure QRS duration. One of the signs of toxicity is prolongation of the QRS complex[22]; therefore, if it is prolonged greater than 25% from baseline, treatment should be stopped and plasma quinidine concentrations measured. Therapeutic concentrations are 2 to 5 μg/ml.[21]

Quinidine is also used to convert horses with supraventricular tachycardia. The same dosing regimens as stated earlier can be used.

Quinidine is a very effective drug in converting horses with a variety of supraventricular dysrhythmias; the chief complaint with its use is the incidence of negative side effects.[19] The most common noncardiac adverse effects are gastrointestinal (colitis, colic), anorexia, depression, paraphimosis, laminitis and nasal oedema. The most common cardiac effects are the induction of tachyarrhythmias (both supraventricular and ventricular), hypotension and negative inotropy. For these reasons, quinidine is contraindicated in horses with congestive heart failure or hypotension, and if the ventricular rate is rapid in horses with AF, and cannot be controlled.

Digoxin

Horses in AF that have elevated or very labile ventricular rates often benefit from digoxin therapy prior to starting quinidine. This will help to slow and control the heart rate and may be needed for one to several days. Digoxin is a cardiac glycoside that functions, at least in part, by inhibiting the sodium-potassium ATPase, resulting in increased intracellular calcium concentrations.[16] This increases the contractility of the heart. Digoxin also affects heart rhythm, by slowing conduction and increasing the refractory period in specialised conducting tissue.[16] It is given orally, every 12 hours, at a dose of 0.011 mg/kg. Plasma concentrations of digoxin should be monitored, as it has a narrow therapeutic range (1–2 ng/ml).[39] Signs of toxicity are primarily related to the gastrointestinal system (i.e., anorexia, depression, colic), although dysrhythmias can develop.[40,41] Once quinidine is started, it is very important to monitor plasma concentrations of digoxin, as quinidine displaces digoxin from its binding sites, resulting in a decreased volume of distribution. It may also decrease renal clearance of digoxin.[23] This can increase plasma concentrations; thus the frequency of digoxin administration may need to be decreased to once per day and/or the dose decreased. It is sometimes beneficial to start the horse on digoxin on day 2 of quinidine treatment (once on the every 6-hour frequency), if the horse has not converted with the every 2-hour quinidine regimen. Again, monitoring of plasma digoxin levels should be done, as well as monitoring for signs of toxicity.

Table 9.2. Treatment of quinidine-induced dysrhythmias

Stop quinidine!
Determine whether supraventricular or ventricular rhythm

Dysrhythmia	Treatment	Dose
Supraventricular		
Heart rate 100–150 bpm	Digoxin	0.0022 mg/kg IV
		0.011 mg/kg PO
Heart rate > 150 bpm	Digoxin	0.0022 mg/kg IV
	$NaHCO_3$	1 mEq/kg IV
	Propranolol	0.03 mg/kg IV
If blood pressure poor	Phenylephrine	0.1–0.2 mg/kg/min IV, total dose ≤0.01 mg/kg
Ventricular		
Torsades de pointes	$MgSO_4$	1–2.5 g/450 kg/min IV, total dose ≤25 g
Ventricular tachycardia	Lidocaine	0.5–1 mg/kg IV; 20–50 μg/kg/min IV CRI
	$MgSO_4$	1–2.5 g/450 kg/min IV, total dose ≤25 g
	Procainamide	1 mg/kg/min IV, total dose ≤20 mg/kg
	Propafenone	0.5–1 mg/kg IV over 5–10 min
	Bretylium	3–5 mg/kg IV, total dose ≤10 mg/kg

Procainamide

Procainamide can be used to convert horses with supraventricular tachyarrhythmias (both AF and SVT). It is administered intravenously, 1 mg/kg/min IV infusion, up to a maximum of 20 mg/kg, or orally, 25 to 35 mg/kg every 8 hours, as described earlier, under ventricular dysrhythmias.

Propafenone

Propafenone has been advocated in people with AF and chronic renal failure, because of its primarily hepatic metabolism. However, there are no published reports of its use clinically in horses. The same doses as described under ventricular dysrhythmias are used.

Propranolol

Propranolol can be tried in horses with rapid SVT, particularly if quinidine induced, to slow the ventricular response rate. In general, it is administered IV, 0.03 mg/kg. Because of hepatic first-pass effects, the oral administration is thought to be less effective.[15]

Phenytoin

Phenytoin is recommended for correction of supraventricular dysrhythmias secondary to digitalis glycoside toxicity. It is given as described above under ventricular dysrhythmias.

Newer drugs

Several newer drugs have been evaluated for the treatment of AF, but they require further investigation and are only mentioned here.

Flecainide has been evaluated in studies on both acute and chronic AF.[42–44] While it was efficacious in treating induced, acute AF, it was not found to be useful in chronic AF and had significant adverse effects; therefore, it cannot be recommended at this time. Further studies on proper dosing regimens may be helpful.

Amiodarone has also been evaluated as a treatment for AF, but at this time, its use in horses requires further study.[45]

The calcium channel blocker diltiazem has been evaluated experimentally as an adjunctive treatment for AF, to slow the accelerated atrioventricular conduction and supraventricular tachycardia that often occurs with quinidine.[46] Its primary use would be in place of digoxin, to help slow the ventricular response rate. Although it shows promise, its use at this time is still experimental.

Transvenous cardioversion

Transvenous cardioversion has been used successfully to treat AF in horses.[47] This treatment appears to be a viable alternative to medical treatment of AF, but it does require general anaesthesia and right heart catheterisation, with their attendant risks and expense. This is an elective procedure and would not be performed as an emergency treatment in an ICU.

Bradydysrhythmias

Horses are very prone to bradydysrhythmias because of their high resting vagal tone. Most bradydysrhythmias are considered normal if abolished by stimulation such as exercise, excitement, fright, or pharmaceutical agents such as parasympatholytics or sympathomimetics. These include sinus block and first- and second-degree atrioventricular block. Advanced second- and third-degree atrioventricular block are rare in horses, and usually indicative of myocardial disease, although they can be secondary to electrolyte disturbances such as hyperkalaemia.

Atropine and glycopyrolate

Agents such as atropine or glycopyrrolate can be administered, but if degeneration or disease of the conducting pathway is present, they are not likely to be helpful.[4] In addition, these drugs cannot be given long term, because of their undesirable side effects.[18]

Corticosteroids

Anti-inflammatory doses of corticosteroids can be tried if an inflammatory cause is suspected, but treatment is unlikely to be successful if there is significant permanent damage to conducting pathways.

Pacemaker implantation

If the horse is unresponsive to corticosteroids or parasympatholytics (e.g., atropine or glycopyrrolate), the only definitive treatment is a pacemaker. This has been reported on several occasions,[48–52] but it is uncommonly instituted compared with its use in small-animal medicine.

Drugs to treat congestive heart failure and/or improve cardiac performance

Horses with congestive heart failure require specific supportive care to improve cardiac output and decrease oedema (particularly pulmonary oedema). This can be attempted by improving myocardial function with positive inotropic agents, decreasing afterload on the heart, and diuretics. In addition, intranasal oxygen should be administered to horses with significant pulmonary oedema.

Digoxin

The most commonly used positive inotropes include β-receptor agonists and digitalis glycosides.[4] Digoxin is one of the oldest and most commonly used drugs in the treatment of equine cardiac diseases.[16,18,40,41,53–55] It has several beneficial effects, including a decrease in heart rate (slows atrioventricular node conduction), a positive inotropic effect and a diuretic effect (from improvement in renal blood flow).[15,16,18,56] It improves cardiac contractility by inhibiting sodium-potassium ATPase, an enzyme associated with the sodium pump, resulting in increased intracellular Ca^{2+} concentrations.[18] It has a weak inotropic effect compared with β-agonists; however, it also helps to improve cardiac function by slowing the heart rate, allowing more time for ventricular filling. Digoxin can be administered either intravenously or orally; often it is first given intravenously, followed by maintenance oral dosing. It is given at a dose of 0.0022 mg/kg IV or 0.011 mg/kg PO.[39] Digoxin has a very narrow margin of safety, with a therapeutic range of approximately 1 to 2 ng/ml.[41] The mean half life of digoxin is 17 hours, but it can be quite variable between horses, so dose and frequency of drug administration depend on plasma concentrations attained.

Digoxin toxicity is influenced by hydration status, electrolyte concentrations, degree of protein binding and renal function, along with concurrent administration of certain other drugs. Hypokalaemia is thought to potentiate digoxin toxicity, and many horses on digoxin for congestive heart failure also receive concurrent furosemide, which has a kaliuretic effect; therefore, these horses should receive adequate potassium in their diet, and plasma potassium concentrations should be monitored. Bioavailability of the oral formulation, volume of distribution and renal excretion will affect plasma concentrations, so peak and trough levels should be used to regulate dose and frequency of drug administration. Once a maintenance dose has been determined, the oral formulation should not be changed, as there can be differences between different products.[15] Noncardiac adverse effects are related primarily to the gastrointestinal tract and include anorexia and colic.[16] Cardiac adverse effects are the induction of dysrhythmias.[57]

Dobutamine

β-Receptor agonists can be used for rapid, acute correction of myocardial failure. Drugs such as dobutamine, with primarily β_1-agonist properties, have a pronounced effect on arterial blood pressure and cardiac contractility.[58–61] However, these drugs cannot be used long term in adult horses and are primarily reserved for increasing cardiac output in horses under anaesthesia, neonates or emergency situations. Dobutamine is typically given at a dosage of 1 to 5 μg/kg/min constant rate infusion, to effect. Adverse effects are related primarily to induction of dysrhythmias and excitement. It increases myocardial oxygen consumption and can damage myocardial cells, particularly in high doses or with prolonged use,[62,63] but it is usually only used short term, in an emergency situation.

Milrinone

The type III phosphodiesterase inhibitor milrinone improves cardiac output, arterial blood pressure and contractility while decreasing systemic vascular resistance; however, it has only been studied in anaesthetised horses.[64] Its effects in horses with cardiac disease have not been reported.

Arterial vasodilators

Arterial vasodilators, used to decrease afterload and peripheral vascular resistance, allow the heart to more efficiently pump blood. By increasing stroke volume and decreasing the regurgitant fraction in horses with valvular diseases, organ perfusion should be improved and pulmonary oedema decreased. Hydralazine is a vasodilator that affects afterload much more than preload and has been shown to decrease pulmonary artery pressures in horses.[65] The recommended dosage is 0.5 to 1.5 mg/kg every 12 hours. Angiotensin-converting enzyme (ACE) inhibitors have been well studied in people, and are commonly used in both people and small animals. The ACE inhibitor enalapril has been used in horses to improve cardiac output in the presence of severe valvular (mitral and aortic) insufficiencies. While intravenous enalaprilat is effective in inhibiting ACE activity in horses,[66] pharmacokinetics of oral enalapril have recently been studied and suggest that at the dose used in healthy horses, effective drug levels are not attained.[67] No studies have been published of its efficacy in horses with cardiac disease. Further studies to determine the optimal dose and dosing interval are needed; however, anecdotally, a dose of 0.5 to 1 mg/kg every 12 to 24 hours has been used.

Furosemide (frusemide)

The most commonly used diuretic in horses is furosemide. Furosemide is a loop diuretic, acting by inhibition of the Na-K-2Cl cotransporter in the thick ascending portion of the loop of Henle.[68] It has a rapid onset of action if administered intravenously, peaking by 30 minutes. Furosemide increases urine volume and decreases plasma and extracellular fluid volume and concentrations of electrolytes (primarily Na, K, Cl and Ca).[68–71] It is used to decrease oedema formation (particularly pulmonary oedema) in horses in congestive heart failure. Furosemide is typically used at a dose of 0.5 to 2 mg/kg IV every 6 to 12 hours. Horses receiving furosemide should have their electrolyte and acid-base status monitored, as it can induce abnormalities that require correction. In addition, horses on digoxin concurrently should be monitored carefully, as hypovolaemia and electrolyte disturbances, particularly hypokalaemia, can predispose to digitalis intoxication.[16]

Recently, continuous rate infusion (CRI) of furosemide to decrease some of the negative side effects has been evaluated in horses.[72] In people it has been shown to be more effective than bolus dosing to promote diuresis, without some of the electrolyte aberrations seen with intermittent dosing. In horses there was a similar urine volume produced over 24 hours, with a more uniform urine flow rate and plasma volume compared with intermittent dosing. Higher concentrations of K, Cl and Ca were lost in the urine; therefore, electrolyte replacement may be more likely to be required if CRI furosemide is used. Furosemide has also been advocated as an oral maintenance treatment in horses requiring more long-term diuresis. Its efficacy given orally in healthy horses was examined recently.[73] The absorption was found to be variable and poor, with minimal diuretic effect compared with intravenous administration; therefore, this route was not recommended.

Treatment of miscellaneous conditions

Bacterial endocarditis

Bacterial endocarditis is bacterial invasion and colonisation of the valves or wall of the endocardium, and it most commonly affects the mitral valve, followed by the aortic, tricuspid and, least commonly, pulmonic valves.[74,75] In order to be successful, aggressive, prolonged treatment is required. Blood cultures should be obtained, and ideally antimicrobial therapy guided by bacterial culture and sensitivity results. In the absence of positive blood cultures, or while awaiting results, broad-spectrum, bactericidal intravenous antibiotics with excellent tissue penetration should be used (Chapter 6.3). Treatment is usually needed for a minimum of 4 to 6 weeks, and should be guided by the echocardiographic appearance of the vegetative lesion(s), as well as complete blood count, fibrinogen and globulin concentrations.[75,76] Ancillary treatment such as aspirin or heparin therapy can be combined with antimicrobials to try to limit additional thrombus formation, although no controlled studies in horses indicating benefits have been reported.[77] Although a bacteriological cure may be obtained, residual scarring of the valve by the lesion can permanently damage its function, causing chronic valvular insufficiency. Prognosis depends on the valve(s) affected and how severely they have been damaged. The prognosis for left-sided valvular lesions is worse than for right-sided lesions because of the higher pressures in the left side of the heart, and the more dire consequences of significant mitral regurgitation.

Pericarditis

Pericarditis is uncommon in horses, but with early recognition and prompt aggressive treatment the prognosis is good.[78] Echocardiography is essential for determining the amount and character of fluid (see Chapter 1.25). A sample for laboratory analysis should be submitted for cytological evaluation, culture and sensitivity, and other diagnostics such as viral isolation and titres. Pericardiocentesis and lavage of the pericardial sac are the mainstays of treatment if the effusion is moderate and compromising cardiac function (cardiac tamponade). This can be performed with either an indwelling catheter or intermittent pericardiocentesis (see Chapter 1.27). Sterile, warmed, isotonic fluids should be used for lavage, and 1 L of sterile, isotonic, polyionic fluid containing bactericidal antimicrobials such as sodium penicillin or gentamicin can be instilled if a septic pericarditis is suspected or confirmed.[78–80] Direct infusion of potassium penicillin should be avoided, because of the potential for potassium-induced dysrhythmias. Drainage and lavage should continue until less than 1 L of fluid is drained from the pericardial sac per day, and minimal fluid is visible on echocardiography. Systemic antibiotics should also be administered if a septic pericarditis exists, and ideally specific drug choice guided by bacterial culture and sensitivity of the fluid. If an infectious component is ruled out, and an idiopathic or immune-mediated pericarditis is suspected, corticisteroids can be beneficial.[81,82] Nonsteroidal anti-inflammatory drugs should be given for their analgesic, antipyretic and anti-inflammatory effects.

References

1. Hilwig RW: Cardiac arrhythmias, in Robinson NE (ed): Current Therapy in Equine Medicine. Philadelphia, WB Saunders, 1983, pp 131-141
2. Holmes JR: Prognosis of equine cardiac conditions. Equine Vet J 9:181-182, 1977
3. Reef VB: Frequency of cardiac arrhythmias and their significance in normal horses, in Proceedings of the Annual Veterinary Medical Forum (ACVIM), San Diego, CA, pp 570-572
4. Marr CM: Treatment of cardiac arrhythmias and cardiac failure, in Robinson NE (ed): Current Therapy in Equine Medicine, ed 4. Philadelphia, WB Saunders, 1997, pp 250-255
5. Piercy RJ, Marr CM: Collapse, in Marr CM (ed): Cardiology of the Horse. London, WB Saunders, 1999, pp 268-288
6. Reef VB: Arrhythmias, in Marr CM (ed): Cardiology of the Horse. London, WB Saunders, 1999, pp 179-209
7. McGuirk SM, Muir WW: Diagnosis and treatment of cardiac arrhythmias. Vet Clin N Am: Equine Pract 1:353-370, 1985
8. Zipes DP: Management of Cardiac Arrhythmias: pharmacological, electrical, and surgical techniques, in Braunwald E (ed): Heart Disease: A textbook of Cardiovascular Medicine, ed 3. Philadelphia, WB Saunders, 1988, pp 621-642
9. Cornick JL, Seahorn TL: Cardiac arrhythmias identified in horses with duodenitis/proximal jejunitis: six cases (1985-1988). J Am Vet Med Assoc 197:1054-1059, 1990
10. Marr CM, Reef VB, Brazil TJ, et al.: Aorto-cardiac fistulas in seven horses. Vet Radiol Ultrasound 39:22-31, 1998
11. Garber JL, Reef VB, Reimer JM, et al.: Postsurgical ventricular tachycardia in a horse. J Am Vet Med Assoc 201:1038-1039, 1992
12. Reimer JM, Reef VB, Sweeney RW: Ventricular arrhythmias in horses: 21 cases (1984-1989). J Am Vet Med Assoc 201:1237-1243, 1992
13. Schwarzwald CC, Hardy J, Buccellato M: High cardiac troponin I serum concentration in a horse with multiform ventricular tachycardia and myocardial necrosis. J Vet Int Med 17:364-368, 2003
14. Sleeper MM, Durando MM, Miller M, et al.: Aortic root disease in four horses. J Am Vet Med Assoc 219:491-496, 2001
15. Baggot JD: The pharmacological basis of cardiac drug selection for use in horses. Equine Vet J Suppl 19:97-100, 1995
16. Muir WW, McGuirk SM: Pharmacology and pharmacokinetics of drugs used to treat cardiac disease in horses. Vet Clin N Am: Equine Pract 1:335-352, 1985
17. McGuirk SM, Muir WW, Sams RA: Pharmacokinetic analysis of intravenously and orally administered quinidine in horses. Am J Vet Res 42:938-942, 1981

18. Muir WW, McGuirk S: Cardiovascular drugs. Their pharmacology and use in horses. Vet Clin N Am: Equine Pract 3:37-57, 1987
19. Deem DA, Fregin GF: Atrial fibrillation in horses: a review of 106 clinical cases, with consideration of prevalence, clinical signs, and prognosis. J Am Vet Med Assoc 180:261-265, 1982
20. Morris DD, Fregin GF: Atrial fibrillation in horses: factors associated with response to quinidine sulfate in 77 clinical cases. Cornell Vet 72:339-349, 1982
21. Reef VB, Reimer JM, Spencer PA: Treatment of atrial fibrillation in horses: new perspectives. J Vet Int Med 9:57-67, 1995
22. Muir WW, Reed SM, McGuirk SM: Treatment of atrial fibrillation in horses by intravenous administration of quinidine. J Am Vet Med Assoc 197:1607-1610, 1990
23. Parraga ME, Kittleson MD, Drake CM: Quinidine administration increases steady state serum digoxin concentration in horses. Equine Vet J Suppl 19:114-119, 1995
24. Reef VB, Levitan CW, Spencer PA: Factors affecting prognosis and conversion in equine atrial fibrillation. J Vet Int Med 2:1-6, 1988
25. Ellis EJ, Ravis WR, Malloy M, et al.: The pharmacokinetics and pharmacodynamics of procainamide in horses after intravenous administration. J Vet Pharmacol Ther 17:265-270, 1994
26. Puigdemont A, Riu JL, Guitart R, et al.: Propafenone kinetics in the horse. Comparative analysis of compartmental and noncompartmental models. J Pharmacol Methods 23:79-85, 1990
27. Fogoros RN: Phenytoin, in Messerli FH (ed): Cardiovascular Drug Therapy, ed 2. Philadelphia, WB Saunders, 1996, pp 1338-1341
28. Fogoros RN, Fiedler SB, Elson JJ: Efficacy of phenytoin in suppressing inducible ventricular tachyarrhythmias. Cardiovasc Drugs Ther 2:171-176, 1988
29. Smith PA, Aldridge BM, Kittleson MD: Oleander toxicosis in a donkey. J Vet Int Med 17:111-114, 2003
30. Wijnberg ID, van der Kolk H, Hiddink EG: Use of phenytoin to treat digitalis-induced cardiac arrhythmias in a miniature Shetland pony. Vet Rec 144:259-261, 1999
31. Wijnberg ID, Verves FF: Phenytoin sodium as a treatment for ventricular dysrhythmia in horses. J Vet Int Med 18:350-353, 2004
32. Kowalczyk DF, Beech J: Pharmacokinetics of phenytoin (diphenylhydantoin) in horses. J Vet Pharmacol Ther 6:133-140, 1983
33. Soma LR, Uboh CE, Guan F, et al.: Disposition, elimination, and bioavailability of phenytoin and its major metabolite in horses. Am J Vet Res 62:483-489, 2001
34. Banai S, Tzivoni D: Drug therapy for torsade de pointes. J Cardiovasc Electrophysiol 4:206-210, 1993
35. Muir WW: Clinical pharmacodynamics and pharmacokinetics of beta-adrenoceptor blocking drugs in veterinary medicine. Compend Contin Educ Pract Vet 6:156-167, 1984
36. Reef VB: Electrocardiography and echocardiography in the exercising horse, in Robinson NE (ed): Current Therapy in Equine Medicine, ed 4. Philadelphia, WB Saunders, 1997, pp 234-239
37. Reef VB: Ambulatory and exercise electrocardiography and post-exercise echocardiography, in Marr CM (ed): Cardiology of the Horse. London, WB Saunders, 1999, pp 150-160
38. Bowen IM: Cardiac dysrhythmias, in Robinson NE (ed): Current Therapy in Equine Medicine, ed 5. St. Louis, MO, Saunders, 2003, pp 602-613
39. Sweeney RW, Reef VB, Reimer JM: Pharmacokinetics of digoxin administered to horses with congestive heart failure. Am J Vet Res 54:1108-1111, 1993
40. Brumbaugh GW, Thomas WP, Hodge TG: Medical management of congestive heart failure in a horse. J Am Vet Med Assoc 180:878-883, 1982
41. Button C, Gross DR, Johnston JT, et al.: Digoxin pharmacokinetics, bioavailability, efficacy, and dosage regimens in the horse. Am J Vet Res 41:1388-1395, 1980
42. Ohmura H, Nukada T, Mizuno Y, et al.: Safe and efficacious dosage of flecainide acetate for treating equine atrial fibrillation. J Vet Med Sci 62:711-715, 2000
43. Ohmura H, Hiraga A, Aida H, et al.: Determination of oral dosage and pharmacokinetic analysis of flecainide in horses. J Vet Med Sci 63:511-514, 2001
44. van Loon G, Blissitt KJ, Keen JA, et al.: Use of intravenous flecainide in horses with naturally-occurring atrial fibrillation. Equine Vet J 36:609-614, 2004
45. De Clercq D, van Loon G, Baert K, et al.: Intravenous amiodarone treatment in horses with chronic atrial fibrillation. Vet J 172:129-134, 2006
46. Schwarzwald CC, Bonagura JD, Luis-Fuentes V: Effects of diltiazem on hemodynamic variables and ventricular function in healthy horses. J Vet Intern Med 19:703-711, 2005
47. McGurrin MK, Physick-Sheard PW, Kenney DG, et al.: Transvenous electrical cardioversion in equine atrial fibrillation: technique and successful treatment of 3 horses. J Vet Intern Med 17:715-718, 2003
48. Hamir AN, Reef VB: Complications of a permanent transvenous pacing catheter in a horse. J Comp Pathol 101:317-326, 1989
49. Reef VB, Clark ES, Oliver JA, et al.: Implantation of a permanent transvenous pacing catheter in a horse with complete heart block and syncope. J Am Vet Med Assoc 189:449-452, 1986
50. Taylor DH, Mero MA: The use of an internal pacemaker in a horse with Adams-Stokes syndrome. J Am Vet Med Assoc 151:1172-1176, 1967
51. van Loon G, Fonteyne W, Rottiers H, et al.: Dual-chamber pacemaker implantation via the cephalic vein in healthy equids. J Vet Intern Med 15:564-571, 2001
52. van Loon G, Fonteyne W, Rottiers H, et al.: Implantation of a dual-chamber, rate-adaptive pacemaker in a horse with suspected sick sinus syndrome. Vet Rec 151:541-545, 2002
53. Brumbaugh GW, Thomas WP, Enos LR, et al.: A pharmacokinetic study of digoxin in the horse. J Vet Pharmacol Ther 6:163-172, 1983
54. Pedersoli WM, Belmonte AA, Purohit RC, et al.: Pharmacokinetics of digoxin in the horse. J Equine Med Surg 2:384-388, 1978
55. Pedersoli WM, Ravis WR, Belmonte AA, et al.: Pharmacokinetics of a single, orally administered dose of digoxin in horses. Am J Vet Res 42:1412-1414, 1981
56. Smith TW: Digitalis. Mechanisms of action and clinical use. N Engl J Med 318:358-365, 1988

57. Ma G, Brady WJ, Pollack M, et al.: Electrocardiographic manifestations: digitalis toxicity. J Emerg Med 20:145-152, 2001
58. Gasthuys F, de Moor A, Parmentier D: Influence of dopamine and dobutamine on the cardiovascular depression during a standard halothane anaesthesia in dorsally recumbent, ventilated ponies. Zentralbl Veterinarmed A 38:494-500, 1991
59. Hellyer PW, Wagner AE, Mama KR, et al.: The effects of dobutamine and ephedrine on packed cell volume, total protein, heart rate, and blood pressure in anaesthetized horses. J Vet Pharmacol Ther 21:497-499, 1998
60. Hinchcliff KW, McKeever KH, Muir WW: Hemodynamic effects of atropine, dobutamine, nitroprusside, phenylephrine, and propranolol in conscious horses. J Vet Int Med 5:80-86, 1991
61. Young LE, Blissitt KJ, Clutton RE, et al.: Temporal effects of an infusion of dobutamine hydrochloride in horses anesthetized with halothane. Am J Vet Res 59:1027-1032, 1998
62. Todd GL, Baroldi G, Pieper GM, et al.: Experimental catecholamine-induced myocardial necrosis. II. Temporal development of isoproterenol-induced contraction band lesions correlated with ECG, hemodynamic and biochemical changes. J Mol Cell Cardiol 17:647-656, 1985
63. Todd GL, Baroldi G, Pieper GM, et al.: Experimental catecholamine-induced myocardial necrosis. I. Morphology, quantification and regional distribution of acute contraction band lesions. J Mol Cell Cardiol 17:317-338, 1985
64. Muir WW: The haemodynamic effects of milrinone HCl in halothane anaesthetised horses. Equine Vet J Suppl. 19:108-113, 1995
65. Bertone JJ: Cardiovascular effects of hydralazine HCl administration in horses. Am J Vet Res 49:618-621, 1988
66. Muir WW, 3rd, Sams RA, Hubbell JA, et al.: Effects of enalaprilat on cardiorespiratory, hemodynamic, and hematologic variables in exercising horses. Am J Vet Res 62:1008-1013, 2001
67. Gardner SY, Atkins CE, Sams RA, et al.: Characterization of the pharmacodynamic properties of the angiotensin-converting enzyme inhibitor, enalapril, in horses, in Proceedings of the Annual Veterinary Medical Forum (ACVIM), Denver, CO, p 889
68. Hinchcliff KW, Muir WW 3rd: Pharmacology of furosemide in the horse: a review. J Vet Intern Med 5:211-218, 1991
69. Hinchcliff KW, McKeever KH, Muir WW 3rd: Furosemide-induced changes in plasma and blood volume of horses. J Vet Pharmacol Ther 14:411-417, 1991
70. Muir WW, Kohn CW, Sams R: Effects of furosemide on plasma volume and extracellular fluid volume in horses. Am J Vet Res 39:1688-1691, 1978
71. Muir WW, Milne DW, Skarda RT: Acute hemodynamic effects of furosemide administered intravenously in the horse. Am J Vet Res 37:1177-1180, 1976
72. Johansson AM, Gardner SY, Levine JF, et al.: Furosemide continuous rate infusion in the horse: evaluation of enhanced efficacy and reduced side effects. J Vet Intern Med 17:887-895, 2003
73. Johansson AM, Gardner SY, Levine JF, et al.: Pharmacokinetics and pharmacodynamics of furosemide after oral administration to horses. J Vet Intern Med 18:739-743, 2004
74. Bonagura JD, Reef VB: Cardiovascular diseases, in Reed SM, Bayly WM (eds): Equine Internal Medicine. Philadelphia, WB Saunders, 1998, pp 290-370
75. Maxson AD, Reef VB: Bacterial endocarditis in horses: ten cases (1984-1995). Equine Vet J 29:394-399, 1997
76. Sage AM, Worth LT: Fever: endocarditis and pericarditis, in Marr CM (ed): Cardiology of the Horse. London, WB Saunders, 1999, pp 256-267
77. Mogg TD: Equine cardiac disease. Clinical pharmacology and therapeutics. Vet Clin North Am Equine Pract 15:523-534, vii, 1999
78. Worth LT, Reef VB: Pericarditis in horses: 18 cases (1986-1995). J Am Vet Med Assoc 212:248-253, 1998
79. Bernard W, Reef VB, Clark ES, et al.: Pericarditis in horses: six cases (1982-1986). J Am Vet Med Assoc 196:468-471, 1990
80. Reef VB, Gentile DG, Freeman DE: Successful treatment of pericarditis in a horse. J Am Vet Med Assoc 185:94-98, 1984
81. Freestone JF, Thomas WP, Carlson GP, et al.: Idiopathic effusive pericarditis with tamponade in the horse. Equine Vet J 19:38-42, 1987
82. Robinson JA, Marr CM, Reef VB, et al.: Idiopathic, aseptic, effusive, fibrinous, nonconstrictive pericarditis with tamponade in a standardbred filly. J Am Vet Med Assoc 201:1593-1598, 1992

9.2.2 Treatments aimed at improving tissue perfusion

Kevin Corley

Early aggressive fluid resuscitation

Fluid therapy (see Chapter 6.5) is the mainstay of improving tissue perfusion. Early descriptions of fluid therapy in foals and horses were relatively conservative, chiefly because of concerns of causing pulmonary oedema.[1–3] However, pulmonary oedema appears to be extremely rare in horses and neonatal foals despite aggressive initial fluid therapy.[4] More recently, authors have been recommending bolus fluid therapy in horses with hypovolaemia, with repeated boluses of 10 to 20 ml/kg of crystalloids given as fast as possible. A maximum of approximately 60 to 80 ml/kg fluids is recommended before additional treatments, such as inotropes or vasopressors, are considered.[5–7]

No primary evidence exists for this aggressive fluid therapy in the horse. However, a retrospective study in septic human children showed markedly better survival in those that received greater than 40 ml/kg fluids in the first hour of treatment, compared to those receiving less than 20 ml/kg.[8] A prospective study in human adult septic patients showed that early goal-directed therapy (EGDT) decreased hospital mortality from 46.5% with conventional treatment to 30.5%. One major difference between the treatment groups was the total amount of fluids administered in the first 6 hours of treatment (5 L for the EGDT group and 3.5 L for the conventional group). In the period between 7 and 72 hours, the conventional group received 10.6 L, compared to 8.6 L in the EGDT group, suggesting that it was the timing of fluid therapy, rather than the total amount given that was important.[9] It is essential to note that there is no evidence for, and no author recommends, continued aggressive fluid therapy once hypovolaemia has been reversed.

Uncontrolled haemorrhage

As noted in Chapter 6.5, uncontrolled haemorrhage is an important exception to aggressive fluid therapy for hypovolaemia.[10,11] Fluids should be administered at a rate of 2 to 3 ml/kg/hr until the haemorrhage has been controlled (usually by surgical intervention). Where arterial blood pressure can be measured, therapy should be titrated to a moderate mean arterial pressure (60 mm Hg).

Fluid challenge

The change in CVP in response to a "fluid challenge" (bolus of fluids) is a method of reversing hypovolaemia[12] that has not been formally evaluated in the horse. The "fluid challenge" method of monitoring fluid therapy may prove particularly useful in acute renal failure or pulmonary oedema. In horses without pulmonary oedema, a "fluid challenge" without measuring central venous pressure can also be useful in the assessment of the fluid status of the horse.

In horses with signs of inadequate tissue perfusion including tachycardia, hypotension or oliguria, the purpose of the "fluid challenge" is to determine whether further fluids alone may reverse the abnormality or if another intervention is required. If there is no improvement after a 10 to 20 ml/kg bolus of crystalloids or a 2 to 5 ml/kg bolus of colloids, it is unlikely that fluids alone will be successful. The author uses this form of "fluid challenge" routinely in hypotensive individuals prior to starting a dobutamine infusion, as the latter drug may cause significant tachycardia in cases resuscitated with insufficient fluid.[13]

Vasoactive therapy

Mean arterial pressure can be raised by increasing cardiac output or systemic vascular resistance (SVR). The aim of therapy for hypotension, however, is not to increase mean arterial pressure *per se*, but to improve organ perfusion. For this reason, treatment strategies that increase cardiac output and therefore blood flow are usually attempted prior to therapies specifically aimed at increasing SVR (Figure 9.17).

Cardiac stroke volume is the difference between end-diastolic volume and end-systolic volume of the ventricle. Fluids increase stroke volume by increasing end-diastolic volume. Inotropes, on the other hand, decrease end-systolic volume by increasing myocardial contraction. In horses that do not respond to fluid therapy, inotropes represent a further way of increasing cardiac output and thus blood flow. However, inotropes increase cardiac work and thus oxygen consumption, which may be important when oxygen delivery is marginal. Inotropes may also cause tachycardia in under fluid-resuscitated animals.[13]

Pressor agents act to increase vascular tone. Markedly decreased vascular tone, resulting in decreased SVR, is a feature of human adult sepsis.[13] Decreased SVR has been documented in septic foals[4] and horses following colic surgery. Although SVRs less than the normal value may be desirable in critical illness,[14] some foals remain hypotensive and oliguric despite aggressive support of cardiac output.[15] In these foals, moderately increasing vascular tone with pressor agents has resulted in improved haemodynamics and urine output.[15]

Pressor agents must be used with caution and their effects monitored closely. Excessive vasoconstriction leads to increased cardiac afterload, resulting in increased cardiac work and decreased stroke volume. The effects of pressor agents may also not be equivalent in all tissues, especially in disease, resulting in excessive vasoconstriction and reduced blood flow in some organs despite improved systemic haemodynamics. The kidney and gastrointestinal tract are particularly at risk. Decreased urine output in response to increases in pressor therapy usually indicates excessive renal vasoconstriction, and should trigger an urgent review of the therapy. Gastrointestinal perfusion is difficult to assess with currently available clinical tools. Excessive gastrointestinal vasoconstriction may lead to ileus, but gastrointestinal motility is also directly affected by the catecholamines, irrespective of perfusion.[16,17] Increased circulating blood lactate concentrations due to inadequate perfusion may result from excessive vasoconstriction of any tissue or organ but are not a constant finding.

Inotropes

Dobutamine

Dobutamine is a catecholamine with strong affinity for the β_1-adrenoceptor and weak affinity for the β_2- and α-adrenergic receptors. The main clinical use of dobutamine is as an inotrope to increase oxygen delivery to the tissues. For this reason, specific indications for dobutamine therapy are low cardiac output or decreased central venous oxygen tension despite adequate fluid therapy.

In a canine model of endotoxaemia, dobutamine (5–10 μg/kg/min) had a beneficial effect on splanchnic perfusion and urine output, compared to fluid therapy alone.[18] In a rat model of endotoxaemia, dobutamine maintained intestinal villi blood flow at preendotoxic levels.[19] This beneficial effect on splanchnic perfusion is also seen with dobutamine therapy in human septic patients, but not with dopamine therapy.[20] All of this evidence suggests a possible benefit if low-dose dobutamine infusion in endotoxic horses, especially those where the primary lesion is of the gastrointestinal tract. The author has used low dose dobutamine (1–2 μg/kg/kg) in horses following surgery for strangulating intestinal lesions, to support the splanchnic

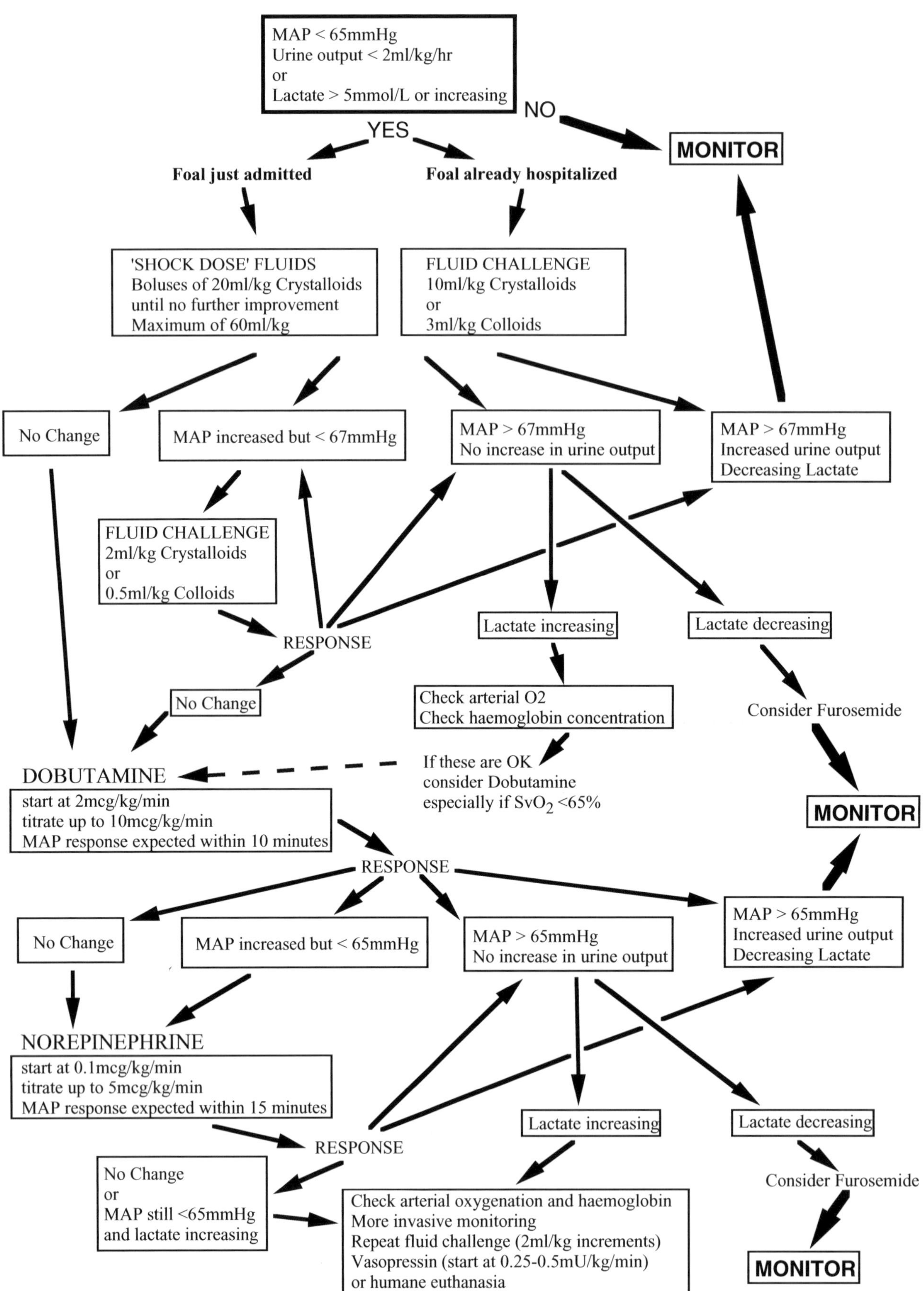

Figure 9.17 Algorithm for treatment of hypotension in neonatal foals. Intended as a guide only. Treatment should always be tailored to the individual case. Adapted from Corley KTT: Monitoring and treating haemodynamic disturbances in critically ill neonatal foals. Part II: assessment and treatment. Equine Vet Educ 14:328-336, 2002. Used with permission.

circulation. In my experience, infusion rates higher than these have been associated with mean arterial pressures above the normal range. Maintenance of splanchnic perfusion may also be important in horses and foals, as it may prevent bacterial translocation across the intestinal wall and establishment or worsening of septicaemia.[21]

Dobutamine may also have a role in improving splanchnic perfusion when vasopressors such as norepinephrine or epinephrine are used,[22–24] presumably through its action on β_2-receptors. Therefore, low-dose dobutamine (up to 5 µg/kg/min) is probably indicated during vasopressor therapy.

It may also be advisable to assess the response to dobutamine before starting vasopressor therapy, to ensure adequate cardiac output when it cannot be measured. However, dobutamine can decrease SVR and mean arterial pressure, probably through its action on β_2-adrenergic receptors,[25] and therefore is rarely suitable as monotherapy in hyperdynamic shock.

Dobutamine should be diluted in isotonic saline, 5% glucose or dextrose, or lactated Ringer's solution. The dose should be carefully titrated from a starting point of 0.5 to 1 µg/kg/min in adult horses and 1 to 3 µg/kg/min in foals (Table 9.3).

Isoproterenol

Isoproterenol is a β_1- and β_2-adrenergic agonist. In humans with septic shock, isoproterenol has been found to be a suitable alternative to dobutamine.[26] However, in normal horses, administration of the drug results in significant tachycardia and decreased arterial pressure.[27] This tachycardia and vasodilation are likely to limit its clinical utility in the horse.

Vasopressors

Norepinephrine

Norepinephrine (noradrenaline) is a strong α-adrenergic agonist with affinity for β_1-receptors and no demonstrable β_2 activity. Norepinephrine is used clinically to restore adequate organ perfusion pressure in vasodilatory shock. The specific clinical indications for norepinephrine are markedly decreased SVR or decreased mean arterial pressure, which responds to neither fluids nor an inotrope, such as dobutamine. The β_1-adrenergic effects of norepinephrine help to offset the negative effects on cardiac output of the increased cardiac afterload associated with vasoconstriction. Indeed, cardiac output may be increased by 10% to 20%, as a result of increased stroke volume.[28] An increase in cardiac output was found with norepinephrine administration in anaesthetised neonatal foals[29] but not in conscious neonatal foals.[30] However, inappropriately high doses of norepinephrine may result in decreased stroke volume due to increased afterload, and reduced end-organ perfusion. Blood pressure, urine output and other cardiovascular parameters should therefore be carefully monitored during norepinephrine infusion.

In human septic shock, norepinephrine is a more effective vasopressor than dopamine.[31] Furthermore, in septic humans requiring greater than 15 µg/kg/min dopamine, the addition of norepinephrine results in significantly higher hospital survival (38%) than increasing the dopamine infusion rate (18%).[32] Previous concerns that norepinephrine might have adverse effects on renal function, based on work in normal subjects, has been shown not to be the case in sepsis and endotoxaemia.[15,33] In sheep with experimental hyperdynamic sepsis, infusion of 0.4 µg/kg/min norepinephrine resulted in significantly increased mean arterial pressure, myocardial performance, stroke volume and creatinine clearance and no change in renal and mesenteric blood flow, which were already significantly increased by onset of sepsis.[34] Furthermore, at a dose of 0.1 µg/kg/min, no effect of norepinephrine was seen on urine output or renal indices in conscious neonatal foals.[30]

The addition of low-dose dobutamine (5 µg/kg/min) to norepinephrine has been demonstrated to result in better splanchnic perfusion in human septic patients, possibly due to splanchnic vasodilation mediated by β_2-adrenergic agonism by dobutamine.[22] In a sheep model of peritonitis, combination of norepinephrine and dobutamine was

Table 9.3. Guideline for diluting and preparing inotropes and pressors. Example starting rates for a 50-kg foal are given as an aid to double-checking calculations. At high dose rates, the amount of drug diluted in 500 ml or 60 ml will need to be increased.

Drug	Starting rate	Maximum rate	Dilute in:			Electronic infusion pump		Syringe driver	
			LRS	NaCl	G5W	Usual amount to dilute in 500 ml	Starting rate (50-kg foal)	Usual amount to dilute in 60 ml	Starting rate (50-kg foal)
Dobutamine	2 µg/kg/min	≈20 µg/kg/min	Yes	Yes	Yes	250 mg	13 ml/hr	125 mg	2.9 ml/hr
Norepinephrine	0.1 µg/kg/min	≈5 µg/kg/min	No	No	Yes	8 mg	19 ml/hr	8 mg	2.3 ml/hr
Vasopressin	0.25 mU/kg/min	? ~8 mU/kg/min	?	Yes	Yes	20 U	19 ml/hr	20 U	2.3 ml/hr
Epinephrine	0.1 µg/kg/min	≈2 µg/kg/min	Yes	Yes	Yes	5 mg	30 ml/hr	5 mg	3.6 ml/hr
Dopamine	5 µg/kg/min	≈25 µg/kg/min	Yes	Yes	Yes	400 mg	19 ml/hr	400 mg	2.3 ml/hr

LRS, lactated Ringer's solution; NaCl, 0.9% sodium chloride solution; G5W, 5% glucose or 5% dextrose solution.

superior to norepinephrine, in terms of survival time, measures of splanchnic perfusion, urine output and histological alterations in pulmonary and intestinal tissue. Combination of dopamine and norepinephrine was also superior to norepinephrine alone, but in some parameters, such as urine output and intestinal pathology, was inferior to the norepinephrine-dobutamine combination.[24] In normal, conscious neonatal foals, addition of 5 μg/kg/min dobutamine to 0.1 μg/kg/min norepinephrine resulted in increased arterial blood pressure, but did not reverse the decrease in cardiac output.[30] Norepinephrine early in resuscitation, at the same time as fluid administration, was superior to delayed norepinephrine administration in a rat model of endotoxic shock.[35]

We investigated concurrent norepinephrine and low dose dobutamine infusions in seven critically ill foals that remained hypotensive despite dobutamine or dopamine therapy. We found an increase in mean arterial pressure in six of seven foals and an increase in urine output in all foals, coincident with the start of the norepinephrine infusion.[15] Three of the seven foals survived to compete as racehorses. The indications for norepinephrine use in adult horses are less clear, as hyperdynamic shock is less frequently recognised.

Norepinephrine should be diluted in 5% glucose or 5% dextrose. Once diluted, the drug only remains fully active for approximately 24 hours. The dose should be carefully titrated from a starting dose of 0.1 μg/kg/min (Table 9.3). Effects may be seen in some patients at doses as low as 0.01 μg/kg/min. The highest dose of norepinephrine we have used in a foal that ultimately survived is 1.5 μg/kg/min.[15]

Vasopressin and terlipressin

Arginine-vasopressin and terlipressin are noncatecholamine vasopressors that have recently been the subject of intense research in human patients and animal models. Vasopressin acts on V1a receptors in the periphery to cause vasoconstriction and on V2 receptors in the collecting tubule of the nephron, to cause water resorption.

Vasopressin increased mean arterial pressure in normal foals anaesthetised with isoflurane.[29] Interestingly, vasopressin is approximately 5 times more potent a vasopressor in endotoxaemia and septic shock, than in normal subjects.[36,37] This may be explained, at least in part, by indirect actions to counteract the vasodilation of shock. Vasopressin restores some of the vasoconstrictor effect of circulating catecholamines,[38] which is reduced in septic shock,[39,40]

Vasopressin and terlipressin are powerful vasoconstrictors and may result in decreased cardiac output and oxygen delivery,[41–43] presumably due to baroceptor mediated reflex reduction in cardiac output. This reduction in cardiac output was also seen in anaesthetised neonatal foals.[29] This reduction in cardiac output may be reversed by the addition of dobutamine[41] or norepinephrine[42]. Of these two, dobutamine may be the more logical choice and concurrent infusion of dobutamine with vasopressin, as opposed to vasopressin on its own, is recommended. In endotoxic sheep, administration of vasopressin resulted in decreased cardiac output, reduced oxygen delivery and increased pulmonary vascular resistance. Addition of norepinephrine resulted in significant increases in cardiac output, towards the values found in normal sheep.

A major concern with vasopressin and terlipressin is that they reduce gastrointestinal perfusion.[44–46] In anaesthetised foals, vasopressin, in contrast to dobutamine and norepinephrine, appeared to reduce gastric perfusion.[29] Evidence in a rat endotoxaemia model demonstrated that terlipressin improved ileal microcirculation in aggressively fluid-resuscitated animals, but was detrimental in animals receiving only 10 ml/kg/hr of crystalloid fluids.[47] Skin necrosis is also a possibility.[48] Therefore these drugs should only be used following fluid resuscitation. A potential interaction between vasopressin (which activates platelets via V1 receptors) and heparin, leading to platelet aggregation and potential organ dysfunction has been noted in human patients.[49]

Anecdotal evidence suggests that vasopressin is useful as a pressor agent in foal septic shock and has similar properties to those seen in human patients. The suggested starting dose is 0.25 to 0.5 mU/kg/min for vasopressin[50] (Table 9.3). Terlipressin has been administered to humans as a bolus of 1 to 2 mg, which resulted in a progressive increase in mean arterial pressure which was maintained for at least 5 hours.[51] Continuous infusion of terlipressin appears to avoid some of the negative side effects (decreases in heart rate and cardiac output and increase in pulmonary vascular resistance) associated with intermittent bolus administration.[52] It is vital to ensure adequate fluid resuscitation prior to administration of these drugs.[47]

Epinephrine

Epinephrine is a strong agonist for both α- and β-adrenergic receptors, with no dopaminergic activity. Although epinephrine is an effective vasopressor, its negative effects on the splanchnic circulation may limit its clinical usefulness.[53] In contrast to norepinephrine, epinephrine decreased mesenteric blood flow relative to aortic blood flow in a rat model of endotoxaemia.[54] In human patients with severe sepsis, the splanchnic blood flow was found to be lower with epinephrine than with norepinephrine.[53] The clinical relevance of these observations regarding the splanchnic circulation is debated.[55]

In human medicine, the main clinical use of epinephrine is as a "rescue" vasopressor agent, when dopamine or norepinephrine is inadequate to restore adequate organ perfusion pressure. Survival is very poor when epinephrine is used for this purpose.[32] Patients may be refractory to norepinephrine because of alteration in the binding capacity of α-adrenergic receptors (see earlier).[56,57] The vasopressor action of epinephrine is also mediated by α-adrenergic receptors. For this reason, V1 agonists such as vasopressin (see later) may be a more logical choice than epinephrine for norepinephrine refractory shock, because they act on a totally different class of receptors.

Epinephrine should be diluted in isotonic saline, 5% glucose or dextrose, or lactated Ringer's solution. The dose should be carefully titrated from a starting dose of 0.1 μg/kg/min (Table 9.3).

Dopamine

Dopamine is an α-, β_1-, and β_2-adrenergic receptor agonist and an agonist for dopaminergic receptors. This results in a complicated drug profile, where different effects predominate at different doses. At high doses, the α-adrenergic effects predominate, and dopamine is principally a vasopressor. At lower doses, the β-adrenergic effects predominate, and dopamine is principally an inotrope. Some clinicians recommend dopamine as a first line vasopressor, because they believe that the action on β_2- and dopaminergic receptors may prevent excessive vasoconstriction in vulnerable vascular beds, such as the splanchnic circulation. However, available evidence from humans and experimental animals suggests that dopamine may actually impair rather than improve gastrointestinal perfusion.[58,59] Furthermore, the plasma concentration of dopamine with a given infusion rate is extremely variable between individual human subjects,[60] and therefore the effects of a given infusion rate of dopamine are unpredictable.

Dopamine has other potentially adverse effects. Infusion of dopamine results in suppression of all anterior pituitary dependent hormones, with the exception of cortisol, in adult human patients. Furthermore, cessation of dopamine infusion results in rebound hypersecretion of some of these hormones.[61] Dopamine also may suppress chemoreflex sensitivity to hypoxia, resulting in a decreased ventilatory response,[62] which may have relevance in horses that are marginal for requiring mechanical ventilation.

Low-dose dopamine does not increase creatinine clearance in normal adult horses,[63] and low-dose (or "renal dose") dopamine has no benefit in prevention or treatment of renal failure in human patients.[64–66] High-dose dopamine is not as effective as norepinephrine for restoring haemodynamics in human hyperdynamic shock.[31] Based on a single case, this may also be true in foals. Norepinephrine successfully reversed hypotension in a foal which had failed to respond to high dose dopamine (24 μg/kg/min).[15]

If used, dopamine should be diluted in isotonic saline, 5% glucose or dextrose, or lactated Ringer's solution. If being used as an inotrope, the starting dose should be 2 to 5 μg/kg/min. If being used as a vasopressor, the starting dose should be 5 to 10 μg/kg/min (Table 9.3).

Choice of vasopressor

There is insufficient evidence to recommend any of the currently used vasopressors over another. A recent randomised clinical trial did not find a difference in mortality between epinephrine and the combination of norepinephrine and dobutamine in human septic patients.[67]

There is no current evidence that vasopressin is either superior or inferior to norepinephrine for reversal of hypotension in septic shock.[68,69] However, in a subset of human septic patients requiring lower doses of vasopressors, there was a slight decrease in mortality when vasopressin was used as the vasopressor, compared to when norepinephrine was used.[69] The incidence of cardiac arrest was slightly more common in the norepinephrine group, and digital ischaemia was slightly more common in the vasopressin group.[69] None of these differences in human patients was sufficient to influence the choice between norepinephrine and vasopressin in horses.

For these reasons, the choice should be based on clinician experience and preference. It is probably wise to use one vasopressor or vasopressor/inotrope combination as a first line treatment in each clinic. This allows the whole staff to become familiar with the treatment, including usual dose rates, dilutions and expected and adverse effects. In my hospital, we use the combination of dobutamine and norepinephrine as our first line treatment for fluid refractory hypotension.

Other drugs that result in decreased vasodilation

Corticosteroids

In a large randomised clinical trial of low-dose steroid therapy (hydrocortisone and 9-α-fludrocortisone) in human septic shock, the median time until vasopressors could be withdrawn was shorter in the treatment group (7 days) than the placebo group (9 days). This effect was limited to patients that did not respond to a corticotrophin test in both drug and placebo groups. Nonresponders were defined as patients that showed an increase of less than 9 μg/dl in cortisol over baseline at both 30 and 60 minutes after administration of 250 μg of tetracosactrin. Nonresponders treated with steroids also had a survival benefit at 28 days, over nonresponders treated with placebo. Of patients in this study, 77% were nonresponders, and there were no negative effects of treatment in responders, resulting in benefits in terms of withdrawal of vasopressors and survival when responders and nonresponders were considered together.[70] The decreased requirement for vasopressors with corticosteroids in this study fits with previous data showing increased sensitivity to norepinephrine in patients administered hydrocortisone.[71,72] It is interesting that corticosteroids may also improve the response to vasopressin.[73] Little is known about the response to ACTH stimulation in septic and endotoxic horses or their response to corticosteroids. The response to ACTH in normal foals has been studied,[74] as has the ACTH and cortisol concentrations in septic foals.[75] At the time of writing, several groups were studying the ACTH responses of septic foals, but these were yet to be published.

One possible concern about the use of corticosteroids in septic patients is that immunosuppression might hinder bacterial clearance mediated by the endogenous immune system. However, if corticosteroids reduced circulating proinflammatory cytokines in sepsis and endotoxaemia, this could possibly be beneficial. New evidence from human septic patients demonstrated that infusion of hydrocortisone inhibited some cytokine expression (interleukin [IL]-6 and IL-8) and neutrophil and endothelial cell activation, but *in vitro* phagocytosis by monocyte-lineage cells was increased.[76] The net effect of these changes on bacterial clearance is unclear but may not be detrimental.

There are no published reports of the use of low-dose hydrocortisone to reverse vasodilation in the horse. Administration of hydrocortisone (100 mg loading dose, followed by 0.18 mg/kg/hr) by the author to a septic foal resulted in a rapid rise in the plasma sodium concentration (increase of 11 mmol/L in 12 hours), such that the infusion had to be discontinued. Post-mortem examination of this foal, 8 days after hydrocortisone therapy, revealed a fungal pneumonia.

Haemoglobin

Administration of haemoglobin-based oxygen-carrying solutions (HBOC) results in increased SVR.[77] Ponies in which normovolaemic anaemia was induced had decreased SVR. Administration of 15 ml/kg polymerised ultrapurified bovine haemoglobin solution resulted in a significant increase in SVR, whereas administration of the same volume of hetastarch did not.[78] In a case report, administration of an HBOC to a Miniature horse with cyclic ovarian haemorrhage resulted in increases in pulmonary artery pressure and central venous pressure.[79]

The mechanism of HBOC-mediated vasoconstriction is still controversial.[77] Possible mechanisms include scavenging of nitric oxide[80,81] or upregulation of expression of endothelin-1, a local vasoconstrictor.[82,83]

Therapeutic goals

The ultimate goal of treatment is to provide oxygen delivery sufficient to meet demand in all tissues in the body. The relationship between oxygen delivery to individual tissues and the elements of the cardiovascular system is a complex one and is not the same for all tissues. This difference between tissues becomes magnified in disease states, and therefore the optimal inotrope and vasopressor combination may be different for different individual animals, depending on the effects on different tissue beds.

For these reasons, several indicators of cardiovascular status should be considered together as a trigger or goal for therapy, as isolated parameters are unlikely to accurately reflect haemodynamics across a range of different tissues. In neonatal foals, this is further complicated by the apparent lack of some appropriate physiological responses, which may mask disturbances. An example is the failure of some foals to increase their heart rate to maintain cardiac output when stroke volume is decreased by hypovolaemia.

Another consideration, when setting goals and thresholds for therapy, is that optimal haemodynamics are not necessarily the same in the critically ill horse as the normal animal. Although normal values are useful to interpret haemodynamic data, they are not always appropriate goals. Particular examples are cardiac output and SVR. Cardiac outputs of 1.5 times the normal value allow for increased oxygen delivery and therefore may be beneficial in some horses. It is important that the increase in cardiac output is a result of increased stroke volume, rather than heart rate. Increased heart rates may result in inadequate cardiac oxygen supply. When coupled with an increased cardiac output, SVR just below the normal range may allow better organ perfusion in some septic patients.[14] It should be noted that the combination of decreased SVR offset by increased cardiac output would result in a mean arterial pressure within the normal range.

When considering starting inotrope or vasopressor therapy, all the available haemodynamic data should be considered. Techniques for monitoring haemodynamics in horses are described in Chapter 9.1.2 and the relevant sections in Chapters 1 and 2. Arterial blood pressure is one of the most important parameters to monitor the haemodynamic status of the animal. Measuring arterial blood pressure is described in Chapters 1.21, 1.22 and 2.7. Decreased arterial pressure is associated with poor survival in horses with acute abdominal disease[84,85] and critically ill neonatal foals[86].

In general, the cardiovascular system should be reviewed and supportive treatments considered if the mean arterial pressure falls below 70 mm Hg. This allows a buffer zone, in which different therapeutic strategies may be formulated and assessed, before the mean arterial pressure falls below 60 mm Hg. However, simply increasing mean arterial pressure is not an appropriate therapeutic goal. This is most starkly illustrated by a trial of L-N^G-methylarginine hydrochloride, a nonselective nitric oxide inhibitor, in human septic shock. This drug increased blood pressure, but also markedly decreased survival.[87] If vasopressors are required for therapy, they should be titrated to maintain blood pressure within the low end of the normal range, because their effects on different organs may be uneven. Limited evidence from human critical care suggests there may be no additional advantage of titrating therapies to achieve a blood pressure of 75 or 85 mm Hg over 65 mm Hg.[88]

Heart rate is an indicator of response to treatment but should not be a target for specific therapy. Therapeutic interventions that result in a reduction in heart rate towards or within the normal range are likely to be beneficial. However, therapies specifically aimed to reduce the heart rate (for example, β-adrenergic blockade) are highly likely to be detrimental and should be avoided without specific indication.

Urine output can be a very useful guide to end-organ perfusion. In many horses, it may be a more useful indicator of cardiovascular status than blood pressure alone. Urine output can be accurately measured by attaching a closed collection system to an indwelling urinary catheter and measuring the urine produced hourly.[86] This is a commonly done procedure in recumbent foals, but less practical in adult conscious horses.

The response in urine output to changes in the cardiovascular system is not direct because of the many interacting feedback control mechanisms. Therefore, urine output only provides a gross indication of cardiovascular status. Changes in mean arterial pressure across the normal physiological range are damped by intrinsic autoregulatory mechanisms resulting in little change in renal blood flow and glomerular filtration rate and urine output. However, in the failing circulation, renal blood flow is decreased both directly and via neuroendocrine feedback mechanisms, resulting in decreased urine output.[89]

Decreased urine output may be the first sign of impending hypovolaemia, and may occur very early in cardiovascular shock from any cause. It is important to note that many variables other than circulatory status can decrease urine output. Acute renal failure may result in oliguria, anuria or polyuria. Measuring the urine specific gravity can help distinguish haemodynamic (prerenal) renal insufficiency from renal failure. The specific gravity is expected to be close to isotonic (1.010) in renal failure and is usually higher than this with significant dehydration or hypovolaemia. Other causes of decreased urine output include blocked urinary catheters and defects in bladder wall integrity.

The cardiovascular system should be reviewed if the urine output is less than two-thirds of the volume of fluid delivered (including all infusates and enteral feeding). Large decreases in urine output demand immediate attention. Urine output can be especially useful to evaluate a change in therapy. For example, a treatment that increases mean arterial pressure but decreases urine output has almost certainly not improved tissue perfusion.

Blood lactate concentrations can be a very useful guide to the adequacy of tissue oxygen delivery and thus help guide haemodynamic therapy. Therapy should be considered if the blood lactate concentration is above the normal range (>1.5 mmol/L for adults; >2.5 mmol/L for foals).

Practical use of inotropes and pressors

Inotrope and vasopressor choice and infusion rate must always be tailored to the individual animal, and reassessed in context of the observed response. This is true even when sophisticated haemodynamic monitoring equipment is available, because treatment strategies are always a compromise between opposing therapies that might be optimal for different vascular beds. Therefore, the response to treatment should always be measured, not assumed, and the treatment plan adjusted accordingly. With these caveats in mind, a possible treatment algorithm for neonatal foals is presented in Figure 9.17. The broad principles for treating adult horses are likely to be similar. My experience of haemodynamic management with horses with presumed endotoxaemia suggests that this order of approach (fluids, dobutamine, norepinephrine) is correct in the adult horse. However, I have far less experience of measuring haemodynamic responses to interventions in non-anaesthetised adult horses than in foals, and so setting comparable guidelines is not yet possible. Furthermore, whereas placement of indwelling urinary catheters and measurement of hourly urine volume is routine in recumbent foals, this is an uncommon technique in adult horses. This limits one of the most useful assessments of changes in end-organ perfusion in response to inotrope and pressor therapy in the adult.

The first response to haemodynamic derangements should be to assess the animal's fluid balance, and ensure that the animal is fluid replete. This is best achieved by means of a "fluid challenge" (Figure 9.17). Inotropes may cause tachycardia in under–fluid-resuscitated animals,[13] resulting in increased myocardial oxygen demand and reduced coronary perfusion. Inadequate circulating volume results in reduced cardiac preload, and therefore reduced cardiac stroke volume. Inappropriately high doses of vasopressors may increase cardiac afterload. The combination of hypovolaemia and high doses of vasopressors can result in marked reductions in cardiac output,[86] reducing blood flow to the tissues. In horses with known renal insufficiency, head trauma and in foals with perinatal asphyxia syndrome, fluid overload is either more likely (renal failure) or carries more serious consequences (cerebral oedema). In these animals, fluid challenges should be done less aggressively (2–3 ml/kg of crystalloids or 0.5 ml/kg colloid) but still represent an effective way of carefully titrating fluid input to the animals needs.

If animals are hypotensive, and no further improvements in haemodynamic status can be achieved with fluid therapy, inotropes or vasopressors should be employed. Vasopressors increase cardiac afterload, and therefore can decrease cardiac output. For this reason, unless cardiac output can be measured and demonstrated to be increased, it is safest to start with inotropes. Current evidence and experience suggests that dobutamine is the inotrope of choice in the horse. If the animal remains hypotensive, vasopressors should be employed.

Response to therapy should always be measured, and no single haemodynamic parameter should be viewed in isolation. Decreased urine output or increased blood lactate concentrations in response to changes in treatment should trigger an urgent review of the therapy.

References

1. Spurlock SL, Furr M: Fluid therapy, in Koterba AM, Drummond WH, Kosch PC (eds): Equine clinical neonatology). Philadelphia, Lea and Febiger, 1990, pp 671-700

2. Waterman A: A review of the diagnosis and treatment of fluid and electrolyte disorders in the horse. Equine Vet J 9:43-48, 1977
3. Seahorn TL, Cornick-Seahorn J: Fluid therapy. Vet Clin N Am: Equine Pract 10:517-525, 1994
4. Corley KTT: Monitoring and treating haemodynamic disturbances in critically ill neonatal foals. Part II – Assessment and treatment. Equine Vet Educ 14:328-336, 2002
5. Corley KT, Axon JE: Resuscitation and emergency management for neonatal foals. Vet Clin North Am Equine Pract 21:431-455, 2005
6. Palmer JE: Fluid therapy in the neonate: not your mother's fluid space. Vet Clin North Am Equine Pract 20:63-75, 2004
7. Corley KTT: Fluid therapy, in Bertone JJ, Horspool LL (eds): Equine Clinical Pharmacology. London, WB Saunders, 2004, pp 327-364
8. Carcillo JA, Davis AL, Zaritsky A: Role of early fluid resuscitation in pediatric septic shock. J Am Med Assoc 266:1242-1245, 1991
9. Rivers E, Nguyen B, Havstad S, et al.: Early goal-directed therapy in the treatment of severe sepsis and septic shock. N Engl J Med 345:1368-1377, 2001
10. Burris D, Rhee P, Kaufmann C, et al.: Controlled resuscitation for uncontrolled hemorrhagic shock. J Trauma 46:216-223, 1999
11. Soucy DM, Rudé M, Hsia WC, et al.: The effects of varying fluid volume and rate of resuscitation during uncontrolled hemorrhage. J Trauma 46:209-215, 1999
12. Webb AR: Fluid management in intensive care—avoiding hypovolaemia. Br J Intensive Care 7:59-64, 1997
13. Hollenberg SM, Ahrens TS, Astiz ME, et al.: Practice parameters for hemodynamic support of sepsis in adult patients in sepsis. Crit Care Med 27:639-660, 1999
14. Shoemaker WC: Diagnosis and treatment of shock and circulatory dysfunction, in Grenvik A, Ayres SM, Holbrook PR, et al. (eds): Textbook of Critical Care, ed 4. Philadelphia, WB Saunders, 2000, pp 92-114
15. Corley KTT, McKenzie HC, Amoroso LM, et al.: Initial experience with norepinephrine infusion in hypotensive critically ill foals. J Vet Emerg Crit Care 10:267-276, 2000
16. Fruhwald S, Scheidl S, Toller W, et al.: Low potential of dobutamine and dopexamine to block intestinal peristalsis as compared with other catecholamines. Crit Care Med 28:2893-2897, 2000
17. King JN, Gerring EL: Biphasic disruption of fasting equine gut motility by dopamine—a preliminary study. J Vet Pharmacol Ther 11:354-361, 1988
18. De Backer D, Zhang H, Manikis P, et al.: Regional effects of dobutamine in endotoxic shock. J Surg Res 65:93-100, 1996
19. Secchi A, Wellmann R, Martin E, et al.: Dobutamine maintains intestinal villus blood flow during normotensive endotoxemia: an intravital microscopic study in the rat. J Crit Care 12:137-141, 1997
20. Nevière R, Mathieu D, Chagnon JL, et al.: The contrasting effects of dobutamine and dopamine on gastric mucosal perfusion in septic patients. Am J Respir Crit Care Med 154:1684-1688, 1996
21. Fink MP, Kaups KL, Wang HL, et al.: Maintenance of superior mesenteric arterial perfusion prevents increased intestinal mucosal permeability in endotoxic pigs. Surgery 110:154-160, 1991
22. Duranteau J, Sitbon P, Teboul JL, et al.: Effects of epinephrine, norepinephrine, or the combination of norepinephrine and dobutamine on gastric mucosa in septic shock. Crit Care Med 27:893-900, 1999
23. Levy B, Bollaert PE, Lucchelli JP, et al.: Dobutamine improves the adequacy of gastric mucosal perfusion in epinephrine-treated septic shock. Crit Care Med 25:1649-1654, 1997
24. Sun Q, Tu Z, Lobo S, et al.: Optimal adrenergic support in septic shock due to peritonitis. Anesthesiology 98:888-896, 2003
25. Shoemaker WC, Appel PL, Kram HB: Hemodynamic and oxygen transport effects of dobutamine in critically ill general surgical patients. Crit Care Med 14:1032-1037, 1986
26. Leone M, Boyadjiev I, Boulos E, et al.: A reappraisal of isoproterenol in goal-directed therapy of septic shock. Shock 26:353-357, 2006
27. Vischer CM, Foreman JH, Constable PD, et al.: Hemodynamic effects of thyroidectomy in sedentary horses. Am J Vet Res 60:14-21, 1999
28. Martin C, Perrin G, Saux P, et al.: Effects of norepinephrine on right ventricular function in septic shock patients. Intensive Care Med 20:444-447, 1994
29. Valverde A, Giguère S, Sanchez LC, et al.: Effects of dobutamine, norepinephrine, and vasopressin on cardiovascular function in anesthetized neonatal foals with induced hypotension. Am J Vet Res 67:1730-1737, 2006
30. Hollis AR, Ousey JC, Palmer L, et al.: Effects of norepinephrine and a combined norepinephrine and dobutamine infusion on systemic hemodynamics and indices of renal function in normotensive neonatal thoroughbred foals. J Vet Intern Med 20:1437-1442, 2006
31. Martin C, Papazian L, Perrin G, et al.: Norepinephrine or dopamine for the treatment of hyperdynamic septic shock? Chest 103:1826-1831, 1993
32. Martin C, Viviand X, Leone M, et al.: Effect of norepinephrine on the outcome of septic shock. Crit Care Med 28:2758-2765, 2000
33. Bellomo R, Kellum JA, Wisniewski SR, et al.: Effects of norepinephrine on the renal vasculature in normal and endotoxemic dogs. Am J Respir Crit Care Med 159:1186-1192, 1999
34. Di Giantomasso D, May CN, Bellomo R: Norepinephrine and vital organ blood flow during experimental hyperdynamic sepsis. Intensive Care Med 29:1774-1781, 2003
35. Sennoun N, Montemont C, Gibot S, et al.: Comparative effects of early versus delayed use of norepinephrine in resuscitated endotoxic shock. Crit Care Med 35:1736-1740, 2007
36. Baker CH, Sutton ET, Zhou Z, et al.: Microvascular vasopressin effects during endotoxin shock in the rat. Circ Shock 30:81-95, 1990
37. Landry DW, Levin HR, Gallant EM, et al.: Vasopressin pressor hypersensitivity in vasodilatory septic shock. Crit Care Med 25:1279-1282, 1997
38. Bartelstone HJ, Nasmyth PA: Vasopressin potentiation of catecholamine actions in dog, rat, cat, and rat aortic strip. Am J Physiol 208, 1965
39. Tsuneyoshi I, Kanmura Y, Yoshimura N: Nitric oxide as a mediator of reduced arterial responsiveness in septic patients. Crit Care Med 24:1083-1086, 1996

40. Chernow B, Roth BL: Pharmacologic manipulation of the peripheral vasculature in shock: clinical and experimental approaches. Circ Shock 18:141-155, 1986
41. Ertmer C, Morelli A, Bone HG, et al.: Dobutamine reverses the vasopressin-associated impairment in cardiac index and systemic oxygen supply in ovine endotoxemia. Crit Care 10: R144, 2006
42. Westphal M, Stubbe H, Sielenkamper AW, et al.: Effects of arginine vasopressin on hemodynamic variables and oxygen transport in healthy and endotoxemic sheep. Crit Care Med 31:1502-1508, 2003
43. Albanese J, Leone M, Delmas A, et al.: Terlipressin or norepinephrine in hyperdynamic septic shock: a prospective, randomized study. Crit Care Med 33:1897-1902, 2005
44. Hiltebrand LB, Krejci V, Jakob SM, et al.: Effects of vasopressin on microcirculatory blood flow in the gastrointestinal tract in anesthetized pigs in septic shock. Anesthesiology 106:1156-1167, 2007
45. Di Giantomasso D, Morimatsu H, Bellomo R, et al.: Effect of low-dose vasopressin infusion on vital organ blood flow in the conscious normal and septic sheep. Anaesth Intensive Care 34:427-433, 2006
46. Westphal M, Bone H-G, Van Aken H, et al.: Terlipressin for haemodynamic support in septic patients: a double-edged sword? Lancet 360:1250-1251, 2002
47. Asfar P, Pierrot M, Veal N, et al.: Low-dose terlipressin improves systemic and splanchnic hemodynamics in fluid-challenged endotoxic rats. Crit Care Med 31:215-220, 2003
48. Kim EH, Lee SH, Byun SW, et al.: Skin necrosis after a low-dose vasopressin infusion through a central venous catheter for treating septic shock. Korean J Intern Med 21:287-290, 2006
49. Angstwurm M: Vasopressin: A tool as rescue therapy? Take care of dosages and adverse effects! Crit Care Med 33:2713-2714, 2005
50. Palmer JE: Foal Cardiopulmonary Resuscitation, in Orsini JA, Divers TJ (eds): Manual of Equine Emergencies, ed 2. Philadelphia, Saunders, 2003, pp 581-614
51. O'Brien A, Clapp L, Singer M: Terlipressin for norepinephrine-resistant septic shock. Lancet 359:1209-1210, 2002
52. Lange M, Morelli A, Ertmer C, et al.: Continuous versus bolus infusion of terlipressin in ovine endotoxemia. Shock, 2007
53. De Backer D, Creteur J, Silva E, et al.: Effects of dopamine, norepinephrine, and epinephrine on the splanchnic circulation in septic shock: Which is best? Crit Care Med 31:1659-1667, 2003
54. Levy B, Mansart A, Bollaert PE, et al.: Effects of epinephrine and norepinephrine on hemodynamics, oxidative metabolism and organ energetics in endotoxemic rats. Intensive Care Med 29:292-300, 2003
55. Levy B: Epinephrine in septic shock: Dr. Jekyll or Mr. Hyde? Crit Care Med 31:1866-1867, 2003
56. Takakura K, Taniguchi T, Muramatsu I, et al.: Modification of alpha1-adrenoceptors by peroxynitrite as a possible mechanism of systemic hypotension in sepsis. Crit Care Med 30:894-899, 2002
57. Zingarelli B, Day BJ, Crapo JD, et al.: The potential role of peroxynitrite in the vascular contractile and cellular energetic failure in endotoxic shock. Br J Pharmacol 120:259-267, 1997
58. Meier-Hellmann A, Sakka SG, Reinhart K: Catecholamines and splanchnic perfusion. Schweiz Med Wochenschr 130:1942-1947, 2000
59. Segal JM, Phang PT, Walley KR: Low-dose dopamine hastens onset of gut ischemia in a porcine model of hemorrhagic shock. J Appl Physiol 73:1159-1164, 1992
60. MacGregor DA, Smith TE, Prielipp RC, et al.: Pharmacokinetics of dopamine in healthy male subjects. Anesthesiology 92:338-346, 2000
61. Van den Berghe G, de Zegher F: Anterior pituitary function during critical illness and dopamine treatment. Crit Care Med 24:1580-1590, 1996
62. van de Borne P, Oren R, Somers VK: Dopamine depresses minute ventilation in patients with heart failure. Circulation 98:126-131, 1998
63. Trim CM, Moore JN, Clark ES: Renal effects of dopamine infusion in conscious horses. Equine Vet J Suppl. 7:124-128, 1989
64. Denton MD, Chertow GM, Brady HR: "Renal-dose" dopamine for the treatment of acute renal failure: scientific rationale, experimental studies and clinical trials. Kidney Int 50:4-14, 1996
65. Australian and New Zealand Intensive Care Society Clinical Trials Group: Low-dose dopamine in patients with early renal dysfunction: a placebo-controlled randomised trial. Lancet 356:2139-2143, 2000
66. Kellum JA, Decker JM: Use of dopamine in acute renal failure: a meta-analysis. Crit Care Med 29:1526-1531, 2001
67. Annane D, Vignon P, Renault A, et al.: Norepinephrine plus dobutamine versus epinephrine alone for management of septic shock: a randomised trial. Lancet 370:676-684, 2007
68. Lauzier F, Levy B, Lamarre P, et al.: Vasopressin or norepinephrine in early hyperdynamic septic shock: a randomized clinical trial. Intensive Care Med 32:1782-1789, 2006
69. Russell JA: Hemodynamic support of sepsis. Vasopressin versus norepinephrine for septic shock, presented at the Society of Critical Care Medicine 36th Critical Care Congress, Orlando, FL, February 17-21, 2007
70. Annane D, Sebille V, Charpentier C, et al.: Effect of treatment with low doses of hydrocortisone and fludrocortisone on mortality in patients with septic shock. JAMA 288:862-871, 2002
71. Annane D, Bellissant E, Sebille V, et al.: Impaired pressor sensitivity to noradrenaline in septic shock patients with and without impaired adrenal function reserve. Br J Clin Pharmacol 46:589-597, 1998
72. Briegel J, Forst H, Haller M, et al.: Stress doses of hydrocortisone reverse hyperdynamic septic shock: a prospective, randomized, double-blind, single-center study. Crit Care Med 27:723-732, 1999
73. Ertmer C, Bone HG, Morelli A, et al.: Methylprednisolone reverses vasopressin hyporesponsiveness in ovine endotoxemia. Shock 27:281-288, 2007
74. Hart KA, Ferguson DC, Heusner GL, et al.: Synthetic adrenocorticotropic hormone stimulation tests in healthy neonatal foals. J Vet Intern Med 21:314-321, 2007
75. Gold JR, Divers TJ, Barton MH, et al.: Plasma adrenocorticotropin, cortisol, and adrenocorticotropin/cortisol ratios in septic and normal-term foals. J Vet Intern Med 21:791-796, 2007

76. Keh D, Boehnke T, Weber Cartens S, et al.: Immunologic and hemodynamic effects of "low-dose" hydrocortisone in septic shock: a double-blind, randomized, placebo-controlled, crossover study. Am J Respir Crit Care Med 167:512-520, 2003
77. Day TK: Current development and use of hemoglobin-based oxygen-carrying (HBOC) solutions. J Vet Emerg Crit Care 13:77-93, 2003
78. Belgrave RL, Hines MT, Keegan RD, et al.: Effects of a polymerized ultrapurified bovine hemoglobin blood substitute administered to ponies with normovolemic anemia. J Vet Int Med 16:396-403, 2002
79. Maxson AD, Giger U, Sweeney CR, et al.: Use of a bovine hemoglobin preparation in the treatment of cyclic ovarian hemorrhage in a minature horse. J Am Vet Med Assoc 203:1308-1311, 1993
80. Migita R, Gonzales A, Gonzales ML, et al.: Blood volume and cardiac index in rats after exchange transfusion with hemoglobin-based oxygen carriers. J Appl Physiol 82:1995-2002, 1997
81. Martin W, Villani GM, Jothianandan D, et al.: Selective blockade of endothelium-dependent and glyceryl trinitrate-induced relaxation by hemoglobin and by methylene blue in the rabbit aorta. J Pharmacol Exp Ther 232:708-716, 1985
82. Gulati A, Sharma AC, Singh G: Role of endothelin in the cardiovascular effects of diaspirin crosslinked and stroma reduced hemoglobin. Crit Care Med 24:137-147, 1996
83. Gulati A, Sen AP, Sharma AC, et al.: Role of ET and NO in resuscitative effect of diaspirin cross-linked hemoglobin after hemorrhage in rat. Am J Physiol 273:H827-836, 1997
84. Parry BW, Anderson GA, Gay CC: Prognosis in equine colic: a comparative study of variables used to assess individual cases. Equine Vet J 15:211-215, 1983
85. Parry BW, Anderson GA, Gay CC: Prognosis in equine colic: a study of individual variables used in case assessment. Equine Vet J 15:337-344, 1983
86. Corley KTT: Monitoring and treating haemodynamic disturbances in critically ill neonatal foals. Part I: haemodynamic monitoring. Equine Vet Educ 14:270-279, 2002
87. Grover R, Lopez A, Lorente J, et al.: Multi-center, randomized, placebo-controlled, double blind study of the nitric oxide synthase inhibitor 546C88: effect on survival in patients with septic shock. Crit Care Med 27:33A, 1999
88. LeDoux D, Astiz ME, Carpati CM, et al.: Effects of perfusion pressure on tissue perfusion in septic shock. Crit Care Med 28:2729-2732, 2000
89. Vander AJ: Renal blood flow and glomerular filtration, in Vander AJ (ed): Renal Physiology, ed 5. New York, McGraw Hill, 1995, pp 24-50

10

Monitoring and treating the respiratory system

Harold C. McKenzie III

10.1 Monitoring the respiratory system
10.2 Management of horses with respiratory disorders

10.1 Monitoring the respiratory system

Patients at risk of developing respiratory disorders during hospitalisation

There are a number of groups of equine patients at risk of developing respiratory disease while hospitalised. Fundamentally, this susceptibly results from impairment or overwhelming of the normal defence mechanisms protecting the lower respiratory tract. These normal defence mechanisms consist of the barrier represented by the upper respiratory tract, which physically limits access of infectious organisms to the lower respiratory tract, and the innate and specific immune responses that eliminate or inactivate infectious organisms that reach the lower respiratory tract. Transport represents a well described risk factor for lower respiratory infections, due to the combined effects of prolonged periods of head elevation, impairing clearance, with the immunosuppressive effects of physiological stress.[1] Individuals undergoing anaesthesia are at risk of lower respiratory infections, due to the temporary loss of the filtering function of the upper respiratory tract and the immunosuppressive effects of general anaesthesia.[2] Another group of susceptible individuals are hospitalised neonatal foals, as they are often immunocompromised and systemically ill. In addition, clinically ill neonates are frequently recumbent, resulting in impaired clearance of respiratory secretions and pulmonary atelectasis. Adult horses suffering from dysphagia or immune compromise are also susceptible to lower respiratory tract infections. Animals suffering from pulmonary hypersensitivities, such as recurrent airway obstruction (RAO), are also at risk of clinical exacerbation due to exposure to noxious or immunogenic stimuli in the hospital environment.

Auscultation and rebreathing examination

Respiratory rate should be monitored by observation, rather than auscultation, to minimise the effect of patient nervousness on rate. A normal respiratory rate in an adult horse is 8 to 16 breaths per minute, while the respiratory rate in foals is higher and more variable (20–40 breaths per minute), with both patient excitement and age. Attention should be paid to the respiratory pattern and the degree of respiratory effort, with increased effort indicative of upper respiratory obstruction or pulmonary dysfunction.

Bronchovesicular sounds are the normal soft, rustling sounds heard over the lung fields in foals and thin horses, or over the central lung field in most horses. Adventitious sounds are the abnormal respiratory sounds. These include crackles, which are primarily inspiratory and are associated with the separation of fluid/air interfaces. Wheezes are primarily expiratory, arising from intrathoracic airways in association with airway narrowing. Airway narrowing is caused by bronchial constriction, oedema of the airway wall and/or intraluminal fluid (mucus, inflammatory exudate). Rattles occur as air vibrates over the surface of fluid exudate adhered to the airway lining and are associated with large airways (trachea, large bronchi). Pleural friction rubs are produced when normal lubrication of pleural surfaces is lost and usually occur in coordination with respirations, while pericardial friction rubs are associated with cardiac contraction/relaxation. These sounds are lost when fluid accumulates within the pleural space or adhesions form between pleural surfaces.

The rebreathing examination facilitates a thorough examination of the equine respiratory tract by allowing for the rebreathing of carbon dioxide (CO_2) leading to increased respiratory depth and rate. To perform this examination a large, stiff plastic bag should be placed over the horse's muzzle and maintained in place for 1 to 3 minutes or until the patient becomes intolerant of rebreathing. Ensure that horse's nostrils are not occluded and that bag is well sealed around the muzzle. In a horse with normal lungs, placement of the rebreathing bag will result in no appreciable increase in respiratory effort for the first 60 to 90 seconds. The duration of rebreathing should be adequate to achieve prolonged deep respirations but should cease immediately if the horse becomes distressed. In a horse with lower airway inflammation, there may be increased respiratory effort and/or coughing. While abnormal lung sounds are often detected, their absence does not eliminate the possibility of lower respiratory disease. Findings of auscultation with rebreathing include: normal vesicular sounds, adventitious sounds and areas of increased or decreased intensity of respiratory sounds. Increased intensity of airway sounds may be associated with atelectasis, while decreased intensity may be associated with pulmonary consolidation or fluid, air or a space-occupying lesion within the pleural cavity. Attention should be paid to the horse's ability to tolerate the rebreathing bag and to recover once the bag has been removed, as poor tolerance and/or prolonged recovery is often indicative of impaired pulmonary function. Horses with pleuropneumonia will often resist rebreathing, and will only take rapid, shallow breaths, likely due to the presence of thoracic pain (pleurodynia).

Collection of samples from the respiratory tree

Tracheal aspirate

The transtracheal aspirate is a useful diagnostic procedure that is relatively easy to perform. It provides a sample of fluid collected under sterile conditions from the lower airways that is suitable for culture, unlike aspirates collected by bronchoalveolar lavage (BAL). Useful cytological assessments can be made regarding lower airway inflammation, but one cannot differentiate large airway inflammation from small airway inflammation using this method alone. The technique for transtracheal aspiration is described in Chapter 1.33.

Clinically significant complications associated with transtracheal aspiration are rare, but subcutaneous emphysema may occur, and mild mediastinal emphysema is not uncommonly noted on thoracic radiography following this procedure. Subcutaneous emphysema should be addressed by placing a bandage over the aspiration site, such that firm pressure is maintained, in order to minimise the escape of further air into the subcutaneous region. The emphysema will gradually resolve spontaneously, and this process typically occurs within 3 to 7 days. Subcutaneous infection may also occur, possibly due to leakage of respiratory tract exudate through the insertion site in the tracheal wall or as a result of external contamination.[3] On occasion the catheter may be inadvertently cut by the insertion needle during the procedure or when the catheter is being withdrawn, but the catheter fragment within the trachea is rapidly expelled by coughing.[4]

An alternative procedure for collection of a tracheal aspirate involves the use of a guarded sampling catheter via a fiberoptic endoscope,[5] also described in Chapter 1.33. This technique is much less invasive than the percutaneous technique, but may not provide an ideal sample for bacterial culture and sensitivity testing. This is due to the fact that the endoscope is introduced via the upper respiratory tract and is therefore susceptible to contamination by resident bacteria comprising the normal flora in that region. The use of a double- or triple-lumen guarded catheter* reduces the risk of contamination and has been shown to provide equivalent microbiological results to those obtained following transtracheal aspiration.[5,6] The diagnostic yield is improved by performing the procedure expediently, using a relatively small volume of infusate (10–15 ml) and by ensuring that only the inner catheter is introduced into the fluid puddle within the trachea.[7]

Sample processing is as crucial as collection of the sample. Samples should be collected for cytology in an EDTA tube and for culture in a sterile plain tube. Samples that cannot be processed rapidly following collection (30–60 minutes), or that have a low cellularity, should be preserved using an equal volume of sample and 50% ethanol in a plain sterile tube, thereby preventing lysis of the cells.[8] Alternatively, air-dried slides can be prepared by either the direct smear or cytocentrifugation techniques. These slides are then stable and can be stained at a later time for cytological examination. Cytocentrifugation is very useful in processing samples of low cellularity, as it concentrates the cellular material and provides a much higher yield of cells for cytological interpretation. Cytology slides are typically stained using Giemsa techniques, such as the Diff-Quik† stain.[9] Examination for bacteria is facilitated by preparing an additional slide using the Gram stain technique. Samples for microbial culture should be processed immediately, or held under refrigeration until processed, to limit the possibility of secondary bacterial overgrowth.

Interpretation of tracheal aspirate cytology

The cellular population is normally mononuclear, consisting primarily of macrophages and lymphocytes, with a moderate number of neutrophils[3,10] (Figure 10.1 and Appendix, Table 19.12). The presence of more than 20% to 40% neutrophils indicates active inflammation, either non-septic (Figure 10.2) or septic (Figure 10.3). Infection can be presumed if there are increased numbers of degenerate neutrophils and intracellular bacteria. The presence of eosinophils also indicates active inflammation but is not specific for allergic inflammation, as these cells can be present with chronic inflammation in the horse, as well as with parasitic inflammation (*Dictyocaulus arnfieldi*). The presence of large numbers of bacteria characterises septic samples but does not differentiate acute infection from secondary bacterial growth associated with chronic inflammation. The presence of small numbers of bacteria is not considered abnormal in tracheal aspirate samples, especially if squamous epithelial cells are present. Identification

* Double-lumen (EMAC700) or triple-lumen (EMAC800) guarded endoscopic sample collection catheters; MILA International, Inc., Florence, KY, USA.

† Diff-Quik; Baxter, Deerfield, IL, USA.

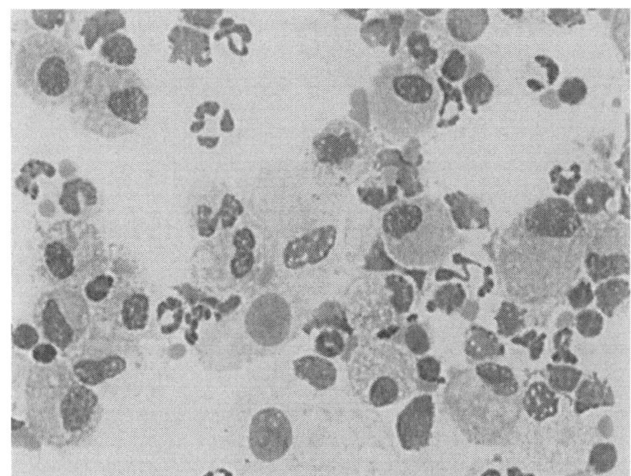

Figure 10.1 Normal tracheal aspirate cytology. ©Harold C. McKenzie III 2006.

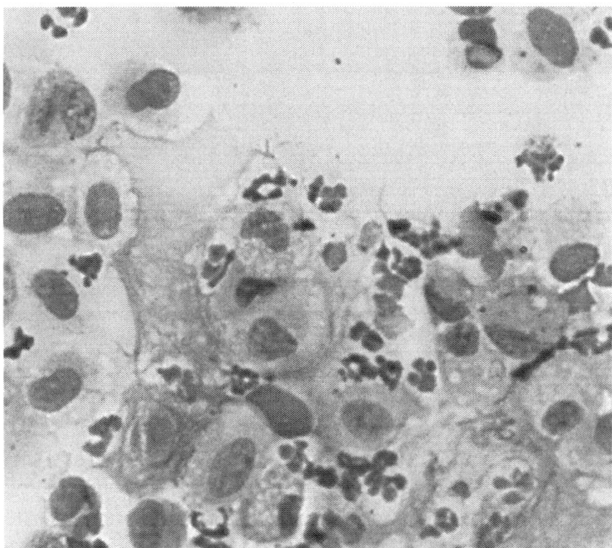

Figure 10.2 Nonseptic inflammatory tracheal aspirate cytology with increased mucus and increased numbers of neutrophils. ©Harold C. McKenzie III 2006.

of phagocytosed bacteria within the inflammatory cells (neutrophils, macrophages) is supportive of the presence of infection, rather than sample contamination. The presence of moderate numbers of ciliated respiratory epithelial cells is normal. Large numbers of degenerative neutrophils also indicate active inflammation and are usually associated with infection, while nondegenerate neutrophils are typically associated with chronic inflammation such as RAO. Mucus is always present, although it is normally found in small amounts, and appears as an amorphous stranded material. Increased amounts of mucus are suggestive of lower respiratory inflammation, and spirals of inspissated mucus (Curschmann's spirals) are often seen in horses with longstanding small airway inflammation, such as RAO (Figure 10.4). The presence of plant material (pollen) or crystalline material is usually the result of contamination.

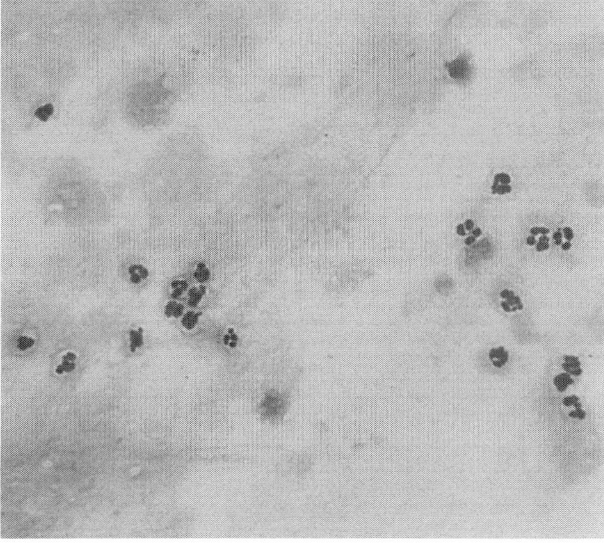

Figure 10.3 Septic tracheal aspirate cytology consisting entirely of degenerate neutrophils and mucus. ©Harold C. McKenzie III 2006.

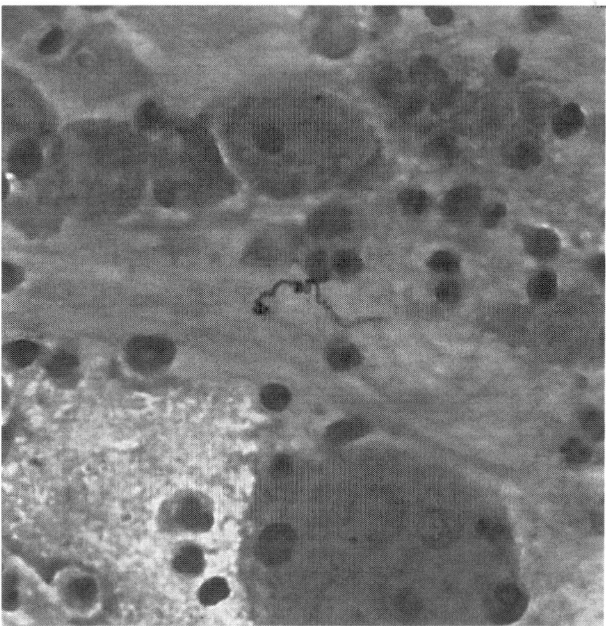

Figure 10.4 Curschmann's spiral. ©Harold C. McKenzie III 2006.

The presence of fungal elements is rarely indicative of fungal pneumonia, as this is a rare condition typically occurring secondary to immunosuppression. The results of microbial culture should always be interpreted in light of the cytology findings. Positive culture results may occur secondary to sample contamination during or after collection or as a result of tracheal contamination due to coughing during the procedure. The presence of a neutrophilic exudate, often with degenerate neutrophils present, along with increased amounts of mucus and intracellular bacteria is supportive of a diagnosis of bacterial lower respiratory disease.

Bronchoalveolar lavage

BAL is a very useful diagnostic technique that provides excellent recovery of small airway and alveolar cells for cytological examination.[11] BAL cytology provides insight into the character and extent of small airway and alveolar inflammation and/or infection. The information obtained from BAL cytology is different from that obtained from tracheal aspirate cytology, and the results of the two techniques are often complementary.[12] Comparing the findings of these two techniques may allow for differentiation between large airway and small airway inflammation or infection. BAL is typically not useful for the purposes of bacterial culture, due to the potential for upper respiratory tract contamination as the tube or endoscope is passed through the nares and pharynx. In some cases it may be useful to obtain culture samples from focal areas of drainage within the bronchial tree using endoscopically guided BAL; however, the results must be interpreted in light of the possibility of contamination.[13,14]

Procedure

BAL should always be performed following completion of the transtracheal aspirate (if one is to be performed), as the BAL procedure will result in contamination of the trachea with cellular debris and bacteria from the upper respiratory tract. The technique for BAL is given in Chapter 1.34. The endoscopically guided technique has the advantage that if an area of focal drainage (Figure 10.5) is identified, the endoscope may be directed to that area and a lavage sample obtained. This procedure may be of therapeutic benefit as well, in that it allows for removal for inflammatory debris and reduces the bacterial load.[13–15]

Sample processing for cytological examination is the same as that described for tracheal aspirate samples. Cytocentrifugation is commonly used due to the low cellularity of BAL fluid samples.

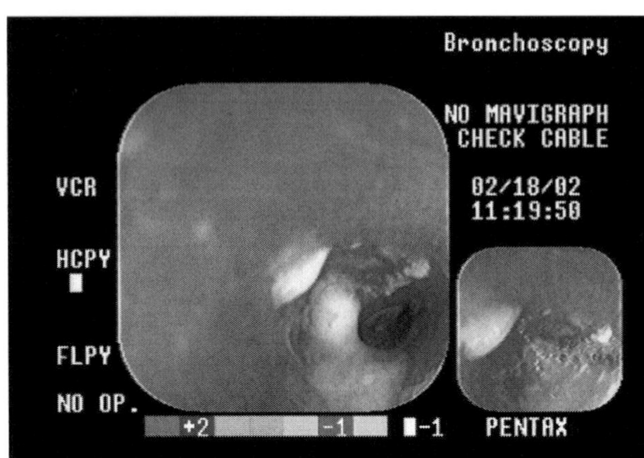

Figure 10.5 Focal purulent drainage identified on bronchoscopic examination. ©Harold C. McKenzie III 2006.

Interpretation of bronchoalveolar lavage cytology

The cellular population is normally mononuclear, consisting of alveolar macrophages (65%) and lymphocytes (30%)[15] (Figure 10.6 and Appendix, Table 19.12). The presence of more than 3% neutrophils indicates active inflammation, either septic (degenerate) or nonseptic (nondegenerate) (Figure 10.7). Higher percentages of neutrophils (up to 15%) are reported to be within normal limits for mature horses over 6 years of age.[15] The presence of eosinophils indicates active inflammation, but is not specific for allergic inflammation, as parasitic pneumonia and idiopathic pulmonary eosinophilia may occur. The presence of even small numbers of bacteria is abnormal in BAL samples, therefore their presence characterises septic samples. The presence of ciliated respiratory epithelial cells is considered normal, as they are typically dislodged due to the disturbance of the respiratory mucosa as a result of the

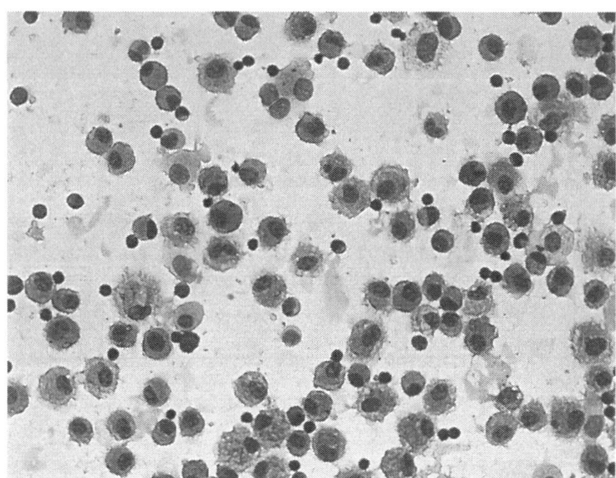

Figure 10.6 Normal bronchoalveolar lavage cytology consisting entirely of mononuclear cells (lymphocytes and macrophages) ©Harold C. McKenzie III 2006.

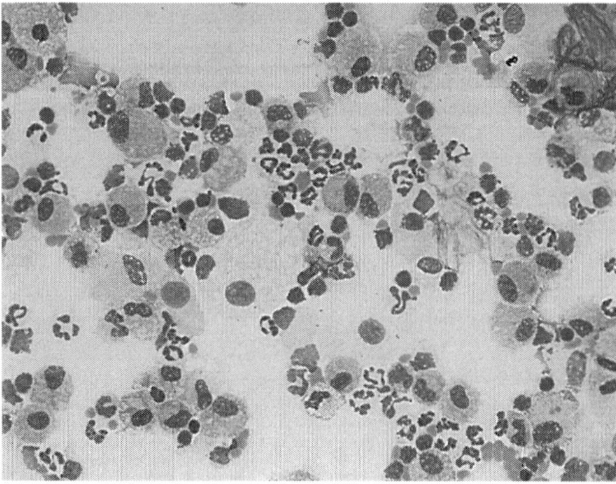

Figure 10.7 Inflammatory bronchoalveolar lavage cytology with increased numbers of neutrophils present. ©Harold C. McKenzie III 2006.

wedging of the BAL catheter. Large numbers of ciliated respiratory epithelial cells, especially if abnormal in appearance, may be consistent with viral respiratory infection. Ciliocytophthoria has been described in horses with suspected viral respiratory disease and is characterised by the presence of both spherical denuded respiratory epithelial cells and isolated ciliated tufts.[16] Horses that have suffered from exercise-induced pulmonary haemorrhage (EIPH) will have increased numbers of haemosiderophages seen on cytological examination of the BAL fluid, and this technique is reported to be more sensitive for identification of horses with EIPH than postexertional endoscopy.[17] Increased amounts of mucus are suggestive of small airway inflammation, and Curschmann's spirals are often seen in horses with chronic small airway inflammation. The presence of pharyngeal contamination is confirmed by the presence of squamous epithelial cells.

Collection of pleural fluid

When accumulation of pleural fluid is identified on thoracic radiographs or ultrasound a sample of this fluid should be collected for both cytological analysis and bacterial culture and sensitivity testing. The exception to this would be when only a very small amount of fluid is present. This procedure is performed on the standing animal on one or both sides of the thorax, as indicated by ultrasonographic examination. This technique allows for the sterile collection of pleural fluid for cytological examination and culture and for drainage of accumulated fluid and inflammatory material.[18,19]

Procedure

Selection of the site for pleurocentesis is ideally based upon ultrasonographic examination, as this allows for the confirmation of the presence of fluid within the pleural space, as well as the identification of structures to be avoided when performing the procedure. Generally, pleurocentesis is performed at the sixth to ninth intercostal space approximately 4 to 6 cm above the olecranon on the left side of the thorax, or at the sixth or seventh intercostal space up to 10 cm above the olecranon on the right side. The technique is described in Chapter 1.35. A sample of fluid should be aspirated in a sterile manner and aliquots submitted for cytological and microbiological analysis. Complications of pleurocentesis are not common but can include cellulitis at the insertion site, pneumothorax, haemothorax, cardiac dysrhythmias and laceration or puncture of the lung, heart, liver or bowel.[20] It is not uncommon for small amounts of air to enter the pleural cavity during placement of the cannula or catheter, and this is usually of no clinical significance and the air is rapidly absorbed by the body.[18]

Samples should be collected for cytology in an EDTA tube, as enough protein may be present for clotting to occur if an anticoagulant is not used. A sample for bacterial culture should be collected in a sterile plain tube. For samples that cannot be processed rapidly following collection (30–60 minutes), air-dried slides should be prepared by either the direct smear or cytocentrifugation technique. These slides are then stable and can be stained at a later time for cytological examination. Cytology slides are processed as described for transtracheal aspirate samples. Samples for aerobic and anaerobic culture should be processed immediately, or held under refrigeration until processed, to limit the possibility of secondary bacterial overgrowth.

Interpretation of cytology

Complete laboratory analysis should be performed on all pleural fluid samples, consisting of total nucleated cell count, total protein determination and cytological evaluation (see Appendix, Table 19.12). Substantial information may be gained, however, simply by visual assessment of the sample. Normal pleural fluid is clear to slightly hazy and straw yellow in colour. Turbidity may occur secondary to elevations in cell count or protein concentration. Discolouration of the fluid is typically due to increased numbers of red blood cells or inflammatory cells. Reddish discolouration may be due to blood contamination during sample collection or existing haemothorax. Orange discolouration is usually associated with inflammation of the pleura, and is likely due to the presence of haemoglobin in combination with inflammatory cells. Yellow discolouration is usually associated with purulent exudates.

The total nucleated cell count of pleural fluid is typically less than 8000 cells/μl, and the total protein concentration is normally less than 25 g/L (2.5 g/dl), with values above these ranges being consistent with inflammation.[21] The normal cytological appearance of pleural fluid consists predominantly of mononuclear cells (macrophages and mesothelial cells) with lower percentages of nondegenerate neutrophils present.[21] In the presence of inflammation the percentage of neutrophils will increase, while infection is often associated with the presence of degenerate neutrophils. Additional abnormalities may include the presence of neoplastic cells or bacteria.

Blood gas collection and analysis

Arterial blood gas collection

Arterial blood gas sampling is performed primarily for evaluation of pulmonary function, although insight into the patient's acid-base status is also obtained. Arterial blood gas sampling is most readily performed in the conscious adult horse using the transverse facial artery. Arterial samples may also be obtained from the facial, carotid or dorsal metatarsal arteries, but these sites are considerably more challenging to utilise in the conscious horse. The technique is described in Chapter 1.20. Collection of arterial blood samples in the foal is described in Chapter 2.8. Samples analysed for pH and $Paco_2$ determination are fairly stable and can be held at room temperature for up to 1 hour.[22] Arterial samples for determination of Pao_2 are less stable, and must be collected in glass syringes and stored on ice (for up to 2 hours) if not immediately processed.[22]

Venous blood gas collection

The most common sites for collection of venous blood gas samples are the jugular vein and cephalic vein. Samples should be collected into a heparinised syringe and one should not allow air to aspirate into the syringe following withdrawal from the skin. Eliminate any visible air bubbles and cap the needle using a rubber stopper, and if samples cannot be run immediately, place them on ice, as discussed for arterial blood gas samples.

Respiratory function testing

Blood gas analysis

Blood gas analysis is the most readily performed form of pulmonary function testing and can be extremely helpful in evaluating the severity of respiratory dysfunction and the response to therapy.[23] This technique provides information regarding the lung's ability to exchange oxygen (O_2) and carbon dioxide (CO_2) between the bloodstream and the atmosphere.

Arterial and venous partial pressures of oxygen and carbon dioxide

Normal Pao_2 values in the standing adult horse at rest are 85 to 105 mm Hg.[24] Slightly lower values may be observed in the recumbent foal, with the Pao_2 of foals in lateral recumbency increasing from 61 ± 2.7 mm Hg at 1 hour of age to 70 to 80 mm Hg at 24 hours of age.[24] When interpreting arterial hypoxaemia in the clinical patient, one must consider that there are four basic causes of arterial hypoxaemia (Box 10.1). Hypoventilation can be caused by decreased respiratory rate or decreased tidal volume (due to decreased respiratory effort or increase in effort required for respiration arising from intrapulmonary or extrapulmonary abnormalities). Ventilation-perfusion mismatching occurs secondary to disease that causes some regions of lung to receive increased or decreased ventilation and/or blood flow compared to the normal lung, where these are finely balanced. The most common cause of arterial hypoxaemia in horses is ventilation-perfusion mismatching.[25] Extrapulmonary right-to-left shunts occur with persistent foetal circulation or intracardiac abnormalities (ventricular septal defect, etc.), and a poor response to administration of O_2 supplementation is classically seen with extrapulmonary shunts. Diffusion impairment results from pulmonary oedema, which increases the distance between the alveolus and the alveolar capillary over which O_2 must diffuse.

Box 10.1. Underlying causes of hypoxaemia in horses

1. Hypoventilation
2. Ventilation-perfusion ($\dot{V}/\dot{Q}$) mismatching
3. Right-to-left shunt
4. Diffusion impairment

Normal resting $Paco_2$ values are 42 to 46 mm Hg in adult horses, and 45 to 50 mm Hg in neonatal foals in lateral recumbency.[24] When interpreting alterations of the $Paco_2$, one must keep in mind the fact that CO_2 is much more soluble than O_2 and more readily overcomes the diffusion barrier.[26] Hypoventilation (due to a decrease in tidal volume and/or respiratory rate) causes accumulation of CO_2 in the bloodstream. This results in an increase in hydrogen ion concentration, thereby lowering pH (respiratory acidosis). Hyperventilation has the opposite effect, resulting in increased pH (respiratory alkalosis). The high solubility of CO_2 and the shape of the oxyhaemoglobin dissociation curve are responsible for the initial appearance of hypoxia with impairment of pulmonary function, followed by hypercapnia. Often, animals with impaired pulmonary function will have relatively normal $Paco_2$ at rest but will have increased $Paco_2$ after exercise.

Blood gas indices

To obtain further insight into pulmonary function, one can determine the blood gas indices of physiological shunt fraction and deadspace ventilation.[27] This requires that one obtain both arterial and venous blood gas samples and also determine peak end-tidal CO_2, by facemask or intratracheal needle collection of expired gases and CO_2 measurement by infrared capnography. These blood gas indices give additional insight into the degree of ventilation–perfusion mismatching. The effect of ventilation–perfusion mismatching is the result of two fundamental processes. Firstly, if poorly ventilated alveoli are perfused, the net effect is an intrapulmonary right-to-left shunt, as the blood is exposed to air with a low O_2 tension and a high CO_2 tension. This blood does not participate in gas exchange, leading to decreased arterial O_2 and increased arterial CO_2. The extent of this effect is assessed by determining the shunt fraction ($\dot{Q}t$ [cardiac output; L/min]/$\dot{Q}s$ [shunt flow; L/min]) (Box 10.2), with normal values in adult horses reported as 0.37% ± 0.98%.[27] Secondly, if poorly perfused alveoli are well ventilated, then this results in relative overventilation of these alveoli. The alveolar gas does not participate in gas exchange with the bloodstream, thereby resulting in accumulation of CO_2 leading to hypercapnia and decreased O_2 uptake leading to hypoxia. The extent of this effect is assessed by determining the deadspace ventilation (Vd/Vt) (Box 10.2). Normal values for deadspace ventilation in adult horses are reported as −18.2% ± 3.1%.[27]

Pulmonary mechanics

The most clinically useful assessment of pulmonary mechanics is the change in transpleural pressure (ΔPpl).[23] This is assessed by placing an esophageal balloon catheter into the thoracic portion of the esophagus and connecting the output to a physiological recorder.[23] Increases in ΔPpl

Box 10.2. Deadspace ventilation and physiological shunt fraction equations[27]

Deadspace ventilation equation:

$$\frac{Vd}{Vt} = \frac{Paco_2 - ETCO_2}{Paco_2}$$

Vd = deadspace volume (ml)
Vt = tidal volume (ml)
$Paco_2$ = arterial partial pressure of carbon dioxide
$ETCO_2$ = end-tidal CO_2
Physiological shunt fraction equation:

$$\frac{\dot{Q}s}{\dot{Q}t} = \frac{Cco_2 - Cao_2}{Cco_2 - Cvo_2}$$

$\dot{Q}t$ = cardiac output (L/min)
$\dot{Q}s$ = shunt flow (L/min)
Cco_2 = end capillary oxygen content (theoretical ideal)
Cao_2 = arterial oxygen content
Cvo_2 = (mixed) venous oxygen content

are associated with increasing small airway narrowing resulting in increased pulmonary resistance (RL) and with chronic inflammation-associated decreases in pulmonary dynamic compliance (Cdyn).[25] Forced oscillometry has been investigated as a noninvasive alternative to more traditional techniques of pulmonary function testing.[28,29] This is a technique that utilises forced oscillation to measure respiratory resistance (Rrs) and reactance (Xrs) during spontaneous breathing in horses and is effective in identifying horses with RAO. The forced oscillation technique is specialised, however, and is only available in a few referral centres.

Ultrasonography of the lungs

The indications for thoracic ultrasonography include abnormalities on auscultation, percussion or radiographs that are suggestive of pleural irregularities, pleural fluid accumulation, pulmonary consolidation and intrathoracic abscesses or masses.[30] The primary limitation of pulmonary ultrasonography results from the inability of the ultrasound waves to penetrate aerated lung, but this technique is often able to provide information not obtainable with other diagnostic modalities, and is particularly useful for localisation of fluid and/or masses for the purpose of thoracocentesis or biopsy. Thoracic ultrasonography in combination with thoracic radiography provides a thorough assessment of the aerated and nonaerated lung tissues as well as the pleural space.[31]

Procedure

An ultrasound machine with a 3- to 7.5-MHz probe is required, with a 5-MHz probe being most commonly used, along with clippers, ultrasound coupling gel and/or isopropyl alcohol. In thin-coated animals, the application of alcohol is often sufficient for ultrasound transmission and can provide diagnostic quality images, with the benefit of not requiring clipping (often appreciated by owners/trainers). In heavier-coated animals, the area of interest should be clipped and cleaned with alcohol, then thoroughly covered with coupling gel. The ultrasound probe is placed in the intercostal space, with the index marker positioned dorsally. Both hemithoraces should be fully examined, with each intercostal space being interrogated, proceeding from the cranial thorax caudally, and examining each space dorsally to ventrally. Rotation of the scan head 90° can provide additional information regarding the three-dimensional structure of the area of interest. The cranial thoracic region is best visualised from the right side, with the right forelimb well advanced. Particular attention should be paid to the ventral most portions of the lung caudal to the heart, as this area is commonly involved with inflammatory and infectious disorders, due to the effects of gravity on pulmonary drainage.

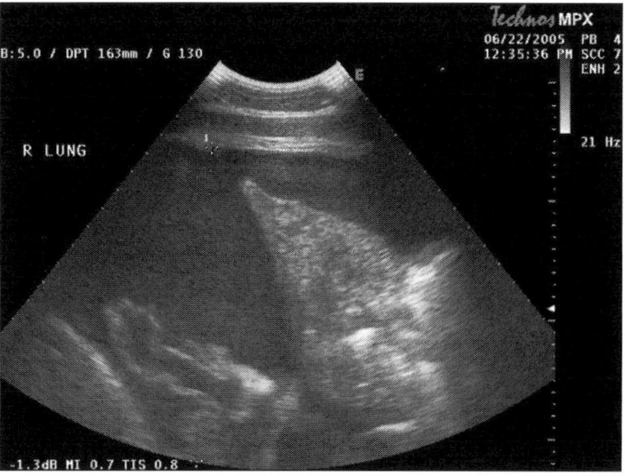

Figure 10.8 Pleural effusion in right ventral thorax, with consolidation of the tip of the lung. ©Harold C. McKenzie III 2006.

Interpretation

The normal thorax will contain minimal free fluid, which is most commonly imaged in the ventral region, with the remainder of the thorax demonstrating only a normal pleural reflection, which appears as a bright white line just deep to the intercostal muscles and the parietal pleura with parallel reverberation artifacts deep to the pleural surface.[31] A few pleural irregularities or "comet tails" are commonly seen even in normal horses, but their number is typically increased in horses with lower respiratory inflammation, and the frequency and severity of this change are fairly well correlated with the degree of inflammation present.[32] Increased amounts of pleural fluid are commonly seen in association with pleuropneumonia (Figure 10.8). Normal pleural fluid is anechoic, but it is not uncommon to see an increased echogenicity due to the presence of cellular material associated with inflammation. Fibrin may be present, and this usually assumes a filamentous appearance, although it may assume a loculated pattern as well. Gas echoes within the pleural fluid are suggestive of infection with anaerobic gas-producing bacteria.[33] Areas of pulmonary consolidation may range from very small focal areas to extensive involvement of an entire lung lobe. Consolidated lung resembles the ultrasonographic appearance of the liver, and the normal anatomic structures of the lung are usually detectable[30] (Figures 10.8 and 10.9). Abscesses may be detected either in the pleural space or within the lung parenchyma itself, and are characterised by a circumscribed area, usually with a thick capsule, containing variably echogenic material[31] (Figures 10.10 and 10.11).

Radiography of the respiratory tract

The indications for thoracic radiography include findings on clinical examination suggestive of significant pulmonary disease, especially in those cases where definitive abnormalities are not identified on thoracic ultrasonography.[34] Thoracic radiography should be performed prior to invasive procedures, such as transtracheal aspiration, endoscopy or BAL, as these may alter the radiographic appearance of the lungs.

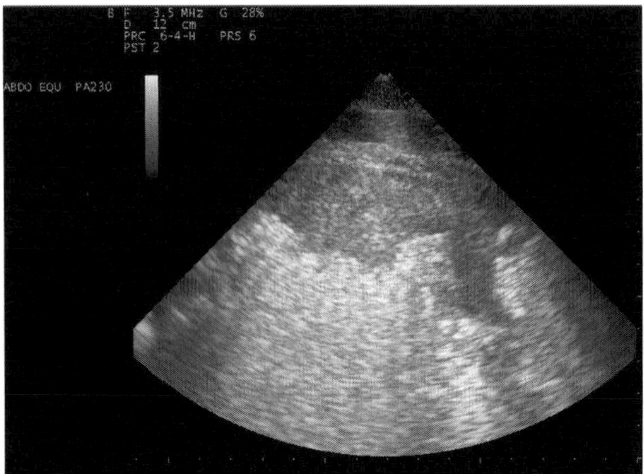

Figure 10.9 Consolidation of the lung parenchyma, with hepatisation. ©Kevin Corley 2007.

Procedure

Thoracic radiography in adults requires a powerful x-ray unit and a 10 : 1 to 12 : 1 grid to reduce the effects of scatter. The use of a short exposure time and a high kV, low mA technique will minimise the effects of breathing or patient motion.[35] In the author's experience using a computed radiography system, kV values of 60 to 70 in foals and 90 to 100 in adults, combined with mA values of 15 to 20 for foals or adults, provide good results. These output requirements preclude obtaining thoracic radiographs on adult horses using portable radiographic equipment, but most neonatal foals can be adequately imaged with portable equipment by using a higher kV of 90 and a mA of 4. The exposure should be made on inspiration to improve visualisation, with the cassette placed against the thoracic wall to minimise magnification artifact. A series of three or four large format films should be obtained to provide a thorough assessment of the thoracic structures in an adult horse, with the regions of interest being the caudodorsal, craniodorsal, caudoventral and cranioventral. Complete characterisation of suspected intrathoracic masses should include obtaining views from both the left and right side, to allow for correction for the magnifying effect that occurs when lesions are at a distance from the plate. This may allow for improved determination of the lesion location within the thorax (left vs right side). Thoracic radiography in foals usually requires only one to two lateral exposures to fully visualise the lung fields. Ventrodorsal views may be obtained in some recumbent foals, if indicated.

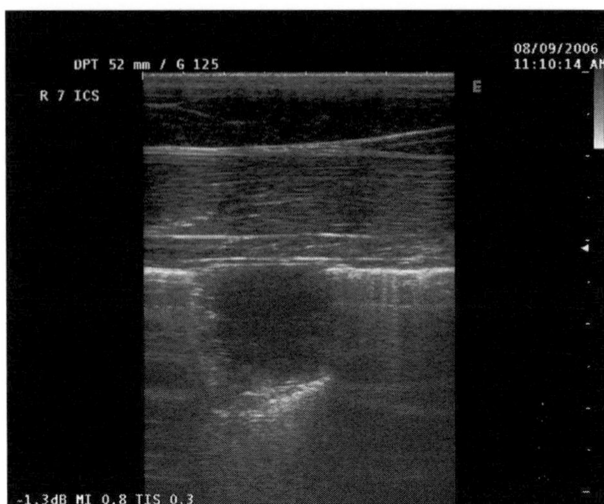

Figure 10.10 Focal pulmonary abscessation detected on ultrasonographic examination. ©Harold C. McKenzie III 2006.

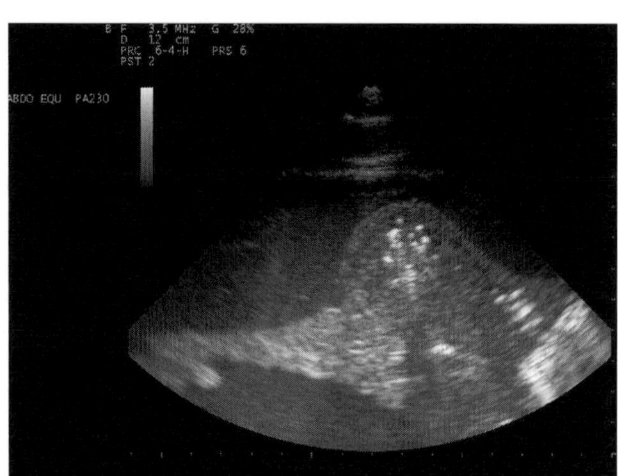

Figure 10.11 Pleural effusion in the right ventral thorax, with consolidation and abscessation of the tip of the lung. The abscess contains hyperechoic material, which is often associated with anaerobic infections. Bacteroides was cultured from a trans-tracheal aspirate. ©Kevin Corley 2007.

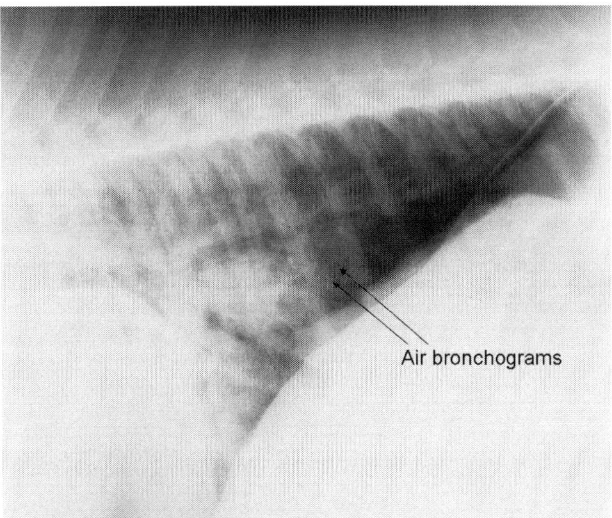

Figure 10.12 Diffuse interstitial pattern with some patchy areas of alveolar density (note air bronchograms). ©Harold C. McKenzie III 2006.

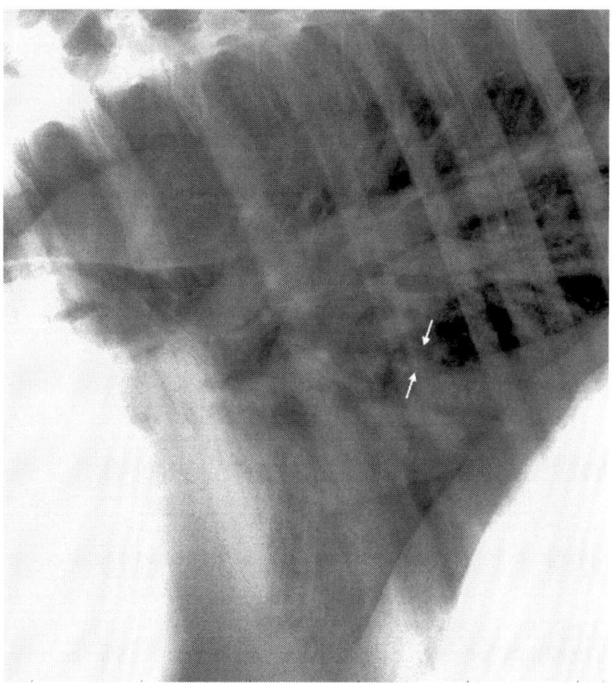

Figure 10.13 Bronchial pattern. The arrows mark some prominent bronchial walls. ©Harold C. McKenzie III 2006.

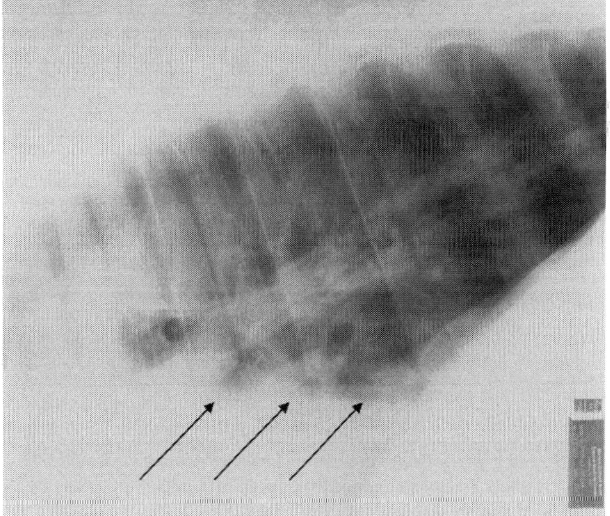

Figure 10.14 Pleural effusion causing a 'fluid line' (marked with arrows) on a thoracic radiograph. ©Harold C. McKenzie III 2006.

Interpretation

The lung tissue, blood vessels, airways, ribs, diaphragm, mediastinum and heart should be examined. One should identify any changes in tissue density, presence of pleural fluid lines, displacement of the trachea, presence of tissue masses, as well as irregularities of the diaphragm, heart, vertebra or ribs. Diseases of the lung tissue are usually characterised by increased tissue density. The increased density is typically observed in patterns termed alveolar, interstitial and bronchial, with hybrids such as bronchointerstitial and interstitial-alveolar occurring frequently. The alveolar pattern results from the filling of the alveoli with fluid, and is characterised by the presence of fluffy, patchy areas of increased density at the mildest, with progression to greatly increased density of the parenchyma resulting in the silhouetting of the bronchi (air bronchograms)[35] (Figure 10.12). The interstitial pattern is frequently observed early in the progression of pulmonary disease. It results from fluid accumulation and/or cellular infiltration of the pulmonary interstitium. This pattern results in a hazy, or "ground glass", appearance to the parenchyma, and can progress to an alveolar pattern.[35] A nodular interstitial pattern may also be observed, often secondary to the presence of many small abscesses or tumours throughout the lung parenchyma. The bronchial pattern results from thickening of the airway walls secondary to inflammation, with resultant oedema of the wall, cellular infiltration (in or around the airway wall) and intraluminal exudate accumulation. [35] The classic pattern is that of "railroad tracks", where prominent airway walls are observed coursing in parallel through the pulmonary parenchyma (Figure 10.13). Additional findings on thoracic radiographs can include: fluid lines associated with pleural fluid accumulation (Figure 10.14) or pleural or pulmonary abscess formation (Figure 10.15), pneumothorax characterised by partial collapse of one or both lungs (Figures 10.16 and 10.17), pneumomediastinum resulting in increased visualisation of mediastinal structures due to the presence of air outlining these structures and mediastinal masses which may present as soft tissue density structures superimposed upon or displacing normal mediastinal structures.

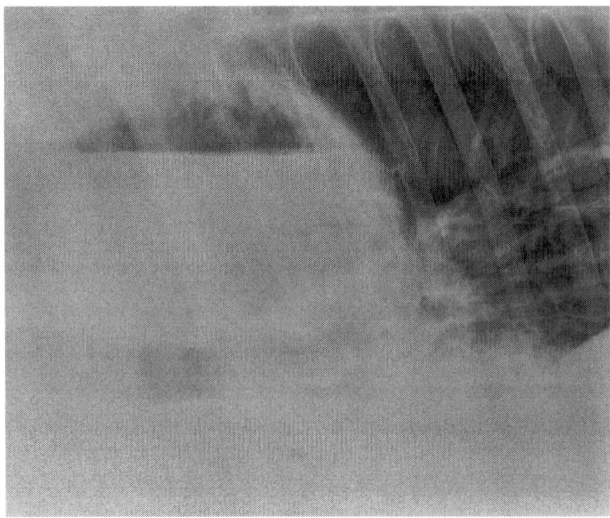

Figure 10.15 Very large cranial abscess (with a fluid line) on a cranio-dorsal radiographic view of the thorax. ©Kevin Corley 2006.

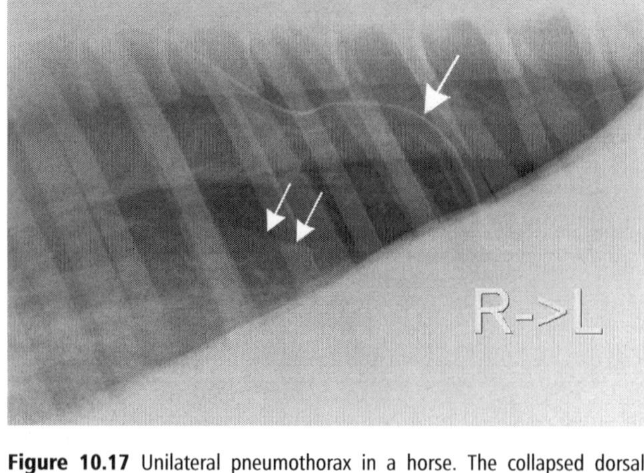

Figure 10.17 Unilateral pneumothorax in a horse. The collapsed dorsal border of the side with the pneumothorax is labelled with the two white arrows. The single white arrow marks the radio-opaque line within an indwelling thoracic drain. ©Kevin Corley 2003.

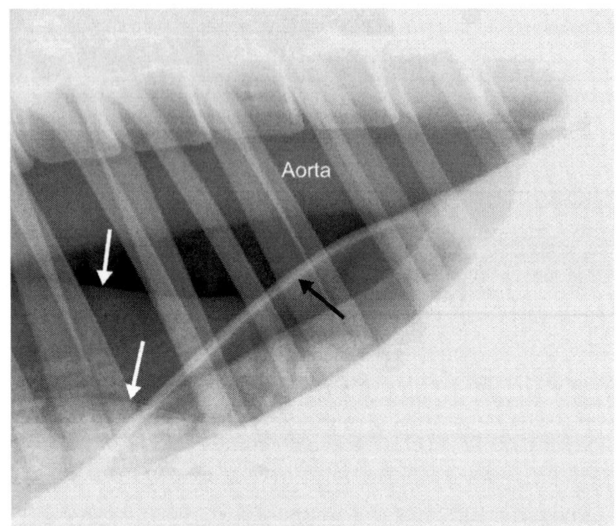

Figure 10.16 Bilateral pneumothorax in a horse. The collapsed dorsal borders of the lungs are marked with white arrows. The diaphragm is marked with a black arrow. ©Kevin Corley 2003.

10.2 Management of horses with respiratory disorders

Metered-dose inhalers and nebulisation

The treatment of lower respiratory disease is complicated by the fact that the respiratory epithelium represents a substantial barrier to the diffusion of drugs from the systemic circulation into the respiratory compartment. This can result in an impaired response to treatment with systemically administered medications, potentially requiring that large dosages be used in order to achieve therapeutic levels within the respiratory tract and increasing the likelihood of adverse side effects. Aerosol administration overcomes these limitations by achieving high drug concentrations within the airway lumen, allowing a decrease in the total dose administered, avoidance of systemic side effects and a rapid onset of action.[36,37] These advantages are particularly valuable with drugs such as bronchodilators and corticosteroids, where the therapeutic index for systemic administration is narrow. Aerosol administration does have limitations, however, including potential problems with drug delivery and pulmonary irritation, as well as the expense of the required equipment and the time required for administration. A detailed discussion of aerosol therapy is given in Chapter 6.4.

Aerosol administration

Aerosol delivery of therapeutic substances presents several challenges. The substance to be delivered must be available in a formulation that can be delivered to the respiratory tract as an aerosol. The therapeutic agent should be nonirritating and nonallergenic and lack local toxicity.[38] The therapeutic substance must be capable of exerting its action on the mucosal surface or of being absorbed into the respiratory mucosa, but if the therapeutic substance has the potential for systemic toxicity it should be poorly absorbed.[38] The delivery method must be capable of producing particles that are of an appropriate size to deliver the medication to the desired portion of the respiratory tract, and the delivery method should be able to deliver the total dose in a reasonable period of time with reasonable efficiency.

The generation of therapeutic aerosols is accomplished using several different inhalation drug delivery systems. None of these systems, however, is capable of delivering aerosolised medication with high efficiency, with less than

10% of the original dose being deposited in the lower respiratory tract regardless of delivery system.[39–43] Two of the most commonly used aerosol delivery devices in human medicine are metered-dose inhalers (MDIs) and dry powder inhalers (DPIs), which generate small volume aerosols of liquids and powders, respectively. These devices have the advantages of being preformulated, prepackaged and capable of delivering multiple doses; however, they do require some dexterity during administration to ensure that administration is correlated with inhalation.[44] Their prepackaged nature also decreases the risk of introducing microorganisms into the respiratory tract during drug administration, which is a concern when using nebulisers for aerosol generation. The most commonly used aerosol delivery device in the horse is the MDI, and the efficacy of these devices for the administration of therapeutic aerosols to horses has been extensively examined.[45–52] The difficulty of coordinating administration with inhalation is addressed in the horse by the use of a closely fitting valved facemask‡ (Figure 10.18) or intranasal delivery device§ (Figure 10.19).

Devices

Nebulisers

Aerosols are generated from liquids by nebulisers, either ultrasonic or compressed-gas driven (jet). Nebulisation is considered to be the optimal method of administration when the dose to be delivered exceeds 200 μg,[44] and does not require coordination of administration and inhalation, depending only on normal tidal breathing.[53] Nebulisers must be used with a facemask in the conscious animal patient, with attendant aerosol wastage on the face, facemask and in the nasal passages and nasopharynx.[54] Nebulisers are attached to the facemask using plastic aerosol tubing (Figure 10.20).

Jet nebulisers (Figure 10.21) are more widely used than ultrasonic nebulisers (Figure 10.20) in human medicine, because they are inexpensive and relatively easy to use. Jet nebulisers are usually limited to reservoir volumes of 6 ml or less, however, and the time required to aerosolise this volume of fluid is anywhere from 10 to 15 minutes.[55] This means that the time required to deliver a large volume of solution (10–20 ml) may become excessive with adult horses. Ultrasonic nebulisers are generally capable of producing more aerosol per unit time than jet nebulisers, resulting in shorter treatment times and greater ease of use.[56] Larger fill volumes (up to 30 ml or more) also allow convenient administration of larger doses. These devices

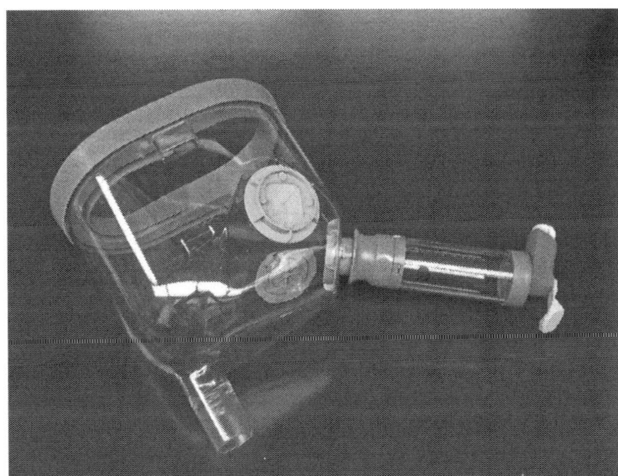

Figure 10.18 Equine valved facemask for delivery of aerosolised medications, with spacer for delivering drugs by metered dose inhaler. ©Harold C. McKenzie III 2006.

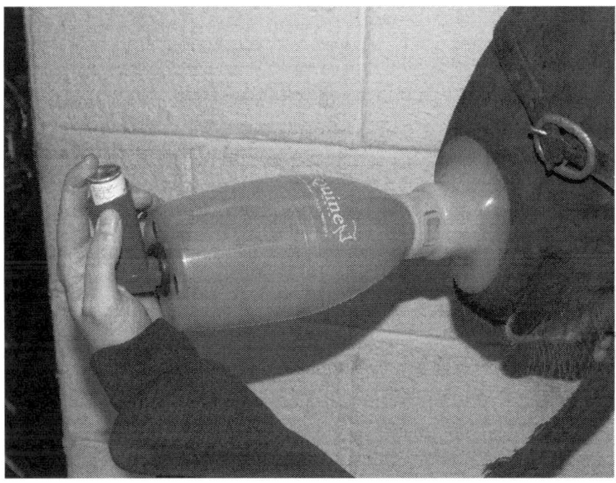

Figure 10.19 Single nostril delivery device for metered dose inhalers. ©Kevin Corley 2007.

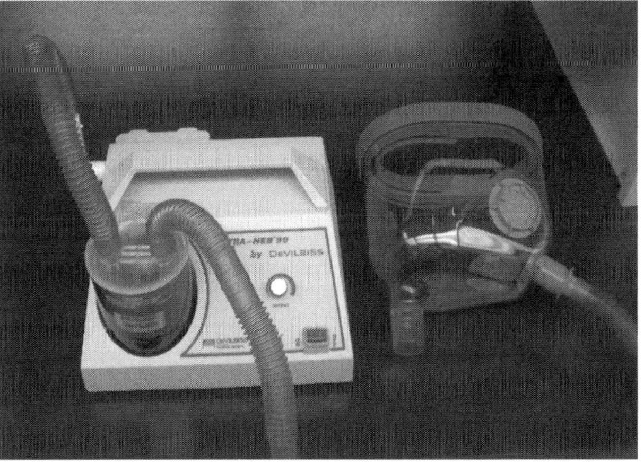

Figure 10.20 Facemask connected to ultrasonic nebuliser. ©Harold C. McKenzie III 2006.

‡ Equine Aeromask; Canadian Monaghan Ltd., London, Ontario, Canada.

§ Equine Haler; Equine HealthCare ApS, Copenhagen, Denmark.

are expensive and fragile, though, limiting their clinical application outside of referral institutions.[54]

Metered-dose and dry powder inhalers

MDIs are self-contained devices, consisting of a canister with an integral metering valve. The canister contains the drug and a liquid propellant.[57] The propellant serves as a dispersion medium for the drug, and as an energy source to expel the formulation from the valve as large droplets that rapidly evaporate following exposure to the air, leaving a drug-containing particle of respirable size.[57] Due to the high velocity of the aerosol as it leaves the actuation valve, these devices have been associated with high levels of oral and upper respiratory deposition in human patients.[58] In an effort to avoid this effect, a spacer device is used, with the MDI being actuated into the device, where the particle velocity dissipates, the propellant evaporates further and the nonrespirable particles impact onto the device, resulting in a decrease in particle size, allowing for increased pulmonary deposition and decreased oropharyngeal deposition[42,44] (Figure 10.18). An intranasal device was developed and marketed specifically for the administration of albuterol to adult horses**, and this device was clinically effective. Acceptance of the device was limited due to client cost concerns, however, and it is no longer marketed.

DPIs are available as either unit-dose or multiple-dose devices.[44] These devices have the advantage of not requiring a propellant for dispersion of the drug, and they do not require coordination of inhalation and actuation, because they are breath actuated.[55] Relatively high inspiratory airflows (30–60 L/min) are required to aerosolise the powder

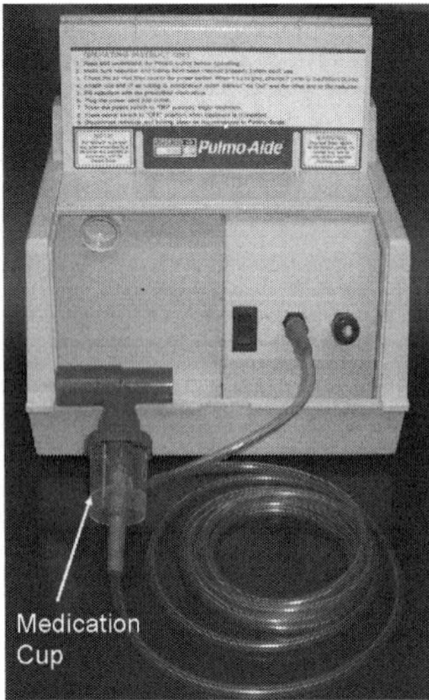

Figure 10.21 Pneumatic (jet) nebuliser system. ©Harold C. McKenzie III 2006.

** Torpex Equine Inhaler; 3M Animal Care Products, St. Paul, MN, USA; and Boehringer Ingleheim Vetmedica, Inc., St. Joseph, MO, USA.

formulations, however, and may be difficult to achieve in the face of pulmonary disease or when using a facemask for aerosol administration.[42,44] The facemask†† marketed for administering aerosols to horses can be used to administer DPI medications, but this facemask system is not very efficient with these devices.[59] Efficiency can be improved by modifications to the mask,[59] but to the author's knowledge, a revised mask is not commercially available.

The use of MDIs has been extensively investigated in the horse. The pulmonary deposition of radioaerosol generated using an MDI with a spacer and facemask was examined by Viel and Tesarowski,[60] and it was demonstrated that significantly more (up to 5 times) of the dose of radioaerosol was deposited in the lung using this device combination than was observed with jet or ultrasonic nebulisers. The therapeutic administration of β_2-agonist bronchodilators to horses by MDI has been validated,[46–48,61,62] and these drugs are commonly used in the treatment of equine lower respiratory disease. While the administration of the anticholinergic bronchodilator ipratropium bromide by DPI has also been validated,[63] this drug is not as commonly used as the β_2-agonists. The aerosol administration of corticosteroids has also been validated, using both beclomethasone and fluticasone MDIs.[45,64–70]

Clinical application of inhaled bronchodilators

β_2-Adrenoreceptor agonists

The most commonly used inhaled medications in horses are the bronchodilators, and of these the β_2-agonists are the most widely used. These compounds achieve rapid bronchodilation following aerosol administration[47,62] and are very effective in relieving bronchospasm in equine patients, or in preventing bronchospasm associated with delivery of other aerosolised medications, such as antimicrobials.[71] Two types of β_2-agonists are available, and they are characterised by their duration of effect. Short-acting β_2-agonists include salbutamol (albuterol), pirbuterol and fenoterol, while the long-acting compounds include salmeterol and formoterol. The short acting compounds are typically faster acting, with onset of clinical effect within as little as 5 minutes, but typically are only active for 1 to 3 hours.[47,61] The long-acting compounds are slower to onset of effect, with salmeterol requiring 30 to 60 minutes to achieve full effect, while clinical efficacy persists for at least 6 hours.[62] While administering these drugs via the aerosol route lessens the likelihood of side effects by decreasing the dosage requirement, the risk is not entirely eliminated. High dosages of these compounds (4–6 times the therapeutic dosage) can lead to sweating, trembling and excitement.[72]

Paradoxical bronchoconstriction is a possible complication when administering β_2-agonists to horses, and this

†† Equine Aeromask; Canadian Monaghan Ltd., London, Ont., Canada.

effect appears to be related to the *S*-isomer of salbutamol (albuterol), which has the potential to exacerbate airway hyperreactivity and may exert a proinflammatory effect.[73,74] The *R*-isomer is responsible for the desired bronchodilatory effect of salbutamol and other β_2-agonists, but most commercially available preparations consist of racemic mixtures containing 50:50 mixtures of the *S*- and *R*-isomers. A single isomer preparation of *R*-albuterol (levalbuterol)‡‡ is commercially available, and this compound has been shown in humans to be up to 4 times more potent in terms of bronchodilation than racemic salbutamol, while at the same time exhibiting a marked reduction in side effects.[74] Although the use of levalbuterol has not been specifically investigated in the horse it has been suggested to be a reasonable alternative to racemic albuterol that may exhibit fewer side effects.[73]

The recommended dosage of salbutamol when using an MDI is 360 to 720 μg, while the reported optimal dose of pirbuterol§§ is 600 μg.[61] Due to the limited duration of activity of the short-acting β_2-agonists, it is difficult to maintain effective bronchodilation, and their use is best limited to the treatment of acute bronchoconstriction or intermittent therapy as needed in the management of chronic lower respiratory conditions, such as RAO. Prolonged administration of β_2-agonists results in the development of tolerance, with a resultant loss of clinical efficacy. Numerous studies in human medicine have documented this effect, which can occur after as little as 1 week of treatment and the effect appears to be similar in horses.[73,75] For this reason long-term dependence upon β_2-agonists in the treatment of chronic lower respiratory inflammatory conditions, such as human asthma, is associated with poor disease control and increased patient fatality rates.[73,75,76] By limiting the use of β_2-agonists to short periods of time, or an as-needed basis, one can avoid the loss of efficacy associated with long-term administration. In the clinical setting the efficacy of β_2-agonist therapy can also serve as a useful indicator of the effectiveness of the overall treatment regimen, as increasing dependence on this therapy indicates that the disease process is poorly controlled and overall management should be reassessed.[76]

Long-acting β_2-agonists, while not as extensively evaluated in the horse as the short acting compounds, have some potential advantages. Firstly, as would be expected, the duration of clinical effect is longer than that observed with the short acting compounds, being on the order of 6 to 12 hours. Perhaps more importantly, however, the development of tolerance appears to be slowed with these compounds, although the mechanisms underlying this effect are unclear.[73,77] This may allow for these compounds to retain clinical efficacy when used for longer periods of time (1–3 weeks). Longer-term therapy is again discouraged, however, as discussed earlier. Salmeterol xinafoate*** has been utilised in horses with RAO at a dosage of 210 μg, and this dosage resulted in a similar bronchodilatory response as is seen with inhaled albuterol, although the 6-hour duration of action was shorter than that observed in humans.[62]

‡‡ Xopenex; Sepracor, Inc., Marlborough, MA, USA.

§§ Maxair; 3M Pharmaceuticals, Northridge, CA, USA.

Parasympatholytics

Given the fact that the bronchoconstrictive response is autonomically mediated, being under the control of the parasympathetic system,[78] it is logical to consider the potential application of anticholinergic medications in the control of bronchoconstriction. As has long been known, atropine is a potent bronchodilator in the horse, even in the face of clinical exacerbations of RAO.[79,80] Clinical application is unfortunately limited by the fact that the therapeutic index of atropine is very narrow, with atropine administration potentially inducing profound ileus, predisposing to the development of colic. Due to their narrow therapeutic index, parasympatholytic medications are good candidates for aerosol administration, particularly if a drug form is available that exhibits poor systemic bioavailability. Ipratropium bromide is a synthetic parasympatholytic bronchodilator that meets these criteria, with only 6% reported respiratory tract absorption and 2% gastrointestinal absorption.[73] This compound has been demonstrated to be efficacious in horses suffering from RAO,[49,63,81] and is clinically effective in the author's experience. As ipratropium acts by interfering with acetylcholine activity at the level of the smooth muscle M3 muscarinic receptors, rather than by stimulating the receptor, the development of tolerance does not appear to be a significant problem.[82,83] Longer-acting anticholinergic bronchodilators, such as tiotropium bromide and oxitropium bromide, have demonstrated excellent efficacy and safety profiles in human patients and may have clinical utility in equine patients, although appropriate dosage regimens remain to be defined.[73]

As the β_2-agonists and anticholinergics act by different mechanisms their combined use may result in additive or synergistic effects. This phenomenon has been demonstrated in human patients, where the β_2-agonist induces a rapid bronchodilatory response that is subsequently maintained by the anticholinergic compound.[84] There is some suggestion of a synergistic effect in human patients, wherein the combination therapy is more effective in improving pulmonary function both acutely and over time than either compound alone.[84] A combination product containing albuterol sulfate and ipratropium bromide is commercially available as a nebulization solution or MDI, and is clinically effective in equine patients†††.

*** Serevent; GlaxoSmithKline, Research Triangle Park, NC, USA.

††† Combivent; Boehringer Ingelheim International GmbH, Ingleheim, Germany.

Clinical application of inhaled corticosteroids

Due to concerns regarding the narrow therapeutic index associated with systemic corticosteroid administration in horses, particularly associated with the potential risk of laminitis, there has been a great deal of interest in aerosolised corticosteroids for the treatment of chronic lower respiratory inflammation. Due to the fact that these medications are delivered directly to the site of inflammation at the level of the respiratory epithelium, far lower dosages are typically required to achieve a therapeutic effect.[64,65] While low dosages of aerosolised corticosteroids are utilised, typically in the 0.5- to 2-mg range, the high potency of these compounds results in measurable systemic effects, primarily consisting of adrenocortical suppression.[69,85,86] In addition to this concern, there are several limitations to this therapeutic approach. The first is that drug delivery is impaired by the presence of bronchoconstriction and inflammatory exudate within the airways, with the result that the corticosteroid is primarily delivered to the best-ventilated, yet least-affected regions of the lungs. This effect can be minimised by pretreatment with a bronchodilator such as albuterol, as the degree of bronchoconstriction is lessened and peripheral distribution improved.[87] The second limitation of aerosolised corticosteroids is that with patients in respiratory distress the respiratory pattern is not conducive to inhalation therapy, as it is characterised by rapid, shallow respirations that prevent deep penetration of aerosolised medications. For these reasons, aerosolised corticosteroids are not rapidly effective and should not constitute a first-line therapy for severe lower respiratory inflammation. An additional concern is that aerosolised corticosteroids are relatively expensive on a per-dose basis, which results in poor owner compliance with long-term treatment plans. Despite all of these concerns inhaled corticosteroid therapy can be clinically useful, primarily with the moderately affected patient or in patients where there is a predisposition to laminitis. Systemic corticosteroid administration remains the preferred therapy, however, in horses with severe RAO.

Inhaled corticosteroid therapy utilises either fluticasone propionate‡‡‡ or beclomethasone dipropionate§§§ MDIs, with the recommended dosage of fluticasone being 1000 to 2500 μg administered every 12 to 24 hours,[68,70] while beclomethasone has been administered at dosages of 500 to 3750 μg every 12 to 24 hours.[45,64,85] Improvement in pulmonary function and in markers of pulmonary inflammation has been reported with these therapies. An additional benefit that may be associated with aerosolised corticosteroid administration is the preservation of activity of the β_2-adrenergic bronchodilators, as this has been consistently demonstrated in human patients. Corticosteroids appear to modulate the activity of the β_2-adrenoceptor by protecting against desensitization and the development of tolerance.[88] It is possible, however, that the same beneficial effects may occur when corticosteroids are administered systemically.

‡‡‡ Flovent; GlaxoSmithKline, Research Triangle Park, NC, USA.

§§§ Qvar; IVAX Laboratories, Inc., Miami, FL, USA.

Oxygen therapy

Intranasal oxygen administration

The provision of supplemental O_2 is easily accomplished in adults and foals by means of nasal O_2 insufflation. The placement of a nasal catheter is required for nasal O_2 insufflation, and these are available commercially. A 14 Fr × 41-cm O_2 catheter**** is most commonly utilised in foals, but these are often too flexible to easily maintain in adults. Alternatively, a 14 Fr to 18 Fr red rubber feeding tube†††† can be used in adults, as these are slightly stiffer than the catheters used in foals. It is important that the nasal catheter be positioned deep within the nasal passages but rostral to the pharynx, and this can be estimated by setting the length of the catheter to reach from the external nares to the level of the medial canthus of the eye. In foals the catheter can be maintained in position by taping it to a 4- to 5-cm segment of tongue depressor, then taping the catheter around the rounded portion of the tongue depressor such that the catheter is directed up the nasal passages. The external portion of the catheter and the tongue depressor can then be affixed to the foal's face by means of a circumferential band of elastic tape‡‡‡‡. In some cases it is helpful to secure the catheter to the external nares using a "butterfly" of tape placed around the catheter that is then secured with a single simple interrupted suture using non-absorbable suture material. In adults the catheter is typically sutured to the external nares and taped to the halter for stabilisation.

Prior to administering O_2 to the patient the O_2 must pass through a humidification device§§§§ in order to prevent the inhalation of dry gas that would result in respiratory tract injury. Delivery of the humidified O_2 to the patient is readily achieved using flexible O_2 tubing***** to connect the output port of the humidifier to the nasal catheter of the patient. Ambulatory patients can present a challenge, as this tubing will become tangled, but this can be minimised by delivering the O_2 through a coiled fluid administration set†††††. Administration rates are generally

**** Allegiance Healthcare Corp., McGaw Park, IL, USA.

†††† Kendall Sovereign; Tyco Healthcare Group, LP, Mansfield, MA, USA.

‡‡‡‡ Elastoplast; Beiersdorf AG, Hamburg, Germany; Elastikon; Johnson & Johnson, Somerville, NJ.

§§§§ Examples include Airlife prefilled humidifier; Allegiance Healthcare Corp., McGaw Park, IL, USA.

***** Examples include 6.4-m-length Airlife oxygen tubing; Allegiance Healthcare Corp., McGaw Park, IL, USA.

††††† Coiled extension set; International Win, Ltd., Kennett Square, PA, USA.

limited by the delivery system to ~10 to 15 L/min, which is adequate for most foals but may not be adequate in adults. In cases where higher flow rates are desired, two separate systems can be utilised to deliver O_2 into both nostrils, thereby further increasing the FIO_2.

Bronchoscopic lavage

The treatment of bacterial pneumonia in horses primarily depends on the administration of systemic broad-spectrum antimicrobials and anti-inflammatory drugs, in combination with rest. The majority of cases respond well to this approach, but complications including pleuropneumonia and pulmonary or pleural abscessation can occur. The prognosis for horses with complicated pneumonia is considered to be guarded,[89,90] although those that survive and return to racing are reported to return to their previous level of performance.[91] The technique of directed bronchoscopic lavage of the affected regions of the equine lung may have utility as a diagnostic and therapeutic aid in the treatment of patients with complicated pneumonia.[13,14,92]

Traditionally, bronchoscopy has been considered to be a purely diagnostic technique in equine medicine, having been utilised as a means of collecting samples from the airways for cytological analysis by means of BAL. This can be very useful, as tracheal aspirate samples do not always reflect abnormalities present in more distal areas of the lungs, and BAL has been shown to provide accurate information regarding diffuse lung diseases in horses.[21] Additional indications for bronchoscopy include visual inspection of the airways for the presence of foreign bodies or for evidence of focal disease, such as the presence of exudate or focal inflammation. BAL of such suspect areas does not always provide useful information, however, and it has been shown that tracheobronchial aspirates provide more consistent results for investigation of horses with suspected pneumonia or pleuropneumonia.[93] In addition, BAL may not provide useful samples for bacterial culture and sensitivity, due to the potential for contamination of the equipment during insertion.[93] For this reason samples for culture should be obtained by transtracheal aspiration prior to performing bronchoscopy. Despite these limitations there are situations where culture of BAL fluid may be useful, as BAL has been shown to be more sensitive than a protected catheter brush technique for the recovery of pathogens from the lower respiratory tract of foals receiving antibiotic treatment.[94] In the author's experience the utility of this technique for culture is enhanced by definitive localization of the affected region and by collection of a grossly abnormal sample. Interpretation of these culture results must always be made in light of the cytological pattern observed and should include consideration of the possibility of contamination.

Additional indications for bronchoscopy in human medicine have long included therapeutic interventions, such as the removal of foreign bodies or respiratory secretions, or the placement of drugs or other therapeutic materials into the airways. A more recent report states that one of the primary uses of bronchoscopy in human critical care units is the removal of airway secretions which cannot be adequately mobilised by other means, with the primary advantage of bronchoscopy being the ability to target specific areas of concern within the bronchial tree.[95] The author is only aware of a single report of the therapeutic use of BAL in equine pneumonia.[13] The lack of appropriate endoscopic equipment until fairly recent times may explain the paucity of reports detailing these types of interventions in equine patients.

Bronchoscopy technique

The technique of equine bronchoscopy has been well described, and involves the use of a flexible fiberoptic endoscope of 2 to 3 metres length with an outer diameter of less than 10 mm.[96] It is very important that the horse to be examined is well sedated to minimise movement during the examination. The combination of detomidine (0.01–0.02 mg/kg IV) and butorphanol (0.02 mg/kg IV) typically provides excellent sedation that is of adequate duration to allow for a thorough examination. The use of butorphanol also provides a beneficial antitussive effect. Horses with substantial lower respiratory inflammation or hyperreactive airways benefit from bronchodilator pretreatment with inhaled albuterol.[4] The endoscope must be thoroughly cleansed and processed to eliminate any potential pathogens from the external or internal surfaces of the endoscope, even though the bronchoscopy procedure is not sterile. Removal of organic debris with an enzymatic cleanser should be followed by disinfection with a glutaraldehyde solution and rinsing with sterile water. Knowledge of equine bronchial anatomy is useful in attempting to correlate the anatomic location of the tip of the endoscope to the area of suspected involvement identified on ultrasonographic or radiographic examination. In most cases, however, detailed anatomic knowledge is unnecessary, as there is a trail of exudate leading to the affected area.

When introducing the endoscope into the respiratory tract a dilute local anesthetic solution (40–60 ml of 0.2% lidocaine) is infused through the biopsy channel onto the laryngeal and tracheal mucosa and upon reaching the affected region of the lung, to decrease patient discomfort and facilitate the examination by minimizing coughing. Upon reaching the area of interest a further 10 to 20 ml of dilute local anesthetic is infused. The tip of the endoscope is then guided into the affected airway until wedged. Sterile saline solution is then infused via the biopsy channel into the area, usually in increments of 120 to 240 ml and then aspirated. While various automated systems have been devised the author typically uses 60 ml syringes for infusion and aspiration. The yield of fluid can be quite variable, often depending on how well wedged the endoscope is and whether the patient coughs during the procedure. In some cases substantial amounts of exudate can be removed by this approach (as much as 60 ml). The yield may improve with subsequent examinations as the degree of airway oedema decreases. In some cases the airways may be occluded by firm plugs of mucous or purulent material, and this can often be dislodged by repeated lavage or by manipulation with endoscopic biopsy forceps. Pulmonary abscesses present more of a challenge, although the author has found that cautious probing with the biopsy forceps has been rewarding in establishing drainage in a few cases.

Following the removal of exudate from the affected region of the lung one can infuse therapeutic agents into the affected area in order to achieve high concentrations at the site of infection. While endobronchial antimicrobial administration is not reported in the horse, this route of administration has been utilised in human medicine for both antibacterials and antifungals, with reported efficacy and safety.[97–99] Consideration must be given, however, to the possibility of local irritation or toxicity when using this route of administration. The author has used injectable solutions of amikacin, gentamicin, ceftiofur and metronidazole as local infusions without apparent untoward effects, at dosages representing less than 25% to 33% of the systemic dosage and with dilution rates of 100 to 300%. Endobronchially administered drugs may be systemically absorbed, potentially interfering with the pharmacokinetics of systemically administered antimicrobials.[100] This is of greatest concern with the aminoglycosides, due to their potential ototoxic and nephrotoxic effects, especially in patients with impaired renal function.[98,100] The author has found that administering endobronchial aminoglycosides at or near the time of systemic administration minimises their influence on clinical pharmacokinetics.

Potential complications

It is important to monitor the total volume of local anesthetic infused while performing bronchoscopy to avoid the possibility of systemic toxicity.[95] The author rarely uses more than 80 to 100 ml of a 0.2% solution during a procedure, which results in the administration of much less lidocaine than would be administered as a loading dose in the treatment of ileus.[101] While it is possible that the bronchial lavage procedure itself could induce an inflammatory response, the literature is conflicting on this point and this does not appear to be an issue clinically.[11,13,102–104] One should be cautious regarding the total volume of fluid infused when lavaging affected segments of the lung as there is the possibility of causing further damage to the lavaged area due to excessive pressure. Infusion of fluid in 60- to 120-ml increments, as opposed to the larger volumes (240–300 ml) traditionally utilised when performing BAL, appears to be safe and effective. An additional concern is that the establishment of intrabronchial drainage will result in the dissemination of exudate more widely throughout the lungs. We have observed fever spikes and radiographic changes suggestive of increased inflammation following dramatic release of exudate in a few patients, but these effects have been transient and were not associated with clinical deterioration. Provision of appropriate antimicrobial therapy is likely to lessen the risk of disseminated intrapulmonary infection, and many of our patients receive concurrent aerosolised antimicrobial therapy to ensure that high levels of antimicrobial are present within the airway lumen.[71,87,104] Patients with hyperreactive airways may be at risk of severe brochoconstriction, which could result in impaired pulmonary function, but this risk can be minimised by prior treatment with inhaled albuterol. It is wise, however, to have a readily available source of supplemental O_2 for patients with impaired pulmonary function.

Efficacy

The best evidence in support of the efficacy of this technique comes from the report by Ito et al. describing the use of BAL in the treatment of uncomplicated transport-associated pneumonia.[13] In that report therapeutic BAL was utilised in 36 Thoroughbred racehorses presenting with transport associated pneumonia. BAL was utilised from the time of admission, prior to the development of complicated pneumonia. BAL was repeated 1 to 7 times at 3- to 8-day intervals until no mucopurulent exudate was detectable on bronchoscopic examination (5–40 days). Significant differences were seen when these cases were compared to 42 cases treated with conventional therapy alone, with 100% survival in the BAL treated horses versus 81% in the conventionally treated horses. The duration of treatment was shorter in BAL treated horses (median 17 days) as compared to conventionally treated horses (median 22 days), and 10% of the conventionally treated horses required thoracic drainage, while none of those treated with BAL required thoracic drainage. Of the BAL treated horses 78% returned to racing, as compared with 50% of those treated conventionally.

Pleural drainage

When accumulation of pleural fluid is identified on thoracic radiographs or ultrasound a sample of this fluid should be collected for both cytological analysis and bacterial culture and sensitivity testing. This technique allows for the sterile collection of pleural fluid for cytological examination and culture, and for drainage of accumulated fluid and inflammatory material.[18,19] The technique for pleurocentesis is described in Chapter 1.35. A sample for bacterial culture should be collected in a sterile plain tube. Samples for aerobic and anaerobic culture should be processed immediately, or held under refrigeration until processed, to limit the possibility of secondary bacterial overgrowth. Complications of pleurocentesis are not common, but can include cellulitis at the insertion site, pneumothorax, haemothorax, cardiac dysrhythmias and laceration or puncture of the lung, heart, liver or bowel.[20]

It is not uncommon for small amounts of air to enter the pleural cavity during placement of the cannula or catheter, and this is usually of no clinical significance and the air is rapidly absorbed by the body.[18]

If pleural drainage is indicated the drainage catheter should be sutured into place using nonabsorbable suture in a Chinese finger trap pattern. The lumen of the catheter should be occluded using a catheter tip syringe or a Heimlich valve should be placed to allow continual drainage. The catheter insertion site should be covered with a non-adherent sterile bandage to prevent contamination of the site. When large amounts of fluid are present one should consider placing the patient on intravenous fluid therapy, as hypovolaemia can occur when the fluid is drained from the pleural cavity. Persistent large volume drainage may result in hypoproteinaemia as well, due to loss of proteinaceous fluid, and this can be addressed by administering intravenous equine plasma. Indwelling drainage catheters are prone to occlusion due to the accumulation of exudate and fibrin plugs, and this can be minimised by instilling 10 to 30 ml of sterile fluid with 5000 to 10,000 IU of heparin sulfate added. This should be repeated 3 to 4 times daily. The removal of large amounts of inflammatory exudate from within the pleural cavity can be facilitated by the implementation of pleural lavage, wherein 5 to 10 L of warmed isotonic fluids are infused through the drainage catheter, allowed to stand for 10 to 30 minutes, then drained by gravity flow. Some clinicians will add antimicrobials to this lavage solution, or instill small volumes of antimicrobial solution following lavage. Appropriate dosages for antimicrobial administration by this route are not established, however.

Mechanical ventilation

A basic guide to operating a mechanical ventilator is given in Chapter 2.3. Further information is given in the section below.

Ventilatory support

The goals of mechanical ventilatory support are to achieve and maintain adequate pulmonary gas exchange, reduce the work of breathing, and to minimise patient discomfort and distress.[105] Mechanical ventilation provides pressure and volume support to ensure that adequate minute ventilation is achieved, and also provides control over the composition of the inspired gases in order to provide sufficient O_2 to support arterial oxygenation. In equine medicine it is generally not practical to mechanically ventilate patients larger than 200 kg, due to the limitations of most ventilators and the difficulty of maintaining recumbent large animals for prolonged periods of time. For that reason this discussion will be focused primarily on mechanical ventilation of foals.

Patients requiring mechanical ventilation typically are suffering from arterial hypercapnia and/or arterial hypoxaemia. Hypercapnia is fundamentally due to hypoventilation, but can be exacerbated by excessive administration of exogenous carbohydrates and lipids, resulting in increased CO_2 production. Hypoxaemia is due to alveolar hypoventilation, impaired O_2 diffusion, ventilation–perfusion mismatching, decreased inspired O_2 tension or extrapulmonary shunts. Of these the most clinically important is ventilation–perfusion mismatching, followed in importance by alveolar hypoventilation and impaired O_2 diffusion. Decreased inspired O_2 tension is unlikely to be a relevant cause of hypoxaemia in the spontaneously ventilating patient, but should be considered a possibility in a patient that becomes hypoxemic while being mechanically ventilated. Extrapulmonary shunts should be considered in a patient profoundly refractory to O_2 supplementation.

Treatment of hypercapnia is fundamentally to increase the patient's alveolar ventilation by increasing the rate and/or depth of breathing. Arterial hypercapnia for the purposes of this discussion is defined as a $Paco_2$ of greater than 60 mm Hg, and some form of treatment is indicated when clinical values exceed this level. For initial therapy some clinicians will utilise respiratory stimulants, such as doxapram hydrochloride (loading dose of 0.5 mg/kg, followed by a continuous rate infusion of 0.03–0.08 mg/kg/min)[106] or caffeine (10 mg/kg PO or per rectum loading, 2.5 mg/kg prn),[107] to increase the patient's ventilatory efforts and try to avoid the need for mechanical ventilation. Doxapram effectively reduced CO_2 concentrations, in an isoflurane-induced model of hypercapnia in foals. Caffeine had no effect in this model.[106] Undesirable side-effects of these drugs can include tachycardia, and increased O_2 consumption. These side-effects appear more likely with doxapram. If respiratory stimulant therapy is unsuccessful at resolving the hypercapnia, or if the hypercapnia is more severe ($PaCO_2$ > 70 mm Hg) one should consider instituting mechanical ventilation. Early intervention is preferable, as there is no benefit to the patient resulting from prolonged hypercapnia and the duration of the requirement for mechanical ventilation is usually shorter with early intervention.

Treatment of hypoxaemia, defined here as a PaO_2 of less than 60 mm Hg, is initially by increasing the fraction of inspired oxygen (Fio_2) through the provision of supplemental O_2 by intranasal insufflation, but this will be inadequate in patients with significant hypoventilation or ventilation–perfusion mismatching. Mechanical ventilation allows for much higher Fio_2 than can be achieved with insufflation, up to 100%, thereby dramatically increasing alveolar O_2 tension. Mechanical ventilation is also useful in terms of increasing minute ventilation through controlled respiratory rate and volume, and also in recruitment of alveoli for participation in gas exchange. An additional benefit is the decrease in the effort required for respiration, which can be dramatically increased in the face of pulmonary disease, which allows for a substantial decrease in the patient's energy and O_2 needs. This can also ease patient distress and increase patient comfort. The use of recruitment manoeuvres, such as increased baseline airway pressure and sigh manoeuvres can further aid in restoration of lung volumes.

Indications

In equine patients the provision of mechanical ventilatory support is indicated in only a few basic situations. First of these is the patient lacking normal respiratory drive, such as the obtunded or comatose neonatal foal, or the patient with impaired ventilatory effort, such as a patient with botulism. These types of patients are fairly easy to ventilate, as the lungs are not diseased and pulmonary function is relatively normal. A fundamentally different situation is present in the patient with severe pulmonary disease resulting in respiratory failure, such as a foal with severe sepsis, ARDS, meconium aspiration or severe pneumonia. In these patients the presence of pulmonary disease results in profound alterations in pulmonary function, primarily in the form of increased pulmonary resistance and decreased dynamic compliance, making these patients much more challenging to ventilate.

Decision to ventilate

The decision to initiate mechanical ventilation can be an agonising one, due to concerns regarding prognosis, client cost, potential complications and the intimidation factor associated with managing the ventilator. Unfortunately this can result in delays in initiation of therapy that can dramatically decrease the likelihood of a successful outcome. The development of some familiarity with the process of mechanical ventilation on the part of the neonatal intensive care team often results in a willingness to use mechanical ventilation earlier. Training sessions that provide familiarity with ventilator setup and initial settings are extremely useful, as is a pictorial guide to setting up a circuit and attaching it to the patient.

Basic objective guidelines for the decision to ventilate would be persistent hypoxaemia despite nasal insufflation with O_2 ($PaO_2 < 60$ mm Hg), hypercapnia that is severe ($PaCO_2 > 70$ mm Hg), or persistent hypercapnia ($PaCO_2 > 60$ mm Hg) despite pharmacological support of ventilation (caffeine therapy). More subjective criteria include the clinician's assessment of respiratory effort, whether due to muscular exhaustion or worsening central nervous system depression, as well as the clinician's assessment of the patient's degree of respiratory distress. These are important indicators, as many foals will benefit from respiratory support prior to the time that blood gas evaluation makes that clinically obvious. The presence of rib fractures due to birthing trauma can result in a flail chest, which impairs the patient's attempts to generate negative pressure during inspiration, and mechanical ventilation is appropriate in these cases as long as the rib fractures are stabilised and not likely to lacerate the lung. The presence of upper respiratory tract swelling or decreased pharyngeal and laryngeal tone can result in dramatic increases in resistance to airflow, and these cases will benefit from intubation to establish and maintain a patent airway. Unfortunately the endotracheal tube itself is the source of substantial resistance, and this may dramatically increase the work of breathing. The use of mechanical ventilation to support the patient's respiratory efforts can alleviate this effect and decrease the likelihood of respiratory failure.

Initiation of mechanical ventilation

The fundamental concept underlying mechanical ventilation is that gas flows along a pressure gradient from an area of high pressure to an area of low pressure. There are two basic means of generating this pressure gradient using mechanical ventilation, termed negative pressure ventilation and positive pressure ventilation. Negative pressure ventilation consists of enclosing the thorax of the patient in an airtight vessel and generating negative pressure within the vessel. This allows for chest wall expansion as atmospheric pressure provides the positive pressure which forces air into the airways and lungs. This type of ventilator is the classic "iron lung" used primarily half a century ago in human medicine. Positive pressure ventilation (PPV) functions by generating a positive pressure within the patient's airways which is used to overcome the resistance to airflow arising from the airways themselves, the lungs and the thoracic wall. Two types of positive pressure ventilation are commonly used in human medicine, and these are characterised as noninvasive and invasive. Noninvasive PPV relies on a sealed facemask to deliver the positive pressure from the ventilator to the patient's respiratory tract. This avoids the risks associated with tracheal intubation, which include intubation-related trauma, plugging of the endotracheal tube with exudate and increased risk of ventilator associated pneumonia. Unfortunately, noninvasive PPV technology has not yet been adapted for clinical application in equines, primarily due to the difficulty of achieving a tight seal with a facemask. Invasive PPV relies upon intubation for the establishment of an airway for gas exchange, and aids in preventing the aspiration of upper respiratory secretions or refluxed stomach contents.

Intubation is described in Chapter 2.1 for foals, and Chapter 1.1 for adult horses. Nasotracheal intubation is greatly preferred for mechanical ventilation, as it reduces the risk of damage to the tube by the teeth. Care should be taken to ensure that the tip of the tube is located in the cervical portion of the trachea, as it is possible to insert the tube too deeply resulting in placement within a mainstem bronchus and ventilation of only one lung. After final positioning of the tube the cuff should be inflated with only enough pressure to maintain a seal during PPV. Excessive cuff pressure can cause tracheal injury and necrosis. The tube should be anchored to the patient's head to prevent inadvertent removal resulting from patient movement, and this can be done by tying a section of umbilical tape to the hub of the tube and anchoring the ends of the tape to an elastic tape bandage placed around the muzzle or to a soft cotton halter around the patients head (Figure 10.22).

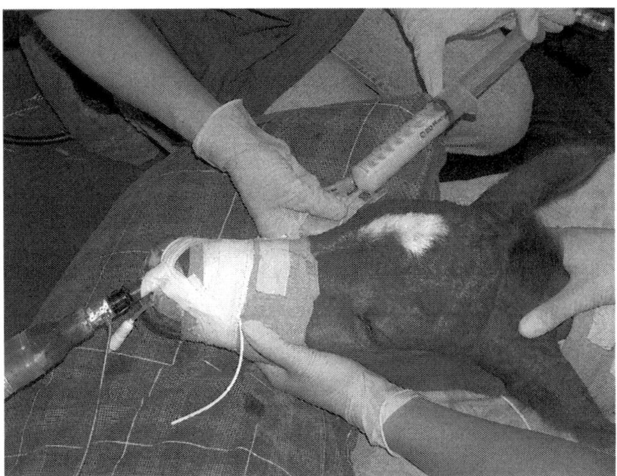

Figure 10.22 Attachment of the nasotracheal tube to an elastic tape bandage placed around the muzzle, to prevent displacement during mechanical ventilation. The foal is also being administered oral drugs via an indwelling stomach tube in this picture. ©Kevin Corley 2005.

Endotracheal tubes should be changed frequently, as respiratory secretions and exudate will accumulate within the lumen of the tube, impeding gas flow and potentially causing obstruction of the tube. While a tube changing interval of 24 hours is generally appropriate, the presence of large amounts of pulmonary exudate may require even more frequent changing of the tube. Suctioning of the endotracheal tube can be performed to remove some of this accumulated material, but is not highly rewarding and causes substantial negative airway pressure resulting in small airway and alveolar collapse and loss of recruited functional capacity.

One must ensure that the ventilator gases will be appropriately pretreated prior to delivery to the patient, in order to ensure that the gases are humidified and warmed and avoid injury to the respiratory mucosa. This can be achieved with an active humidifier, which is typically a component of the mechanical ventilator, and these devices are very effective in humidifying and warming the large volumes of gases involved. Unfortunately the gases tend to cool as they pass through the tubing from the ventilator to the patient, resulting in substantial condensation within the circuit that must be periodically drained. This effect is accentuated if the hospital environmental temperature is low, but can be minimised by using a warming wire in the inspiratory tubing.

Alternatively a passive humidifier can be used, and these consist of a heat-moisture exchange (HME) filter device that is placed in between the ventilator circuit and the patient.[108] These devices are effective with small foals, but may not be adequate for foals over 70 kg, and may need to supplemented with a cold active humidifier in the ventilator circuit.[108] The primary limitation to these HME filters is that they tend to clog with airway discharge, which can result in obstruction and failure of mechanical ventilation.[107,109] For these reasons, the author typically uses HME filters only for short periods of time, such as when first initiating mechanical ventilation, and relies on active humidification for the duration of ventilation.

The settings on the ventilator should be established prior to attaching the patient to the ventilator, in order to avoid inadvertent overinflation of the lungs. Although there are several different ventilator modes to select from on most ventilators, there are some basic settings that are fairly universal. These include the FiO_2, tidal volume, peak flow and breath rate. The FiO_2 should be set to the minimum level required to maintain an adequate PaO_2, but should not be set below 0.21 (the FiO_2 of room air). The tidal volume is the volume of gas delivered with each machine-controlled breath, and this should be set such that the peak inspiratory pressure does not exceed 25 to 35 cm H_2O, in order to avoid trauma to the pulmonary tissues. Peak flow is the maximal gas flow rate delivered by the ventilator during the inspiratory phase of ventilation. Excessive peak flow rates will result in overly rapid inflation of the lungs and high peak airway pressures. Low peak flow rates will result in an overly long inspiratory phase, resulting in a loss of synchrony with the ventilator, especially at high respiratory rates. Reasonable initial settings for these parameters are an FiO_2 of 0.5 (0.3–1.0), a tidal volume of 5 ml/kg (up to 10 ml/kg), a peak flow of 70 L/min (60–80 L/min) and a breath rate of 20 breaths/minute[108] (see also Chapter 2.3). These values may require adjustment once ventilation is instituted, and the response to ventilation should be closely monitored. Additional variables that may be controlled with the ventilator are positive end-expiratory pressure (PEEP), trigger sensitivity, pressure support, base flow and flow trigger. Not all of these variables will be available in the different modes of ventilator function, so they will be discussed where appropriate.

Modes

When considering mechanical ventilation one encounters a bewildering array of modes of ventilation, but it should be kept in mind that the ideal mode is one that maintains consistent and adequate tidal volume and minute ventilation at moderate airway pressures, is synchronised to the patient's respiratory efforts, responds to patient demands and allows for the lowest possible work of breathing.[105] By considering these goals one can more effectively evaluate these modes as they are discussed, and thereby determine which mode may be most appropriate for a particular clinical patient. Fundamentally, there are two basic modes of inspiratory gas delivery in PPV, termed volume controlled and pressure controlled.[110]

In volume controlled ventilation, the desired tidal volume is set, and the pressure delivered by the ventilator is varied in order to achieve the desired volume. This approach risks trauma to the lungs if the desired tidal volume is too large for the patient. In pressure controlled ventilation, the desired peak inspiratory pressure is set, and the tidal volume achieved will vary depending on lung compliance. This approach decreases the risk of pulmonary trauma, but may not achieve adequate tidal volumes for effective ventilation. Once the desired inspiratory gas has been delivered, the ventilator must determine when to cycle from inspiration to expiration. This is determined based upon a set inspiratory phase duration (time cycled), a decrease in inspiratory flow, usually to 25% of peak (flow cycled) or once a set tidal volume is achieved (volume cycled). Once expiration has occurred, the ventilator must be triggered to provide another inspiration, and this is accomplished based upon time, pressure or flow. Time triggering is where a mandatory breath rate per minute has been set, and inspiration will occur at the interval required to achieve that rate. Pressure triggering depends upon a decrease in airway pressure resulting from the patient's own inspiratory effort. Flow triggering is used in ventilatory modes wherein a base flow of gas is always circulating through the circuit, and the trigger is an increase in flow rate that results from the patient's inspiratory effort. When considering different ventilator modes, it is also useful to consider what type of breathing pattern is utilised, and these include mandatory breaths which are completely determined by the set breath rate, assisted breaths which are initiated by the patient and supported by the ventilator, and spontaneous breaths which are completely patient driven, with only enough pressure provided by the ventilator to maintain positive airway pressure during inspiration.

With an understanding of these different aspects of breath control, one can consider the actual modes that can be selected on the mechanical ventilator. While different models of ventilator will have different selections of modes, in general the modes consist of controlled mandatory ventilation (CMV), assist-control ventilation (ACV), synchronised intermittent mandatory ventilation (SIMV), pressure support ventilation (PSV) and continuous positive airway pressure (CPAP).[108] In CMV, the ventilator exerts complete control over breathing and does not allow any spontaneous patient initiated breaths. This mode is very unforgiving and is poorly tolerated in the conscious patient, rendering it useful only in comatose or anesthetised patients. In general, it is preferred to allow the patient as much control over ventilation as possible, and CMV is rarely used by the author for these reasons. In ACV, there is a mandatory baseline breath rate of machine-delivered breaths; however, the patient can trigger additional breaths that are then delivered in the same manner as the mandatory breaths. The rigid control of volume, inspiratory time and flow rate in each breath is unforgiving to the patient, however, and is often poorly tolerated in the conscious patient.

SIMV is a modification of assist-control ventilation that still delivers a set minimum rate of mandatory breaths, which are rigidly controlled; however, the ventilator attempts to synchronise these breaths with the patient's inspiratory efforts if possible. The primary advantage of this mode is that it is well tolerated by the patient due to the synchronisation of mandatory breaths with patient effort (Figure 10.23). In addition, SIMV ensures a minimum breath rate in patients with variable respiratory efforts or that are exhibiting periods of apnoea. The limitation of SIMV is that the spontaneous breaths are not supported by the ventilator and require a large degree of patient inspiratory effort. PSV allows the patient complete control over all aspects of the ventilatory cycle except for the pressure limit. In this mode, each patient breath is supported by a preset assist pressure, which is stopped when the flow rate decreases below a set fraction of peak flow at end inspiration. This allows the patient to determine the size of the breath and the inspiratory flow rate, substantially decreasing the work of breathing. The risk of PSV is that there is no mandatory minimal breath rate guaranteed by the ventilator. The limitations of SIMV and PSV can be overcome by using them together, which is possible on many ventilators, with the SIMV providing a guaranteed minimal breath rate and the PSV providing pressure support of the patient-initiated breaths to overcome the inherent resistance of the ventilator circuit and endotracheal tube.

CPAP is used only with a spontaneously breathing patient, and provides for a positive airway pressure throughout the ventilatory cycle. The pressure that is provided is typically the clinician selected PEEP (positive end-expiratory pressure) level. The primary limitation to CPAP is that it may not provide adequate support to overcome the resistance of the ventilator circuit and endotracheal tube, although if used inappropriately it can substantially worsen pulmonary compliance and resistance and decrease cardiac output.[108] It is often beneficial to combine CPAP with PSV to aid in overcoming the resistance of the circuit and thereby decrease the work of breathing. This can be

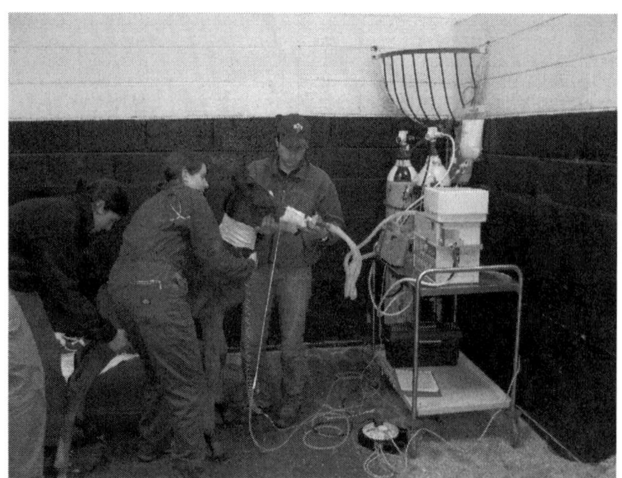

Figure 10.23 Ventilation of a conscious foal with Synchronised Intermittent Mandatory Ventilation (SIMV). The foal is not sedated, and is being supported to stand. ©Kevin Corley 2007.

achieved on many ventilators by setting the breath rate to zero in the SIMV/PSV mode.

The progression of modes from CMV to PSV as discussed earlier may in some cases constitute the clinical progression for the ventilated patient, especially in foals with profound central nervous system dysfunction or severe pulmonary disease, as they require a great deal of external control over ventilation initially but can be weaned to support modes as their clinical condition improves. However, while CMV can certainly be used, a preferable initial mode is arguably ACV, as this provides as much control as CMV but allows for patient-initiated breaths. In ACV the available settings are tidal volume, breath rate, peak flow and assist sensitivity. Assist sensitivity is the pressure trigger setting that determines when a patient-initiated breath should be supported, and this should be set to 2 to 3 cm H_2O initially.[108] Too low a setting will result in inadvertent triggering due to patient motion, while too high a setting may prevent the recognition of any patient's inspiratory efforts. As the patient's condition improves, the assist sensitivity setting can be increased gradually to assess the patient's capability of ventilating spontaneously and to challenge the inspiratory muscles and prepare them better for when ventilatory support is discontinued.

Due to the rigid restrictions of CMV and ACV on the parameters of ventilation, the most frequently used initial mode in the author's clinic is SIMV/PSV. This combined mode allows for complete control of ventilation if there are no spontaneous respiratory efforts by the patient but will provide pressure support if inspiratory efforts occur. Initial settings are tidal volume, breath rate, peak flow and assist sensitivity, with the addition of a pressure support setting (see Box 2.4). The pressure support required is dependent upon the pulmonary compliance of the patient, and patients without substantial pulmonary disease may require as little as 8 to 12 cm H_2O, while the presence of pulmonary disease may increase the required level to 20 to 25 cm H_2O or higher.[108] A typical initial setting for pressure support is 15 to 18 cm H_2O, with subsequent adjustment based upon clinical monitoring of the response to ventilation. If the tidal volume generated is too low, then higher pressures will be required. In general, care should be taken that the peak inspiratory pressure does not exceed 25 to 30 cm H_2O, as this substantially increases the risk of barotrauma. Pressure support may not be appropriate in patients with severe pulmonary dysfunction, as inadequate levels of pressure support may inappropriately shorten or prolong the inspiratory phase, resulting in further impairment of pulmonary function.[108] This mode, however, has excellent utility in the patient without severe pulmonary dysfunction, is generally well tolerated and lends itself to a process of gradually decreasing ventilatory support prior to discontinuing mechanical ventilation.

As mechanical ventilation is used with greater frequency, the clinician will find it useful for support of patients that previously would not have been considered candidates for ventilation, and these patients are typically conscious and only require support to decrease the work of breathing until they are strong enough to adequately ventilate themselves. In this situation, there is no need to begin with rigid modes such as CMV or ACV, as pressure support may be all that is required. Starting with CPAP with pressure support in these patients will alleviate the distress associated with impaired respiration and typically is well tolerated. As the patient's strength returns, the degree of pressure support can be decreased and the trigger sensitivity can be increased prior to discontinuing ventilatory support.

Recruitment manoeuvres

It is generally desirable when ventilating a patient to not only provide for the minimal ventilatory needs of the patient but also utilise the ventilator to recruit poorly ventilated regions of the lung back into participation in gas exchange. The most commonly utilised recruitment manoeuvre (RM) is PEEP, which functions to maintain positive pressure within the ventilatory circuit during exhalation and between breaths to prevent alveolar collapse that might result during periods of negative pressure. Over time, the presence of PEEP will keep open the alveoli that are "recruited" during the inspiratory cycle, and this allows for gradual improvement in the functional capacity of the lungs. This can result in substantial increases in PaO_2, and may allow for a decrease in the FIO_2.[111] By preventing cyclical alveolar collapse and reopening PEEP may also decrease the amount of shear stress–induced pulmonary injury.[111] The use of PEEP is not always benign, however, as it can cause compression of the intrathoracic venous system and impair cardiac return, with detrimental effects on cardiac output. A typical initial PEEP setting is from 3 to 5 cm H_2O, although this may require adjustment based upon clinical response. When first initiating mechanical ventilation it is reasonable to use PEEP in most patients, especially at moderate settings, as the benefits appear to outweigh the potential negative effects. Care should be taken to avoid routine use of settings above 5 cm H_2O, as this can impair venous return or contribute to high airway pressures and pressure and/or volume associated trauma to the lungs. In some circumstances, however, PEEP may be judiciously used up to settings of 10 cm H_2O. It has been demonstrated in human patients with acute respiratory distress syndrome that high PEEP levels (>12 cm H_2O) in combination with low tidal volume ventilation (6 ml/kg) is associated with improved recruitment and improved outcome.[112]

Without additional recruitment, PEEP may over inflate the functional airspaces in the lung and actually increase the severity of ventilation–perfusion mismatching.[113] For this reason the effectiveness of PEEP may be enhanced if other techniques are used to recruit injured lung units, which can then be kept patent by the presence of PEEP. These recruitment manoeuvres consist of the intermittent application of high levels of airway pressure, with the goal of "prying open" nonventilated lung units.[113] There are a variety of recruitment manoeuvres, but the most commonly used is the "sigh" manoeuvre. The sigh manoeuvre is the intermittent application of volume-controlled breaths where the tidal volume is up to 150% greater than the normal tidal volume, which will also result in higher peak airway pressures. This is generally well tolerated but may not be extremely effective in the face of substantial pulmonary disease. Sighs may be more effective when using low tidal volume ventilation, as there can be a tendency toward alveolar derecruitment with that ventilator strategy.[114] More complicated and aggressive recruitment techniques involving stepwise increases in pressure or sustained periods of high pressure are used in human medicine; however, these are beyond the scope of the current discussion. Interestingly, a recent study performed in experimental animals found that the most important determining factor in the efficacy of these manoeuvres was the postrecruitment level of PEEP and suggested that RMs achieved little more than the use of PEEP alone.[113] There is also evidence that RMs can be deleterious by inducing volume trauma and that they are not indicated in cases of bacterial pneumonia.[113,115] Due to these concerns, the author rarely uses RMs other than the sigh manoeuvre in the clinical setting.

Monitoring

The provision of mechanical ventilation is a very dynamic process requiring substantial involvement of the clinician in the supervision of ventilator setup and adjustment. Appropriate monitoring is critical to effective mechanical ventilation, and this cannot be overemphasised. The two most important aspects of monitoring are the assessment of pulmonary mechanics and pulmonary function. When considering the assessment of pulmonary mechanics one is really analysing the interaction of the mechanical ventilator and the patient, and the three most important parameters are the driving pressure, the tidal volume and tidal airflow. The primary parameters of ventilator function and ventilator/patient interaction are the peak inspiratory pressure (PIP) and tidal volume (V_T). These parameters are interrelated, as increasing pressures will be associated with increasing tidal volume in normal lungs within normal physiological limits. In ventilated patients, especially those with substantial pulmonary disease, one will often find that this relationship is abnormal, with normal pressures resulting in inadequate tidal volumes, or excessively high pressures being required to achieve a desired V_T. Continuous monitoring of PIP is extremely important, as sudden decreases may indicate a circuit leak, ventilator failure, inadequate gas supply or a leak in the endotracheal tube cuff.[108] Increases in PIP may indicate obstruction of the endotracheal tube due to kinking or accumulation of exudate, bronchospasm or pneumothorax.[108] When one is actually assessing the effectiveness of ventilation, the value of greatest interest is the driving pressure (P_{Dr}), which is the pressure gradient between the PIP and the PEEP setting, as this is the pressure required to overcome the resistance of the circuit, endotracheal tube and respiratory system. By examining the relationship between P_{Dr} and V_T one can derive an indirect approximation of the total respiratory compliance, which is fundamentally the change in volume (ml) per 1 cm H_2O change in P_{Dr}.[116] A decrease in compliance will occur with worsening pulmonary disease, as the lungs become less elastic. Assessment of the effective respiratory compliance is facilitated with some ventilators, as they will dynamically calculate and display this value, and in some cases the ventilator will also graphically display pressure-volume loops for each breath.

The other critical aspect of monitoring involves monitoring of pulmonary function, which fundamentally consists of the evaluation of pulmonary ventilation, in the form of elimination of CO_2, and pulmonary oxygenation, in the form of arterial O_2 tension. The monitoring of ventilation requires knowledge of the patients $Paco_2$, as the degree of alveolar ventilation is inversely proportional to $Paco_2$. The other important value is V_T, as this value provides important insight into the degree of alveolar ventilation. Alveolar ventilation is fundamentally derived by multiplying the breath rate by the difference between V_T and the deadspace ventilation (V_D). As deadspace ventilation can be difficult to accurately determine one must realise that in the presence of a constant Vd any changes in breath rate or V_T will result in proportional changes in $Paco_2$.[116] Given this relationship one can infer that inadequate ventilation can be addressed by increases in breath rate and/or V_T. Additional information can be derived from knowledge of the exhaled CO_2 concentration ($ETCO_2$), which is measured using capnography. The $ETCO_2$ is representative of the $Paco_2$ in patients with normal pulmonary function, usually having a value 2 to 5 mm Hg less than the $Paco_2$.[108] This relationship does not hold up in the presence of pulmonary disease, and the changes observed provide valuable information regarding the ventilation-perfusion relationship within the lungs. Specifically, given the $ETCO_2$ and the $Paco_2$ one can determine the V_D, simply by the equation $Paco_2 - ETCO_2/Paco_2$ (see Chapter 10.1). Increases in V_D can occur with decreased pulmonary perfusion secondary to decreases in cardiac output or increases in pulmonary vascular resistance.[108]

Assessment of pulmonary oxygenation relies primarily upon the measured Pao_2, as the Fio_2 is known. In the patient with normal pulmonary function there should be a linear increase in Pao_2 with increasing Fio_2, but this relationship breaks down in the presence of pulmonary disease, due to ventilation–perfusion mismatching. The presence of intrapulmonary shunts, resulting from the perfusion of poorly ventilated regions of the lungs, will cause the Pao_2 to be lower than expected. This physiological shunt fraction can be calculated (see Chapter 10.1), but this is rarely required in the clinical setting. The clinical import derives from the appreciation that the measured PaO_2 is lower than expected given the delivered FIO_2. This information alerts the clinician that areas of the lung are not participating in gas exchange, indicating a possible worsening of pulmonary disease and potentially indicating the need for increased PEEP or the use of other recruitment manoeuvres. A reasonable target for PaO_2 is 80 to 100 mm Hg or slightly higher, as values above 150 mm Hg are not beneficial and are an indication to decrease the FIO_2. The goal is to use the FIO_2 closest to room air (0.21) that achieves the desired PaO_2, and one should keep in mind that FIO_2 values above 60% are associated with O_2 toxicity to the respiratory mucosa.

An important aspect of clinical monitoring is to check the endotracheal tube for exudate accumulation when the tube is changed, which should be done at least daily (more often if copious exudate is present). An increase in the amount of exudate within the tube, or a change in the character of the exudate to a more purulent appearance, may be early indications of ventilator-associated pneumonia. A haemorrhagic appearance to the tube exudate may suggest ventilator-associated lung injury (VILI) or worsening of pulmonary inflammation due to other insults.

Weaning

The discontinuation of mechanical ventilation ("weaning") can be the most challenging part of the entire process, and in human patients this phase may constitute as much as 50% of the time the patient is being mechanically ventilated.[117] Arguably, the process of weaning begins as soon as the patient is placed on the ventilator, as the clinician constantly strives to identify the minimum level of support required to maintain adequate ventilation and oxygenation. By minimising the degree of support one can accelerate the patient's recovery of strength and stamina in the muscles of respiration (or minimise its loss), while also increasing the clinician's ability to identify when the patient no longer requires ventilatory support. Progressive challenge of the patient's ability to ventilate on its own can be accomplished by gradually decreasing the level of pressure support provided and increasing the trigger sensitivity level. Prior to weaning, machine-delivered breaths should be discontinued, and support provided with PSV or CPAP. Ultimately however the determination of readiness to be removed from the ventilator is a subjective one, and the question can only be answered by an extubation challenge. This is preferable to simply removing the patient from the ventilator while leaving the endotracheal tube in place, as the tube causes significant resistance to airflow and increases the patient's work of breathing. Intranasal O_2 insufflation should be provided immediately following tube removal in most cases, unless the patient has been maintaining normal oxygenation at an FIO_2 of 0.21 while on the ventilator. Care must also be taken that one is fully prepared to *immediately* reintubate the patient if the challenge is not successful and mechanical ventilation must be reinstituted. The primary endpoints of the challenge are respiratory rate, respiratory effort and arterial blood gas evaluation and some patients may fail within minutes while others fail over several hours. Several challenges may be required over a period of hours to days before one is certain that the patient is able to maintain itself without ventilatory support.

Complications

The administration of mechanical ventilation is inherently unnatural and unphysiological, and has the potential to disrupt the normal functioning of many body systems. The provision of PPV, especially in the form of excess PEEP, has the potential to substantially decrease venous return, leading to impaired cardiac output. This is a serious concern, especially in the critically ill patient where cardiac output is likely already impaired. The presence of an endotracheal tube has a number of potential adverse effects. Firstly, the tube causes an increase in airway resistance due to a long narrow lumen, and increases the work of breathing associated with spontaneous respirations. Secondly, the presence of the endotracheal tube results in a bypass of the normal protective functions of the upper respiratory tract, and can allow access to the respiratory tract for pathogenic organisms. Infections arising by this route are termed ventilator-associated pneumonia (VAP), and the likelihood of VAP developing is increased with prolonged duration of mechanical ventilation. The presence of inflammation secondary to the process of mechanical ventilation itself will also increase the likelihood of VAP, as will impairment of the patient's immune function associated with systemic illness. The organisms involved in VAP are often nosocomial in nature, which can be associated with a pattern of increased resistance to antimicrobials, complicating treatment of the condition. Aerosolised ceftazidime has been shown to be effective in the prevention of VAP in human patients, while also attenuating the proinflammatory response in the lung.[118] The author has subjectively observed a decreased rate of VAP in mechanically ventilated foals when aerosolised amikacin is nebulised into the ventilator circuit once daily (8 mg/kg) starting within 24 hours of the initiation of mechanical ventilation. One significant clinical manifestation of this effect is a substantial reduction in the amount of exudate that accumulates within the endotracheal tube.

VILI should be considered to be inevitable, and the clinicians goal is fundamentally to minimise the severity of this effect. There are three fundamental types of VILI: barotrauma, volutrauma and atelectotrauma.[119] Barotrauma is typically monitored for using PIP, although a more clinically relevant assessment would come from monitoring the transpulmonary pressure (alveolar minus pleural pressure), however this is not routinely done.[119] Interestingly there is some evidence that the pulmonary injury associated with barotrauma may actually be the result of excessive volume (volutrauma), rather than the pressure itself, as limitation of chest wall expansion prevents barotrauma in the experimental setting.[120] In patients with poor pulmonary compliance and areas of pulmonary atelectasis high PIP may be required to achieve adequate ventilation, and this causes overdistension of the ventilated regions of the lung (local volutrauma).[111] Volutrama results from exceeding the normal physiological functional residual capacity of the ventilated regions of the lung, and results in the development of pulmonary oedema and initiation/amplification of the local inflammatory response. PEEP is somewhat protective in that it appears to slow the development of pulmonary oedema unless it too is excessive, at which point it contributes to overinflation and causes further harm.[121] Atelectotrauma is due to the repeated opening and closing of lung units during tidal ventilation, and essentially represents a syndrome of low-volume injury resulting in the initiation of an inflammatory response.[119] By appreciating that the lungs are susceptible to both high and low volume injury it is apparent that optimal mechanical ventilation is achieved within a fairly narrow range of tidal volumes, and that this range may vary dramatically from patient to patient.

References

1. Raidal SL, Bailey GD, Love DN: Effect of transportation on lower respiratory tract contamination and peripheral blood neutrophil function. Aust Vet J 75:433-438, 1997
2. Ciepichal J, Kubler A: Effect of general and regional anesthesia on some neutrophil functions. Arch Immunol Ther Exp (Warsz) 46:183-192, 1998
3. Whitwell KE, Greet TR: Collection and evaluation of tracheobronchial washes in the horse. Equine Vet J 16:499-508, 1984
4. Hoffman A, Viel L: Techniques for sampling the respiratory tract of horses. Vet Clin North Am 13:463-475, 1997
5. Darien BJ, Brown CM, Walker RD, et al.: A tracheoscopic technique for obtaining uncontaminated lower airway secretions for bacterial culture in the horse. Equine Vet J 22:170-173, 1990
6. Sweeney CR, Sweeney RW III, Benson CE: Comparison of bacteria isolated from specimens obtained by use of endoscopic guarded tracheal swabbing and percutaneous tracheal aspiration in horses. J Am Vet Med Assoc 195:1225-1229, 1989
7. Hodgson JL, Hodgson DR: Tracheal aspirates: Indications, technique and interpretation, in Hoffman AM (ed): Current Therapy in Equine Medicine, ed 5. St Louis, WB Saunders, 2003, pp 401-406
8. Powers CN: Diagnosis of infectious diseases: a cytopathologist's perspective. Clin Microbiol Rev 11:341-365, 1998
9. Zinkl JG: Lower respiratory tract, in Cowell RL, Tyler RD (eds): Cytology and Hematology of the Horse. St Louis, Mosby, 2002, pp 73-86
10. Beech J: Cytology of tracheobronchial aspirates in horses. Vet Pathol 12:157-164, 1975
11. Fogarty U: Evaluation of a bronchoalveolar lavage technique. Equine Vet J 22:174-176, 1990
12. Derksen FJ, Brown CM, Sonea I, et al.: Comparison of transtracheal aspirate and bronchoalveolar lavage cytology in 50 horses with chronic lung disease. Equine Vet J 21:23-26, 1989
13. Ito S, Hobo S, Eto D, et al.: Bronchoalveolar lavage for the diagnosis and treatment of pneumonia associated with transport in Thoroughbred racehorses. J Vet Med Sci 63: 1263-1269, 2001
14. McKenzie HC: Bronchial lavage for the treatment of focal pneumonia, Proceedings of the 23rd Annual ACVIM Forum, Baltimore, 2005
15. Viel L, Hewson J: Bronchoalveolar lavage, in Robinson NE (ed): Current Therapy in Equine Medicine, ed 5. St. Louis, WB Saunders, 2003
16. Hodgson JL, Hodgson DR: Inflammatory airway disease, in Lekeux P (ed): Equine Respiratory Diseases. Ithaca, NY, International Veterinary Information Service (www.ivis.org), 2002
17. Doucet MY, Viel L: Alveolar macrophage graded hemosiderin score from bronchoalveolar lavage in horses with exercise-induced pulmonary hemorrhage and controls. J Vet Intern Med 16:281-286, 2002
18. Schott HC, II, Mansmann RA: Thoracic drainage in horses. Compend Contin Educ Pract Vet 12:251-256, 258-261, 1990
19. Raidal SL: Equine pleuropneumonia. Br Vet J 151:233-262, 1995
20. Chaffin MK, Carter GK, Relford RL: Equine bacterial pleuropneumonia. II. Clinical signs and diagnostic evaluation. Comp Cont Educ Pract Vet 16:362-379, 1994
21. Bain FT: Cytology of the respiratory tract. Vet Clin North Am Equine Pract 13:477-486, 1997
22. Deane JC, Dagleish MP, Benamou AE, et al.: Effects of syringe material and temperature and duration of storage on the stability of equine arterial blood gas variables. Vet Anaesth Analg 31:250-257, 2004
23. Roy M-F, Lavoie JP: Tools for the diagnosis of equine respiratory disorders. Vet Clin North Am Eq Pract 19:1-17, 2003
24. Van Erck E, Art T, Lekeux P: Normal respiratory values, in Lekeux P (ed): Equine Respiratory Diseases. Ithaca, NY, International Veterinary Information Service (www.ivis.org), 2005
25. Derksen FJ, Robinson NE: Overview of the equine respiratory system, in Lekeux P (ed): Equine respiratory Diseases. Ithaca, NY, International Veterinary Information Service (www.ivis.org), 2002
26. George SC, Hlastala MP, Souders JE, et al.: Gas exchange in the airways. J Aerosol Med 9:25-33, 1996
27. Davis MS, Murray MJ, Donaldson LL: Clinical assessment of gas exchange in mature horses. Equine Vet J 30:396-400, 1998
28. Van Erck E, Votion D, Art T, et al.: Measurement of respiratory function by impulse oscillometry in horses. Equine Vet J 36:21-28, 2004
29. Mazan MR, Hoffman AM, Manjerovic N: Comparison of forced oscillation with the conventional method for histamine bronchoprovocation testing in horses. Am J Vet Res 60:174-180, 1999

30. Reef VB: Ultrasonographic evaluation, in Beech J (ed): Equine Respiratory Disorders. Philadelphia, Lea and Febiger, 1991, pp 69-88
31. Rantanen NW: Thoracic ultrasound, in Rantanen NW, McKinnon AO (eds): Equine Diagnostic Ultrasonography. Baltimore, Williams and Wilkins, 1998, pp 41-46
32. Gross DK, Morley PS, Hinchcliff KW, et al.: Pulmonary ultrasonographic abnormalities associated with naturally occurring equine influenza virus infection in standardbred racehorses. J Vet Intern Med 18:718-727, 2004
33. Reimer JM, Reef VB, Spencer PA: Ultrasonography as a diagnostic aid in horses with anaerobic bacterial pleuropneumonia and/or pulmonary abscessation: 27 cases (1984-1986). J Am Vet Med Assoc 194:278-282, 1989
34. Reef VB, Boy MG, Reid CF, et al.: Comparison between diagnostic ultrasonography and radiography in the evaluation of horses and cattle with thoracic disease: 56 cases (1984-1985). J Am Vet Med Assoc 198:2112-2118, 1991
35. Anonymous: The thorax, in Colles CM, Dyson SJ, Kold SE, et al. (eds): Clinical Radiology of the Horse. Oxford, Blackwell Publishing Professional, 2000, pp 483-528
36. Duvivier DH, Votion D, Vandenput S, et al.: Aerosol therapy in the equine species. Vet J 154:189-202, 1997
37. Lipworth BJ: Pharmacokinetics of inhaled drugs. Br J Clin Pharmacol 42:697-705, 1996
38. Gough PA, Jordan NS: A review of the therapeutic efficacy of aerosolized and endotracheally instilled antibiotics. Pharmacotherapy 2:367-377, 1982
39. Newman SP, Clarke SW: Therapeutic aerosols, 1: physical and practical considerations. Thorax 38:881-886, 1983
40. Newman SP: Aerosol deposition considerations in inhalation therapy. Chest 88:152S-160S, 1985
41. Gupta P, Hickey A: Contemporary approaches in aerosolized drug delivery to the lung. J Control Release 17:129-148, 1991
42. Smith SJ, Bernstein JA: Therapeutic uses of lung aerosols, in Hickey AJ (ed): Inhalation Aerosols: Physical and Biological Basis for Therapy. New York, Marcel Dekker, 1996, pp 233-269
43. Hall CB, McBride JT: Pulmonary infections, in Moren F, Dolovich MB, Newhouse MT, et al (eds): Aerosols in medicine. Principles, diagnosis and Therapy. London, Elsevier Science Publishers, 1993, pp 291-301
44. Atkins PJ, Barker NP, Mathisen D: The design and development of inhalation drug delivery systems, in Hickey AJ (ed): Pharmaceutical Inhalation Aerosol Technology. New York, Marcel Dekker, 1992, pp 155-185
45. Ammann VJ, Vrins AA, Lavoie JP: Effects of inhaled beclomethasone dipropionate on respiratory function in horses with chronic obstructive pulmonary disease (COPD). Equine Vet J 30:152-157, 1998
46. Mazan MR, Hoffman AM: Effects of aerosolized albuterol on physiologic responses to exercise in standardbreds. Am J Vet Res 62:1812-1817, 2001
47. Derksen FJ, Olszewski M, Robinson NE, et al.: Use of a hand-held, metered-dose aerosol delivery device to administer pirbuterol acetate to horses with "heaves." Equine Vet J 28:306-310, 1996
48. Tesarowski DB, Viel L, McDonell WN, et al.: The rapid and effective administration of a beta 2-agonist to horses with heaves using a compact inhalation device and metered-dose inhalers. Can Vet J 35:170-173, 1994
49. Bayly WM, Duvivier DH, Votion D, et al.: Effects of inhaled ipratropium bromide on breathing mechanics and gas exchange in exercising horses with chronic obstructive pulmonary disease. Equine Vet J 34:36-43, 2002
50. Bayly WM, Slocombe RF, Schott HC 2nd, et al.: Effects of inhalation of albuterol sulphate, ipratroprium bromide and frusemide on breathing mechanics and gas exchange in healthy exercising horses. Equine Vet J 33:302-310, 2001
51. Bailey J, Colahan P, Kubilis P, et al.: Effect of inhaled beta 2 adrenoceptor agonist, albuterol sulphate, on performance of horses. Equine Vet J Suppl 30:575-580, 1999
52. Robinson NE, Derksen FJ, Berney C, et al.: The airway response of horses with recurrent airway obstruction (heaves) to aerosol administration of ipratropium bromide. Equine Vet J 25:299-303, 1993
53. Hardy JG, Newman SP, Knoch M: Lung deposition from four nebulizers. Respir Med 87:461-465, 1993
54. Votion D, Ghafir Y, Munsters K, et al.: Aerosol deposition in equine lungs following ultrasonic nebulisation versus jet aerosol delivery system. Equine Vet J 29:388-393, 1997
55. Hickey AJ: Summary of common approaches to pharmaceutical aerosol administration, in Hickey AJ (ed): Pharmaceutical Inhalation Aerosol Technology. New York, Marcel Dekker, 1992, pp 255-288
56. Faurisson F, Dessanges JF, Grimfeld A, et al.: Nebulizer performance: AFLM study. Respiration 62(Suppl 1):13-18, 1995
57. Dalby RN, Tiano SL, Hickey AJ: Medical devices for the delivery of therapeutic aerosols to the lungs, in Hickey AJ (ed): Pharmaceutical Inhalation Aerosol Technology. New York, Marcel Dekker, 1992, pp 441-473
58. Martonen T, Yang Y: Deposition mechanics of pharmaceutical particles in human airways, in Hickey AJ (ed): Pharmaceutical Inhalation Aerosol Technology. New York, Marcel Dekker, 1992, pp 57-68
59. Duvivier DH, Votion D, Vandenput S, et al.: Technical validation of a face mask adapted for dry powder inhalation in the equine species. Equine Vet J 29:471-476, 1997
60. Viel L, Tesarowski D: Radioaerosol deposition in equids. Proceedings of the American Association of Equine Practitioners, Vancouver, 1994
61. Derksen FJ, Olszewski MA, Robinson NE, et al.: Aerosolized albuterol sulfate used as a bronchodilator in horses with recurrent airway obstruction. Am J Vet Res 60:689-693, 1999
62. Henrikson SL, Rush BR: Efficacy of salmeterol xinafoate in horses with recurrent airway obstruction. J Am Vet Med Assoc 218:1961-1965, 2001
63. Duvivier D, Votion D, Vandenput S, et al.: Airway response of horses with COPD to dry powder inhalation of ipratroprium bromide. Vet Jour 154:149-153, 1997
64. Rush BR, Raub ES, Rhoads WS, et al.: Pulmonary function in horses with recurrent airway obstruction after aerosol and parenteral administration of beclomethasone dipropionate and dexamethasone, respectively. Am J Vet Res 59:1039-1043, 1998
65. Rush BR, Flaminio MJ, Matson CJ, et al.: Cytologic evaluation of bronchoalveolar lavage fluid from horses with recurrent airway obstruction after aerosol and parenteral

administration of beclomethasone dipropionate and dexamethasone, respectively. Am J Vet Res 59:1033-1038, 1998
66. Couetil LL, Art T, de Moffarts B, et al.: Effect of beclomethasone dipropionate and dexamethasone isonicotinate on lung function, bronchoalveolar lavage fluid cytology, and transcription factor expression in airways of horses with recurrent airway obstruction. J Vet Intern Med 20:399-406, 2006
67. Ammann V, Lavoie J, Vrins A: Effects of beclomethasone dipropionate in horses with chronic obstructive pulmonary disease (COPD). Proceedings of the 13th ACVIM Forum, Lake Buena Vista, FL, 1995 (available from ACVIM)
68. Couetil LL, Chilcoat CD, DeNicola DB, et al.: Randomized, controlled study of inhaled fluticasone propionate, oral administration of prednisone, and environmental management of horses with recurrent airway obstruction. Am J Vet Res 66:1665-1674, 2005
69. Laan TT, Westermann CM, Dijkstra AV, et al.: Biological availability of inhaled fluticasone propionate in horses. Vet Rec 155:361-364, 2004
70. Giguère S, Viel L, Lee E, et al.: Cytokine induction in pulmonary airways of horses with heaves and effect of therapy with inhaled fluticasone propionate. Vet Immunol Immunopathol 85:147-158, 2002
71. McKenzie HC, 3rd, Murray MJ: Concentrations of gentamicin in serum and bronchial lavage fluid after once-daily aerosol administration to horses for seven days. Am J Vet Res 65:173-178, 2004
72. Derksen FJ, Robinson NE, Berney CE: Aerosol pirbuterol: bronchodilator activity and side effects in ponies with recurrent airway obstruction (heaves). Equine Vet J 24:107-112, 1992
73. Rush BR: Treatment of inflammatory airway disease: aerosol delivery devices and medications. Proceedings of the 48th AAEP Annual Convention, Orlando, FL, 2002 (available from AAEP)
74. Handley D: The asthma-like pharmacology and toxicology of (S)-isomers of beta agonists. J Allergy Clin Immunol 104: 1999
75. Salpeter SR, Ormiston TM, Salpeter EE: Meta-analysis: respiratory tolerance to regular beta2-agonist use in patients with asthma. Ann Intern Med 140:802-813, 2004
76. Cockcroft DW: As-needed inhaled beta2-adrenoceptor agonists in moderate-to-severe asthma: current recommendations. Treat Respir Med 4:169-174, 2005
77. Johnson M: Molecular mechanisms of beta(2)-adrenergic receptor function, response, and regulation. J Allergy Clin Immunol 117:18-24; quiz 25, 2006
78. Robinson NE, Derksen FJ, Olszewski MA, et al.: The pathogenesis of chronic obstructive pulmonary disease of horses. Br Vet J 152:283-306, 1996
79. Pearson EG, Riebold TW: Comparison of bronchodilators in alleviating clinical signs in horses with chronic obstructive pulmonary disease. J Am Vet Med Assoc 194:1287-1291, 1989
80. Murphy JR, McPherson EA, Dixon PM: Chronic obstructive pulmonary disease (COPD): effects of bronchodilator drugs on normal and affected horses. Equine Vet J 12:10-14, 1980
81. Duvivier DH, Bayly WM, Votion D, et al.: Effects of inhaled dry powder ipratropium bromide on recovery from exercise of horses with COPD. Equine Vet J 31:20-24, 1999
82. Beeh KM, Welte T, Buhl R: Anticholinergics in the treatment of chronic obstructive pulmonary disease. Respiration 69:372-379, 2002
83. Rennard SI, Serby CW, Ghafouri M, et al.: Extended therapy with ipratropium is associated with improved lung function in patients with COPD. A retrospective analysis of data from seven clinical trials. Chest 110:62-70, 1996
84. Auerbach D, Baughman R, Boyars M, et al.: Routine nebulized ipratropium and albuterol together are better than either alone in COPD. The COMBIVENT Inhalation Solution Study Group. Chest 112:1514-1521, 1997
85. Rush BR, Raub ES, Thomsen MM, et al.: Pulmonary function and adrenal gland suppression with incremental doses of aerosolized beclomethasone dipropionate in horses with recurrent airway obstruction. J Am Vet Med Assoc 217:359-364, 2000
86. Rush BR, Trevino IC, Matson CJ, et al.: Serum cortisol concentrations in response to incremental doses of inhaled beclomethasone dipropionate. Equine Vet J 31:258-261, 1999
87. McKenzie HC: Characterization of antimicrobial aerosols for administration to horses. Vet Ther 4:110-119, 2003
88. Sin DD, Man SF: Corticosteroids and adrenoceptor agonists: the compliments for combination therapy in chronic airways diseases. Eur J Pharmacol 533:28-35, 2006
89. Lavoie JP, Fiset L, Laverty S: Review of 40 cases of lung abscesses in foals and adult horses. Equine Vet J 26:348-352, 1994
90. Raphel CF, Beech J: Pleuritis secondary to pneumonia or lung abscessation in 90 horses. J Am Vet Med Assoc 181:808-810, 1982
91. Ainsworth DM, Erb HN, Eicker SW, et al.: Effects of pulmonary abscesses on racing performance of horses treated at referral veterinary medical teaching hospitals: 45 cases (1985-1997). J Am Vet Med Assoc 216:1282-1287, 2000
92. Hewson J, Viel L: Sampling, microbiology and cytology of the respiratory tract, in Lekeux P (ed): Equine Respiratory Diseases. Ithaca, NY, International Veterinary Information Service, 2002
93. Rossier Y, Sweeney CR, Ziemer EL: Bronchoalveolar lavage fluid cytologic findings in horses with pneumonia or pleuropneumonia. J Am Vet Med Assoc 198:1001-1004, 1991
94. Hoffman AM, Viel L, Staempfli HR, et al.: Sensitivity and specificity of bronchoalveolar lavage and protected catheter brush methods for isolating bacteria from foals with experimentally induced pneumonia caused by Klebsiella pneumoniae. Am J Vet Res 54:1803-1807, 1993
95. Liebler JM, Markin CJ: Fiberoptic bronchoscopy for diagnosis and treatment. Crit Care Clin 16:83-100, 2000
96. Sweeney CR, Weiher J, Baez JL, et al.: Bronchoscopy of the horse. Am J Vet Res 53:1953-1956, 1992
97. Arthur RR, Drew RH, Perfect JR: Novel modes of antifungal drug administration. Expert Opin Investig Drugs 13:903-932, 2004
98. Badia JR, Soy D, Adrover M, et al.: Disposition of instilled versus nebulized tobramycin and imipenem in ventilated intensive care unit (ICU) patients. J Antimicrobial Chemother 54:508-514, 2004
99. Bennett MR, Weinbaum DL, Fiehler PC: Chronic necrotizing pulmonary aspergillosis treated by endobronchial amphotericin B. South Med J 83:829-832, 1990

100. Crosby SS, Edwards WA, Brennan C, et al.: Systemic absorption of endotracheally administered aminoglycosides in seriously ill patients with pneumonia. Antimicrobial Agents Chemother 31:850-853, 1987
101. Brianceau P, Chevalier H, Karas A, et al.: Intravenous lidocaine and small-intestinal size, abdominal fluid, and outcome after colic surgery in horses. J Vet Intern Med 16:736-741, 2002
102. Sweeney CR, Rossier Y, Ziemer EL, et al.: Effect of prior lavage on bronchoalveolar lavage fluid cell population of lavaged and unlavaged lung segments in horses. Am J Vet Res 55:1501-1504, 1994
103. Clark CK, Lester GD, Vetro T, et al.: Bronchoalveolar lavage in horses: effect of exercise and repeated sampling on cytology. Aust Vet J 72:249-252, 1995
104. McKenzie HC, 3rd, Murray MJ: Concentrations of gentamicin in serum and bronchial lavage fluid after intravenous and aerosol administration of gentamicin to horses. Am J Vet Res 61:1185-1190, 2000
105. Donn SM, Sinha SK: Newer techniques of mechanical ventilation: an overview. Semin Neonatol 7:401-407, 2002
106. Giguére S, Sanchez LC, Shih A, et al.: Comparison of the effects of caffeine and doxapram on respiratory and cardiovascular function in foals with induced respiratory acidosis. Am J Vet Res 68:1407-1416, 2007
107. Wilkins PA: Lower respiratory problems of the neonate. Vet Clin North Am Equine Pract 19:19-33, 2003
108. Palmer JE: Ventilatory support of the critically ill foal. Vet Clin North Am Equine Pract 21:457-486, vii-viii, 2005
109. Morgan-Hughes NJ, Mills GH, Northwood D: Air flow resistance of three heat and moisture exchanging filter designs under wet conditions: implications for patient safety. Br J Anaesth 87:289-291, 2001
110. Neligan P: Critical care medicine tutorials, 2005. Available at: http://www.ccmtutorials.com
111. Tobin MJ: Mechanical ventilation. N Engl J Med 330:1056-1061, 1994
112. Barbas CS, de Matos GF, Pincelli MP, et al.: Mechanical ventilation in acute respiratory failure: recruitment and high positive end-expiratory pressure are necessary. Curr Opin Crit Care 11:18-28, 2005
113. Lim SC, Adams AB, Simonson DA, et al.: Intercomparison of recruitment maneuver efficacy in three models of acute lung injury. Crit Care Med 32:2371-2377, 2004
114. Bigatello LM, Davignon KR, Stelfox HT: Respiratory mechanics and ventilator waveforms in the patient with acute lung injury. Respir Care 50:235-245; discussion 244-235, 2005
115. Piacentini E, Villagra A, Lopez-Aguilar J, et al.: Clinical review: the implications of experimental and clinical studies of recruitment maneuvers in acute lung injury. Crit Care 8:115-121, 2004
116. Bhutani VK: Clinical applications of pulmonary function and graphics. Semin Neonatol 7:391-399, 2002
117. MacIntyre NR: Respiratory mechanics in the patient who is weaning from the ventilator. Respir Care 50:275-286; discussion 284-276, 2005
118. Wood GC, Boucher BA, Croce MA, et al.: Aerosolized ceftazidime for prevention of ventilator-associated pneumonia and drug effects on the proinflammatory response in critically ill trauma patients. Pharmacotherapy 22:972-982, 2002
119. Attar MA, Donn SM: Mechanisms of ventilator-induced lung injury in premature infants. Semin Neonatol 7:353-360, 2002
120. Dreyfuss D, Soler P, Basset G, et al.: High inflation pressure pulmonary edema. Respective effects of high airway pressure, high tidal volume, and positive end-expiratory pressure. Am Rev Respir Dis 137:1159-1164, 1988
121. Dreyfuss D, Saumon G: Role of tidal volume, FRC, and end-inspiratory volume in the development of pulmonary edema following mechanical ventilation. Am Rev Respir Dis 148:1194-1203, 1993

11

Monitoring and treating the gastrointestinal system

11.1 Monitoring the gastrointestinal system

11.2 Management of horses with gastrointestinal disorders

11.1 Monitoring the gastrointestinal system

11.1.1. Patients at risk, auscultation, examination per rectum and blood analysis

Emma Rowe

Patients at risk of developing gastrointestinal disorders during hospitalisation

The hospital environment is quite unnatural for the equine patient. The horse is a grazing animal and therefore the equine gastrointestinal system is designed to digest small quantities of feed 24 hours per day. Many horses are hospitalised following acute trauma or illness, which changes their routine dramatically. This change is significant for an animal that thrives on routine and can result in stress and subsequent gastrointestinal disorders such as gastric ulceration or diarrhoea. Thus, it is not only the horse admitted to hospital for abdominal pain that is at risk for gastrointestinal disease, but also horses with musculoskeletal or other medical problems. Every horse in hospital should be monitored very closely for gastrointestinal disorders as some are associated with subtle clinical signs and can be very serious or fatal.

Change of environment

Horses in hospital have limited exercise and usually a change in feeding regimen, and this situation alone can predispose even a healthy horse to colic. A change in feeding regimen can disrupt the horse's gastrointestinal system. For example, a recent change in the batch of hay, decreased exposure to pasture and a recent change in the type of grain or concentrate feed have been shown to be a risk factor for colic.[1] In addition to the feeding changes, which may not be drastic as most hospitals have a variety of hay and concentrate to accommodate the horse's usual diet, the increased hours of confinement are a problem. Stabling for 24 hours per day, a recent change in exercise program and travel within the previous 24 hours have all been shown to be risk factors for simple colonic obstruction and distension colic.[2] The hospital environment may be a drastic change for a race-fit Thoroughbred normally housed in pasture that is in hospital for an orthopaedic injury.

Postoperative ileus

Postoperative ileus has long been recognised in human patients and can follow any operation, not only abdominal surgery. There are two types of human postoperative ileus recognised: postoperative and paralytic.[3] Postoperative ileus will resolve spontaneously in 2 to 3 days and is most likely large bowel inhibition. Paralytic ileus is more severe, lasting more than 3 days, and may involve small bowel.[3] There are many factors that reduce gastrointestinal tract activity in humans and many of these will be common to the horse. Some of these factors include sympathetic stimulation, pain, increased endogenous catecholamines, vasopressin, administration of catecholamines, inhalational anaesthetics, nitrous oxide or opiods.[4] Results of a recent study found that there is an intermediate clinical phase after a horse has undergone surgery in which there is reduced faecal output before any signs of colic. [5] This finding backed up other anecdotal reports suggesting that colic can be a complication of horses that have had surgery for nonrelated abdominal problems. This syndrome in horses may be similar to the uncomplicated postoperative ileus in human patients.

Stable confinement and large colon impactions

Stall confinement after musculoskeletal injury and hospitalisation for problems not related to the gastrointestinal tract have been linked to the development of large colon impactions. In a retrospective study investigation of equine large colon impaction, 53.7% of horses in the study had recent increases in stall confinement prior to the development of the large colon impaction.[6] The authors of this study postulated that there were several possibilities for this association, including inadequate water intake, changing in feeding practices upsetting the normal intestinal motility patterns and a decrease in exercise (adequate exercise may be important in maintaining normal function of the equine large intestine).

Caecal impactions

Caecal impactions have been recognised to be particularly associated with hospitalisation or to develop after surgery (that is, surgery unrelated to the gastrointestinal tract). The caecal impactions can develop very quickly, and there is a condition associated with hospitalisation in which the caecum ruptures acutely. It is possible for the horse to be clinically normal and then found acutely endotoxic with a ruptured caecum in less than 12 hours. Often the only warning is reduced faecal output or mild depression. They often do not show overt signs of colic or may display very mild colic signs that can go unnoticed even with hourly colic checks. It is possible that caecal perforation is a secondary event that occurs subsequent to altered caecal motility and abnormal accumulation of ingesta in the caecum.[7] In one study that looked at caecal disease in horses, 13% of horses suffered caecal rupture associated with concurrent unrelated disease and another 5% suffered rupture with no associated disease.[8] General anaesthesia, *Anoplocephala perfoliata* and phenylbutazone have been implicated in the pathophysiology of acute caecal rupture, but in the aforementioned study only 42% of horses had had general anaesthesia and at necropsy there were no tapeworms identified.[8] The definitive cause for acute caecal rupture is to date elusive, but the high-risk patient appears to be the fit Thoroughbred in training that has been hospitalised for an orthopaedic injury, is confined to the stall and is being treated with nonsteroidal anti-inflammatory drugs (NSAIDs).

A relationship between NSAIDs and caecal perforation has been identified and was thought to be a result of these drugs masking the signs of mild abdominal pain rather than a primary ulcerogenic effect.[9,7,10] It is possible that NSAIDs directly inhibit the caecal motility, as it has been shown *in vitro* that they inhibit contractility of large colon taenia.[11] However, administration of NSAIDs is not all bad; while some evidence suggests hospitalised horses receiving phenylbutazone are at an increased risk for gastrointestinal problems, other evidence indicates a beneficial effect. In a study that assessed pain and analgesia in horses administered phenylbutazone or placebo after arthroscopic surgery, the placebo group did develop signs of abdominal pain more frequently than the horses in the phenylbutazone group but these results were not significant.[12] Results from an investigation into reduced faecal output in horses undergoing general anaesthesia for reasons unrelated to the gastrointestinal tract, indicated that horses 5 years or older that underwent orthopaedic procedures of more than 60 minutes' duration and that did not receive phenylbutazone after surgery were at significant risk for developing reduced faecal output.[5] Therefore, it is possible that phenylbutazone can either have a protective effect for horses following surgery through its analgesic effects or cause alterations in gastrointestinal motility due to inhibition of prostaglandin.[5] Early recognition of reduced faecal output and appropriate treatment may be important in the survival of horses with caecal or large colon impaction following surgery.

Nonsteroidal anti-inflammatory drug toxicity

Excessive administration of NSAIDs above the recommended dose rate can result in toxicity, and specifically right dorsal colitis. This colitis is characterised by mucosal ulceration of variable severity localised to the right dorsal colon and is associated with experimental and clinical administration of NSAIDs. The NSAIDs cause ulceration through inhibition of the cyclooxygenase and suppression of prostaglandin production.[13] Experimentally giving a high dose of phenylbutazone (6 g PO daily for 5 days) and halving the horse's maintenance fluid intake has created the disease; however, in the clinical setting different horses have different susceptibilities.[13] Some horses will be susceptible at lower doses, even when well hydrated, whereas other horses may be only susceptible at higher than the recommended dose or to the recommended dose when dehydrated. The sick horse in hospital should be having its hydration monitored closely (see Chapter 6.5), and this is definitely the case for any patient receiving NSAIDs because they are always at risk for developing right dorsal colitis in addition to other problems such as nephrotoxicity.

Anaesthesia and surgery

Horses that have had any surgical procedure are therefore at risk for gastrointestinal problems when hospitalised. This may be due to the stress of the surgery itself or may be related to the general anaesthesia. In humans, it has been questioned whether the severity or duration of surgery influences the postoperative ileus that may occur following the procedure. Surgery time of longer than 1 hour was shown to be a risk factor for reduced faecal output in the horse.[5] It is thought that the following factors may predispose to ileus after surgery—severity of the surgical procedure, duration of exposure to anaesthetic agents and perfusion of the gastrointestinal tract during surgery.[5] General anaesthesia has been shown to affect gastrointestinal motility and the extent to which motility is affected depends on the anaesthetic drugs used. For example, horses previously treated with glycopyrrolate who are then induced with the xylazine/ketamine combination have a reduction in gastrointestinal motility and it can take up to 3 to 6 hours for this motility to return to normal.[14]

Atropine

Atropine has been shown to be a risk factor for gastrointestinal problems following surgery. Atropine is administered topically to the eye following ophthalmic procedures.

The recommended dose is 1 to 2 drops of 1% atropine solution applied to the eye 3 or 4 times daily until mydriasis is achieved.[5] This is the dose that is recommended to avoid systemic events such as ileus. A horse with a severe corneal ulcer may be hospitalised for longer than 2 weeks and may be treated with atropine for the entire hospital period and after discharge. These horses need very careful monitoring for attitude, appetite and faecal production as they are at risk for impactions secondary to ileus. These horses are also often being treated with flunixin meglumine, which decreases ocular inflammation and which may mask gastrointestinal pain. If abdominal pain is masked, it may mean the impaction is quite severe before clinical signs are evident. Decreased faecal production is often the first sign of a problem.

Diarrhoea

The development of diarrhoea is also a potential complication of any horse in hospital. There are certain situations in which the horse may be more predisposed to diarrhoea, but it can affect any horse in hospital. A horse may be hospitalised for diarrhoea as the primary disease or diarrhoea can develop in hospital secondary to other conditions such as sepsis, toxaemia or disease unrelated to the gastrointestinal tract. The endotoxaemic horse with Gram-negative sepsis is at risk of developing diarrhoea, as is the horse that has had abdominal surgery or has peritonitis. Certain colic conditions may predispose to diarrhoea. For example, a horse treated for either a sand or gravel impaction may have a very irritated large colon mucosa. These horses may develop diarrhoea following successful medical or surgical treatment to relieve the impaction. Diarrhoea is also commonly associated with small colon impactions. In some cases, colitis will develop secondary to a small colon impaction, and in other circumstances, colitis may then lead to a small colon impaction forming due to altered intestinal motility with the inflamed mucosa. Horses with impaction of the small colon, especially those treated surgically, are at an increased of salmonellosis. In one study, bacteriological culture was positive for *Salmonella* spp. in 43% of horses treated surgically for small colon impaction.[15] Of the horses that cultured positive to *Salmonella*, only some had diarrhoea.[15] Some also had fevers and were leukopenic.[15] This is important—it means that postoperative horses should be monitored very closely and horses with endotoxaemia or inflammation should be tested for *Salmonella* spp. *Salmonella* is highly contagious, and therefore if one horse is shedding the organism, others may become infected. It is possible for horses to contract infectious diarrhoea from the hospital environment. *Salmonella* spp. and *Clostridium difficile* would be the most common causes of nosocomial diarrhoea.

Immunocompromised horses are obviously going to be at higher risk of contracting an infectious organism, and thus a critically ill equine patient is at risk. Any stressed horse in the hospital environment is also at risk for shedding *Salmonella* spp. or developing clinical salmonellosis. The risk factors that have been associated with *Salmonella* shedding in hospitalised horses are given in Box 11.1. In a study that investigated the shedding of *Salmonella* in adult horses with gastrointestinal disease, the most important risk factors identified by means of logistic regression were a history of exposure to antimicrobial drugs prior to hospitalisation and abdominal surgery during hospitalisation.[26]

Box 11.1. Risk factors that have been associated with *Salmonella* shedding amongst hospitalised horses

- Lower respiratory tract disease[16]
- Colic at the time of admission[17,18]
- Long-distance transport[18,19]
- A change in diet while hospitalised[20]
- Withholding of feed[21,22]
- Use of common instruments such as nasogastric tubes and rectal thermometers[22–24]
- Antimicrobial administration[17,21,25,26]

Hospitals should have a protocol in place to ensure effective isolation of horses that present to the hospital with diarrhoea or that develop diarrhoea during their stay (see Chapter 3.3). It is this author's policy that any horse developing diarrhoea in the hospital irrespective of whether there is also fever (>38.5° C [>101.3° F]) and leukopaenia (white cell count <5.0 × 10^9/L [<5000 cells/μL]) present must be placed in an isolation ward. Any horse with fever (>38.5° C [>101.3° F]) and leukopaenia (white cell count <5.0 × 10^9/L [<5000 cells/μL]) without diarrhoea should also be placed in isolation. It is very important that all staff are consistent and follow a standard protocol to ensure horses are appropriately isolated to prevent spread of infectious disease. Complete blood counts should be performed on hospitalised horses within 24 hours of the development of fever of unknown origin or diarrhoea without fever present. If a leukopenia is known to be related to another clinical disease such as metritis, pleuritis, peritonitis or neonatal sepsis and the horse or foal does not have diarrhoea, then isolation may not be required. For horses that have had an exploratory laparotomy diarrhoea may be possible within the first 24 hours following surgery as a direct result of the procedure. For example, if a pelvic flexure enterotomy has been performed and the contents of the large colon removed with the aid of lavage, isolation for these horses is not necessary for the first 24 hours post-operatively unless there is fever or leukopenia.

Gastric ulceration

The hospitalised horse is also at risk for gastrointestinal ulceration, which is due in part to the associated stress and, in some cases, anorexia. Many horses that are hospitalised for gastrointestinal problems are held off feed when the transit of ingesta is a problem, and this imposed feed deprivation can result in erosion and ulceration of the gastric squamous mucosa.[27] Other horses are anorecic due to a gastrointestinal problem or other disease or sepsis, which can also result in the development of ulceration in their gastric mucosa. Feeding changes can place the horse at risk for colic and can also influence gastric acidity and peptic injury to the gastric squamous mucosa.[27] Horses moved from pasture to stall confinement and free-choice timothy hay for 7 days had erosion and ulceration of the gastric squamous mucosa in one study.[28] There can also be a negative feedback cycle created where the horse is consuming less roughage in hospital, which results in mild ulcerative lesions within the stomach and then discomfort, subsequently decreasing roughage or feed consumption further.[27] The development of gastric ulceration in the neonatal foal is a concern for clinicians, and many clinicians treat critically ill neonatal foals prophylactically with antiulcer medications. This prophylactic treatment is now controversial. It has been postulated that the pathogenesis of gastric ulceration in the critically ill neonate may be due to hypoxic-ischaemic injury to the gastric mucosa rather than as a direct result of the gastric acid.[29] It has also been shown that critically ill foals often have different intragastric pH profiles from those reported for healthy foals. Many critically ill foals have continuously alkaline intragastric pH profiles, questioning the need for prophylactic administration of acid suppressors in all critically ill foals.[30] There is the concern that an increased pH may actually predispose to sepsis as there is some evidence in humans that airway colonisation by new pathogens occurs more frequently in patients receiving agents that increased gastric pH compared with those receiving sulcralfate.[30] On the other hand, there is anecdotal evidence that the gastric ulceration seen at examination *post mortem* in foals that did not receive prophylactic acid suppression is of greater severity than those in which this treatment was given. Thus careful consideration must be given prior to prophylactic treatment for gastric ulcers in critically ill neonates and it will be clinician preference whether it is administered or not. Foals that are older than neonates (>30 days) will usually be treated the same as for an adult hospitalised horse in regard to the prophylactic ulcer medication, and again opinions will differ and clinician preference will be important in the decision for treatment.

Oesophageal obstruction (choke)

Another gastrointestinal consideration for the hospitalised horse is choke, or oesophageal obstruction. This can occur if the horse is fed too soon after recovering from general anaesthesia or sedation. Many hospitals have a policy that horses are to be muzzled in the hospital stall for 45 minutes to 1 hour after heavy sedation (detomidine/butorphanol, for example) and 1 hour after coming back in the stall following general anaesthesia. However, the incidence of choke in hospitals that do not enforce this policy is anecdotally extremely small. If glycopyrrolate has been administered, the anaesthetist may recommend a longer period of time without food as this particular drug is an anticholinergic and can decrease the motility of the oesophagus. It is important that horses are checked when their muzzles are removed to ensure that they have recovered sufficiently to chew and swallow their food, especially if there is hay in the stall.

Auscultation

Abdominal auscultation is an important part of the brief clinical examination performed regularly on hospitalised horses. Borborygmi will be an indication of the status of the gastrointestinal system. Quiet borborygmi may be indicative of decreased motility, abdominal pain or abdominal disease. Very active borborygmi may be indicative of pending diarrhoea or spasmodic type abdominal pain. However, borborygmi cannot be relied on solely to detect problems with the gastrointestinal system, as one study showed borborygmi were not a reliable indicator of reduced faecal output in the hospitalised horses.[5] Other studies have indicated the same concern: in one study, only 31% of horses with caecal perforations secondary to caecal impaction had reduced borborygmi,[7] and in another, only 24% of horses with large colon impaction had reduced or absent borborygmi.[6]

To auscultate the abdomen, the stethoscope is placed on the four major sites that include the left and right lower and upper paralumbar regions. The ventral midline of the abdomen should also be auscultated, especially in regions, such as Australia and California, where sand colic is prevalent. Sounds should be heard in all four quadrants and will be more frequent on the left side, where most of the large colon (left ventral and dorsal colons) is located, compared to the right side, where the caecum is located close to the body wall. The characteristic borborygmi sound like gurgling fluid and are produced by the interface and mixing of gas and fluid in both the large colon and caecum.[31] The small intestine can be very motile but may not create referred sounds; thus, the borborygmi auscultated are a good indication of large bowel motility but not always of small intestinal motility, which needs to be evaluated with ultrasound.

The frequency of borborygmi is quite consistent between horses, with the mixing sounds normally occurring 2 to 4 times a minute.[31] The frequency will vary depending on whether the horse is eating at the time of auscultation, as does the amplitude. There is more variation between horses in amplitude than frequency of sounds.[32] When the horse has not recently eaten, progressive sounds will be heard only once every 2 to 4 minutes, and thus the veterinarian must be diligent and take this time to auscultate each site for this period of time for all hospitalised horses, as many will not be eating. The progressive sounds will become more intense when the horse is eating, with the amplitude

Box 11.2. Some commonly used drugs that decrease or abolish propulsive gastrointestinal sounds

- Atropine[34–36]
- Xylazine[35,37,38]
- Romifidine[39]
- Detomidine[38]
- Butorphanol[38,40]
- Morphine[41]

and frequency both increasing.[32,33] This results in borborygmi that are a long progressive rush of gurgling heard on both the left and right side for 6 to 10 seconds.[32,33] Borborygmi may be affected by certain commonly used drugs (Box 11.2). Xylazine and butorphanol have a short-term effect on intestinal motility, whereas atropine can have a longer duration of affect, causing marked ileus, reduced faecal output and possibly impaction.

In most cases of abdominal pain, the propulsive sounds are decreased, and in cases of severe intestinal disease such as strangulated bowel, ruptured bowel or severe peritonitis, the borborygmi will be absent. Even with small intestinal disease, the propulsive motility of the large colon and caecum is usually absent due to the sympathetic response to pain and the inflammatory response affecting the entire intestine causing a generalised ileus.[31] Static, distended large intestine or small intestine that is filled with gas and fluid may make bubbling or pinging sounds if the horse is moved, and it is important to recognise the difference between this and normal propulsive motility.[31] In spasmodic colic, excessive borborygmi are heard and are suspected to be due to intestinal spasms from ischaemia, parasite irritation or contraction against an impaction.[31] Increased borborygmi will also be audible prior to the onset of diarrhoea and may sound "fluidy" with a lot of slushing noises. In foals, these increased gastrointestinal sounds may be accompanied by pain before the onset of enteritis or colitis. It is also possible that borborygmi may increase after a period of ileus and tympanic or simple obstructive colic that has resolved, and with this type of increase there is usually no pain but the horse may appear tired or depressed.[31]

Examination per rectum

Horses hospitalised for gastrointestinal problems such as diarrhoea or colic, urogenital problems such as uroliths, reproductive problems such as a mare with placentitis and miscellaneous problems such as retroperitoneal or abdominal abscess may require rectal examinations as part of the disease-monitoring process. Horses hospitalised for diseases other than that of gastrointestinal or abdominal origin may also require a rectal examination if they develop clinical signs of colic, reduced faecal output or depression and there is concern of reduced intestinal motility and transit of ingesta. The rectal examination is one of the most important parts of the diagnostic work-up of the acute abdomen. The examination per rectum is described in Chapter 1.4.

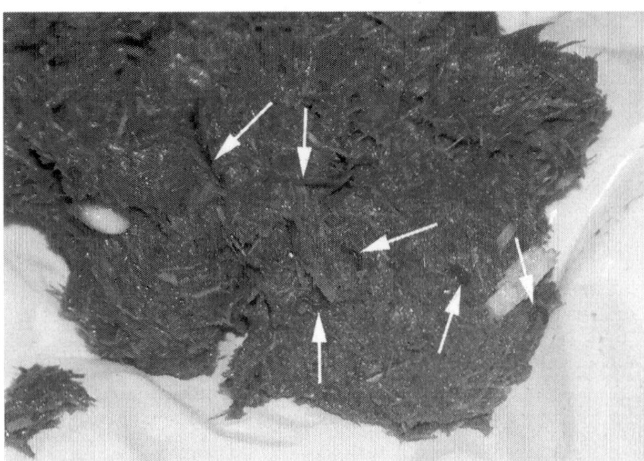

Figure 11.1 Larval cyathostomes (*arrows*) in a faecal sample from a yearling. ©Kevin Corley 2007.

During the rectal examination, the examiner should take notice of the gross appearance of the faecal balls. The faecal contents should be examined for a dry or hard consistency (which indicate increased transit time or dehydration), mucus covering, the presence of sand, gravel, undigested feed material, watery consistency (decreased transit time), mineral oil that may have been administered previously (can be indicative of transit time) and parasites (Figure 11.1). Sand may not always be visible grossly. To assess its presence and quantity, the faeces should be placed in a rectal sleeve filled with water. The sleeve can be tied up to allow the sand to sediment out. This is particularly useful for assessing whether a sand impaction is resolving in response to medical treatment. This simple test can be performed daily and is much simpler, cheaper and easier than abdominal radiographs, which are usually taken after 7 to 10 days of medical treatment to confirm the large colon is empty of sand.

Cytological (to evaluate parasite burden), biochemical, bacteriological (to test for *Salmonella* spp. and *Clostridium* spp.), immunological and electron microscopic evaluations can be performed on faecal samples if necessary. Daily cultures of faecal samples are performed on many horses with diarrhoea (see Chapter 3.3). Faecal occult blood can also be tested. However, the interpretation of this test can be difficult as there may be contamination from previous rectal examinations where there has been some minor bleeding from the mucosa.[31] This test can be useful for diagnosing ulceration in the gastrointestinal tract (e.g., right dorsal colitis), but available tests are not very sensitive or specific for digested blood.[42]

Abnormal findings

Stomach and small intestine

Gastric problems are rarely diagnosed on rectal examination because the stomach is so cranial and is therefore out of reach. A very distended stomach, as found in severe gastric impaction, may displace the spleen caudally. However, the spleen can also displace caudally if there is primary splenic enlargement. Very rarely, with very great distension of the stomach, it can be directly felt on examination per rectum.

The duodenum cannot usually be palpated in the right dorsal quadrant, and therefore abnormalities may be missed with the rectal examination. However, if it is very distended, as in the case of a small intestinal obstruction or duodenitis-proximal jejunitis, the duodenum can be palpated as a tubular structure over the base of the caecum, just ventral to the aorta.[31,43,44] Distended small intestine resulting from small intestinal obstruction, enteritis or ileus palpates like several soft tubes. The tubes will vary in diameter and tautness depending on the severity of the distension. The distended loops of small intestine will often be located on midline but can be located in any quadrant of the abdomen. Even if there are multiple distended loops of small intestine, only one or two may be felt. In cases of severe small intestinal distension, the loops of distended bowel may take up the space of almost the entire abdomen so that the distended small intestine is the first and only structure that can be felt on rectal palpation.

Abnormalities of the ileum (impaction, for example) may be palpated, but the ileum may be out of reach of the examiner. Ileal pain, or pain and tension associated with its mesentery, may cause a painful response to palpation of the normal ventral and medial caecal ligaments and can occur with conditions such as epiploic foramen entrapment.[45] However, this painful response can also occur with other small intestinal diseases.[31] If small intestine is trapped within the inguinal canal, a strand of mesentery not normally attached to the inguinal canal may be palpated. This is usually quite painful when manipulated. The small intestine itself may be palpable in close proximity to the inguinal ring. Another specific small intestinal abnormality, which may be palpable, is a jejunojejunal intussusception—the intussusception itself is a sausage-like structure, which can feel like a thickened tubular structure on rectal palpation.

Caecum

Caecal distension is usually quite obvious on rectal examination. The caecum displaces from its normal position on the right to a more central position and the caecal bands become taut as the caecum enlarges. When the caecum distends with gas (as can occur with a primary caecal disease or a large colon obstruction), it often moves back in the pelvic inlet and feels like a tight gas filled viscus in the right dorsal quadrant. In these cases it is often very difficult to distinguish between a right dorsal displacement and caecal distension. When the caecum fills with ingesta (caecal impaction) or fluid (caecal dysfunction), it will tend to be pulled cranially and ventrally due to the weight and will be palpable in the right ventral quadrant. If a caecal impaction extends above the caecocolic orifice, there is complete obstruction. The caecal base fills with fluid, resulting in the distended caecum filling the right dorsal and ventral abdominal quadrants.[46] If a mass or oedematous bowel is palpable in the right dorsal quadrant, it may indicate the presence of a caecocolic intussusception.[47] If the caecum feels thickened on palpation, it may indicate that the viability is questionable.

Large colon

When the pelvic flexure becomes impacted, it moves and extends from the left ventral quadrant to the right ventral quadrant. When the impaction is very large and there is a large amount of gas distension, the pelvic flexure is often pushed up towards the pelvic inlet. In some cases, the impacted colon can enter the pelvic inlet and fill the entire caudal abdomen. Failure to palpate an impaction does not rule out cranial impactions, such as those in the right dorsal colon impaction. These are out of reach in a rectal examination. When an impaction is palpated, it needs to be determined whether the large colon is displaced or not. The large colon may also be displaced without the presence of an impaction.

A left dorsal displacement or nephrosplenic entrapment can be diagnosed if the large colon is found over the nephrosplenic ligament. It is often possible to follow the taenia of the ventral colon as it traverses left and dorsally towards the nephrosplenic space. This displacement can also be suspected if there is large colon between the spleen and body wall or if the spleen is displaced medially.[48] In these cases, ultrasound can be used to support the diagnosis (see Chapter 11.1.3). If there is a large amount of large colon distension, it may not be possible to feel the nephrosplenic entrapment, as the space may be obscured. Several different conditions of the colon can cause marked colonic distension, and it may not always be possible to distinguish between them on the rectal examination. In one retrospective study, rectal examination was diagnostic for nephrosplenic entrapment in 72% cases.[49]

The position of the large colon may vary with right dorsal displacement. With the most common presentation, the large colon retroflexes and passes between the caecum and the right body wall.[46] The large colon and the taenia are felt cranial to the pelvic rim coursing from the right caudal abdomen transversely towards the left cranial abdomen.[46] The pelvic flexure cannot normally be felt because it is in the left cranial abdomen and the caecum is often difficult to palpate because it displaces medially and cranially.[46] Cranial displacements can also occur and the large colon can be found to be against the diaphragm at surgery. In these cases, the pelvic flexure cannot be felt, and in some cases no large colon at all can be felt during the rectal examination because it is out of reach, even when distended. A diaphragmatic hernia may also result in the caudal abdomen being quite empty if there is a large amount of intestine within the thoracic cavity, and in some cases there will be no large colon or caecum palpable.

Large colon volvulus generally produces more severe clinical signs and gas distension than does a more simple displacement, but in the early stages the distension may not be as severe. The pelvic flexure may be palpable on the right side and when there is at least a volvulus of 180° and the ventral colon haustra will be palpable dorsally. In some cases the large colon and caecum are displaced cranially and are not palpable. If the large colon volvulus is 360° or greater, there is usually severe gas distension. In this case, the large colon may be pushed so far back into the pelvic inlet that the examiner cannot manipulate the arm past the gas distended viscus cranial to the pelvic rim. As the large colon fills with blood and fluid, the haustrae become more prominent and the large colon may be quite thick on palpation.[31]

Small colon

Many obstructions of the small colon will be out of the examiner's reach. If faecaliths or enteroliths, for example, are located in a more proximal area of the small colon or within the transverse colon, they are not palpable. Enteroliths are not commonly palpated on rectal examination.[31] Complete obstructions of the small colon do not allow passage of gas and can result in severe large colon and caecal distension that is palpable on rectal examination and evident as gross abdominal distension.

Small colon impactions can usually be palpated as they most often occur in the distal segments of the small colon. They are palpated as a long, thick tubular structure. The tubular structure is identified as small colon by recognition of the antimesenteric band. In some cases, the tubular structure (impaction) will extend beyond the reach of the examiner. In severe small colon impactions, the entire small colon can be filled with ingesta and the rectal ampulla may be pulled ventrally and to the left of midline because of the weight of the ingesta and the tension on the mesentery.[46]

Miscellaneous abnormalities

Abscesses within the abdominal cavity may be palpable in various locations and then ultrasound examination (transrectal or transabdominal) can confirm the definitive diagnosis (see Chapter 11.1.3). Abscesses can occur in the small intestinal mesentery and may be associated with adhered loops of small intestine.[31] Neoplastic masses may also be palpable in some cases. Abnormalities with the spleen may be palpable; for example, with splenomegaly, the spleen will extend medially and push caudally.[31] With tumours of the spleen, the surface may feel irregular or nodular. Adhesions may be difficult to palpate. Usually, when the adhesions have been present for a period of time, the small intestine will be chronically distended and thickened. If the adhesion is adhered to the inguinal rings, small colon, abdominal wall or in the pelvic canal, it may be felt.[31] Adhesions adherent to the large colon and abdominal wall or those associated with the omentum are not usually palpable, but in some cases adhesions from an enterotomy site to the pelvic rim can be felt.[31]

Late gestational mares

Mares with a large gravid uterus present a problem for rectal palpation. Many structures cannot be reached due to the size of the uterus. Distended large colon and caecum can be felt around the gravid uterus, but it can be difficult to differentiate whether one (and which one) or both are distended. The small intestine cannot normally be palpated, and if distension is suspected, it must be confirmed with the ultrasound (see Chapter 11.1.3). In the last trimester of pregnancy uterine torsion should be considered as a differential for colic.[31] With a uterine torsion the broad ligaments will be taut, crossing the caudal abdomen below and above the cervix. In most cases the direction of the uterine torsion can be determined by relative displacement and asymmetry of the left and right broad ligaments.[50,51] If the uterine torsion has been chronic, the broad ligaments may not be palpable and the rectal findings may be inconclusive; diagnosis is sometimes made at exploratory laparotomy.[52]

Other findings

In some cases, the examiner can develop a feel for the status of the general abdominal condition. For example, if the horse is very dehydrated and the abdomen has very little peritoneal fluid, it may feel a bit dry with the intestines not characteristically slipping over each other, as in the case when they are well lubricated with peritoneal fluid. In some cases, when there is excessive peritoneal fluid, the intestine may feel that it is moving through fluid.[31] If there is fibrin deposition over the serosal surfaces, the intestinal surfaces may feel rough to the examiner.[31] When a part of the intestine ruptures, gas escapes into the peritoneal cavity and the examiner may palpate emphysema such as crepitus in the caecal wall or crepitus in the fibrin covering an area of rupture in the bowel wall.[31] With certain ruptures, there will be faecal contamination throughout the abdomen and there may be a rough, granular feel to the intestines on rectal examination.

Haematology and biochemistry

Laboratory investigations can be extremely useful to monitor, diagnose and treat gastrointestinal disorders. Infectious and inflammatory disorders of the intestine can cause increases or decreases in the peripheral white cell count. In general, diseases that result in a large release of endotoxins, such as salmonellosis, result in decreased white cell count, due to margination of the neutrophils in capillaries. There may be a brief period of leukocytosis before the leukopaenia in these horses, and a leukocytosis may return during the recovery phase. In clostridial diarrhoea, there is generally a moderate leukocytosis. Monitoring the white cell count in horses at risk for infectious diarrhoea may help identify disease early, and therefore allow earlier institution of increased biosecurity measures (see Chapter 3.3). The packed cell volume is often monitored during gastrointestinal disease to monitor fluid status. This may not be the most accurate way of determining fluid status and other parameters such as lactate and urine output should be monitored in conjunction with packed cell volume (see Chapter 6.5). Electrolyte disturbances are extremely common in gastrointestinal disease, and these should be monitored closely during acute disease and in horses after colic surgery, to allow prompt supplementation when required (see Chapter 6.5).

Gastrointestinal disease can result in secondary damage to other organs, such as the kidney and liver. Intermittent monitoring of enzyme activities and metabolite concentrations associated with these organs (see Chapters 12.1 and 13.1) can allow early identification and treatment of secondary organ damage or dysfunction. Lastly, coagulopathies in hospitalised horses are highly associated with endotoxaemia and therefore, in turn, with severe gastrointestinal disorders. Monitoring the coagulation system is advised in at risk patients (see Chapter 8.1).

References

1. Hudson JM, et al.: Feeding practices associated with colic in horses. J Am Vet Med Assoc 219:1419-1425, 2001
2. Hillyer MH, et al.: Case control study to identify risk factors for simple colonic obstruction and distension colic in horses. Equine Vet J 34:455-463, 2002
3. Livingston E, Passaro EJ: Postoperative ileus. Dig Dis Sci 35:121-132, 1990
4. Steinbrook R: Epidural anesthesia and gastrointestinal motility. Anesth Analg 86:837-844, 1998
5. Little D, Redding W, Blikslager A: Risk factors for reduced postoperative fecal output in horses: 37 cases (1997-1998). J Am Vet Med Assoc 218:414-420, 2001
6. Dabareiner R, White N: Large colon impaction in horses: 147 cases (1985 1991). J Am Vet Med Assoc 206:679-685, 1995
7. Ross MW, Martin BB, Donawick WJ: Cecal perforation in the horse. J Am Vet Med Assoc 187:249-253, 1985
8. Dart AJ, Hodgson DR, Snyder JR: Caecal disease in equids. Aust Vet J 75:552-557, 1997
9. Collatos C, Romano S: Cecal impaction in horses: causes, diagnosis, and medical treatment. Compend Contin Educ Pract Vet 15:976-981, 1992
10. Ross MW, Hansen RR: Large intestine, in Auer JA (ed): Large Intestine. Philadelphia, WB Saunders, 1992, pp 386-390
11. Van Hoogmoed L, et al.: In vitro effects of nonsteroidal anti-inflammatory agents and prostaglandins I2, E2, and F2alpha on contractility of taenia of the large colon of horses. Am J Vet Res 60:1004-1009, 1999
12. Raekallio M, Taylor P, Bennett RC: Preliminary investigations of pain and analgesia assessment in horses administered phenylbutazone or placebo after arthroscopic surgery. Vet Anaesth 26:150-155, 1997
13. Karcher L, et al.: Right dorsal colitis. J Vet Intern Med 4:247-253, 1990
14. Singh S, et al.: Cardiopulmonary and gastrointestinal motility effects of xylazine/ketamine-induced anesthesia in horses previously treated with glycopyrrolate. Am J Vet Res 57:1762-1770, 1996
15. Rhoads WS, Barton MH, Parks A: Comparison of medical and surgical treatment for impaction of the small colon in horses: 84 cases (1986-1996). J Am Vet Med Assoc 214:1042-1047, 1999
16. Alinovi C, et al.: Risk factors for fecal shedding of *Salmonella* from horses in a veterinary teaching hospital. Prev Vet Med 60:307-317, 2003
17. Hird D, et al.: Risk factors for salmonellosis in hospitalized horses. J Am Vet Med Assoc 188:173-177, 1986
18. Kim L, et al.: Factors associated with *Salmonella* shedding among equine colic patients at a veterinary teaching hospital. J Am Vet Med Assoc 218:740-748, 2001
19. Owen R, Fullerton J, Barnum D: Effects of transportation, surgery, and antibiotic therapy in ponies infected with *Salmonella*. Am J Vet Res 44:46-50, 1983
20. Traub-Dargatz JL, Salman M, Jones R: Epidemiologic study of salmonellae shedding in the feces of horses and potential risk factors for development of the infection in hospitalized horses. J Am Vet Med Assoc 196:1617-1622, 1990
21. Smith B, Reina-Guerra M, Hardy A: Prevalence and epizootiology of equine salmonellosis. J Am Vet Med Assoc 172: 353-356, 1978
22. Hird D, Pappaioanou M, Smith B: Case-control study of risk factors associated with isolation of *Salmonella saintpaul* in hospitalized horses. Am J Epidemiol 120:852-864, 1984
23. Tillotson K, et al.: Outbreak of *Salmonella infantis* infection in a large animal veterinary teaching hospital. J Am Vet Med Assoc 211:1554-1557, 1997
24. Hartmann F, et al.: Control of an outbreak of salmonellosis caused by drug-resistant *Salmonella anatum* in horses at a veterinary hospital and measures to prevent future infections. J Am Vet Med Assoc 209:629-631, 1996
25. House J, et al.: Risk factors for nosocomial *Salmonella* infection among hospitalized horses. J Am Vet Med Assoc 214: 1511-1516, 1999
26. Ernst N, et al.: Risk factors associated with fecal *Salmonella* shedding among hospitalized horses with signs of gastrointestinal tract disease. J Am Vet Med Assoc 225:275-281, 2004
27. Murray MJ: Disorders of the stomach, in Smith B (ed): Disorders of the Stomach. St. Louis, Mosby, 2002, pp 617-624
28. Murray MJ, Eichorn E: Effects of intermittent feed deprivation, intermittent feed deprivation with ranitidine administration, and stall confinement with ad libitum access to hay on gastric ulceration in horses. Am J Vet Res 57:1599-1603, 1996
29. Navab F, Steingrub J: Stress ulcer: is routine prophylaxis necessary? Am J Gastroenterol 90:708-712, 1995
30. Sanchez LC, Lester GD, Merritt AM: Intragastric pH in critically ill neonatal foals and the effect of ranitidine. J Am Vet Med Assoc 218:907-911, 2001
31. White NA: Examination and diagnosis of the acute abdomen, in White NA (ed): Examination and Diagnosis of the

Acute Abdomen. Malvern, PA, Lea and Febiger, 1990, pp 102-142
32. Ehrhardt EE, Lowe JE: Lengthy electronic auscultation of the equine abdomen to monitor the effects of analgesics, sedtaives and other drugs. Proc AAEP Annu Conv 525-538, 1987
33. Adams SB: Equine intestinal motility: an overview of normal acitvity, changes in disease and effects of drug administration. Proc AAEP Annu Conv 539-556, 1980
34. Williams M, et al.: Systemic effects of topical and subconjunctival ophthalmic atropine in the horse. Vet Ophthalmol 3:193-199, 2000
35. Adams S, Lamar C, Masty J: Motility of the distal portion of the jejunum and pelvic flexure in ponies: effects of six drugs. Am J Vet Res 45:795-799, 1984
36. Ducharme N, Fubini S: Gastrointestinal complications associated with the use of atropine in horses. J Am Vet Med Assoc 182:229-231, 1983
37. Rutkowski JA, Eades SC, Moore JN: Effects of xylazine butorphanol on cecal arterial bloodflow, cecal mechanical activity, and systemic hemodynamics in horses. Am J Vet Res 52:1153-1158, 1991
38. Merritt AM, Burrow JA, Hartless CS: Effect of xylazine, detomidine, and a combination of xylazine butorphanol on equine duodenal motility. Am J Vet Res 59:619-623, 1998
39. Freeman SL, England GCW: Effect of romifidine on gastrointestinal motility, assessed by transrectal ultarsonography. Equine Vet J 33:570-576, 2001
40. Sellon D, et al.: Pharmacokinetics and adverse effects of butorphanol administered by single intravenous injection or continuous intravenous infusion in horses. Am J Vet Res 62:183-189, 2001
41. Kohn C, Muir WR: Selected aspects of the clinical pharmacology of visceral analgesics and gut motility modifying drugs in the horse. J Vet Intern Med 2:85-91, 1988
42. Cohen ND, Mealey RH, Carter GK: The recognition and medical management of right dorsal colitis in horses. Vet Med 90:687-692, 2000
43. Huskamp B: Diagnosis of gastroduodenitis and its surgical treatment by a temporary duodenocaecostomy. Equine Vet J 17:314-316, 1985
44. White NA, et al.: Hemorrhagic fibrinonecrotic duodenitis-proximal jejunitis in horses: 20 cases (1977-1984). J Am Vet Assoc 190:311-315, 1987
45. Kopf N: Rectal findings in horses with intestinal obstruction. Proc Equine Colic Res Symp 236-260, 1982
46. Mueller POE, Moore JN: Rectal examination of horses with acute abdominal pain. Compend Continu Educ Pract Vet 22:606-615, 2000
47. Martin BBJ, et al.: Cecocolic and cecocecal intussusception in horses: 30 cases (1976-1996). J Am Vet Med Assoc 214:80-84, 1999
48. Burba DJ, Moore RM: Renosplenic entrapment: a review of clinical presentation and treatment. Equine Vet Educ 9:180-184, 1997
49. Hardy J, et al.: Nephrosplenic entrapment in the horse: a retrospective study of 174 cases. Equine Vet J 32:95-97, 2000
50. Pascoe JR, Meagher DM, Wheat JD: Surgical managament of uterine torsion in the mare: a review of 26 cases. J Am Vet Med Assoc 179:351-354, 1981
51. Vasey JR: Uterine torsion, in Mckinnon AO, Voss JL (eds): Uterine Torsion. Philadelphia, Lea and Febiger, 1993, pp 456-460
52. Doyle AJ, et al.: Clinical signs and treatment of chronic uterine torsion in two mares. J Am Vet Med Assoc 220:349-353, 2002

11.1.2. Interpretation of peritoneal fluid

Jennifer O. Stephen

Peritoneal fluid is relatively easy to obtain from horses and can be very useful in the investigation of abdominal disease. The technique for collection is described in Chapter 1.8.

Effect of age, surgery and foaling

When interpreting the results of peritoneal fluid analysis, the age and immediate clinical history of the animal must be taken into account. The normal reference range for foals is different to adults[1] (see Appendix, Table 19.11). Normal foaling has no effect on peritoneal fluid values.[2,3] A complicated dystocia may increase total protein and the percentage neutrophils.[2] Therefore, in a postpartum mare with significantly increased peritoneal protein, white blood cell count and percentage neutrophils, intestinal compromise must be suspected. Abdominal exploratory surgery without resection caused an increase in nucleated cell counts (>13.7×10^9/L [13,700 cells/µl]), the percentage of neutrophils, total protein and fibrinogen within 1 day of surgery, these values remaining increased until the sixth day postoperatively.[4] Castration has also been shown to increase the nucleated cell counts in horses to greater than 10×10^9/L (>10,000 cells/µl) within 1 day of surgery, remaining increased for 5 days in 74% of horses examined.[5] Post castration peritoneal fluid was obviously blood tinged in 21 of 24 horses in this study and red blood cell counts peaked on day 3 ($0–9 \times 10^{12}$/L [$0–9 \times 10^6$/µl]), then sharply declined after day 5.[5]

Determination of medical versus surgical colic

Abdominal fluid analysis does not provide definitive guidance in determining the appropriate management of horses with colic. It must be taken in context with other signs. A wide range of cytokines, enzymes and cytology have been analysed to help to determine medical from surgical lesions. Colour and protein concentration have been consistently identified as the most useful variables for this purpose.[6–11] Clear, pale-yellow, transparent fluid is considered normal. Dark yellow/orange fluid has been associated with equine grass sickness.[12] Red/serosanguinous fluid is commonly seen with surgical lesions, and dark red/black lesions, with necrotic bowl or rupture. A green sample with solid material in it is suggestive of enterocentesis. However, plant material may also be present after the rupture of a piece of bowel. The clinician should look at a slide of the sample

Table 11.1. Peritoneal and serum phosphate concentrations in horses with colic (SI units)[13]

	Normal horse	Medical colic	Surgery: no resection	Surgery: resection
Peritoneal fluid phosphate concentration (mmol/L)	0.9 ± 0.07	0.94 ± 0.09	0.96 ± 0.09	1.48 ± 0.11
Serum phosphate concentration (mmol/L)	0.88 ± 0.07	0.9 ± 0.07	0.9 ± 0.07	1.24 ± 0.1

Table 11.2. Peritoneal and serum phosphate concentrations in horses with colic (U.S. units)[13]

	Normal horse	Medical colic	Surgery: no resection	Surgery: resection
Peritoneal fluid phosphate concentration (mg/dl)	2.78 ± 0.21	2.92 ± 0.27	2.98 ± 0.28	4.58 ± 0.34
Serum phosphate concentration (mg/dl)	2.73 ± 0.22	2.80 ± 0.21	2.78 ± 0.22	3.87 ± 0.3

that has been Gram-stained. Intracellular bacteria are suggestive of true bowel rupture, rather than enterocentesis. A peritoneal fluid protein greater than 20 g/L strongly suggests the horse has a surgical lesion.[6]

Serum inorganic phosphate and peritoneal inorganic phosphate are significantly different in normal horses, horses with medical colic, horses undergoing surgery with no resection and those undergoing surgery with resection (see Table 11.1 or 11.2). A peritoneal phosphate greater than 1.16 mmol/L (3.6 mg/dl) was associated with the horse undergoing a resection or euthanasia (sensitivity 77%, specificity 73%). In cases where a peritoneal sample cannot be obtained, serum phosphate greater than 1.07 mmol/L (3.3 mg/dl) is a predictor of major intestinal injury (sensitivity 60%, specificity 73%).[13]

The appearance of the sample is the most reliable predictor of intestinal injury. The red colour of peritoneal fluid is associated with haemolysed and whole red blood cells that have been released into peritoneum via diapedisis. Spectrophotometric assessment of peritoneal fluid allows early detection of this. Horses with greater than 0.01 mmol/L haemoglobin were predicted to have surgical colic (sensitivity 80%, sensitivity 82%).[14]

Peritoneal lactate has a normal range of 0.60±0.19 mmol/L. Clinical colic cases had a mean lactate of 4.0±4.63 mmol/L; horses with a nonstrangulating obstruction had a mean lactate of 2.09 mmol/L, and horses with a strangulating obstruction had a level of 8.45 mmol/L.[15]

Total nucleated cell count

The range for normal values in nucleated cell count is very wide and variable. The cell population of peritoneal fluid can also vary widely and should be interpreted as indicative of a range of diseases not a definitive diagnosis. Only in certain neoplasms such as melanoma or lymphosarcoma can a definitive diagnosis be made from peritoneal fluid. Identification of degenerative cell changes, bacteria or ingesta by cytology is more important than the total cell count.

Septic peritonitis

Diagnosis of horses with septic peritonitis after surgery can be difficult, as peritoneal total nucleated cell count (TNCC) and total protein will increase even in normal horses postoperatively.[4] Horses with septic peritonitis, however, will have significantly lower peritoneal fluid pH (range 6.43–7.59) and glucose concentrations (<4.7 mmol/L [<85 mg/dl]) than horses with nonseptic peritonitis or healthy horses. Measuring both serum and plasma glucose concentrations has been shown to be very helpful in the detection of septic peritonitis. Serum/peritoneal glucose concentration differences greater than 2.8 mmol/L (50 mg/dl) have the highest diagnostic use for detection of septic peritonitis. A peritoneal fluid pH less than 7.3, glucose concentration less than 1.67 mmol/L (30 mg/dl) and fibrinogen concentration greater than 2 g/L (200 mg/dl) are all highly indicative of septic peritonitis.[15]

Grass sickness

The peritoneal fluid of subacute grass sickness cases has a higher specific gravity (1.018 ± 0.006; range 1.010–1.041) and protein content (22.4 ± 11.6 g/L [2.24 ± 1.16 g/dl]; range 9.3–50.5 g/L) than medical colics (specific gravity: 1.014 ± 0.008; range 1.008–1.038/protein: 10.6 ± 4.1 g/L [1.06 ± 0.41 g/dl]; range 6.2–20.6 g/L).[12] Acute grass sickness cases may be distinguishable from cases of surgical colic on the basis of appearance of peritoneal fluid. Samples from acute and subacute grass sickness have a deep yellow to orange colour, whilst surgical cases have a red to brown colour. The peritoneal fluid in acute grass sickness cases has also been reported to have a lower alkaline phosphatase activity (175.4±139.9; range 8.0–531.5 IU/L) compared to surgical colic cases (936.8 ± 696.8; range 209–1833 IU/L).[12]

References

1. Grindem CB, Fairley NM, Uhlinger CA, et al.: Peritoneal fluid values from healthy foals. Equine Vet J 22:359, 1990
2. Frazer GS, Burba D, Paccamonti D, et al.: Diagnostic value of peritoneal fluid changes in the post-partum mare. Proc Am Assoc Equine Pract 1996, p 266
3. Van Hoogmead L, Synder JR, Christopher M, et al.: Peritoneal fluid analysis in peripartum mares. J Am Vet Med Assoc 209:1280, 1996
4. Santschi EM, Grindem CB, Tate LP, et al.: Peritoneal fluid analysis in ponies after abdominal surgery. Vet Surg 17:6-9, 1988
5. Schumacher J, Spano JS, McGuire J, et al.: Effects of castration on peritoneal fluid in the horse. J Vet Intern Med 2:22-25, 1988
6. Matthews S, Dart AJ, Reid SW: Predictive values, sensitivity and specificity of abdominal fluid variables in determining the need for surgery in horses with an acute abdominal crisis. Aust Vet J 80:132-136, 2000
7. Puotunen-Reinert A: Study of variables commonly used in examination of equine colic cases to assess prognostic value. Equine Vet J 18:275-277, 1986
8. Parry BW: Use of clinical pathology in evaluation of horses with colic. Vet Clin North Am Equine Pract 3:529-542, 1987
9. Nelson AW: Analysis of equine peritoneal fluid. Vet Clin North Am Large Anim Pract 1:267-274, 1979
10. Brownlow MA: Abdominal paracentesis in the horse: basic concepts. Aust Vet Pract 11:60-67, 1981
11. Freden GO, Provost PJ, Rand WM: Reliability of using results of abdominal fluid analysis to determine treatment and predict lesion type and outcome for horses with colic: 218 cases (1991-1994). J Am Vet Med Assoc 213:1012-1015, 1998
12. Milne EM, Doxey DL, Gilmour JS: Analysis of peritoneal fluid as a diagnostic aid in grass sickness (equine dysautonomia). Vet Rec 127:162-165, 1990
13. Arden WA, Stick JA: Serum and peritoneal fluid phosphate concentrations as predictors of major intestinal injury associated with equine colic. J Am Vet Med Assoc 193:927-931, 1988
14. Weimann CD, Thoefner MB, Jensen AL: Spectrophotometric assessment of peritoneal fluid haemoglobin in colic horses: an aid to selecting medical vs. surgical treatment. Equine Vet J 34:523-527, 2002
15. Latson KM, Nieto JE, Beldomenico PM, et al.: Evaluation of peritoneal fluid lactate as a marker of intestinal ischaemia in equine colic. Equine Vet J 37:342-346, 2005
16. Van Hoogmoed L, Rodger LD, Spier SJ, et al.: Evaluation of peritoneal fluid pH, glucose concentration, and lactate dehydrogenase activity for detection of septic peritonitis in horses. J Am Vet Med Assoc 214:1032-1036, 1999

11.1.3. Ultrasonography of the gastrointestinal system

Kevin Corley

Ultrasonography is an extremely useful tool for diagnosing and monitoring gastrointestinal tract conditions, especially when used to complement the examination per rectum in adult horses. However, in adult horses presenting in acute abdominal pain, ultrasonography is only necessary if a determination whether surgery is required cannot be made from the rectal examination, physical examination and results from passage of a nasogastric tube and immediate laboratory investigations. In animals that are physically too small to perform a rectal examination, especially foals, ultrasonography may be the only way to make a definitive diagnosis apart from an exploratory celiotomy.

In adult horses, a 2.5- to 3.5-MHz sector or linear array probe is most useful for transabdominal imaging of the intestines. In foals, a 5-MHz sector or linear array probe gives greater detail and sufficient depth than a 3.5-MHz probe. Transrectal imaging of the intestine in the adult horse is best carried out with a 5- to 8-MHz linear probe (Box 3.2).

Stomach

The stomach is imaged in the 10th and 11th intercostal spaces, caudal to the liver and medial to the spleen in the left abdomen. It may often also be imaged one rib space in front or behind this.[1] It has a smooth semicircular wall, which has a thickness of up to 7.5 mm in the adult horse[2] (Table 11.3). In foals with a duodenal stricture (secondary to a duodenal ulceration) and adult horses with a gastric impaction, the stomach can be greatly increased in size. An enlarged stomach can be followed caudally as a continuous structure from its normal position into the abdomen (Figure 11.2).

Small intestine

The duodenum can be imaged in the 16th to 17th right intercostal space, ventral to the right kidney. It may often also be followed cranially from here as it courses medial to the right lobe of the liver. It is a small circular structure, with a hypoechoic or echogenic wall, and a fluid lumen.[1] In normal horses, the jejunum often cannot be imaged by

Table 11.3. Normal wall thickness and diameter of sections of the intestine, as measured by ultrasound[1,2,8,12]

Section	Wall thickness	Diameter
Stomach	4–7.5 mm	—
Duodenum	3 mm	Up to 4.5 cm during distension phase
Jejunum	3 mm	Up to 4 cm
Ileum	4–5 mm	Up to 4 cm
Caecum	Up to 4 mm	—
Large colon	Up to 4 mm	—
Right ventral colon	2.3–5.1 mm	—
Right dorsal colon	2–6 mm	—
Small colon	Up to 4 mm	7–10 cm

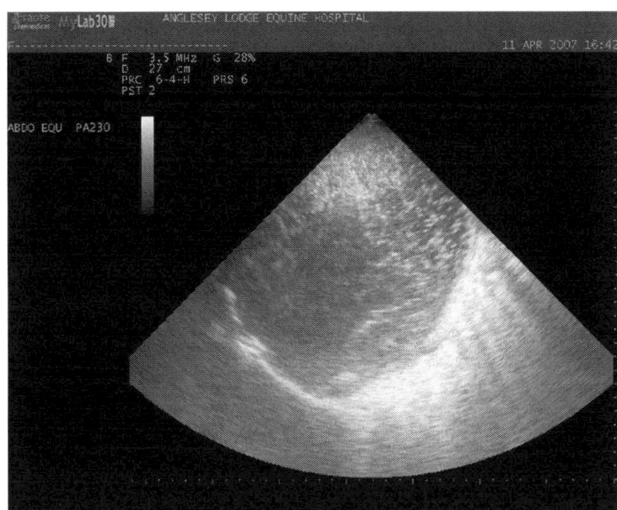

Figure 11.2 Transabdominal ultrasound image of an enlarged stomach in a 4-month-old foal with a duodenal stricture. This image was made ventrally in the midabdomen. In the real-time ultrasound image, there was a swirling motion of the stomach contents. ©Kevin Corley 2007.

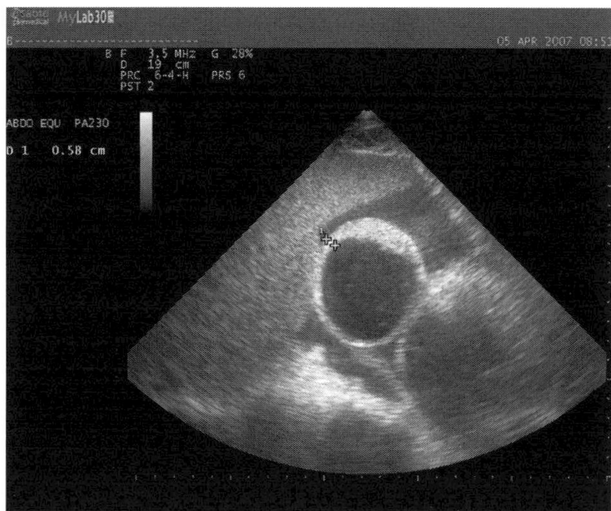

Figure 11.4 A distended loop of small intestine adjacent to the spleen in a horse after resection and anastomosis of the jejunum. The wall thickness of this loop is 0.58 cm, and the echogenicity of the wall is increased, suggesting inflammatory infiltrates. ©Kevin Corley 2007.

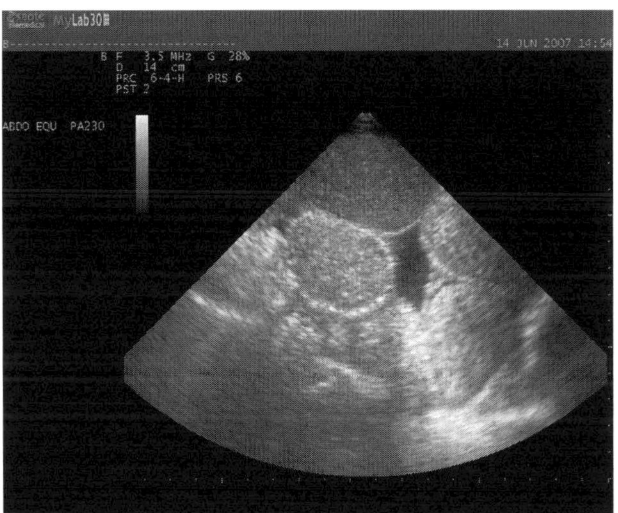

Figure 11.3 Multiple loops of moderately distended, amotile small intestine in a horse with ileus 1 day after surgery for a small intestinal volvulus. ©Kevin Corley 2007.

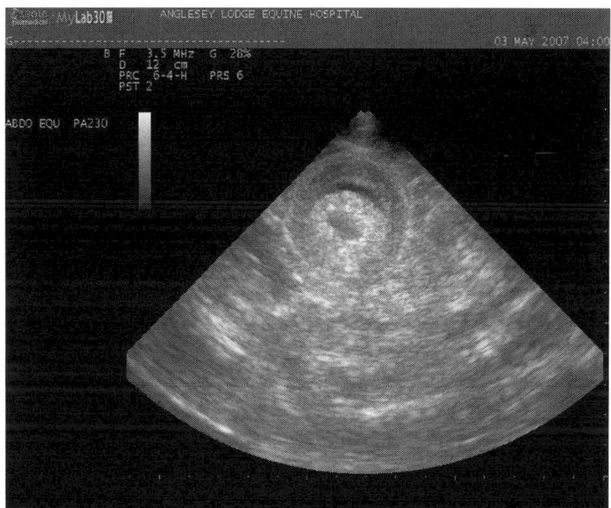

Figure 11.5 Small intestinal intussusception in a 4-month-old foal. There is a classic "target" appearance to the lesion, which consists of a hyperechoic thick-walled inner piece of intestine, surrounded by a hypoechoic thick-walled middle piece of intestine. The outer piece of intestine, whilst markedly increased in diameter, has a relatively normal echogenicity and wall thickness. ©Kevin Corley 2007.

transabdominal ultrasound. In one study, the jejunum could only be imaged in 1 of 10 normal-fed horses and 6 of 10 fasted horses.[3] If it is found, it is usually just caudal to the xiphisternum or just in front of the mammary gland or prepuce. The wall thickness of the normal duodenum and jejunum is 3 mm, and of the ileum is 4 to 5 mm[2] (Table 11.3).

Strangulated small intestine appears as nonmotile loops of intestine (Figure 11.3), which may have an increased wall thickness (Figure 11.4). The loops may be very distended, with a diameter of up to 13.5 cm.[4] Ultrasonography can be particularly useful in diagnosis of small intestine strangulated in the epiploic foramen, particularly when the animal is not showing signs of pain.[5] Small intestinal intussusception lends itself to diagnosis by ultrasound. The affected piece of intestine is heavier than surrounding intestine and often can be imaged at or close to the ventral midline. The classic ultrasound appearance is a "target" or "bull's-eye" type pattern, with a thick hypoechoic rim[6] (Figure 11.5). In a few older animals, intussusceptions may be imaged transrectally. *Lawsonia intracellularis* infection of the small intestine results in a markedly thickened and oedematous intestinal wall[7] (Figure 11.6), which at first inspection can appear similar to the image on an intussus-

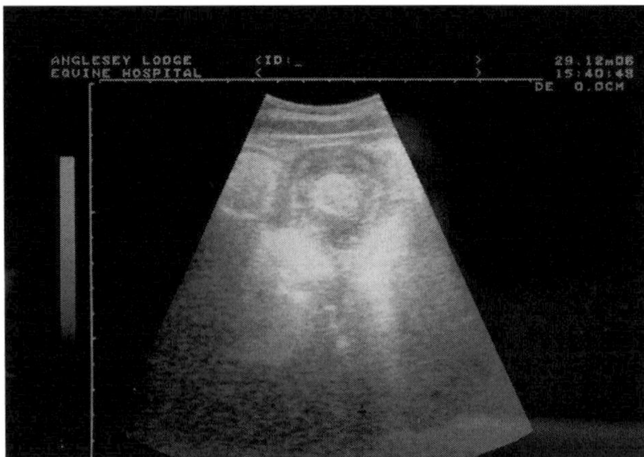

Figure 11.6 A markedly thickened (wall thickness 11 mm) loop of small intestine in an 8-month-old foal, in which *Lawsonia intracellularis* infection was confirmed by serology and faecal PCR. The foal made a full recovery with oxytetracycline and then doxycycline treatment. ©Kevin Corley 2007.

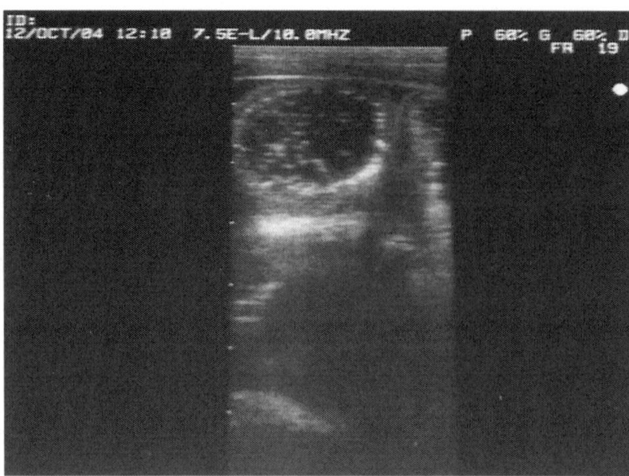

Figure 11.8 A cross-sectional image of small intestine in a 3-week-old foal with clostridial enteritis. Note the hyperechoic rim, representing gas formation by the bacteria, just inside the wall of the intestine. ©Kevin Corley 2004.

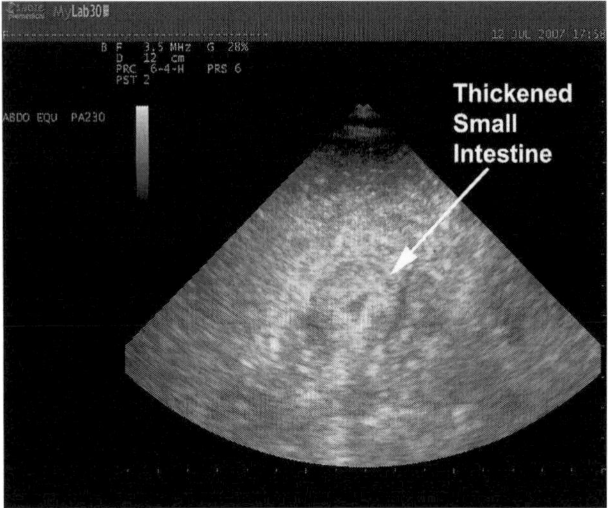

Figure 11.7 A loop of markedly thickened small intestine in a 3-month-old foal with enteric *Rhodococcus equi*. The foal made a full recovery with azithromycin and rifampicin treatment. ©Kevin Corley 2007.

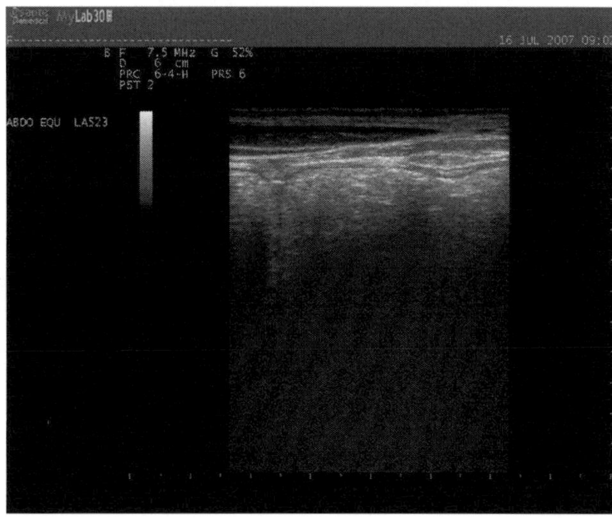

Figure 11.9 Normal haustrated left ventral colon imaged transabdominally in a 3-month-old foal. ©Kevin Corley 2007.

ception. However, there is only one layer of intestine in *Lawsonia* infection, compared to the two or three seen with an intussusception. The small intestine may be thickened with conditions other than *Lawsonia* infection, such as other infections (Figure 11.7), infiltrative bowel disease and compromise to the blood supply including strangulations. Enteritis can also result in moderately distended small intestine, which may be hypermotile. When gas-forming bacteria are responsible for the enteritis, there may be a rim of hyperechoic gas bubbles on the inside of the intestinal wall (Figure 11.8).

Peritonitis results in increased peritoneal fluid, often with an increased echogenicity, and may also result in increased small intestinal wall thickness (0.5–1.3 cm) and moderate increases in diameter (2–5 cm). The small intestine usually shows some motility.[4]

Caecum and colon

The normal wall thickness of the colon and caecum is 0.1 to 0.3 mm.[8] The caecum is on the right flank, in the paralumbar fossa, and in two to three intercostal spaces cranial to it. Caecal tympany can be detected as an increase in size of the caecum, a decrease in the number of haustrations and a hyperehoic line indicating gas accumulation.

The colon normally has a wall thickness of less than 4 mm (Table 11.3, Figure 11.9). An increase in wall thickness of greater than 9 mm in the colon wall measured at the ventral midline was diagnostic for colon torsion in 8 of 12 horses in one study. None of the 28 horses without a colon torsion that were examined in this study had a wall thickness greater than 9 mm at this site.[9] Increased colon

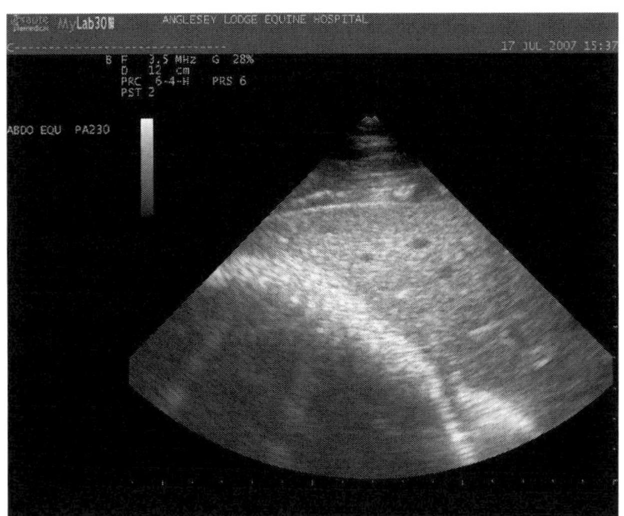

Figure 11.10 Normal right dorsal colon in an adult horse. ©Kevin Corley 2007.

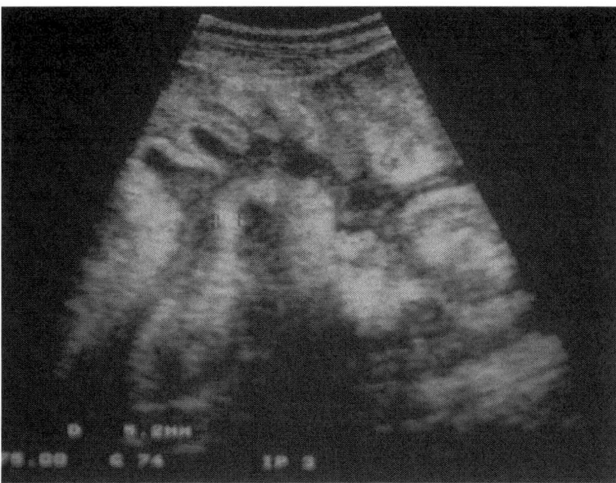

Figure 11.11 Small and large intestine adhered to a large abdominal *Rhodococcus equi* abscess in a 6-month-old foal. The real-time image did not change with breathing. The foal was treated with azithromycin and rifampicin, but succumbed to intractable colic 4 weeks later, at which time the diagnosis was confirmed. ©Kevin Corley 2007.

wall thickness is also found in horses with colitis. An alternative method for detecting colon torsions by ultrasound has been proposed, in which the nonsacculated left dorsal colon is found in the area normally occupied by the sacculated left ventral colon. The left ventral colon is normally imaged on the ventral left flank, below the ribcage, in an area with the cranial border level with the 11th intercostal space, and the caudal border with the 17th intercostal space.[10] Many clinicians, however, will question the need for either technique to diagnose colon torsions, especially given that they apparently take up to 15 minutes to perform. Colon torsions usually can be diagnosed by a combination of history, assessment of pain, examination per rectum findings and physical examination. In hospitals without a large staff, there are likely to be other priorities to stabilise and prepare the patient for surgery. Ultrasonography of these patients is probably only feasible in hospitals where there is someone dedicated to imaging who is not required for other tasks.

Ultrasonography of colon in the midventral abdomen can support a diagnosis of sand colic. The following findings are considered suggestive of sand accumulation in the intestine: poor motility, direct contact between the colon and the ventral body wall and a hyperechoic appearance to the ventral aspect of the colon.[11] However, if available, abdominal radiography is superior for detecting sand accumulations in the colon.[11]

The right dorsal colon can be imaged on the right flank, in the 11th, 12th and 13th intercostal spaces, below the ventral lung margin and axial to the liver (Figure 11.10). The normal thickness of the wall of the right dorsal colon is 0.2 to 0.6 cm. In horses with right dorsal colitis, the wall is thickened (0.7–1.6 cm) with a prominent hypoechoic line.[12]

The small colon has a normal diameter of 7 to 10 cm and a normal wall thickness up to 4 mm.[2] Strangulation of the small colon was identified by an increased wall thickness with transrectal ultrasound.[13] Small colon strangulations have also been diagnosed transabdominally in Miniature horses.[1]

Abscesses

Intra-abdominal abscesses can often be imaged with ultrasound. They appear as an approximately spherical, thick-walled structure. The echogenicity and fluidity of the purulent material within the abscess can vary among abscesses, but usually there is some movement of the material within the abscess distinguishing them from solid masses.[1] Abscesses can often be found in the midventral abdomen by transabdominal ultrasonography. They may also occur in the inguinal rings, if they are associated with castration of the animal. Abscesses in the root of the mesentery are also relatively common and can often be imaged with transrectal ultrasound.

When abscesses are found, they should be carefully observed with real-time ultrasound to check for adhesions to the surrounding intestine.[1] In some animals, a mass of unmoving intestine adhered to an abscess may be imaged (Figure 11.11).

References

1. Reef VB, Whittier M, Allam LG: Sonographic evaluation of the adult abdomen. Clin Tech Equine Pract 3:294-307, 2004
2. Reef VB: Adult abdominal ultrasonography, in Equine Diagnostic Ultrasound. Philadelphia, WB Saunders, 1998, pp 273-363
3. Mitchell CF, Malone ED, Sage AM, et al.: Evaluation of gastrointestinal activity patterns in healthy horses using B mode and Doppler ultrasonography. Can Vet J 46:134-140, 2005

4. Klohnen A, Vachon AM, Fisher AT: Use of diagnostic ultrasonography in horses with signs of acute abdominal pain. J Am Vet Med Assoc 209:1597-1601, 1996
5. Vachon AM, Fischer AT: Small intestinal herniation through the epiploic foramen: 53 cases (1987-1993). Equine Vet J 27:373-380, 1995
6. Bernard WV, Reef VB, Reimer JM, et al.: Ultrasonographic diagnosis of small-intestinal intussusception in three foals. J Am Vet Med Assoc 194:395-397, 1989
7. Schumacher J, Rolsma M, Brock KV, et al.: Surgical and medical treatment of an Arabian filly with proliferative enteropathy caused by *Lawsonia intracellularis*. J Vet Intern Med 14:630-632, 2000
8. Hendrickson EH, Malone ED, Sage AM: Identification of normal parameters for ultrasonographic examination of the equine large colon and cecum. Can Vet J 48:289-291, 2007
9. Pease AP, Scrivani PV, Erb HN, et al.: Accuracy of increased large-intestine wall thickness during ultrasonography for diagnosing large-colon torsion in 42 horses. Vet Radiol Ultrasound 45:220-224, 2004
10. Abutarbush SM: Use of ultrasonography to diagnose large colon volvulus in horses. J Am Vet Med Assoc 228:409-413, 2006
11. Korolainen R, Ruohoniemi M: Reliability of ultrasonography compared to radiography in revealing intestinal sand accumulations in horses. Equine Vet J 34:499-504, 2002
12. Jones SL, Davis J, Rowlingson K: Ultrasonographic findings in horses with right dorsal colitis: five cases (2000-2001). J Am Vet Med Assoc 222:1248-1251, 2003
13. Freeman SL, Boswell JC, Smith RK: Use of transrectal ultrasonography to aid diagnosis of small colon strangulation in two horses. Vet Rec 148:812-813, 2001

11.1.4. Gastroscopy and duodenoscopy

Tim Brazil

Gastroscopy is indicated in the examination and monitoring of animals presented for investigation of recurrent low-grade abdominal pain, weight loss or anorexia and animals with unexplained poor appetite during recovery from major surgery or systemic disease. However, it should be remembered that there is a high incidence of gastric ulceration in performance horses, particularly racehorses,[1,2] so a thorough diagnostic investigation must be completed to avoid over interpretation of the effect of any gastric ulcers identified.

The technique for gastroscopy is described in Chapter 1.10. Each region of the gastric mucosa that is examined can be graded—squamous fundus, greater curvature, lesser curvature/cardia, margo plicatus right side and glandular mucosa/pylorus—using the grading system recommended by the Equine Gastric Ulcer Council (Box 11.3) and an overall grade ascribed.[3] The position and extent of unusual lesions can be recorded in the medical record.

Grades 0 and 1 are considered normal. Grades 3 and 4 require treatment. Localised Grade 2 lesions on the squamous mucosa may not be clinically significant and careful review of the clinical history is necessary to correlate such lesions with presenting clinical picture. The glandular mucosa of the gastric antrum and pylorus must be examined in detail as even relatively mild lesions (Grade 2) are highly significant and can cause affected animals significant discomfort. Patience may be required whilst viewing the antrum to allow gastric motility to reveal all aspects of the antral rugal folds.

Box 11.3. Equine Gastric Ulcer Council lesion grading system[3]

Grade	Description
0	The epithelium is intact and there is no mucosal erythema or yellow hyperkeratosis (squamous only)
1	The mucosa is intact but there are areas of mucosal erythema or hyperkeratosis.
2	Small, single or multifocal ulcers
3	Large, single or multifocal ulcers or extensive superficial lesions
4	Extensive ulceration with areas of apparent deep ulceration

Suspected gastric impaction is readily confirmed endoscopically and gastroscopy facilitates monitoring of the response to therapy. Care should be exercised not to overdiagnose gastric impaction in donkeys as large, residual, dry, rounded food/bedding masses are common in donkeys' stomachs following overnight starvation for gastroscopy. In contrast to clinical gastric impaction, these feed masses are smaller, smoother and rarely associated with significant gastric ulceration.

Gastric squamous cell carcinoma can be readily diagnosed by gross identification of a raised inflammatory mass originating from the squamous mucosa and confirmed by transendoscopic biopsy or at post mortem. Although clinical presentations are variable, weight loss, hypoalbuminaemia and hyperglobulinaema are consistent.[4]

Duodenoscopy is a highly valuable technique because, although only rarely is any gross pathology identified, it facilitates collection of a number of diagnostic samples. Occasionally, there may be gross evidence of parasitic disease, gastroduodenal ulceration and rare cases of duodenal neoplasia or granuloma formation. Although as yet unreported, aspiration and bacteriological culture of duodenal contents or bile from the major duodenal papilla[5] (see Figure 1.27) may be useful in the investigation of animals with suspected duodenitis-proximal enteritis or septic cholangiohepatitis, respectively. Similarly transendoscopic proximal duodenal mucosal biopsies can be readily harvested. Biopsy is indicated in animals with clinical and laboratory evidence of small intestinal malabsorption, protein losing enteropathy and thickened small intestine on transabdominal ultrasonography. Little is known about the anatomical distribution of mucosal pathology in equine inflammatory infiltrative enteritis cases, but preliminary data suggest a positive diagnostic yield in approximately 20% of cases (T. J. Brazil, unpublished data). Although less useful than full-thickness intestinal biopsy samples harvested at exploratory celiotomy, the minimally invasive nature of transendoscopic biopsy makes it a viable preliminary approach.

References

1. Jonsson H, Egenvall A: Prevalence of gastric ulceration in Swedish Standardbreds in race training. Equine Vet J 38:209-213, 2006
2. Murray MJ, Grodinsky C, Anderson CW, et al.: Gastric ulcers in horses: a comparison of endoscopic findings in horses with and without clinical signs. Equine Vet J Suppl 7:68-72, 1989
3. Equine Gastric Ulcer Syndrome Council: Recommendations for the diagnosis and treatment of Equine Gastric Ulcer Syndrome (EGUS). Equine Vet Educ 11:262-272, 1999
4. Deegen E, Venner M: Diagnosis of stomach carcinoma in the horse. Dtsch Tierarztl Wochenschr 10:472-476, 2000
5. Bain FT, Petrizzi L, Valbonetti L, Muttini A: Gastroscopy and duodenoscopy, in Slovis NM (ed): Atlas of Equine Endoscopy. St. Louis, Mosby, 2004, pp 147-168

11.2 Management of horses with gastrointestinal disorders

Emma Rowe

Ileus

Pathophysiology of ileus

Intestinal stasis or ileus is a serious complication in the hospitalised horse. Postoperative ileus is a common complication in horses that undergo surgery for colic, especially when there is involvement of the small intestine. The reported incidence of ileus in horses ranges from 14% to as high as 47%.[1–4] Postoperative ileus also has a high mortality rate, which can be 83% to 86%.[2,5]

The intestinal motility is reduced when there is disruption of the complex pathways leading to aboral movement of feed material. This disruption can be explained as loss of intrinsic or extrinsic electrical activity, incoordination of contractile activity from regional stimuli, and dissociation between electrical and mechanical activity.[6] When this occurs, there is failure in intestinal propulsive contractile activity and this results in the intestine distending with fluid, ingesta and gas causing gastric reflux and abdominal pain. Many factors contribute to the cause of this disruption in intestinal motility and transit. Endotoxaemia, sympathetic stimulation, inflammation and distension are all thought to contribute to the cause of ileus.[7–10] Sympathetic stimulation has been thought to be a major contributor to ileus as it inhibits motility within the gastrointestinal system, while the parasympathetic system is excitatory. Recently it has been shown experimentally that the predominant inhibitory innervation to the gastrointestinal smooth muscle comes from the intrinsic, nonadrenergic, noncholinergic inhibitory neurons.[11] This explains why prokinetic drugs directed towards decreasing the adrenergic inhibition have been unsuccessful in alleviating motility disorders.[11] There is research being done constantly in order to understand these inhibitory pathways and to investigate drugs that may be able to target these pathways. For example, recent data suggest that drug interactions with *ether-a-go-go* potassium channels in the equine intestine are important for the prokinetic effects of cisapride,[12] and there are now efforts being made to develop and market noncardiotoxic versions of cisapride.[13] Substance P has also been found to be an important neurotransmitter and may also provide a therapeutic option for motility disorders of horses that are unresponsive to adrenergic and cholinergic drugs.[14]

Treatment of ileus

Decompression of the stomach and fluid therapy

The mainstays of treatment of ileus are intermittent decompression of the stomach, and fluid therapy. To decompress the stomach, a nasogastric tube is passed (see Chapter 1.7). If reflux does not flow spontaneously from the tube (which is not that common), attempts should be made to siphon the stomach. The tube is filled via a funnel with a small amount of water, and then the end is placed into a discard bucket, which should be considerably lower than the level of the horse's stomach. Several attempts should be made, with the tube advanced and retracted slightly, to maximise the chance of obtaining reflux if it is present. It is important to keep track of the amount of water used to try and obtain reflux, and this should be subtracted from the final amount of reflux in the bucket. The reflux should be treated as potentially infectious material, and appropriate precautions taken. The interval between refluxing attempts should vary with the amount of reflux obtained, and should probably be at least every 2 hours if more than 2 L of reflux per hour is being obtained.

Horses lose a large quantity of fluid through reflux, and it is important to take this into account when considering fluid therapy for these patients. Initially refluxing horses may become hypochloraemic and alkalotic due to loss of hydrochloric acid from the stomach. However, lactic acidosis associated with fluid loss–induced hypovolaemia will the major acid-base abnormality in many patients with reflux. With chronicity, refluxing horses tend to become hyponatraemic and acidotic, as they lose sodium bicarbonate from the proximal duodenum. Deliberately under–fluid-resuscitating refluxing animals to try and reduce reflux is a very dangerous practice. The physiological response to hypovolaemia is to divert blood away from the gastrointestinal tract, to other essential organs such as the brain and heart (this is also seen in the so-called fight-or-flight reaction). Diverting blood away from the gastrointestinal tract will reduce the amount of fluid that can pass into the lumen as reflux, because much of this will be drawn from plasma. However, it also will markedly reduce oxygen delivery to an already damaged organ, with potentially serious long-term consequences. Fluid therapy is discussed in detail in Chapter 6.5.

Nonsteroidal anti-inflammatory drugs

Endotoxaemia is important in the pathophysiology of ileus. Infusions of endotoxin have been shown to disrupt intestinal motility, and administration of both phenylbutazone and flunixin meglumine have been shown to attenuate this motility disruption in the stomach, small intestine and large colon.[15] These nonsteroidal drugs attenuate or reduce the effects of endotoxaemia, reduce inflammatory mediators and provide analgesia (reduce sympathetic stimulation) and therefore can protect against ileus through several different mechanisms. Thus this anti-inflammatory and analgesic therapy is very important to protect against ileus and is the first line of defence.

Prokinetic drugs

In the hospitalised horse, prokinetic drugs may be required in cases of intestinal stasis. Examples of conditions where they are commonly used include postoperative colic and proximal duodenitis-jejunitis. Prokinetic drugs have been used for several years with varying success. There have been many inconsistent results with the various drugs used in horses clinically affected with ileus. Examples of the drugs that have been used are given in Box 11.4.[16–18] Each of the common prokinetics used in equine hospitals will be discussed separately with a summary of when to use the various drugs being addressed at the end.

Lidocaine (Lignocaine)

Lidocaine (lignocaine) is one of the most common prokinetic drugs being used in equine hospitals. It was the most popular choice for treatment of ileus in horses following surgery for a small intestinal lesion in the recent prokinetic survey.[19] In our hospital, it is frequently used postoperatively and also during general anaesthesia for horses with significant intestinal inflammation. Intravenous lidocaine may also have a role in equine anaesthesia as it has been shown to decrease halothane minimal alveolar concentrations in anaesthetised ponies, in a dose-dependent fashion[20] (see also Chapter 4). Lidocaine is thought to act via several different mechanisms to stimulate gut motility. These mechanisms include direct stimulation of smooth muscle, blockade of sympathetic inhibitory reflexes, reduction in concentrations of circulating catecholamines and a decrease of inflammation.[21] It has been shown to increase contractile amplitude of the proximal duodenum *in vitro* in normal equine intestine but did not have an effect on pyloric antrum or mid jejunum. However, the ability to reduce inflammation and block inhibitory reflexes may be more important than the direct stimulation of smooth muscle, and thus it may be a lot more effective in clinically affected animals which have significant bowel and peritoneal inflammation. Lidocaine also has a central effect at the level of the spinal cord that may be the major site of antinociceptive action.[22] Intravenous lidocaine has been shown to have a dose-dependent inhibitory effect on neuronal populations in the spinal cord involved with visceral pain.[23] The prokinetic effects have also been well documented in humans, with bowel function returning quicker and days in the hospital being decreased with lidocaine treatment following radical surgeries such as retropubic prostatectomy.[24] Lidocaine has also been successful in the treatment of postoperative ileus or duodenitis-jejunitis in horses.[25,26] Lidocaine is the author's choice of prokinetic drug in most situations.

The anti-inflammatory effects of lidocaine could be of great benefit in horses with ischaemia-reperfusion injury and marked inflammation of the gastrointestinal tract. It is also useful in medical colics for which surgery is not an option. For example, if a horse in which surgery is not an option has a severe large colon impaction, no borborygmi, marked gas distension of the large colon and pain that is not responding to analgesics given, lidocaine administered intravenously can provide very good analgesia and may possibly stimulate motility allowing the impaction to begin resolving. The analgesic effect can be profound and it is possible to mask moderate-severe pain with horses remaining comfortable with severe conditions such as large colon volvulus. Thus lidocaine should be reserved for postoperative cases, proximal duodenitis-jejunitis or in cases for which surgery is not an option. The accepted dose rate is 1.3 mg/kg bolus to be administered over 15 minutes and then a constant rate infusion (CRI) of 0.05 mg/kg/min. This should be administered with an electronic infusion pump (see Chapter 1.17) to avoid accidental overdosing and toxicity. If the CRI is discontinued for a period of time greater than 45 minutes to 1 hour, the bolus should be given again and the CRI then restarted as the drug has a very short half-life. Signs of toxicity have been observed with serum concentrations between 1.85 and 4.53 µg/ml.[27]

Box 11.4. Examples of prokinetic drugs that have been used in the horse[16–18]

- Lidocaine
- Erythromycin
- Metoclopramide
- Cisapride
- Neostigmine
- Bethanechol
- Acepromazine
- Yohimbine
- Propanolol
- Phenoxybenzamine
- Naloxone

This serum concentration is 2 to 3 times higher than the target therapeutic level used in the treatment of ileus. In the horse, neurological side effects with toxicity are more marked than cardiovascular changes. In a study investigating toxicity, one horse developed rapid and profound ataxia, which progressed to collapse, and the serum concentration was 2.86 μg/ml.[27] The lidocaine was immediately discontinued, and there were no cardiovascular or cardiopulmonary effects and no seizure activity. The horse stood in 10 minutes and could walk.[27] This has also been the author's experience with a small number of horses clinically showing some neurological signs such as depression or ataxia, while being treated with a CRI of lidocaine. When the drug is discontinued, the improvement is rapid. This is due to the drug's short half-life. Intravenous lidocaine should not be administered with intravenous cimetidine as the two drugs are both metabolised by the same pathway in the liver and signs of toxicity may occur.

Erythromycin

Erythromycin is a macrolide antibiotic that is used to treat infections in horses, but also at low doses stimulates intestinal motility by binding to motilin receptors. Motilin receptors have been identified in the duodenum, jejunum, pelvic flexure and caecum of horses.[28] The highest number of these receptors is in the duodenum and then the numbers decrease distally along the bowel segments.[28] Erythromycin lactobionate has been shown to compete with motilin, binding to the motilin receptors located throughout the equine gastrointestinal tract.[28] Experimental work suggests that erythromycin has an effect on myoelectric activity of the ileum, caecum and pelvic flexure in horses, but the prokinetic effect when it is administered during the immediate postoperative period is not the same as when it is administered 8 days after surgery.[29] In this study, erythromycin was administered at 0.5 mg/kg IV over 1 minute; it did not have an effect for the first 24 hours after surgery, but a significant effect was recorded on day 8.[29] The magnitude of the effect was greatest at the pelvic flexure compared with the ileum and caecum. The authors concluded that erythromycin may be most effective for large colon ileus rather than decreased motility of the caecum or small intestine. In the recent prokinetic survey, it was the most common drug used for caecal impaction and was the second choice of prokinetic for horses following surgery for a small intestinal lesion and refluxing greater than 5 L before surgery and for 24 hours postoperatively.[19] Prolonged use of erythromycin or high doses can result in down regulation of the motilin receptors and the intestine becoming refractory to this treatment. Therefore, lower doses should be used in preference to the higher doses. A significant effect of erythromycin, compared to saline controls, on the myoelectric activity of the caecum and right ventral colon, and caecal emptying has been documented. The doses used in this study were 0.10, 1.0, and 10 mg/kg IV over 60 minutes with a 0.10 mg/kg bolus.[30] When given to horses over 60 minutes, doses greater than 0.10 mg/kg increased activity.[30] Clinically, a dose of 2.2 mg/kg in 1 L of saline infused over 60 minutes every 6 hours has been used.[31] The most common side effect of this drug is abdominal pain.

Metoclopramide

This drug promotes the release of acetylcholine from post-synaptic cholinergic neurons via activation of 5-hydroxytryptamine receptors. Metoclopramide also antagonises the inhibitory influence of dopamine on intestinal smooth muscle and blocks the α_2-adrenergic receptors.[32–36] *In vitro* it has been shown to increase the contractile amplitude of both longitudinal and circular smooth muscle in the small intestine, with muscle strips located in more proximal regions responding to lower doses.[18] *In vivo* models have shown that it may restore gastroduodenal coordination.[33,37] The drug, unfortunately, has some undesirable side effects. It is able to penetrate the blood-brain barrier and produce central nervous system signs such as muscle spasms, motor restlessness and aggression.[38] However, despite these side effects, the drug has been used successfully in equine hospitals as a prokinetic agent. In a retrospective study, metoclopramide administered as a CRI decreased the incidence and severity of ileus following small intestinal resection and anastomosis.[39] In this study, the horses that received metoclopramide as a CRI (0.04 mg/kg/h diluted in 5 L 0.9% sodium chloride solution) had a reduced total volume, shorter duration and slower rate of gastric reflux and a shorter postoperative hospital stay when compared to horses receiving no metoclopramide and to horses receiving intermittent doses (40–60 mg diluted in 1 L 0.9% sodium chloride IV administered over 1 hour).[39] There are various other doses reported. It can be administered at a dosage of 0.25 mg/kg diluted in 500 ml saline IV over 30 to 60 minutes.[31] In the recent survey of prokinetics, there was a variety of doses used by the respondents including 0.1 mg/kg in 1 L crystalloids IV over 45 minutes every 6 hours; 0.04 mg/kg/hr CRI; 0.05 mg/kg intramuscularly every 6 hours; 0.1 mg/kg subcutaneously 3 to 4 times daily; 0.005 g/kg orally 3 times daily; 0.175 mg/kg/hr IV as CRI; 0.25 mg/kg/hr IV as CRI; and 0.25 mg/kg subcutaneously 4 times daily.[19]

Cisapride

This second-generation substituted benzamide is a serotonin receptor agonist, which, unlike metoclopramide, does not have any dopamine-blocking activity.[36] It has been documented that cisapride can coordinate progressive gastrointestinal motility throughout the equine gastrointestinal tract and may reduce the incidence of postoperative ileus.[40–44] In a clinical trial, cisapride significantly decreased the incidence of postoperative ileus when administered at 0.1 mg/kg IM every 8 hours. The prokinetic effect is not entirely due to its stimulatory effects on serotonin receptors as there is evidence to suggest that it is a partial agonist of the 5-hydroxytryptamine receptors.[43] Cisapride has also been shown to attenuate the endotoxin-induced delayed gastric emptying through a possible mechanism that involves *ether-a-go-go* (ERG) potassium channel blocks.[45] In addition to this, ERG protein has been identified in all segments of the intestinal tract of horses and these ERG channels were found to modulate the motility of the intestinal muscles.[12] In this study, the interactions of cisapride with these ERG channels were found to be important for the prokinetic effects of the drug.[12]

Unfortunately, cisapride has been taken off the market in most countries and is therefore no longer available to equine practitioners, due to events associated with cardiotoxicosis in humans.[46] With the findings of this recent research there is a need to develop a noncardiotoxic version of cisapride, or another drug, which can target these ERG potassium channels. Prior to cisapride coming off the market, administration was difficult as it was only available in an oral preparation that is obviously not suitable for the horse with gastric reflux. It was shown to have poor absorption per rectum.[47,48]

Neostigmine

Neostigmine enhances intestinal motility by inhibiting cholinesterase activity and therefore prolongs the presence of acetylcholine in the neuromuscular junction.[49] Neostigmine has been found to increase premature phase III contractions in the ileum of clinically normal ponies.[50] However, in one experimental model, neostigmine was found to decrease jejunal myoelectric activity and delay gastric emptying.[51] Neostigmine is usually used for large intestinal ileus,[19] although it has also been reported clinically as being successful in treating small intestinal ileus when other prokinetic agents have failed.[52] Neostigmine can be given at a dose rate of 0.022–0.044 mg/kg subcutaneously or intravenously. The usual dose given clinically is 0.044 mg/kg subcutaneously or intravenously and is repeated in 20 to 60 minutes, if there is no clinical response (abdominal cramping or restlessness) the amount can be increased by 2 mg every hour to a total of 10 mg per treatment.[49]

Bethanechol

Bethanechol chloride is a muscarinic cholinergic agonist that stimulates acetylcholine receptors on the intestinal smooth muscle. It has been shown to increase the rate of gastric and caecal emptying in normal ponies.[33] Some studies have also suggested that the effect of bethanechol is enhanced when administered in combination with yohimbine.[33] Yohimbine hydrochloride is an α-adrenergic competitive antagonist and may be useful for postoperative ileus associated with endotoxaemia.[31] Bethanechol has been used successfully as a prokinetic for treating horses with delayed gastric emptying. Even though this drug is classically reported as a successful prokinetic, in a recent survey of prokinetic use in horses it was used by very few clinicians.[19] The dose rate for bethanechol is 0.025 mg/kg subcutaneously every 3–4 hours, with a dose of 2.5 mg/500 kg at 2 and 5 hours after surgery.[49] Because this drug increases parasympathetic tone there may be some side effects such as abdominal cramps, diarrhoea, salivation and gastric secretion.[31] Bethanechol can be used for horses with postoperative ileus, but is usually not the first choice. However, anecdotally positive clinical responses have been seen with administration of this drug.

Acepromazine and yohimbine

Like yohimbine, acepromazine is an α-adrenergic antagonist. The objective of these drugs is to suppress the sympathetic nervous system, which has an inhibitory effect on intestinal smooth muscle. It can be given intramuscularly at the time of surgery and then every 4 to 6 hours using the 0.01 mg/kg dose rate. Acepromazine is a nonselective α-blocker that can produce hypotension, and thus the horse should be well hydrated if acepromazine is to be administered.[31] Some clinicians believe it may be beneficial to administer acepromazine in the postoperative period not only for its prokinetic effect but also to protect against potential laminitis.[52] It has been shown that acepromazine does increase blood flow to the foot.[53] Yohimbine is a more selective α_2-antagonist and therefore may be more effective than acepromazine. Yohimbine, 0.075 mg/kg administered over a 10-minute period, has been shown to induce a significant increase in spiking activity of the upper intestinal tract with a more mild and transient response in the large intestine.[50] There is another α_2-antagonist, atipamezole, which has been evaluated in rats but not yet in horses, which has minimal α_1 action and does not bind dopamine or serotonin receptors and therefore may even be more effective than yohimbine.[25]

Naloxone

Naloxone is a narcotic antagonist that has been shown to induce contractile activity in the caecum and left colon.[54,55] Naloxone is administered intravenously at 0.05 mg/kg and defaecation often follows the administration within approximately 15 to 20 minutes.[56]

Choice of prokinetic drug

The choice of prokinetic will depend on the intestinal lesion, where it is located in the gastrointestinal tract, the systemic status of the horse, duration of reflux, personal preference, hospital management strategies, availability of drug, ease of administration and financial considerations. The most effective therapy is most likely going to be a combination of agents as the causes of ileus are multifactorial and quite complex. As the use of prokinetics has produced inconsistent results in clinically affected animals, treatment should not really be based on the administration of one drug.[18] Appropriate surgical treatment followed by aggressive medical therapy is essential in horses at risk for developing postoperative ileus.[18] The prophylactic use of

Box 11.5. Possible choices for prokinetic drugs based on the condition or site of lesion

Postoperative small intestinal ileus
- Lidocaine
- Erythromycin
- Metoclopramide
- Lidocaine and erythromycin

Endotoxaemia causing or contributing to the ileus
- Acepromazine
- Yohimbine

Large intestinal stasis or obstruction
- Lidocaine
- Erythromycin
- Neostigmine
- Naloxone

During surgery (any lesion)
- Lidocaine (note that the infusion is halved during anaesthesia)

prokinetics is warranted in horses at risk for ileus and lidocaine is a very good choice for this purpose. The use of prokinetic drugs may also be of help in duodenitis/proximal jejunitis to possibly shorten the duration of the disease, in combination with gastric decompression, intravenous fluid administration and anti-inflammatory drugs. Intravenous lidocaine has the most potential in reducing inflammation and increasing intestinal motility in horses with this disease.[57]

The final selection of drug or combination treatment will depend on the individual case and the clinical status of the horse but clinicians can follow the rough guide given in Box 11.5.

There are varying opinions on when it is necessary to change the prokinetic drug if no effect is noticed after administration. The mucosal barrier is restored quite quickly, but will take between 3 and 5 days to heal sufficiently for return of function, and the clinical signs of endotoxaemia to reduce; therefore, it may be wise to continue a treatment for at least 72 hours before concluding that a drug is not efficacious. These decisions will often be based on the clinician's experience with the promotility agent being used. Horses with sustained ileus will often also require parenteral nutrition (see Chapter 5). Adequate nutrition is essential for wound healing and immune function and therefore is very important for postoperative patients in hospital. The horse with ileus may not be able to tolerate enteral nutrition for several days and optimally should receive parenteral nutrition.

Box 11.6. Clinical features of endotoxaemia[31]

- Pain
- Tachycardia
- Congested mucous membranes
- Peripheral oedema
- Gastrointestinal hypomotility
  - Intestinal distension
  - Nasogastric reflux
- Thrombosis or bleeding tendencies

Treatments for endotoxaemia, sepsis and systemic inflammatory response syndrome (SIRS)

Endotoxaemia is the presence of endotoxin in the bloodstream, and the term is used clinically to describe the clinical signs the equine patient demonstrates when there is circulating endotoxin. Endotoxaemia is of great importance in the hospitalised horse or neonate as it is a major cause of mortality and morbidity. As well as mortality, it also results in the development of many potentially life-threatening sequelae in critically ill patients,[58–60] including laminitis.[61,62]

Endotoxin is the lipopolysaccharide part of the outer cell wall of Gram-negative bacteria. In the normal horse, there is a large amount of endotoxin in the large intestine. However, it is primarily in the form of Gram-negative bacteria and is normally prevented from entering the bloodstream. If small amounts of endotoxin enter the portal circulation, they are rapidly neutralised. In certain circumstances the defences may be breached, and endotoxin can enter the bloodstream. Examples include the lipopolysaccharide clearing capacity of the liver being overwhelmed with very large amounts (surgical gastrointestinal conditions, severe colitis, hypovolaemia)[63] and when the lipopolysaccharide bypasses the portal circulation entering the systemic circulation directly from the peritoneal cavity, pleural cavity or uterus.[62] Once in the bloodstream the endotoxin induces widespread effects, the most severe being on the cardiovascular system. It causes decreased circulating vascular volume, increased capillary permeability, ileus and coagulation disorders.[31] The clinical features of endotoxaemia is given in Box 11.6. Gastrointestinal stasis and reflux, increased capillary permeability and maldistribution of fluids with venous pooling all contribute to the massive fluid losses and hypovolaemia seen with endotoxaemia.[31] The increased capillary permeability usually also results in significant protein loss. Thus one of the most important parts of treatment for endotoxaemia is fluid therapy and careful adjustments and additional treatments may be necessary to prevent significant hypoproteinaemia (see Chapter 6.5).

Box 11.7. Treatments for endotoxaemia

Current treatments
- Fluid therapy
- Antibiotics
- Polymixin B
- Hyperimmune plasma*
- Pentoxifylline*
- Nonsteroidal anti-inflammatory drugs
- Low-molecular-weight heparin (dalteparin or enoxaparin)

Possible future treatments
- Competitive inhibitors of endotoxin
- Platelet-activating factor agonists
- Omega-3 fatty acids

*The effectiveness of these treatments is debated.

Other treatments for endotoxaemia are based on preventing the absorption of the endotoxin molecule, chelating and eliminating the endotoxin molecule and pharmacological management of the cascade of inflammatory mediators triggered by the endotoxin.[31] Possible treatments for endotoxaemia are listed in Box 11.7.

Polymixin B

Polymixin B has been used for several years as a treatment for endotoxaemia. It is a cationic polypeptide antibiotic that forms a stable complex with the lipid A component of the lipopolysaccharide.[64,65] By forming this complex it neutralises the lipopolysaccharide and alters the release of mediators and the response of target cells.[66–68] The drug when used in high concentrations is a bactericidal antibiotic. Care must be taken when administering this drug in the clinical setting as it has the potential side effect of nephrotoxicity. There have been several studies to evaluate the efficacy of polymixin B in horses with endotoxaemia. In one study in foals, a dose of 6000 IU of polymixin B/kg was more effective than antiendotoxin antibodies for the treatment of endotoxaemia, and the foals did not show any signs of toxicity including nephrotoxicity[69] or neurotoxicity.[64,68] Pretreatment of horses with polymixin B–dextran 70 combination prior to administration of endotoxin prevented signs of endotoxaemia, although this treatment was associated with mild adverse side effects (transient tachypnoea, sweating and increased plasma thromboxane concentration).[70] All of the adverse affects associated with administration of polymixin B–dextran 70 were eliminated when it was given in combination with ketoprofen, and thus it was concluded that it was a potential treatment for horses with endotoxaemia, if coadministered with a cyclooxygenase-inhibiting drug.[70] Recently the effects of polymixin B on experimentally induced endotoxaemia have been evaluated.[71] Treatment with polymixin B before or after administration of endotoxin significantly reduced fever, tachycardia and serum tumour necrosis factor, compared to horses receiving saline. The greatest difference between treatment groups was found between the horses receiving saline compared with those receiving 5000 IU/kg polymixin B prior to administration of endotoxin. In this study, the urine γGT-to-creatinine ratio did not change significantly and thus there were no signs of nephrotoxicity and it was concluded that polymixin B is a safe and effective treatment of endotoxaemia, even when administered after onset.[71] The recommended dose is 1000 to 5000 IU/kg 2 to 3 times daily, starting as early in the clinical disease process as possible.[72] Based on the *in vivo* studies, 5000 IU/kg appears to be a safe and effective dose.[71] Horses with endotoxaemia receiving this drug are most likely going to be on intravenous fluid therapy and should be well hydrated; however, in some cases (colitis, postoperative ileus with high volume reflux, for example) the horse may be hypovolaemic despite fluid therapy and these horses should be very closely monitored as they are potentially at risk for renal damage. All horses receiving polymixin B should have their serum creatinine levels checked regularly and close attention paid to their hydration status. Neonatal foals with concurrent azotaemia will be more susceptible to the nephrotoxic side effects of polymixin B and therefore must be monitored extremely carefully for renal function.[72]

Antiendotoxic plasma and antiendotoxic antibodies

The use of antiendotoxic antibody containing products is controversial, with conflicting reports on their efficacy. The theory behind their use is that the anti–lipid A antibodies will bind the lipopolysaccharide and then will prevent interaction with and activation of the mononuclear phagocyte system. The commercially available antiendotoxin antibodies are harvested from horses vaccinated against the core regions of mutant strains of Gram-negative bacteria, such as the rough strains of J5 *Escherichia coli*.[73] This gives one of the plasma products its name: "J5 plasma". These antibodies have been used in clinical and experimental trials. Initial studies in foals and horses found no significant difference in the parameters studied when comparing J5 plasma to normal plasma.[74,75] In a double-blinded trial evaluating hyperimmune lipopolysaccharide core antigen plasma as a treatment for horses with clinicopathological evidence of endotoxic shock, the horses receiving plasma had a significantly improved clinical appearance 48 hours after administration and a shorter period of recovery than did the control horses.[76] There are other studies evaluating the affects of hyperimmune plasma, with conflicting results. In some of these, the plasma used contained antibodies directed against the lipopolysaccharide of *Salmonella* spp. There are possible reasons for discrepancies between studies and clinical trials with the use of hyperimmune plasma. The interaction between endotoxin and the horses' inflammatory cells occur rapidly and thus in some studies the antibody may be administered too late to block initiation of the inflammatory cascade and clinical signs of endotoxaemia to develop.[73] If this is the case, then the clinical utility will be limited, as often any treatments must be administered considerably after the onset of endotoxaemia. Other possible reasons for the failure of these products in some trials are that the anti-core antibodies may be unable to penetrate the O-antigenic chains of intact smooth endotoxin to neutralise the core region[77] or that the host's compromised inflammatory system may not be able to opsonise or phagocytose bacteria.[78]

Based on the current literature, hyperimmune J5 plasma may be beneficial in the treatment of early endotoxaemia in adult horses. Anti–endotoxic antibody–containing preparations should, however, be avoided in foals as in one study there was worsening of clinical signs and increases in certain inflammatory mediators following administration.[64] More clinical trials need to be performed evaluating administration of J5 plasma early on in the course of the disease. In the hospitalised horse, the J5 plasma can provide an available source of protein for the hypoproteinaemic horse, such as the colitis case or the postoperative large colon volvulus. Maintaining colloidal pressure in these patients is very important (see Chapter 6.5), and thus administration of this product may be of benefit not only for the antiendotoxic effects but also for maintaining vascular volume. It should definitely be considered in the endotoxic horse, especially those horses with low total solids.

Competitive inhibition of endotoxin binding

Novel lipid A portions from plant bacteria, such as *Rhodobacter spheroides* and *Rhizobium* spp., can act as endotoxin antagonists. These molecules competitively inhibit interaction of lipopolysaccharides with its binding protein or other receptors.[79,80] The lipid A–like portion of these products binds to human monocytes but does not activate them, thus competitively blocking binding of endotoxin.[81] A related synthetic compound (E5531), based on the structure of *R. spheroides*, has also shown promise in humans.[82,83] However, the action of these drugs may be host species dependent. Investigations *in vitro* have shown activation of equine monocytes, leading to cytokine release, which could potentially exacerbate clinical signs.[84] It is thought that this difference is related to species differences in Toll-like receptor 4,[85] which is involved in monocyte activation in response to endotoxin. Work continues to produce synthetic lipid A derivatives that block endotoxin without activating monocytes,[86] and it is possible that one of these molecules will be suitable for use in the horse.

Pentoxifylline

Pentoxifylline has become popular recently for treatment of endotoxaemia. Pentoxifylline is a member of the methylxanthine class of drugs and is a haemorrheological drug that improves flexibility and deformity of rigid erythrocytes by inhibiting phosphodiesterase and increasing cAMP.[87–89] It is used in human medicine to treat peripheral vascular diseases, cerebrovascular disease and sepsis. *In vitro* and *ex vivo* experimental studies have demonstrated that pentoxifylline reduces endotoxin-induced production of cytokines, thromboxane and expression of tissue factor while simultaneously increasing plasma concentrations of prostaglandin I_2.[90,91] Specifically, pentoxyfylline inhibits tumour necrosis factor, interleukin-6 and tissue factor activity in a dose-dependent manner when equine whole blood is exposed to lipopolysaccharides.[91] When oral pentoxifylline has been administered to endotoxic horses *in vivo*, the beneficial effects have been limited. There has been no effect on tumour necrosis factor or interleukin-6 *in vivo*, although lower respiratory rates and rectal temperatures were associated with its administration.[92,93] When pentoxifylline has been administered in combination with flunixin meglumine the deleterious haemodynamic effects of endotoxin are offset more effectively than either drug administered on their own.[93] Even though pentoxifylline is widely used in equine hospitals, there as yet are no clinical studies documenting its effects. Pentoxifylline has also been used in the treatment of laminitis because of the possible effects on blood flow in the microvasculature. However, it was recently shown that pentoxifylline does not increase blood flow to the digit or dorsal laminae in healthy horses.[53]

There is also a question over the bioavailability and current recommended doses of pentoxifylline. There is evidence that it is poorly and erratically absorbed after oral administration and affected by food consumption around the time of dosing.[94,95] It also is unlikely to have any significant effect when given intravenously at the current recommended dose rates based on pharmacokinetic studies.[63] Thus, there are serious questions over is efficacy in the treatment of endotoxaemia, SIRS or sepsis in the clinical setting. Further investigation is warranted.

Nonsteroidal anti-inflammatory drugs

Nonsteroidal anti-inflammatory drugs (NSAIDs) are commonly used as part of a treatment regimen for horses with endotoxaemia.[96] The popularity of NSAIDs is linked to their dual function as analgesic and anti-inflammatory drugs.[97] The drugs most commonly used include flunixin meglumine*, phenylbutazone† and ketoprofen‡.[96]

*Examples include Finadyne (UK, Australia), Banamine (USA) (Schering Plough), Norixin (UK) (Norbrook), Flumav (Australia) (Mavlab).

†Examples include Equipalazone (UK) (Arnolds), Butazolidin (USA) (Schering Plough), Solvabute (Australia) (Fort Dodge).

‡Examples include Ketofen (UK, Australia) (Merial), Ketofen (USA) (Fort Dodge).

Carprofen§, eltenac**, vedaprofen††, ketorolac‡‡, meclofenamic acid§§, suxibuzone***, ibuprofen††† and meloxicam‡‡‡ are alternative NSAIDs for which pharmacokinetic studies have been performed in the horse or foal.[98–101] Flunixin and phenylbutazone have been most extensively studied with regard to endotoxaemia.

Flunixin has long been documented to ameliorate the cardiovascular effects of endotoxin, including hypotension, peripheral perfusion and vasodilatation, when administered shortly after endotoxin.[102] Administration of flunixin meglumine or phenylbutazone, prior to endotoxin, also reduces endotoxin associated respiratory signs, colic, diarrhoea, hypoxaemia, hyperglycaemia, prolonged coagulation times, haemoconcentration and lactic acidosis.[103–106] The profound neutropenia and leukopenia associated with endotoxin administration was not altered by a single dose of flunixin,[104] but was lessened by repeated doses.[107] Pretreatment with flunixin or phenylbutazone ameliorated endotoxin induced changes in gastric and left dorsal colon contraction. Phenylbutazone was more effective than flunixin.[108] Flunixin, phenylbutazone, ketoprofen, carporfen, meloxicam and eltenac have all been demonstrated to reduce the endotoxin-induced expression of a number of prostaglandins and thromboxane, demonstrating cyclooxygenase inhibition as their mode of action against endotoxaemia.[109–113]

Although NSAIDs clearly have beneficial actions in endotoxaemia, there are important side effects and potential toxicities, which may result in changes in their use in horses over the next several years. Classically described toxicities include gastrointestinal ulceration (gastric ulceration and right dorsal colitis), nephropathy and hepatopathy.[100,114] Toxic effects are more likely to occur when NSAIDs are given to hypovolaemic animals, a risk in horses with endotoxaemia, and when inappropriately large doses are given.[114] The potential to cause toxic effects differs between individual NSAIDs, and there is some evidence that ketoprofen is less toxic than flunixin, which, in turn, is less toxic than phenylbutazone.[115] Suxibuzone has also been shown to cause gastric ulcers of less severity and in fewer horses than phenylbutazone.[116] In addition to these classic toxicities, NSAIDs have been shown to retard the recovery of equine jejunum after ischaemic injury.[117] The delayed healing results in a prolonged period of impaired intestinal epithelial layer barrier function, but importantly does not promote LPS absorption.[118]

The analgesic and cardiovascular effects of flunixin have caused concern that this drug may mask the signs of surgical colic. For this reason, and to reduce the risk of the toxicities outlined above, experiments were performed to find a dose of flunixin that significantly decreased endotoxin mediated prostaglandin release, without significant effect on clinical signs.[107,119] This dose is 0.25 mg/kg of flunixin every 8 hours, and has been termed "the antiendotoxic" dose. This term is perhaps misleading, as higher doses of flunixin ameliorate clinical signs as well as decrease prostaglandin production. It should be noted that 0.25 mg/kg dose provides less analgesia than a standard 1.1 mg/kg dose. There is some evidence that providing good analgesia after surgery for colic can improve outcome, at least in terms of duration of hospitalisation.[120] For these reasons, the standard dose of flunixin (1.1 mg/kg every 12 hours) may be preferable. It may be prudent to delay the first dose until hypovolaemia has been reversed (see Chapter 6.5), if possible.

Despite the apparent positive effects of NSAIDs in endotoxaemia, there is no evidence that they improve survival in horses. In humans, a very large clinical trial of ibuprofen in septicaemia (which has many features in common with endotoxaemia) showed no difference in mortality between the treatment and placebo groups.[121] Interestingly, there was improved survival in a subset of people with hypothermic sepsis.[122] Although an equivalent subgroup is not immediately apparent for equine endotoxaemia, it is increasingly becoming apparent that targeted use of drugs for subgroups with a particular disease spectrum yields better results than blanket administration.[123,124] The use of NSAIDs for endotoxaemia, which has become dogma in equine medicine, may change over the next few years.

Low-molecular-weight heparin

The cytokine release associated with endotoxaemia results in activation of the extrinsic coagulation pathway, leading to microthrombi formation.[125] This microthrombi formation may prevent blood flow through the microcirculation in the affected tissue, resulting in decreased local oxygen supply and ultimately tissue or organ failure. Low-molecular-weight heparins might be effective prophylactically to prevent this microthrombi formation. Low-molecular-weight heparins and other treatments for coagulopathies are discussed in Chapter 8.2.

Platelet-activating factor antagonists

Platelet-activating factor (PAF) has been shown to be involved in many of initial clinical signs of endotoxaemia,

§Examples include Rimadyl (UK, Australia), Rimadyl (USA—licensed for dogs only) (Pfizer).

**Examples include Telzenac (UK, Australia) (Schering Plough).

††Examples include Quadrisol (UK), Vedaprofen (Australia) (Intervet).

‡‡No products licensed for horses in USA, UK or Australia at time of writing.

§§Examples include Arquel (UK, Australia, USA) (UK: Pharmacia. Australia: Bioniche. USA: Fort Dodge).

***Examples include Danilon Equilos (UK) (Esteve).

†††No products licensed for horses in USA, UK or Australia at time of writing.

‡‡‡Metacam (Boehringer) licensed for dogs in UK, Australia and USA.

including hypotension, platelet aggregation, increased vascular permeability and ileus.[126,127] PAF antagonists have been shown to reduce the endotoxin-mediated increase in heart rate, packed cell volume and reduction of abnormal gastrointestinal motor activity in ponies,[15] and to delay onset of fever, tachycardia, leucopenia and lactic acidaemia in horses given endotoxin.[128] In rat endotoxaemia models, it has been shown that survival was improved when high doses of various PAF antagonists were administered. Lower doses improved hypotension, but not survival.[129–131] However, as with many drugs trialed in human sepsis, PAF antagonists failed to improve outcome in two separate clinical trials. There was no improvement in survival with administration of either a PAF receptor antagonist[132] or a PAF acetylhydrolase, which rapidly degrades PAF.[133] These human trials provide some doubt that these drugs will be effective in our clinical patients.

Omega-3 fatty acids

Arachidonic acid, the precursor of the prostaglandins, thromboxane and leukotrienes, is an omega-6 fatty acid. Feeding diets rich in omega-3 fatty acids leads to a decrease in the content of arachidonic acid and its metabolites in plasma, and a shift of these fatty acids from the phospholipid portion in a tissue to the triacylglycerol and/or cholesterol ester pools.[134,135] Feeding omega-3 fatty acid–rich substances has been shown to have a beneficial effect on experimental murine endotoxaemia and clinical human sepsis.[136,137] Results in horses have been mixed. Horses fed an omega-3 rich diet for 8 weeks prior to endotoxin challenge showed no beneficial effect in their response compared to horses fed a regular diet.[138] In an equine *ex vivo* model, horses were administered omega-3 fatty acids as an infusion. Peripheral blood monocytes taken from these horses were demonstrated to have reduced endotoxin induced production of the inflammatory mediators thromboxane B2/thromboxane B3 and tumour necrosis factor-α.[139] Infusion of omega-3 fatty acids at the time of endotoxin challenge, therefore, may be a future antiendotoxic treatment in the horse.

Special considerations for medical colic patients

Monitoring

One of the most critical factors in the management of the medical colic patient is close monitoring. Horses hospitalised for colic may have a problem that can be treated medically or may have a possible surgical problem that is being monitored closely for deterioration that would warrant surgical intervention, or the horse may have a surgical problem being treated medically with financial restraints and no option for surgery. In any of these scenarios, it is extremely important that the horse is kept as comfortable as possible and is closely observed for any deterioration as a colic condition can worsen and become surgical at any time. In general, deterioration is most likely in the first 24 hours of treatment, when the horse is first given some food, and when the amount of food is increased towards a normal ration.

Monitoring for degree of pain is extremely important. Some colic patients may be extremely painful and if surgery is not an option may deteriorate to the point of requiring euthanasia for humane reasons. Analgesia is discussed in Chapter 6.2. Regular walking outside the stall can help reduce pain and encourage intestinal motility. It may also help prevent a horse damaging itself by rolling within the box. In certain conditions walking the horses may help correct the problem; for example, walking a horse, with a nephrosplenic entrapment, up and down a hill or lunging that horse following treatment with phenylephrine may help move the large colon off the spleen.

While hospitalised for a medical colic the horse will require constant walk-bys, especially in the early stages of an undiagnosed condition, or a condition that may progress and require surgery. When fluids are being administered the horse must be checked regularly to ensure the fluids are flowing at the correct rate, and that there are no fluid line or catheter complications (see Chapter 6.5). The horses need to be monitored for attitude, appetite, abdominal pain and distension, faecal production and consistency, water intake or hydration status and urination. These findings can be recorded on a specially designed form (see Figure 3.33).

Regular instructions for monitoring usually include hourly heart rate checks until the clinician is comfortable that medical treatment is being effective and the horse has improved to a point that these checks may be extended. Checking the heart rate is important as it can be an indicator of the severity of the condition and the cardiovascular status of the patient and can be an indicator of prognosis with certain conditions of the abdomen. Tachycardia is one of the indicators that surgery may be required, and generally a heart rate greater than 60 beats/min is of concern. The medical colic with a simple obstruction or displacement will usually have a heart rate between 40 and 70 beats/min, but if this increases it may indicate that the condition has progressed to a surgical lesion. However, heart rates can be deceiving. Severe conditions can be associated with a low heart rate, especially in old stoical ponies. Mild displacements can be associated with heart rates above 60 beats/min. Tachycardia is an indicator of pain and therefore may alert the clinician to the fact that more analgesia is required (see Chapter 6.2). A persistent tachycardia in the absence of a worsening abdominal problem or pain may indicate electrolyte abnormalities. Electrolyte disturbances such as hypocalcaemia, hypokalaemia and hypomagnaesemia may be present in medical colics and these horses may require intravenous supplementation (see Chapter 6.5).

Even when heart rate checks have been extended to every 2 to 3 hours or when they are limited to being recorded when the regular physical examinations are performed every 4 to 6 hours, hourly walk-bys should always be carried out (the medical colic can deteriorate at any time) and the attitude/pain status and character and volume of faeces should be recorded on the medical record. Medical colics will require regular physical examinations (known often as "flows" within the hospital setting) to be performed every 6 hours which include temperature, heart rate, respiratory rate, gastrointestinal sounds (see Chapter 11.1.1), mucous membrane colour, moisture and capillary refill time, palpation of digital pulses and recorded details of treatments given and fluids that have been administered and recordings of faeces and urine. All of these recordings may give an indication of how the horse is progressing and may give the clinician more information on the disease process present; for example, an elevated temperature may be present in medical conditions such as peritonitis, duodenitis/proximal jejunitis, pending colitis, endotoxaemia or Potomac horse fever. The nature and character of the faeces are important. The faecal contents should be examined for the presence of sand, gravel, undigested feed material, watery consistency (increased transit time), mineral oil that may have been administered previously and parasites (see Figure 11.1). A thorough examination does not need to be performed every time, but volume and character must be marked frequently. In areas where sand colic is prevalent, sand in the faeces should be monitored daily. The faeces can be placed in a rectal sleeve filled with water and tied up to allow the sand to sediment out. This can be a useful monitoring method to determine if sand is being passed during treatment.

A nasogastric tube should be passed if there is pain and/or abdominal distension. For horses that are refluxing, such as in the case of duodenitis/proximal jejunitis, the nasogastric tube should be passed (see Chapter 1.7) and taped in place to the halter and covered with the muzzle. The horse can then be regularly checked for reflux without trauma to the larynx or pharynx with repeated passage of the nasogastric tube. The horse that is refluxing volumes greater than 5 L should be checked and refluxed every hour. The horse with less than 5 L can be checked every 2 to 3 hours depending on the volume collected at each check. When checking for reflux, the clinician or technician should have repeated attempts to ensure that a pocket of fluid is not missed.

The medical colic should have blood taken and submitted regularly for packed cell volume and total solids and electrolytes. Depending on the severity of the condition, the frequency of this blood monitoring will change. In the critically ill case, electrolytes may be monitored every 6 hours and packed cell volume/total protein every 12 hours. This ensures that hydration and electrolyte status are monitored very closely.

A horse with abdominal pain or distension may need repeat rectal examinations as part of the monitoring process (see Chapters 1.4 and 11.1.1). Other diagnostic modalities that may be necessary to monitor the disease process or response to treatment include abdominocentesis (see Chapter 1.8), abdominal ultrasound (see Chapter 11.1.3) and abdominal radiographs. Another consideration for the medical colic, with worsening gas distension and no option for surgery, is percutaneous trocharisation of the distended viscus (see Chapter 1.11). This procedure is cost effective and can be performed in the stable. Releasing the gas distension can allow the large colon to return back to its normal position in some cases or to make the horse more comfortable to allow more time for the medical therapy to work.

Fluid therapy

The mainstay of treatment for the medical colic is fluid therapy. Fluid therapy may be administered by the enteral or intravenous route (see Chapter 6.5). The enteral route will not be appropriate for certain medical colics, such as those horses that have ileus and are refluxing or have severely compromised transit. However, enteral fluids may be extremely effective in medical conditions such as large colon impaction. Nasogastric tubes used to treat horses with colic (see Chapter 1.7) can be used for the administration of enteral fluid therapy for periods less than 2 days in duration and may be taped in place or removed and replaced with each treatment (depending on the frequency of fluid administration). These tubes should not be used for periods longer than 2 days as they may cause significant damage to the upper respiratory tract mucosa. Another option available is to use a commercial enteral feeding tube that has a small outer diameter (4.7 or 6 mm) that produces less pressure on the upper respiratory tract mucosa and thus causes less irritation/discomfort to the horse.[140] Placement of these tubes is described in Chapter 1.7. To ensure that there is no reflux before administering the fluid, the tip of the feeding tube should be placed into the stomach and suction applied. It is also imperative to confirm placement of the tube in the oesophagus and stomach and not in the trachea before fluid administration. The horse should be muzzled when the nasogastric tube is in place to prevent any feed intake and possible aspiration.[140] The small enteral feeding tubes may not be useful for checking for reflux as food particles may occlude the tube. This is an important disadvantage of smaller-bore tubes as in some cases the horse will not tolerate the enteral fluids and the stomach requires drainage. If the stomach needs to be emptied it may be necessary to remove the tube and replace with a larger-bore nasogastric tube.

Recipes for enteral fluids are given in Table 6.13. Usually isotonic or slightly hypotonic sodium-potassium-chloride is administered, unless there are specific electrolyte abnormalities indicating another fluid should be used (see Chapter 6.5). Gravity should be used to deliver fluids through the nasogastric tube or feeding tube to reduce the risk of gastric distension.[140] A funnel can be used if a large-bore nasogastric tube is in place, and is particularly useful if large fluid boluses are to administered rather than continuous infusion. Large volumes up to 10 L can be administered with the funnel through the large bore nasogastric tube in a few minutes.[140] Volumes over 6 L to a 500-kg horse may induce temporary abdominal pain. When administering the fluids through a feeding tube, a container such as a carboy or empty intravenous fluid bag can be attached to the tube via a coiled administration set usually used for intravenous fluids. The coiled lines can be reused as they do not have to be sterile for enteral administration. It is best to start the fluid therapy slowly with continuous infusions and gradually increase the rate of administration over a few hours.[140] High fluid rates have been reported, for example up to 10 L of fluids every 30 minutes, which is 40 ml/kg/hr for a 500-kg horse,[141] but this is not necessary and slower rates will reduce the chance of gastric distension, pain and poor tolerance to the administration.[142]

Large colon impactions are usually treated with intravenous fluids and laxatives such as magnesium sulphate. Magnesium sulphate is an osmotic laxative and appears to be very effective as part of the treatment for impactions. However, overdose of magnesium sulphate can lead to sweating, flaccid paralysis, coma and recumbency due to a blockade of peripheral neuromuscular transmission.[143] For this reason, it is advised that one 1-g/kg dose of magnesium sulphate is given via the nasogastric tube no more frequently than every 12 to 24 hours. Mineral oil is a traditional treatment but is usually not effective in moving impacted ingesta but can provide a crude estimate of fluid transit, with oil first detected in the faeces at approximately 12 to 18 hours after administration. This can give the clinician an idea of whether there is a complete obstruction present. Treatment of an impaction aims at creating systemic overhydration and increased intraluminal osmolality that will promote ingesta rehydration and transit.[144] Recently it has been shown that both enteral fluid therapy and intravenous fluid therapy combined with magnesium sulphate administered through the nasogastric tube can both increase colonic and faecal hydration and produce plasma expansion.[140] Enteral fluids were shown to produce the more marked hydration of ingesta than intravenous fluids. Therefore, for the mild to moderate large colon impaction, enteral fluids may be cheaper and the preferred treatment. When enteral fluids are administered to the medical colic patient, there must be continual monitoring for any intolerance such as abdominal pain due to gastric distension.[140]

Thrombophlebitis and laminitis

Horses that have an intravenous jugular catheter in place for intravenous fluid administration or medication need to have the catheter site monitored closely as there is a risk of thrombophlebitis (see Chapter 7.2). Another possible complication in the critically ill medical colic patient is laminitis (see Chapter 15.2), especially if there is concurrent endotoxaemia present with the intestinal disease, such as in the case of duodenitis/proximal jejunitis. These horses should have "lily pads" or supportive foam taped to their feet and should be on suitable bedding. The digital pulses will be monitored at each flow check, and any increase should be investigated in these high-risk patients. If there is obvious pain in the both front feet, lateral radiographs should be taken to investigate possible rotation or sinking.

Analgesia

Analgesia is very important for the medical colic patient (see also Chapter 6.2). It is essential to provide adequate analgesia without masking a deteriorating condition. Many clinicians will use an α_2-agonist such as xylazine in the mild to moderately painful medical colic. Xylazine provides short-term analgesia that does not mask severe pain. It is a common practice to administer flunixin meglumine at a reduced dose (0.5 mg/kg every 6–12 hours) as an analgesic, in the expectation that this will not mask increasing pain associated with the development of a surgical lesion. However, it is unlikely that a standard dose of flunixin (1.1 mg/kg) would mask severe pain, although many clinicians are not comfortable taking that risk.

Opoids are highly effective analgesics. They are rarely administered to nonsurgical colic patients, for fear of masking escalating pain associated with a surgical lesion. They are occasionally used when surgical intervention has been ruled out on financial or other grounds. The use of these drugs is described in Chapter 6.2. Intravenous lidocaine, originally described as a promotility agent, is gaining popularity as an analgesic agent. It is administered as a CRI (1.3 mg/kg over 15 minutes bolus and then 0.05 mg/kg/min CRI). It is particularly indicated for treatment of peritonitis or duodenitis/proximal jejunitis as a prokinetic and anti-inflammatory agent in addition to the analgesic effects. However, lidocaine infusions may also mask severe pain and should be used with great caution in a patient where surgery is an option. The author has used it in cases where surgery is not an option and the analgesia it has provided has been very good.

Antimicrobials

Antibiotics are not commonly administered to medical colics. However, in certain conditions, such as duodenitis/proximal jejunitis or septic peritonitis, they may be administered. The antibiotic choice will be based on the type of disease being treated (see Chapter 6.3). Antibiotic therapy is usually indicated when there is peripheral leukopenia, fever or degenerate white blood cells in the peritoneal fluid following abdominocentesis.[145]

Special considerations for surgical colic patients

Immediate treatment after surgery

When the postoperative patient returns to the stall following recovery from anaesthesia, the horse should be immediately connected to intravenous fluids (see Chapter 1.16). Surgical colic patients may be significantly hypovolaemic following surgery and recovery from anaesthesia, even if hypovolaemia was reversed prior to surgery. Many clinicians will measure blood electrolytes and lactate as the patient returns to the stall to immediately tailor the fluid therapy to the patient's needs (see Chapter 6.5). If the patient is likely to be or become endotoxic, specific treatment for endotoxaemia should be begun or continued, if it was initiated during surgery (these treatments are described earlier in this chapter).

Particular attention should be paid to keeping the patient warm. Core body temperature will decrease in adult horses anaesthetised in a cool, dry environment and additional body heat can be lost rapidly when anaesthetised horses are placed on cold surfaces during recovery.[146] The abdomen may have been open for prolonged periods, which also contributes to heat loss. The horse should be dried with towels if covered in sweat or otherwise wet and warm blankets should be applied. The horse may be shivering quite dramatically when it returns to the stall. These postanaesthetic tremors are thought to result from uninhibited spinal reflexes, pain, decreased sympathetic activity and a physiological response to hypothermia.[146–148]

Monitoring

Monitoring is as important in the surgical colic as the medical colic. Certain postoperative patients such as those that have undergone correction of a large colon volvulus or large colon resection may be critically ill and endotoxaemic. These horses require intensive care and may require additional cardiovascular monitoring such as blood pressure monitoring (see Chapter 9.1).

Monitoring of horses that have had abdominal surgery is based on restoration of circulating fluid volume, electrolyte and acid-base equilibrium, and the gastrointestinal function.[31] The horse should be monitored carefully with frequent heart rate checks, depending on the status of the horse and the lesion diagnosed at surgery. Horses in which small intestinal resection and anastomosis was performed will require 1 to 2 hourly heart rate and reflux checks, whereas a horse that has had a nephrosplenic entrapment corrected with minimal manipulation and no enterotomy may require less intensive monitoring. The postoperative colic should be monitored for improvement in attitude, appetite, abdominal pain and distension, faecal production and consistency and urination in a similar manner to the medical colic patient.

Physical examinations ("flow checks" or "colic checks") should be performed every 2 to 6 hours depending on the patient status and lesion identified at surgery. These should include temperature, heart rate, respiratory rate, gastrointestinal sounds (see Chapter 11.1.1), mucous membrane colour, moisture and capillary refill time, palpation of digital pulses and recording of faeces and urine. Details of treatments given and fluids that have been administered should also be recorded. Frequently, horses are tachycardic in the first 24 hours following colic surgery. This may be associated with endotoxaemia, hypovolaemia, cortisol release or pain. Severe tachycardia (>70 beats/min), tachycardia that lasts longer than 24 hours after surgery, or dysrhythmias may be associated with pain or electrolyte imbalances and warrants investigation.

This may include passage of a nasogastric tube (if there is not one in place), rectal examination, abdominal ultrasound, blood electrolyte analysis and an electrocardiogram (ECG) to investigate the cause of the high heart rate.

An increased respiratory rate may indicate pain, secondary respiratory tract complications, or acid-base disturbances. However, the respiratory rate will not always be increased with any of these conditions. If an increased rate cannot be explained by pain, then a complete blood count, thoracic auscultation, rebreathing examination and thoracic ultrasound should be performed to rule out postanaesthetic pneumonia (see Chapter 10.1). Monitoring the body temperature is extremely important; the temperature may be moderately increased for the first 24 hours after surgery, but thereafter a fever needs to be investigated. Possible sources of fever are listed in Box 11.8.[150] A fever of unknown origin should be investigated by evaluating the individual body systems (see Chapter 7.1), and if the source is located, then culture and sensitivity should be performed. The mucous membrane colour may be slightly congested following surgery but if the horse is not endotoxaemic they should return to a normal colour, be moist and have a capillary refill time of 2 seconds when the patient is adequately hydrated. It is extremely important to monitor the catheter site in postoperative colics as the patient is at risk for thrombophlebitis expecially if endotoxaemic, suffering from postoperative diarrhoea or is debilitated. The catheter site should be palpated at every flow check and monitored for signs of heat, pain, swelling or any drainage (see Chapter 7.2). If there is any concern, the catheter should be removed immediately. Borborygmi may be reduced following surgery for the first 24 hours; however, they should gradually start increasing and should be present when food is first introduced. Hand walking with or without a small amount of grazing may help stimulate motility. Prolonged absence of borborygmi is concerning and indicates postoperative ileus is present.

Box 11.8. Possible sources of fever in horses following colic surgery[150]

- Endotoxaemia
- Focal ischaemic large colon necrosis
- Colitis
- Peritonitis
- Septic thrombophlebitis
- Incisional infection
- Pneumonia
- Placentitis in broodmares
- Endometritis in broodmares

Nasogastric intubation

The surgical colic may have a nasogastric tube placed when returned to the stall after surgery for a small intestinal lesion or if there is the concern of postoperative ileus and reflux. There is some debate whether an indwelling nasogastric tube should be placed immediately in candidates at risk for ileus and reflux or whether it is better to monitor the horse carefully and place a nasogastric tube only if required. There has been some concern that the presence of the tube itself may contribute to ileus and the production of gastric reflux. It is also possible, however, that the postoperative patient being depressed may not show signs of abdominal pain in response to gastric distension and is at risk for gastric rupture. If a nasogastric tube is in place and the horse is being checked for reflux regularly, this should decrease that chance. However, in a retrospective study of gastric rupture in horses, it was found that at least six horses suffered gastric rupture in the postoperative period with an indwelling nasogastric tube in place, and in addition, the presence or absence of gastric reflux following nasogastric intubation was not a reliable indicator on its own of gastric dilation.[151] It is reasonable to place an indwelling nasogastric tube in a patient at risk for postoperative ileus and check for reflux every 1 to 3 hours in the immediate postoperative period. If less than 2 L reflux is obtained in a 3-hour period, then the tube should be removed. In some hospitals, an indwelling tube will not be placed in patients at risk for ileus, but in this case the horse must be monitored very carefully and the tube replaced if necessary.[5] The efficacy of indwelling nasogastric tubes in humans has been questioned and may in fact delay recovery,[152,153] and thus it may be better in the hospitalised postoperative patient to monitor carefully and pass the tube if indicated by clinical signs such as an increase in heart rate or signs of pain.[5]

Monitoring fluid status

The vast majority of surgical colic patients are treated with intravenous fluid therapy, at least in the immediate postoperative period. They therefore need to be monitored very frequently to ensure that the fluids are flowing in at the correct rate, and their hydration status, catheter and fluid delivery set should be monitored regularly. Packed cell volume and total solid concentration are monitored frequently in many clinics in the immediate postoperative period. It is a bad prognostic indicator if the packed cell volume remains high and the total solids decrease. It is not uncommon for the total solids to be low (<5 g/L [<5 g/dl]) for the first 24 to 48 hours after surgery, and the packed cell volume to be low (associated with some blood loss) or high (>40%–50%) during this time. As the horse improves through the recovery phase, these parameters should normalise. The total solids may become very low in horses with severe lesions and compromised mucosa such as following ischaemia-reperfusion injury to the large colon following large colon torsion. If the total solids are less than 40 g/L (4 g/dL), the horse will almost certainly benefit from supplementation with plasma or a colloid in order to maintain oncotic pressure and reduce or prevent oedema formation in the affected parts of the intestine (see Chapter 6.5). Plasma lactate concentration is also extremely useful to monitor the cardiovascular system in horses after colic surgery. Persistently increased lactate concentrations in the face of adequate fluid therapy portend a poor prognosis (see Chapters 6.5 and 9.1).

Electrolyte concentrations and acid-base status are frequently deranged in horses that have had colic surgery. In a recent study evaluating the prevalence and prognostic importance of hypomagnesaemia and hypocalcaemia after colic surgery, both hypomagnesaemia and hypocalcaemia were common in the perioperative period, especially in horses with strangulating intestinal lesions and ileus.[154] Horses with ileus had a significantly lower serum concentration of ionised magnesium after surgery, but neither serum magnesium nor calcium concentrations were predictors of hospital time or survival.[154] Electrolytes should be corrected as necessary (see Chapter 6.5).

An increased plasma creatinine concentration in the colic patient usually reflects either hypovolaemia or renal dysfunction. If creatinine is increased before surgery due to prerenal azotaemia secondary to hypovolaemia, it should decrease rapidly following fluid therapy after surgery. If persistently high after surgery, it may indicate that the fluid therapy is not adequate or that there is renal damage. Collection of a urine sample for specific gravity may help distinguish between the two[150] (see Chapter 13.2). Urination frequency should also be monitored, and if there is an increased creatinine in conjunction with oliguria or anuria, then specific therapy should be initiated[150] (see Chapter 13.2).

Other laboratory investigations

Many postoperative colics are leukopenic after surgery for a few days. There is often a neutropenia and left shift, and a hyperfibrinogenemia present on a complete blood count taken after abdominal surgery.[150] The neutropenia may be due to margination of neutrophils within the capillaries, as part of the endotoxaemia syndrome. A low fibrinogen or a sudden decrease in fibrinogen can be indicative of a coagulopathy[150] (see Chapter 8).

Antimicrobials

Perioperative antibiotics should be broad spectrum and have minimal effects on the gastrointestinal system. Penicillin combined with gentamicin is the most common choice, regardless of the lesion found at surgery.[155] If there is an increase in the creatinine concentration or a suspicion of renal insufficiency, another drug with good Gram-negative coverage (e.g., ceftiofur, cefquinome or enrofloxacin) may be used in the place of gentamicin (see Chapter 6.3). Common practice is to administer postoperative antibiotics for 24 hours if the surgery was uncomplicated and the bowel lumen was not penetrated. In a recent survey of antimicrobial use in adult surgical colic patients that required an enterotomy or bowel resection, respondents used antimicrobial drugs for 1 to 10 days, with the majority using them for 3 days.[155] Usually the clinician will use objective criteria to decide the appropriate time to discontinue the antibiotics.[31] A normal temperature, absence of abdominal pain, normal surgical incision, normal white blood cell count with no immature neutrophils ("bands") and a normal appetite and faecal production will indicate that it is safe to discontinue antibiotics.

Analgesia

Surgical colic patients require analgesia. The most commonly used analgesic is flunixin meglumine. It is recommended to administer flunixin for at least 24 hours following surgery and then for as long as required. It is either administered at 1.1 mg/kg every 12 hours or 0.5 mg/kg every 6 hours IV. However, flunixin meglumine has been shown to inhibit mucosal recovery at a dose *in vitro* that is comparable to that achieved with the 1.1 mg/kg dose administered intravenously.

The action of NSAIDs, such as flunixin, is to inhibit cyclooxygenase (COX) enzymes. These enzymes catalyze the production of prostaglandin G_2 from arachidonic acid.[156] Prostaglandin G_2 is an unstable intermediate, and is the precursor of many prostaglandins (PG) and thromboxanes (TX). The functions of these mediators are varied, and include gastrointestinal tract protection (PGE_2), changes in vascular tone (PGE_2, PGI_2), control of platelet aggregation (PGI_2, TXA_2) and control of inflammation (TXA_2, PGE_2, PGI_2).[100] Two COX enzymes have been identified: COX-1 is preformed and constituitively expressed, and is responsible for producing PGs required for homeostatic ("housekeeping") functions. COX-2 is largely newly synthesized in response to inflammatory stimuli, such as endotoxin. The PGs produced by COX-2 are mainly proinflammatory.[100] Flunixin inhibits COX-1 and COX-2 pathways.

There are now more selective COX-2 inhibitors (etodolac, eltenac) on the market. Eltenac has been shown to ameliorate endotoxin-associated physical signs and hormone and cytokine production in the horse.[110] It was thought that COX-2–selective inhibitors would reduce excessive prostaglandin production by COX-2 but would still allow production of prostaglandins by COX-1 (such as PGE_2), and therefore preserve mucosal repair. However, in a recent study investigating the effects of flunixin meglumine or etodolac on mucosal recovery of equine jejunum following ischaemic injury, both of the drugs were found to retard the recovery significantly compared to saline controls and there was no difference between the two drugs.[117] Therefore, at the time of writing, flunixin meglumine is still the nonsteroidal of choice in the postoperative colic.

Other analgesics that may be used in postoperative colic include lidocaine and butorphanol. Lidocaine is frequently administered to postoperative colics in an attempt to prevent postoperative ileus in high-risk candidates and for its analgesic and anti-inflammatory effects. Lidocaine is given as a 1.3 mg/kg bolus over 15 minutes and then as a CRI at 0.05 mg/kg/min. Butorphanol may also be administered as a CRI to provide analgesia in the postoperative horse. A 13 µg/kg/hr CRI of butorphanol has been found to decrease plasma cortisol concentrations and result in less weight loss and shorter hospital stays compared with untreated horses.[120] Morphine may also be administered as a CRI (0.3 mg/kg loading dose with an α_2-agonist, then 0.05–0.1 mg/kg/hr). In many countries, it is considerably cheaper than a butorphanol infusion and appears to be clinically highly effective. However, opioids may increase segmentation and decrease peristaltic motility in the large intestine. This could possibly result in large colon impactions or ileus in patients treated with opioids. Although there was a decrease in faecal production, there was no increase in incidence of ileus when a butorphanol infusion was admininstered for 24 hours after surgery.[120]

Feeding back the colic patient

Nutritional management

Feeding is an extremely important part of the management of the colic patient (see Chapter 5). Horses with conditions of the small intestine cannot have any feed or water until there is no gastric reflux, there is no longer distension of the small intestine (confirmed with rectal examination, transabdominal ultrasound), there is motility of the small intestine (confirmed with transabdominal ultrasound) and borborygmi are audible indicating that there is large intestinal motility and the caecum is functioning and emptying into the large colon. In the case of small intestinal lesions treated surgically, feeding can be begun as early as 12 hours after surgery if there is no reflux. However, many clinicians wait longer than 12 hours to start feeding in these patients.

Usually water is offered every hour (only 1 L) for a few times; if that is tolerated, then the water is given free choice for 24 hours. If this is tolerated, then small feeds can be given. Some clinicians will feed small pelleted or hard feeds, where as others will feed horses back with hay, haylage or grass. It is the author's preference to feed back with hay, especially for medical colics when there is not the concern of a narrow anastomosis site. Hay may also not be ideal for feeding back small colon impactions, when there is concern about the integrity of the mucosa and risk of reimpaction. The author usually introduces feed with small periods of grazing grass outside. This should start very gradually with 5 minutes every 6 hours, for example. A haynet can be started tied outside the stall if the stall is fitted with bars through which small amounts of hay can be nibbled. Then hay is offered in small amounts every 3 to 4 hours. It is usually best to start with a quarter flake and increase to a half flake and then a flake, with each increase in 12 to 24 hours to give an adequate amount of time to test whether the horse will tolerate the feed. It must be more gradual with a small intestinal problem. Once the horse is tolerating whole flakes every few hours, then free choice hay can be introduced. Grain and hard feeds should be introduced gradually over 7 to 10 days following, at least 24 hours after introduction of free-choice hay. The choice of type of hay will vary with clinician preference and the region in which the hospital is located. The author prefers to feed alfafa hay (USA) or lucerne hay (Australia) until normal intestinal transit is established. Haylage may be an alternative in Europe.

For large colon problems, a similar regimen can be followed. However, feed can usually be increased quicker once the horse has established good audible gut sounds and is passing faeces. Often the increases in amounts of hay can be made every 12 hours. These time periods can be adjusted depending on the individual case and the period of time over which normal intestinal transit resumes. During the feeding back process, grazing grass should be offered at regular intervals, usually approximately 15 minutes 4 times daily. These time periods can be adjusted depending on the individual case and the period of time over which normal intestinal transit resumes. In postoperative large colon torsions, the feeding may be delayed until there is evidence of mucosal integrity. Ileal, caecal and large and small colon impactions should be closely monitored, and usually laxatives are used in the treatment regimen to assist intestinal transit in the postoperative period and prevent reimpaction.

The pregnant mare

Pregnant mares with colic should be monitored closely. Late-term mares may require daily transabdominal ultrasound examinations to observe foetal heart rate (Figure 11.12). Transrectal ultrasound is useful for examining placental thickness and the echogenicity of the amniotic fluid. This gives information as to the likelihood of placental or uterine infection and is indicated if the mare has a fever or vulval discharge. In a retrospective study of pregnant mares with colic, there was an 18% abortion rate. Most of the abortions were in mares with a surgical lesion; however, 80% of these had a live foal and the type of surgical lesion had no affect on outcome.[157] Hypoxia during surgery was a major factor affecting foetal outcome. If hypoxia occurred during surgery and the mare was in the last 60 days of pregnancy, the mares either aborted or delivered a severely compromised foal that did not survive.[158]

Altrenogest (0.044 to 0.088 mg/kg, by mouth, once daily) should be administered to hospitalised horses in the first 8 weeks of pregnancy.[150] Altrenogest compensates for potentially decreased endogenous progesterone production in clinically ill horses and has been shown to be of benefit in preventing foetal loss.[158] Altrenogest is often

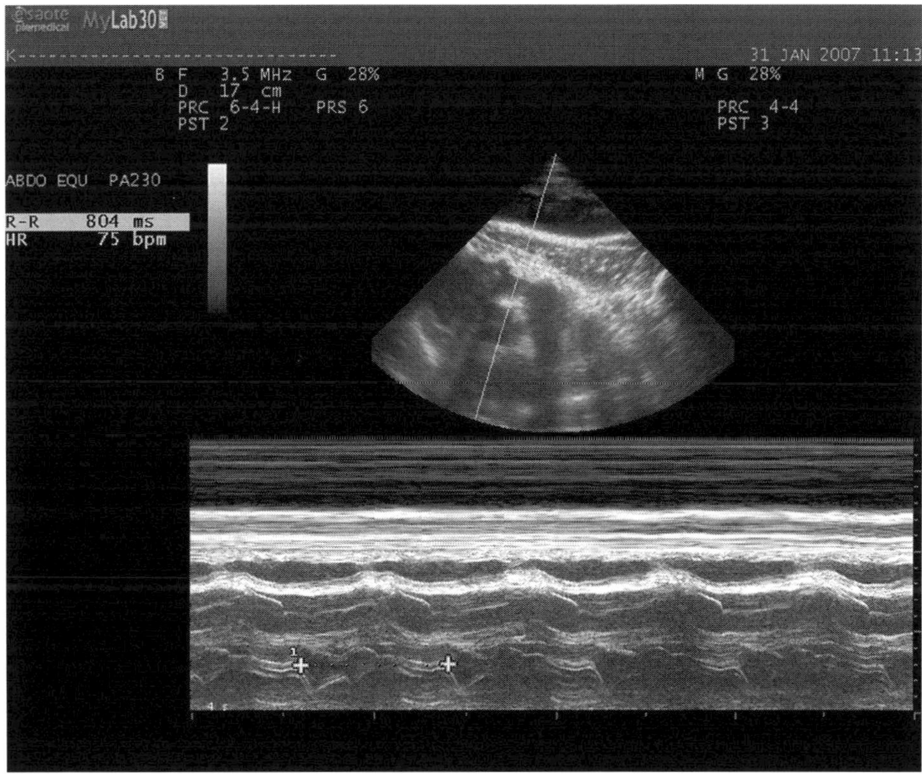

Figure 11.12 Measurement of foetal heart rate in a mare with colic at 8 months of gestation. The foetal heart rate is normal at 75 beats/min. ©Kevin Corley 2007.

administered to hospitalised mares at any time of gestation, even though efficacy at greater than 8 weeks of pregnancy is questionable.

Surgical wound management

Successful wound healing is dependent on the surgical closure and the management in the postoperative period. The incision should be kept as clean as possible in the postoperative period. The most important factors contributing to postoperative incisional infection include preexisting dermatitis, poor intraoperative drape adherence, high numbers of bacterial colony-forming units obtained after recovery and high numbers of bacterial colony-forming units obtained from the surgery room environment.[159] Protection of the wound during anaesthetic recovery with a plastic adhesive drape, antimicrobial surgical incise drape§§§ or gauze sponges and stretchy adhesive dressing (Elastoplast****/Elastikon††††) may help in reducing contamination. Ideally, this bandage should be removed when the horse returns from the recovery room to the stall as it will be contaminated from the recovery room and often there is some mild haemorrhage from the incision during recovery. It is always optimal to maintain a clean and dry incision. In most uncomplicated cases the incision may be left uncovered, and the author prefers to manage the incision without a bandage unless the horse is a mare in the last trimester of pregnancy. In these cases, it may be optimal to apply a supportive abdominal bandage to support the ventral midline incision that has excess weight placed on it. There are commercially available equine abdominal support bandages‡‡‡‡. For mares with nursing foals, it is often wise to apply a bandage to protect the wound from trauma by the foal, if the foal cannot be weaned or transferred to a nurse mare. In cases where the horse itself is traumatising the incision or lying down frequently and contaminating the area with bedding, it may also be necessary to cover the wound. If a bandage is applied, it needs to be changed regularly. Exudate accumulation on the bandage can act as a site for bacterial growth and possibly lead to infection ascending into the wound. The author usually applies abdominal sponges or a similar dressing against the wound and then wraps stretchy adhesive dressing (Elastoplast/Elastikon) in place with minimal tension, but enough to hold the dressing against the wound.

There is usually a ventral plaque of oedema cranial to or around the incision in horses that have had colic surgery. This may enlarge over the postoperative period but should not be hot or painful. The incision should be palpated twice daily with gloved hands to monitor for any heat, swelling, pain or discharge. If there is heat, swelling or pain but no discharge, it is useful to hotpack the incision every 6 hours. In the acute stages of an incisional infection, the signs may not be obvious as the area may not be draining. Ultrasound examination can be useful in determining any small pockets of suspicious exudate/abscesses within the oedematous tissue. In some cases, the infection will be obvious and there will be drainage of serum, fibrin strands or mucopurulent material from the incision. These signs can develop after the horse is discharged but also commonly occur during hospitalisation. In one study, the mean time to incisional drainage was 17 days, which is usually after hospital discharge.[159] Horses older than 1 year and those that weigh more than 300 kg are at a higher risk for infection.[160] Other factors that may increase the risk include an enterotomy being performed,[161] increased fibrinogen concentration in the peritoneal fluid, use of polyglactin 910 to close the linea alba[161] and use of a near-far-far-near closure pattern.[162]

Treatment of these infections involves removal of skin sutures for drainage and cleaning the incision as often as required with a weak antiseptic with or without systemic antibiotics (ideally, following culture and sensitivity testing). The use of antibiotics is questionable, and many incisional infections will heal with drainage alone. The antibiotics may not be effective as there is usually a wide range of organisms cultured from an infected abdominal incision,[159] and an open incision will most likely have a changing bacterial population. Severe incisional infections may lead to dehiscence, but dehiscence can also result from tearing of the body wall. In these cases, the horse needs to be anaesthetised and the suture material remaining is removed and the region is repaired with a secondary closure. There are rare circumstances when there may be an acute dehiscence. In these cases, there may be acute bowel prolapse. Treatment steps for an acute bowel prolapse are given in Box 11.9.

Postoperative rest is critical; anything that stresses the incision should be avoided. For example, if the patient is very fractious when the nasogastric tube is being placed, heavy sedation should be administered to avoid a wound breakdown. Another incisional complication is the development of a hernia, but this usually occurs weeks to months

Box 11.9. Steps to take in the case of acute bowel prolapse through a dehisced surgical wound

- Containment of the intestines with rapid application of a abdominal support bandage
- Immediate immobilisation of the horse
- Rapid induction of anaesthesia
- Lavage of the bowel and replacement into the abdomen
- Secondary closure

§§§Ioban2 Antimicrobial Incise Drape; 3M, St. Paul, MN, USA.

****Beiersdorf AG, Hamburg, Germany.

††††Johnson and Johnson, New Brunswick, NJ, USA.

‡‡‡‡ReWrap BOA; Wire2Wire, Paris, KY, USA.

after the initial surgery, long after the horse has been discharged.

References

1. Blikslager A, et al.: Evaluation of factors associated with postoperative ileus in horses: 31 cases (1990-1992). J Am Vet Med Assoc 205:1748-1752, 1994
2. Roussel AJ, et al.: Risk factors associated with development of postoperative ileus in horses. J Am Vet Med Assoc 219:72-78, 2001
3. Macdonald MH, et al.: Survival after small intestine resection and anastomosis in horses. Vet Surg 18:415-423, 1989
4. Hunt M, Edward G, Clarke K: Incidence, diagnosis and treatment of postoperative complications in colic cases. Equine Vet J 18:264-270, 1986
5. Freeman DE, et al.: Short and long term survival and prevalence of postoperative ileus after small intestinal surgery in the horse. Equine Vet J Suppl 32:42-51, 2000
6. Fenger CK, Bertone AL: Gastrointestinal motility and adynamic ileus, in Reed S, Bayly WN (eds): Equine Internal Medicine. London, WB Saunders, 1998, pp 207-215
7. King J, Gerring EL: The action of low dose endotoxin on equine bowel motility. Equine Vet J 23:11-17, 1991
8. Eades SC, Moore JN: Blockade of endotoxin-induced cecal hypoperfusion and ileus with an alpha 2 antagonist in horses. Am J Vet Res 54:586-590, 1993
9. Clark ES, Collatos C: Hypoperfusion of the small intestine during slow infusion of a low dosage of endotoxin in anesthetized horses. Cornell Vet 80:163-172, 1990
10. Dabareiner R, White NA, Donaldson L: Effects of intraluminal distension and decompression on microvascular permeability and hemodynamics of the equine jejunum. Am J Vet Res 62:225-236, 2001
11. Rakestraw P, et al.: Intracellular microelectrode recording to characterize inhibitory neuromuscular transmission in jejunum of horses. Am J Vet Res 61:362-368, 2000
12. Lillich J, et al.: Expression of the ether-a-go-go (ERG) potassium channel in smooth muscle of the equine gastrointestinal tract and influence on activity of jejunal smooth muscle. Am J Vet Res 64:267-272, 2003
13. Potet F, et al.: Gastrointestinal prokinetic drugs have different affinity for the human cardiac human ether-a-go-go K(+) channel. J Pharmacol Exp Ther 299:1007-1012, 2001
14. Malone E, Kannan M, Brown DR: Evaluation of substance P as a neurotransmitter in equine jejunum. Am J Vet Res 61:1178-1184, 2000
15. King J, Gerring EL: Antagonism of endotoxin-induced disruption of equine gastrointestinal motility with the platelet-activating factor antagonist WEB 2086. J Vet Pharmacol Ther 13:333-339, 1990
16. White NA: Treatment to alter intestinal motility, in White NA (ed): The Equine Acute Abdomen. Philadelphia, Lea and Febiger, 1990, pp 178-184
17. Lester GD: Disorders of equine GI motility and the use of prokinetic drugs. Annual Meeting of the American College of Veterinary Internal Medicine Forum 603-606, 1994
18. Nieto JE, et al.: In vitro effects of erythromycin, lidocaine, and metoclopramide on smooth muscle from the pyloric antrum, proximal portion of the duodenum, and middle portion of the jejunum of horses. Am J Vet Res 61:413-419, 2000
19. Van Hoogmoed LM, et al.: Survey of prokinetic use in horses with gastrointestinal injury. Vet Surg 33:279-285, 2004
20. Doherty TJ, Frazier DL: Effect of intravenous lidocaine on halothane minimum alveolar concentration in ponies. Equine Vet J 30:300-303, 1998
21. Rimback G, Cassuto J, Tollesson P: Treatment of postoperative paralytic ileus by intravenous lidocaine infusion. Anesth Analg 70:414-419, 1990
22. Tsai P, et al.: Lidocaine concentrations in plasma and cerebrospinal fluid after systemic bolus administration in humans. Anesth Analg 87:601-604, 1998
23. Ness T: Intravenous lidocaine inhibits visceral nociceptive reflexes and spinal neurons in the rat. Anesthesiology 92:1685-1691, 2000
24. Groudine S, et al.: Intravenous lidocaine speeds the return of bowel function, decreases postoperative pain, and shortens hospital stay in patients undergoing radical retropubic prostatectomy. Anesth Analg 86:235-239, 1998
25. Dart A, Hodgson DR: Role of prokinetic drugs for treatment of postoperative ileus in the horse. Aust Vet J 76:25-31, 1998
26. Malone ED, Turner T, Wilson J: Intravenous lidocaine for the treatment of ileus in the horse. Presented at the 5th Equine Colic Reserach Symposium 39, 1994
27. Meyer G, et al.: Effects of intravenous lidocaine overdose on cardiac electrical activity and blood pressure in the horse. Equine Vet J 33:434-437, 2001
28. Koenig J, et al.: Binding of radiolabeled porcine motilin and erythromycin lactobionate to smooth muscle membranes in various segments of the equine gastrointestinal tract. Am J Vet Res 63:1545-1550, 2002
29. Roussel AJ, et al.: Prokinetic effects of erythromycin on the ileum, cecum, and pelvic flexure of horses during the postoperative period. Am J Vet Res 61:420-424, 2000
30. Lester G, et al.: Effect of erythromycin lactobionate on myoelectric activity of ileum, cecum, and right ventral colon, and cecal emptying of radiolabeled markers in clinically normal ponies. Am J Vet Res 59:328-334, 1998
31. Hardy J, Rakestraw PC: Postoperative care and complications associated with abdominal surgery, in Auer JA, Stick JA (eds): Equine Surgery, ed 2. Philadelphia, WB Saunders, 1999, pp 294-305
32. Fernandez A, Massingham R: Peripheral receptor populations involved in the regulation of gastrointestinal motility and the pharmacological actions of metoclopramide-like drugs. Life Sci 36:1-14, 1985
33. Gerring EE, Hunt J: Pathophysiology of equine postoperative ileus: effect of adrenergic blockade, parasympathetic stimulation and metoclopramide in an experimental model. Equine Vet J 18:249-255, 1986
34. Hall JA, Washabau RJ: Gastrointestinal prokinetic therapy: dopaminergic antagonist drugs. Compend Contin Educ Pract Vet 19:214-218, 1997
35. Reynolds J, Putman P: Prokinetic agents. Gastroenterol Clin North Am 21:567, 1992
36. Tonini M: Recent advances in the pharmacology of gastrointestinal prokinetics. Pharmacol Res 33:217-226, 1996

37. Hall JA, Washabau RJ: Gastrointestinal prokinetic therapy: motilin-like drugs. Comp Continu Educ Pract Vet 19:281-288, 1997
38. Dowling P: Prokinetic drugs: metoclopramide and cisapride. Can Vet J 36:115-116, 1995
39. Dart A, et al.: Efficacy of metoclopramide for treatment of ileus in horses following small intestinal surgery: 70 cases (1989-1992). Aust Vet J 74:280-284, 1996
40. Gerring E, King J: Cisapride in the prophylaxis of equine post operative ileus. Equine Vet J Suppl 52-55, 1989
41. Kan T, et al.: [The effect of prostaglandin E1 and prostaglandin F2 alpha in the ischemic small intestine of dogs]. Nippon Shokakibyo Gakkai Zasshi 90:114-123, 1993
42. King J, Gerring EL: Actions of the novel gastrointestinal prokinetic agent cisapride on equine bowel motility. J Vet Pharmacol Ther 11:314-321, 1988
43. Nieto J, et al.: In vitro effects of 5-hydroxytryptamine and cisapride on the circular smooth muscle of the jejunum of horses. Am J Vet Res 61:1561-1565, 2000
44. Sasaki N, Yoshihara T: The effect of orally administered cisapride on intestinal motility in conscious horses. J Vet Med Sci 62:211-213, 2000
45. Valk N, et al.: Effect of cisapride on gastric emptying in horses following endotoxin treatment. Equine Vet J 30:344-348, 1998
46. Wysowski D, et al.: Postmarketing reports of qt prolongation and ventricular arrhythmia in association with cisapride and food and drug administration regulatory actions. Am J Gastroenterol 96:1698-1703, 2001
47. Cook G, Papich MG, Roberts MS: Cisapride pharmacokinetics in the horse after iv and rectal administration. Proceedings of the American College of Veterinary Internal Medicine 1997
48. Steel CM, et al.: Unreliable rectal absorption of cisapride in horses. Equine Vet J 31:82-84, 1999
49. Van Hoogmoed L, Snyder J: Adjunctive methods in equine gastrointestinal surgery. Vet Clin North Am Equine Pract 13:221-242, 1997
50. Lester GD, et al.: Effect of alpha 2-adrenergic, cholinergic, and nonsteroidal anti-inflammatory drugs on myoelectric activity of ileum, cecum, and right ventral colon and on cecal emptying of radiolabeled markers in clinically normal ponies. Am J Vet Res 59:320-327, 1998
51. Adams SB, Lamar CH, Masty J: Motility of the distal portion of the jejunum and pelvic flexure in ponies: effects of six drugs. Am J Vet Res 45:795-799, 1984
52. Van Hoogmoed L: Clinical application of prokinetics. Vet Clin N Am: Eq Pract 19:729-740, 2003
53. Ingle-Fehr JE, Baxter GM: The effect of oral isoxsuprine and pentoxifylline on digital and laminar blood flow in healthy horses. Vet Surg 28:154-160, 1999
54. Ruckebusch Y, Roger T: Prokinetic effects of cisapride, naloxone and parasympathetic stimulation at the equine ileo-caeco-colonic junction. J Vet Pharmacol Ther 11:322-329, 1988
55. Roger T, Bardon T, Ruckebusch Y: Colonic motor responses in the pony: relevance of colonic stimulation by opiate antagonists. Am J Vet Res 46:31-35, 1985
56. Lester GD: Gastrointestinal ileus, in Smith B (ed): Large Animal Internal Medicine, ed 3. St. Louis, Mosby, 2002, pp 674-679
57. Paradis M: Prokinetic drugs in the treatment of proximal enteritis. Comp Continu Educ Pract Vet 21:1147-1157, 1999
58. Hunt E, Tennant BC, Whitlock RH: Interpretation of peritoneal fluid erythrocyte counts in horses with abdominal disease. Proc Equine Colic Res Symp 2:168-174, 1986
59. French N, et al.: Equine surgical colic: risk factors for postoperative complications. Equine Vet J 34:444-449, 2002
60. Proudman CJ, et al.: Long-term survival of equine surgical colic cases. Part 2: modelling postoperative survival. Equine Vet J 34:438-443, 2002
61. Baxter G: Equine laminitis caused by distal displacement of the distal phalanx: 12 cases (1976-1985). J Am Vet Med Assoc 189:326-329, 1986
62. Moore JN, White NA: Acute abdominal disease: pathophysiology and preoperative management. Vet Clin North Am Equine Pract 4:61-78, 1982
63. Sykes B, Furr M: Equine endotoxaemia–a state-of-the-art review of therapy. Aust Vet J 83:45-50, 2005
64. Durando M, et al.: Effects of polymixin B and *Salmonella typhimurium* antiserum on horses given endotoxin intravenously. Am J Vet Res 55:921-927, 1994
65. Parviainen A, Barton MH, Norton N: Evaluation of polymixin B in an ex vivo model of endotoxemia in horses. Am J Vet Res 62:72-76, 2001
66. Danner R, et al.: Purification, toxicity, and antiendotoxin activity of polymixin b nonapeptide. Antimicrob Agents Chemother 33:1428-1434, 1989
67. Issekutz A, Biggar W: Effect of methylprednisolone and polymixin B sulfate on endotoxin-induced inhibition of human neutrophil chemotaxis. J Lab Clin Med 92:873-882, 1978
68. Raisbeck M, Garner H, Osweiler G: Effects of polymixin B on selected features of equine carbohydrate overload. Vet Hum Toxicol 31:422-426, 1989
69. Bucklin S, et al.: Therapeutic efficacy of a polymixin B-dextran 70 conjugate in experimental model of endotoxemia. Antimicrob Agents Chemother 39:1462-1466, 1995
70. Mackay R, et al.: Effect of a conjugate of polymixin B-dextran 70 in horses with experimentally induced endotoxemia. Am J Vet Res 60:68-75, 1999
71. Barton MH, Parviainen A, Norton N: Polymixin B protects horses against induced endotoxaemia in vivo. Equine Vet J 36:397-401, 2004
72. Barton MH: Use of polymixin B for treatment of endotoxaemia in horses. Comp Continu Educ Pract Vet 11:1056-1059, 2000
73. Moore JN: A perspective on endotoxaemia. Proceedings of the American Association of Equine Practioners 47:61-74, 2001
74. Morris DD, Whitlock R: Therapy of suspected septicemia in neonatal foals using plasma-containing antibodies to core lipopolysaccharide (LPS). J Vet Intern Med 1:175-182, 1987
75. Morris DD, Whitlock R, Corbeil L: Endotoxemia in horses: protection provided by antiserum to core lipopolysaccharide. Am J Vet Res 47:544-550, 1986
76. Spier S, et al.: Protection against clinical endotoxemia in horses by using plasma containing antibody to an RC mutant *E. coli* (J5). Circ Shock 28:235-248, 1989

77. Morris D: Antiendotoxin serum: therapeutic rationale and clinical perspectives. Compend Continu Educ Pract Vet 11:1096-1099, 1989
78. Tyler J, et al.: Immunity targeting common core antigens of gram-negative bacteria. J Vet Intern Med 4:17-25, 1990
79. Golenbock DT, Hampton RY, Qureshi N, et al.: Lipid A-like molecules that antagonize the effects of endotoxins on human monocytes. J Biol Chem 266:19490-19498, 1991
80. Vaara M: Lipid A: target for antibacterial drugs. Science 274:939-934, 1996
81. Lei MG, Qureshi N, Morrison DC: Lipopolysaccharide (LPS) binding to 73-kDa and 38-kDa surface proteins on lymphoreticular cells: preferential inhibition of LPS binding to the former by *Rhodopseudomonas sphaeroides* lipid A. Immunol Lett 36:245-250, 1993
82. Bunnell E, Lynn M, Habet K, et al.: A lipid A analog, E5531, blocks the endotoxin response in human volunteers with experimental endotoxemia. Crit Care Med 28:2713-2720, 2000
83. Christ WJ, Asano O, Robidoux AL, et al.: E5531, a pure endotoxin antagonist of high potency. Science 268:80-83, 1995
84. Lohmann KL, McNeill BW, Vandenplas M: Lipopolysaccharide from Rhodobacter spheroides is an endotoxin agonist in equine cells. Proceedings of the Twenty-Fourth Annual Conference on Shock, Marco Island, FL, 2001
85. Lien E, Means TK, Heine H, et al.: Toll-like receptor 4 imparts ligand-specific recognition of bacterial lipopolysaccharide. J Clin Invest 105:497-504, 2000
86. Santhanam B, Wolfert MA, Moore JN, Boons GJ: Synthesis and biological evaluation of a lipid a derivative that contains an aminogluconate moiety. Chemistry 10:4798-4807, 2004
87. Dettelbach H: Clinical pharmacology of pentoxifylline with special reference to its hemorrhagic effect for the treatment of intermittent claudication. J Clin Pharmacol 25:8-26, 1985
88. Ehrly AM: The effect of pentoxifylline on the deformability of erythrocytes and on the muscular oxygen pressure in patients with chronic arterial disease. J Med 10:331-338, 1979
89. Schroer R: Antithrombotic potential of pentoxifylline. A hemorheologically active drug. Angiology 36:387-398, 1985
90. Barton M, et al.: The effects of pentoxifylline infusion on plasma 6-keto-prostaglandin F1 alpha and ex vivo endotoxin-induced tumour necrosis factor activity in horses. J Vet Pharmacol Ther 20:487-492, 1997
91. Barton M, Moore J: Pentoxifylline inhibits mediator synthesis in an equine in vitro whole blood model of endotoxemia. Circ Shock 44:216-220, 1994
92. Barton M, Moore JN, Norton N: Effects of pentoxifylline infusion on response of horses to in vivo challenge exposure with endotoxin. Am J Vet Res 58:1300-1307, 1997
93. Baskett A, et al.: Effect of pentoxifylline, flunixin meglumine, and their combination on a model of endotoxemia in horses. Am J Vet Res 58:1291-1299, 1997
94. Crisman M, et al.: Pharmacokinetic disposition of intravenous and oral pentoxifylline in horses. J Vet Pharmacol Ther 16:23-31, 1993
95. Kwong E, Chen F, Young LM: Urinary excretion of pentoxifylline and its metabolites by standardbred mares. Can J Vet Res 53:147-153, 1989
96. Shuster R, Traub Dargatz J, Baxter G: Survey of diplomates of the American College of Veterinary Internal Medicine and the American College of Veterinary Surgeons regarding clinical aspects and treatment of endotoxemia in horses. J Am Vet Med Assoc 210:87-92, 1997
97. Morris DD: Endotoxemia in horses. A review of cellular and humoral mediators involved in its pathogenesis. J Vet Intern Med 5:167-181, 1991
98. Breuhaus BA, DeGraves FJ, Honore EK, Papich MG: Pharmacokinetics of ibuprofen after intravenous and oral administration and assessment of safety of administration to healthy foals. Am J Vet Res 60:1066-1073, 1999
99. Jaraiz V, Rodriguez C, San Andres MD, et al.: Pharmacokinetics and bioequivalence of two suxibuzone oral dosage forms in horses. J Vet Pharmacol Ther 22:247-254, 1999
100. Kollias-Baker C, Cox K: Non-steroidal anti-inflammatory drugs, in Bertone JJ, Horspool LL (eds): Equine Clinical Pharmacology. London, WB Saunders, 2004, pp 247-66
101. Toutain PL, Reymond N, Laroute V, et al.: Pharmacokinetics of meloxicam in plasma and urine of horses. Am J Vet Res 65:1542-1547, 2004
102. Bottoms GD, Fessler JF, Roesel OF, et al.: Endotoxin-induced hemodynamic changes in ponies: effects of flunixin meglumine. Am J Vet Res 42:1514-1518, 1981
103. Burrows GE: Therapeutic effect of phenylbutazone on experimental acute *Escherichia coli* endotoxemia in ponies. Am J Vet Res 42:94-99, 1981
104. Ewert KM, Fessler JF, Templeton CB, et al.: Endotoxin-induced hematologic and blood chemical changes in ponies: effects of flunixin meglumine, dexamethasone, and prednisolone. Am J Vet Res 46:24-30, 1985
105. Fessler JF, Bottoms GD, Roesel OF, et al.: Endotoxin-induced change in hemograms, plasma enzymes, and blood chemical values in anesthetized ponies: effects of flunixin meglumine. Am J Vet Res 43:140-144, 1982
106. Moore JN, White NA, Berg JN, et al.: Endotoxemia following experimental intestinal strangulation obstruction in ponies. Can J Comp Med 45:330-332, 1981
107. Semrad SD, Moore JN: Effects of multiple low doses of flunixin meglumine on repeated endotoxin challenge in the horse. Prostaglandins Leukot Med 27:169-181, 1987
108. King JN, Gerring EL: Antagonism of endotoxin-induced disruption of equine bowel motility by flunixin and phenylbutazone. Equine Vet J Suppl: 38-42, 1989
109. Bottoms GD, Templeton CB, Fessler JF, et al.: Thromboxane, prostaglandin I2 (epoprostenol), and the hemodynamic changes in equine endotoxin shock. Am J Vet Res 43:999-1002, 1982
110. MacKay RJ, Daniels CA, Bleyaert HF, et al.: Effect of eltenac in horses with induced endotoxaemia. Equine Vet J Suppl: 26-31, 2000
111. Moore JN, Hardee MM, Hardee GE: Modulation of arachidonic acid metabolism in endotoxic horses: comparison of flunixin meglumine, phenylbutazone, and a selective thromboxane synthetase inhibitor. Am J Vet Res 47:110-113, 1986
112. Moses VS, Hardy J, Bertone AL, Weisbrode SE: Effects of anti-inflammatory drugs on lipopolysaccharide-challenged

and -unchallenged equine synovial explants. Am J Vet Res 62:54-60, 2001
113. Templeton CB, Bottoms GD, Fessler JF, et al.: Effects of repeated endotoxin injections on prostanoids, hemodynamics, endothelial cells, and survival in ponies. Circ Shock 16:253-264, 1985
114. Karcher LF, Dill SG, Anderson WI, King JM: Right dorsal colitis. J Vet Intern Med 4:247-253, 1990
115. MacAllister CG, Morgan SJ, Borne AT, Pollet RA: Comparison of adverse effects of phenylbutazone, flunixin meglumine, and ketoprofen in horses. J Am Vet Med Assoc 202:71-77, 1993
116. Monreal L, Sabate D, Segura D, et al.: Lower gastric ulcerogenic effect of suxibuzone compared to phenylbutazone when administered orally to horses. Res Vet Sci 76:145-149, 2004
117. Tomlinson JE, Wilder BO, Young KM, Blikslager AT: Effects of flunixin meglumine or etodolac treatment on mucosal recovery of equine jejunum after ischemia. Am J Vet Res 65:761-769, 2004
118. Tomlinson JE, Blikslager AT: Effects of ischemia and the cyclooxygenase inhibitor flunixin on in vitro passage of lipopolysaccharide across equine jejunum. Am J Vet Res 65:1377-1383, 2004
119. Semrad SD, Hardee GE, Hardee MM, Moore JN: Low dose flunixin meglumine: effects on eicosanoid production and clinical signs induced by experimental endotoxaemia in horses. Equine Vet J 19:201-206, 1987
120. Sellon DC, Roberts MC, Blikslager AT, et al.: Effects of continuous rate intravenous infusion of butorphanol on physiologic and outcome variables in horses after celiotomy. J Vet Intern Med 18:555-563, 2004
121. Bernard GR, Wheeler AP, Russell JA, et al.: The effects of ibuprofen on the physiology and survival of patients with sepsis. Ibuprofen in Sepsis Study Group. N Engl J Med 336:912-918, 1997
122. Arons MM, Wheeler AP, Bernard GR, et al.: Effects of ibuprofen on the physiology and survival of hypothermic sepsis. Ibuprofen in Sepsis Study Group. Crit Care Med 27:699-707, 1999
123. Annane D, Sebille V, Charpentier C, et al.: Effect of treatment with low doses of hydrocortisone and fludrocortisone on mortality in patients with septic shock. JAMA 288:862-871, 2002
124. Panacek EA, Marshall JC, Albertson TE, et al.: Efficacy and safety of the monoclonal anti-tumor necrosis factor antibody F(ab′)2 fragment afelimomab in patients with severe sepsis and elevated interleukin-6 levels. Crit Care Med 32:2173-2182, 2004
125. Weiss DJ, Rashid J: The sepsis-coagulant axis: a review. J Vet Int Med 12:317-324, 1998
126. Hardie EM, Kruse-Elliott K: Endotoxic shock. Part I: a review of causes. J Vet Intern Med 4:258-266, 1990
127. Hardie EM, Kruse-Elliott K. Endotoxic shock. Part II: a review of treatment. J Vet Intern Med 4:306-314, 1990
128. Carrick JB, Morris DD, Moore JN: Administration of a receptor antagonist for platelet-activating factor during equine endotoxaemia. Equine Vet J 25:152-157, 1993
129. Etienne A, Hecquet F, Soulard C, et al.: In vivo inhibition of plasma protein leakage and *Salmonella enteritidis*-induced mortality in the rat by a specific PAF-acether antagonist: BN 52021. Agents Actions 17:368-370, 1986
130. Etienne A, Hecquet F, Guilmard C, et al.: Inhibition of rat endotoxin-induced lethality by BN 52021 and BN 52063, compounds with PAF-acether antagonistic effect and protease-inhibitory activity. Int J Tissue React 9:19-26, 1987
131. Terashita Z, Kawamura M, Takatani M, et al.: Beneficial effects of TCV-309, a novel potent and selective platelet activating factor antagonist in endotoxin and anaphylactic shock in rodents. J Pharmacol Exp Ther 260:748-755, 1992
132. Dhainaut JF, Tenaillon A, Hemmer M, et al.: Confirmatory platelet-activating factor receptor antagonist trial in patients with severe gram-negative bacterial sepsis: a phase III, randomized, double-blind, placebo-controlled, multicenter trial. BN 52021 Sepsis Investigator Group. Crit Care Med 26:1963-1971, 1998
133. Opal S, Laterre PF, Abraham E, et al.: Recombinant human platelet-activating factor acetylhydrolase for treatment of severe sepsis: results of a phase III, multicenter, randomized, double-blind, placebo-controlled, clinical trial. Crit Care Med 32:332-341, 2004
134. Croft KD, Beilin LJ, Vandongen R, Mathews E: Dietary modification of fatty acid and prostaglandin synthesis in the rat. Effect of variations in the level of dietary fat. Biochim Biophys Acta 795:196-207, 1984
135. Garg ML, Wierzbicki AA, Thomson AB, Clandinin MT: Omega-3 fatty acids increase the arachidonic acid content of liver cholesterol ester and plasma triacylglycerol fractions in the rat. Biochem J 261:11-15, 1989
136. Mayer K, Gokorsch S, Fegbeutel C, et al.: Parenteral nutrition with fish oil modulates cytokine response in patients with sepsis. Am J Respir Crit Care Med 167:1321-1328, 2003
137. Rosa DM, Spillert CR, Flanagan JJ, Lazaro EJ: Beneficial effect of cod liver oil in murine endotoxemia. Res Commun Chem Pathol Pharmacol 70:125-127, 1990
138. Henry MM, Moore JN, Fischer JK: Influence of an omega-3 fatty acid-enriched ration on in vivo responses of horses to endotoxin. Am J Vet Res 52:523-527, 1991
139. McCann ME, Moore JN, Carrick JB, Barton MH: Effect of intravenous infusion of omega-3 and omega-6 lipid emulsions on equine monocyte fatty acid composition and inflammatory mediator production in vitro. Shock 14:222-228, 2000
140. Lopes M, et al.: Enteral fluid therapy for horses. Compend Contin Educ Pract Vet 25:390-397, 2003
141. Rose R, Gibson K, Suann C: An evaluation of an oral glucose-glycine-electrolyte solution for the treatment of experimentally induced dehydration in the horse. Vet Rec 119:522-525, 1986
142. Lopes M, Pfeiffer C: Functional morphology of the equine pelvic flexure and its role in disease. a review. Histol Histopathol 15:983-991, 2000
143. Henninger RW, Horst J: Magnesium toxicosis in two horses. J Am Vet Med Assoc 211:82-85, 1997
144. White NN, Dabareiner R: Treatment of impaction colics. Vet Clin North Am Equine Pract 13:243-259, 1997
145. White NA: Intensive care, monitoring, and complications of acute abdominal disease, in White NA (ed): The Equine Acute Abdomen. Malvern, PA, Lea and Febiger, 1990, pp 310-333

146. Tomasic M: Temporal changes in core body temperature in anesthetized adult horses. Am J Vet Res 60:556-562, 1999
147. Kurz A, et al.: Heat balance and distribution during the core-temperature plateau in anesthetized humans. Anesthesiology 83:491-499, 1995
148. Nikki P, Rosenberg P: Halothane shivering in mice after injection of catecholamines and 5HT into the cerebral ventricles. Ann Med Exp Biol Fenn 47:197-202, 1969
149. Soliman MG, Gillies D: Muscular hyperactivity after general anaesthesia. Can Anaesth Soc J 19:529-535, 1972
150. Southwood L: Postoperative management of the large colon volvulus patient. Vet Clin North Am Equine Pract 20:167-197, 2004
151. Todhunter R, Erb H, Roth L: Gastric rupture in horses: a review of 54 cases. Equine Vet J 18:288-293, 1986
152. Cheadle W, et al.: Prophylactic postoperative nasogastric decompression. A prospective study of its requirement and the influence of cimetidine in 200 patients. Ann Surg 202:361-366, 1985
153. Cheatham M, et al.: A meta-analysis of selective versus routine nasogastric decompression after elective laparotomy. Ann Surg 221:469-476; discussion 476-478, 1995
154. Garcia-Lopez JM, et al.: Prevalence and prognostic importance of hypomagesemia and hypocalcemia in horses that have colic surgery. Am J Vet Res 62:7-12, 2001
155 Traub-Dargatz JL, et al.: Survey of complications and antimicrobial use in equine patients at veterinary teaching hospitals that underwent surgery because of colic. J Am Vet Med Assoc 220:1359-1365, 2002
156. Ziel R, Krupp P: The significance of inhibition of prostaglandin synthesis in the selection of non-steroidal anti-inflammatory agents. Int J Clin Pharmacol Biopharm 12:186-191, 1975
157. Santschi E, et al.: Types of colic and frequency of postcolic abortion in pregnant mares: 105 cases (1984-1988). J Am Vet Med Assoc 199:374-377, 1991
158. Daels P, et al.: Evaluation of progesterone deficiency as a cause of fetal death in mares with experimentally induced endotoxemia. Am J Vet Res 52:282-288, 1991
159. Galuppo L, et al.: Evaluation of iodophor skin preparation techniques and factors influencing drainage from ventral midline incisions in horses. J Am Vet Med Assoc 215:963-969, 1999
160. Wilson D, Baker G, Boero M: Complications of celiotomy incisions in horses. Vet Surg 24:506-514, 1995
161. Honnas C, Cohen ND: Risk factors for wound infection following celiotomy in horses. J Am Vet Med Assoc 210:78-81, 1997
162. Kobluk C, et al.: Factors affecting incisional complication rates associated with colic surgery in horses: 78 cases (1983-1985). J Am Vet Med Assoc 195:639-642, 1989

12

Monitoring and treating the liver

Andy Durham

12.1 Monitoring the hepatic system
12.2 Management of horses with hepatic disorders

12.1 Monitoring the hepatic system

Patients at risk of developing hepatic disorders during hospitalisation

The vast majority of hospitalised horses with hepatopathy are likely to have been admitted to hospital with preexisting liver disease. However, some clinical conditions may be associated with hepatic insult that may develop during hospitalisation, and early detection of hepatic compromise in such cases is important.

Hepatic lipidosis

Hepatic lipidosis is the most common hepatopathy to develop during hospitalisation. Hyperlipaemia (serum triglyceride >5.6 mmol/L [500 mg/dl]) precedes hepatic lipidosis and is most likely to develop in subjects with the following risk factors in Box 12.1.[1–3]

The energy intake of hospitalised donkeys and ponies should always be carefully monitored and, if insufficient, must be supplemented enterally and/or parenterally. Serum triglyceride concentration should be quantified at least every 24 hours in hospitalised donkeys and ponies without a normal nutritional intake.

Box 12.1. Risk factors for hyperlipaemia in hospitalised equines

- Donkey and pony breeds
- Obesity (including mild obesity)
- Anorexia
- Stress/pain
- Female
- Pregnant
- Lactating
- Older age

Intestinal disease

The close anatomic relationship between the liver and intestine is matched by their relationship in terms of clinical syndromes. Colic and diarrhoea, although suggestive of intestinal disease, are also common clinical signs of hepatopathy.[4–6] Conversely, hyperammonaemic encephalopathy, although suggestive of hepatic disease, is also reported secondary to intestinal disease.[7,8] Furthermore, cases of primary intestinal disease are occasionally seen that develop clinical or clinicopathological evidence of hepatopathy during hospitalisation.[9–13] Physical pressure from distended abdominal viscera such as the colon or stomach may potentially lead to acute biliary obstruction[12] and ischaemia,[9] leading to hepatic compromise and, in chronic cases, hepatic atrophy.[10] Many cases of acute intestinal disease are associated with compromise of the intestinal mucosal barrier and increased leakage of luminal lipopolysaccharide and other noxious substances. It is likely therefore that the liver is exposed to relatively high concentrations of potentially injurious material via the hepatic portal vasculature, especially in cases of inflamed or strangulated bowel.[11] Cholangiohepatitis is suspected to result from reflux of duodenal contents along the hepatic duct,[14] and it is therefore possible that horses affected by conditions associated with duodenitis and/or obstruction of duodenal transit may be at risk of hepatopathy.[9,11,12]

Hepatotoxicity

As the liver is central to the biotransformation of most therapeutic agents in common usage, the potential complication of iatrogenic hepatopathy and altered pharmacokinetics in medicated hospitalised horses always exists. In a study of 294 hospitalised human patients, 28 cases (9.5%) of drug-induced liver injury were recorded.[15] The finding that most cases of drug-induced hepatotoxicity in humans are asymptomatic and diagnosed on the basis of serum biochemistry may mitigate against the seriousness of such events but also may infer that many such cases go undetected in clinical practice. There are very few reports of drugs causing hepatoxicity in horses, although volatile anaesthetic agents, tetracyclines, erythromycin, rifampicin, phenothiazines, diazepam, aspirin and dantrolene are among those with a notable theoretical capacity to do so.[16–18] Nonsteroidal anti-inflammatory drugs (NSAIDs) are well known for their potential hepatotoxicity in humans,[19] although there is little evidence for NSAID hepatotoxicity in horses despite their widespread usage.[20–22]

During hospitalisation, the clinician takes responsibility for general feeding and management of the patient, and the owner will reasonably expect a higher standard of care than that practiced by a reasonably competent stableyard manager. Consequently, extreme care should be taken in selection and sourcing of feed materials with particular consideration of potentially hepatotoxic plants in preserved forage and fungal contamination of stored grains.

Parenteral administration of products of equine origin

Acute hepatitis and necrosis is a well-recognised adverse effect of tetanus antitoxin administration in some geographic locations, primarily in the United States.[23] The condition has also been reported following use of other biologicals of equine origin including plasma transfusion.[24] Disease in foals has not been reported and most cases have occurred in the summer and autumn between 4 and 8 weeks following administration of the suspected product. The condition appears to be very rare in the United Kingdom, although this author has seen an outbreak in a group of recently imported horses.

Biochemical monitoring of the liver

Liver derived serum enzyme concentrations

Increased serum concentrations of several intracellular enzymes have been reported to be useful in establishing the diagnosis and prognosis of hepatopathies in the horse. These include alanine aminotransferase (ALT), alkaline phosphatase (AP), arginase, aspartate aminotransferase (AST), γ-glutamyltranferase (γGT), glutamate dehydrogenase (GLDH), iditol dehydrogenase (IDH) (previously referred to as sorbitol dehydrogenase, or SDH) and lactate dehydrogenase (LDH).[25–27] Relative increases in serum concentrations of liver-derived enzymes may infer the underlying nature of the liver disease in horses.[5,28] A primarily biliary source is suggested for γGT, hepatocellular sources for arginase, ALT, AST, GLDH, IDH and LDH and both biliary and hepatocellular sources for AP.[5,29–32]

The four most commonly assayed liver-derived serum enzymes comprise AP, AST, GLDH and γGT. Of these enzymes, increased AP has the strongest association with failure to survive liver disease,[5,6] although increased AP is neither consistently increased in acute[33] or chronic[34] liver disease nor is it liver specific.[25,34] γGT is the most sensitive biochemical indicator of hepatopathy,[4,34] and marked increases in serum γGT concentration (e.g., 5–10 × upper limit of reference range) are associated with a poor prognosis.[4–6] However, modest increases in γGT (e.g., up to 1.5 times the upper limit of the reference range) should be interpreted with great caution as examination of liver biopsy specimens in such cases often fails to reveal significant underlying liver disease.[34] The pancreas, or even kidneys, could potentially be the source of increased serum γGT in the absence of hepatopathy, although renally derived γGT is widely accepted to appear in urine and not serum.[35] Another possible explanation for the apparently poor specificity of γGT is that increases in serum concentrations of liver-derived γGT may result from insults too minor to result in detectable histopathology. AST is derived from widespread tissue sources and has low specificity for liver disease,[25,34] although the majority of liver disease cases do have increased serum AST.[34] Although increased serum GLDH is considered specific for acute liver disease,[27] only a moderate specificity was found in one study.[34] This may be explained by insignificant hepatic insults resulting in increased serum GLDH concentrations. Prognostic usefulness of AST has not been found in equine hepatopathy cases[5,6] and the prognostic value of GLDH is equivocal.[4,5] This information is summarised in Table 12.1.

Table 12.1. Sources of enzymes commonly measured to assess the liver

Enzyme	Abbreviation	Hepatic origin	Other sources	Specificity for liver disease	Association with prognosis in liver disease
Alanine aminotransferase	ALT	Hepatocellular	Possibly muscle	Low	—
Alkaline phosphatase	AP or ALP	Hepatocellular and biliary system	Bone, intestine	Low	High
Arginase	Ar	Hepatocellular	—	High	—
Aspartate aminotransferase	AST	Hepatocellular	Muscle, kidneys, erythrocytes	Low	Low
Glutamate dehydrogenase	GLDH	Hepatocellular	—	High	Equivocal
γ-Glutamyltransferase	γGT or gGT	Biliary system	Pancreas (possibly kidneys)	High	Fairly good
Iditol dehydrogenase	IDH (or SDH*)	Hepatocellular	—	High	—
Lactate dehydrogenase	LDH	Hepatocellular	Many tissues, including muscle and kidneys	Low	—

*This enzyme was formerly known as sorbitol dehydrogenase.

Serum biochemical evaluation of hepatic function

Serum concentrations of several biochemical substances have been reported to reflect the capability of the liver to perform its normal functions. These are primarily endogenous and exogenous substances that accumulate in the blood as a result of failure of extractive and processing functions normally performed by the liver. It is also possible to monitor other substances whose serum concentrations are normally maintained by hepatic biosynthesis. These "functional parameters" might be more useful in the differentiation of hepatic failure from cases of adequately compensated hepatic disease and consequently have both diagnostic and prognostic value. They include serum concentrations of various amino acids, ammonia, bile acids, bilirubin, fibrinogen, globulins, glucose and urea, in addition to blood clotting times (activated partial thromboplastin time [aPTT] and prothrombin time [PT]) and half-life of plasma bromosulphthalene, indocyanine green and radionuclides.[25–27]

Hyperglobulinaemia is a common finding in association with liver disease[4,6,34,36] and probably results from systemic immunostimulation by intestinal-derived antigenic material following loss of the protective barrier of hepatic Kupffer cells. Serum globulin concentration has been found to have good prognostic value in equine hepatopathies.[5] In the author's experience, serum globulin concentrations greater than 45 g/L (4.5 g/dl) are concerning, and values as high as 60 to 70 g/L (6.0–7.0 g/dl) are occasionally seen and warrant a very guarded prognosis.

Although albumin is synthesised by the liver, hepatic reserve capacity and relatively long serum half-life of albumin explain the rarity of marked hypoalbuminaemia in equine liver disease,[4,6,34,36] which greatly limits its clinical usefulness. Serum albumin concentrations below 20 g/L (2.0 g/dl) are rarely encountered even in severe hepatopathies. Nevertheless, even when present to a moderate degree, hypoalbuminaemia is a useful prognostic indicator in equine hepatopathy cases.[5,36]

Plasma fibrinogen is another liver-derived protein occasionally reported to be decreased in association with liver disease.[25,36] In contrast, one study of equine hepatic disease found that plasma fibrinogen was significantly higher in nonsurvivors than in survivors.[5] This latter finding suggests that hepatic acute phase protein synthesis is common in association with severe liver disease in horses and is consistent with the parallel inflammatory findings of hyperglobulinaemia and neutrophilia in equine hepatic insufficiency[5,6,36] and also the significant association of tumour necrosis factor-α with hepatic insufficiency in human patients.[38]

Serum bile acid concentration is an excellent diagnostic and prognostic indicator of liver disease in the horse,[4,5,32,34,37] although liver disease must be quite severe before increased concentrations are detected.[39] Chronic hepatopathy cases with serum bile acid concentrations greater than 20 μmol/L (7.8 μg/ml) are less likely to survive than those with lower values.[5] In this author's experience, chronic hepatopathy cases with bile acid concentrations above 100 μmol/L (39.3 μg/ml) rarely recover, although much higher values can be seen in nonfatal acute hepatopathies.

Hepatic insufficiency is often associated with increased serum concentrations of unconjugated and/or conjugated bilirubin.[4,6,34] Anorexia[40] and haemolysis[41,42] are additional causes of unconjugated hyperbilirubinaemia. The majority of equine liver disease cases have normal or only moderate increases in serum bilirubin concentration,[4,6,34] and the unconjugated fraction usually greatly exceeds the conjugated fraction,[28] creating interpretive problems in anorexic subjects. Cases of liver disease in the horse in which serum conjugated bilirubin represents greater than 25% of total bilirubin are very likely to be suffering from obstruction of the biliary tract.[43]

Low concentrations of serum urea have been recognised previously in association with liver failure and have been suggested to indicate reduced hepatic synthesis of urea from ammonia,[28,44] although one study found no association between serum urea and ammonia concentration in equine hepatopathies.[4] Although the majority of equine hepatopathy cases have normal serum urea concentrations,[4,6,34] decreased serum urea infers a worse prognosis.[5] Interestingly, a similar association was found in one study between low serum creatinine and a worse prognosis.[5] The association of low urea and low creatinine with a poor prognosis may suggest that polyuria secondary to polydipsia, rather than reduced hepatic synthesis, is the underlying mechanism behind low serum urea in some cases of liver failure. Polydipsia and polyuria have occasionally been reported in horses with liver failure.[27,44] However, clinical experience suggests that polydipsia and polyuria are frequently not recognised by horse owners, and thus may be underreported in liver failure.

Hepatic insufficiency is associated with a decrease in the synthesis and function of the majority of procoagulant, anticoagulant and fibrinolytic proteins in addition to reduced platelet numbers and function.[45] An increase in procoagulant proteins synthesised at nonhepatic sites is often seen including factor VIII, von Willebrand factor and monocyte tissue factor.[45,46] Despite the complexities of effects on individual proteins, the net effect of hepatic failure on haemostasis is invariably impairment of coagulation as determined by increased aPTT and PT.[28] However, it is more common to see laboratory evidence of coagulopathy than clinical bleeding problems in horses with hepatic insufficiency.[4–6]

Derangements in serum concentrations of amino acids is commonly recognised in association with hepatic insufficiency comprising increased concentrations of methionine and the aromatic amino acids (AAAs) tyrosine, tryptophan and phenylalanine and decreased concentrations of the branched chain amino acids (BCAAs) valine, leucine and isoleucine.[47] Increased AAAs result from reduced hepatic clearance, whereas decreased BCAAs result from increased muscular metabolism.[47] Although clinical usefulness of these parameters has been established in the horse,[48,49] limited availability of testing has greatly restricted their employment.

Despite the central gluconeogenic role of the liver, hypoglycaemia is an uncommon consequence of hepatic failure with normoglycaemia to hyperglycaemia being almost invariably found.[4,6] Although plasma ammonia concentration is increased in nearly all cases of hepatic encephalopathy, the concentration does not necessarily correlate with severity of the disease.[4,5] This apparent paradox may be explained by variable permeability of the blood-brain barrier to ammonia in the plasma.[50]

Dynamic testing of liver function has been examined in horses using exogenous agents including bromosulphothalein, indocyanine green and radiopharmaceuticals,[51–53] although none appear to be widely used due to limited availability, in contrast to other simple tests of hepatic function earlier. In human subjects, clearance studies using other exogenous agents such as lidocaine and galactose have been used,[54] although no reports exist of these methods in equine subjects with liver disease.

Other serum biochemical tests

Hepatic fibroplasia quantified by liver biopsy is the single most valuable prognostic indicator in equine liver disease.[55] There are currently no readily available blood tests for the assessment of hepatic fibrosis in the horse, although there are several useful serum markers of fibrosis used in humans including hyaluronan, collagen IV, laminin, procollagen III peptide and α-smooth muscle actin.[56–60] Serum hyaluronan has been measured successfully in horses in experimental studies of joint and lung diseases, and reference ranges are established.[61]

Pyrrolizidine alkaloids (PAs) have been shown to bind to haemoglobin via thiol groups to form a stable compound that can be identified in equine blood samples using chromatographic methods.[62] Further evaluation of this procedure may provide a useful screening and monitoring test in suspected cases of PA toxicosis.

Ultrasonography of the liver

The normal liver has a relatively hypoechoic homogeneity interrupted by anechoic blood vessels (Figure 12.1). Peripheral intrahepatic blood vessels are typically no larger than 8 mm in diameter, although larger vessels are sometimes seen in ponies due to the ability to image relatively deeper hepatic tissue than in horses. The ability to image several dilated blood vessels may be associated with portal hypertension and hepatic fibrosis. Very localised hyperechoic (without acoustic shadows) signals are commonly associated with blood vessels as a result of fibrous perivascular connective tissue. Bile ducts cannot normally be visualised. In larger blood vessels flow can often be visualised in real time with standard B-mode ultrasonography (using a 3.54- to 7.5-MHz transducers), although Doppler can be used to establish active blood flow where doubt exists over the

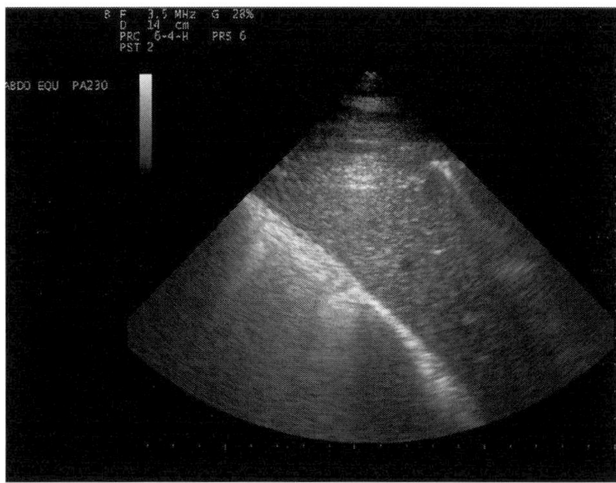

Figure 12.1 Transabdominal ultrasonographic image of a normal liver. The image was taken through the 13th intercostal space on the righthand side, using a 3.5-Mhz probe. ©Kevin Corley 2007.

identity of dilated vessels. Fibrosis, haemosiderosis and lipidosis may increase the echogenicity of hepatic tissue.[5,28,63]

In most horses, examination from the right hemithorax allows imaging of a larger volume of liver than from the left. The right lobe of the liver projects caudoventral to the right lung and may be imaged via several intercostal spaces somewhere between the 6th and 16th ribs. Typically, 10 to 12 cm of liver projects caudoventrally to the expiratory border of the right lung in the 13th intercostal space, enabling semiquantitative assessment of hepatic size. Imaging is frequently possible via more rib spaces in ponies and small horses (e.g., often via 6–8 intercostal spaces) than in larger animals in which liver might only be imaged via as few as 2 or 3 intercostal spaces. The normal hepatic image from the right side is approximately triangular in shape with a convex surface adjacent to the diaphragm laterally and a concave surface against the hyperechoic colonic image medially.

The left lateral lobe of the liver projects caudoventral to the left lung for approximately 2 or 3 intercostal spaces caudal to the palpable cardiac apex beat. When imaged from the left side, a triangular or biconvex shape is often seen and should not be confused with the caudomedially adjacent spleen, which has similar ultrasonographic architecture but is significantly more hyperechoic than the liver and has fewer blood vessels. In cases of hepatic atrophy, the left lobe of the liver can be imaged more consistently than the right. Rarely, hepatopathy cases are seen in which no liver tissue can be imaged ultrasonographically and laparoscopy can then be used to visualise the liver and guide biopsy collection.

Transabdominal ultrasonography should be used to guide liver biopsy (see Chapter 1.13), and a site is usually chosen based on thickness of imaged hepatic tissue, absence of large blood vessels and, occasionally, focal presence of hepatic tissue with an abnormal ultrasonographic appearance. The widespread availability of diagnostic ultrasound makes the ongoing use of unguided biopsy techniques questionable. Although the majority of cases of hepatopathy do not have discernable ultrasonographic abnormalities, images classified as abnormal have a high specificity for the presence of significant liver disease and are associated with poorer outcomes.[5,34] Definition of ultrasonographic abnormalities is frequently subjective with the commonest classifications being changes in general echogenicity and size, although focally abnormal tissue (e.g., hydatid cysts, hepatoliths, neoplasia, abscessation), excessively dilated vessels and rounded liver margins are among the more objective abnormalities occasionally imaged.[5,63]

Biopsy of the liver

If liver disease is suspected on the basis of preliminary noninvasive tests, then liver biopsy remains the "gold standard" technique by which to address key questions, including confirmation of the presence of significant liver disease, determining the aetiology of the condition, selection of specific therapy and determination of prognosis.[28,55] In this author's experience, the technique is benign, especially when performed under ultrasonographic guidance. The frequently purported contraindication of prolonged clotting times appears to have little evidence basis.[28] The technique is described in Chapter 1.13.

Minor hepatopathic changes are frequently encountered in horses without liver disease, and this should be considered when interpreting liver biopsy specimens.[55] Some conditions of the equine liver, such as pyrrolizidine alkaloid toxicity[64] and septic cholangiohepatitis,[14,43] are associated with characteristic histopathological findings. However, it is this author's experience that biopsy specimens commonly fail to identify the inciting cause of liver disease. Frequently, histopathological abnormalities are present in combinations without aetiological specificity, leading to many biopsy specimens being unclassifiable with respect to a recognised named diagnosis.[4,36,65] Furthermore, attempted culture of biopsies from cases of suppurative hepatitis is usually unsuccessful.[43] Although sometimes possible, determination of aetiology should not be a primary aim of liver biopsy in the horse. Nevertheless, certain histopathological findings may serve to guide therapy even in the absence of a specific diagnosis. For example, marked lymphoplasmacytic infiltrates may indicate glucocorticoid therapy, neutrophilic infiltrates may indicate antibacterial therapy and haemosiderosis may require careful dietary advice to limit further iron ingestion.

A score based on the presence and severity of five key histopathological changes in liver biopsies has been found to be the most accurate means of predicting survival in horses with suspected chronic liver disease[55] (Table 12.2). Scores of 0 to 1 were associated with an excellent prognosis (96% survival to 6 months), scores 2 to 6, a guarded prognosis (67% survival to 6 months), and scores of 7 to 14, a poor prognosis (14% survival to 6 months).

Table 12.2. Scores attributable to specific histopathologic findings in liver biopsy specimens

Histopathological finding	Mild	Moderate	Severe
Megalocytosis/necrosis	1	2	2
Fibroplasia	—	2	4
Biliary hyperplasia	—	2	4
Inflammatory infiltrate	—	1	2
Haemosiderin accumulation	—	—	2

Total biopsy score is calculated as the total of each individual score (minimum 0, maximum 14).[55]

12.2 Management of horses with hepatic disorders

Specific fluid therapy considerations

Horses affected by hepatic insufficiency may present with hypovolaemia due to failure to voluntarily consume adequate feed and water, perhaps potentiated by diarrhoea or even gastric reflux. Fluid therapy will, in most cases, not present any particular problems but certain prime considerations should be taken into account when formulating a fluid therapy plan, including serum concentrations of glucose, proteins, electrolytes and acid-base balance.

Despite occasional references to hypoglycaemia,[28] the vast majority of horses presenting with hepatic insufficiency (with or without hepatic encephalopathy [HE]) are normoglycaemic to hyperglycaemic,[4,6] and therefore glucose- or dextrose-containing fluids are usually unnecessary or contraindicated. Should hypoglycaemia be confirmed, then supplementation of intravenous fluids to 2.5% to 5% dextrose (50–100 ml 50% dextrose added to each litre of fluid) is appropriate.[28]

Horses with hepatic insufficiency may often be mildly hypoalbuminaemic and hyperglobulinaemic frequently with a normal total serum protein concentration.[36] In such cases, plasma colloidal osmotic pressure (COP) will be only mildly decreased, although the greater contribution made by albumin to total plasma COP[66] means that some cases affected by more marked hypoalbuminaemia (especially if without hyperglobulinaemia) may be more prone to oedema in response to intravenous fluid loads. Colloidal therapy in the form of plasma, pentastarch or hetastarch should be administered in association with rehydration in such cases. In cases without access to colloidal osmometry, an approximation of COP can be calculated from the following formula[66]:

$$\text{COP (mm Hg)} \approx (0.55 \times \text{albumin g/L}) + (0.25 \times \text{globulin g/L}) - 4.4$$

This author subjectively uses a threshold of approximately 15 mm Hg with which to decide whether or not colloidal therapy is indicated. In subjects with clinical or subclinical coagulopathy, plasma may be preferred to hetastarch due to their respective potentially beneficial and deleterious effects on blood clotting.[67–69] Furthermore, albumin solution, but not synthetic colloid infusion, improves the symptoms of HE in hypovolaemic human patients and increases renal ammonia excretion.[70]

Cases of hepatic lipidosis should be treated with lipid-free parenteral nutrition and insulin.[71,72] Significant decreases of serum triglycerides and liver-derived serum enzyme concentrations should occur promptly within 12 hours of therapy,[71,72] and recovery may also be monitored by a gradual decrease in ultrasonographic echogenicity of hepatic parenchyma as lipid is removed.[28] Heparin therapy is inadvisable due to lack of proved efficacy and potentiation of any hepatogenous clotting disorder. Particular care should be taken to monitor and control hyperglycaemia when parenteral nutrition is administered.[72,73]

Hypokalaemia is common as a result of anorexia associated with hepatic insufficiency and maintenance intravenous fluids can be supplemented with 20 to 40 mmol/L potassium chloride (10 ml 15% KCl = 20 mmol) to restore and maintain normokalaemia. Complex, but usually mild, acid-base disturbances are often seen including lactic acidosis, hypoalbuminaemic alkalosis and respiratory alkalosis.[28,74] Correction of acid-base abnormalities should be performed with great care in subjects with hepatic failure. Whereas acidosis is associated with reduced detoxification of ammonia,[75] alkalosis favours diffusion of ammonia into the central nervous system.[76] Rehydration with lactated Ringer's solution is usually adequate to restore blood pH in acidotic subjects, although doubts must exist over the capacity of a failing liver to convert lactate to bicarbonate, and therefore gradual and carefully monitored corrective therapy with bicarbonate solution (bicarbonate deficit = base deficit × 0.3 × body weight) should be considered in cases where volume expansion has failed to normalise blood pH.

Hepatic encephalopathy

HE reflects a spectrum of neurological signs associated with acute and chronic hepatic insufficiency and portal-systemic bypass.[77] More subtle psychiatric illness that is recognised in human subjects[78] may well go unnoticed in horses. In horses, signs related to cerebral and brain stem dysfunction predominate, although rarer signs such as laryngeal paralysis, dysphagia, gastric impaction, foot stamping and pruritus might result from disturbance of the peripheral nervous system. Clinical signs associated with HE in horses are listed in Box 12.2. Horses with signs of HE have a poorer prognosis than those with liver disease without HE,[5] although the results of two studies indicate that more than 40% of cases showing signs of HE can survive,[5,6] justifying attempted treatment of the condition.

Box 12.2. Clinical signs associated with hepatic encephalopathy in horses[4,5,28,79,80]

- Depression
- Behavioural changes
- Yawning
- Disorientation
- Compulsive walking
- Ataxia
- Pruritus
- Foot stamping
- Circling
- Blindness
- Head pressing
- Dysphagia
- Dyspnoea and inspiratory stertor (bilateral laryngeal paralysis)
- Colic and reflux (gastric impaction)
- Seizure
- Coma

Neurons appear morphologically normal in the brains of subjects affected by HE, although astrocytes frequently demonstrate nuclear enlargement, peripheral chromatin margination and prominent nucleoli (Alzheimer type II degeneration).[81] Astrocytes are the only source of glutamine synthetase (converts ammonia to glutamine) in the brain and also play important regulatory roles in cerebral uptake of various substances from the blood as well as neurotransmitters, electrolytes and nutrients.[82,83] The central pathological feature of HE is disturbance of astrocyte cell volume homeostasis.[82,84,85] Acute hepatic decompensation with HE is characterised by overt brain oedema, increased intracranial pressure and possible cerebral herniation, whereas chronic hepatic failure with HE is associated with chronic low-grade astrocyte swelling in the absence of significantly increased intracranial pressure.[50,82,83,86,87]

Although cases of HE are almost invariably hyperammonaemic,[4,5,88] the finding of a poor correlation between serum ammonia concentration and severity of HE,[4,5,78] along with contrasting clinical effects of experimental administration of ammonia versus HE,[88] has led to doubt regarding the pathogenic role of ammonia. However, there is compelling evidence that increased cerebral ammonia is indeed the key primary pathophysiological event leading to HE and that blood and brain ammonia concentrations are weakly correlated due to increased blood-brain barrier permeability in HE.[50,78,87,89–91] Astrocytic glutamine synthesis from ammonia is greatly increased in HE cases, and glutamine is the likely ultimate cause of astrocyte swelling.[50,82,91]

Additional and sometimes interacting pathogenic roles are proposed for tumour necrosis factor-α, aromatic amino acids, manganese, copper, phenols, benzodiazepine-like substances, mercaptans, short chain fatty acids, monoamines, neurosteroids, bilirubin and electrolytes.[39,78,83,87,88,92,93] Hyperammonaemia is well recognised in horses with HE,[4,5] and one study identified a high concentration of ammonia in the cerebrospinal fluid of a horse with HE.[24] This author has identified increased cerebral manganese and normal copper concentrations in equine HE cases.

Specific therapies for hepatic diseases

Specific therapy is not indicated in all horses with liver disease and should only be applied when a specific diagnosis has been achieved (almost invariably by liver biopsy). Medical therapies are discussed later, although rarely liver disease may indicate surgical treatment.[94] Response to therapy can be judged initially by clinical signs, haematology and clinical chemistry, although confirmation of histopathological status by re-biopsy is always preferable in cases with equivocal results or apparent treatment failure. It is not uncommon to find continuing serum biochemical abnormalities despite reassuring improvements in histopathology of biopsy specimens.[74]

Treatment of hepatic encephalopathy

Sedation is usually required in subjects manifesting moderate to severe signs of HE. This should not pose any particular problems in mature horses in which slightly reduced doses of commonly used sedatives and tranquilisers (e.g., xylazine* 0.5 mg/kg IV; detomidine† 10 µg/kg IV; acepromazine‡ 25 µg/kg IV) are suitable. Diazepam is probably best avoided due to the implication of benzodiazepine-like substances in the pathophysiology of HE, but this will have more practical implications in the treatment of foals.

The orally administered nonabsorbable disaccharide lactulose§ is metabolised by colonic bacteria to acetic and lactic acids, thus acidifying the colon.[78] This leads to ionisation and reduced absorption of ammonia, increased incorporation of ammonia into bacteria and a relative increase in less proteolytic bacterial species.[75,87] Additionally, faecal urease and protease are markedly suppressed even in mildly acidic environments.[95]

In the author's experience, oral lactulose administration almost invariably has a prompt and beneficial effect on the clinical signs of HE in horses, and this product also remains the most popular substance for decreasing intestinal ammonia production in human hepatopathies,[78,87] albeit without a strong evidence basis.[96] In horses, an oral dose of 0.3 ml/kg body weight is given initially every 6 hours and gradually reduced to once or twice daily treatments and is suitable for long-term administration (months to years). The dose and/or frequency should be reduced in the rare event of soft faeces being produced.

An alternative approach to reducing intestinal ammoniagenesis is the use of orally administered antibiotics including neomycin or metronidazole that may kill implicated species of colonic bacteria. One study proposed that oral antibiotics had a subjectively superior influence on HE in horses than did lactulose,[4] although this experience has not been shared by this author. Similar equivocal debate exists in the therapeutic choice for human patients.[78,96] Long-term administration of antibiotics is undesirable due to potential adverse effects, including colitis, ototoxicity and nephrotoxicity.[75] Nevertheless, a short course of oral neomycin** (15 mg/kg every 6 hours) or metronidazole†† (15 mg/kg PO loading dose followed by 7.5 mg/kg PO every 6 hours) could be used in conjunction with lactulose in treatment of acute HE.

Although methods to reduce colonic ammoniagenesis remain central in HE therapy of humans and horses, recent awareness of the small intestine, muscle and kidney as significant additional ammoniagenic organs has lead to increased interest in alternative therapeutic strategies.[91] In human patients, L-ornithine-L-aspartate effectively reduces serum ammonia concentration by providing essential substrates for peripheral conversion of ammonia into urea and glutamine. Indeed, this is one of the very few treatments for HE in humans with an evidence basis from placebo-controlled trials,[97] and is perhaps worthy of investigation in horses. Other ammonia-reducing strategies used in humans include sodium benzoate, which stimulates conversion of ammonia into hippuric acid,[98] and zinc supplementation, which is an essential component of carbamoylphosphate synthetase in the urea cycle.[99] The dopamine receptor agonist bromocryptine and the benzodiazepine receptor antagonist flumazenil are sometimes used in people with HE but are of equivocal value.[75,78,87] Additionally, some experimental studies support the use of glutamate receptor antagonists,[100] nonsteroidal anti-inflammatory drugs[101] and antihistamines[102] in HE cases.

Antifibrotic therapy

Hepatic fibroplasia is a common histopathological finding in liver biopsies, being found in 33 of 73 (45%) cases in one report.[55] Fibrosis is negatively associated with survival, and horses with evidence of moderate or severe fibrosis were, respectively, 17 and 56 times less likely to survive for 6 months than were horses without evidence of fibrosis in their biopsies.[55]

---

* Rompun; Bayer Animal Health, Newbury, Berkshire, UK; Chanazine 10%; Chanelle Animal Health, Liverpool, UK.

† Domosedan; Pfizer, Sandwich, Kent, UK.

‡ ACP; C-Vet, Leyland, Lancashire, UK.

§ Lactugal; Intrapharm Laboratories, Maidstone, Kent, UK.

** Neomycin; Pharmacia & Upjohn, Crawley, West Sussex, UK.

†† Metronidazole 400mg tablets, Ranbaxy Ireland Ltd, Cashel, Tipperary, Ireland.

Hepatic fibrosis is potentially reversible and persists only as a dynamic balance between the activities of degradative matrix metalloproteinases (MMPs) and tissue inhibitors of metalloproteinases (TIMPs) controlled by hepatic stellate cells (HSCs).[103] Although many proposed antifibrotic therapies that target HSCs are likely to be cost-prohibitive, interferons and angiotensin-converting enzyme inhibitors[104] may be worthy of investigation as potential antifibrotic drugs in horses. Additionally, corticosteroid therapy may have a theoretical indication in reducing the activating effects of inflammatory cytokines (e.g., tumour necrosis factor-α) on HSCs.

Antibacterial therapy

Cases of bacterial hepatitis (septic chlolangitis, cholangiohepatitis, cholelithiasis, hepatic abscessation and Tyzzer's disease)[43,105–108] should be treated with antibacterial drugs. Foals with confirmed or suspected Tyzzer's disease should be treated aggressively with ampicillin‡‡ (30 mg/kg IV every 8 hours) and gentamicin§§ (6.6 mg/kg IV every 24 hours).[107] Sodium benzyl penicillin*** (50,000 IU/kg IV every 6 hours) or oxytetracycline††† (10 mg/kg IV every 12 hours) are possible alternatives.[106] Suppurative hepatitides in mature horses may involve a variety of aerobic, anaerobic, Gram-positive and Gram-negative bacterial species,[43,105,108] and therefore broad-spectrum antibacterial therapy is essential. In mature horses, drug selection and dose are influenced by factors including hepatic metabolism and likely target bacterial species, but inevitably the choice of drug is heavily biased by the requirement for prolonged therapy (typically for at least 6–8 weeks),[43] and therefore administration route (and cost). For this reason, antibacterials suitable for enteral administration are preferred, including potentiated sulphonamides‡‡‡ (30 mg/kg combined product PO every 12–24 hours), enrofloxacin§§§ (7.5 mg/kg PO every 24 hours), doxycycline**** (10 mg/kg PO every 12 hours) and metronidazole (15 mg/kg PO loading dose followed by 7.5 mg/kg PO every 6 hours).

Anti-inflammatory therapy

Nonseptic (lymphoplasmacytic) hepatitis is a very common feature of equine liver biopsies[55] and indicates glucocorticoid therapy. This author usually uses prednisolone‡‡‡‡ (1 mg/kg PO every 24 hours) for at least 4 to 6 weeks in cases of mild to moderate lymphoplasmacytic hepatitis. Severe inflammatory infiltrates may benefit from more aggressive therapy commencing with dexamethasone§§§§ (0.05–0.1 mg/kg IV every 24 or 48 hours). NSAIDs are rarely indicated in the treatment of hepatopathies. Horses with cholelithiasis/cholangiohepatitis suffering from pyrexia or colic will probably receive NSAID treatment, and some evidence supports the use of NSAIDs in the treatment of HE.[101]

Anthelmintic therapy

Although hepatic hydatid cysts (*Echinococcus granulosus*) are occasionally found incidentally in horses,[109] they may also be seen in association with hepatic insufficiency and require specific therapy. This author has treated such cases with albendazole***** (10 mg/kg PO every 24 hours) for 7 days, repeated 6 times at 2-week intervals,[110] and also by cyst aspiration and injection of sterile saturated saline into the cyst cavity. Rare cases of liver fluke (*Fasciola hepatica*) are also reported in horses and donkeys, with the treatment of choice being triclabendazole††††† (12 mg/kg PO).[111,112]

Phlebotomy

Iron toxicity and/or iron accumulation in the failing liver is a significant cause of liver injury[113,114] and was found in 75% of equine liver biopsy samples in one report.[55] Regular phlebotomy has been successfully employed in human patients to reduce iron status and reduce ongoing hepatic injury[115] and should be considered in horses found to have severe haemosiderosis in liver biopsy specimens.

Specific diets for hepatic diseases

Hepatic disease in the absence of clinical or clinicopathological signs of insufficiency does not require any specific dietary changes. However, the failing liver will benefit from supportive nutritional strategies. The liver has a central role in many aspects of nutrient metabolism including storage, biotransformation, synthesis, secretion and digestion. Weight loss as a result of protein-caloric malnutrition typifies hepatic failure. It has been proposed that the primary cause of weight loss in humans with hepatic insufficiency is the failure of hepatic glycogen storage leading to reliance on gluconeogenesis from amino acids even during short-term fasting.[116] Additionally, inappetance, nausea and altered taste sensation potentiate the state of protein-calorie malnutrition in humans.[116] Utilisation of lipids as

‡‡ Ampicillin; American Pharmaceutical Partners, Inc. Schaumburg, IL, USA.

§§ Gentamicin sulfate solution; Schering-Plough Animal Health, Union, NY, USA.

*** Crystapen; Schering-Plough, Uxbridge, Middlesex, UK.

††† Engemycin; Intervet, Milton Keynes, Buckinghamshire, UK.

‡‡‡ Duphatrim; Fort Dodge, Southampton, Hampshire, UK.

§§§ Baytril 10% Oral Solution; Bayer, Bury St Edmonds, Suffolk, UK.

**** Doxycycline 100-mg capsules; Chanelle Medical, Ashford, Kent, UK.

‡‡‡‡ Prednisolone 25-mg tablets; Beacon Pharmaceuticals, Tunbridge Wells, Kent, UK.

§§§§ Duphacort Q; Fort Dodge, Southampton, Hampshire, UK.

***** Valbazen; Pfizer, Sandwich, Kent, UK.

††††† Fasinex; Novartis, Litlington, Hertfordshire, UK.

an energy source may also be impaired in subjects with hepatic insufficiency, further potentiating muscle catabolism and limiting energy availability.[117]

Dietary management of subjects with hepatic insufficiency is a delicate balance between provision of adequate nutrients to prevent or limit catabolism but at the same time preventing excess nutrient supply that could precipitate or exacerbate HE. Horses with hepatic insufficiency are likely to require a dietary energy intake of at least that of healthy animals under similar conditions (e.g., approximately 125–150 kJ/kg digestible energy).[118] Free access to fresh grass or grass hay is advisable. Provision of supplementary feed divided into at least four to six daily meals[28] appears sensible in the light of likely compromise of nutrient processing and regulation present in cases of hepatic insufficiency. In addition to providing a less variable nutrient supply, this protocol may also reduce potential peaks of ammoniagenesis.

Dietary protein potentiates ammoniagenesis in the colon, and proteins relatively high in aromatic amino acids may be additionally harmful in subjects with HE. However, a positive nitrogen balance must be maintained in order to avoid catabolism with further undesirable consequences on hyperammonaemia, body mass and metabolism. Therefore, excessive dietary protein should be avoided, but low-protein diets may be equally undesirable.[119] The target for protein intake in human patients with hepatic insufficiency is 1 to 1.5 g protein/kg/day,[75,78,116] and similar targets for crude protein likely apply in sick horses.[118] The failing liver inadequately metabolises aromatic amino acids ([AAAs] tryptophan, phenylalanine, tyrosine). This, combined with increased muscular catabolism of branched chain amino acids ([BCAAs] leucine, isoleucine, valine) as an energy source, leads to an increased AAA : BCAA ratio in serum,[47–49] that is implicated in the pathogenesis of HE.[88] Consequently, protein sources with a low AAA : BCAA ratio are preferable, especially in subjects with HE, or alternatively BCAA supplementation may be offered.[75,116] Wheat, soya, beet pulp and oats are all relatively rich in AAAs and should probably be avoided, whereas wheat bran, maize and milo (sorghum) have a relatively high BCAA content.[28,120] Alfalfa has a suitably low AAA : BCAA ratio (<0.5), although it should be offered with care due to the relatively high protein content.[120] Feeding beet pulp has been reported to reduce the plasma ammonia concentration.[121]

Hepatic and skeletal muscle glycogen synthesis is reduced in cases of liver failure,[116,122] suggesting that a stable and adequate dietary supply of nonstructural carbohydrate is important to reduce gluconeogenesis from endogenous proteins. Additionally, studies in humans have shown that relatively high carbohydrate diets allow higher protein intake in patients with chronic liver disease without increasing plasma amino acid concentrations that may contribute to the pathogenesis of HE.[123] A 10 : 2 : 1 carbohydrate : protein : fat ratio (by weight) has been found to effectively limit plasma amino acid concentrations.[123] Addition of molasses to the diet of horses with hepatic insufficiency is frequently advocated and seems reasonable in the light of this evidence.[28] High-fat diets are associated with deterioration in serum biochemical indices of liver injury in humans.[124] Most equine diets tend to have a low-fat content that is unlikely to present metabolic or digestive problems to a horse with hepatic insufficiency. However, increasing the energy density of an equine ration by the addition of fat is probably unwise in the presence of a failing liver.

Dietary supplementation with vitamins is commonly recommended for horses suffering from hepatic disease,[28,125] but caution is warranted regarding potential hepatotoxins contained in proprietary multivitamin preparations. Micronutrients with a particular capacity for hepatic insult include iron, copper, manganese and vitamin A.[116] Probably the most concerning hepatotoxin in multivitamin preparations is iron owing to its frequent inclusion and its capacity for accumulating in the liver and causing oxidative injury and fibrosis.[113,114,126,127] Excessive iron deposition in the form of haemosiderin is a common finding in the liver of normal horses and occurs to a greater degree in association with various forms of liver disease.[55] Furthermore, increased presence of haemosiderin is associated with a poorer prognosis for recovery from liver disease in horses[55] and in humans.[128] Where vitamin preparations are used in horses with hepatic insufficiency, care should be taken to use an iron-free product‡‡‡‡‡, especially if haemosiderosis has been found on liver biopsy.

The biliary system is the major route of excretion of copper and manganese, and toxic accumulation is frequently recognised in humans with hepatic insufficiency and HE.[116] This author has recognised increased manganese accumulation in horses with hepatic insufficiency. Vitamin A accumulation is a potential cause of hepatotoxicity in humans, although most patients are found to have low plasma vitamin A concentrations.[116] Nevertheless, supplementation should perhaps only be administered in the light of serum concentrations. Mild to severe hepatotoxicity induced by herbal remedies is well recognised in humans.[129] Lack of toxicity studies of many proprietary feed supplements and herbal remedies is concerning with known potential hepatotoxins including germander, gentian, *Asafoetida*, mistletoe, senna, chaparral, valerian, comfrey, pennyroyal, *Dictamnus* and *Paeonia*.[130,131]

Hypozincaemia is common in other species with chronic liver disease and may potentiate the toxic effects of copper and iron.[116,122] Zinc supplementation may also improve the activity of the urea cycle.[99] Vitamin D deficiency is frequently identified in humans with hepatic insufficiency.[132] Vitamin K deficiency is described as the most rapidly developing vitamin deficiency in dogs and cats with liver failure[121] and may therefore merit supplementation in horses.[120] Supplementation of vitamin E and B vitamins is also frequently advocated.[122]

‡‡‡‡‡ Multiplex; TRM, Newbridge, Co. Kildare, Ireland.

References

1. Jeffcott LB and Field JR: Current concepts of hyperlipaemia in horses and ponies. Vet Record 116:461-466, 1985
2. Reid SWJ, Mohammed HO: Survival analysis approach to risk factors associated with hyperlipemia in donkeys. J Am Vet Med Assoc 209:1449-1452, 1996
3. Hughes KJ, Hodgson DR, Dart AJ: Equine hyperlipaemia: a review. Aust Vet J 82:136-142, 2004
4. McGorum BC, Murphy D, Love S, Milne EM: Clinicopathological features of equine primary hepatic disease: a review of 50 cases. Vet Rec 145:134-139, 1999
5. Durham AE, Newton JR, Smith KC, Hillyer MH, Hillyer LL, Smith MR, Marr CM: Retrospective analysis of historical, clinical, ultrasonographic, serum biochemical and haematological data in prognostic evaluation of equine liver disease. Equine Vet J 35:542-547, 2003
6. Amory H, Perron M-F, Sandersen C, Delguste C, Grulke S, Cassart D, Godeau J-M, Detilleux J: Prognostic value of clinical signs and blood parameters in equids suffering from hepatic diseases. J Equine Vet Sci 25:18-25, 2005
7. Peek SF, Divers TJ, Jackson CJ: Hyperammonaemia associated with encephalopathy and abdominal pain without evidence of liver disease in four mature horses. Equine Vet J 29:70-74, 1997
8. Mair TS, Jones RD: Acute encephalopathy and hyperammonaemia in a horse without evidence of liver disease. Vet Record 137:642-643, 1995
9. Davis DM, McClure JR, Bertone AL, Cazayoux CA, Vice JD: Hypoglycemia and hepatic necrosis after small intestinal incarceration through the epiploic foramen in a horse. Cornell Vet 82:173-179, 1992
10. Jakowski RM: Right hepatic lobe atrophy in horses: 17 cases (1983-1993) J Am Vet Med Assoc 204:1057-1061, 1994
11. Vachon AM, Fischer AT: Small intestinal herniation through the epiploic foramen: 53 cases (1987-1993). Equine Vet J 27:373-380, 1995
12. Davis JL, Blikslager AT, Catto K, Jones SL: A retrospective analysis of hepatic injury in horses with proximal enteritis (1984-2002). J Vet Intern Med 17:896-901, 2003
13. Gardner RB, Nydam DV, Mohammed HO, Ducharme NG, Divers TJ: Elevations in serum gamma glutamyl transferase values in horses with right dorsal displacements of the large colon [abstract]. Proceedings of the 22nd Annual ACVIM Forum, Minneapolis, MN, 2004, p 793
14. Peek SF: Cholangiohepatitis in the mature horse. Equine Vet Educ 16:72-75, 2004
15. Tegeder I, Levy M, Muth-Selbach U, Oelkers R, Neumann F, Dormann H, Azaz-Livshits T, Criegee-Rieck M, Schneider HT, Hahn E, Brune K, Geisslinger G: Retrospective analysis of the frequency and recognition of adverse drug reactions by means of automatically recorded laboratory signals. Br J Clin Pharmacol 47:557-564, 1999
16. Engelking LR, Dodman NH, Hartman G, Valdez H, Spivak W: Effects of halothane anesthesia on equine liver function. Am J Vet Res 44:607-615, 1984
17. Engelking LR, Dodman NH, Hartman G, Valdez H: Effects of isofluorane anesthesia on equine liver function. Am J Vet Res 44:616-619, 1984
18. Pearson EG: Chemical and drug hepatotoxins, in Smith BP (ed): Large Animal Internal Medicine. St. Louis, Mosby, 1990, pp 854-856
19. Lacroix I, Lapeyre-Mestre M, Bagheri H, Pathak A, Montastruc JL: Non-steroidal anti-inflammatory drug-induced liver injury: a case-control study in primary care. Fundam Clin Pharmacol 18:201-206, 2004
20. Lees P, Creed RF, Gerring EL, Gould PW, Humphreys DJ, Maitho TE, Michel AR, Taylor JB: Biochemical and haematological effects of phenylbutazone in horses. Equine Vet J 15:158-167, 1983
21. Goodrich LR, Furr MO, Robertson JL, Warnick LD: A toxicity study of eltenac, a non-steroidal anti-inflammatory drug in horses. J Vet Pharmacol Ther 21:24-33, 1998
22. Jaraiz MV, Rodriguez C, San Andres MD, Gonzales F, San Andres MI: Disposition and tolerance of suxibuzone in horses. Equine Vet J 31:411-416, 1999
23. Guglick MA, MacAllister CG, Ely RW, Edwards WC: Hepatic disease associated with administration of tetanus antitoxin in eight horses. J Am Vet Med Assoc 206:1737-1740, 1995
24. Aleman M, Nieto JE, Carr EA, Carlson GP: Serum hepatitis associated with commercial plasma transfusion in horses. J Vet Intern Med 19:120-122, 2005
25. Stockham SL: Interpretation of equine serum biochemical profile results. Vet Clin N Am Equine Pract 11:391-414, 1995
26. Eades SC, Bounous DI: Hepatic diseases, in Eades SC, Bounous DI (eds): Laboratory Profiles of Equine Diseases. London, Mosby, 1997, pp 241-253
27. Barton MH, Morris DD: Diseases of the liver, in Reed SM, Bayly WM (eds): Equine Internal Medicine. Philadelphia, WB Saunders, 1998, pp 707-738
28. Divers TJ, Bernard WV, Reef VB: (1988) Equine liver disease and liver failure—causes, diagnosis and treatment. Proceedings of the 10th Bain-Fallon Memorial Lectures, Adelaide, Australia, 1988, pp 35-46
29. Gopinath C, Ford EJH, Jones RS: The effects of chloroform or halothane on horse liver in the early stage of ragwort poisoning. J Pathol Bacteriol 107:253-263, 1972
30. Leonard TB, Neptun DA, Popp JA: Serum gamma glutamyl transferase as a specific indicator of bile duct lesions in the rat liver. Am J Pathol 116:262-269, 1984
31. Scarratt WK, Saunders GK, Fessler RL: Cholelithiasis and biliary obstruction in a horse. Compend Contin Educ Pract Vet 7:S428-S431, 1985
32. Hoffmann WE, Baker G, Rieser S, Dorner JL: Alterations in selected serum biochemical constituents in equids after induced hepatic disease. Am J Vet Res 48:1343-1347, 1987
33. Bortell R, Asquith RL, Edds GT, Simpson CF, Aller WW: Acute experimentally induced aflatoxicosis in the weanling pony. Am J Vet Res 44:2110-2114, 1983
34. Durham AE, Smith KC, Newton JR: An evaluation of diagnostic data in comparison to the results of liver biopsy in mature horses. Equine Vet J 35:554-559, 2003
35. Rico AG, Braun JP, Benard P, El Hassan AA, Cazieux A: Tissue distribution and blood levels of gamma-glutamyl transferase in the horse. Equine Vet J 9:100-101, 1977
36. Parraga ME, Carlson GP, Thurmond M: Serum protein concentrations in horses with severe liver disease: a retrospective study and review of the literature. J Vet Intern Med 9:154-161, 1995

37. West HJ: Clinical and pathological studies in horses with hepatic disease. Equine Vet J 28:146-156, 1996
38. Odeh M, Sabo E, Srugo I, Oliven A: Serum levels of tumour necrosis factor-α correlate with severity of hepatic encephalopathy due to chronic liver failure. Liver Int 24:110-116, 2004
39. Pearson EG, Craig AM: Serum bile acids for diagnosis of chronic liver disease in horses. Proceedings of the 4th Annual ACVIM Forum, Washington, DC, 1986, pp 1071-1075
40. Gronwall R, Mia AS: Fasting hyperbilirubinemia in horses. Am J Dig Dis 17:473-476, 1972
41. Robbins RL, Wallace SS, Brunner CJ, Gardner TR, Difranco BJ, Speirs VC: Immune-mediated haemolytic disease after penicillin therapy in a horse. Equine Vet J 25:462-465, 1993
42. David JB, Byars TD, Braniecki A, Chaffin MK, Storts RW: Kernicterus in a foal with neonatal isoerythrolysis. Compend Contin Educ Pract Vet 20:517-519, 1998
43. Peek SF, Divers TJ: Medical treatment of cholangiohepatitis and cholelithiasis in mature horses: 9 cases (1991-1998). Equine Vet J 32:301-306, 2000
44. Byars TD: Chronic liver failure in horses. Compend Contin Educ Pract Vet 5:S423-S430, 1983
45. Lisman T, Leebeek FWG, de Groot PG: Haemostatic abnormalities in patients with liver disease. J Hepatol 37:280-287, 2002
46. Kerr R, Newsome P, Germain L, Thomson E, Dawson P, Stirling D, Ludlam CA: Effects of acute liver injury on blood coagulation. J Thromb Haemost 1:754-759, 2002
47. Morgan MY, Marshall AW, Milsom JP, Sherlock S: Plasma amino-acid patterns in liver disease. Gut 23:362-370, 1982
48. Gulick BA, Knight HD, Rogers QR: Use of plasma amino acid patterns in liver disease of the horse. Calif Vet 33:21-23, 1979
49. Gulick BA, Liu IKM, Qualls CW, Gribble DH, Rogers QR: Effect of pyrrolizidine alkaloid-induced hepatic disease on plasma amino acid patterns in the horse. Am J Vet Res 41:1894-1898, 1980
50. Butterworth RF: Role of circulating neurotoxins in the pathogenesis of hepatic encephalopathy: potential for improvement following their removal by liver assist devices. Liver Int 23:5-9, 2003
51. Engelking LR, Anwer MS, Lofstedt J: Hepatobiliary transport of indocyanine green and sulfobromophthalein in fed and fasted horses. Am J Vet Res 46:2278-2284, 1985
52. Buonanno AM, Carlson GP, Kantrowitz B: Clinical and diagnostic features of portosystemic shunt in a foal. J Am Vet Med Assoc 192:387-389, 1988
53. Durando MM, MacKay RJ, Staller GS, Cooper BJ, Ginn PE, Meneghetti N: Septic cholangiohepatitis and cholangiocarcinoma in a horse. J Am Vet Med Assoc 206:1018-1021, 1995
54. Tanaka E, Inomata S, Yasuhara H: The clinical importance of conventional and quantitative liver function tests in liver transplantation. J Clin Pharm Ther 25:411-419, 2000
55. Durham AE, Smith KC, Newton JR, Hillyer MH, Hillyer LL, Smith MR, Marr CM: Development and application of a scoring system for prognostic evaluation of equine liver biopsies. Equine Vet J 35:534-540, 2003
56. Teare JP, Sherman D, Greenfield SM, Simpson J, Bray G, Catterall AP, Murray-Lyon IM, Peters TJ, Williams R, Thompson RP: Comparison of serum procollagen III peptide concentrations and PGA index for assessment of hepatic fibrosis. Lancet 342:895-898, 1993
57. Oberti F, Valsesia E, Pilette C, Rousselet MC, Bedossa P, Aube C, Gallois Y, Rifflet H, Maiga MY, Penneau-Fontbonne D, Cales P: Noninvasive diagnosis of hepatic fibrosis or cirrhosis. Gastroenterology 113:1609-1616, 1997
58. Castera L, Hartmann DJ, Chapel F, Guettier C, Mall F, Lons T, Richardet JP, Grimbert S, Morassi O, Beaugrand M, Trinchet JC: Serum laminin and type IV collagen are accurate markers of histologically severe alcoholic hepatitis in patients with cirrhosis. J Hepatol 32:412-418, 2000
59. Guechot J, Serfaty L, Bonnand AM, Chazouilleres O, Poupon RE, Poupon R: Prognostic value of serum hyaluronan in patients with compensated HCV cirrhosis J Hepatol 32:447-452, 2000
60. Lindqvist U: Is serum hyaluronan a helpful tool in the management of patients with liver diseases? J Intern Med 242:67-71, 1997
61. Tulamo RM, Saari H, Konttinen YT: Determination of concentration of hyaluronate in equine serum. Am J Vet Res 51:740-742, 1990
62. Seawright AA, Hrdlicka J, Wright JD, Kerr DR, Mattocks AR, Jukes R: The identification of hepatotoxic pyrrolizidine alkaloid exposure in horses by the demonstration of sulphur-bound pyrrolic metabolites on their hemoglobin. Vet Hum Toxicol 33:286-287, 1991
63. Rantanen NW: Diseases of the liver. Vet Clin N Am Equine Pract 2:105-114, 1986
64. Mendel VE, Witt MR, Gitchell BS, Gribble DN, Rogers QR, Segall HJ, Knight HD: Pyrrolizidine alkaloid-induced liver disease in horses: an early diagnosis. Am J Vet Res 49:572-578, 1988
65. Smith MRW, Stevens KB, Durham AE, Marr CM: Equine hepatic disease: the effect of patient- and case-specific variables on risk and prognosis. Equine Vet J 35:549-552, 2003
66. Brown SA, Dusza K, Boehmer J: Comparison of measured and calculated values for colloidal osmotic pressure in hospitalized animals. Am J Vet Res 55:910-915, 1994
67. Jones PA, Tomasic M, Gentry PA: Oncotic, hemodilutional, and hemostatic effects of isotonic saline and hydroxyethyl starch solutions in clinically normal ponies. Am J Vet Res 58:541-548, 1997
68. Belgrave RL, Hines MT, Keegan RD, Wardrop KJ, Bayly WM, Sellon DC: Effects of a polymerized ultrapurified bovine hemoglobin blood substitute administered to ponies with normovolemic anemia. J Vet Intern Med 16:396-403, 2002
69. Haldane S, Roberts J, Marks S L, Raffe M R: Transfusion Medicine. Compend Contin Educ Pract Vet 26:502, 2004
70. Jalan R, Kapoor D: Reversal of diuretic-induced hepatic encephalopathy with infusion of albumin but not colloid. Clin Sci 106:467-474, 2004
71. Durham AE: How to use parenteral nutrition in equine practice. Proceedings of the 43rd British Equine Veterinary Association Annual Congress, Birmingham, UK, 2004, p 237

72. Durham AE: Clinical application of parenteral nutrition in the treatment of five ponies and one donkey with hyperlipaemia. Vet Rec 158:159-164, 2006
73. Durham AE, Phillips TJ, Walmsley JP, Newton JR: Nutritional and clinicopathological effects of post operative parenteral nutrition following small intestinal resection and anastomosis in the mature horse. Equine Vet J 36:390-396, 2004
74. Durham AE, unpublished observations, 2005
75. Kircheis G, Häussinger D: Management of hepatic encephalopathy. J Gastroenterol Hepatol 17:S260-S267, 2002
76. Eades SC, Booth AJ, Hansen TO, Mueller POE, Williamson L: Liver disease in horses, in Higgins AJ, Wright IM (eds): The Equine Manual. London, WB Saunders, 1995. pp 523-537
77. Ferenci P, Lockwood A, Mullen K, Tarter R, Weissenborn K, Blei AT: Hepatic encephalopathy-definition, nomenclature, diagnosis, and quantification: final report of the working party at the 11th World Congresses of Gastroenterology, Vienna, 1998. Hepatology 35:716-721, 2002
78. Blei AT, Cordoba J: Hepatic encephalopathy. Am J Gastroenterol 96:1968-1976, 2001
79. Milne EM, Pogson DM, Doxey DL: Secondary gastric impaction associated with ragwort poisoning in three ponies. Vet Rec 126:502-504, 1990
80. Pearson EG: Liver failure attributable to pyrrolizidine alkaloid toxicosis and associated with inspiratory dyspnea in ponies: three cases (1982-1988). J Am Vet Med Assoc 198:1651-1654, 1991
81. Butterworth RF, Giguère J-F, Michaud J, Lavoie J, Layrargues GP: Ammonia: key factor in the pathogenesis of hepatic encephalopathy. Neurochem Pathol 6:1-12, 1987
82. Häussinger D, Kircheis G, Fischer R, Schliess F, vom Dahl S: Hepatic encephalopathy in chronic liver disease: a clinical manifestation of astrocyte swelling and low grade cerebral oedema? J Hepatol 32:1035-1038, 2000
83. Häussinger D, Schliess F, Kircheis G: Pathogenesis of hepatic encephalopathy. J Gastroenterol Hepatol 17:S256-S259, 2002
84. Norenberg MD: Astroglial dysfunction in hepatic encephalopathy. Metab Brain Dis 13:319-336, 1998
85. Balata S, Damink SW, Ferguson K, Marshall I, Hayes PC, Deutz NE, Williams R, Wardlaw J, Jalan R: Induced hyperammonemia alters neuropsychology brain MR spectroscopy and magnetization transfer in cirrhosis. Hepatology 37:931-939, 2003
86. Kato MD, Hughes RD, Keays RT, Williams R: Electron microscopic study of brain capillaries in cerebral edema from fulminant hepatic failure. Hepatology 15:1060-1066, 1992
87. Butterworth RF: Pathogenesis of hepatic encephalopathy: new insights from neuroimaging and molecular studies. J Hepatol 39, 278-285, 2003
88. Maddison JE: Hepatic encephalopathy: current concepts of the pathogenesis. J Vet Intern Med 6:341-353, 1992
89. Strauss GI, Knudsen GM, Kondrup J, Moller K, Larsen FS: Cerebral metabolism of ammonia and amino acids in patients with fulminant hepatic failure. Gastroenterology 121:1109-1119, 2001
90. Butterworth RF: Pathophysiology of hepatic encephalopathy: a new look at ammonia. Metab Brain Dis 17:221-227, 2002
91. Shawcross D, Jalan R: Dispelling myths in the treatment of hepatic encephalopathy. Lancet 365:431-433, 2005
92. Basile AS, Saito K, Li Y, Heyes MP: The relationship between plasma and brain quinolinic acid levels and the severity of hepatic encephalopathy in animal models of fulminant hepatic failure. J Neurochem 64:2607-2614, 1995
93. Layrargues GP, Spahr L, Butterworth RF: Increased blood manganese in cirrhotic patients: relationship to pallidal magnetic resonance signal hyperintensity and neurological symptoms. Hepatology 24:1112-1120, 1995
94. Green DS, Davies JV: Successful choledocholithotomy in a horse. Equine Vet J 21:464-467, 1989
95. Alexander T, Thomas K, Cherian AM, Kanakasabapathy I. Effect of three antibacterial drugs in lowering blood & stool ammonia production in hepatic encephalopathy. Indian J Med Res 96:292-296, 1992
96. Als-Nielsen B, Gluud LL, Gluud C: Non-absorbable disaccharides for hepatic encephalopathy: systematic review of randomized trials. Br Med J 328, 1046-1050, 2004
97. Kircheis G, Wettstein M, Dahl S, Haussinger D: Clinical efficacy of L-ornithine-L-aspartate in the management of hepatic encephalopathy. Metab Brain Dis 17:453-462, 2002
98. Sushma S, Dasarathy S, Tandon RK: Sodium benzoate in the treatment of acute hepatic encephalopathy: a double-blind randomized trial. Hepatology 16:138-144, 1992
99. Bresci G, Parisi G, Banti S: Management of hepatic encephalopathy with oral zinc supplementation: a long term treatment. Eur J Med 2:414-416, 1993
100. Vogels BA, Maas MA, Daalhuisen J, Quack G, Chamuleau RAFM: Memantine, a non-competitive NMDA receptor antagonist improves hyperammonemia-induced encephalopathy and acute hepatic encephalopathy in rats. Hepatology 25:820-827, 1997
101. Chung C, Gottstein J, Blein AT: Indomethacin prevents the development of experimental ammonia-induced brain edema in rats after portocaval anastomosis. Hepatology 34:249-254, 2001
102. Lozeva V, Tuomisto L, Soal D, Plumed C, Hippelainen N, Butterworth RF: Increased density of brain histamine H1 receptors in rats with portocaval anastomosis and in cirrhotic patients with chronic hepatic encephalopathy. Hepatology 33:1370-1376, 2001
103. Zhou X, Hovell CJ, Pawley S, Hutchings MI, Arthur MJP, Iredale JP, Benyon RC: Expression of matrix metalloproteinase-2 and -14 persists during early resolution of experimental liver fibrosis and might contribute to fibrolysis. Liver Int 24:492-501, 2004
104. Iredale JP: Cirrhosis: new research provides a basis for rational and targeted treatments. Br Med J 327:143-147, 2003
105. Johnston JK, Divers TJ, Reef VB, Acland H: Cholelithiasis in horses: ten cases (1982-1986). J Am Vet Med Assoc 194:405-409, 1989
106. Peek SF, Byars T D, Rueve E: Neonatal hepatic failure in a Thoroughbred foal: successful treatment of a case of presumptive Tyzzer's disease. Equine Vet Educ 6:307-309, 1994
107. Borchers A, Magdesian KG, Halland S, Pusterla N, Wilson WD: Successful treatment and polymerase chain reaction (PCR) confirmation of Tyzzer's disease in a foal and clinical

and pathologic characteristics of 6 additional foals (1986-2005). J Vet Intern Med 20:1212-1218, 2006
108. Sellon DC, Spaulding K, Breuhaus BA, Katz L, Mealey R: Hepatic abscesses in three horses. J Am Vet Med Assoc 216:882-887, 2000
109. Binhazim AA, Harmon BG, Roberson EL, Boerner M: Hydatid disease in a horse. J Am Vet Med Assoc 200:958-960, 1992
110. Summerhays GES, Mantell JAR: Ultrasonography as an aid to diagnosis and treatment of a retrobulbar hydatid cyst in a horse. Equine Vet Educ 7:39-42, 1995
111. Rubilar L, Cabreira A, Giacaman L: Treatment of Fasciola hepatica infection in horses with triclabendazole. Vet Record 123:320-321, 1988
112. Trawford AF, Tremlett JG: Efficacy of triclabendazole against Fasciola hepatica in the donkey (*Equus asinus*). Vet Record 139:142-143, 1996
113. Lavoie JP, Teuscher E: Massive iron overload and liver fibrosis resembling haemochromatosis in a racing pony. Equine Vet J 25:552-554, 1993
114. Stal P, Hultcrantz R: Iron increases ethanol toxicity in rat liver. J Hepatol 17:108-115, 1993
115. Yano M, Hayashi H, Wakusawa S, Sanae F, Takikawa T, Shiono Y, Arao M, Ukai K, Ito H, Watanabe K, Yoshioka K: Long term effects of phlebotomy on biochemical and histological parameters of chronic hepatitis C. Am J Gastroenterol 97:133-137, 2002
116. Jurewitsch B, Kim Y: Nutritional issues in the management of advanced liver disease. Nutr Clin Care 4:87-93, 2001
117. Marks SL, Rogers QR, Strombeck DR: Nutritional support in hepatic disease. Part I: metabolic alterations and nutritional considerations in dogs and cats. Compend Contin Educ Pract Vet 16:971-978, 1994
118. Naylor JM: Feeding the sick horse. Proceedings of the BEVA Specialist Days on Behaviour and Nutrition, 1999, pp 97-99
119. Mullen KD, Dasarathy S: Protein restriction in hepatic encephalopathy: necessary evil or illogical dogma? J Hepatol 41:147-148, 2004
120. Ralston SL: Equine clinical nutrition: specific problems and solutions. Compend Contin Educ Pract Vet 10:356-363, 1988
121. Olsman AF, Huurdeman CM, Jansen WL, et al.: Macronutrient digestibility, nitrogen balance, plasma indicators of protein metabolism and mineral absorption in horses fed a ration rich in sugar beet pulp. J Anim Physiol Anim Nutr (Berl) 88:321-331, 2004
122. Rutgers HC: Nutritional support of hepatic disease. Eur J Comp Gastroenterol 4:13-20, 1999
123. IlanY, Sobol T, Sasson O, Ashur Y, Berry EM: A balanced 5:1 carbohydrate:protein diet: a new method for supplementing protein to patients with chronic liver disease. J Gastroenterol Hepatol 15:1436-1441, 2000
124. Deems RO, Friedman LS, Friedman MI, Munoz SJ, Deems DA, Maddrey WC: Relationship between liver biochemical tests and dietary intake in patients with liver disease. J Clin Gastroenterol 18:304-308, 1994
125. Savage CJ, Diseases of the liver, in Colahan PT, Mayhew IG, Merritt AM, Moore JN (eds): Equine Medicine and Surgery, vol 1, ed 5. St. Louis, Mosby, 1999. pp 816-862
126. Mullaney TP, Brown CM: Iron toxicity in neonatal foals. Equine Vet J 20:119-124, 1988
127. Riley TR, Smith JP: Preventive care in chronic liver disease. J Gen Intern Med 14:699-704, 1999
128. Di Bisceglie AM, Axiotis CA, Hoofnagle JH, Bacon BR: Measurements of iron status in patients with chronic hepatitis. Gastroenterology 102:2108-2113, 1992
129. McCarthy M, Wilkinson ML: Recent advances—hepatology. Br Med J 318:1256-1259, 1999
130. Bashir RM, Lewis JH: Hepatotoxicity of drugs used in the treatment of gastrointestinal disorders. Gastroenterol Clin N Am 24:937-967, 1995
131. Kane JA, Kane SP, Jain S: Hepatitis induced by traditional Chinese herbs: possible toxic components. Gut 36:146-147, 1995
132. Shiomi S, Masaki K, Habu D, Takeda T, Nishiguchi S, Kuroki T, Tanaka T, Ochi H: Calcitriol for bone disease in patients with cirrhosis of the liver. J Gastroenterol Hepatol 14:547-552, 1999

13

Monitoring and treating the urogenital system

Anna Hollis and Kevin Corley

13.1 Monitoring the urogenital system
13.2 Treating the urogenital system

13.1 Monitoring the urogenital system

Patients at risk of developing urogenital disorders during hospitalisation

Renal insufficiency and acute renal failure

The incidence of renal insufficiency and acute renal failure in the equine hospital population has not been reported. In the human intensive care unit, up to 15% of patients suffer from renal insufficiency or acute renal failure.[1–4] Critically ill foals may have a similarly high rate of renal insufficiency.[5] However, clinical experience suggests that nephropathy is relatively uncommon in mature horses. Acute renal failure can result from decreased renal perfusion, an ischaemic, toxic or obstructive insult to the renal tubule, a tubulointerstitial process with inflammation and oedema, or a primary reduction in the filtering capacity of the glomerulus.[6] Prerenal failure and intrinsic renal failure due to ischaemia and nephrotoxins are responsible for most cases of acute renal failure in humans,[6] with prerenal azotaemia accounting for approximately 40% of hospital-acquired cases.[7]

Disease states increasing the risk of renal insufficiency

The highest risk factor for developing acute renal failure appears to be primary gastrointestinal diseases in both adult horses[8,9] and foals.[10] The systemic inflammatory response syndrome (SIRS) may predispose to nephropathy. Acute renal failure was reported in foals with sepsis, perinatal asphyxia syndrome and enterocolitis,[5] all of which has been associated with SIRS. In adult horses, endotoxaemia may cause acute renal failure. Endotoxaemia also results in SIRS. It is thought that SIRS mainly causes nephropathy through renal hypoperfusion, as a result of haemodynamic disturbances.[11] This certainly seems the case in critically ill human patients, in which sepsis and SIRS are important predisposing factors in the development of acute renal failure.[12,13]

Other disease states associated with renal insufficiency include rhabdomyolysis and postanaesthetic myopathy, which cause renal problems secondary to pigmenturia[14–18] and leptospirosis.[19–22]

Postrenal failure is unusual in the adult horse, although ruptured bladders have been reported following trauma during the birthing process in mares, and with and without a history of trauma in both sexes.[23,24] Postrenal failure may also be seen with urinary tract obstructions secondary to urolithiasis in the adult.[25] In contrast, ruptured bladders are relatively common in the neonatal foal, where they may be the presenting complaint, or may occur during the course of hospitalisation.[26,27]

Drugs increasing the risk of renal insufficiency

It is well recognised that certain drugs are potentially nephrotoxic in the horse, including the aminoglycoside antibiotics[28–33] and nonsteroidal anti-inflammatory drugs (NSAIDs).[34–38] Renal insufficiency has also been reported following high doses of oxytetracycline.[39] Polymyxin B is potentially nephrotoxic, although the risk appears to be low at the dose rates used for its antiendotoxic effects.[40,41] In patients with prerenal azotaemia, the administration of these potentially nephrotoxic drugs may increase the risk of renal injury.[42–45]

The administration of vasopressors such as norepinephrine may increase the risk of renal insufficiency. Norepinephrine has been shown to decrease renal blood flow and/or urine output in normotensive humans[46,47] and dogs,[48] although norepinephrine caused no change in urine output in normotensive foals.[49] In addition, norepinephrine-induced renal vasoconstriction appears to be less of a problem in hyperdynamic shock, where the addition of norepinephrine improved urine output in septic humans[50–54] and foals.[55] All animals receiving vasopressor support should have their renal function closely monitored. A decreased urine output in response to an initiation of or increase in pressor support may indicate excessive renal vasoconstriction.[56]

Toxic causes of renal insufficiency

Renal insufficiency may be seen following a variety of toxic insults, and animals with a history of exposure to these substances should be carefully monitored. Vitamin D intoxication may cause renal insufficiency following renal mineralisation, which has been reported in the horse following supplementation and the ingestion of certain plants.[57–59] Heavy metals (including mercury, zinc and cadmium) may cause renal insufficiency, amongst other clinical signs.[60–65] Cantharidin toxicosis may cause renal insufficiency in areas where blister beetles are prevalent (chiefly southern and midwest states of the United States, Central and South America and sub-Saharan Africa).[66,67]

Urinary tract infections

Mares are at greater risk of developing ascending infections than are geldings as a result of their shorter urethra. Urinary tract infections (UTIs) are also a potential consequence of urethral catheterisation. The risk of ascending infections is increased in animals with indwelling urinary catheters. This can be minimised by aseptic placement, clean management and maintaining a totally closed urine collection system. Silver- or antimicrobial-impregnated urinary catheters have been developed to reduce infection rates in humans but have not been evaluated in horses. Urinary catheterisation under anaesthesia also increases the risk of UTI development and should therefore be treated as an aseptic procedure. Animals with urethral damage, such as mares with trauma following foaling, are at increased risk of developing UTIs. UTIs are more common in animals with urinary retention or decreased urethral sphincter tone, which are usually associated with other neurological deficits.

Infections of the upper urinary tract are uncommon in horses. In neonatal foals, septicaemia may predispose to the development of pyelonephritis.[68]

Urolithiasis

Males are at greater risk of developing urolithiasis than are females, as the shorter, more distensible urethra of the female allows passage of any calculi that may develop. The factors increasing the risk of urolithiasis are not fully ascertained but may include urinary retention, urinary tract infections, and the use of nonsteroidal anti-inflammatory drugs. There is a possible association with high-calcium diets and the development of urolithiasis, so in horses prone to this condition, it may be advisable to avoid a legume-based diet.

Genital disorders

The periparturient mare is at risk of developing genital disorders during hospitalisation. All mares immediately postpartum should have full reproductive tract examinations.

Any stallion with colic should have its testicles carefully examined, as inguinal hernias are a potential cause of strangulating intestinal lesions. The other major consideration is care with the use of phenothiazines, such as acepromazine, in the intact male. Phenothiazine administration may cause paraphimosis and priapism, which, if not recognised and treated, is potentially disastrous in the breeding male.[69]

Collecting urine

The two most common methods of urine collection are a midstream catch of spontaneously voided urine and bladder catheterisation. Although a free catch sample is not an invasive procedure, encouraging the horse to urinate is not always easy. Placing a horse on fresh bedding often encourages urination. There are patented horse "nappy" systems* available for urine and/or faecal collection. For male horses, it is possible to secure a 2-L water bottle, cut in half, to the sheath as a cheap and relatively easy method of collecting urine.

Free catch samples are less suitable for urine culture as there will be contamination of the urine from the external genitalia.[70] It may therefore be desirable to obtain a sample via urethral catheterisation. This is a straightforward procedure that yields a sterile sample suitable for full urinalysis, including culture. Restraint of adult horses in suitable stocks will make the process safer and easier. Foals can usually be restrained in lateral recumbency (see Chapter 2.4). Catheterisation of the urinary tract in the adult animal is described in Chapter 1.42, and in the foal, in Chapter 2.9.

Urinalysis

General appearance

Equine urine is normally straw-yellow to pale brown in colour and can have a turbid appearance due to the mucus and calcium carbonate crystals that are commonly present. Naturally voided urine may change in appearance during the course of micturition, so the whole urination should be observed. Where discolouration is noted, the timing of the discolouration during micturition may aid lesion localisation. Consistent discolouration is more indicative of myoglobinuria, haemoglobinuria or a bladder or renal lesion, whereas discolouration at the beginning or end of micturition may be more likely with a lesion in the urethra or, in the male, the accessory sex glands.

Urine output

The normal, nursing, neonatal foal produces large quantities of urine, in the order of 148 ml/kg/day (6.17 ml/kg/hr).[71] In contrast, the normal adult horse produces 1.24 ml/kg/hr (approximately 30 ml/kg/day).[72] Urine output can be measured by urethral catheterisation with a closed collection system†.The urethral catheter can be connected to a

---

* Equisan Marketing Pty Ltd, South Melbourne, Victoria, Australia.

† Simpla drainable 2-L bag; Coloplast A/S, Humleback, Denmark.

commercially available urine collection bag, which, in foals, can be secured to the animal's hind legs with an adhesive bandage if it is not recumbent. Alternatively, an empty fluid bag with a giving set attached to the urethral catheter works well, although emptying the bag requires detachment from the urethral catheter. These collection systems are well tolerated by the neonatal foal but may be more difficult to maintain in the adult horse.

Specific gravity

Urine specific gravity is a measure of the number of particles present in the urine and is thus a measure of urine concentration. This is usually measured with a refractometer. The presence of large molecules in the urine (e.g., glucose or protein) will lead to overestimation of the urine specific gravity by the refractometer, so where glucosuria or proteinuria is suspected, a more accurate measure of urine concentration is by measuring urine osmolarity in the laboratory. The description of urine concentration is given in Box 13.1.

The urine of the adult horse is normally concentrated, and the mean urine specific gravity in the normal horse given free access to feed and water is 1.028.[72] In contrast, the normal foal will be hyposthenuric due to their large fluid intake. The mean urine specific gravity in normal foals is 1.004 to 1.008,[71,73] and urine specific gravities of 1.000 to 1.004 are common in foals treated with intravenous fluids. Normal foals may also have more concentrated urine in the first 2 days of life, up to 1.032. A dehydrated or hypovolaemic foal will increase its urine specific gravity in response to its hydration status, provided that its renal function is normal.

Isosthenuria, or urine specific gravity of 1.008 to 1.012, will be seen irrespective of hydration status in some types of renal failure. Inability to concentrate the urine in the face of dehydration may also result from diabetes insipidus, an unusual disease in the horse.

Reagent strips

Reagent strips are quick and easy to use and require a small urine sample.

Box 13.1. Description of urine concentration

- Hyposthenuria
  - Urine more dilute than serum
  - Urine specific gravity <1.008
- Isosthenuria
  - Urine and serum concentrations similar
  - Urine specific gravity 1.008–1.012
- Hypersthenuria
  - Urine more concentrated than serum
  - Urine specific gravity >1.012

pH

The normal pH of adult horse urine is 7.0 to 9.0,[74–76] and 5.5 to 8.0 in normal foal urine.[71] Aciduria in adult horses may be seen after exertion, after prolonged fasting, with bacterial infections, with hypovolaemia and in response to metabolic acidosis. Hypokalaemia and/or hypochloraemia may result in paradoxical aciduria. Renal tubular acidosis is a rare condition in the horse, which may lead to the production of alkaline urine despite systemic acidosis.

Occult blood

A positive reaction to blood on urine reagent strips indicates the presence of haematuria, haemoglobinuria or myoglobinuria. Centrifugation of the urine aids differentiation—red blood cells will collect in the sediment if haematuria is present. Haemoglobin and myoglobin do not separate following centrifugation, and the urine will remain discoloured. Haematology will aid differentiation of the two—haemoglobinaemia is accompanied by discoloured plasma, which is not a feature of myoglobinaemia. Myoglobinaemia can also be differentiated from haemoglobinaemia by the ammonium sulphate precipitation test, performed in a laboratory.

Glucose

Glucose is not normally found in equine urine. If the blood glucose exceeds the renal threshold (10 mmol/L [180 mg/dL] in adult horses), glucosuria may be seen. Hyperglycaemia and glucosuria may be seen with pituitary pars intermedia dysfunction (Cushing's disease, pituitary adenoma) and diabetes mellitus. Other potential causes of hyperglycaemia leading to glucosuria include stress and administration of dextrose-containing fluids. Glucosuria in the absence of hyperglycaemia suggests primary tubular dysfunction.

Protein

Protein is not normally present in equine urine; however, false-positive results are common with reagent strips due to the alkalinity of equine urine. A positive result on a dipstick should be confirmed with an acid precipitation procedure. Proteinuria may be seen with haemorrhage or inflammation in the urogenital tract or may be transiently present following strenuous exercise. The differential diagnoses for haemorrhage include cystic or renal calculi, neoplasia, coagulopathy and traumatic urine collection. Inflammation may be seen with pyelonephritis, cystitis, genital infections and vasculitis.

Persistent proteinuria without evidence of haemorrhage or inflammation may occur with glomerular diseases such as glomerulonephritis and amyloidosis, which are rare in the horse.

Ketones

Ketones are rare in equine urine. Ketonuria may be seen following protein catabolism. In addition, ketonuria has been anecdotally reported following administration of intravenous ceftiofur.

Bilirubin
Bilirubinuria may be seen following intravascular haemolysis, hepatic necrosis and obstructive hepatopathies. Bilirubinuria is normally accompanied by abnormal blood biochemistry.

Sediment examination
Sediment examination can provide useful information and has been used in humans to aid the differential diagnosis of and severity of acute renal failure.[77] Sediment examination should be performed as soon as possible following urine collection, and within 1 hour, as urinary casts are unstable in alkaline urine. Following collection, 5 ml urine should be centrifuged at 700*g* for 5 minutes. All but 0.5 ml of the supernatant urine can be discarded, and the sediment resuspended. This can be placed on a slide and covered with a coverslip. Staining with a commercial stain (e.g., Sedistain) is not necessary, but may facilitate evaluation. Urine should be evaluated using both low-power (×100) and high-power (×400) fields.

Casts
Urinary casts are cylindrical accumulations of Tamm-Horsfall glycoprotein and cellular debris that form in the renal tubules and pass into the bladder with urine. This cellular debris may consist of white blood cells, red blood cells or renal tubular epithelial cells. Casts are usually associated with inflammation and/or infection, but a small number per high-power field may be normal. Hyaline casts may also be seen, which are formed from mucoprotein as a result of glomerulonephritis or severe nephropathy. In humans, a higher number of casts indicate acute tubular necrosis and thus aids differential diagnosis of the cause of renal insufficiency.[77] This may also be true in horses with aminoglycoside toxicity. However, the number of casts seen does not always correlate with the severity of the disease process.

Epithelial cells
Epithelial cells seen may be squamous, transitional or renal tubular, and the presence of small numbers on sediment examination is normal, especially following urethral catheterisation. Large numbers of epithelial cells may be seen as a result of inflammation or neoplasia of the renal tubules or urinary tract.

Red blood cells
It is normal to see 5 or fewer red blood cells, assuming the sample was atraumatically collected. Urethral catheterisation may cause a small amount of trauma and account for the slightly increased number of red blood cells seen in samples from catheterisation compared to free catch samples. An increased number of red blood cells indicate haematuria, which may occur with inflammation, infection, neoplasia, coagulopathy, renal calculi, cystic calculi, toxaemia and acute tubular disease.

Leucocytes
Five or fewer white blood cells should be seen per high-power field in normal horses. Increased numbers indicate inflammation in the urogenital tract.

Crystals
Equine urine is normally rich in crystals. These are usually calcium carbonate, but calcium phosphate and oxalate may also be seen. A small amount of 10% acetic acid may be added to the sediment to dissolve these crystals to facilitate sediment examination.

Mucus
Mucus is commonly seen and is normal in equine urine.

Bacteria
Spontaneously voided urine may contain bacteria that are normal constituents of the genitalia. These should not be present in a sample collected aseptically by catheter.

Assessment of renal function

Measurement of glomerular filtration rate
The glomerular filtration rate (GFR) is the volume of plasma filtered by the kidneys per unit of time. The clearance of a substance is the volume of plasma from which that substance is completely cleared by the kidneys per unit time. If a substance is freely filterable, not reabsorbed, secreted, synthesised or broken down by the renal tubules, it can be used to calculate the GFR.[78] GFR is a measure of renal function, as a reduction in the GFR signifies a reduction in the ability of the kidney to filter the substrate measured. Decreases in GFR therefore indicate a reduction in renal function.

Creatinine is formed from muscle creatine and is released into the blood at a relatively constant rate; thus its blood concentration changes little over a 24-hour period. Endogenous creatinine clearance is used to estimate the GFR as it is freely filterable. Creatinine is secreted by the renal tubules, and thus endogenous creatinine clearance may slightly overestimate the actual GFR.[78] However, plasma creatinine concentration may be overestimated if the Jaffe method is used for laboratory analysis of plasma creatinine, in which case the GFR may be underestimated.[79,80]

Other methods of measuring GFR are available and include the clearance of inulin, iohexol and technetium-diethyletneaminopentacetic acid (Tc-DTPA). These methods have been used in both adult horses[79,81–86] and foals[80,87,88] but are not used in the clinical setting due to their impracticality and/or expense. Inulin clearance is often considered the "gold standard" for measurements of GFR. There are conflicting results regarding the accuracy of endogenous creatinine clearance compared with inulin clearance in the horse and foal.[79–82,87] However, these discrepancies do not appear to be clinically important, and endogenous creatinine clearance is used to estimate GFR in the clinical situation.

Endogenous creatinine clearance is a simple, relatively noninvasive procedure to perform in the neonatal foal and is also possible in the mature horse. A urinary catheter should be placed and attached to a closed collection system, and a blood sample collected into a plain tube at this time. A second blood sample should be taken a set amount of time later, at which point the urine collection bag is emptied, the volume of urine accurately measured, and a representative urine sample collected to measure the creatinine concentration. The minimum time period over which these measurements should be performed is 1 hour, and the ideal is to perform this test over 24 hours. The creatinine clearance can then be calculated from the equation given in Box 13.2. Reported values for the normal endogenous creatinine clearance in the adult equine are 1.20 to 2.38 ml/min/kg,[79,81,82,89–93] and 1.78 to 2.17 ml/min/kg in the foal.[80,87,88]

Fractional excretion of electrolytes

The fractional excretion of electrolytes is used to evaluate the secretory and reabsorptive function of the renal tubules. The fractional excretion of electrolytes will be affected by renal tubular function, dietary intake, hormones and the administration of certain drugs. The fractional excretions in the normal horse are listed in Table 13.1. In general, an increase in the fractional excretion of an electrolyte represents a degree of renal tubular damage and can thus give information regarding the prognosis for recovery of renal function. Where the renal tubules have been damaged, recovery of normal renal function is less likely. As phosphate is almost entirely reabsorbed in the proximal tubule,[94] and potassium primarily secreted in the distal tubule,[95] the fractional excretion of these may provide the most useful information as to the location of any tubular damage. Other causes of increased fractional excretions include the administration of sodium-rich intravenous fluids (sodium) and hyperparathyroidism (phosphorus).

The fractional urinary excretion of electrolytes can be calculated following simultaneous collection of urine and blood, with the measurement of urinary and serum creatinine and electrolyte concentrations. These are usually expressed as a percentage of endogenous creatinine clearance. The formula for calculating the fractional excretion of an electrolyte is given in Box 13.3. The normal values are given in Table 13.1.

Urinary enzyme activity

Enzymes are found in the epithelial cells lining the renal tubules. Turnover of proximal renal tubular cells leads to active enzyme present in the urine, and increases in the amount of enzyme occur with inflammation, necrosis or sloughing of the epithelium secondary to renal tubular damage.[101] An increase in urinary enzymes (measured by their activity) provides evidence for renal tubular damage which may be seen prior to other signs, allowing prompt institution of treatment.[101,102] Urinary enzyme activities are measured by the collection of a urine sample and analysis of enzyme activity and creatinine concentrations. Various urinary enzymes have been measured in the horse, including γ-glutamyltransferase (γGT), alkaline phosphatase, lactate dehydrogenase, kallikrein and *N*-acetyl-β-D-gluosaminidase (NAD).[71,103–105] There is increasing interest

Box 13.2. Equation for endogenous creatinine clearance

$$\text{Creatinine clearance (ml/min/kg)} = \frac{(\text{Urine [creatinine]/plasma [creatinine]}) \times (\text{Urine output [ml]/Time [min]})}{\text{Body weight (kg)}}$$

Box 13.3. Equation for calculation of fractional excretion of an electrolyte (*x*)

$$\text{Fractional excretion of an electrolyte, } x = \left\{\frac{\text{Plasma [creatinine]} \times \text{Urine } [x]}{\text{Urine [creatinine]} \times \text{Plasma } [x]}\right\} \times 100$$

Table 13.1. Normal fractional excretion of electrolytes in the mature and neonatal horse

Electrolyte	Fractional excretion in adults (%)	Fractional excretion in foals (%)
Sodium	0.0002–0.87[74,90,96]	0.31 ± 1.8[71]
Potassium	1–75.1[74,90,96]	13.26 ± 4.49[71]
Chloride	0.012–3.47[74,90,96]	0.42 ± 0.32[71]
Phosphorus	0.023–5.53[74,90,97,98]	3.11 ± 3.81[71]
Calcium	–0.158–6.723[96,97]	2.85 ± 3.26[71]
Magnesium	20.8–43.1[99,100]	—

Box 13.4. Equation for calculation of urinary γGT : creatinine ratio

$$\text{Urinary } \gamma\text{GT : creatinine} = \left\{\frac{\text{Urinary } \gamma\text{GT}}{\text{Urinary creatinine}}\right\} \times 0.01$$

Note: Creatinine must be in mg/dl for comparison with normal values.
The value in μmol/L is converted to mg/dl by dividing by 88.4.

in NAD excretion in the human field,[106] and this technique may gain popularity in the horse. At the present time, the most widely available urinary enzyme assay is γGT, which is commonly used in the clinical setting. The activity is usually expressed as a ratio of γGT to urinary creatinine (to account for the concentration or dilution of the urine), and is calculated following collection of a urine sample. The calculation is given in Box 13.4.

The normal γGT-to-creatinine ratio is less than 25 IU/g Cr in the adult horse[103–105,107] and 8.2 ± 5.7 IU/g Cr in the normal foal.[71] This ratio assumes a measurement of creatinine in mg/dl. In order to convert the creatinine from SI units (μmol/L), and thus use these reference ranges, the creatinine value in μmol/L should be divided by 88.4. The γGT-to-creatinine ratio may be increased in renal proximal tubular disease and renal azotaemia, and mildly increased with dehydration where renal blood flow is decreased. Monitoring the γGT-to-creatinine ratio may be useful in animals at risk of developing acute renal failure with gentamicin (or other potentially nephrotoxic drug) administration, as an increase in the ratio may represent early renal tubular damage. This information allows the clinician to make an informed decision to increase the dosing interval or cease administration of the nephrotoxic drug.

Measurement of renal blood flow

Renal blood flow measurements are expensive and time consuming and require multiple samples. They are therefore rarely measured in the clinical setting. However, they may be more useful than creatinine clearance as they measure the actual renal blood flow, as opposed to GFR, which only estimates the volume of plasma filtered per unit time. The clearance of *para*-aminohippuric acid (PAH) is used as a measure of renal blood flow. The PAH clearance measures the effective renal plasma flow and is approximately 85% to 90% of the total renal plasma flow.[78] This technique has been used in the adult horse[82,83,85,108] and the foal.[80,87] Other techniques have been described in the horse, including the clearance of radionuclides[85,109,110] and microsphere injections.[111–113] Renal blood flow has also been measured by Doppler blood flow, which can detect a change in flow rather than an absolute measurement.[114]

Renal ultrasound

Renal ultrasound is a simple procedure to perform and is well established as a useful diagnostic tool in the human intensive care unit.[115] In humans with unexplained renal failure, 50% of ultrasonographic examinations revealed some renal abnormality, and a definitive diagnosis of the cause was discovered in 25% of patients.[116,117] Changes in the size, shape, echogenicity and architecture of the kidneys can be detected on ultrasonographic examination and may provide valuable information as to the cause of the renal insufficiency and the prognosis for the horse with renal disease.[118–120]

Image acquisition

The kidneys are usually imaged transcutaneously. In the adult horse, the right kidney may be imaged with a 3- or 5-MHz probe, and the left with a 2.5- to 3-MHz probe.[121,122] Both kidneys are imaged with a 5-MHz probe in the foal.[122] Ideally, a sector or curvilinear probe should be used, as it enables a small transducer/patient contact area with a wide field of view, so a more complete examination can be performed than with a straight linear array probe.[120] Clipping of the hair in the region of the scan should be performed to gain better images, but if this is not possible reasonable images can usually be obtained if a large amount of surgical spirit is applied to the area. The right kidney can be found ventral to the transverse processes in the 16th intercostal space, at the level of the tuber coxae, closely apposed to the abdominal wall.[118–120,123,124] The left kidney is more caudally located, and is found in the paralumbar fossa to the 17th intercostal space, medial to the spleen.[118–120,123,124] The left kidney is imaged using the spleen as an acoustic window and usually requires a 20-cm field of view compared to the 15-cm field used for the right kidney.[120] The deeper location and attenuation of the ultrasound beam by the spleen lead to less anatomical detail of the left kidney compared to the right.[125]

Gas-filled bowel may obstruct the view of the kidney. Transrectal ultrasonography of the left kidney with a linear array 5- to 7.5-MHz probe can easily be performed in the majority of horses.[120] This technique provides far greater detail than transabdominal imaging. Placing the probe into a glove filled with ultrasound gel prior to rectal examination will aid evaluation.[122] However, transrectal ultrasonography of the right kidney is not normally possible due to its more cranial location. If gas-filled bowel is obstructing the view of the right kidney, imaging should be repeated at a later time.

The normal kidney

The normal right kidney is heart shaped or triangular, with a prominent hilar notch.[124] In the adult Thoroughbred, it is 15 to 18 cm wide, 13 to 15 cm long and 5 cm thick[124] (Figure 13.1). The normal left kidney is longer and narrower than the right kidney and is normally bean-shaped[125] (Figure 13.2). It is 11 to 15 cm wide, 15 to 18 cm long and

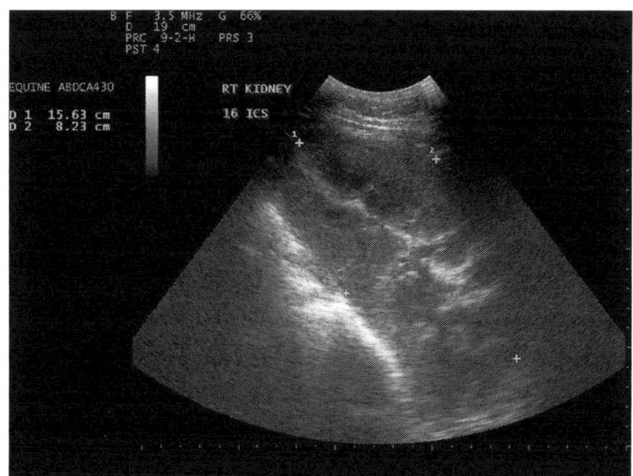

Figure 13.1 Transabdominal ultrasonographic image of a normal right kidney. This image was made with a 3.5-Mhz probe through the right 16th intercostal space, with the field set to a depth of 19 cm. © Anna Hollis 2007.

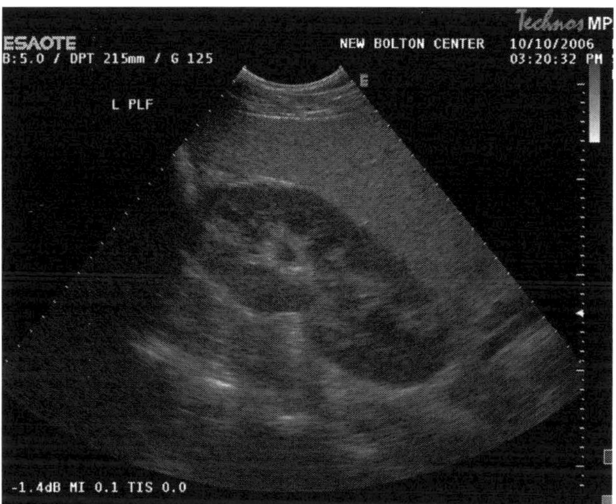

Figure 13.2 Transabdominal ultrasonographic image of a normal left kidney in a weanling. This image was made with a 5-Mhz probe just caudal to the left 18th rib (in the paralumbar fossa), with the field set to a depth of 21.5 cm. © Anna Hollis 2007.

5 to 6 cm thick.[125] The normal kidneys of the neonatal foal are found in the same location as in the adult. The sizes have been reported as 6.7 to 10.4 cm wide by 8.8 to 10.3 cm long in the normal, neonatal Thoroughbred foal.[126]

The renal capsule is not distinct on these images,[124] although the surface of the kidneys should appear smooth.[120] The cortex and medulla of the equine kidney are normally distinct.[125] The cortex is hypoechoic compared to the surrounding tissues, with a homogeneous, slightly mottled appearance, and is 1 to 2 cm thick.[118,120] The medulla is less echogenic than the cortex.[118–120,124] At the cranial and caudal extremities, the cortex and medulla are more echogenic due to acoustic anisotropy.[124] The normal renal pelvis is very echogenic due to fibrous tissue and intrapelvic fat[125] and appears as a homogeneous rim.[123]

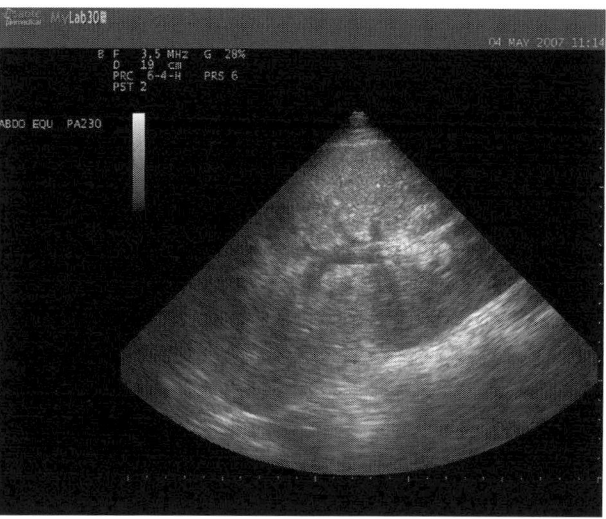

Figure 13.3 Transabdominal ultrasonographic image of a right kidney from a 19-year-old "Teaser" with chronic renal failure showing general increased echogenicity, and loss of distinction between the cortex and medulla. This image was made with a 3.5-Mhz probe through the right 16th intercostal space, with the field set to a depth of 19 cm. © Kevin Corley 2007.

It contains connective tissue that may cast a small shadow that allows imaging of deeper structures.[123] The proximal portion of the right ureter may be visible as an echogenic structure,[125] but the left ureter is not normally visible.[120,125]

The abnormal kidney

Echogenicity

Normal renal echogenicity does not preclude the presence of renal disease, and kidneys of normal echogenicity have been reported in horses with acute renal failure.[118,120] Poor echogenic distinction between the cortex and medulla is usually associated with chronic renal failure[120,123] (Figure 13.3).

An increase in renal echogenicity is a common finding in horses with renal insufficiency.[125] Traditionally, it is stated that the normal kidney is less echogenic than the normal liver. However, in 72% of humans, the echogenicity of the kidney was equal to that of the liver in patients with no evidence of renal disease.[127] A diagnosis of hyperechogenicity where the kidney and liver are equally echogenic should thus be made with caution. Hyperechogenicity may suggest a cellular infiltrate into the renal parenchyma,[128] fibrosis[123] or amyloidosis[129] and is often associated with chronic renal failure,[123] and thus a worse prognosis. Renal tubular damage may result in an increase in renal parenchymal echogenicity.[125]

Renal papillary necrosis may be seen as an elliptical, echogenic focus with acoustic shadowing[130] or as echogenic debris in the renal pelvis with hyperechogenic renal papillae.[125] This has been associated with the administration of phenylbutazone in the horse.[37,38,125,131] An echogenic line in the outer renal medulla that is parallel to the corticomedullary junction is known as the medullary rim

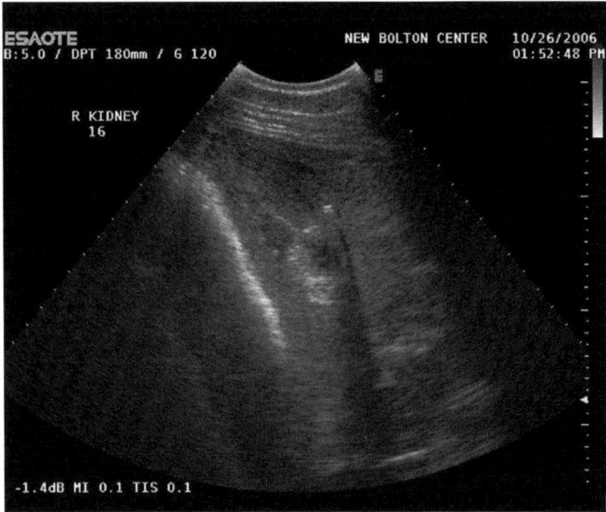

Figure 13.4 Transabdominal ultrasonographic image of a right kidney from a horse with chronic renal failure; small hyperechoic structures in the medulla casting echogenic shadows. This image was made with a 5-Mhz probe through the right 16th intercostal space, with the field set to a depth of 18 cm. © Anna Hollis 2007.

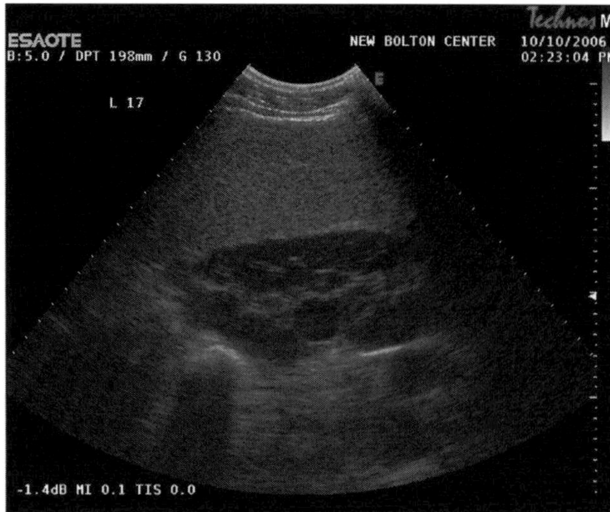

Figure 13.5 Transabdominal ultrasonographic image of a hypoechoic renal cyst in the left kidney. This is unlikely to be of clinical significance. This image was made with a 5-Mhz probe through the left 17th intercostal space, with the field set to a depth of 19.8 cm. © Anna Hollis 2007.

sign.[132] This may indicate primary renal disease but is a nonspecific indicator and gives no prognostic information.[132] In dogs, the medullary rim sign has been found in patients with no apparent renal dysfunction.[133] Its presence should therefore be interpreted with caution, although it has been reported in the horse following phenylbutazone toxicity.[36]

An accumulation of echoic to hyperechoic debris in the renal pelvis, which may cast an acoustic shadow, is associated with pyelonephritis.[125] Focal glomerulosclerosis-like disease may produce hyperechogenicity, and has been reported with nephrotic syndrome in the horse.[134]

Mineralised areas may be seen with chronic renal disease[123] and are seen as bright reflections with acoustic shadows[135] (Figure 13.4). Renal calculi will cast a bright, complete acoustic shadow deep to the area.[123,135] The most mineralised calculi will have an acoustic shadow that originates at the near surface of the calculus, whereas more proteinaceous calculi will have shadows originating on the deeper side.[125] Renal calculi have been found incidentally on post mortem examination[136] and in horses with no evidence of renal impairment[125] but are usually associated with renal disease.[137–139]

Hypoechogenicity is consistent with a diagnosis of renal oedema.[125] Hydronephrosis is seen as an enlarged, hypoechoic centre to the kidney and is associated with chronic renal disease[123] and with nephrolithiasis and ureterolithiasis.[120,128,139] Dilation of the renal pelvis and a thin cortex are other features of hydronephrosis.[125] Where hydronephrosis is suspected, images of the ureters should be sought. Transrectal ultrasonography with a 7.5-MHz probe will provide good images of both ureters[120] and may reveal the presence of ureterolithiasis and/or hydroureter.[125]

Cystic structures may be associated with disease or may be a congenital abnormality.[125] A single, circumscribed renal cyst may be an incidental finding[118,123] (Figure 13.5), whereas multiple cysts have been associated with renal dysfunction in the horse.[140,141] Renal and perirenal abscesses are uncommon in the horse and will appear as a hypoechoic to echogenic, fluid-filled cavity.[125] Renal or perirenal haematomas will appear as echoic structures and may be seen following renal biopsy or abdominal trauma.[125] Focal abnormalities in echogenicity may also be detected, but histopathological correlation with the ultrasonographic appearance is not fully established[125]; thus, their significance is uncertain.

Size

Kidney size is an important factor in clinical assessment and may help to differentiate acute and chronic renal insufficiency.[115] The kidney size is usually normal in patients with prerenal causes of renal insufficiency but may increase in the acute stages of primary renal disease.[120,142] Bilateral renal enlargement has been reported in horses with acute renal failure[11] (Figures 13.6 and 13.7). A differential diagnosis for renal enlargement in the horse is renal neoplasia.[120,143–149] Enlarged kidneys may also be seen with obstructive nephrolithiasis.[125]

Small kidneys are usually associated with chronic renal failure in the horse[120,123,150] and may also be seen with obstructive nephrolithiasis and ureterolithiasis.[151] Congenital, bilateral renal hypoplasia has been reported in the horse and is associated with clinical signs of renal dysfunction.[152] A small kidney with a thin cortex usually indicates irreversible damage.[153] Horses with acute renal failure may have enlarged renal cortices.[120]

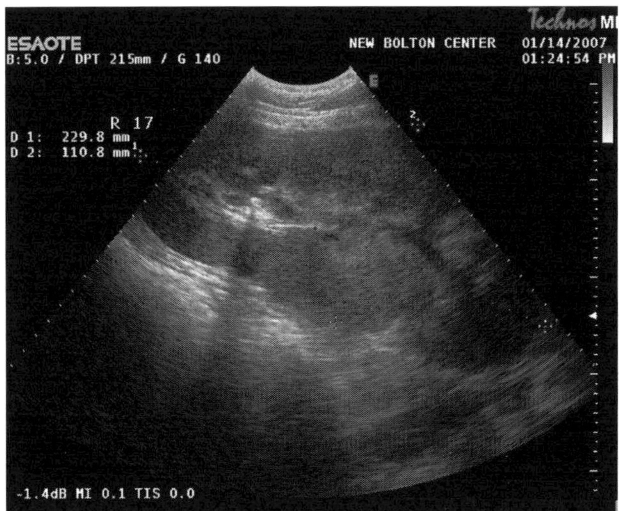

Figure 13.6 Acute renal failure; transabdominal ultrasonographic image of an enlarged right kidney. This image was made with a 5-Mhz probe through the right 17th intercostal space, with the field set to a depth of 21.5 cm. © Anna Hollis 2007.

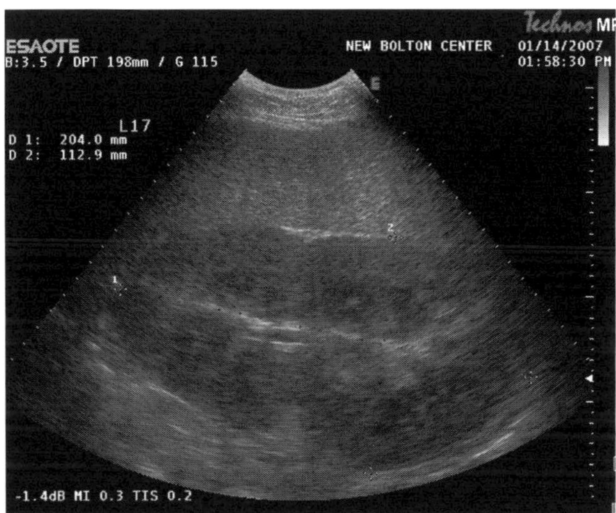

Figure 13.7 Acute renal failure; transabdominal ultrasonographic image of an enlarged left kidney, measuring 20.4 cm in length, and 11.3 cm in width. This image was made with a 3.5-Mhz probe through the left 17th intercostal space, with the field set to a depth of 19.8 cm. © Anna Hollis 2007.

Other abnormalities

Perirenal oedema may be detected in some horses with oliguric or anuric renal failure.[60,120] This has been described as a hypoechoic, homogeneous band running outside the periphery of the renal cortex.[60] Perirenal oedema has also been seen with renal rupture,[125] which has been reported with a renal calculus,[136] and with retroperitoneal rupture of the ureter.[125]

The kidneys may have an irregular shape with chronic renal disease from any cause, including due to nephrolithiasis,[151,154] and with congenital abnormalities such as renal hypoplasia.

Renal biopsy

Where abnormalities have been detected on ultrasonographic examination of the kidneys, renal biopsy can be an invaluable tool for definitive diagnosis of the disease process and can provide important prognostic information.[123] However, renal biopsy is not generally necessary in the evaluation and treatment of patients with acute renal failure where prerenal causes are suspected. Where bilateral renal disease is suspected, it is preferable, for practical reasons, to perform biopsies of the right kidney. However, penetration of the spleen to gain access to the left kidney does not appear to be associated with major complications.[155] Renal biopsy is described in Chapter 1.46.

Ultrasound of the bladder

Ultrasonography of the bladder is best performed per rectum with a linear array 5- to 7.5-MHz probe in the adult horse and may be performed transcutaneously in the foal. The bladder size, contents and wall integrity can be imaged, and any cystic calculi will be identified as hyperechoic structures that cast a complete acoustic shadow.[123] An amorphous echogenic area at the bottom of the bladder is usually associated with sludging of calcium carbonated crystals, which may be secondary to bladder atony.[123]

Endoscopy of the urinary tract

Endoscopy of the bladder is described in Chapter 1.43. Indications for urinary tract endoscopy include clinical findings of haematuria and suspected neoplasia or infection/inflammation of the kidneys, bladder or urethra.[123] The endoscope should be disinfected prior to use to avoid the risk of introducing infection. The endoscope is introduced into the urethra in the same way as a urinary catheter. The urethra and bladder can be visualised, as well as the ureters where they enter the bladder. The mucosa should be pale and salmon-pink and becomes reddened with cystitis or urethritis. Large calculi are normally readily visualised.

Urine samples can be collected from each individual ureter as described in Chapter 1.43. Urine is produced in pulses and can be collected by applying gentle suction to the tubing with a syringe. Urine production from each kidney can be subjectively assessed by watching the ureters; however, normal values of the number of pulses per minute are not established.

Investigating the male and female genital tract

Female

Careful examination of the external genitalia should be undertaken in the mare postpartum and in any animal in which genital disease is suspected. This should include conformation of the external vulva, especially in relation to the anus.

A manual vaginal and cervical examination should be performed, which will allow detection of any damage and any cervical abnormalities. A full examination should include palpation per rectum and transrectal ultrasonography. The introduction of a speculum will allow direct visualisation of the cervix and vagina and should be combined with digital palpation of these areas to allow identification of trauma or other abnormalities. With the exception of ultrasonography and palpation per rectum, the vulva should be thoroughly cleansed with a dilute povidone-iodine or chlorhexidine solution, the tail bandaged or placed in a rectal sleeve and the possibility of pregnancy ruled out prior to any diagnostic techniques.

Ultrasonography of the female genital tract
A linear, B-mode, 5- to 7.5-MHz ultrasound probe will allow imaging of the ovaries, uterine horns, uterine body and the cervix per rectum.[123] Scanning should be systematically performed to examine all areas of the reproductive tract. Abnormalities of the uterus that may be detected are cysts, debris such as retained placentae or foetal remains and intraluminal air or fluid. The ovaries should be evaluated for size and shape and should be of approximately the same size. The normal ovary is bean-shaped. During anoestrus both ovaries are small, and during dioestrus and pregnancy both are large. The presence of one large and one small ovary is abnormal and warrants further investigation. Ovaries greater than 10 cm in diameter are generally considered abnormal.

Endoscopy of the female genital tract
This may be performed with a disinfected endoscope. It is possible to visualise the vagina, external cervical os, the uterine body and horns to the uterotubeal junctions. This is most easily performed during dioestrus.[123] Following introduction of the endoscope, the uterus should be distended with air or saline.[123] The uterus can be evaluated for the presence of inflammation, fluid and debris. This can provide useful information aiding diagnosis and can be used to gain samples for cytology and culture.[156–162]

Uterine swab
Ideally, samples should be collected during oestrus. There are several commercially available designs of uterine swabs‡, and the exact technique varies slightly between designs, although the principles are the same. The swab should be introduced in a sterile manner into the cervix before the inner sleeve is pushed through the outer sleeve and advanced into the uterus. Once contact with the endometrium is achieved, the swab should be held still for 15 to 30 seconds to absorb uterine secretions. Rotation of the swab through 360° for 30 to 60 seconds will aid collection of cells suitable for cytology.[163] Following removal of the swab, the cells can be transferred onto a sterile slide for microscopic examination, and the swab submitted for culture. If sterile slides are not available, two swabs should be obtained—one for culture and one for cytology. Cytology slides should be stained for analysis§.[163]

It is not advisable to use a vaginal speculum for this procedure, as contamination of the sample may occur and culture results are difficult to interpret.[164] Culture is useful to determine the aetiology of genital infections,[165,166] although it may be preferable to culture endometrial biopsy samples.[167]

Endometrial biopsy
Endometrial biopsies may be part of breeding soundness examination and allow more detailed cytology to be performed. The technique is described in Chapter 1.44. The biopsy is usually taken from the base of a uterine horn, and for breeding purposes, one biopsy is usually considered representative of the whole uterus. If a particular area is of interest, the biopsy can be performed concurrent with ultrasonographic examination per rectum, which requires two operators. Alongside cytology, these biopsies should be cultured to maximise the information gained.[167]

Uterine lavage
Lavaging the uterus may be performed to obtain cellular material or as a technique to aid cleansing the uterus by removing fluid, pus and debris. The technique is described in Chapter 1.45.

Evaluating endometrial cytology
Endometrial cells can be stained with Diff-Quick and evaluated under both low (×40) and high (×400 and ×1000 with oil) power. The cells present include endometrial cells, neutrophils, monocytes, erythrocytes and squames.[163] A minimum of 100 cells should be counted under high-power magnification with oil (×1000).[163] There are various criteria that have been used to define the presence of inflammation. These include the presence of more than 2 inflammatory cells per high-power field, more than 1 neutrophil per high-power field, a ratio of endometrial to inflammatory cells less than 40:1 and the presence of greater than 5% neutrophils.[163,168–171] If the sample has low total cellularity, the endometrial cell population may not be accurately reflected and such results should be interpreted with care.

Bacteria are evaluated based on the number per high-power field with oil. A scoring system has been identified according to severity, which involves evaluating the number of bacteria per 30 high-power fields.[163] Any bacteria can be further evaluated by the preparation of a second slide with Gram's stain. Gram-negative cocci are likely to be

‡Guarded Culture Instrument; Kalayjian Industries Inc, Long Beach, CA, USA.

§Diff-Quik; Baxter, Deerfield, IL, USA.

contaminants, whereas rods and coccobacilli may be pathogenic organisms.[163]

Male

The majority of the male genitalia can be examined externally. The scrotum, testicles and spermatic cord should be examined and be symmetrical in size and consistency. Careful palpation of the scrotum should be undertaken in any stallion demonstrating signs of colic to rule out inguinal/scrotal herniation. The testicle and epididymis are normally palpable and their size, symmetry and consistency can be determined. The testicle should be 8 to 12 cm long × 5 cm wide in the Thoroughbred stallion, and the total scrotal width should be at least 8 cm to pass a breeding soundness examination.[172]

Ultrasonography of the scrotum and testicles will aid examination and can be performed with a 5- to 10-MHz linear transducer.

The penis and sheath are best examined under sedation, when the majority of animals will extrude the penis, allowing full assessment. The penis should be evaluated manually and visibly, inspecting the urethral process, glans, and shaft and moving on to examine the prepuce for any lesions.

13.2 Treating the urogenital system

Specific treatment for renal failure

Despite the frequency of acute renal insufficiency in the human intensive care unit, morbidity and mortality remain high.[1–4,173] Evidence for the efficacy of commonly recommended therapies is variable, and the mainstay of therapy remains supportive care. The management priorities for patients with acute renal failure are given in Box 13.5.[174]

Correct underlying conditions, prerenal and/or postrenal factors

Treating underlying conditions and the cause of acute renal failure, for example, by reversing hypovolaemia and treating sepsis or endotoxaemia, will prevent further damage to the kidney. Where postrenal factors are contributing, stabilisation of the acute electrolyte and fluid derangements must take place prior to correction of the cause (e.g., surgery for a ruptured bladder).

Avoid administration of nephrotoxins

Combinations of nephrotoxic drugs (e.g., nonsteroidal anti-inflammatory drugs [NSAIDs] with aminoglycoside antibiotics) should be avoided in animals with acute renal failure. Alternatives should be sought where possible, such as the use of opioids for analgesia rather than NSAIDs, and a change in antibiotic therapy. The risk of nephrotoxicity following aminoglycoside administration can be reduced by monitoring the serum peak and trough concentrations, in order to optimise the dosing interval (see Chapter 6.3).

Treat acute complications

Acute complications of acute renal failure are usually treated symptomatically. The most common potential complications are summarised in Table 13.2.

Optimising cardiac output and renal blood flow, restore and/or increase urine output

At low mean arterial pressure, renal vasoconstriction may occur,[175,176] which will reduce renal blood flow. The mainstay of improving cardiac output and renal blood flow is providing appropriate fluid therapy. There is limited evidence as to the effectiveness of pharmacological methods of improving renal blood flow and cardiac output in acute renal failure.

Dobutamine

Dobutamine is a β_1-adrenergic agonist with weak β_2- and α-adrenergic affinity and thus acts predominantly as a positive inotrope.[177] In patients where blood pressure is low despite appropriate fluid resuscitation, dobutamine

Box 13.5. Management priorities for patients with acute renal failure

- Correct underlying conditions, prerenal and/or postrenal factors.
- Avoid/stop administration of nephrotoxins.
- Treat acute complications.
- Optimise cardiac output and renal blood flow.
- Restore and/or increase urine output.
- Monitor fluid input and output.
- Provide early nutritional support.

Table 13.2. Complications of acute renal failure

Metabolic	Cardiovascular	Neurological	Gastrointestinal	Haematological	Infectious
Hyperkalaemia	Dysrythmias	Somnolence	Ileus	Anaemia	Urinary tract infections
Acidosis		Seizures	Anorexia	Platelet dysfunction	
				Factor VII dysfunction	

may be a valuable addition to the treatment protocol, improving cardiac output and blood pressure.

In addition, with its β_2 activity, dobutamine may dilate the microcirculation, which may improve renal blood flow. Dobutamine may be given at a dose rate of 1 to 20 µg/kg/min, with the starting rate recommended as 2 to 5 µg/kg/min.[177] Potential side effects of dobutamine include tachycardia, which is usually associated with hypovolaemia, and dysrhythmias, usually seen at doses of 10 µg/kg/min and above, so the patient must be closely monitored.[178]

Loop diuretics

Loop diuretics have a number of properties that make them potentially useful in the treatment of acute renal failure. Loop diuretics induce cyclooxygenases, leading to prostaglandin release and vasodilation, increasing renal blood flow.[179–181] The diuresis may increase distal tubular flow and thus pressure, dislodging any material obstructing the tubules, and may cause an increase in glomerular filtration rate due to tubuloglomerular feedback.[182] In addition to these effects, the reduction in active sodium transport in the medullary tubules reduces oxygen demand by the kidney, reducing the potential for ischaemic damage.[183,184]

There has been controversy regarding the use of diuretics in acute renal failure, as studies have shown variable effects on renal function. Some studies suggest that diuretics may increase mortality in acute renal failure, and converting oliguric renal failure to nonoliguric renal failure does not appear to alter the course of the disease.[185–194] However, a large, multicentre, multinational study showed no increase in mortality associated with the use of diuretics in acute renal failure.[195] Although there are no randomised, controlled trials of diuretics in acute renal failure, loop diuretics such as furosemide (frusemide) reduce the severity of acute renal failure in experimental animal models.[181,182,196–199] They may therefore be useful in the treatment of acute renal failure in the horse. Furosemide is usually given intravenously for the treatment of acute renal failure in the horse, at intravenous dose rates of 0.5 to 2 mg/kg every 4 to 8 hours or as a constant rate infusion of 0.5 to 4.2 µg/kg/min. Oral bioavailability is poor, erratic and variable in the horse.[200]

Osmotic diuretics

Mannitol is an osmotic diuretic that may increase urine output. It is thought that mannitol increases renal blood flow by releasing intrarenal vasodilating prostaglandins and atrial natriuretic peptides.[201] However, the osmotic effects may increase renal oxygen demand, which is potentially deleterious by increasing the risk of further ischaemic injury to the kidney. There are no studies demonstrating a beneficial effect of mannitol in acute renal failure in excess of the effect of fluid loading, and some studies show detrimental effects, thus mannitol is not recommended.[202,203]

Dopamine

Dopamine was traditionally used as a vasopressor that was thought to improve renal blood flow at a low, or "renal", dose rate. Recent evidence suggests that dopamine actually worsens renal blood flow in acute renal failure.[204] This, combined with its lack of proven efficacy and potentially deleterious side effects, means that dopamine is no longer recommended to prevent or treat acute renal failure.[189,204–210]

Fenoldopam mesylate

Unlike dopamine, fenoldopam is a selective dopamine-1 receptor agonist, and thus preferentially vasodilates the renal, mesenteric, coronary and cerebral vasculature. It has a rapid onset of action and a short half-life and is administered as a constant rate infusion. A low dose of fenoldopam increases renal blood flow in normotensive humans and dogs, without affecting systemic haemodynamics.[211–213] Results of early clinical trials suggest that fenoldopam may have a place in the prevention and treatment of acute renal failure.[214,215]

In normotensive foals, a low dose (0.04 µg/kg/min) of fenoldopam increased urine output without affecting systemic haemodynamics.[216] Fenoldopam at 0.04 µg/kg/min has been used in a small number foals showing signs of acute renal failure.[5] At the present time, fenoldopam is financially viable for use in foals but cost prohibitive in adult horses.

Potential therapies for the future

Several promising new therapies are currently undergoing evaluation in human medicine and may have some future role in the treatment of horses. These include atrial natriuretic peptide,[217,218] calcium channel blockers (e.g., diltiazem),[219,220] antioxidants (e.g., acetylcysteine)[221,222] and prostaglandins (e.g., prostacylcin).[223,224]

A potentially exciting therapy for the future is the use of stem and endothelial progenitor cells,[225–232] although there is a long way to go before this could be considered as a therapy for acute renal failure in human or equine patients. It is also important to remember that some therapies may be detrimental and this may not be discovered until large-scale clinical trials are performed. Thyroxine has been reported to promote protection and recovery from acute renal failure in animals, but increased mortality in humans with acute renal failure when a double-blind, prospective, placebo-controlled study was carried out.[233–238]

Other treatment options

Renal replacement therapy is commonly used in the human field. Haemodialysis is not widely available for use in the horse, although it has been used in the foal.[39] However, peritoneal dialysis is a simple and practical alternative that can be performed. Peritoneal dialysis involves infusing an isotonic electrolyte solution with dextrose into the abdominal cavity. The solution reaches equilibrium with the plasma by osmosis across the peritoneal membrane. Draining this solution thus leads to clearance of abnormal concentrations of solutes from the body. Although small molecules and water pass rapidly through the membrane, larger molecules such as creatinine will take longer to diffuse across.[239] Peritoneal dialysis is widely used in the treatment of acute renal failure in human medicine as it is safe, simple and effective.[240–247] The technique has been described for the treatment of acute renal failure in small animals.[239,248–250] In the horse, peritoneal lavage is well described for the treatment of peritonitis and the prevention of intra-abdominal adhesions[251–256] but has been less commonly reported for the treatment of acute renal failure. However, intermittent and continuous peritoneal dialysis have been used for acute renal failure in the horse, with the intermittent technique described in the foal[257] and continuous flow in the adult horse.[14] Intermittent peritoneal dialysis is probably more practical. In the foal, a specially designed peritoneal lavage catheter may be placed, but in the adult horse, temporary placement of a thoracic drainage tube (e.g., a 32Fr thoracic drain) into the ventral abdomen is a practical alternative that can be introduced in the same manner as a tube for peritoneal lavage (see Chapter 1.9). A large volume (10–15 L for a 500-kg horse) of warm, isotonic fluids is introduced via an infusion pump (e.g., an arthroscopic irrigation pump) or by gravity flow, and the drain clamped or removed. The horse should be walked around to aid contact of the infused fluid with the peritoneum. After a minimum of 30 minutes, and preferably 2 to 3 hours, the fluid can be removed by replacing or unclamping the drain, and allowing the fluid to drain by gravity. In the foal, repeating peritoneal dialysis 9 times over a 36-hour period returned all its electrolyte abnormalities to within the normal range.[257] Continuous flow peritoneal dialysis is described briefly:[14] A 28Fr indwelling thoracic tube can be placed into the ventral abdomen, and a T-fluted catheter placed in the left flank. A standard diasylate solution (1.5% glucose in isotonic fluid) is continuously infused at a rate of 3 L/hr, and fluid collected from the ventral abdomen into a closed collection system. This technique was reportedly well tolerated, and more effective than intermittent dialysis in the patient, with creatinine concentrations almost halving in 72 hours.[14] Both techniques carry a risk of causing peritonitis,[242] so absolute sterility must be maintained during the procedure. Other reported complications of peritoneal dialysis in animals include hypoproteinaemia, overhydration and catheter obstruction.[248,250]

Peritoneal dialysis is generally considered useful in cases where fluid and pharmacological therapy have not been sufficient to resolve the azotaemia associated with acute renal failure. It may also be useful in cases where hyperkalaemia is not responsive to the therapies discussed below.

Early nutritional support

In humans with acute renal failure, nutritional support is considered an important part of the treatment protocol.[174] The nutritional requirements of these patients are high, and a hypercatabolic state is common.[174] This is likely to be true for the equine patient, so enteral (where appropriate) or parenteral nutrition should be instituted in all patients with acute renal insufficiency or failure. In addition to nutritional support, there is evidence to suggest that hyperglycaemia in the critically ill is detrimental and that tight control of blood glucose with the administration of insulin reduces mortality and morbidity in such patients.[258–263] Intensive insulin therapy has been shown to reduce the incidence of acute renal failure requiring dialysis in mechanically ventilated human patients,[264] suggesting that it may have a role in the prevention and/or treatment of acute renal failure. Close control of blood glucose by the use of constant rate infusions of insulin to effect should thus be considered.

Special considerations for fluid therapy

Fluid therapy is the cornerstone of resuscitation of critically ill patients.[265,266] The kidneys play a critical role in fluid haemostasis, and renal dysfunction leads to disturbances in these mechanisms.[266] Patients with renal dysfunction require special attention to issues of fluid balance and fluid overload.[266] The major goal of fluid therapy in acute renal failure is to achieve and maintain normal effective circulating volume.[267]

Patients with acute renal failure with intravascular volume depletion require prompt and carefully monitored fluid resuscitation.[267] In order to achieve this, any horse with suspected acute renal failure should have its urine output monitored to determine if there is anuric, oliguric or polyuric renal failure. Fluid replacement must be carefully monitored in animals with anuric or oliguric renal failure, as overhydration is a risk. Although pulmonary oedema is unusual in the horse with normal renal function, it may occur with overzealous fluid therapy in those with renal insufficiency. Close monitoring of the fluid input versus the fluid output is thus necessary. Where polyuric renal failure is seen, care must be taken to ensure adequate fluid rates to avoid the development of hypovolaemia, which will further compromise renal function.

Where sophisticated monitoring techniques are not available, alongside a full physical examination, monitoring the packed cell volume, total solids and serum lactate concentration will help assess the patient's hydration status. The patient should also be weighed daily. Further assessment includes monitoring skin turgor and checking for the development of peripheral oedema. Once normal intravascular volume is achieved, its maintenance depends on balancing fluid intake and fluid losses.[267] This can be usefully monitored by estimating the urine output, preferably by the maintenance of a closed urine collection system, and measuring the fluid intake.

Central venous pressure (CVP) gives an indication of right ventricular preload. Preload may increase with fluid overload, and decrease with hypovolaemia. Thus measuring CVP can be extremely useful in balancing fluid requirements in renal failure. The technique for measuring central venous pressure is described in Chapter 1.23. Central venous pressure is normally between 8 and 10 cm H_2O in the adult horse. Where central venous pressure is equal to or greater than 8 to 10 cm H_2O, measures other than fluid therapy should be considered to improve renal perfusion and urine output in the oliguric or anuric patient.

Where the technology is available, cardiac output monitoring will give a more thorough evaluation of the patient's haemodynamic status. Cardiac output determination by lithium dilution has been described and validated in the adult and neonatal foal, and cardiac output by pulse contour analysis has been validated in the adult equine.[268–270] Cardiac output determination by lithium dilution has been reported in the conscious foal[216] and used in the clinic with conscious adult horses. Briefly, a bolus of a known amount of lithium chloride is given into a central vein and blood withdrawn from a peripheral artery at a constant rate (via a peristaltic pump), past a lithium-specific sensor. A computer calculates the lithium time-concentration curve, and from this the cardiac output, stroke volume and systemic vascular resistance are determined (Chapter 1.26). The cardiac output and stroke volume give information about hydration status in the patient. In addition, the systemic vascular resistance provides some idea of perfusion. If the systemic vascular resistance is very low, organ perfusion (including renal perfusion) will be poor, and administration of a vasopressor (such as norepinephrine) may be appropriate.

Electrolytes and acid-base balance

Horses with renal failure often show acid-base derangements, the most common of which are hyperchloraemic and mixed metabolic acidoses.[11] As the administration of 0.9% sodium chloride induces a hyperchloraemic acidosis in normal ponies,[271] this fluid seems a poor choice for animals in renal failure, in which hyperchloraemic acidosis may be a feature.

Sodium regulation is frequently poor in acute renal failure, with both hyponatraemia and hypernatraemia being recognised. If the changes in sodium concentration are subclinical, isotonic electrolyte solutions are likely to be the most appropriate choice for fluid therapy.

Hyperkalaemia is a potentially life-threatening consequence of acute renal failure, and thus serum potassium should be closely monitored. The effects of hyperkalaemia on the cardiac conduction pathways are exacerbated by hypocalcaemia and hypomagnesaemia, both of which are common in acute renal failure.[242,244] If hyperkalaemia becomes apparent, supplementation and the use of potassium-containing fluids should cease.[240] If the hyperkalaemia is symptomatic or over 7 mmol/L, specific treatment should commence. Treatment involves administration of 40% calcium gluconate at 0.5 ml/kg over 10 minutes. If this is unsuccessful or unavailable, 50% dextrose can be administered at 2 ml/kg IV over 5 minutes, which may be followed by a bolus of regular insulin at 0.1 IU (unit)/kg IV. If these treatments are unsuccessful, sodium bicarbonate at 1 to 2 mEq/kg IV over 15 minutes should be given. These treatments should be combined with diuresis with at least 5 ml/kg/hr Hartmann's solution, provided that the animal is not volume overloaded. Diuresis should also be given to animals with potassium above the normal range, but less than 7 mmol/L. If the animal is well hydrated, the administration of furosemide (frusemide) at 1 mg/kg IV or as a constant rate infusion of 0.5 to 4 μg/kg/min may reduce the hyperkalaemia. If these measures do not work, peritoneal dialysis should be considered.

Conversely, hypokalaemia may be seen with polyuric renal failure. Potassium should not be supplemented at rates greater than 0.5 mmol/kg/hr because of possible adverse effects on cardiac electrical activity. Careful calculation of the maximum rate of supplementation is required (including the potassium concentration of any balanced electrolyte solution administered) when high fluid rates are being administered. Oral supplementation of potassium chloride (at 0.1–0.2 g/kg) can be particularly useful in these cases.

Calcium homeostasis may be disrupted with acute renal failure, and both hypocalcaemia and hypercalcaemia have been reported in horses with acute renal failure.[11,272] Hypercalcaemia is usually seen with chronic renal failure.[273] Hypercalcaemia may be treated with diuresis and intravenous magnesium sulphate, 4 to 16 mg/kg. Hypocalcaemia is often seen with hyperphosphataemia and may be treated with 0.1 to 0.5 ml/kg 20% calcium gluconate solution over 2 to 3 hours. When treating hypocalcaemia, other disease states should be taken into account. There is experimental evidence to suggest that calcium supplementation is detrimental in endotoxaemia,[274,275] so unless hypocalcaemia is symptomatic, calcium supplementation should be avoided in patients with endotoxaemia.

Conclusions

Treatment of acute renal failure is difficult, and very few therapies have been proved to be of benefit. The priorities for management of acute renal failure should be to ensure that fluid therapy is adequate, to normalise electrolyte abnormalities and to provide nutritional support. Other therapeutic options include optimising cardiac output with dobutamine, improving urine output with fenoldopam (in foals) and/or furosemide, and considering peritoneal lavage where fluid therapy alone is not enough to reduce high creatinine, urea and potassium concentrations.

Urinary tract infections

Cystitis

Where urinary tract infections are diagnosed, culture and sensitivity of the urine should guide therapy where possible. However, antimicrobial therapy should commence prior to receiving these results. The ideal antibiotic choice is one that is excreted in high concentrations in the urine, so trimethoprim-sulphadiazine or penicillin G may be sensible choices. Traditionally, this course is a week long, but in the case of recurrent or persistent infections, prolonged therapy may be required (4–6 weeks).[276] Where fungal elements are seen or cultured, antibiotic therapy should be discontinued and antifungal therapy (e.g., fluconazole) should be considered.[276]

Cystic lavage can be an effective adjunct to the treatment of cystitis. This process is most safely performed in stocks and may require sedation. Following sterile passage of a urinary catheter into the bladder, the bladder can be lavaged with very dilute povidone-iodine solution. This can be achieved with catheter-tipped syringes or, more efficiently, a small amount of povidone-iodine can be added to a bag of isotonic fluids. This can be introduced into the bladder via a giving set and, once empty, the bag with giving set inverted to allow drainage by gravity. This can be repeated daily until the cystitis clears.

Pyelonephritis and ureteritis

Upper urinary tract infections are rare in the adult horse and uncommon in the foal. Recurrent lower urinary tract infections may be a predisposing factor for the development of upper urinary tract infections; however, the link is unproved. The treatment of pyelonephritis may prove difficult and may require prolonged antimicrobial therapy (4–6 weeks) following culture and sensitivity of the inciting organisms.[276] In the absence of culture and sensitivity results, penicillin G and trimethoprim-sulphadiazine are again logical choices. If pyelonephritis is unilateral and does not respond to antimicrobial therapy, unilateral nephrectomy with further antibiotic therapy is a potential option.

Urolithiasis

The treatment of urolithiasis depends on the location of the concretion. Urethral stones are far more common in the male horse, and one of two surgical approaches may be necessary. Passing a urethral catheter may allow retropulsion of the calculus into the bladder, from which the calculus can be surgically removed. Alternatively, an urethrostomy may be required. Urethral calculi are unusual in the female and can usually be carefully removed manually under standing sedation with epidural anaesthesia. Following a diagnosis of cystic calculi in the male horse, surgical removal from the bladder should be combined with systemic antibiotic and anti-inflammatory therapy. In the adult female, the distensible urethra means that manual removal following heavy sedation and epidural anaesthesia may be possible. This process may be aided by transrectal ultrasonographic guidance, or cystoscopy. It may also be possible to break down the calculus in the bladder either with a lithotripsy instrument or a pulse-dye laser under ultrasonographic or endoscopic guidance. Flushing or manual removal can follow this procedure. Nephrolithiasis or ureterolithiasis usually requires nephrectomy where the condition is unilateral.

Retained foetal membranes

The foetal membranes are expelled from the majority of mares within 90 minutes of parturition. If the foetal membranes are retained for longer than 3 hours, veterinary intervention is very likely to be necessary. However, there is no universal agreement on a time period after which the membranes should be considered to be retained. Retained foetal membranes have been reported to occur following 2% to 10.5% of foalings, with the incidence higher in certain breeds (e.g., draft and Friesian mares) and following dystocia, caesarean section and prolonged gestation times.[277–280] The mainstay of treatment is oxytocin. This can be administered as a slow intravenous infusion (30–100 IU in 1 L saline over 30–60 minutes) or as intravenous (10–40 IU) or intramuscular (10–120 IU) bolus injections. The oxytocin may be repeated at 0.5- to 2-hourly intervals until the foetal membranes are passed. Oxytocin administration can be associated with signs of abdominal discomfort. If this occurs, the mare should be lightly sedated to reduce the risk of rolling, which may endanger the foal.[281]

Other treatments include large-volume uterine lavage, saline distension of the chorioallantoic cavity to stimulate uterine contractions and manual removal. Manual removal is not generally advisable, as there is a risk of breaking part of the placenta off and leaving part behind, making removal even more difficult.[281] Distension of the chorioallantoic sac is performed by passing a sterile stomach tube between the membranes. Whilst holding the membranes around the tube, 10 to 15 L sterile saline is infused into the sac, and the tube removed. The ends are then tied off (e.g., with umbilical tape). This is a simple technique that may be extremely effective but is best performed when the membranes are fairly fresh. If the membranes have been retained for a long period, they are likely to tear when the fluid is infused, worsening the situation. Uterine lavage may be performed by passing a sterile stomach tube in between the wall of the uterus and the foetal membranes, and infusing 10 to 15 L sterile saline or dilute povidone-iodine solution into the uterus. This may be used in combination with uterine infusion of a broad-spectrum antibiotic, preferably povidone-based oxytetracycline.[281]

The presence of a retained placenta carries a risk of septic metritis, which frequently leads to endotoxaemia and its sequelae, most commonly laminitis. The mare with a retained placenta of greater than 6 hours duration should thus be treated with broad-spectrum antibiotics (e.g., penicillin and gentamicin), anti-inflammatory agents (e.g., flunixin meglumine) and supportive care for any complications that may result. In addition, the tetanus status of the mare should be checked, and tetanus antitoxin administered if required.[281]

Lost uterine swab

If a uterine swab breaks off in the uterus, it must be removed. Uterine lavage with large volumes (5–10 L) sterile saline may be sufficient to flush out the swab. If this is not successful, removal under endoscopic guidance is required. This can be achieved by using a biopsy instrument passed down the biopsy channel of a sterilely prepared endoscope to grasp the swab, which is then pulled out together with the endoscope.

Priapism

Priapism is persistent erection of the penis not associated with sexual arousal. The penis cannot be retracted into the prepuce, leading to discomfort and difficulty with urination.[282] In contrast to a normal erection, priapism results from selective engorgement of the corpus cavernosum penis (CCP).[282] It may be seen in stallions or geldings. Most reports of priapism in the horse are associated with administration of phenothiazine derivatives or severe debilitation.[282–290] Conservative treatment options include hydrotherapy, massage, lubrication and support in a sling. A useful sling can be made with stockings, passed around the caudal abdomen and underneath the penis.[290] A purpose-built device has also been successfully used for support.[289] It may also be helpful to attempt to place a pressure bandage to encourage venous drainage. An indwelling catheter may be required to allow urine voiding. Pharmacological therapies described include diuretics, corticosteroids, diphenhydramine, terbutaline and benztropine mesylate, which have been used with varying success.[282,287–290] If medical management is unsuccessful, more aggressive intervention should be considered. Lavage of the CCP can be achieved with placement of a 14-gauge needle into the CCP 6 cm proximal to the glans penis, attached with a fluid-giving set to heparinised, sterile intravenous fluids (such as 0.9% NaCl, with 10,000 IU heparin/L), and a further 14-gauge needle placed into the CCP, 16 cm caudal to the scrotum.[290] The fluids should be infused at a rate high enough to produce a steady stream of the partially coagulated blood in the CCP from the second needle site. This may be attempted in the standing, sedated animal or performed under general anaesthesia. This procedure may result in detumescence, in which case the penis should be replaced into the prepuce and sutured in place with umbilical tape in a purse-string pattern around the prepuce. Where medical management fails, salvage procedures have been described and successfully attempted in valuable breeding animals;[286,289,291] however, partial or total phallectomy may be warranted.[292]

Paraphimosis

Paraphimosis is the inability to retract the penis into the preputial sheath. Paraphimosis is most often seen following trauma and debilitation; however, it may be seen following priapism and with reserpine toxicosis.[290,293–296] Paraphimosis can be distinguished from priapism as it is a flaccid paralysis. Treatment involves massage, hydrotherapy, lubrication and support in a sling. If the penis can be replaced in the prepuce, it should be sutured in place with umbilical tape in a purse-string pattern around the prepuce. Placement of an indwelling urinary catheter may be required. The penis should not be removed from the prepuce until it regains normal function. Where conservative management fails, the progressive oedema and vascular compromise of the penis may eventually necessitate partial or total phallectomy.

Conclusions

Prompt recognition and treatment of urogenital abnormalities can avoid morbidity and mortality in the hospitalised equine patient.

References

1. Menashe PI, Ross SA, Gottlieb JE: Acquired renal insufficiency in critically ill patients. Crit Care Med 16:1106-1109, 1988
2. Brivet FG, Kleinknecht DJ, Loirat P, et al.: Acute renal failure in intensive care units—causes, outcome, and prognostic factors of hospital mortality; a prospective, multicenter study. French Study Group on Acute Renal Failure. Crit Care Med 24:192-198, 1996
3. Uchino S, Kellum JA, Bellomo R, et al.: Acute renal failure in critically ill patients: a multinational, multicenter study. JAMA 294:813-818, 2005
4. Nash K, Hafeez A, Hou S: Hospital-acquired renal insufficiency. Am J Kidney Dis 39:930-936, 2002
5. Corley K, Axon J, Herron C, et al.: Acute renal failure in critically-ill neonatal foals. J Vet Intern Med 19:446, 2005
6. Thadhani R, Pascual M, Bonventre JV: Acute renal failure. N Engl J Med 334:1448-1460, 1996
7. Hou SH, Bushinsky DA, Wish JB, et al.: Hospital-acquired renal insufficiency: a prospective study. Am J Med 74:243-248, 1983
8. Seanor JW, Byars TD, Boutcher JK: Renal disease associated with colic in horses. Mod Vet Pract 65:A26-29, 1984
9. Groover ES, Woolums AR, Cole DJ, et al.: Risk factors associated with renal insufficiency in horses with primary gastrointestinal disease: 26 cases (2000-2003). J Am Vet Med Assoc 228:572-577, 2006
10. Divers T, Perkins G: Urinary and hepatic disorders in neonatal foals. Clin Tech Equine Pract 2:67-78, 2003
11. Divers TJ, Whitlock RH, Byars TD, et al.: Acute renal failure in six horses resulting from haemodynamic causes. Equine Vet J 19:178-184, 1987
12. Gehr T, Schoolwerth A: Adult acute and chronic renal failure, in Textbook of Critical Care. Philadelphia, WB Saunders, 2000, pp 1648-1659
13. Schrier RW, Wang W: Acute renal failure and sepsis. N Engl J Med 351:159-169, 2004
14. Gallatin LL, Couetil LL, Ash SR: Use of continuous-flow peritoneal dialysis for the treatment of acute renal failure in an adult horse. J Am Vet Med Assoc 226:756-759, 732, 2005

15. Sprayberry KA, Madigan J, LeCouteur RA, et al.: Renal failure, laminitis, and colitis following severe rhabdomyolysis in a draft horse-cross with polysaccharide storage myopathy. Can Vet J 39:500-503, 1998
16. Andrews FM: Acute rhabdomyolysis. Vet Clin North Am Equine Pract 10:567-573, 1994
17. Perkins G, Valberg SJ, Madigan JM, et al.: Electrolyte disturbances in foals with severe rhabdomyolysis. J Vet Intern Med 12:173-177, 1998
18. Taylor P, Clarke K: Anaesthetic problems, in Handbook of Equine Anaesthesia. Philadelphia, WB Saunders, 2003, pp 95-143
19. Bernard WV: Leptospirosis. Vet Clin North Am Equine Pract 9:435-444, 1993
20. Divers TJ, Byars TD, Shin SJ: Renal dysfunction associated with infection of *Leptospira interrogans* in a horse. J Am Vet Med Assoc 201:1391-1392, 1992
21. Hogan PM, Bernard WV, Kazakevicius PA, et al.: Acute renal disease due to *Leptospira interrogans* in a weanling. Equine Vet J 28:331-333, 1996
22. Frazer ML: Acute renal failure from leptospirosis in a foal. Aust Vet J 77:499-500, 1999
23. Higuchi T, Nanao Y, Senba H: Repair of urinary bladder rupture through a urethrotomy and urethral sphincterotomy in four postpartum mares. Vet Surg 31:344-348, 2002
24. Walesby HA, Ragle CA, Booth LC: Laparoscopic repair of ruptured urinary bladder in a stallion. J Am Vet Med Assoc 221:1737-1741, 1715, 2002
25. Newton SA, Cheeseman MT, Edwards GB: Bilateral renal and ureteral calculi in a 10-year-old gelding. Vet Rec 144:383-385, 1999
26. Dunkel B, Palmer JE, Olson KN, et al.: Uroperitoneum in 32 foals: influence of intravenous fluid therapy, infection, and sepsis. J Vet Intern Med 19:889-893, 2005
27. Kablack KA, Embertson RM, Bernard WV, et al.: Uroperitoneum in the hospitalised equine neonate: retrospective study of 31 cases, 1988-1997. Equine Vet J 32:505-508, 2000
28. Riviere JE, Coppoc GL, Hinsman EJ, et al.: Species dependent gentamicin pharmacokinetics and nephrotoxicity in the young horse. Fundam Appl Toxicol 3:448-457, 1983
29. Hinchcliff KW, McGuirk SM, MacWilliams PS, et al.: Phenolsulfonphthalein pharmacokinetics and renal morphologic changes in adult pony mares with gentamicin-induced nephrotoxicosis. Am J Vet Res 50:1848-1853, 1989
30. Schumacher J, Wilson RC, Spano JS, et al.: Effect of diet on gentamicin-induced nephrotoxicosis in horses. Am J Vet Res 52:1274-1278, 1991
31. Sweeney RW, Divers TJ, Rossier Y: Disposition of gentamicin administered intravenously to horses with sepsis. J Am Vet Med Assoc 200:503-506, 1992
32. van der Harst MR, Bull S, Laffont CM, et al.: Gentamicin nephrotoxicity—a comparison of in vitro findings with in vivo experiments in equines. Vet Res Commun 29:247-261, 2005
33. Riviere JE, Traver DS, Coppoc GL: Gentamicin toxic nephropathy in horses with disseminated bacterial infection. J Am Vet Med Assoc 180:648-651, 1982
34. Baggot JD: Drug therapy in the neonatal foal. Vet Clin North Am Equine Pract 10:87-107, 1994
35. MacAllister CG, Morgan SJ, Borne AT, et al.: Comparison of adverse effects of phenylbutazone, flunixin meglumine, and ketoprofen in horses. J Am Vet Med Assoc 202:71-77, 1993
36. Ramirez S, Seahorn TL, Williams J: Renal medullary rim sign in 2 adult quarter horses. Can Vet J 39:647-649, 1998
37. Gunson DE: Renal papillary necrosis in horses. J Am Vet Med Assoc 182:263-266, 1983
38. Gunson DE, Soma LR: Renal papillary necrosis in horses after phenylbutazone and water deprivation. Vet Pathol 20:603-610, 1983
39. Vivrette S, Cowgill LD, Pascoe J, et al.: Hemodialysis for treatment of oxytetracycline-induced acute renal failure in a neonatal foal. J Am Vet Med Assoc 203:105-107, 1993
40. Barton M: Use of polymyxin B for treatment of endotoxaemia in horses. Compend Contin Educ Pract Vet 22:1056-1059, 2000
41. Morresey P, Mackay R: Endotoxin-neutralizing activity of polymyxin B in blood after IV administration in horses. Am J Vet Res 67:642-647, 2006
42. Moore RD, Smith CR, Lietman PS: Predicting aminoglycoside nephrotoxicity. JAMA 256:864-866, 1986
43. Moore RD, Smith CR, Lipsky JJ, et al.: Risk factors for nephrotoxicity in patients treated with aminoglycosides. Ann Intern Med 100:352-357, 1984
44. Shankel SW, Johnson DC, Clark PS, et al.: Acute renal failure and glomerulopathy caused by nonsteroidal anti-inflammatory drugs. Arch Intern Med 152:986-990, 1992
45. Abuelo JG: Diagnosing vascular causes of renal failure. Ann Intern Med 123:601-614, 1995
46. Hoogenberg K, Smit AJ, Girbes AR: Effects of low-dose dopamine on renal and systemic hemodynamics during incremental norepinephrine infusion in healthy volunteers. Crit Care Med 26:260-265, 1998
47. Richer M, Robert S, Lebel M: Renal hemodynamics during norepinephrine and low-dose dopamine infusions in man. Crit Care Med 24:1150-1156, 1996
48. Bellomo R, Kellum JA, Wisniewski SR, et al.: Effects of norepinephrine on the renal vasculature in normal and endotoxemic dogs. Am J Respir Crit Care Med 159:1186-1192, 1999
49. Hollis A, Ousey J, Palmer L, et al.: Effects of norepinephrine and a combined infusion of norepinephrine and dobutamine on systemic hemodynamics and indices of renal function in the normotensive neonatal thoroughbred foal. J Vet Intern Med 20:1437-1442, 2006
50. Desjars P, Pinaud M, Bugnon D, et al.: Norepinephrine therapy has no deleterious renal effects in human septic shock. Crit Care Med 17:426-429, 1989
51. Desjars P, Pinaud M, Potel G, et al.: A reappraisal of norepinephrine therapy in human septic shock. Crit Care Med 15:134-137, 1987
52. Hesselvik JF, Brodin B: Low dose norepinephrine in patients with septic shock and oliguria: effects on afterload, urine flow, and oxygen transport. Crit Care Med 17:179-180, 1989
53. Martin C, Eon B, Saux P, et al.: Renal effects of norepinephrine used to treat septic shock patients. Crit Care Med 18:282-285, 1990

54. Martin C, Papazian L, Perrin G, et al.: Norepinephrine or dopamine for the treatment of hyperdynamic septic shock? Chest 103:1826-1831, 1993
55. Corley KTT, McKenzie HC, Amoroso LM, et al.: Initial experience with norepinephrine infusion in hypotensive critically ill foals. J Vet Emerg Crit Care 10:267-276, 2000
56. Corley KTT: Monitoring and treating haemodynamic disturbances in critically ill neonatal foals. Part 2: assessment and treatment. Equine Vet Educ 14:328-336, 2002
57. Harmeyer J, Schlumbohm C: Effects of pharmacological doses of vitamin D3 on mineral balance and profiles of plasma vitamin D3 metabolites in horses. J Steroid Biochem Mol Biol 89-90:595-600, 2004
58. Harrington DD, Page EH: Acute vitamin D3 toxicosis in horses: case reports and experimental studies of the comparative toxicity of vitamins D2 and D3. J Am Vet Med Assoc 182:1358-1369, 1983
59. Krook L, Wasserman RH, Shively JN, et al.: Hypercalcemia and calcinosis in Florida horses: implication of the shrub, *Cestrum diurnum*, as the causative agent. Cornell Vet 65:26-56, 1975
60. Bayly WM, Elfers RS, Liggitt HD, et al.: A reproducible means of studying acute renal failure in the horse. Cornell Vet 76:287-298, 1986
61. Guglick MA, MacAllister CG, Chandra AM, et al.: Mercury toxicosis caused by ingestion of a blistering compound in a horse. J Am Vet Med Assoc 206:210-214, 1995
62. Markel MD, Dyer RM, Hattel AL: Acute renal failure associated with application of a mercuric blister in a horse. J Am Vet Med Assoc 185:92-94, 1984
63. Schuh JC, Ross C, Meschter C: Concurrent mercuric blister and dimethyl sulphoxide (DMSO) application as a cause of mercury toxicity in two horses. Equine Vet J 20:68-71, 1988
64. Casteel SW: Metal toxicosis in horses. Vet Clin North Am Equine Pract 17:517-527, 2001
65. Gunson DE, Kowalczyk DF, Shoop CR, et al.: Environmental zinc and cadmium pollution associated with generalized osteochondrosis, osteoporosis, and nephrocalcinosis in horses. J Am Vet Med Assoc 180:295-299, 1982
66. Ray AC, Tamulinas SH, Reagor JC: High pressure liquid chromatographic determination of cantharidin, using a derivatization method in specimens from animals acutely poisoned by ingestion of blister beetles, *Epicauta lemniscata*. Am J Vet Res 40:498-504, 1979
67. Schmitz DG: Cantharidin toxicosis in horses. J Vet Intern Med 3:208-215, 1989
68. Robinson JA, Allen GK, Green EM, et al.: A prospective study of septicaemia in colostrum-deprived foals. Equine Vet J 25:214-219, 1993
69. Taylor P, Clarke K: Sedation, analgesia and premedication, in Handbook of Equine Anaesthesia. Edinburgh, WB Saunders, 2003, pp 15-31
70. MacLeay JM, Kohn CW: Results of quantitative cultures of urine by free catch and catheterization from healthy adult horses. J Vet Intern Med 12:76-78, 1998
71. Brewer BD, Clement SF, Lotz WS, et al.: Renal clearance, urinary excretion of endogenous substances, and urinary diagnostic indices in healthy neonatal foals. J Vet Intern Med 5:28-33, 1991
72. Rumbaugh GE, Carlson GP, Harrold D: Urinary production in the healthy horse and in horses deprived of feed and water. Am J Vet Res 43:735-737, 1982
73. Edwards DJ, Brownlow MA, Hutchins DR: Indices of renal function: values in eight normal foals from birth to 56 days. Aust Vet J 67:251-254, 1990
74. Edwards DJ, Brownlow MA, Hutchins DR: Indices of renal function: reference values in normal horses. Aust Vet J 66:60-63, 1989
75. Kohn CW, Chew DJ: Laboratory diagnosis and characterization of renal disease in horses. Vet Clin North Am Equine Pract 3:585-615, 1987
76. Wood T, Weckman TJ, Henry PA, et al.: Equine urine pH: normal population distributions and methods of acidification. Equine Vet J 22:118-121, 1990
77. Marcussen N, Schumann J, Campbell P, et al.: Cytodiagnostic urinalysis is very useful in the differential diagnosis of acute renal failure and can predict the severity. Ren Fail 17:721-729, 1995
78. Vander AJ: Renal clearance. In: Renal Physiology. New York, McGraw-Hill, 1995, pp 51-61
79. Knudsen E: Renal clearance studies on the horse. I. Inulin, endogenous creatinine and urea. Acta Vet Scand 1:52-66, 1959
80. Holdstock NB, Ousey JC, Rossdale PD: Glomerular filtration rate, effective renal plasma flow, blood pressure and pulse rate in the equine neonate during the first 10 days post partum. Equine Vet J 30:335-343, 1998
81. Finco DR, Groves C: Mechanism of renal excretion of creatinine by the pony. Am J Vet Res 46:1625-1628, 1985
82. Zatzman ML, Clarke L, Ray WJ, et al.: Renal function of the pony and the horse. Am J Vet Res 43:608-612, 1982
83. Brewer BD, Clement SF, Lotz WS, et al.: Single injection inulin/PAH method for the determination of renal clearances in adult horses and ponies. J Vet Pharmacol Ther 11:409-412, 1988
84. Gleadhill A, Marlin D, Harris PA, et al.: Use of a three-blood-sample plasma clearance technique to measure GFR in horses. Vet J 158:204-209, 1999
85. Matthews HK, Andrews FM, Daniel GB, et al.: Comparison of standard and radionuclide methods for measurement of glomerular filtration rate and effective renal blood flow in female horses. Am J Vet Res 53:1612-1616, 1992
86. Walsh DM, Royal HD: Evaluation of a single injection of 99mTc-labeled diethylenetriaminepentaacetic acid for measuring glomerular filtration rate in horses. Am J Vet Res 53:776-780, 1992
87. Brewer BD, Clement SF, Lotz WS, et al.: A comparison of inulin, para-aminohippuric acid, and endogenous creatinine clearances as measures of renal function in neonatal foals. J Vet Intern Med 4:301-305, 1990
88. Gonda KC, Wilcke JR, Crisman MV, et al.: Evaluation of iohexol clearance used to estimate glomerular filtration rate in clinically normal foals. Am J Vet Res 64:1486-1490, 2003
89. Rawlings C, Bisgard G: Renal clearance and excretion of endogenous substances in the small pony. Am J Vet Res 36:45-48, 1975
90. Kohn CW, Strasser SL: 24-hour renal clearance and excretion of endogenous substances in the mare. Am J Vet Res 47:1332-1337, 1986

91. McKenzie EC, Valberg SJ, Godden SM, et al.: Comparison of volumetric urine collection versus single-sample urine collection in horses consuming diets varying in cation-anion balance. Am J Vet Res 64:284-291, 2003
92. Bickhardt K, Deegen E, Espelage W: [Kidney function tests in horses—methods and reference values in healthy animals]. Dtsch Tierarztl Wochenschr 103:117-122, 1996
93. Gronwall R: Effect of diuresis on urinary excretion and creatinine clearance in the horse. Am J Vet Res 46:1616-1618, 1985
94. Rose BD, Post TW: Proximal tubule, in Clinical Physiology of Acid-Base and Electrolyte Disorders, ed 5. New York, McGraw-Hill, 2001, pp 71-122
95. Rose BD, Post TW: Potassium homeostasis. in Clinical Physiology of Acid-Base and Electrolyte Disorders, ed 5. New York, McGraw-Hill, 2001, pp 372-403
96. Morris DD, Divers TJ, Whitlock RH: Renal clearance and fractional excretion of electrolytes over a 24-hour period in horses. Am J Vet Res 45:2431-2435, 1984
97. Caple I, Doake P, Ellis P: Assessment of the calcium and phosphorous nutrition in horses by analysis in urine. Aust Vet J 58:125-131, 1982
98. Lane V, Merritt A: Reliability of single-sample phosphorous fractional excretion determination as a measure of daily phosphorous renal clearance in equids. Am J Vet Res 44:500-502, 1983
99. Toribio RE, Kohn CW, Hardy J, et al.: Alterations in serum parathyroid hormone and electrolyte concentrations and urinary excretion of electrolytes in horses with induced endotoxemia. J Vet Intern Med 19:223-231, 2005
100. Stewart AJ, Hardy J, Kohn CW, et al.: Validation of diagnostic tests for determination of magnesium status in horses with reduced magnesium intake. Am J Vet Res 65:422-430, 2004
101. Raab WP: Diagnostic value of urinary enzyme determinations. Clin Chem 18:5-25, 1972
102. Bayly WM, Brobst DF, Elfers RS, et al.: Serum and urinary biochemistry and enzyme changes in ponies with acute renal failure. Cornell Vet 76:306-316, 1986
103. Brobst DF, Carroll RJ, Bayly WM: Urinary enzyme concentrations in healthy horses. Cornell Vet 76:299-305, 1986
104. Rossier Y, Divers TJ, Sweeney RW: Variations in urinary gamma glutamyl transferase/urinary creatinine ratio in horses with or without pleuropneumonia treated with gentamicin. Equine Vet J 27:217-220, 1995
105. Adams R, McClure JJ, Gossett KA, et al.: Evaluation of a technique for measurement of gamma-glutamyltranspeptidase in equine urine. Am J Vet Res 46:147-150, 1985
106. Skalova S: The diagnostic role of urinary N-acetyl-beta-D-glucosaminidase (NAG) activity in the detection of renal tubular impairment. Acta Medica (Hradec Kralove) 48:75-80, 2005
107. Rudolph WG, Corvalan EO: Urinary and serum gamma glutamyl transpeptidase in relation to urinary pH and proteinuria in healthy thoroughbred horses in training. Equine Vet J 24:316-317, 1992
108. Hinchcliff KW, McKeever KH, Schmall LM, et al.: Renal and systemic hemodynamic responses to sustained submaximal exertion in horses. Am J Physiol 258:R1177-1183, 1990
109. Woods PR, Drost WT, Clarke CR, et al.: Use of 99mTc-mercaptoacetyltriglycine to evaluate renal function in horses. Vet Radiol Ultrasound 41:85-88, 2000
110. Held JP, Daniel GB: Use of nonimaging nuclear medicine techniques to assess the effect of flunixin meglumine on effective renal plasma flow and effective renal blood flow in healthy horses. Am J Vet Res 52:1619-1621, 1991
111. Staddon GE, Weaver BM, Webb AI: Distribution of cardiac output in anaesthetised horses. Res Vet Sci 27:38-45, 1979
112. Manohar M, Goetz TE: Cerebral, renal, adrenal, intestinal, and pancreatic circulation in conscious ponies and during 1.0, 1.5, and 2.0 minimal alveolar concentrations of halothane-O_2 anesthesia. Am J Vet Res 46:2492-2497, 1985
113. Manohar M, Goetz TE, Saupe B, et al.: Thyroid, renal, and splanchnic circulation in horses at rest and during short-term exercise. Am J Vet Res 56:1356-1361, 1995
114. Trim CM, Moore JN, Clark ES: Renal effects of dopamine infusion in conscious horses. Equine Vet J Suppl:124-128, 1989
115. Huang SW, Lee CT, Chen CH, et al.: Role of renal sonography in the intensive care unit. J Clin Ultrasound 33:72-75, 2005
116. Chang VH, Cunningham JJ: Efficacy of sonography as a screening method in renal insufficiency. J Clin Ultrasound 13:415-417, 1985
117. Noone TC, Semelka RC, Chaney DM, et al.: Abdominal imaging studies: comparison of diagnostic accuracies resulting from ultrasound, computed tomography, and magnetic resonance imaging in the same individual. Magn Reson Imaging 22:19-24, 2004
118. Kiper M, Traub-Dargatz J, Wrigley R: Renal ultrasonography in adult horses. Compend Contin Educ Pract Vet 12:993-1000, 1990
119. Penninck D, Eisenberg H, Teuscher E, et al.: Equine renal ultrasonography: normal and abnormal. Vet Radiol 3:81-84, 1986
120. Rantanen NW: Diseases of the kidneys. Vet Clin Equine 2:89-103, 1986
121. Reimer J: The abdomen, in Atlas of Equine Ultrasonography. St. Louis, Mosby-Year Book, 1998, pp 172-242
122. Divers T, Yeager A: The value of ultrasonographic examination in the diagnosis and management of renal diseases in the horse. Equine Vet Educ 7:334-341, 1995
123. Traub-Dargatz JL, McKinnon AO: Adjunctive methods of examination of the urogenital tract. Vet Clin Equine 4:339-358, 1988
124. Hoffman K, Wood A, McCarthy P: Sonographic-anatomic correlation and imaging protocol for the kidneys of horses. Am J Vet Res 56:1403-1412, 1995
125. Reef VB: Adult abdominal ultrasonography, in Equine Diagnostic Ultrasound. Philadelphia, WB Saunders, 1998, pp 273-363
126. Hoffmann KL, Wood AK, McCarthy PH: Ultrasonography of the equine neonatal kidney. Equine Vet J 32:109-113, 2000
127. Platt JF, Rubin JM, Bowerman RA, et al.: The inability to detect kidney disease on the basis of echogenicity. AJR Am J Roentgenol 151:317-319, 1988
128. Rantanen N: Diseases of the abdomen. Vet Clin Equine 2:67-88, 1986

129. Jakob W: Spontaneous amyloidosis of mammals. Vet Pathol 8:292-306, 1971
130. Braden GL, Kozinn DR, Hampf FE Jr., et al.: Ultrasound diagnosis of early renal papillary necrosis. J Ultrasound Med 10:401-403, 1991
131. Read WK: Renal medullary crest necrosis associated with phenylbutazone therapy in horses. Vet Pathol 20:662-669, 1983
132. Biller D, Bradley G, Partington B: Renal medullary rim sign: ultrasonographic evidence of renal disease. Vet Radiol Ultrasound 33:286-290, 1992
133. Mantis P, Lamb CR: Most dogs with medullary rim sign on ultrasonography have no demonstrable renal dysfunction. Vet Radiol Ultrasound 41:164-166, 2000
134. Wimberly HC, Antonovych TT, Lewis RM: Focal glomerulosclerosis-like disease with nephrotic syndrome in a horse. Vet Pathol 18:692-694, 1981
135. Taylor F, Hillyer M: Urinary diseases, in Diagnostic Techniques in Equine Medicine. Philadelphia, WB Saunders, 1997, pp 93-108
136. Laverty S, Pascoe JR, Ling GV, et al.: Urolithiasis in 68 horses. Vet Surg 21:56-62, 1992
137. Hope WD, Wilson JH, Hager DA, et al.: Chronic renal failure associated with bilateral nephroliths and ureteroliths in a two-year-old Thoroughbred colt. Equine Vet J 21:228-231, 1989
138. Hillyer M, Mair T, Lucke V: Bilateral renal calculi in an adult horse. Equine Vet Educ 2:117-120, 1990
139. Divers TJ: Nephrolithiasis and ureterolithiasis in horses and their association with renal disease and failure. Equine Vet J 21:161-162, 1989
140. Bertone JJ, Traub-Dargatz JL, Fettman MJ, et al.: Monitoring the progression of renal failure in a horse with polycystic kidney disease: use of the reciprocal of serum creatinine concentration and sodium sulfanilate clearance half-time. J Am Vet Med Assoc 191:565-568, 1987
141. Aguilera-Tejero E, Estepa JC, Lopez I, et al.: Polycystic kidneys as a cause of chronic renal failure and secondary hypoparathyroidism in a horse. Equine Vet J 32:167-169, 2000
142. Mucelli RP, Bertolotto M: Imaging techniques in acute renal failure. Kidney Int Suppl 66:S102-S105, 1998
143. Berggren PC: Renal adenocarcinoma in a horse. J Am Vet Med Assoc 176:1252-1253, 1980
144. Brown PJ, Holt PE: Primary renal cell carcinoma in four horses. Equine Vet J 17:473-477, 1985
145. Haschek WM, King JM, Tennant BC: Primary renal cell carcinoma in two horses. J Am Vet Med Assoc 179:992-994, 1981
146. Owen RA, Haywood S, Kelly DF: Clinical course of renal adenocarcinoma associated with hypercupraemia in a horse. Vet Rec 119:291-294, 1986
147. Pomroy W: Renal adenocarcinoma in a horse. Equine Vet J 13:198-200, 1981
148. Rumbaugh ML, Latimer FG, Porthouse KR, et al.: Renal carcinoma with osseous and pulmonary metastases in an Arabian gelding. Equine Vet J 35:107-109, 2003
149. Van Amstel SR, Huchzermeyer D, Reyers F: Primary renal cell carcinoma in a horse. J South Afr Vet Assoc 55:35-38, 1984
150. Rebhun WC, Tennant BC, Dill SG, et al.: Vitamin K3-induced renal toxicosis in the horse. J Am Vet Med Assoc 184:1237-1239, 1984
151. Ehnen SJ, Divers TJ, Gillette D, et al.: Obstructive nephrolithiasis and ureterolithiasis associated with chronic renal failure in horses: eight cases (1981-1987). J Am Vet Med Assoc 197:249-253, 1990
152. Andrews FM, Rosol TJ, Kohn CW, et al.: Bilateral renal hypoplasia in four young horses. J Am Vet Med Assoc 189:209-212, 1986
153. O'Neill WC: Sonographic evaluation of renal failure. Am J Kidney Dis 35:1021-1038, 2000
154. Divers T: Chronic renal failure in horses. Compend Contin Educ Pract Vet 5:S310-S317, 1983
155. Barrat-Boyes S, Spensley M, Nyland T, et al.: Ultrasound localization and guidance for renal biopsy in the horse. Vet Radiol 32:121-126, 1991
156. Allen WR, Bracher V: Videoendoscopic evaluation of the mare's uterus: III. Findings in the pregnant mare. Equine Vet J 24:285-291, 1992
157. Bracher V, Allen WR: Videoendoscopic evaluation of the mare's uterus: I. Findings in normal fertile mares. Equine Vet J 24:274-278, 1992
158. Bracher V, Mathias S, Allen WR: Videoendoscopic evaluation of the mare's uterus: II. Findings in subfertile mares. Equine Vet J 24:279-284, 1992
159. Rambags BP, Stout TA: Transcervical endoscope-guided emptying of a transmural uterine cyst in a mare. Vet Rec 156:679-682, 2005
160. Ricketts SW: Endometrial biopsy as a guide to diagnosis of endometrial pathology in the mare. J Reprod Fertil Suppl:341-345, 1975
161. Berezowski C: Diagnosis of a uterine leiomyoma using hysteroscopy and a partial ovariohysterectomy in a mare. Can Vet J 43:968-970, 2002
162. Burns TE, Card CE: Fetal maceration and retention of fetal bones in a mare. J Am Vet Med Assoc 217:878-880, 845, 2000
163. Card C: Post-breeding inflammation and endometrial cytology in mares. Theriogenology 64:580-588, 2005
164. Allen WE, Newcombe JR: Aspects of genital infection and swabbing techniques in the mare. Vet Rec 104:228-231, 1979
165. Newcombe JR: Comparison of the bacterial flora of three sites in the genital tract of the mare. Vet Rec 102:169-170, 1978
166. Brook D: Uterine culture in mares. Mod Vet Pract 65:A3-8, 1984
167. Nielsen JM: Endometritis in the mare: a diagnostic study comparing cultures from swab and biopsy. Theriogenology 64:510-518, 2005
168. Ball B, Shin S, Patten V, et al.: Use of low-volume uterine flush for microbiologic and cytologic examination of the mare's endometrium. Theriogenology 29:1269-1283, 1988
169. Dascanio J: Endometrial cytology, in Current Therapy in Equine Medicine, ed 5. Philadelphia, WB Saunders, 2003, pp 226-228
170. LaCoeur A, Sprinkle T: Relationship of endometrial cytology and fertility in the broodmare. Equine Pract 7:28-36, 1985

171. Purswell B, Ley W, Sriranganathan N, et al.: Aerobic and anaerobic bacterial flora in postpartum mare. Equine Vet Sci 9:141-144, 1989
172. Available at: http://www.uky.edu/Ag/AnimalSciences/extension/pubpdfs/asc117.pdf
173. Esson ML, Schrier RW: Diagnosis and treatment of acute tubular necrosis. Ann Intern Med 137:744-752, 2002
174. Lameire N, Van Biesen W, Vanholder R: Acute renal failure. Lancet 365:417-430, 2005
175. Adams PL, Adams FF, Bell PD, et al.: Impaired renal blood flow autoregulation in ischemic acute renal failure. Kidney Int 18:68-76, 1980
176. Kelleher SP, Robinette JB, Conger JD: Sympathetic nervous system in the loss of autoregulation in acute renal failure. Am J Physiol 246:F379-F386, 1984
177. Corley KT: Inotropes and vasopressors in adults and foals. Vet Clin North Am Equine Pract 20:77-106, 2004
178. Lee YH, Clarke KW, Alibhai HI, et al.: Effects of dopamine, dobutamine, dopexamine, phenylephrine, and saline solution on intramuscular blood flow and other cardiopulmonary variables in halothane-anesthetized ponies. Am J Vet Res 59:1463-1472, 1998
179. Mackay IG, Muir AL, Watson ML: Contribution of prostaglandins to the systemic and renal vascular response to frusemide in normal man. Br J Clin Pharmacol 17:513-519, 1984
180. Passmore AP, Copeland S, Johnston GD: The effects of ibuprofen and indomethacin on renal function in the presence and absence of frusemide in healthy volunteers on a restricted sodium diet. Br J Clin Pharmacol 29:311-319, 1990
181. Kramer HJ, Schuurmann J, Wassermann C, et al.: Prostaglandin-independent protection by furosemide from oliguric ischemic renal failure in conscious rats. Kidney Int 17:455-464, 1980
182. Bayati A, Nygren K, Kallskog O, et al.: The effect of loop diuretics on the long-term outcome of post-ischaemic acute renal failure in the rat. Acta Physiol Scand 139:271-279, 1990
183. Brezis M, Agmon Y, Epstein FH: Determinants of intrarenal oxygenation. I. Effects of diuretics. Am J Physiol 267:F1059-1062, 1994
184. Heyman SN, Rosen S, Epstein FH, et al.: Loop diuretics reduce hypoxic damage to proximal tubules of the isolated perfused rat kidney. Kidney Int 45:981-985, 1994
185. Mehta RL, Pascual MT, Soroko S, et al.: Diuretics, mortality, and nonrecovery of renal function in acute renal failure. JAMA 288:2547-2553, 2002
186. Girbes AR: Prevention of acute renal failure: role of vasoactive drugs, mannitol and diuretics. Int J Artif Organs 27:1049-1053, 2004
187. Schetz M: Should we use diuretics in acute renal failure? Best Pract Res Clin Anaesthesiol 18:75-89, 2004
188. Dybedock L, Kane K: Are diuretics helpful in acute renal failure? J Fam Pract 52:188, 190, 2003
189. Gambaro G, Bertaglia G, Puma G, et al.: Diuretics and dopamine for the prevention and treatment of acute renal failure: a critical reappraisal. J Nephrol 15:213-219, 2002
190. Shilliday IR, Quinn KJ, Allison ME: Loop diuretics in the management of acute renal failure: a prospective, double-blind, placebo-controlled, randomized study. Nephrol Dial Transplant 12:2592-2596, 1997
191. Shilliday I, Allison ME: Diuretics in acute renal failure. Ren Fail 16:3-17, 1994
192. Kleinknecht D, Ganeval D, Gonzalez-Duque LA, et al.: Furosemide in acute oliguric renal failure. A controlled trial. Nephron 17:51-58, 1976
193. Minuth AN, Terrell JB, Jr., Suki WN: Acute renal failure: a study of the course and prognosis of 104 patients and of the role of furosemide. Am J Med Sci 271:317-324, 1976
194. Kellum JA: Use of diuretics in the acute care setting. Kidney Int Suppl 66:S67-S70, 1998
195. Uchino S, Doig GS, Bellomo R, et al.: Diuretics and mortality in acute renal failure. Crit Care Med 32:1669-1677, 2004
196. Kurtz TW, Hsu CH: Effects of furosemide diuresis on mercuric chloride-induced acute renal failure in the rat. Nephron 43:279-282, 1986
197. Heyman SN, Brezis M, Greenfeld Z, et al.: Protective role of furosemide and saline in radiocontrast-induced acute renal failure in the rat. Am J Kidney Dis 14:377-385, 1989
198. Ward JM, Grabin ME, Berlin E, et al.: Prevention of renal failure in rats receiving cis-diamminedichloroplatinum(II) by administration of furosemide. Cancer Res 37:1238-1240, 1977
199. Burke TJ, Malhotra D, Shapiro JI: Effects of enhanced oxygen release from hemoglobin by RSR13 in an acute renal failure model. Kidney Int 60:1407-1414, 2001
200. Johansson AM, Gardner SY, Levine JF, et al.: Pharmacokinetics and pharmacodynamics of furosemide after oral administration to horses. J Vet Intern Med 18:739-743, 2004
201. Gelman S: Does mannitol save the kidney? Anesth Analg 82:899-901, 1996
202. Solomon R, Werner C, Mann D, et al.: Effects of saline, mannitol, and furosemide to prevent acute decreases in renal function induced by radiocontrast agents. N Engl J Med 331:1416-1420, 1994
203. Reddy VG: Prevention of postoperative acute renal failure. J Postgrad Med 48:64-70, 2002
204. Lauschke A, Teichgraber UK, Frei U, et al.: "Low-dose" dopamine worsens renal perfusion in patients with acute renal failure. Kidney Int 69:1669-74, 2006
205. Jones D, Bellomo R: Renal-dose dopamine: from hypothesis to paradigm to dogma to myth and, finally, superstition? J Intensive Care Med 20:199-211, 2005
206. Kellum JA, J MD: Use of dopamine in acute renal failure: a meta-analysis. Crit Care Med 29:1526-1531, 2001
207. Bellomo R, Chapman M, Finfer S, et al.: Low-dose dopamine in patients with early renal dysfunction: a placebo-controlled randomised trial. Australian and New Zealand Intensive Care Society (ANZICS) Clinical Trials Group. Lancet 356:2139-2143, 2000
208. Argalious M, Motta P, Khandwala F, et al.: "Renal dose" dopamine is associated with the risk of new-onset atrial fibrillation after cardiac surgery. Crit Care Med 33:1327-1332, 2005
209. Trim CM, Moore JN, White NA: Cardiopulmonary effects of dopamine hydrochloride in anaesthetised horses. Equine Vet J 17:41-44, 1985

210. Debaveye YA, Van den Berghe GH: Is there still a place for dopamine in the modern intensive care unit? Anesth Analg 98:461-468, 2004
211. Mathur VS, Swan SK, Lambrecht LJ, et al.: The effects of fenoldopam, a selective dopamine receptor agonist, on systemic and renal hemodynamics in normotensive subjects. Crit Care Med 27:1832-1837, 1999
212. Girbes AR, Smit AJ, Meijer S, et al.: Renal and endocrine effects of fenoldopam and metoclopramide in normal man. Nephron 56:179-185, 1990
213. Lass NA, Glock D, Goldberg LI: Cardiovascular and renal hemodynamic effects of intravenous infusions of the selective DA1 agonist, fenoldopam, used alone or in combination with dopamine and dobutamine. Circulation 78: 1310-1315, 1988
214. Brienza N, Malcangi V, Dalfino L, et al.: A comparison between fenoldopam and low-dose dopamine in early renal dysfunction of critically ill patients. Crit Care Med 34:707-714, 2006
215. Tumlin JA, Finkel KW, Murray PT, et al.: Fenoldopam mesylate in early acute tubular necrosis: a randomized, double-blind, placebo-controlled clinical trial. Am J Kidney Dis 46:26-34, 2005
216. Hollis A, Ousey J, Palmer L, et al.: Effects of fenoldopam mesylate on systemic hemodynamics and indices of renal function in normotensive neonatal foals. J Vet Intern Med 20:595-600, 2006
217. Mitaka C, Hirata Y, Habuka K, et al.: Atrial natriuretic peptide infusion improves ischemic renal failure after suprarenal abdominal aortic cross-clamping in dogs. Crit Care Med 31:2205-2210, 2003
218. Sward K, Valsson F, Odencrants P, et al.: Recombinant human atrial natriuretic peptide in ischemic acute renal failure: a randomized placebo-controlled trial. Crit Care Med 32:1310-1315, 2004
219. Bergman AS, Odar-Cederlof I, Westman L, et al.: Diltiazem infusion for renal protection in cardiac surgical patients with preexisting renal dysfunction. J Cardiothorac Vasc Anesth 16:294-299, 2002
220. Epstein M: Diltiazem and renal hemodynamics: implications for renal protection. J Cardiovasc Pharmacol 18(Suppl 9):S21-S25, 1991
221. Shyu KG, Cheng JJ, Kuan P: Acetylcysteine protects against acute renal damage in patients with abnormal renal function undergoing a coronary procedure. J Am Coll Cardiol 40:1383-1388, 2002
222. Tepel M, van der Giet M, Schwarzfeld C, et al.: Prevention of radiographic-contrast-agent-induced reductions in renal function by acetylcysteine. N Engl J Med 343:180-184, 2000
223. Morgera S, Woydt R, Kern H, et al.: Low-dose prostacyclin preserves renal function in high-risk patients after coronary bypass surgery. Crit Care Med 30:107-112, 2002
224. Nielsen CB, Bech JN, Pedersen EB: Effects of prostacyclin on renal haemodynamics, renal tubular function and vasoactive hormones in healthy humans. A placebo-controlled dose-response study. Br J Clin Pharmacol 44:471-476, 1997
225. Arriero M, Brodsky SV, Gealekman O, et al.: Adult skeletal muscle stem cells differentiate into endothelial lineage and ameliorate renal dysfunction after acute ischemia. Am J Physiol Renal Physiol 287:F621-F627, 2004
226. Bates CM, Lin F: Future strategies in the treatment of acute renal failure: growth factors, stem cells, and other novel therapies. Curr Opin Pediatr 17:215-220, 2005
227. Herrera MB, Bussolati B, Bruno S, et al.: Mesenchymal stem cells contribute to the renal repair of acute tubular epithelial injury. Int J Mol Med 14:1035-1041, 2004
228. Lange C, Togel F, Ittrich H, et al.: Administered mesenchymal stem cells enhance recovery from ischemia/reperfusion-induced acute renal failure in rats. Kidney Int 68:1613-1617, 2005
229. Lin F: Stem cells in kidney regeneration following acute renal injury. Pediatr Res 59:74R-78R, 2006
230. Morigi M, Imberti B, Zoja C, et al.: Mesenchymal stem cells are renotropic, helping to repair the kidney and improve function in acute renal failure. J Am Soc Nephrol 15:1794-1804, 2004
231. Patschan D, Plotkin M, Goligorsky MS: Therapeutic use of stem and endothelial progenitor cells in acute renal injury: CA IRA. Curr Opin Pharmacol 6:176-183, 2006
232. Togel F, Hu Z, Weiss K, et al.: Administered mesenchymal stem cells protect against ischemic acute renal failure through differentiation-independent mechanisms. Am J Physiol Renal Physiol 289:F31-F42, 2005
233. Acker CG, Singh AR, Flick RP, et al.: A trial of thyroxine in acute renal failure. Kidney Int 57:293-298, 2000
234. Cronin RE, Brown DM, Simonsen R: Protection by thyroxine in nephrotoxic acute renal failure. Am J Physiol 251: F408-416, 1986
235. Michael UF, Logan JL, Meeks LA: The beneficial effects of thyroxine on nephrotoxic acute renal failure in the rat. J Am Soc Nephrol 1:1236-1240, 1991
236. Negri AL, Alvarez C, Fernandez MC, et al.: Accelerated recovery from toxic acute renal failure with thyroxin: stimulation of renal phospholipid biosynthesis. Ren Fail 16:19-26, 1994
237. Siegel NJ, Gaudio KM, Katz LA, et al.: Beneficial effect of thyroxin on recovery from toxic acute renal failure. Kidney Int 25:906-911, 1984
238. Sutter PM, Thulin G, Stromski M, et al.: Beneficial effect of thyroxin in the treatment of ischemic acute renal failure. Pediatr Nephrol 2:1-7, 1988
239. Dzyban L, Labato M, Ross L, et al.: Peritoneal dialysis: a tool in veterinary critical care. J Vet Emerg Crit Care 10:91-102, 2000
240. Moghal NE, Embleton ND: Management of acute renal failure in the newborn. Semin Fetal Neonatal Med 11:207-213, 2006
241. McNiece KL, Ellis EE, Drummond-Webb JJ, et al.: Adequacy of peritoneal dialysis in children following cardiopulmonary bypass surgery. Pediatr Nephrol 20:972-976, 2005
242. Andreoli SP: Acute renal failure in the newborn. Semin Perinatol 28:112-123, 2004
243. Shostak A, Smilovich L, Mogilner G, et al.: Peritoneal dialysis and recovery from acute renal failure in a 847-gram newborn infant. Peritoneal Dial Int 10:183-184, 1990
244. Haycock GB: Management of acute and chronic renal failure in the newborn. Semin Neonatol 8:325-334, 2003
245. Ash SR: Peritoneal dialysis in acute renal failure of adults: the safe, effective, and low-cost modality. Contrib Nephrol:210-221, 2001

246. Pastan S, Bailey J: Dialysis therapy. N Engl J Med 338:1428-1437, 1998
247. Coles GA, Williams JD: What is the place of peritoneal dialysis in the integrated treatment of renal failure? Kidney Int 54:2234-2240, 1998
248. Labato MA: Peritoneal dialysis in emergency and critical care medicine. Clin Tech Small Anim Pract 15:126-135, 2000
249. Lew S, Kuleta Z, Pomianowski A: Peritoneal dialysis in dogs and cats. Pol J Vet Sci 8:323-327, 2005
250. Crisp MS, Chew DJ, DiBartola SP, et al.: Peritoneal dialysis in dogs and cats: 27 cases (1976-1987). J Am Vet Med Assoc 195:1262-1266, 1989
251. Valdez H, Scrutchfield WL, Taylor TS: Peritoneal lavage in the horse. J Am Vet Med Assoc 175:388-391, 1979
252. Easter JL, Hague BA, Brumbaugh GW, et al.: Effects of postoperative peritoneal lavage on pharmacokinetics of gentamicin in horses after celiotomy. Am J Vet Res 58:1166-1170, 1997
253. Hague BA, Honnas CM, Berridge BR, et al.: Evaluation of postoperative peritoneal lavage in standing horses for prevention of experimentally induced abdominal adhesions. Vet Surg 27:122-126, 1998
254. Eggleston RB, Mueller PO: Prevention and treatment of gastrointestinal adhesions. Vet Clin North Am Equine Pract 19:741-763, 2003
255. Nieto JE, Snyder JR, Vatistas NJ, et al.: Use of an active intra-abdominal drain in 67 horses. Vet Surg 32:1-7, 2003
256. Smith CL, Dowling BA, Dart AJ: Recent advances in equine abdominal surgery. Vet J 170:41-51, 2005
257. Kritchevsky JE, Stevens DL, Christopher J, et al.: Peritoneal dialysis for presurgical management of ruptured bladder in a foal. J Am Vet Med Assoc 185:81-82, 1984
258. Ellger B, Debaveye Y, Vanhorebeek I, et al.: Survival benefits of intensive insulin therapy in critical illness: impact of maintaining normoglycemia versus glycemia-independent actions of insulin. Diabetes 55:1096-1105, 2006
259. Krinsley J: Perioperative glucose control. Curr Opin Anaesthesiol 19:111-116, 2006
260. Nasraway SA Jr.: Hyperglycemia during critical illness. J Parenter Enteral Nutr 30:254-258, 2006
261. Pittas AG, Siegel RD, Lau J: Insulin therapy for critically ill hospitalized patients: a meta-analysis of randomized controlled trials. Arch Intern Med 164:2005-2011, 2004
262. Schetz M, Van den Berghe G: Glucose control in the critically ill. Contrib Nephrol 144:119-131, 2004
263. Van den Berghe G, Wouters PJ, Bouillon R, et al.: Outcome benefit of intensive insulin therapy in the critically ill: Insulin dose versus glycemic control. Crit Care Med 31:359-366, 2003
264. van den Berghe G, Wouters P, Weekers F, et al.: Intensive insulin therapy in the critically ill patients. N Engl J Med 345:1359-1367, 2001
265. Bellomo R, Ronco C, Kellum JA, et al.: Acute renal failure—definition, outcome measures, animal models, fluid therapy and information technology needs: the Second International Consensus Conference of the Acute Dialysis Quality Initiative (ADQI) Group. Crit Care 8:R204-R212, 2004
266. Mehta RL, Clark WC, Schetz M: Techniques for assessing and achieving fluid balance in acute renal failure. Curr Opin Crit Care 8:535-543, 2002
267. Feld LG, Cachero S, Springate JE: Fluid needs in acute renal failure. Pediatr Clin North Am 37:337-350, 1990
268. Corley KT, Donaldson LL, Durando MM, et al.: Cardiac output technologies with special reference to the horse. J Vet Intern Med 17:262-272, 2003
269. Corley KT, Donaldson LL, Furr MO: Comparison of lithium dilution and thermodilution cardiac output measurements in anaesthetised neonatal foals. Equine Vet J 34:598-601, 2002
270. Hallowell GD, Corley KT: Use of lithium dilution and pulse contour analysis cardiac output determination in anaesthetized horses: a clinical evaluation. Vet Anaesth Analg 32:201-211, 2005
271. Gossett KA, French DD, Cleghorn B, et al.: Effect of acute acidemia on blood biochemical variables in healthy ponies. Am J Vet Res 51:1375-1379, 1990
272. Elfers RS, Bayly WM, Brobst DF, et al.: Alterations in calcium, phosphorus and C-terminal parathyroid hormone levels in equine acute renal disease. Cornell Vet 76:317-329, 1986
273. Tennant B, Lowe JE, Tasker JB: Hypercalcemia and hypophosphatemia in ponies following bilateral nephrectomy. Proc Soc Exp Biol Med 167:365-368, 1981
274. Carlstedt F, Eriksson M, Kiiski R, et al.: Hypocalcemia during porcine endotoxemic shock: effects of calcium administration. Crit Care Med 28:2909-2914, 2000
275. Malcolm DS, Zaloga GP, Holaday JW: Calcium administration increases the mortality of endotoxic shock in rats. Crit Care Med 17:900-903, 1989
276. Jose-Cunilleras E, Hinchcliff KW: Renal pharmacology. Vet Clin North Am Equine Pract 15:647-664, ix, 1999
277. Sevinga M, Barkema HW, Stryhn H, et al.: Retained placenta in Friesian mares: incidence, and potential risk factors with special emphasis on gestational length. Theriogenology 61:851-859, 2004
278. Vandeplassche M, Spincemaille J, Bouters R: Aetiology, pathogenesis and treatment of retained placenta in the mare. Equine Vet J 3:144-147, 1971
279. Freeman DE, Hungerford LL, Schaeffer D, et al.: Caesarean section and other methods for assisted delivery: comparison of effects on mare mortality and complications. Equine Vet J 31:203-207, 1999
280. Watkins JP, Taylor TS, Day WC, et al.: Elective cesarean section in mares: eight cases (1980-1989). J Am Vet Med Assoc 197:1639-1645, 1990
281. Perkins NR, Frazer GS: Reproductive emergencies in the mare. Vet Clin North Am Equine Pract 10:643-670, 1994
282. Rochat MC: Priapism: a review. Theriogenology 56:713-722, 2001
283. Pearson H, Weaver BM: Priapism after sedation, neuroleptanalgesia and anaesthesia in the horse. Equine Vet J 10:85-90, 1978
284. Lucke JN, Sansom J: Penile erection in the horse after acepromazine. Vet Rec 105:21-22, 1979
285. Gerring EL: Priapism and ACP in the horse. Vet Rec 109:64, 1981
286. Schumacher J, Harden DK: Surgical treatment of priapism in a stallion. Vet Surg 16:193-196, 1987
287. Wilson DV, Nickels FA, Williams MA: Pharmacologic treatment of priapism in two horses. J Am Vet Med Assoc 199:1183-1184

288. Sharrock AG: Reversal of drug-induced priapism in a gelding by medication. Aust Vet J 58:39-40, 1982
289. Boller M, Furst A, Ringer S, et al.: Complete recovery from long-standing priapism in a stallion after propionylpromazine/xylazine sedation. Equine Vet Educ 17:305-311, 2005
290. Feary DJ, Moffett PD, Bruemmer JE, et al.: Chemical ejaculation and cryopreservation of semen from a breeding stallion with paraphimosis secondary to priapism and haemorrhagic colitis. Equine Vet Educ 17:299-304, 2005
291. Schumacher J, Varner DD, Crabill MR, Blanchard TL: The effect of a surgically created shunt between the corpus cavernosum penis and corpus spongiosum penis of stallion on erectile and ejaculatory function. Vet Surg 28:21-24, 1999
292. Van Herreveld PD, Gaughan EM: Partial phallectomy to treat priapism in a horse. Aust Vet J 77:167-169, 1999
293. Taylor NR: Traumatic balanoposthitis in a yearling Appaloosa colt. Vet Rec 107:154-155, 1980
294. Simmons HA, Cox JE, Edwards GB, et al.: Paraphimosis in seven debilitated horses. Vet Rec 116:126-127, 1985
295. Love CC, McDonnell SM, Kenney RM: Manually assisted ejaculation with erectile dysfunction subsequent to paraphimosis. J Am Vet Med Assoc 200:1357-1359, 1992
296. Lloyd KC, Harrison I, Tulleners E: Reserpine toxicosis in a horse. J Am Vet Med Assoc 186:980-981, 1985

14

Monitoring and treating the neurological system

Martin Furr

14.1 Monitoring the neurological system
14.2 Management of horses with neurological disorders

14.1 Monitoring the neurological system

Horses at risk of developing neurological disorders

Horses with a variety of conditions are at risk of developing neurological disorders during hospitalisation. Relative risk rates associated with these various conditions are not quantified, but risk factors are recognised. Conditions that do not primarily involve the nervous system but that may have neurological sequelae are listed in Box 14.1. Such animals should be carefully monitored during hospitalisation to ensure that neurological signs do not develop or are found early in case that they do occur.

Clinical examination of the nervous system

The clinical examination is the most important means of evaluating the nervous system. A quick assessment of the neurological system can be accomplished each day during the normal physical examination and assessment. A full gait analysis may not be required on each horse each day, but observation of the horse's demeanour, ability to prehend, masticate and swallow food, and ability to move around the stall is easily and quickly performed and will usually detect some abnormality, which may then be more fully evaluated if necessary. To perform the neurological examination properly requires knowledge of the mechanics of the examination, as well as experience in interpreting the observations of the exam. In general, examination of the nervous system involves observation of reflexes that are associated with the sensory and motor systems, as well as the conscious and general proprioceptive system. These systems are examined by observation of the horse at rest and while in motion, and when performing specific movements that challenge the nervous system. Proper interpretation of the results requires knowledge of the range of normal, which is developed from experience. Hence, it is important that the procedures of the nervous system examination be incorporated into the routine physical examination of any horse, such that the range of normal responses is understood and appreciated by the examiner when challenged with a horse with nervous system disease.

The nervous system examination should include an assessment of the horse's mental alertness, head and body position (Figure 14.1), stance and muscle development. Abnormal behaviours, such as excessive yawning, head tilt, or muscle fasciculations, should be observed prior to handling the horse, as this may obscure subtle abnormalities.

Box 14.1. Conditions that may have neurological sequelae in hospitalised horses*

- Internal carotid mycosis and/or guttural pouch disease
- Vascular diseases and coagulopathies
- General anaesthesia leading to:
  - Recumbency myopathy
  - Peripheral neuropathies
  - Spinal cord degeneration
- Hepatic disease
- Patients receiving intravenous injections
- Mares with dystocia
- Foals following dystocia or caesarean section

*This is not an all-inclusive list.

Cranial nerves

The cranial nerves are often examined first, although this is not required. Vision is assessed by observation of the horse's movements in an unfamiliar environment or failure to demonstrate a menace response. It should be noted, however, that cerebellar disease can result in a loss of the menace response in a visual horse. Other signs of cerebellar disease (such as intention tremors or hypermetric gait) should be present if this is the cause of the altered menace response. The menace response can be difficult to elicit in

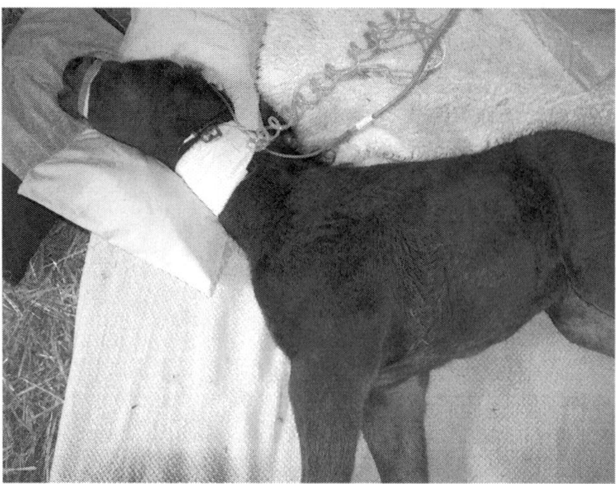

Figure 14.1 Opisthotonus in a foal with severe hyponatraemia. The foal's sodium concentration was 103 mmol/L, as a sequel to renal disease. The foal was also showing seizure activity, characterised by rapid mouth and tongue movements. © Kevin Corley 2007.

some circumstances and should be repeated several times if questionable. Pupil size, position and symmetry should be evaluated, and the direct and consensual pupillary light response evaluated. In the normal animal, a bright light directed into one eye should result in constriction of both pupils. A widely dilated pupil in a visual eye suggests oculomotor nerve damage and there will be no direct or consensual light response. The oculomotor nerve also innervates the extraocular muscles of the eye, along with the trochlear (cranial nerve [CN] 4) and abducens nerves (CN 6), which control eye position. These nerves are tested by observation of eye position and motion. Spontaneous or positional nystagmus is always abnormal.

The head should be examined for facial symmetry (reflecting function of CN 7), and the presence of a head tilt, reflecting vestibular disease. The masseter and temporal muscles should also be examined. These muscles atrophy if CN 5 is damaged. Swallowing can be evaluated by observation of normal mastication and swallowing, the "gag" reflex, or by passing a stomach tube. Dysfunction of CN 9 and CN 10 can result in swallowing abnormalities. Pharyngeal function and the swallowing reflex can also be tested by observation with an endoscope. Tongue tone is dependent upon the function of the hypoglossal nerve (CN 12), and can be tested by grasping the tongue and applying gentle traction. Inability to resist or withdraw the tongue suggests hypoglossal nerve damage.

Limb placement and panniculus tests

Limb placement and panniculus tests can be easily performed in the stable and can detect muscular weakness and proprioceptive deficits. For limb placement, one front hoof is lifted and then placed across the other front leg. Horses should quickly move the hoof back into normal position or vigorously resist placement into an abnormal position. An abnormal response is to leave the hoof in this crossed position for a prolonged period (usually more than several seconds) or to attempt to move the foot back to a normal position but have difficulty in doing so. The demeanour and training of the horse must be carefully considered: A slow response in a 3-year-old Thoroughbred in race training is abnormal, but a similar response in an aged gelding may be normal. Placing the foot in a base-wide position can also be performed, and the expected response is for the horse to quickly replace it into a normal position.

The panniculus reflex is tested by stimulating the skin over the trunk, then observing for a "skin-flick" response.

Tail and anal tone evaluation

Tail and anal tone evaluation can also be performed in the stable, and detect muscular weakness. Tail tone should be evaluated by grasping the tail and assessing the strength of the tail clamp, and anal tone and response tested by stimulating the anus and observing a contraction. Perianal skin reactions should also be evaluated.

Gait analysis

The horse should be examined in motion at a walk and possibly trot and asked to perform certain manoeuvres that "challenge" specific functions of the nervous system. These include walking with the head elevated, downhill, backing, turning in tight circles or moving over or around obstacles. Specific neurological abnormalities that are observed during this phase of the examination include proprioceptive deficits, ataxia, paresis and dysmetria or spasticity.

Clinical signs that are associated with proprioceptive loss include a base-wide stance, stumbling, dragging a hoof, abnormal position of the limbs after coming to a stop and truncal sway (if severe). When spun in a tight circle, the outside limb may be abducted, the horse may pivot on the affected limb or the horse cross the rear limb over the other. Extending (elevating) the head often increases the degree of incoordination and deficit. Horses with muscular weakness have a low foot flight arc, stumble and have a poor response to the sway test. The sway test demonstrates an animal's ability to resist being pushed off balance and can be performed on the front limbs or the rear limbs. When pushed at the withers, most adult horses should be able to resist or quickly step sideways if pushed off balance. Weak horses cannot resist and recover poorly after being pushed sideways. A similar procedure is used in the rear limbs and is referred to as the "tail-pull". In this test, the horse is pulled sideways using the tail. Most adult horses can easily resist even a strong pull and if pulled off balance will quickly recover. This test can and should also be done when the horse is walking, and as in the standing test, the horse should quickly correct rear limb position with the next stride.

Dysmetria refers to a gait in which the limb movements are either too long (hypermetria) or too short (hypometria). *Hypometria* is due to stiffness and decreased flexion,

Box 14.2. Grading system for gait analysis

Grade	Description
0	No neurological deficits detected.
1	Neurological deficits just detected at a normal gait but worsened by backing, turning, loin pressure or neck extension.
2	Neurological deficits easily detected at the walk, and exaggerated by backing, turning, loin pressure or neck extension.
3	Neurological deficits prominent at the walk, with a tendency to buckle or fall with backing, turning, loin pressure or neck extension. Postural deficits noted at rest.
4	Stumbling, tripping and falling spontaneously at a normal gait.
5	Horse recumbent.

Modified from Mayhew, I., deLahunta, A., Whitlock, R., et al.: Spinal cord disease in the horse. Cornell Vet 68(Suppl 6):24–29, 1978.

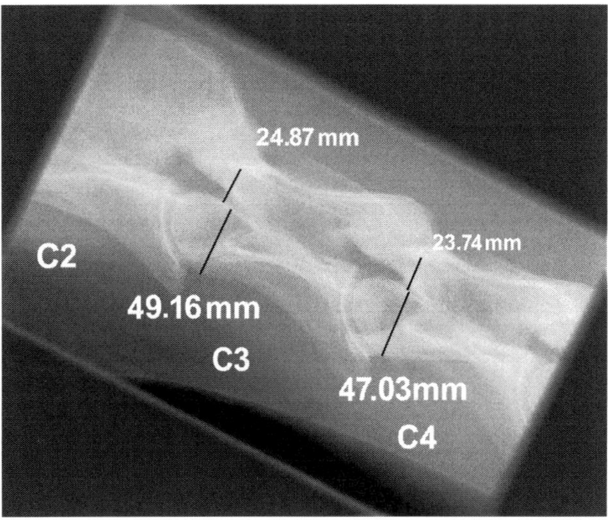

Figure 14.2 Sagittal ratio measurements on cervical radiographs. The narrowest part of the spinal column and the widest part of the head of the vertebrae are measured. The sagittal ratios for this radiograph are 0.506 for C3 and 0.505 for C4. © Kevin Corley 2007.

whereas *hypermetria* is associated with an increased range of motion. *Spasticity* is an expression of dysmetria in which the limbs are hypometric.

Each examiner can establish his or her own approach to performing the gait analysis, but the author generally first observes the horse being led at a walk from the front, back and side. It is helpful to walk alongside the horse, matching speed, and concentrate on detecting the various gait deficits. Each limb should be observed independently and is scored using a standardised scoring system as described by Mayhew. In this system, normal horses are given a score of 0 (Box 14.2).

Next, standing and walking tail pulls are performed, followed by backing the horse. Backing will exacerbate proprioceptive deficits and ataxia, which are demonstrated by abnormal (usually base-wide) limb placement and dragging of the hooves. Limb placement, panniculus tests and anal tone are evaluated next, and the horse is spun in a tight circle. It is important not to spin the horse for prolonged periods, as this confuses the evaluation by potentially making the horse dizzy. I try to spin the horse about 3 times around, then stop and give it a few seconds' break. If you need to see more, the test can be repeated. The final test is to lead the horse down an incline with the head in a neutral position, then again with the head elevated. Passive and active flexion of the neck should also be evaluated.

Once the neurological examination has been completed, a determination should be made regarding the neuroanatomic location of the lesion (central or peripheral disease, spinal cord segment involved), symmetry versus asymmetry, and if there is one (unifocal) or more (multifocal) lesions present. One should attempt to explain all neurological deficits by the presence of a single lesion. In general, horses with a lesion of the cervical region (C2-T2) will demonstrate caudal weakness and proprioceptive deficits that are one grade worse in the rear limbs than the front. Horses that demonstrate neurological deficits of the pelvic limbs but normal thoracic limb responses have a lesion that is caudal to T2. If neurological signs are worse in the front limbs than the rear, yet both are involved, a lesion in the region of C7-T1 is suggested. The presence of cranial nerve signs confirms that the lesion is cranial to the foramen magnum.

Ancillary tests

Ancillary tests are procedures such as cervical radiographs, cerebrospinal fluid (CSF) evaluation, Western blot (WB) testing for equine protozoal myeloencephalopathy (EPM) and haematology and clinical chemistry evaluation.

Cervical radiography

All horses with evidence of ataxia localised to the cervical spine should have radiographs to rule out cervical compressive disease or fractures. Using modern portable radiographic machines and rare earth screens, cervical films of diagnostic quality can be taken of adult horses in the field. The intravertebral sagittal ratio of the spinal canal can be determined (Figure 14.2), and horses with a ratio of less than 0.50 have a (roughly) 90% chance of having cervical stenosis.[1] Evidence of cervical pain, or sudden onset of ataxia should also be an indication that cervical radiographs are necessary (Figures 14.3 and 14.4). It must be recognised, however, that in the author's experience, many horses with cervical orthopaedic disease do not demonstrate neck pain.

Cerebrospinal fluid analysis

The methods for collection of CSF are described in detail in Chapters 1.39 and 1.40. Collection and evaluation of the

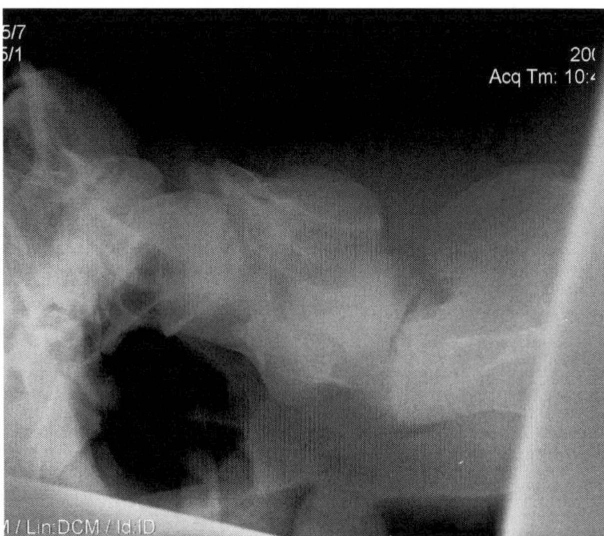

Figure 14.3 Cranial cervical radiograph showing a fractured dens of C2. This 4-month-old foal became acutely ataxic and then recumbent in the field. There was evidence of trauma around the foal's head. © Kevin Corley 2007.

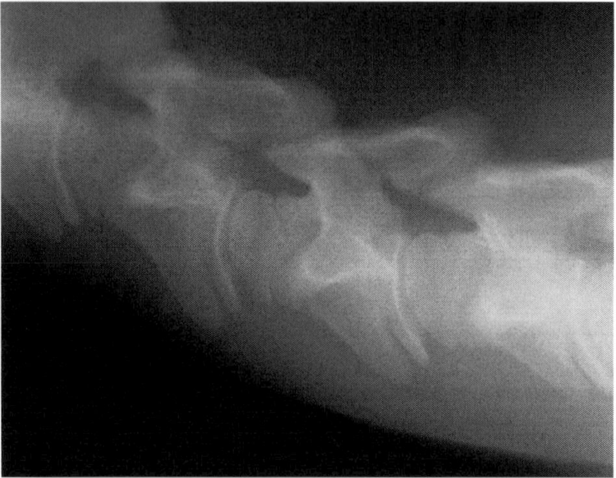

Figure 14.4 Mid cervical radiograph showing fractures of C3 and C4. This 5-week-old foal was observed to run into a fence post. The foal was mildly ataxic in all four limbs. Radiograph courtesy of Scone Veterinary Hospital, NSW, Australia. © Kevin Corley 2004.

CSF is indicated in any horse that demonstrates central nervous system (CNS) disease. Repeat analysis is useful in equivocal cases or cases in which the horse's clinical condition deteriorates significantly. The fluid is evaluated for cell count and various biochemical elements, which routinely include total protein and glucose concentration. Additional biochemical parameters that have been described in the horse include the enzymes lactate dehydrogenase,[2] aspartate transaminase (AST)[2] and creatine kinase (CK).[3] Normal values for CSF are given in the Appendix (see Chapter 19).

Red blood cells

CSF is clear and colourless and becomes turbid when the total protein or cell counts are substantially increased. There should be no red blood cells in normal CSF; however, a few cells are often present due to the collection process. This has lead to the number of cells in a "normal CSF sample" to be reported higher (up to 0.6×10^9/L cells [600 cells/μl])[4] than is likely to be true. The presence of red blood cells in the fluid renders it pink to red, and haemorrhage into the CSF that has occurred previously leads to a yellow discolouration of the fluid referred to as *xanthochromia*. Mild xanthochromia has been reported to be normal in foals less than 10 days of age and hence should not be overinterpreted in neonates.[5] Increased red blood cells are found with haemorrhage within the CNS, associated with trauma or vascular tumours, as well as with severe inflammation and tissue necrosis, as may be seen with fumonisin B1 toxicosis, bacterial abscessation and verminous meningoencephalitis. It is important to quantitate red blood cell concentrations, as substantial amounts of blood can be present in the CSF without an obvious change in the gross appearance of the fluid.[6]

White blood cells

White blood cell counts increase in response to infection and inflammation, with nucleated cells generally predominating in bacterial infection and mononuclear cells predominating in viral disease. There is, however, a significant range of responses possible within this general paradigm, and distinguishing between the two conditions is often not clearcut. CSF cell counts in cases of West Nile virus encephalitis have been reported and a mononuclear pleocytosis was seen in 16 of 30 confirmed cases.[7] A predominance of lymphocytes and large mononuclear cells was uniformly seen in these cases; normal cell counts were found in 8 of 30 horses. In horses with EHV-1 myeloencephalopathy, cell counts usually remain normal, while the total protein is elevated.[8] In other viral disease of the CNS, such as rabies, the CSF cells counts are often normal, while a lymphocytic pleocytosis was observed in the CSF of horses with neurological equine infectious anaemia (EIA).[9] Hence, a wide range of cellular responses can be seen in the CSF of horses with viral disease, and fluid may be normal in the presence of severe nervous system disease. The cellular reactions associated with bacterial infection appear to be much less variable and are predominantly neutrophilic. However, the magnitude of the increase in neutrophil count can be quite variable in bacterial infection, ranging from near normal to grossly elevated.[10,11] Verminous infections usually result in increased numbers of eosinophils, although this too is variable.[12]

Glucose, lactate and enzyme concentration

Glucose concentrations decrease in infection of the CNS, while lactate concentrations have been reported to increase.[4] CSF concentrations of various enzymes have been described in horses, including creatine kinase (CK), lactate dehydrogenase (LDH) and aspartate transferase (AST). In humans, increased CSF AST concentrations have been associated with CNS infections, haemorrhage and neoplasia,[13] although no studies evaluating either AST or LDH in horses have been performed. In horses with CNS inflammation, CSF concentrations of CK have been reported to be increased, particularly in cases of EPM.[3] Other investigators have reported that CK concentrations can be significantly altered by epidural fat, making them difficult to interpret.[14] This study also demonstrated that considerations regarding the presence of peripheral blood contamination and the amount of difficulty collecting the sample apply to the interpretation of enzyme concentrations, just as they do in the interpretation of CSF WB tests for EPM.

Equine protozoal myeloencephalopathy

In countries where it is prevalent, testing for EPM can also be performed on the CSF. However, many horses that appear neurologically normal have been found to have a positive EPM WB test. Weak positive test results should be very cautiously interpreted as evidence of active infection. If the WB EPM test is performed, it must be coupled with CSF red blood cell counts to ensure that there is no blood contamination present. Counts less than 0.01×10^9/L cells (10 cells/μl) confirm that there is no peripheral contamination with blood. In countries where EPM is not reported, it is important to remember that the positive predictive value of a test for any very rare disease is always low. Test results from horses that have no history of having been in the United States therefore need to be interpreted with caution.

Haematology and biochemistry

In horses with evidence of systemic disease, such as fever, depression or dehydration, for example, routine serum clinical chemistry and haematology tests should be performed, and all results interpreted in conjunction with all other data, not individually. Increased activities of liver enzymes may support a diagnosis of hepatic encephalopathy (see Chapter 12.2). Decreased sodium concentrations can cause marked neurological signs in neonatal foals (see Figure 14.1). However, horses with CNS disease commonly have normal clinical chemistry and complete blood cell results.

Electroencephalography

Electroencephalography (EEG) is an electrical recording of the cumulative discharge of superficial cortical neurons. It has value in localising degenerative or inflammatory conditions but requires specialised equipment and significant experience to interpret. EEG also has value in confirming the presence of organic disease. Few reports of the use of EEG in the horse exist, but its value as a diagnostic tool has been validated.[15] Normal horses demonstrate a primary wave frequency of 8 to 13 cycles/second and a voltage of 25 to 50 mV. In 20 horses with a variety of intracranial abnormalities, EEG demonstrated a sensitivity of 100 and specificity of 70 and was considered to be a valuable adjunct in the diagnosis of intracranial disorders.[15]

14.2 Management of horses with neurological disorders

Horses with neurological disease present unique problems related to safe and effective management in the hospital setting. Animals that are severely compromised or are ill enough to require hospitalisation usually have problems in which normal equine housing and management may need to be altered. In addition, the specific nature of the neurological illness dictates, in some cases, specific management modalities that differ from case to case. The clinician's primary concerns are to provide an environment in which the horse can be safely treated and to protect the safety of human caretakers in the process. These issues may require consideration of the physical size of the stall, proper footing, use of restraints and slings, and head protectors.

Housing and husbandry

Horses with neurological problems may have difficulty standing due to weakness and hence may require more room than a normal horse to "lunge" forward, using their momentum to help them stand. It is important that the stall is of adequate size to allow the horse to do this, as well as to provide adequate room for human caretakers to move about freely without placing themselves into a corner. Preferably, there should be two methods to exit the stall in case the horse becomes excited or manic or has seizures during treatment or physical manipulations. In addition, adequate stall space is required for horses that are down, such that caretakers can move around the horse freely without placing themselves in tight corners (too near the legs, which may flail wildly) where they can be kicked or knocked against a wall. Padding of the walls is of value in horses that may fall or need to lean against something for stability (Figure 14.5). Cinder block or rough wood partitions can cause severe abrasions of the skin or ocular damage if the horse leans or falls against the wall. The stall should be equipped with, or capable of being equipped with, an overhead winch or pulley system (Figure 14.5). If an electric winch is used, it should be fully rated to carry the weight of the animal, and the rate of travel of the winch should be fairly rapid. Winches that move slowly are of little to no value in assisting a horse to rise, and an old-fashioned block and tackle, using "people power," may be a better alternative.

Flooring

As horses with neurological weakness or ataxia often have difficulty standing, the nature of the flooring is important in the overall care. Weak horses are at increased risk to slip

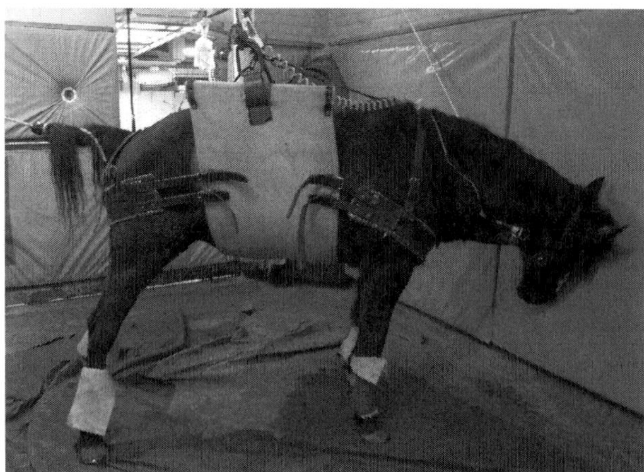

Figure 14.5 Padding of the walls can be extremely useful in the management of horses with severe neurological injury. This horse is head-pressing due to intestinal hyperammonaemia. © Anna Hollis 2005.

when standing or stumble and fall when moving and may have catastrophic fracture. Even if catastrophic injury does not occur, less severe injuries complicate the care and increase morbidity associated with myopathies, skin wounds, bruising, ocular damage and head trauma.

The ideal footing for horses, in the author's opinion, is a dry grassy area that is smooth, level and free of holes and ruts. This provides the optimum combination of traction and padding. However, in many, if not most cases, outdoor housing on grass is not an option for horses requiring hospital care. It is a useful option to remember, however, in the horse that may have trouble standing but can walk into the barn after they get on their feet. The choice of hospital stable flooring is not straightforward and must be carefully considered. Padded floors, as are used in anaesthetic induction/recovery areas, are often good choices, but it must be remembered and considered that the animals may spend prolonged periods in these stalls, and cleaning of the flooring becomes an issue. A floor that retains some traction even when wet is ideal; however, these types of floors often are more difficult to disinfect. Finally, flooring and mats that are too soft can increase the risk of falling. If the flooring is too soft, the animal can catch its hooves and stumble because it is too weak to pick the foot up quickly when it trips. There are a variety of both permanent and portable padded flooring systems available from a number of vendors. Portable pads can be used, which have the advantage of being able to be cleaned and disinfected after they have been used, as well as to be moved from stall to stall as needed. The final choice depends upon the individual hospital circumstances of design, stall locations and staffing.

Stable environment

Another important concept to realise is that horses with neurological illness may not respond to environmental situations would as a normal horse. These events must be anticipated and guarded against. Feed and water buckets in the box (stall) are normal, and almost all horses are accustomed to their presence, However, a horse with neurological disease may have difficulty eating or drinking from certain types of feeders or waterers. These may have to be placed on the floor or at a higher than normal position to allow access. Horses with cerebral and/or pharyngeal disease have a tendency to immerse their head deeply into water to drink. In the compromised horse, this can lead to their getting a bucket stuck over their head, perhaps with catastrophic results. If the horse is anxious or nervous, it is important keep things quiet around them. The author has observed weak/neurological horses startle at a sudden noise, stumble and fall, and break a leg. Cotton can be placed into the horse's ears to deaden sounds, but the effectiveness of this practice is unknown. Finally, the stall in which a horse with neurological disease is kept should be readily accessible to remove a horse that is recumbent.

Padded head covers can be used to protect horses head and eyes from trauma during seizures or severe neurological episodes. While beneficial, it is important to ensure that the device fits properly, as it can become twisted and traumatise the eye.

Slings

Slings can be useful in caring for the horse with neurological disease, but it is not appropriate in all circumstances, and it is fully contraindicated in some. The precise nature of the horse's illness, as well as its demeanour, influence whether a sling is useful or not. Slings are useful with the horse that can stand and almost support itself but not completely; that needs the sling for stability; or that needs to have intermittent periods of rest, during which the sling is supporting a large proportion of its weight, but for only short periods of time. The sling should not be supporting more 25% of the animal's weight for any extended periods of time (hours). Horses cannot be wholly supported in most slings, as doing so compresses the chest and abdomen, limiting respiration. Horses that simply "hang" limply in a sling will not survive. Furthermore, the demeanour of some horses precludes the use of the sling. This includes those that are frantic, convulsive or simply temperamentally unsuited.

The down horse

Down horses represent an immense challenge to the clinician, although horses have recovered following prolonged recumbency. There is no efficient and labour-saving method of caring for a down horse. A large amount of physical work is involved, often requiring more than one person, and it must be continued around the clock for a favourable outcome. The prognosis depends upon the precise cause of the neurological illness, as well as the animal's size. Mature adult horses cannot be maintained in recumbency for as long as can yearlings and small ponies, due to the inevitable complications that arise. Careful consideration should be given to the diagnosis, the horse's demeanour and willingness to tolerate recumbency, the nature of any complications that may be present and, not least, the owner's commitment to the process. Complications of recumbency should be expected and commonly include ocular and head trauma, decubital ulceration, peripheral neuropathies, colic and pneumonia.

The most common complication is, of course, decubital ulceration. These will begin over the bony prominences of the hip, shoulder and lateral aspects of the antebrachium and will be observed within 2 days in adults. With appropriate care, young foals and neonates can be maintained in recumbency for prolonged periods without the development of skin ulcers. Whilst pressure is a major component of the pathophysiology of these wounds, abrasions from movement are also important; hence, keeping the horse quiet and still becomes important. Moisture associated with sweating and urine scalding are also important factors in the development of skin ulcers, as the constant moisture macerates the skin, breaking down tight junctions and allowing bacterial colonisation. For these reasons, it is important in the management of recumbent horses to change the side down as frequently as possible, followed by careful drying of the skin. This can be done by towel drying, followed by hair dryers on low setting, and application of cornstarch or baby powder. If sores are present, antibiotic creams such as silver sulphadiazine should be used liberally. In neonates, the side that they are lying on should be changed every 1 to 2 hours. Whilst this is often difficult, if not impossible, in adult horses, they should be rolled to the opposite side 2 to 4 times per day. In addition to skin lesions, changing the animal from side to side minimises the risk of lung atelectasis and pneumonia, myopathy and peripheral neuropathy, while helping to minimise the horse's pain and discomfort.

To minimise pressure sores, heavy padding should be placed under horses that are down. Deep bedding of the stall with normal materials can and should be done. However, these materials usually compact very quickly, the result being that the horse is lying on hard bedding. Padding such as towels and pillows are inadequate, as they are not cushioning enough, and are difficult to maintain in position. Thick mats (12 inches) are much better but should be covered with material that is impermeable to moisture and can be disinfected. The downside of mats that are substantial enough to support the weight of an adult horse is that they are often fairly firm and, when the horses flail, they tend to slide off.

Waterbeds have been advocated for recumbent foals. They have also been used for fully grown, mature adult horses. A king-sized waterbed will support a mature adult horse and provides a very effective protective mattress. The waterbed can be cleaned and stored away in a small space when not used. A waterbed heater can be employed and will increase the horse's comfort. The horse should be placed on the mattress when it is empty; then the mattress is filled with warm water to a point that the horse's hip is lifted off the floor by an inch or so. Avoid overfilling the mattress, and only fill it enough to get the horse off the ground, as this makes it harder for the horse to wriggle off the mattress as it moves. These mattresses will need to have water added on occasion, as they tend to stretch.

Nonpurposeful movements are common in horses that are down. These horses often flail, trying to raise their head or paddling with their limbs. Although these movements may be beneficial in allowing the horse to shift their position and perhaps remove pressure from a painful spot, constant movements are usually problematic for the caretaker and the horse's care overall. In addition to moving the horse off any protective padding, the movements lead to severe skin abrasions and massive skin damage. Hence, it is often beneficial in some cases to minimise movement. Sedatives that are useful include the α_2-antagonists xylazine and detomidine, chloral hydrate, diazepam and phenobarbital. The sedative used will depend upon the degree of sedation required and the animal's specific condition (see Chapter 6.1). The drug with the least potent depressive effects, at the lowest dosage possible, should be used.

Specific conditions and treatments

Dysphagia

Dysphagia can result from a number of clinical neurological conditions, which can be categorised as either causing pain, obstruction, or arising from diseases of the nervous system. Neurological conditions that may lead to dysphagia are listed in Box 14.3.

Regardless of the cause, if the dysphagia is severe enough that the horse cannot eat and drink, or risks aspiration pneumonia, then the horse must be withheld from food and water, and supportive nutrition provided until the horse can safely consume food. For nutritional support during periods of dysphagia, an indwelling nasogastric tube can be passed for giving water or feed slurry. Alterna-

Box 14.3. Neurological conditions that may lead to dysphagia*

- Guttural pouch mycosis or empyema
- Encephalitis
  - Viral, mycotic, verminous or bacterial
- Botulism
- Tetanus
- Toxicity
  - Yellow star thistle
  - Lead
  - Herbicides
  - Leukoencephalomalacia
  - Locoweed

*This is not an all-inclusive list.

tively, intravenous nutrition and fluids can be given. Nutritional support is further described in Chapter 5.

The ability to swallow can be assessed by visualising the pharynx with an endoscope and observing for swallowing or by challenging the horse with feed and closely observing for the ability to swallow. Once the horse can swallow, water, and then feed, can be reintroduced. Pelleted feeds may be easier for the slightly dysphagic horse to consume than hay.

Seizures

Seizures can arise from a wide variety of CNS conditions including equine protozoal myeloencephalopathy, bacterial, viral, mycotic or verminous encephalitis, bacterial abscessation, tumours, trauma and toxicity (Boxes 14.4 and 14.5). Seizures in the horse can vary in severity from mild alterations in consciousness to grand mal tonic-clonic seizure activity. Horses that are severely painful or are struggling to stand can be confused with seizure activity, but a true seizure should be associated with some other signs of cerebral disease, such as nystagmus, or altered mentation.

Fundamental objectives for treatment of seizures in the horse include (1) immediate control of the seizure event, (2) specific treatment of the primary cause, (3) protecting the safety of human caretakers, and (4) protecting the horse from self-induced injury (Table 14.1). Effective short- and long-term seizure control are essential for safe management of the horse. Acute management of a seizure event in an adult horse must be carefully attempted, as significant injury can occur to the veterinarian. Abrupt and startling movements and loud noises, such as running, shouting and approaching the animal too quickly should be avoided, as these may stimulate further seizure activity.

Box 14.4. Causes of seizures in the neonatal foal*

Vascular disorders
- Hypoxic-ischemic encephalopathy
- Intracranial haemorrhage

Metabolic disorders
- Hyponatraemia
- Hypernatraemia
- Hypocalcaemia
- Hypoglycaemia
- Hyomagnesaemia
- Metabolic acidosis

Drug-Associated
- Theophylline toxicity
- Intracarotid injection

Trauma

Infection
- Generalised sepsis
- Meningitis
- Cerebral abscessation
- Tyzzer's disease
- Viral encephalitis

Other
- Hydrocephalus
- Congenital brain malformations
- Acute hepatic necrosis

*This is not an all-inclusive list.

Box 14.5. Causes of seizures in the older foal and adult horse*

Vascular disorders
- Cerebral thromboembolism
- Intracranial haemorrhage
- Verminous thrombosis

Metabolic disorders
- Hypocalcaemia
- Hypoglycaemia
- Hypomagnesaemia
- Hyperlipidaemia
- Metabolic acidosis

Infection
- Meningitis
- Cerebral abscessation
- Viral encephalitis
- Rabies
- Arboviral encephalitis
- Equine protozoal myeloencephalitis
- Mycotic encephalitis
- Verminous encephalitis
- Halicepholobus
- Aberrant strongyle

Trauma

Toxic
- Organophosphates
- Strychnine
- Metaldehyde
- Fumonison B (leukoencephalomalacia)
- Locoweed
- Bracken fern
- Intracarotid injection
- "Grove" poisoning

Other
- Hydrocephalus
- Congenital brain malformations
- Hepatoencephalopathy
- Neoplasia
- Cholesterol granuloma
- Pancreatic tumour
- Benign epilepsy of Arabian foals

*This is not an all-inclusive list.

Table 14.1. Treatment goals for seizures in horses

Objective	Treatment	Dose
Control seizures (acute)	Diazepam	0.01–0.4 mg/kg q30min
	Phenobarbitol	4–11 mg/kg IV
	Pentobarbitol	2–20 mg/kg IV q4h or as needed
Control seizures (maintenance)	Phenobarbitol	2–11 mg/kg PO q12h
	Phenytoin	1–2 mg/kg PO q8h
Control cerebral oedema	DMSO	0.5–1 g/kg as a 10% solution IV q12h
	Mannitol	0.25–2 g/kg as 20% solution IV q12–24h
Correct metabolic derangements (if present)	Oxygen supplementation Glucose supplementation Electrolyte supplementation	
Provide nutritional support	Tube feeding Intravenous nutrition	
Minimise trauma	Bedding, head protectors	

Horses may have altered vision and awareness, so they should be approached cautiously so they are not startled. If the horse is standing, anticonvulsant drugs can be given in the conventional manner. It is sometimes most prudent to observe the horse and first determine if the seizure is passing and if medication is required. If the horse is recumbent, it should be approached from the dorsal side to avoid the legs, and injections of anticonvulsant made carefully. Veterinarians should ensure that they are not placing themselves in a position in which they cannot get away from the horse if it has sudden violent movements. An exit strategy should be planned before entering the stall. It is sometimes not possible to get close enough to the horse to give anticonvulsants, and you may have to wait until it stops on its own. One should avoid the temptation to try to physically restrain the horse from their muscular activity. This is almost always futile and can lead to injury of the horse or person. Owners in particular want the veterinarian to "rush in and hold his head" to keep the horse from hurting itself and must be firmly advised to stay back to avoid injury.

Treatment of acute seizures

Little primary literature exists regarding the treatment of seizure disorders in the horse. Currently, diazepam (0.01–0.04 mg/kg IV) is considered to be the drug of choice for treatment of seizures in either adult horses or foals. The elimination and clinical effects of diazepam in the horse have been investigated. Following administration of various doses (0.05, 0.1, 0.2 and 0.4 mg/kg IV) of diazepam to normal adult horses, there was no observed effect upon heart rate, cardiac output, mean pulmonary artery pressure, respiratory rate or arterial pH.[16] Mild sedation was noted at doses greater than 0.2 mg/kg, persisting for up to 2 hours.[16] In the foal, the metabolism and elimination of diazepam differ from those of the adult. At less than 21 days of age, the clearance of diazepam was decreased when compared to adults or older foals, and the half-life was slightly prolonged.[17] In addition, it was found that the free fraction of diazepam in the foals was greater than that reported from adults.[17] These considerations led the authors to suggest that multiple doses of diazepam to foals younger than 21 days of age might lead to accumulation and increased blood concentrations. Diazepam is considered to be very safe for use in compromised patients, as there are no reported cardiovascular effects, even in people with myocardial infarction.[18]

If diazepam is ineffective in terminating the seizure or if seizures recur, then treatment with phenobarbitol is recommended. Intravenous administration of phenobarbital (12 mg/kg) to adult horses resulted in a mean half-life of 18.8 hours, with a range of 14.1 to 24 hours.[19] From this, an IV loading dosage of 12 mg/kg, followed by 6.6 mg/kg every 12 hours, is anticipated to result in a blood concentration within the desired therapeutic range of 15 to 40 μg/ml.[19] The dose should be given slowly, over 20 minutes, as more rapid administration leads to more profound sedation. Excessive sedation and respiratory depression are concerns in critical horses and foals, and the lowest dosage possible to achieve the desired effect should be employed. In the author's experience, this dose (6.6 mg/kg IV twice daily) does not result in excessive respiratory depression in most foals.

α_2-Agonists (such as xylazine and detomidine) are not recommended in the treatment of acute seizures. Xylazine decreases cerebral blood flow and increases intracranial pressure, which is probably contraindicated in the convulsive horse.[20] Ketamine increases cerebral blood flow and intracranial pressure and may exacerbate seizures.[20] The promazine derivative tranquilisers (specifically, acetylpromazine) lower the seizure threshold and also should be avoided.[8] It may be necessary in some situations, however, to administer these drugs to control or immobilise animals until more appropriate treatment can be provided.

Long-term treatment for seizures

Long-term treatment with anticonvulsants is usually recommended if horses are noted to have seizures more frequently than once every 2 months, clusters of seizures 3 or 4 times per year or several seizures over a few days' period. Prior to beginning long-term maintenance anticonvulsant therapy, the diagnosis, prognosis, safety considerations and owner compliance issues should be considered. Oral absorption and pharmacokinetic evaluation of phenobarbitol have been determined in adult horses resulting in a recommended oral dose of 11 mg/kg once per day.[21] With repeated dosing, however, there is an increase in clearance of the drug, presumably due to induction of liver enzymes.[22] This effect was observed by day 42 of treatment and required increasing the dose to 25 mg/kg PO once per day to maintain a desired blood concentration of 20 μg/ml.[22] This observation dictates that blood concentrations of horses being administered phenobarbital for prolonged periods be monitored every 2 to 4 weeks to ensure that the recommended therapeutic range is being maintained. Dosage should be adjusted as necessary; however, control of seizures may be achieved at lower blood concentrations.[8] Potential drug interactions must be considered also, and it is therefore recommended that tetracyclines, chloramphenicol and ivermectin not be given to horses on phenobarbital treatment.

Botulism

Horses with botulism often require nutritional support due to dysphagia, but additional clinical manifestations that must be managed include ileus and an inability to pass faeces, as well as bladder paralysis. The bladder should be evacuated several times per day by rectal palpation. It is preferable in most situations, however, to simply catheterise the bladder for continuous drainage. A urinary catheter* can be placed and left indwelling, and connected to a sterile urinary collection bag† with an antireflux valve or caped with a Heimlich valve‡. The catheter should be placed and handled aseptically to minimise ascending infections. Urinary catheter disinfection should be performed every other day and can be performed by infusing 100 ml of 30% dimethylsulphoxide (DMSO) solution in the catheter and allowing it to be retained for several minutes. In addition, it may be beneficial to prophylactically administer antibiotics that are eliminated by renal excretion, such as penicillin or trimethoprim-sulphadiazine, to horses with urinary catheters. Aminoglycosides (e.g, gentamicin) should be avoided in horses with botulism, as they can cause a neuromuscular blockade that can exacerbate clinical signs. Primary treatment of botulism is best achieved with specific *C. botulinum* antiserum, which is commercially available in the USA§.

Rectal impactions

Rectal impactions can occur in horses experiencing a number of different neurological conditions affecting the caudal spinal cord, such as equine herpesvirus-1 (EHV-1) myeloencephalitis. In such cases, manual evacuation of the rectum is necessary, usually twice per day. The faeces usually are very dry and firm, and therefore large amounts of lubricant are necessary. Failure to achieve adequate evacuation can result in obstruction and colic.

Antibacterial treatment (see also Chapter 6.3)

Bacterial infections of the nervous system are relatively infrequent in the horse. When they occur, successful treatment requires the consideration of several factors. A variety of bacteria have been isolated from the CNS of adult horses and foals. These include *Staphylococcus aureus*,[23] *Actinomyces* spp.[24] and *Streptococcus zooepidemicus*.[10,11] In the foal, *Escherichia coli* has also been isolated.[11] An important factor in considering antimicrobial drugs to be used in horses with bacterial infection of the CNS is the fact that the nervous system is contained within the blood-brain barrier, a tissue barrier that sequesters the nervous system from the peripheral circulation. The ability of xenobiotics to cross the blood-brain barrier and achieve adequate concentration within the CNS is directly related to their lipid solubility and molecular size. Also, drugs that are highly protein bound are less able to enter the CNS, as most plasma proteins are too large to cross the blood-brain barrier.

There are few antibiotics used in the horse that readily achieve antibacterial concentrations in the equine CNS or CSF. Most information known about CSF antibiotic concentrations is extrapolated from work in humans and laboratory animals.

Penicillins

Penicillin achieves concentrations in the CSF that are roughly 10% of corresponding serum concentrations.[25] Whilst meningeal inflammation does increase the proportion of penicillin that can cross the blood-brain barrier, this is variable and may not be adequate to result in therapeutic concentrations. Ampicillin achieves higher concentrations within the CSF than does penicillin, but only in the presence of meningeal inflammation.[26]

* Cook Urinary Catheter; Cook Veterinary Products, Bloomington, IN, USA.

† The Kendall Company, Mansfield, MA, USA.

‡ Bard-Parker, Rutherford, NJ, USA.

§ Veterinary Dynamics, San Louis Obispo, CA, USA.

Cephalosporins

The third- and fourth-generation cephalosporins cefquinome, ceftazidime, cefotaxime and cefepime achieve good CSF concentrations following peripheral administration and have favourable spectrum of activity. Proper dosages and dose intervals for many of these drugs have not been established in the horse at this time. Ceftriaxone has been investigated in the horse, and a dose of 50 mg/kg IV resulted in a CSF concentration of 0.6 ± 0.14 µg/ml at 3 hours after dosage and 0.4 ± 0.31 µg/ml at 8 hours after dosage.[27] This concentration exceeds the MIC for many equine pathogens, making ceftriaxone an attractive choice for the treatment of bacterial meningitis in horses. Due to the cost, however, this may be limited to use in foals and small ponies. Cefotaxime has been used with success in foals with meningitis at a dose of 40 mg/kg QID.[28] Cefquinome has been shown to reach adequate concentrations in the CSF 12 hours after a single dose of 2 mg/kg in pigs.[29] Whether this is also true in horses remains to be elucidated. Dosages for other cephalosporins must be extrapolated from those used in humans and may or may not be appropriate. The expense of many of these antibiotics limits their use to the neonate in most cases.

Chloramphenicol

Chloramphenicol has been extensively evaluated in the horse, and it has been used for the treatment of a number of equine infectious conditions.[30] Chloramphenicol has a favourable spectrum of activity for equine pathogens, and in humans achieves almost 60% of serum concentrations when administered orally.[31] CSF concentrations in horses are similar.[32] The half-life of chloramphenicol in the horse is short,[33] and metabolism and excretion in neonatal foals have been demonstrated to be similar to adult horses.[34] This short half-life makes frequent dosing necessary and limits its intravenous use. Dose recommendations vary widely but are commonly reported as 25 to 59 mg/kg orally every 6 hours.[35] Chloramphenicol can cause aplastic anaemia in a very small number of humans (see Chapter 6.3).

Potentiated sulphonamides

Trimethoprim-sulphamethoxazole concentrations are commonly used in the treatment of equine infections. At a dose of 2.5 mg/kg trimethoprim (TMP) and 12.5 mg/kg sulphamethoxazole (SMZ), CSF concentrations in one horse were 0.15 µg/ml TMP (28% of corresponding serum concentration) and 4.8 µg/ml SMZ (43% of corresponding serum concentration).[36] These concentrations were not adequate to be effective against a number of equine pathogens reported by the authors. Although the authors suggested that there was evidence of accumulation of SMZ in the CSF, this was not confirmed. Meningeal inflammation does not appear to enhance the CSF concentration of TMP-SMZ.[37,38] Hence use of this drug in CNS infections of the horse should be considered carefully and may not be optimal. Sulphadimethoxine does not appear to achieve as high a concentration in the CSF as does sulphamethoxazole, although ormetoprim concentration achieved 47% of corresponding serum concentrations.[39]

Fluoroquinolones

Fluoroquinolones are highly lipid soluble and have been reported to achieve high concentrations in the CNS following parenteral administration.[40] In dogs treated with enoxacin, good CSF concentrations were reported, and concentrations of pefloxacin in healthy dogs resulted in CSF concentrations that were 55% of those in serum.[41] The most commonly used fluoroquinolone in horses is enrofloxacin, and CSF concentrations following administration have been evaluated. The CSF concentration was approximately 15% and 25% of corresponding serum concentrations at 74 and 84 hours, respectively, following treatment.[42] The concentration achieved at a dosage of 5 mg/kg PO every 12 hours exceeded the MIC for most equine pathogens (0.5 µg/ml).[42]

Rifampicin and metronidazole

Rifampicin (rifampin) achieves high CSF concentrations. However, it must be administered concurrently with other antibiotics due to the rapid development of resistance.[43]

Metronidazole is highly lipophylic and it achieves high concentrations in the CSF.[44] However, metronidazole has a limited spectrum of activity and is almost exclusively active against anaerobic infections. There are no reports of CNS infections with anaerobes in horses.

Other antimicrobials

Parenteral administration of aminoglycosides or macrolide antimicrobials does not result in measurable concentrations within the CNS. Administration of doxycycline at 10 mg/kg body weight did not result in measurable concentrations of the drug within the CSF of horses.[45] Hence, these drugs have little value in the treatment of CNS infections in the horse.

Clinical choice of antimicrobial

The optimal antimicrobial to use in equine CNS infections has not been established. The choice of antimicrobial used should therefore be determined based upon culture and sensitivity of the organism, if available, as well as knowledge of the pharmacology of the drug and its ability to enter the CNS in an adequate concentration. In one study describing the treatment of human meningitis, antimicrobial combinations were most commonly used, including one or more third-generation cephalosporins, penicillin, ampicillin and chloramphenicol.[46] It is reasonable to assume that due to the limited penetration of most antibiotics into the CSF of the horse, combination therapy would be of value. However, this should ideally be determined on a case-by-case basis accompanied by culture and sensitivity data.

One means to achieve high CSF concentrations of antibiotics is by direct injection into the CSF. This method of treatment has been utilised in humans, particularly when treating resistant organisms, and high concentrations of antibiotics result.[47,48] No reports using intrathecal antibiotics in horse could be found. This may be a useful route in cases with specific resistant organisms, but the dose and frequency of treatment are totally unknown. Anecdotally, seizures have been reported in horses from this procedure, likely associated with the carrier and formulation of the compounds used.

Antiviral drugs

Acyclovir has been proposed for the treatment of EHV-1 myeloencephalopathy. Acyclovir is an acyclic nucleoside analogue that has a high activity against herpes simplex virus types 1 and 2.[49] Acyclovir has been shown to inhibit the replication of EHV-1 in Syrian hamsters at a dose of 100 mg/kg.[50] *In vitro* evaluation of the effectiveness of acyclovir against EHV-1 isolates has been performed, and good activity was demonstrated against some strains, although significant strain variation in susceptibility was demonstrated.[49] Absorption following oral administration of 10 mg/kg BID was also demonstrated, with blood concentrations of about 0.25 to 0.85 μg/ml reported, with most horses being below 0.4 μg/ml at 30 minutes after treatment. Significant interindividual variability was demonstrated. These concentrations were effective for some, but not all, EHV-1 isolates *in vitro*.[49] Acyclovir has been used clinically at a dose of 20 mg/kg every 8 hours in one EHV-1 myeloencephalitis outbreak.[51] A clear benefit was not demonstrated in this outbreak, and the value of acyclovir in such situations remains unclear.

Anti-inflammatory drugs

The CNS is considered an "immune privileged site", in that response to infection and inflammation of the CNS is less robust than that noted in other tissues. This restriction upon the degree of inflammation likely has survival benefit. In the treatment of CNS infections and inflammation, therefore, control of inflammation is of paramount importance. Prostaglandins and thromboxanes are produced in the CNS in a number of clinical conditions, including seizures, inflammation, traumatic brain injury and cerebral vascular disease.[52,53] The relative concentrations of and ability to generate eicosanoids appear to vary depending upon the region of the CNS affected.[52] While this topic has not been evaluated in the horse, it is presumed that a similar increase in prostanoid products would be found. From the preceding observations, a number of nonsteroidal anti-inflammatory drugs (NSAIDs) have been recommended in neuroinflammatory disease.

Nonsteroidal anti-inflammatory drugs

The NSAIDs ibuprofen, aspirin and indomethacin increase survival in mice with Sandhoff's disease, an inflammatory neurodegenerative disorder,[54] and NSAIDs have a protective effect in Alzheimer's disease, in which chronic brain inflammation is a significant contributor to neuropathology.[55] These findings suggest that the NSAIDs should be useful in horses with neuroinflammation, as well as attenuating fever, myalgia and perhaps improving appetite. No specific recommendations can be made at this time, however, in regard to the specific NSAID to use or dosages. These should be determined on a case-by-case basis.

Corticosteroids

The use of corticosteroids in horses with neuroinflammation is controversial, as it is in people. Concern has been expressed regarding the potential for the immunosuppression associated with dexamethasone administration to allow infection to progress. However, it is well recognised that corticosteroids are effective in the treatment of cerebral oedema and that they attenuate tissue injury by inhibiting host mediators at several steps in the inflammatory process.[56] Extensive research has been conducted in humans and laboratory animals. In one study of bacterial meningitis in adults, treatment with dexamethasone was found to reduce the relative risk of death (0.48, 95% confidence interval 0.24–0.96, $P = .04$) when compared to placebo.[57] Another study found that the use of corticosteroids in human patients with bacterial meningitis reduced death, hearing loss and neurological sequelae.[58] A meta-analysis of randomised clinical trials also found that treatment with dexamethasone in people was beneficial and associated with low risk of side effects.[59] No comparable studies are reported in horses; however, it is assumed that the general beneficial effects upon cerebral inflammation would exist. In horses, the possible risk of laminitis associated with corticosteroid use must be considered and assessed on an individual case basis, although a short-term course of corticosteroids in horses with bacterial meningitis seems warranted.

The use of corticosteroids in viral disease is also controversial, although corticosteroids have been used successfully in people with West Nile Virus encephalitis[60] and have been proved beneficial in acute viral meningitis.[61] Furthermore, glucocorticoids have been found to be beneficial in people and experimental animals with herpes simplex encephalitis, and the use of glucocorticoids did not increase viral load.[62] In fact, in another study, the use of corticosteroids alone was associated with a reduction in viral load by 63% (±13%).[63] As in bacterial meningitis, similar studies have not been reported for equine viral encephalitis. However, these data suggest that the use of corticosteroids in horses with encephalitis is not contraindicated and may in fact be desirable. In horses with neurological deficits due to viral encephalitis that are severe enough to require hospitalisation, a short course of corticosteroids is probably indicated.

Dimethylsulphoxide

Another commonly used anti-inflammatory drug in horses is DMSO. It is commonly recommended for the treatment of horses with neuroinflammation. However, there is little to no controlled evaluation of its use in the horse. Clinical experience suggests that it does have an anti-inflammatory effect, but this is difficult to establish conclusively. There is, however, a large body of work describing the effects of DMSO in neurological disease in laboratory animal species, as well as its clinical use in humans. Calcium flux as a result of excitotoxic amine release is a well-recognised cause of neuronal cell death. It has been demonstrated that DMSO at clinical concentrations decreases excitotoxic cell death of neurons.[64] Further, DMSO has been shown to enhance the drug-induced blockade of calcium channels.[65] Intravenous DMSO at 1 mg/kg body weight, given as a 10% solution, has been shown to decrease intracranial pressure by 45% in a model of brain oedema in rabbits.[66] In addition, DMSO reduced neuronal cell death in an *in vivo* model of ischaemia-reperfusion.[67] It was further shown to rapidly decrease intracranial pressure in patients suffering head trauma[68] and improve cerebral perfusion pressure and neurological outcomes.[69] It is expected that horses would have a similar response to DMSO, and a dose of 0.5 to 1 g/kg as a 10 % solution (IV) 2 times per day is recommended in cases of anticipated neuroinflammation. The drug should not be given at greater than a 20% solution, as haemolysis can be seen at concentrations greater than this. Dosages of 4 g/kg IV were associated with toxic signs in three of six treated horses. Signs included muscle trembling, loose faeces and colic, and they abated quickly after cessation of the drug infusion.[70]

Cerebral oedema

Other compounds used to combat CNS oedema include mannitol and hypertonic saline. Hypertonic saline reduces cerebral oedema, apparently due to its hyperosmolar effects. Various concentrations of hypertonic saline have been investigated in cases of brain oedema, with improvement noted in intracranial pressure following treatment with as low as 1.8% NaCl.[71] The beneficial effects of hypertonic saline persist even when followed by normal crystalloid solutions[72] and appear to be due to its ability to draw water from the cell, decreasing tissue pressure.[72] The recommended dose of hypertonic saline for horses with head trauma is 4 to 6 ml/kg of 5% or 7% NaCl as a bolus,[73] which can then be followed by normal crystalloid solutions at a maintenance dose. Isotonic fluids should not be given to horses with head trauma at high dose rates, such as that used for circulatory shock, as this is likely to increase cerebral oedema and intracranial pressure.[74]

References

1. Moore BR, Reed SM, Biller DS, et al.: Assessment of vertebral canal diameter and bony malformations of the cervical part of the spine in horses with cervical stenotic myelopathy. Am J Vet Res 55:5-13, 1994
2. Mayhew IG, Whitlock RH, Tasker JB: Equine cerebrospinal fluid: reference values of normal horses. Am J Vet Res 38:1271-1274, 1977
3. Furr MO, Tyler RD: Cerebrospinal fluid creatine kinase activity in horses with central nervous system disease: 69 cases (1984-1989). J Am Vet Med Assoc 197:245-248, 1990
4. Green E, Constantinescu G, Kroll R: Equine cerebrospinal fluid: analysis. Compend Contin Educ Pract Vet 15:288-301, 1993
5. Furr M, Bender H: Cerebrospinal fluid variables in clinically normal foals from birth to 42 days of age. Am J Vet Res 55:781-784, 1994
6. Miller MM, Sweeney CR, Russell GE, et al.: Effects of blood contamination of cerebrospinal fluid on Western blot analysis for detection of antibodies against Sarcocystis neurona and on albumin quotient and immunoglobulin G index in horses. J Am Vet Med Assoc 215:67-71, 1999
7. Wamsley H, Alleman R, Porter M, et al.: Findings in cerebrospinal fluids of horses infected with West Nile virus: 30 cases (2001). J Am Vet Med Assoc 221:1303-1305, 2002
8. Mayhew IG: Large Animal Neurology. Philadelphia, Lea and Febiger, 1989
9. McClure JJ, Lindsey WA, Taylor W, et al.: Ataxia in four horses with equine anemia virus. J Am Vet Med Assoc 180:279-283, 1982
10. Raphel C: Brain abscess in three horses. J Am Vet Med Assoc 180:874-877, 1982
11. Foreman JH, Santschi E: Equine bacterial meningitis: part II. Compend Cont Educ Pract Vet 11:640-644, 1989
12. Mayhew IG, Brewer BD, Reinhard MK, et al.: Verminous (Strongylus vulgaris) myelitis in a donkey. Cornell Vet 74:30-37, 1984
13. Kjeldsberg C, Krieg A: Cerebrospinal fluid and other body fluids, in Henry J (ed): Clinical Diagnosis and Management by Laboratory Methods. Philadelphia, WB Saunders, 1984, pp 459-490
14. Jackson C, DeLahunta A, Divers TJ, et al.: The diagnostic utility of cerebrospinal fluid creatine kinase activity in the horse. J Vet Intern Med 10: 246-251, 1996
15. Lacombe VA, Podell M, Furr M, et al.: Diagnostic validity of electroencephalography in equine intracranial disorders. J Vet Intern Med 15:385-393, 2001
16. Muir W, Sams R, Huffman R, et al.: Pharmacodynamic and pharmacokinetic properties of diazepam in horses. Am J Vet Res 43:1756-1762, 1982
17. Norman W, Court M, Greenblatt M: Age-related changes in the pharmacokinetic disposition of diazepam in foals. Am J Vet Res 58:878-880, 1997
18. Melsom M, Andreassen P, Melsom H: Diazepam in acute myocardial infarction, clinical effects and effects on catecholamine, free fatty acids and cortisol. Br Heart Jr 38:804-810, 1976
19. Duran S, Ravis W, Pedersoli W, et al.: Pharmacokinetics of phenobarbitol in the horse. Am J Vet Res 48:807-810, 1987
20. Andrews F, Mathews H: Seizures, narcolepsy, and cataplexy, in Reed S, Bayly W (eds): Equine Internal Medicine. Philadelphia, WB Saunders, 1998, pp 451-457
21. Ravis W, Duran S, Pedersoli W, et al.: A pharmacokinetic study of phenobarbital in mature horses after oral dosing. J Vet Pharmacol Ther 10:283-289, 1987

22. Knox D, Ravis W, Pedersoli W, et al.: Pharmacokinetics of phenobarbital in horses after single and repeated oral administration of the drug. Am J Vet Res 53:706-710, 1992
23. Mitchell E, Mackenzie H, Furr M: Bacterial meningitis in five mature horses. Equine Vet Educ 18:249-255, 2006
24. Rumbaugh G: Disseminated septic meningitis in a mare. J Am Vet Med Assoc 171:452-454, 1977
25. Barling R: The penetration of antibiotics into cerebrospinal fluid and brain tissue. J Antimicrobial Chemother 4:203-227, 1978
26. Thea D: Use of antibacterial agents in infections of the central nervous system. Infect Dis Clin North Am 3:553-570, 1989
27. Ringger N, Pearson E, Gronwall R, et al.: Pharmacokinetics of ceftriaxone in healthy horses. Equine Vet J 28:476-479, 1996
28. Morris D, Rutkowski J, Lloyd K: Therapy in two cases of neonatal foal septicemia and meningitis with cefotaxime sodium. Equine Vet J 19:151-154, 1987
29. Thomas E, Allan M, Boettner A: Pharmacokinetics of cefquinome in porcine cerebrospinal fluid. Proceedings of the International Pig Veterinary Society, Ames, IA, June 2-5. 2002
30. Page S: Chloramphenicol, 3: clinical pharmacology of systemic use in the horse. Aust Vet J 68:5-8, 1991
31. Friedman C: Chloramphenicol disposition in infants and children. J Pediatr 95:1071-1077, 1979
32. Gronwall R, Brown M, Merritt A, et al.: Body fluid concentrations and pharmacokinetics of chloramphenicol given to mares intravenously or by repeated gavage. Am J Vet Res 47:2591-2595, 1986
33. Brown M, Kelly R, Gronwall R, et al.: Chloramphenicol sodium succinate in the horse: serum, synovial, peritoneal and urine concentrations after single-dose intravenous administration. Am J Vet Res 45:578-580, 1984
34. Brumbaugh G, Martens R, Knight H, et al.: Pharmacokinetics of chloramphenicol in the neonatal horse. J Vet Pharmacol Ther 6:219-227, 1983
35. Knight H: Antimicrobial agents used in the horse. Proc Annu Meet Am Assoc Equine Pract 21:131-145, 1975
36. Brown M, Gronwall R, Castro L: Pharmacokinetic and body fluid and endometrial concentrations of trimethoprim-sulfamethoxazole in mares. Am J Vet Res 49:918-922, 1988
37. Levitz R Quintaliani R: Trimethoprim-sulfamethoxazole for bacterial meningitis. Ann Intern Med 100:881-890, 1984
38. Dudley M, Levitz R, Quintaliani R, et al.: Pharmacokinetics of trimethoprim-sulfamethoxazole in serum and cerebrospinal fluid of adult patients with normal meninges. Antimicrob Agents Chemother 26:811-814, 1984
39. Brown M, Gronwall R, Houston E: Pharmacokinetics and body fluid and endometrial concentrations of ormetoprim-sulfadimethoxine in mares. Can J Vet Res 53:12-16, 1989
40. Cottagnoud P, Tauber M: Fluoroquinolones in the treatment of meningitis. Curr Infect Dis Rep 5:329-336, 2003
41. Neer T: Clinical pharmacologic features of fluoroquinolone antimicrobial drugs. J Am Vet Med Assoc 193:577-580, 1988
42. Giguère S, Sweeney R, Belanger M: Pharmacokinetics of enrofloxacin in adult horses and concentration of the drug in serum, body fluids, and endometrial tissues after repeated intragastrically administered doses. Am J Vet Res 57:1025-1030, 1996
43. Farr M: Rifampin. Med Clin North Am 66:157-168, 1982
44. Anonymous: Metronidazole, in McEvoy G (ed): AHFS Drug Information. Bethesda, MD, American Society of Health System Pharmacists, 2004, pp 848-857
45. Bryant J, Brown M, Gronwall R, et al.: Study of intragastric administration of doxycyline: pharmacokinetics including body fluid, endometrial and minimum inhibitory concentrations. Equine Vet J 32:233-238, 2000
46. Nau R: Pharmacokinetic optimization of the treatment of bacterial central nervous system infections. Clin Pharmacokinet 35:223-246, 1998
47. Corpus K, Weber K, Zimmerman C: Intrathecal amikacin for the treatment of pseudomonal meningitis. Ann Pharmacother 38:992-995, 2004
48. Matsubara H, Makimoto A, Higa T, et al.: Successful treatment of meningoencephalitis caused by methicillin-resistant *Staphylococcus aureus* with intrathecal vancomycin in an allogenic peripheral blood stem cell transplant recipient. Bone Marrow Transplant 31:65-67, 2003
49. Wilkins PA, Papich M, Sweeney RW: Pharmacokinetics of acyclovir in adult horses. J Vet Emerg Crit Care 15:174-178, 2005
50. Rollinson R, White G: Relative activities of acyclovir and BW 759 against Aujeskys disease and equine rhinopneumonitis viruses. Antimicrob Agents Chemother 24:221-226, 1983
51. Friday P, Scarrat W, Elvinger P, et al.: Ataxia and paresis with equine herpesvirus type 1 infection in a herd of riding school horses. J Vet Intern Med 14:197-201, 2000
52. Wolfe L, Horrocks L: Eicosenoids, in Siegel C, et al. (eds): Basic Neurochemistry. New York, Raven Press, 1994, pp 475-490
53. Boje K, Jaworowicz D, Raybon J: Neuroinflammatory role of prostaglandins during experimental meningitis: evidence suggestive of an in vivo relationship between nitric oxide and prostaglandins. J Pharmacol Exp Ther 304:319-325, 2003
54. Jeyakumar M, Smith D, Williams I, et al.: NSAIDs increase survival in the Sandhoff disease: synergy with N-butyldeoxynorimycin. Ann Neurol 57:642-649, 2004
55. Scali C, Prosperi C, Vannucchi M, et al.: Brain inflammatory reaction in an animal model of neuronal degeneration and its modulation by an anti-inflammatory drug: implications in Alzheimer's disease. Eur J Neurosci 12:1900-1912, 2000
56. Jafari H, McCracken G: Dexamethasone therapy in bacterial meningitis. Pediatr Ann 23:82-88, 1994
57. de Gans J, van de Beek D: Dexamethasone in adults with bacterial meningitis. N Engl J Med 347:1549-1556, 2002
58. Morris A: Review: adjuvant corticosteroid therapy reduces death, hearing loss, and neurologic sequelae in bacterial meningitis. Evid Based Med 9:48, 2004
59. McIntyre P, Berkey C, King S, et al.: Dexamethasone as adjunctive treatment in bacterial meningitis. A meta-analysis of randomized clinical trials since 1988. JAMA 278:925-931, 1997
60. Pyrgos V, Younus F: High-dose steroids in the management of acute flaccid paralysis due to West Nile virus infection. Scand J Infect Dis 36:509-512, 2004
61. Nakano A, Yamasaki R, Miyazaki S, et al.: Beneficial effect of steroid pulse therapy on acute viral encephalitis. Eur Neurol 50:225-229, 2003
62. Meyding-Lamande U, Oberlinner C, Seyfer S, et al.: Experimental herpes simplex virus encephalitis: a combination

therapy of acyclovir and glucocorticoids reduces long-term magnetic resonance imaging abnormalities. J Neurovirol 9:118-125, 2003

63. Thompson K, Blessing W, Wesselingh S: Herpes simplex replication and dissemination is not increased by corticosteroid treatment in a rat model of focal herpes encephalitis. J Neurovirol 6:25-32, 2000
64. Lu C, Mattson M: Dimethyl sulfoxide suppresses NMDA and AMPA-induced ion currents and calcium influx and protects against excitotoxic death in hippocampal neurons. Exp Neurol 170:180-185, 2001
65. Wu L, Karpinski E, Wang R, et al.: Modification by solvents of the action of nifedipine on calcium channel currents in neuroblastoma cells. Naunyn Schmiedebergs Arch Pharmacol 345:478-484, 1992
66. James H, Camp P, Harbaugh R, et al.: Comparison of the effects of DMSO and pentobarbitone on experimental brain oedema. Acta Neurochir 60:245-255, 1982
67. Phillis J, Estevez A, O'Regan M: Protecxtive effects of the free radical scavengers, dimethyl sulfoxide and ethanol, in cerebral ischemia in gerbils. Neurosci Lett 244:109-111, 1998
68. Karaca M, Bilgin U, Akar M, et al.: Dimethyl sulfoxide lowers ICP after closed head trauma. Eur J Pharmacol 40:113-114, 1991
69. Kulah A, Akar M, Baykut L: Dimethyl sulfoxide in the management of patients with brain swelling and increased intracranial pressure after severe closed head injury. Neurochirurgica 33:177-180, 1990
70. Appell L, Blythe L, Lassen E, et al.: Adverse effects of rapid intravenous DMSO administration in horses. J Equine Vet Sci 12:215-218, 1992
71. Shackford S, Zhuang J, Schmoker J: Intravenous fluid tonicity: effect on intracranial pressure, cerebral blood flow, and cerebral oxygen delivery in focal brain injury. J Neurosurg 74:43-48, 1992
72. Gunnar W, Jonasson O, Merlotti G: Head injury and haemorrhagic shock: studies of the blood brain barrier and intracranial pressure after resuscitation with normal saline solution, 3% saline solution and dextran-40. Surgery 103:398-402, 1988
73. Bertone J: Hypertonic saline in the management of shock in horses. Compend Cont Educ Pract Vet 13:665-670, 1991
74. Crowe D: Triage and trauma management, in Murtaugh R, Kaplan P (eds): Veterinary Emergency and Critical Care Medicine. St. Louis, Mosby-Year Book, 1992, p 77

15

Monitoring and treating common musculoskeletal problems in hospitalised horses

15.1 Monitoring the musculoskeletal system
15.2 Laminitis
15.3 Biochemical monitoring of the muscles
15.4 Management of rhabdomyolysis and myopathy
15.5 Monitoring horses with implants
15.6 Monitoring surgical incisions
15.7 Ultrasonography of surgical incisions
15.8 Management of surgical site infections
15.9 External coaptation (splinting)
15.10 Application of casts

15.1 Monitoring the musculoskeletal system

Louise L. Southwood

Patients at risk of developing musculoskeletal disorders during hospitalisation

Musculoskeletal disorders can develop in hospitalised horses as a result of their primary illness, general anaesthesia or treatment or as a complication of being confined to a stall. Some of the more serious musculoskeletal disorders that can develop in hospitalised horses include laminitis/founder, septic arthritis, rhabdomyolysis, vascular thrombosis as well as specific complications associated with surgery, bandages and casts. Patients that are at an increased risk of developing these complications include draft breeds, geriatric horses and neonatal foals. Horses with colic, diarrhoea or primary musculoskeletal diseases or that have previously had problems are also at increased risk. Horses having undergone musculoskeletal surgery and horses with bandages or casts should be monitored particularly closely for complications associated with the primary disease or arising as a result of bandaging or casting.

Patients at risk of laminitis and founder

Laminitis is inflammation of the digital laminae. *Founder* is the term used in the United States to describe when the hoof begins to fail mechanically. There appear to be two general mechanisms of laminitis in hospitalised horses:

1. Local mechanical (support-limb)
2. Systemic or metabolic disease (bilateral or quadrilateral)

Any horse that has a non–weight-bearing lameness is predisposed to developing support-limb laminitis in the contra-lateral hoof. Types of lesions that would predispose horses to support-limb laminitis include septic arthritis, bursitis, or tenosynovitis, flexor tendon lacerations, osteomyelitis or osteitis and complicated long-bone fractures. Horses that are reluctant to lie down are especially prone to develop support-limb laminitis. The duration of lameness is associated with the risk of developing support-limb laminitis.[1] Body weight is not a risk factor for the development of support-limb laminitis.[1] Any horse that is hospitalised for a musculoskeletal problem should be monitored for signs of laminitis (see later). While foals do not develop support-limb laminitis, they may develop carpal or tarsal varus as a consequence of prolonged unilateral weight-bearing.

Bilateral fore limb and/or hind limb laminitis can develop in any critically ill horse. Endotoxaemia has been shown experimentally to cause laminitis via digital hypoperfusion[2,3] induced by release of 5-hydroxytryptamine (5-HT), thromboxane (TX)A_2 and TXB_2, from white cells, platelets and endothelial cells.[2] Therefore, any disease process that causes endotoxaemia will predispose the horse to laminitis. Endotoxin is released from Gram-negative bacteria during rapid proliferation or death and any horse with a Gram-negative infection or disruption of the gastrointestinal tract barrier function could develop laminitis. More recently, the role of Gram-positive bacteria exotoxin in systemic inflammatory response syndrome (SIRS) and the development of laminitis has been investigated, with *in vitro* demonstration of a laminar inflammatory response and destruction.[4] In critically ill horses, laminitis can occur as a consequence of SIRS and may be one manifestation of multiple organ dysfunction syndrome (MODS).[5] There have been several vascular and "laminitic trigger factors" proposed to be involved in the development of laminitis in critically ill horses, particularly septic horses and horses with gastrointestinal tract disease; however, the exact role of these factors in clinical patients is still unknown.[6]

Predisposition to laminitis

Specific lesions that predispose to laminitis are listed in Box 15.1. The general incidence of laminitis in horses undergoing abdominal surgery was 1% (3 of 311 horses),[11] and in horses with duodenitis-proximal jejunitis (DPJ) or colitis, approximately 30%.[7,8] Horses with DPJ that were particularly predisposed to developing laminitis had a body weight greater or equal to 550 kg and haemorrhagic reflux at admission.[7] In the latter study,[7] treatment with heparin decreased the occurrence of laminitis (heparin-treated, 0 of 12 [0%]; no heparin, 31 of 104 [30%]); however, other studies have failed to demonstrate a benefit of heparin treatment in laminitis prevention.[13] Similarly, draft horses were more predisposed compared to non–draft horses to developing complications of laminitis associated with retained foetal membranes.[12] Horses that were between 5 to 7 years old and between 13 to 31 years of age were more likely to develop acute laminitis compared to horses younger than 5 years.[14] Mares were more likely than geldings to develop acute laminitis, and non–Quarter Horse/non–Thoroughbred horses were more likely to develop laminitis compared to Quarter Horses or Thoroughbreds.[14] Compared to Thoroughbreds, Quarter Horses and ponies were more likely to develop acute laminitis.[14] Interestingly, neonatal foals, although often suffering from sepsis and predisposed to gastrointestinal tract disruption, do not appear to be susceptible to laminitis.

Glucocorticoids appear to predispose horses to developing laminitis, and various mechanisms have been proposed for the association between glucocorticoids and laminitis.[5] Horses with excessive endogenous glucocorticoid release (Cushing's disease, pituitary pars intermedia dysfunction)[5] and horses administered exogenous corticosteroids appear to be predisposed to developing laminitis.[5] Additionally, laminitis has also been associated with middle-aged obese horses with "equine metabolic syndrome".[15] However, the vascular and metabolic aberrations leading to laminitis in these horses are likely to be due to hyperinsulinaemia and abnormal glucose regulation rather than excessive endogenous glucocorticoids.[15] While the association between laminitis and Cushing's syndrome has been demonstrated, the association with exogenous corticosteroid administration is controversial and studies have failed to induce laminitis with corticosteroid administration.[5,16] Any overweight (equine metabolic syndrome) or geriatric (pituitary pars intermedia dysfunction) horse or horse receiving exogenous corticosteroids should be monitored closely for signs of laminitis. Particular attention should be paid to horses with a previous history of laminitis[15] and owners or trainers should be questioned regarding this at the time of hospital admission.

Box 15.1. Specific lesions associated with laminitis

- Duodenitis-proximal jejunitis (anterior enteritis)[7]
- Colitis[8]
    - particularly Potomac horse fever[9,10]
- Horses having undergone abdominal surgery[11]
- Mares with retained foetal membranes and metritis postpartum[12]

Patients at risk of septic arthritis

The most common causes of septic arthritis in horses are articular wounds, inoculation during intra-articular injection, postsurgical infection, haematogenous localisation and idiopathic.[17] Therefore, patients with trauma, who undergo lameness workup or who have evidence of a systemic bacterial disease should be monitored closely for signs of septic arthritis.

Monitoring for signs of septic arthritis is particularly important in hospitalised neonatal foals. It is important to always remember that septic arthritis is the most common cause of lameness in foals.[18] Septic arthritis is the cause of death in 12.5% of foals between 8 and 31 days of age.[19] The occurrence rate of this disease in foals with failure of passive transfer is extremely high (78%).[20] Neonatal foals with failure of passive transfer and sepsis are particularly prone to develop septic arthritis and osteomyelitis, and this can occur hours to days following the onset of signs of sepsis.[18] Foals with higher sepsis scores had more joint infections compared to foals with lower sepsis scores.[21] Septic arthritis and osteomyelitis is a result of localisation of bacteria from the blood (septicaemia) in the synovial membrane (type S), epiphyseal subchondral bone (type E), metaphyseal aspect of the physis (type P) or tarsal/carpal bones in premature foals (type T).[18] Because of the presence of functional transphyseal vessels in young foals (<7 days of age), type S and E infections usually occur in these patients. Older foals (>10 days of age) are more likely to develop type P infection.[18,22] Sources of bacteria in septicaemia are listed in Box 15.2.

Other types of hospitalised horses that are predisposed to the development of septic arthritis are postoperative arthroscopy and trauma cases. Interestingly, the carpal joint is most commonly infected postoperatively.[17] The fetlock joint is the joint most commonly affected by trau-

Box 15.2. Sources of bacteria in septicaemia

- Gastrointestinal tract
- Respiratory tract
- Umbilicus
- Accidental or iatrogenic trauma

matic wounds.[17] In equine arthroscopy patients, the infection rate is very low (0.08%)[23]; however, these patients should still be monitored closely for any signs of infection postoperatively. Horses that are admitted to the hospital with a laceration involving a joint, bursa or sheath, or because of septic synovitis, should be monitored for the signs of worsening or recrudescence of the infection.

Patients at risk of other musculoskeletal disorders

Myopathies

Horses under going general anaesthesia are predisposed to developing rhabdomyolysis (tying-up). With improved anaesthetic, surgical and recovery techniques, complications associated with rhabdomyolysis are becoming less common. Other types of musculoskeletal injuries associated with general anaesthesia include fracture, neuropathy/myopathy and ligamentous injury. In one study,[24] the overall mortality rate for horses undergoing general anaesthesia between 1991 and 1994 was 6.7% (including euthanasia because of a poor prognosis associated with the primary disease), with 32% of deaths attributed to fractures or myopathies. The occurrence rate of postanaesthetic myopathy following arthroscopic surgery was 0.66% and was correlated with the duration of general anaesthesia.[25] Myopathies/neuropathies are diagnosed based on physical examination with the horse being unable to bear weight and collapsing on the affected limb. Myopathies/neuropathies can generally be managed with phenylbutazone, dimethylsulphoxide (DMSO) and by splinting the limb.

Thrombophlebitis

Rarely, horses can develop signs of lameness associated with a thrombophlebitis or arteritis. Horses with signs of endotoxaemia and coagulopathy are predisposed to this type of lesions. Clinical signs include an acute onset of severe lameness. Ultrasound examination can be used to confirm the diagnosis as shown in Figures 15.1, A and B.

Bandage- or cast-related problems

Horses in bandages or casts are predisposed to develop complications. Horses in casts should be monitored for any signs of lameness, and the cast limb should be monitored at least twice daily for signs of swelling proximal to the cast and drainage from the cast. If there are signs of lameness, the limb should be undergo radiography to determine if there has been further bone damage or damage to the fracture repair. The decision to remove the cast should be based on the degree and suspected cause of lameness. Complications associated with bandages are less common compared to casts. Tendinitis or peritendinitis ("bandage bow") can occur as a complication of bandaging too tight or unevenly or from the bandage slipping. An ultrasound examination should be performed on any horse that has swelling and/or lameness following removal of a bandage. Bandages that slip or are applied inappropriately can also cause pressure necrosis of the skin over bony prominences such as the accessory carpal bone or of other areas of skin.

Confinement

Horses that are confined to a stall for prolonged periods of time without walking can develop distal limb oedema ("stocking up"). Distal limb oedema is associated with a lack of venous and lymphatic drainage as a result of relative immobility and is usually a benign musculoskeletal problem. Regular walking and distal limb bandages can be used to manage distal limb oedema.

Monitoring lameness in the hospitalised horse

Hospitalised horses should be evaluated at least twice daily for signs of lameness. The horse should be observed from

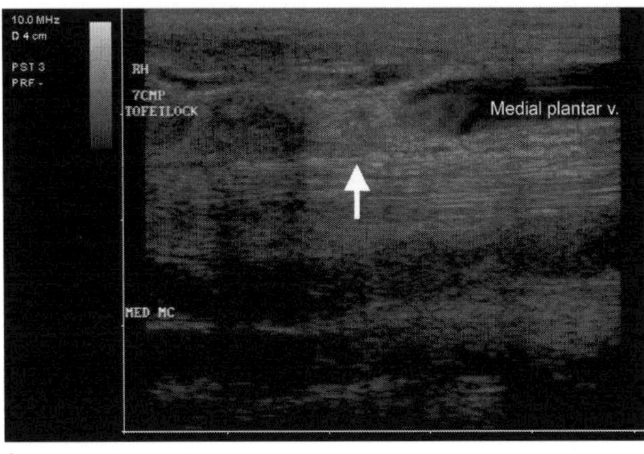

A

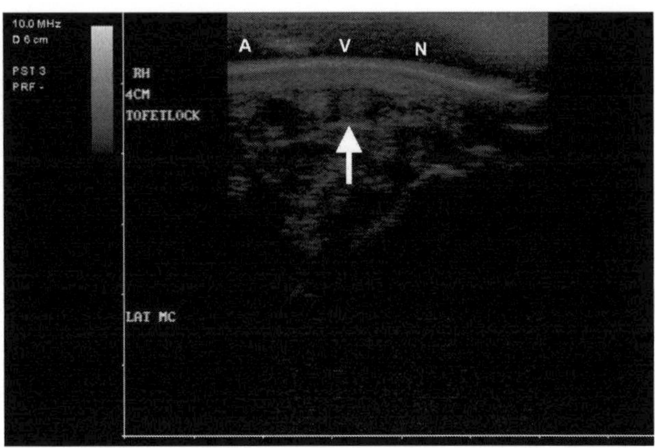

B

Figures 15.1A-B Ultrasonographic image of a thrombosed medial plantar artery (arrow). (15.1A) Longitudinal and (15.1B) cross-sectional image. The horse had had abdominal surgery for correction of a large colon volvulus and had developed an acute severe lameness in the right hindlimb. Ultrasound examination was used to confirm the diagnosis of thrombophlebitis. a = artery, v = vein, n = nerve. Image provided by Dr. Diana Short, New Bolton Center, University of Pennsylvania. © Dr. Diana Short 2006.

outside the stall for changes in stance, weight shifting between limbs, holding one limb forward or backward and signs of lameness. Lameness examination should consist of walking the horse around the stall in circles toward the left and right as well as walking forward and backward. Depending on the horse's problem, the horse can also be walked up and down the hospital isle to identify any new lameness or changes in existing lameness. Usually, the clinician is looking for obvious signs of lameness in hospitalised horses (i.e., lame at a walk or non–weight-bearing lame). If signs of lameness are observed, the cause should be localised within the limb using physical examination and occasionally peripheral nerve blocks. Hoof testers should always be applied to the hoof of any horse with unexplained lameness. Once the lameness has been localised, radiographic and ultrasonographic examination can be performed to obtain a diagnosis and to determine the degree of damage. Laboratory analysis of synovial fluid and blood is useful in cases suspected of having infection. Rarely, more sophisticated imaging modalities such as nuclear scintigraphy, computerised tomography or magnetic resonance imaging are needed.

Physical examination

Physical examination of the musculoskeletal system should always begin with the hoof. The hooves should be palpated for an increase in warmth and the coronary band palpated for swelling or softening. The digital pulses should be palpated and any increases compared to normal noted. If laminitis is suspected based on findings of bilateral or quadrilateral lameness and/or an increase in hoof warmth and digital pulses compared to normal, a more thorough examination should be performed (see Chapter 15.2.1). Other causes of lameness associated with the hoof that can develop in hospitalised horses include abscessation and fracture of the third phalanx (P_3 or coffin bone). Clinical signs associated with these causes of lameness are usually unilateral, and a diagnosis can be made using hoof testers, examination of the sole and radiographs.

The fore and hind limbs should be examined and palpated for signs of heat, pain or swelling. In particular, the joints and sheaths should be palpated for synovial effusion and the flexor tendons for swelling and pain that may be associated with tendonitis. If the limb is bandaged, palpation should be performed when the bandage is changed. Radiography and synoviocentesis (see "Synoviocentesis and cytological evaluation of synovial effusion") should be performed on any horse predisposed to septic arthritis or tenosynovitis with an acute onset of moderate to severe lameness and synovial effusion. Radiography and ultrasonography should be performed on any horse with swelling and pain associated with tendons or other nonspecific areas. The muscles, particularly the gluteal and lumbar muscles, should be palpated for firmness in any horse showing signs of stiffness or an abnormal gait that is predisposed to rhabdomyolysis.

Horses or foals that are predisposed to developing septic synovitis should be monitored closely for lameness, synovial effusion and periarticular oedema, heat and pain. Rectal temperature, total white cell count, differential white cell count and fibrinogen should be also be monitored. Often, horses with septic arthritis or osteomyelitis will have a mild fever, leucocytosis, neutrophilia and hyperfibrinogenaemia. If the horse has had arthroscopic surgery, the surgical site should be checked regularly for swelling, pain, redness, drainage and wound dehiscence. In horses with lacerations involving synovial structures, following the initial wound repair and joint lavage, the horse should be treated with parenteral antimicrobials and a low dose of phenylabutazone so that early signs of worsening lameness can be detected. The wound and affected synovial structure should also be evaluated, at the time that the bandage is changed, for signs of infection.

Monitoring the joints in neonatal foals

Foals with failure of passive transfer or sepsis should be monitored at least every 6 hours for signs of septic arthritis. Early signs may be subtle in foals and include mild periarticular oedema and stiffness and difficulty or reluctance to rise. All joints should be examined for periarticular swelling, synovial effusion, pain on palpation or flexion, and heat. Because multiple joints are commonly affected (50% of cases),[17] it is critical to assess and monitor all joints. If the foal is showing signs of lameness and there is no obvious synovial effusion, arthrocentesis of the shoulder, elbow or hip joints should be considered (see "Synoviocentesis and cytological evaluation of synovial effusion").[18] Femorotibial joint effusion may not be obvious in many cases. The medial femorotibial joint usually communicates with the femoropatellar joint; therefore, femoropatellar joint effusion is usually present in cases of sepsis involving the medial femorotibial joint. Lateral femorotibial joint effusion, however, may be more difficult to palpate. In some cases, lateral femorotibial joint effusion may be associated with effusion of the long digital extensor pouch.[18] Swollen joints should undergo radiography to look for signs of bone lysis as an indication of osteomyelitis. Ultrasonography can also be performed to look for an increase in the amount or echogenicity of synovial fluid, as well as the presence of periarticular oedema, cellulitis and osteomyelitis. If the joint is thought to be septic, arthrocentesis should be performed (see "Synoviocentesis and cytological evaluation of synovial effusion"). Measurement of fibrinogen can also provide evidence of development of osteomyelitis; foals with osteomyelitis can have a fibrinogen concentration > 9 g/L (>900 mg/dl) (J. E. Palmer, personal communication). Other diagnostic tests that can be used to localise sepsis include nuclear scintigraphy using either technetium-99m oxidronate, white cells, or ciprofloxacin; magnetic resonance imaging; and computed tomography.

Synoviocentesis ("joint tap") and cytological evaluation of joint fluid

Synoviocentesis (arthocentesis) is most commonly performed in hospitalised horses to evaluate septic joints, sheaths or bursae. Synoviocentesis should be performed when there is moderate to severe lameness (grade 4/5 to 5/5) that can be localised to a particular joint based on the presence of synovial effusion, peri-articular oedema or cellulitis, heat, redness and pain on palpation or flexion. It is also indicated in any horse that has a wound in close proximity to a joint, sheath or bursa. Radiographic and/or ultrasonographic examination should be performed prior to synoviocentesis to assess the joint for signs of intra-articular gas, boney abnormalities or a change in the echogenicity of the synovial fluid.

Synoviocentesis should always be performed aseptically and atraumatically. Adult horses can be restrained with a halter and lead-rope, with a twitch, in stocks or by using sedation (xylazine 0.3–0.4 mg/kg IV and butorphanol 0.01–0.02 mg/kg IV), and foals can be restrained by holding the limbs and head and sedated with butorphanol (0.01–0.1 mg/kg IV or IM) or diazepam (0.1–0.2 mg/kg IV). While there is evidence that the arthrocentesis site can be adequately prepared without clipping the hair,[26] it is recommended to clip and aseptically prepare the arthrocentesis site. The equipment needed is listed in Box 15.3.

When there is a wound associated with the synovial structure, it is useful to have a 20- to 60-ml syringe with sterile isotonic fluid available to distend the joint and assess communication between the wound and synovial structure following joint fluid collection. If the synovial structure is likely to be infected and standing lavage performed, it is best to be prepared to lavage following synovial fluid collection. The synovial structure can be lavaged with 1 to 6 L of polyionic isotonic fluid. Therefore, in addition to the previous mentioned supplies, you will need a bag of sterile polyionic isotonic fluid, fluid pump or pressurising bag, drip set, and extension tubing. Synoviocentesis should be performed with an 18-gauge 3.75-cm (1.5-inch) needle because a smaller needle may not yield adequate fluid, particularly if there is a high concentration of fibrin or white cells. Antimicrobials, such as amikacin (500 mg), are usually placed in the joint, sheath or bursa following collection of synovial fluid or lavage (see Chapter 16).

It is important to learn multiple sites for synoviocentesis for each joint. Often a wound is near a site commonly used for synoviocentesis, and if this occurs, an alternate site should be used. Additionally, when lavaging a joint, an ingress-egress technique is used, and having needles inserted at sites on the medial and lateral and/or dorsal/cranial and palmar/plantar/caudal aspect of the joint will facilitate the lavage.

Box 15.3. Equipment for synoviocentesis

Required:
Clippers with a fine (#40) blade
Small gauze swabs (4 ± 4) soaked in chlorhexidine* or povidone iodine solution
Small gauze swabs (4 ± 4) soaked in surgical spirit (alcohol)
Sterile surgery gloves
18- or 16- gauge 3.75 cm (1.5 inch) needle
2–10 ml syringes
Collection tube containing EDTA for cytological analysis
Sterile collection tube for protein analysis and bacteriological culture

If there is an associated wound:
20- to 60 ml syringe containing sterile saline

Optional:
Sedation
Twitch
Stocks to restrain the horse

*Hibiscrub, Mölnlycke Health Care, Dunstable, UK.

Distal interphalangeal joint (coffin joint)

Synoviocentesis of the distal interphalangeal (coffin) joint can be performed with the limb in a weight-bearing position using a dorsal or lateral approach.[27] The dorsal aspect of the joint is approached by inserting a needle 1 to 1.5 cm proximal to the hoof wall just above the palpable edge of the coronary cushion and 1 cm lateral or medial to the long axis of the limb at a 90° angle to the ground and at a 45° angle to the sagittal plane (Figure 15.2, A). The needle can also be inserted on midline at a 90° angle to the ground. The needle is inserted less than 3.8 cm to enter the joint.[27] Alternatively, the coffin joint can be approached laterally. For the lateral approach, the needle is inserted above the collateral cartilages of the hoof, midway between the dorsal and palmar/plantar aspect of the second phalanx (P_2) and angled toward the centre of the frog[27] (Figure 15.2, B). This approach can also be easily performed with the limb in a non–weight-bearing position.

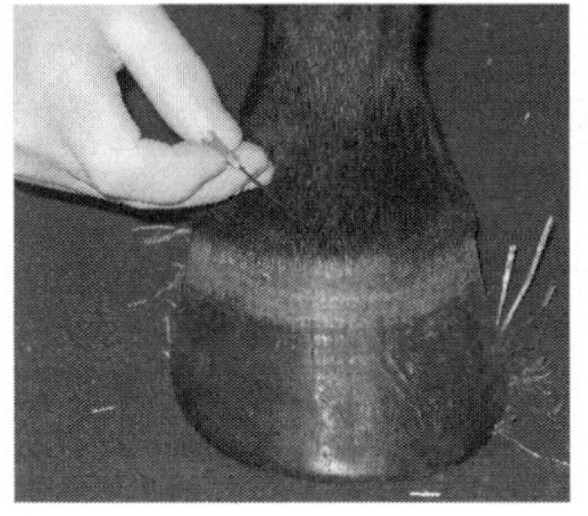
A

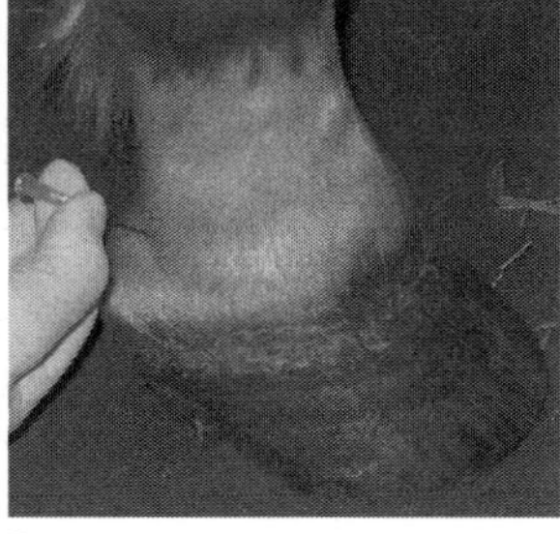
B

Figures 15.2A-B Approaches to the coffin joint for synoviocentesis. (15.2A) Dorsal and (15.2B) lateral approach. © Louise Southwood 2006.

Proximal interphalangeal joint (pastern joint)

The proximal interphalangeal (pastern) joint can also be approached from a dorsal or palmar/plantar site.[27] The dorsal approach is most easily made with the limb in a weight-bearing position. The palpable eminence on the first phalanx (P_1; boney prominence in the pastern region) is palpated and the needle inserted about 1 cm distal to the palpable eminence on the dorsal aspect of the limb. The needle can be positioned parallel to the ground at a 90° angle to the sagittal plane and is inserted deep to the common digital extensor tendon (Figure 15.3, A). The needle can also be inserted on midline at a 90° angle to the ground. Alternatively, the pastern joint can be approached using a palmar/plantar approach with the horse in a non–weight-bearing (slightly flexed) position. The plantar/palmar P_2 eminence is palpated and the needle is inserted immediately proximal to the eminence and dorsal to the deep flexor tendon (Figure 15.3, B).

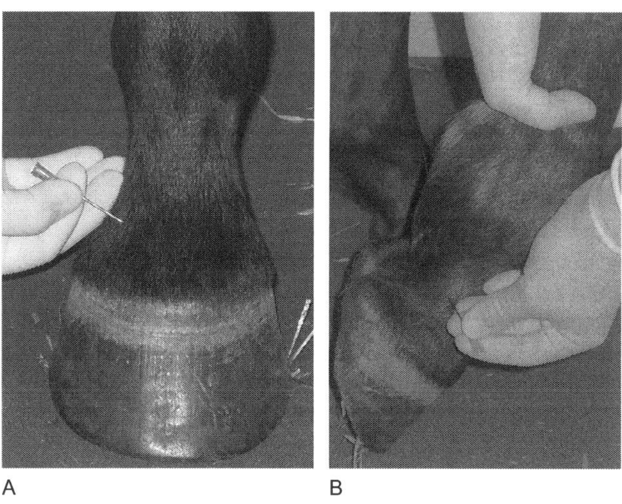

Figures 15.3A-B Approaches to the pastern joint for synoviocentesis. (15.3A) Dorsal and (15.3B) lateral approach. © Louise Southwood 2006.

Metacarpophalangeal joint (fetlock joint)

The metacarpophalangeal (fetlock) joint can be approached using several techniques.[27] The lateral approach, through the collateral sesamoidean ligaments that is commonly used for fetlock joint injections, is not practical for assessing the communication between the fetlock joint and a wound or for joint lavage because the limb needs to be maintained in flexion. Fetlock joint approaches that can be used with the limb in a weight-bearing or near weight-bearing position are the proximal and distal palmar/plantar pouch and dorsal pouch approaches. A proximal palmar/plantar pouch approach to the fetlock joint is made immediately palmar/plantar to the third metacarpus/metatarsus (MC III/MT III), dorsal to the suspensory ligament, distal to the palpable ends of the splint bones (MC/MT II or IV) and proximal to the proximal sesamoid bones and collateral sesamoidean ligaments The needle is inserted at a 90° angle to the limb. (Figure 15.4, A). The proximal palmar/plantar pouch is commonly distended with synovial fluid and easily palpated. The landmarks for the distal palmar/plantar pouch approach are the distal aspect of the sesamoid bones and the palmar/plantar eminence of the first phalanx (P_1). Using this approach, synoviocentesis should be performed with the limb in a weight-bearing position and either dorsal or palmar/plantar to the palmar/plantar digital vessels. The needle should be inserted with the point directed slightly dorsad and proximad to enter the joint (Figure 15.4, B). Alternatively, if there is considerable effusion, the fetlock joint can be approached by inserting a needle in the dorsal pouch (Figure 15.4, C).

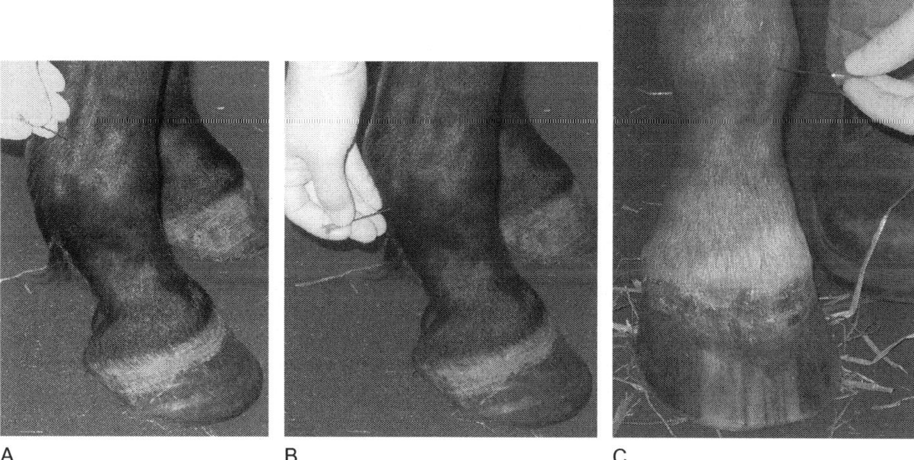

Figures 15.4A-C Approaches to the fetlock joint for synoviocentesis. (15.4A) Proximal palmar/plantar pouch, (15.4B) distal palmar/plantar, and (15.4C) dorsal approaches. © Louise Southwood 2006.

Carpal joints

Synoviocentesis of the carpal joints is generally easy to perform. The cranial approach to the radiocarpal or middle carpal joint, which communicates with the carpometacarpal joint, is performed with the carpus flexed (flexion may not be necessary if there is a large volume of synovial fluid) and the needle is inserted in the palpable space between the carpal bones either medial or lateral to the extensor carpi radialis tendon (Figure 15.5, A). The medial approach may be easier because the common digital extensor tendon results in a smaller space on the lateral aspect of the joint. The carpal joints can also be approached from the caudolateral aspect with the limb in a weight-bearing position. Using a caudolateral approach for the radiocarpal joint, the depression between the distal end of the vestigial ulna (lateral distal aspect of the radius) and the ulna carpal bone is palpated. The needle is inserted perpendicular to the skin at this site[27] (Figure 15.5, B). The middle carpal joint can also be approached from a caudolateral site palmar to the ulnar carpal bone proximally and the fourth carpal bone distally[27] (Figure 15.5, C).

Tibiotarsal, intertarsal and tarsometatarsal joints (hock joints)

The tibiotarsal joint is also easily approached for synoviocentesis, particularly if it is distended. Synoviocentesis of the tibiotarsal joint is performed with the limb in a weight-bearing position by inserting the needle on either side of the saphenous vein into the medial aspect of the dorsal pouch (Figure 15.6, A). The dorsal pouch of the

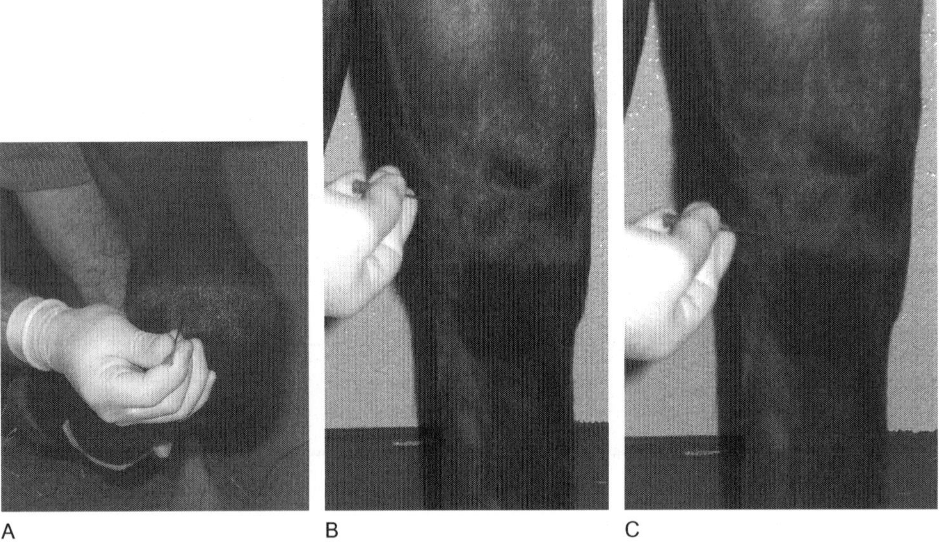

A B C

Figures 15.5A-C Approaches to the carpal joints for synoviocentesis. (15.5A) Dorsal approach to the radiocarpal joint. Note that a similar approach is used for the middle carpal joint. Palmarolateral approach to the radiocarpal (15.5B) and middle carpal (15.5C) joints. © Louise Southwood 2006.

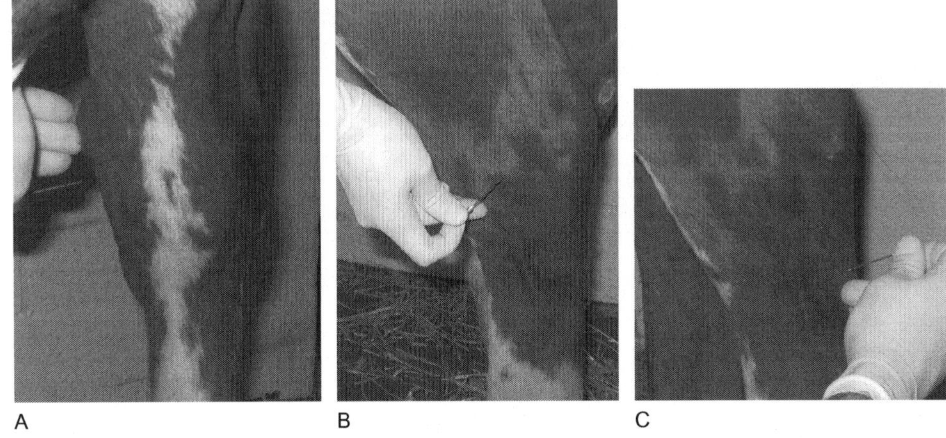

A B C

Figures 15.6A-C Approaches to the tarsal joints for synoviocentesis. (15.6A) Dorsal approach to the tibiotarsal joint. Note the finger is palpating the medial malleolus and injection is performed 2 to 4 cm below the medial malleolus. (15.6B) Approach to the lateral plantar pouch of the tibiotarsal joint. (15.6C) Plantarolateral approach to the tarsometatarsal joint. Note the finger is palpating the proximal aspect of metatarsal IV (MTIV) and the needle is inserted approximately 0.5 cm proximal to the proximal aspect of MTIV. © Louise Southwood 2006.

tibiotarsal joint can also be approached from the lateral aspect. Synoviocentesis of the medial and lateral plantar pouches of the tibiotarsal joint can also be performed easily when there is joint effusion (Figure 15.6, B). The proximal intertarsal joint communicates with the tibiotarsal joint and synoviocentesis of this joint is unnecessary. It is considerably more difficult to insert a needle into the distal intertarsal joint compared to the other tarsal joints, and it is rare to obtain synovial fluid from either the distal intertarsal or the tarsometatarsal joints. However, distension of these joints with sterile polyionic isotonic fluid can assess communication between the joint and a wound. The distal intertarsal and tarsometatarsal joints are approached with the limb in a weight-bearing position. The distal intertarsal joint is approached by inserting a needle on the medial aspect of the distal tarsus, midway between the dorsal and plantar aspect of the tarsus, distal to the palpable cunean tendon and in the notch created between the central, third and first-second tarsal bones.[27] The tarsometatarsal joint is approached by palpating the head of MTIV and inserting the needle 0.5 cm proximal to the head of MTIV and directing it distad and dorsad (Figure 15.6, C).

Digital sheath

Synoviocentesis of the digital sheath is difficult if there is no effusion. However, if there is a septic tenosynovitis or if the sheath has been penetrated by a laceration, moderate to marked effusion is usually present. The digital sheath can be approached with the limb in a weight-bearing position. The digital sheath extends from the distal third of the metacarpal/metatarsal region to the pastern and an approach can be made proximal or distal to the fetlock joint. The proximal approach is made several centimetres above the sesamoid bones between the lateral or medial aspect of the superficial and deep digital flexor tendons. The needle is inserted off the edge of the superficial digital flexor tendon and with the point of the needle directed distad. The distal approach is performed in the palmar or plantar pastern region with the needle directed horizontal to the ground and inserted superficial to the deep digital flexor tendon.

Bursae

Synoviocentesis of the various bursae has been described[28]; however, the need for injection of these sites is uncommon and if there is a problem in a hospitalised horse, there is usually considerable effusion and the needle can be inserted at the site of effusion for sample collection.

Humoradial (elbow), scapulohumeral (shoulder), femoropatellar and femorotibial (stifle) and coxofemoral (hip) joints

Synoviocentesis of the joints in the proximal limb is less commonly performed. Lacerations or wounds affecting these joints are less common because of the large amount of soft tissue surrounding these joints. Synoviocentesis of these joints is indicated, however, in foals with signs of severe lameness that cannot be localised to another site, particularly in foals with failure of passive transfer and/or sepsis.[18] An 18-gauge 8.9-cm spinal needle is needed for synoviocentesis of some of these joints (elbow, shoulder, hip) in older animals; however, 3.8-cm needle may be adequate for neonatal foals and for more superficial joints (femoropatella joint).[18] The humeroradial (elbow) joint can be approached from the lateral aspect of the limb, cranial or caudal to the palpable lateral collateral ligament. The needle is inserted two thirds of the distance between the lateral epicondyle of the humerus and the lateral tibial tuberosity.[18,29,30] Synoviocentesis of the scapulohumeral (shoulder) joint is performed by inserting a needle between the cranial and caudal prominences of the lateral tuberosity of the humerus and directing the needle in a caudomedial direction at a 45° angle to the body.[18,29,30] The femoropatellar joint is approached by inserting a needle either lateral or medial to the middle patella ligament. The femorotibial joint has a medial and lateral pouch. While the medial pouch often communicates with the femoropatellar joint, it should be evaluated and treated separately.[18] The medial femorotibial joint is approached by inserting a needle between the medial patella ligament and the medial collateral ligament and the lateral femorotibial joint lateral to the lateral patella ligament and immediately proximal to the tibia.[18] Synoviocentesis of the coxofemoral (hip) joint is difficult and is performed by palpating the greater trochanter, which is the prominent bony eminence in the hip region. The trochanteric notch between the greater and lesser trochanter is immediately caudal to the greater trochanter. An 18- or 16-gauge 8.9-cm spinal needle is inserted in the trochanteric notch perpendicular to the long axis of the limb and at 45° in a craniomedial direction.[29]

Synovial fluid analysis

Cytology

Normal synovial fluid is pale yellow, clear and viscus. A large volume of cloudy fluid with low viscosity is the first indication of a septic joint. Normal synovial fluid has a nucleated cell count less than 0.5×10^9/L cells (<500 cells/µl) with less than 10% neutrophils and total solids less than 0.2 g/L (<2 g/dl).[31] Sepsis should be suspected in a joint with total solids greater than 0.35 g/L (>3.5 g/dl) and/or a synovial fluid cell count greater than 30×10^9/L cells (>30,000 cells/µl) with greater than 90% neutrophils.[32] Sepsis cannot be ruled out in cases where the white cell count is less than 30×10^9/L (<30,000 cells/µl) (see Appendix, Table 19.16). In foals, synovial effusion with a moderate increase in cell count and protein may be associated with septic physitis.[18] A mucin precipitate should also be performed to assess the synovial fluid viscosity. Bacteria may be observed using a Gram stain of the synovial fluid in up to 25% of cases.[17]

Bacteriology

A sample of the synovial fluid should always be collected for culture and sensitivity in horses or foals suspected of having septic arthritis. The sample can be collected in a sterile plain tube or in a culture vial.[32] A positive culture is generally obtained in approximately 50% of cases.[33] Overall, Gram-negative organisms were isolated in 63% and Gram-positive organisms in 61% of septic arthritis cases, with Gram-positive organisms isolated more commonly from adult horses compared to foals. Foals were more likely compared to adults to have multiple and Ggram-negative organisms isolated.[17] The most common bacteria isolated from equine septic joints were Enterbacteriaceae (26%) and *Escherischia coli* (11.5%).[17] The most common microorganisms isolated from septic arthritis in foals are *Actinobacillus* spp., *E. coli*, *Klebsiella* spp., *Pseudomonas* spp. and *Salmonella* spp.[18] *Staphylococcus* spp. were most commonly isolated from equine septic joints associated with an intra-articular injection (69%)[17] or surgery (86%).[34] While antimicrobial choice should be made based on the results of culture and sensitivity, these results take several days to obtain. Antimicrobials that can be used while culture results are pending include penicillin and gentamicin or enrofloxacin.[17,34] Penicillin was effective against β-haemolytic streptococci.[16,33] Gentamicin was effective against 70% to 85% of isolates, including *Staphylococcus* spp., *Salmonella* spp., *Pseudomonas* spp. and *Actinobacillus* spp.[17,34] Amikacin was very effective against most isolates (>85%).[17] Amikacin is expensive to use systemically in the adult horse, and there are often concerns with nephrotoxicity in the septic neonate; however, it can be used locally (intra-articular or regional limb perfusion).

Synoviocentesis can be performed to monitor resolution of septic arthritis; however, monitoring the degree of lameness and amount of synovial effusion can be just as useful and less invasive.

References

1. Peloso JG, Cohen ND, Walker MA, et al.: Case-control study of risk factors for the development of laminitis in the contralateral limb in Equidae with unilateral lameness. J Am Vet Med Assoc 290:1746-1749, 1996
2. Menzies-Gow, NJ, Bailey SR, Katz LM, et al.: Endotoxin-induced digital vasoconstriction in horses: associated changes in plasma concentrations of vasoconstrictor mediators. Equine Vet J 36:273-278, 2004
3. Ingle-Fehr JE, Baxter GM: Evaluation of digital and laminar blood flow in horses given a low dose of LPS. Am J Vet Res 59:192-196, 1998
4. Mungall BA, Kyaw-Tanner M, Pollitt CC: In vitro evidence for a bacterial pathogenesis of equine laminitis. Vet Microbiol 79:209-223, 2001
5. Johnson PJ, Slight SH, Ganjam VK, et al.: Glucocorticoids and laminitis in the horse. Vet Clin N Am Equine Pract 18:219-236. 2002
6. Moore RM, Eades SC, Stokes AM: Evidence for vascular and enzymatic events in the pathophysiology of acute laminitis: which pathway is responsible for initiation of this process in horses? Equine Vet J 36:204-209, 2004
7. Cohen ND, Parson EM, Seahorn TL, Carter GK: Prevalence and factors associated with development of laminitis in horses with duodenitis/proximal jejunitis: 33 cases (1985-1991). J Am Vet Med Assoc 204:250-254, 1994
8. Stewart MC, Hodgson JL, Kim H, et al.: Acute febrile diarrhea in horses: 86 cases (1986-1991). Aust Vet J 72:41-44, 1995
9. Palmer JE, Whitlock RH, Benson CE: Equine ehrlichial colitis (Potomac horse fever): recognition of the disease in Pennsylvania, New Jersey, New York, Ohio, Idaho, and Connecticut. J Am Vet Med Assoc 189:197-199, 1986
10. Mulville P: Equine monocytic ehrlichiosis (Potomac horse fever): a review. Equine Vet J 23:400-404, 1991
11. Proudman CJ, Smith JE, Edwards GB, French NP: Long-term survival of equine surgical colic cases. Part 1: patterns of mortality and morbidity. Equine Vet J 34:432-437, 2002
12. Blanchard T, Varner D, Scrutchfield W, et al.: Management of dystocia in mares: Retained placenta, metritis and laminitis. Compend Contin Educ Pract Vet 12:563-569, 1990
13. Belknap JK, Moore JN. Evaluation of heparin for prophylaxis of equine laminitis: 71 cases (1980-1986). J Am Vet Med Assoc 195:505-507, 1989
14. Alford P, Geller S, Richardson B, et al.: A multicenter, matched case-control study of risk factors for equine laminitis. Prev Vet Med 49:209-222, 2001
15. Johnson PJ: The equine metabolic syndrome: peripheral Cushing's syndrome. Vet Clin N Am Equine Pract 18:271-294. 2002.
16. McCluskey MJ, Kavenagh PB: Clinical use of triamcinolone acetonide in the horse (205 cases) and the incidence of glucocorticoid-induced laminitis associated with its use. Equine Vet Educ 16:86-89, 2004
17. Schneider RK, Bramlage LR, Moore RM, et al.: A retrospective study of 192 horses affected with septic arthritis/tenosynovitis. Equine Vet J 24:436-442, 1992
18. Hardy J, Latimer F: Orthopaedic disorders in the neonatal foal. Clin Tech Equine Pract 2:96-119, 2003
19. Cohen ND. Causes of and farm management factors associated with disease and death in foals. J Am Vet Med Assoc 204:1644-1651, 1994
20. Robinson JA, Allen GK, Green EM, et al. A prospective study of septicaemia in colostrums-deprived foals. Equine Vet J 25:214-219, 1993
21. Martens RJ, Auer JA, Carter GK: Equine pediatrics: septic arthritis and osteomyelitis. J Am Vet Med Assoc 188:582-585, 1986
22. Firth E. Current concepts of infectious polyarthritis in foals. Equine Vet J 15:5-9, 1983
23. McIlwraith CW: Problems and complications of diagnostic and surgical arthroscopy, in McIlwraith CW (ed): Diagnostic and Surgical Arthroscopy in the Horse, ed 2, Philadelphia, Lea & Febiger, 1990, pp 213-218
24. Johnston GM, Eastment JK, Wood JLN, Taylor PM: The Confidential Enquiry into Perioperative Equine Fatalities (CEPEF): mortality results of phases 1 and 2. Vet Anesth Analg 29:159-170, 2002

25. Toniato M, Torre F: Anaesthesiologic characteristics and perioperative complications during arthroscopic surgery in the horse: 763 cases (1990-1997). Ippologia 10:5-18, 1999
26. Hague BA, Honnas CM, Simpson RB, Peloso JG: Evaluation of skin bacterial flora before and after aseptic preparation of clipped and nonclipped arthrocentesis sites in horses. Vet Surg 26:121-125, 1997.
27. Moyer W, Carter GK: Techniques to facilitate intra-articular injection of equine joints. Proc Am Assoc Equine Pract 48-54, 1996
28. Grant BD: Bursal injections. Proc Am Assoc Equine Pract 42:64-68, 1996
29. Stashak TS: Diagnosis of lameness, in Stashak TS (ed): Adam's Lameness in Horses, ed 4. Philadelphia, Lea & Febiger, 1987, pp 100-156.
30. Lewis RD: Techniques for arthrocentesis of equine shoulder, elbow, stifle, and hip joints. Proc Am Assoc Equine Pract 55-63, 1996
31. Trotter GW, McIlwraith CW: Clinical features and diagnosis of equine joint disease, in McIlwraith CW, Trotter GW (eds): Joint Disease in the Horse. Philadelphia, WB Saunders, 1996, pp 120-145
32. Bertone AL: Infectious arthritis, in McIlwraith CW, Trotter GW (eds): Joint Disease in the Horse. Philadelphia, WB Saunders, 1996, pp 397-409
33. Madison JB, Sommer M, Spencer PA: Relations among synovial membrane histopathologic findings, synovial fluid cytologic findings, and bacterial culture results in horses with suspected infectious arthritis: 64 cases (1979-1987). J Am Vet Med Assoc 198:1655-1661, 1991
34. La Pointe JM, Laverty S, LaVoie JP: Septic arthritis in 15 standardbred racehorses after intra-articlar injection. Equine Vet J 24:430-434, 1992

15.2 Laminitis

15.2.1 Detection and treatment of laminitis

Louise L. Southwood

Any hospitalised horse should be monitored closely for signs of laminitis and founder. At admission to the hospital, the hooves should be examined for signs of previous or chronic laminitis, such as broken back hoof-pastern axis, concave dorsal hoof walls, thick white line and divergent growth rings.[1] While laminitis is much more common in the fore compared to the hind limbs, it is critical to monitor the hind limbs for any signs of laminitis. Hind limb laminitis can go unrecognised or misdiagnosed as rhabdomyolysis, weakness or a neurological problem. Digital pulses should be palpated in all four limbs at least 2 to 8 times a day, depending on the presence of predisposing factors. Digital pulses can be described subjectively as normal, palpably increased compared to normal, or bounding. The hooves should be palpated for warmth and the coronary band for softening or a depression. Horses that are sinking have a depression that extends the full length of the coronary band.[1] The sole of the hoof should be examined for bulging of the horny sole at the toe region, or for prolapse, which is when the solar corium becomes visible protruding through the horny sole.[1]

The horse should be walked around the stall toward the left and right to identify any lameness and observed from outside the stall for abnormal stance and weight shifting. Horses with laminitis commonly shift weight back and forth between left and right fore or hind limbs, and horses with fore limb laminitis will stand with the hind limbs under the body to take the weight off the fore limbs and use a heel-loading and toe-relieving stance. Support-limb laminitis should be suspected in any horse with a severe lameness on one limb that acutely begins to increase weight-bearing on the affected limb. If any of these signs are observed, the development of laminitis should be suspected and further diagnostics and treatment pursued.

Hoof testers should be applied to the sole of the hoof to identify painful areas, particularly in the area just in front of the apex of the frog (Figure 15.7). In laminitic horses, the dorsal hoof wall is usually painful when percussed with hoof testers (Figure 15.8). If a diagnosis of laminitis is suspected but the clinician is unsure that this is the source of lameness, a unilateral abaxial sesamoid nerve block can be performed. Following the nerve block, a horse with bilateral laminitis will become lame in the unblocked limb. It is recommended to perform an abaxial sesamoid nerve block on the other limb to prevent excessive weight-bearing on one laminitic hoof. Clinical signs of laminitis can be graded, using a modification of the grading system developed by Obel[2] as shown in Box 15.4.[1] Horses with signs consistent with laminar damage have been classified as laminitis, acute founder, sinker and chronic founder as shown in Box 15.5.[1] This classification was significantly associated with outcome; horses that were classified as

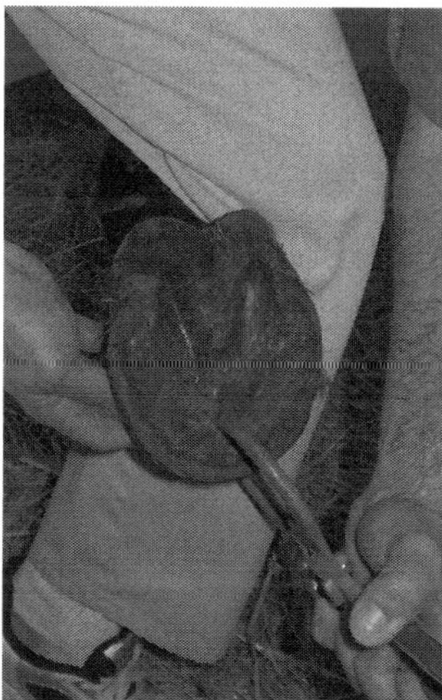

Figure 15.7 Hoof testers applied to the sole of the hoof just in front of the apex of the frog. Hoof testers can be applied at this site for detection of laminitis. Horses with laminitis often develop abscesses in the toe region and will be particularly painful when hoof testers are applied to the affected area. © Louise Southwood 2006.

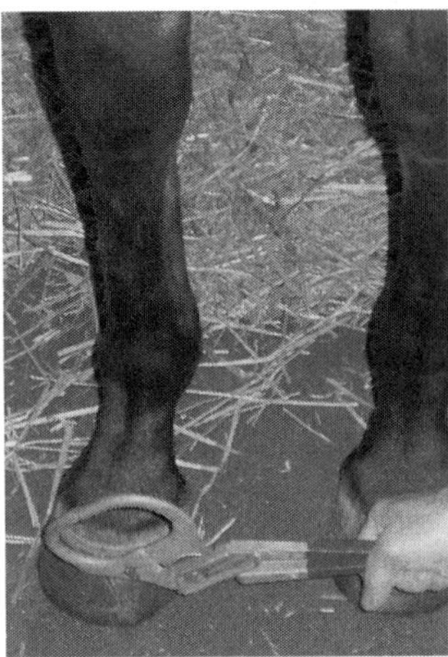

Figure 15.8 Percussion of the dorsal hoof wall can be used in the early diagnosis of laminitis. © Louise Southwood 2006.

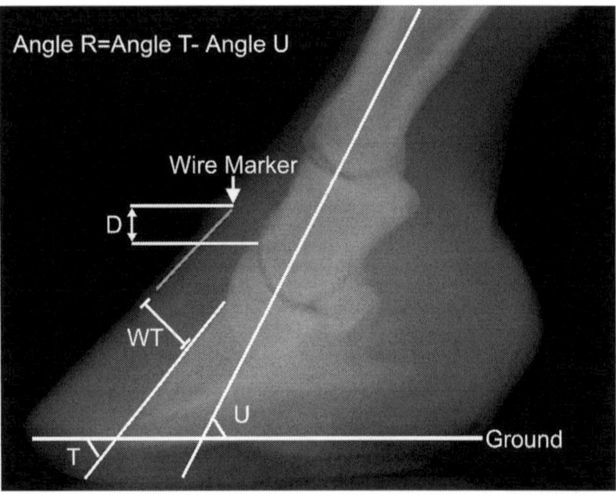

Figure 15.9 Lateral radiograph of a horse with founder. The horse was a post-operative colic patient (strangulating small intestinal lesion requiring resection and jejunocaecostomy that developed postoperative ileus) that had a previous history of laminitis and founder. Adapted from Cripps and Eustace.[1] WT = wall thickness, D = founder distance, T = angle T, and U = angle U. © Louise Southwood 2006.

Box 15.4. A grading system for horses with laminitis[1]

Grade	Description
0	No lameness at walk nor at a trot in a straight line on a hard surface
1	No lameness at a walk and moved freely. Lameness at a trot in a straight line on a hard surface. Animal turned carefully.
2	Animal did not move freely at a walk and had a "stiff" gait. May have overt lameness in one limb at a walk. Reluctant to trot on a hard surface. Difficulty turning.
3	Reluctant to move at a walk on any surface. Difficult to lift a limb. May be non–weight bearing on one limb.
4	Animal will not move without encouragement. Reluctant to move from a soft to a hard surface. Impossible to lift a limb.
5	Recumbent most of the time. Can only stand for a few minutes.

Box 15.5. Classification of horses with hoof laminar damage[1]

Classification	Description
Laminitis	Normal hooves, increased compared to normal digital pulses, heel-loading toe-relieving stance, may have pain with hoof testers, shifting weight.
Acute Founder	Similar to laminitis except there was a depression part but not all of the way around the coronary band.
Sinker	Bounding digital pulse, depressions around the full length of the coronary band. Reluctant to move or have the limb lifted. May have serous discharge at the coronary band.
Chronic Founder	Changes in the hoof wall consistent with previous or chronic founder.

having laminitis had 100% success, as acute founder 81% had success, as sinker had 20% success and as chronic founder had 79% success, where success was defined as alive and sound.[1]

Radiography

Radiographs (lateral, weight-bearing view) should then be taken of the affected hooves, and preferably all four hooves, depending on economical constraints. Radiographs should be taken with the horse unshod and standing on a flat ground using a wooden block under the hoof with a metal ground line.[1] A wire marker, of known length, should be taped to the dorsal hoof wall with the proximal aspect of the wire marker just below the coronary band at the point where the wall began to yield to moderate digital pressure.[3]

The radiographic beam should be parallel to the ground and the long axis of the navicular bone, and aimed at the centre of the third phalanx.[1] The hoof should be cleaned and the frog trimmed. Radiographs should be evaluated for the hoof wall thickness (WT), the "founder" distance (D) and degree of rotation (angle T) as shown in Figure 15.9.[1,3] Radiographic measurements in normal horses of various breeds have been performed.[3] There is variability between breeds and between horses in radiographic measurements.[3] Normal values (mean ± standard deviation) for the front feet in Thoroughbred horses were 16.3 ± 1.8 mm, 5.2 ± 2.0 mm and 47.6 ± 2.1° for WT, D and angle T, respectively.[3] In Thoroughbred horses, a hoof wall thickness greater than 16.6 mm was indicative of laminitis (mean normal of 14.6 mm).[4] The front foot wall thickness was greater in Hanoverians (18 mm) and less in ponies (13.2 mm) compared to Thoroughbreds.[3] The front foot D was less in both Hanoverians (3.3 mm) and ponies (3.1 mm) and the angle T greater in Hanoverians (50.5°) and ponies (53°) compared to Thoroughbreds.[3]

Predictors of outcome

Classification (Box 15.2) was the best predictor of outcome (81% accuracy).[1] However, the grade of lameness (Box 15.1), D, angle T (angle between the dorsal cortex of the distal phalanx and the ground) and angle R (angle T minus the angle between a line connecting the centres of curvature of the proximal and distal interphalangeal joints and the ground [angle U]) were able to correctly predict success in 94% and failure in 43% of horses, with an overall accuracy of 82%. *Success* was defined as the horse returning to an athletic career at the original or higher level, and failure where animals were euthanised or were unable to be ridden.[1] In horses with support-limb laminitis, the WT was greater than 29% of the palmar cortical length of P_3 and there was only one horse with rotation of P_3.[1]

Treatment and prevention

Unfortunately, laminitis has usually progressed by the time signs are detected; hence, prevention is critical. Horses that are at risk of developing laminitis associated with systemic disease can be treated prophylactically with cryotherapy.[5] The proposed mechanism for prevention of laminitis using cryotherapy is thought to involve vasoconstriction, which prevents delivery of "laminitic trigger factors" in the circulation to the digit, and hypometabolism, which is thought to reduce the activity of inflammatory mediators and enzymes that are thought to be important in the development of laminitis.[5] The fore and/or hind limbs can be continuously cooled in an ice/water mixture using boots made from rubber inner tube, plastic or commercially available boots*†.[5,6]

The opposing theory is that laminitis is a result of ischaemic necrosis secondary to vasoconstriction (arterial as well as venous) and vascular thrombosis and there have been numerous studies to demonstrate a decrease in digital blood flow with various factors and mediators.[2,3,7] Endotoxin, in particular, has been shown to decrease digital perfusion,[1,2] emphasising the importance of treatment of endotoxaemia in laminitis prevention and supporting the theory of digital hypoperfusion. Based on this theory, mechanisms that cause vasodilation would be important in the treatment and prevention of laminitis. Isoxsuprine hydrochloride (0.6 mg/kg IV or 1.2 mg/kg PO every 12 hours), acepromazine (0.066 mg/kg IV every 4–6 hours) and nitroglycerine (30–60 mg/foot/450-kg horse/topical application) have been used to create digital vasodilation and pentoxifylline (4.4 mg/kg PO every 8 hours) and heparin (40–80 IU IV or SQ every 8–12 hours) have also been used to increase digital perfusion by increasing red cell deformability and inhibiting thrombosis, respectively.[8] *In vitro* and *in vivo* studies have demonstrated conflicting results, and there are limited studies to support the use of these drugs in the treatment of laminitis.[8] Isoxsuprine hydrochloride caused dilation of digital vessels *in vitro*[9,10] and had a beneficial effect in an equine experimental model of laminitis[11]; however, intravenous administration of isoxsuprine hydrochloride did not increase laminar blood flow[12] and oral administration did not increase digital or laminar blood flow.[13] While intravenous acepromazine increased digital blood flow,[13] it only increased laminar blood flow slightly[13] or not at all.[12] Studies investigating the use of nitroglycerine have been controversial.[8,14] Nitroglycerine tolerance is likely to develop in horses as in other species and an 8- to 12-hour drug-free period is recommended.[8,14] Oral administration of pentoxifylline did not increase laminar blood flow[13]; however, it may be useful in preventing laminitis in endotoxaemic horses because it has been shown to decrease tumour necrosis factor-α expression.[8] As mentioned previously, studies investigating the use of heparin in laminitis prevention have been contradictory.[7,13] While the results of these treatments in laminitis prevention are controversial, a survey study in the early 1990s reported that phenylbutazone (68%), acepromazine (34%), dimethylsulphoxide (DMSO, 27%) and flunixin meglumine (19%) were the most commonly used drugs in treating laminitis, with acepromazine, DMSO and flunixin meglumine used more commonly in acute compared to chronic laminitis.[15] The majority of cases in the latter study were horses with gastrointestinal tract disease.[15] Regardless of the mechanisms of laminitis development, the use of phenylbutazone (2–4 mg/kg every 12–24 hours IV or PO) and flunixin meglumine (0.5–1 mg/kg every 12–24 hours IV) as anti-inflammatory analgesic drugs are important in managing horses with laminitis.

Treatment of support-limb laminitis

Support-limb laminitis can be prevented by early and effective treatment of the underlying disease and by providing appropriate analgesia so that the horse is as comfortable as possible on the affected limb. The reported mortality rate in horses with support-limb laminitis is 50%, emphasising the importance of prevention.[1] Types of analgesia that can be used include phenylbutazone (2–4 mg/kg every 12–24 hours PO or IV), lidocaine (lignocaine) (1.3 mg/kg bolus IV over 15 minutes followed by 0.05 mg/kg/min constant rate infusion [CRI] IV),[16] butorphanol (13 μg/kg/h CRI IV),[17] transdermal fentanyl (30 to 110 μg/kg; 2 x 10 ug/hour patches/350–500 kg horse i.e.

* Jack's Whirlpool boot; Jack's Manufacturing Inc, Washington, OH, USA.

† Bigfoot Ice boot; Bigfoot Ice Boots, Esk, Queensland, Australia.

2 x 10 mg patches/350–500 kg horse)[18] and epidural morphine (40–50 mg diluted in 10- to 30-ml sterile saline). Phenylbutazone should not be administered at the high dose for longer than 24 to 48 hours, because horses can develop right dorsal colitis as a consequence of prolonged use of high doses.

While analgesia is critical for a successful outcome in horses with orthopaedic problems, particular attention should be paid to more subtle signs associated with worsening of the primary lesion or development of laminitis. It is important to encourage the horse to lay down by providing adequate bedding and in some instances the use of acepromazine. Often, the cast limb is longer than the supporting limb, which can result in excessive weight-bearing on the support limb and laminitis. To prevent excessive weight-bearing on the support limb, an appropriately sized boot*† with a piece of wood of similar thickness to the built-up cast screwed onto the bottom of the boot can be placed on the opposite foot to make the limbs of equal length.[19] During full weight-bearing, there is a lack of fill in the dorsal laminar vessels as a result of the constant pull of the deep digital flexor tendon on P_3 and the dorsal laminar attachment, suggesting that poor perfusion of the dorsal laminar during constant excessive unilateral weight-bearing may play an important role in the development of support-limb laminitis.[20] Therefore, it has been suggested that raising the heels (10°), setting back the functional breakover point so that the horse stands with a palmar/plantar angle (angle between palmar/plantar margin of P_3 and the ground) of 20° and providing solar support prevent support-limb laminitis by improving perfusion to the dorsal laminar in horses with severe contralateral limb lameness.[20]

References

1. Cripps PJ, Eustace RA: Factors involved in the prognosis of equine laminitis in the UK. Equine Vet J 31:433-442, 1999
2. Obel N: Studies on the Histopathology of Acute Laminitis. Boktryckeri ab Uppsala, Almquist and Wiksells, 1948
3. Cripps PJ, Eustace RA: Radiological measurements from the feet of normal horses with relevance to laminitis. Equine Vet J 31:433-442, 1999
4. Lindford RL: A radiographic, morphometric, histological and ultrastructural investigation of lamellar function, abnormality and the associated radiographic findings for sound and footsore Thoroughbreds, and horses with experimentally induced traumatic and alimentary laminitis. PhD thesis, University of California, 1987
5. Van Eps AW, Pollitt CC: Equine laminitis: cryotherapy reduces the severity of the acute lesion. Equine Vet J 36:255-260, 2004
6. Pollitt CC, Van Eps AW: Prolonged, continuous distal limb cryotherapy in the horse. Equine Vet J 36:216-220, 2004

* Easy Boot; Easy Care, Inc, Oro Valley, AZ.

† Davis Boot; Davis Manufacturing, Inc, Brandon, WI.

7. Bailey SR, Menzies-Gow NJ, Marr CM, Elliott J: The effects of vasoactive amines found in the equine hindgut on digital blood flow in the normal horse. Equine Vet J 36:267-272, 2004
8. Belknap J: Medical treatment options in equine laminitis. Compend Cont Educ 23:918-921, 2001
9. Baxter GM, Tackett RL, Moore JN: Reactivity of equine palmar digital arteries and veins to vasodilating agents. Vet Surg 18:221-226, 1989
10. Galey FD, Beasley VR, Schaeffer DJ, Davis LE: Antagonism in isolated equine digital vessels of contraction induced by epinephrine in the presence of hydrocortisone and an aqueous extract of black walnut (Juglans nigra). J Vet Pharmacol Ther 12:411-420, 1989
11. Kirker-Head CA, Stephens KA, Toal RL, Goble DO: Circulatory and blood gas changes accompanying the development and treatment of induced laminitis. J Equine Vet Sci 6:293-301, 1986
12. Adair HS, Schmidhammer JL, Goble DO, et al.: Effects of acepromazine maleate, isoxsuprine hydrochloride and prazosin hydrochloride on laminar microcirculatory blood flow in healthy horses. J Equine Vet Sci 17:599-603, 1997
13. Ingle-Fehr JE, Baxter GM: The effect of oral isoxsuprine and pentoxifylline on digital and laminar blood flow in healthy horses. Vet Surg 28:154-160, 1999
14. Ragle CA: Nitroglycerin treatment of equine laminitis. Compend Cont Educ 21:170-174, 1999
15. Slater MR, Hood DM, Carter GK: Descriptive epidemiological study of equine laminitis. Equine Vet J 27:364-367, 1995
16. Rakestraw PC: Modulation of intestinal motility, in White NA, Moore JN (eds): Current Techniques in Equine Surgery and Lameness, ed 2, Philadelphia, WB Saunders, 1998, pp 303-307
17. Sellon DC, Roberts MC, Blikslager A, Ulibarri C: Effects of continuous intravenous infusion of butorphanol in horses after exploratory celiotomy. Proc Int Equine Colic Res Symp 7:21-22, 2002
18. Thomasy SM, Slovis N, Maxwell LK: Transdermal fentanyl combined with non-steroidal antiinflammatory drugs for analgesia in horses. J Vet Int Med 18:550-554, 200
19. Hendrickson DA, Stokes M, Wittern C: Use of an elevated boot to reduce contralateral support limb complications secondary to cast application. Proc Annu Am Assoc Equine Pract 149-150, 1997
20. Redden RF: Preventing laminitis in the contralateral limb of horses with non-weight-bearing lameness. Proc Am Assoc Equine Pract 49:320-327, 2003

15.2.2 Supporting the laminitic foot

Nicola Menzies-Gow

Supporting the foot is an essential part of the management of acute laminitis. The horse naturally adopts a stance that allows most of the weight to be borne over the caudal part of the foot rather than the painful toe region. Providing additional support to this region of the foot will provide pain relief and also help to minimise the mechanical forces on the laminae and hence laminar tearing and pedal bone movement. The simplest strategy is to increase the depth of the bedding and ensure that the bedding extends to the

Table 15.1. Muscle associated enzymes, and increases seen with mild, moderate and severe injury

Parameter	Reference range	Mild increase	Moderate increase	Severe increase
Creatine kinase (CK)	133–738 u/l	740–1000 u/l	1000–3000 u/l	>3000 u/l
Creatine kinase (CK) following general anaesthesia	133–738 u/l	740–5000 u/l	5000–10000 u/l	>10000 u/l
Asparate aminotransferase (AST)	198–476 u/l	500–800 u/l	800–1200 u/l	>1200 u/l
Lactate dehydrogenase (LDH)	Total 225–700 u/l % of total LDH 1: 10–18 LDH 2: 22–30 LDH 3: 34–42 LDH 4: 13–23 LDH 5: 1–7	700–1000 u/l	1000–1500 u/l	>1500 u/l
Cardiac troponin I (cTnI)	0.05–0.2 ng/ml	N/a	N/a	N/a

door. Shavings, sand, peat or hemp-based products are optimal as they pack beneath the feet better than straw or paper.

Extra support can be applied directly to the caudal two-thirds of the foot itself. This can be done in a variety of ways that can be broadly divided into frog-only supports and combined frog and sole supports. Frog-only support can be achieved using rolled up bandaging material of the same length as the frog, placed along the length of the frog and secured in place with adhesive tape. Alternatively, a commercially available product such as the Lily Pad* can be used. To achieve optimal support, the part of the pad that will cover the frog should be trimmed to the same size as the frog. Combined frog and sole support can be provided using, for example, dental impression material that is moulded to the contours of the caudal two-thirds of the foot or styrofoam pads that are crushed by the weight of the horse.

Regardless of which type of support is used, it must be removed intermittently and the feet examined for evidence of softening and thinning of the sole over the toe region suggestive of imminent pedal bone penetration and for evidence of infections such as thrush or white line infection that require additional treatment. The supports should be left in place whilst the horse remains acutely painful. They can be replaced by more permanent alternatives such as heart bar shoes, egg bar shoes or imprint shoes that can be combined with gel or dental impression material sole supports once the horse is comfortable.

15.3 Biochemical monitoring of the muscles

Nicola Menzies-Gow

The parameters most useful in the biochemical monitoring of the muscles in the hospitalised horse include serum activities of the enzymes creatine kinase (CK), aspartate aminotransferase (AST), lactate dehydrogenase (LDH) and troponin I. Increases in the plasma activity of these enzymes can occur due to impaired enzyme clearance or increased synthesis but most commonly occur as a consequence of increased cell membrane permeability and/or cell necrosis.[1] Normal and pathological values for these are shown in Table 15.1.

Creatine kinase

CK is the enzyme that catalyses the breakdown of creatine phosphate to creatine and phosphate, releasing energy for muscle contraction. It is found mainly in skeletal muscle, the myocardium and the brain,[2,3] and the normal range of CK activity is assumed to be due to endogenous turnover of skeletal muscle.[4] There is little exchange of CK between the cerebrospinal fluid and the plasma, so a significant increase in the plasma CK activity is caused by skeletal or cardiac muscle damage. However, no assumption can be made regarding the amount of muscle damaged on the basis of the serum CK activity as muscle cells appear to be able to release significant quantities of CK without necessarily being lysed.[5]

In humans, there are two monomers of CK designated M and B. The enzyme is dimeric and exists in three forms: MM found mainly in the skeletal muscle, BB in the brain and MB in the myocardium. However, isoenzymes do not appear to be useful in the differentiation of skeletal and cardiac muscle damage in the horse.[6–9]

The plasma half-life ($t\frac{1}{2}$) of CK released following muscle injury is approximately 9 hours.[10] Thus, following muscle damage, the plasma enzyme activity increases quickly, peaking at 4 to 6 hours but will return to normal within 48 to 72 hours provided there is no further damage.[11,12]

Aspartate aminotransferase

AST is found primarily in skeletal muscle, liver and heart and is involved in protein metabolism. However, lower

* Therapeutic Equine Products Inc, Shelbyville, KY, USA.

activities are found in several other tissues, making it non–tissue specific.[2,13,14] Two isoenzymes have been identified, mAST (mitochondrial origin) and cAST (cytoplasm or sarcoplasm origin), but there is no tissue specificity for either isoenzyme .[15] The plasma $t\frac{1}{2}$ of AST is 2 to 4 days,[11] so that following muscle damage, the plasma activity will increase slower than that of CK, reaching a peak after approximately 24 to 48 hours and returning to baseline after approximately 7 to 10 days. Thus, concurrent evaluation of plasma CK and AST activities allows determination of the timing of the muscle injury and repeated sampling allows detection of ongoing muscle injury.

Lactate dehydrogenase

LDH is a tetrapeptide made up of combinations of two peptides H (heart) and M (muscle) that form the various isoenzymes. LDH is found in most tissues and so is not tissue specific.[3] However, the isoenzyme profile has been used to identify specific tissue damage. LDH_5 is found in the locomotor muscles,[15,16] the liver contains mainly LDH_3 and the heart contains mostly LDH_1.[6,9] Haemolysis will falsely elevate the LDH concentration as erythrocytes contain large amounts of LDH.

Troponin I

Cardiac troponin I (cTnI) is a myocardial polypeptide that is a highly sensitive and specific biomarker of myocardial injury in people and dogs.[17,18] Plasma cTnI concentrations have been determined in normal horses,[19] and increased plasma concentrations of cTnI have been reported in two horses with myocardial disease.[20,21] Thus, concurrent measurement of cTnI may aid in distinguishing increases in plasma CK and AST activity of cardiac origin from those of skeletal muscle origin.

Assessing the significance of the result

Most clinicians believe that serum CK and AST activities must be high before considering primary disorders of the skeletal system as the cause (see Table 15.1). However, it must be remembered that CK and AST activities may be normal or only mildly increased in some inflammatory or degenerative myopathies such as equine motor neuron disease (EMND)[22] and polysaccharide storage myopathy (PSSM).[23] In addition, many clinicians dismiss slight increases in CK activity in horses that have been transported or lying down excessively. Repeat sampling at 24-hour intervals should show a rapid decrease to normal values if this is true. If AST activity is simultaneously increased in a horse with a history of being transported or lying down of less than 24 hours, due to the kinetics of the enzymes, an underlying myopathy should be considered.[4] Horses undergoing general anaesthesia and surgery often have a moderate postoperative increase in serum CK activity. If this increase is severe and/or the animal is showing clinical signs of painful, firm muscles, then a postanaesthetic myopathy should be considered, and if CK activity does not decrease rapidly, a possibility of an ongoing muscle injury should be evaluated.[15]

References

1. Boyd J: The mechanisms relating to increases in plasma enzymes and isoenzymes in disease of animals. Vet Clin Pathol 12:9-24, 1985
2. Gerber H: The clinical significance of serum enzyme activities with particular reference to myoglobinuria. Proc Am Assoc Equine Prac 14:81, 1968
3. Thornton JR, Lohni MD: Tissue and plasma activity of lactic dehydrogenase and creatine kinase in the horse. Equine Vet J 11:235-238, 1979
4. Valentine B: Serum CK and AST in equine neuromuscular disease: searching for diagnostic approaches. Equine Vet Educ 15:250-252, 2003
5. MacLeay JM: Diseases of the musculoskeletal system, in Reed SM, Bayly WM, Sellon DC (eds): Equine Internal Medicine, ed 2. Philadelphia, WB Saunders, 2004, p 469
6. Anderson MG: The effect of exercise on the LDH and CK isoenzyme composition of horse serum. Res Vet Sci 20:191, 1976
7. Fujii Y, Ikeda S, Watanabe H: Analysis of creatine kinase isoenzymes in racehorse serum and tissues. Bull Equine Res Inst 17:21, 1980
8. Argiroudis SA, Kent JE, Blackmore DJ: Observations on the isoenzymes of creatine kinase in equine serum and tissues. Equine Vet J 14:317-321, 1982.
9. Sighieri C, Longa A, Mariani A: Preliminary observations on the creatine kinase isoenzyme in equine blood serum by polyacrylamide-gel isoelectrofocusing: influence of physical exercise. Arch Vet Ital 36:45, 1985
10. Volfinger L, Lassourd V, Michaux JM, et al.: Kinetic evaluation of muscle damage during exercise by calculation of amount of creatine kinase released. Am J Physiol 266:R434-R441, 1994
11. Cardinet GH, Littrell JF, Freedland RA: Comparative investigations of serum creatine kinase and glutamic-oxaloacetic transaminase activities in equine paralytic myglobinuria. Res Vet Sci 8:219-226, 1967
12. Lindsey WA, Robinson GM, Brunson DB, et al.: Induction of equine postanaesthetic myositis after halothane-induced hypotension. Am J Vet Res 50:404-410, 1989
13. Arighi M, Baird J, Hulland T: Equine exertional rhabdomyolysis. Compend Cont Educ Prac Vet 6:5726, 1984
14. Cornelius C, Burnham L, Hill H: Serum transaminase activities of equine thoroughbred horses in training. J Am Vet Med Assoc 142:639-642, 1963
15. Rej R, Rudofsky U, Magro A, et al.: Effects of exercise on serum amino-transferase activity and pyroxidal phosphate saturation in thoroughbred racehorses. Equine Vet J 22:205-208, 1990
16. Littlejohn A, Blackmore DJ: Blood and tissue content of the isoenzymes of lactate dehydrogenase in the thoroughbred. Res Vet Sci 25:118-119, 1978
17. Cummins B, Auckland ML, Cummins P. (1987) Cardiac-specific troponin-I radioimmunoassay in the diagnosis of acute myocardial infarction. Am Heart J 113:1333-1344, 1987

18. Oyama MA, Sisson DD: Cardiac troponin-I concentration in dogs with cardiac disease. J Vet Intern Med 18:831-839, 2004
19. Phillips W, Giguère S, Franklin RP et al.: Cardiac troponin I in pastured and race-training Thoroughbred horses. J Vet Intern Med 17:597-599, 2003
20. Cornelisse CJ, Schott HC 2nd, Olivier NB, et al.: Concentration of cardiac troponin I in a horse with a ruptured aortic regurgitation jet lesion and ventricular tachycardia. J Am Vet Med Assoc 15:231-235, 2000
21. Schwarzwald CC, Hardy J, Buccellato M: High cardiac troponin I serum concentration in a horse with multiform ventricular tachycardia and myocardial necrosis. J Vet Intern Med 17:364-368, 2003
22. Divers TJ, Mohammed HO, Cummings JF, et al.: Equine motor neuron disease: findings in 28 horses and proposal of a pathophysiological mechanism for the disease. Equine Vet J 26:409-415, 1994
23. Valentine BA: Polysaccharide storage myopathy in draft and draft-related horses and ponies. Equine Pract 21:16-19, 1999

15.4 Management of rhabdomyolysis and myopathy

Nicola Menzies-Gow

Rhabdomyolysis refers to the syndrome of muscle cramping that occurs following physical exertion or exercise. Anaesthetic-related myopathy occurs following poor positioning of the recumbent patient, prolonged surgery or recovery or poor perfusion of the muscles for any reason under general anaesthesia. Exertional rhabdomyolysis may occur in the horse for two main reasons—namely, the horse has an underlying myopathy (chronic rhabdomyolysis) or the horse has been overexerted physically (sporadic exertional rhabdomyolysis). Horses with underlying myopathies usually suffer from repeated bouts of rhabdomyolysis after relatively short bouts of exercise, whereas individuals that are overexerted may only experience a single episode in their lifetime as it is caused by physical circumstances as opposed to an underlying pathological condition of the muscle.

Acute rhabdomyolysis

Acute rhabdomyolysis can be used to refer to either an anaesthetic-induced myopathy or to the one off bout of muscle cramping that occurs in horses with no underlying myopathy that are overexerted physically or to a severe exacerbation of the clinical signs in an individual with chronic rhabdomyolysis.

Clinical signs

The clinical signs of acute rhabdomyolysis vary from relatively mild to severe. The predominant clinical signs are mild to moderate muscle cramping of the hindquarter muscles, associated with mild to severe pain; however other muscles may also be involved. In anaesthesia related myopathy, the muscles affected are typically those on the downside. In lateral recumbency, the triceps or the gluteal muscles on the down side are most frequently affected. In dorsal recumbency, the gluteal muscles are often affected bilaterally. With poor positioning, muscles on the upper side may be affected (for example if a limb on the upper side is not supported during a prolonged procedure in lateral recumbency).

Clinical signs include anxiety, sweating, reluctance to move, tachycardia and tachypnoea. The affected muscles are firm and painful on palpation. Severe cases may progress to recumbency. With moderate to severe muscle necrosis, the myoglobin that is released into the circulation as a consequence is filtered by the kidneys into the urine resulting in pigmenturia due to myoglobinuria.

Diagnosis

The diagnosis of acute rhabdomyolysis is based on the history, clinical signs, biochemistry and possibly urinalysis.

History

If the horse has no underlying myopathy, then the horse will not have experienced similar episodes previously and the clinical signs will have been preceded by a period of relatively intensive physical activity. If the horse has an underlying myopathy, then it may have suffered from numerous episodes previously and the clinical signs will have been preceded by a relatively short bout of exercise. Rhabdomyolysis should be suspected in any postoperative patient showing the clinical signs described above within twelve hours of general anaesthesia.

Biochemistry

Muscle damage is confirmed by moderate to severe increases in the serum activities of creatine kinase (CK), aspartate aminotransferase (AST) and lactate dehydrogenase (LDH) (Chapter 15.3). If the clinical signs are moderate to severe, if there is pigmenturia or if the serum activities of CK and AST are severely moderately to increased, then urea and creatinine concentrations should also be measured in order to detect any decrease in renal function.

Urinalysis

Serum myoglobin has a short half-life such that measuring serum myoglobin concentrations is of limited diagnostic value. Instead it is preferable to measure urine myoglobin concentrations, as acute tubular necrosis and acute renal failure have been associated with myoglobinuria in horses. In addition, urine specific gravity should be measured. The result will need to be interpreted in the light of prior fluid therapy but will aid detection of altered renal function.

Management

The amount of therapy required will depend on the severity of the clinical signs. However, regardless of severity, the goals of therapy for acute rhabdomyolysis are to provide adequate analgesia, limit further muscle damage, restore and maintain fluid and electrolyte balance and prevent acute renal failure due to hypovolaemia and/or myoglobinuria.

Mild cases can be treated with rest and analgesia in the form of nonsteroidal anti-inflammatory drugs (NSAIDs) such as phenylbutazone (4.4 mg/kg IV as single dose or 4.4 mg/kg PO BID) or flunixin meglumine (1.1 mg/kg IV BID). Some clinicians advocate the use of acepromazine (0.03–0.1 mg/kg IV or IM BID) to cause peripheral vasodilation and improve muscle blood flow. However, this is contraindicated in the more severely affected hyovolaemic horse. Horses should be fed good-quality hay with minimal grain supplementation in order to minimise carbohydrate intake. In addition, the use of the antioxidants vitamin E (2000–4000 IU/day PO) and selenium (1 mg/day PO) has been suggested to minimise myocyte damage.

Severe cases require additional therapy in the form of fluid therapy to restore and maintain the fluid and electrolyte balances. Frequently oral fluid therapy is insufficient and intravenous therapy using balanced polyionic fluids (e.g., Hartmann's) is required. The rate of fluid therapy required will depend on the estimate of the initial degree of hypovolaemia and ongoing losses, especially sweating. The fluids can be supplemented with the appropriate electrolytes based on any deficits highlighted by biochemical analysis (see Chapter 6.5). If there is little or no urine production despite correction of hypovolaemia, attempts should be made to invoke diuresis with furosemide (frusemide) (0.5–1.0 mg/kg IV every 6–8 hours) to prevent myoglobin nephrotoxicity (see Chapter 13).

Sedatives such as detomidine (10–20 μg/kg IM or IV) are useful to reduce the associated anxiety and provide analgesia.[1] Additional analgesia in the form of opiate drugs such as butorphanol (0.1 mg/kg IV) may be required. Further muscle damage is limited through exercise restriction. Forced exercise in horses that are reluctant to move should be avoided. Horses should be stabled on a deep bed until they are comfortable moving around, at which time turnout into a paddock is recommended.[1]

Corticosteroids are sometimes used to stabilise cell membranes, but their efficacy is unproved.[2] Dantrolene (800–2000 mg PO SID), a drug that limits the release of calcium from the sarcoplasmic reticulum, has been used in the acute stages of rhabdomyolysis, but its efficacy in this situation has not been assessed.

Horses with the underlying myopathy polysaccharide myopathy (PSSM) can present as an acutely recumbent horse, particularly post general anaesthesia.[3] Therapy of a recumbent PSSM horse should include either oral lipid therapy with administration of vegetable-based oil by nasogastric tube, dose syringe or in the feed or the use of intravenous lipid solutions[4] as this significantly increases the survival rate of such severely affected animals.[5]

Monitoring horses with acute rhabdomyolysis

The serum activities of CK and AST increase rapidly from the reference range, peaking 4 to 6 hours and 24 to 48 hours after the insult, respectively (see Chapter 15.3). If muscle necrosis is not ongoing, the serum activity of CK will decrease rapidly over the next 24 to 48 hours and the serum activity of AST will remain increased for 7 to 10 days. In acute myopathies following general anaesthesia, large changes in CK (>10,000 IU/L) are usually evident on recovery from anaesthesia. More moderate increases (1000–5000 IU/L) may be seen following anaesthesia with no apparent clinical signs. For horses with exertional rhabdomyolysis, and depending on the severity of the situation, it may be most useful to submit blood samples to the laboratory for measurement of the serum activities of these enzymes approximately 4 to 6 hours after the onset of the clinical signs to confirm the diagnosis and determine peak CK activity, 24 to 48 hours after to determine the peak AST activity and that the CK activity is declining and after 7 to 10 days to determine that AST activity has returned to normal. The horse should be rested until the serum activity of AST has returned to within the reference range.

If the clinical signs have been severe, if the horse has pigmenturia or if the serum activities of CK and AST increased moderately to severely, then urine myoglobin concentration and specific gravity and blood urea and creatinine concentrations should be measured daily until the clinical signs have resolved in order to monitor renal function.

Chronic rhabdomyolysis

Recurrent episodes of rhabdomyolysis can occur in horses with an underlying myopathy. Once the acute episode has resolved, the nature of the myopathy needs to be ascertained so that the appropriate dietary and exercise changes can be instituted in order to reduce the frequency of recurrence of clinical episodes. Three specific underlying myopathies—namely, recurrent exertional rhabdomyolysis (RER), PSSM and equine polysaccharide storage myopathy (EPSM)—have been described. However, there are a significant number of individual animals that experience chronic rhabdomyolysis and so would be expected to have an underlying myopathy which to date remains idiopathic.

Recurrent exertional rhabdomyolysis

Pathogenesis

RER occurs in Thoroughbred horses[6] and appears to be due to an abnormality of calcium regulation[7] that is inherited as an autosomal dominant trait. The exact cellular mechanism that leads to RER has yet to be elucidated. It may affect as much as 5% of racing Thoroughbreds. The expression of the disease is multifactorial and depends on the fitness level and exercise schedule of the horse, diet, age, gender, temperament and presence of lameness.[6] There is increased expression of the disease in females compared to males, in younger (2 years old) compared to older (5–6 years old) animals, in individuals with a nervous temperament, in animals fed a high-carbohydrate diet (>4 kg cereals/day) that contains excessive calories, in horses that are gallop trained and in lame animals.

Clinical signs
Affected animals exhibit signs of muscle cramping as previously described (see Acute rhabdomyolysis, above). Animals can also be subclinically affected.

Diagnosis
The diagnosis of RER is based on a history of recurrent episodes of acute rhabdomyolysis following relatively short bouts of exercise in a Thoroughbred. The gold standard for diagnosis RER is the caffeine or halothane muscle contracture test. However, this test is performed on an intercostal muscle biopsy specimen and is only available in the research situation. Instead, a muscle biopsy specimen should be obtained from the hindquarters (see Chapter 1.55) and histological examination should reveal an increased number of central nuclei without evidence of accumulation of abnormal polysaccharide.

Acute management
The management of an acute episode of the disease has been described earlier.

Long-term management
The goal of long-term management of affected horses is to reduce the frequency of recurrence of clinical episodes. Environmental and dietary factors appear to affect the expression of RER; thus, long-term management is based on recommendations that focus on exercise and diet.

Exercise regimen
The exercise regimen should be altered to minimise stress. This will vary according to the individual animal, some preferring to exercise alone, others as part of a group, some requiring a prolonged warm-up. In addition, box rest for more than 24 hours should be avoided.

Dietary management
The diet should be modified to provide adequate, but not excessive, calories according to the amount of work performed. This requires dietary analysis using commercially available computer software or can be achieved through the feed manufacturer. The majority of the calories should be supplied in the form of fat rather than carbohydrate,[8] but the optimal fat source and dietary percentage have yet to be identified. The current recommendation is to feed 1.5% to 2% body weight as fibre, no greater than 20% of digestible energy requirements as nonstructural carbohydrate, and to supply 20% to 25% from fat. The diet should contain no more than 2 kg of cereals, 600 ml of vegetable oil and 2 kg of rice bran per day. Alternatively, a specialised commercially available diet that has been designed for intensely exercised horses with chronic exertional rhabdomyolysis can be fed. One commercial diet* contains 13% fat by weight (rice bran and corn oil) or 20% digestible energy as fat and only 9% as starch. All supplemental feeds should be reduced in amount on days when energy requirements are not as high, particularly if the horse is at risk of weight gain. Other management strategies may help to decrease the intensity of the postprandial glycaemic response and include feeding small meals, providing at least 1.5% to 2.0% body weight per day in forage, and feeding a forage source either 2 hours before or concurrently with any grain. Avoiding high starch supplements such as molasses is also important. The mechanism through which fats decrease creatine kinase activity remains unknown, but they appear to result in a calmer temperament.[9] Because stress has been associated with RER, the calming effect may explain the prophylactic efficacy of the high-fat diet.

Drug therapy
If these measures fail to adequately prevent the clinical signs, dantrolene (800–2000 mg PO 60–90 minutes before exercise) can be used. Studies have shown that preexercise and postexercise serum CK and AST activities were significantly lower in horses treated with oral dantrolene.[10,11] There is no rationale for the once-popular administration of sodium bicarbonate to horses to prevent episodes because most horses do not have underlying acid-base disorders and become alkalotic during exercise.[12] The use of phenytoin (1.4–2.7 mg/kg PO BID) which acts on a number of ion channels within muscle and nerves including sodium and calcium channels has been reported, but it is expensive and may cause sedation, ataxia, focal seizures and recumbency.[13] Thus, until further studies prove the drug's efficacy, it should only be used as a last resort.

Polysaccharide storage myopathy
Pathogenesis
PSSM has been described in Quarter Horses and Appaloosas.[14] It is a heritable myopathy[16] characterised by high muscle glycogen concentrations and the accumulation of abnormal polysaccharide within the myoplasm. There is no defect in the glycolytic or glycogenolytic pathways in affected horses. It has been suggested that there is increased insulin-stimulated glucose uptake by the skeletal muscle and the resultant enhanced glycogen synthesis may be intimately involved in the mechanism responsible for the accumulation of excess glycogen and abnormal polysaccharide.[17] However, the primary defect responsible remains unknown. Longitudinal studies of young horses with PSSM show that when forced to exercise, horses develop muscle

* Re-Leve; Kentucky Equine Research, Versailles, KY, USA (www.Re-Leve.com).

stiffness, cramping and high serum activity of CK prior to the onset of abnormal polysaccharide accumulation.[18]

Diagnosis
PSSM is seen as repeated episodes of muscle cramping induced by little exercise. A genetic test has yet to be developed, so a definitive diagnosis requires histological examination of a gluteal or semimembranosis muscle biopsy specimen (see Chapter 1.55). There is subsarcolemmal accumulation of an abnormal polysaccharide that is visible with a periodic acid–Schiff stain and resistant to amylase digestion.

Acute management
The management of an acute episode of the disease has been described earlier.

Long-term management
As for RER, the goal of long-term management of PSSM is to reduce the frequency of recurrence of clinical episodes through dietary and exercise modification. The diet should be modified to provide adequate calories, with at least 20% of the total calories provide by fat and limited carbohydrate intake (<5% energy from starch). For many horses this can be achieved by feeding 1.5% to 2% of body weight as fibre (i.e., hay), eliminating all grains and adding 0.5 to 1.0 kg rice bran or 0.45 kg (480 ml) vegetable-based oil as fat supplement.[1] Horses in heavy work can be fed up to 2 kg of rice bran with a balanced mineral supplement. Alternatively, a high-fat feed that contains rice bran, which has been developed for rhabdomyolysis*, can be fed in conjunction with the fibre. The horse should be introduced to the higher fat diet over several weeks, and it takes approximately 4 months for full fat adaptation to occur in these horses.[19] Affected animals should be exercised regularly (i.e., daily) and the exercise intensity should be increased gradually. Ideally, horses should be kept at pasture 24 hours a day as the continual low-grade exercise appears to lessen the frequency of episodes of rhabdomyolysis.

Equine polysaccharide storage myopathy
Pathogenesis
EPSM has been described in draft breeds.[15] It is a heritable myopathy characterised by accumulation of abnormal polysaccharide, but the primary defect responsible remains unknown. The incidence of EPSM in the general draft horse population has been estimated to be 45% to 66%.

Clinical signs
The clinical signs of EPSM appear to take two forms. Affected animals may exhibit the traditional exercise-associated muscle cramping. Alternatively, EPSM is associated with a second syndrome characterised by poor performance, progressive muscle wasting, weakness, recumbency and death. Although initially thought to be associated, it appears that even though EPSM and shivers are both common to draft horses, they are unrelated disorders.

Diagnosis
Diagnosis of EPSM is based on the presence of abnormal polysaccharide in muscle biopsy specimens as described for PSSM (see Chapter 1.55).

Acute management
The management of an acute episode of the disease has been described earlier.

Long-term management
The long-term management recommendations for EPSM are identical to those for PSSM.

Monitoring horses with chronic rhabdomyolysis
Monitoring of horses with chronic rhabdomyolysis usually involves evaluating the effect of management recommendations on the frequency of bouts of clinical signs. However, individuals may continue to suffer from subclinical disease. This can be detected by collecting blood samples for the measurement of serum activities of CK and AST before and 4 and 24 hours after a period of submaximal exercise. In the absence of subclinical disease, the baseline serum CK and AST activities should be within the reference range; the serum CK activity should not more than double compared to the baseline value 4 hours after exercise and should have returned to baseline 24 hours after exercise; and the serum AST activity should not increase by more than 50% at 24 hours after exercise.

Electrolyte depletion
Electrolytes play an important role in normal muscle function. In horses with no underlying myopathy, electrolyte imbalances and deficiencies may occasionally cause muscle dysfunction and rhabdomyolysis. In horses predisposed to rhabdomyolysis due to an underlying myopathy, electrolyte imbalances and deficiencies may lead to more frequent and severe bouts of acute rhabdomyolysis.

Detection
Alterations in the intracellular or extracellular concentrations of electrolytes can be due to a dietary deficiency and/or loss in sweat during exercise. The most appropriate method of detection of such deficiencies is through dietary analysis and measurement of urinary fractional excretions (FE).

Dietary analysis
This can be performed using commercially available computer software or by contacting the manufacturer of the feed currently used.

* Re-Leve; Kentucky Equine Research, Versailles, KY, USA (www.Re-Leve.com).

Urinary fractional excretions

A free catch urine sample and a venous blood sample should be obtained at approximately the same time. Urine and blood concentrations of sodium, potassium, chloride, calcium, phosphate and creatinine are measured. The FE is calculated as follows:

$$FE = [(\text{plasma creatinine/urine creatinine}) \times (\text{urine electrolyte/plasma electrolyte})] \times 100$$

A low FE is suggestive of either a dietary deficiency or excessive loss in sweat and should be corrected by oral supplementation.

References

1. De La Corte FD, Valberg SJ: Treatment of polysaccharide storage myopathy. Compend Cont Educ Pract Vet 22:782-788, 2000
2. Piercy RJ, Rivero JL: Muscle disorders of equine atheletes, in Hinchcliff KW, Kaneps AJ, Geor RJ (eds): Equine Sports Medicine and Surgery. Philadelphia, WB Saunders, 2004, pp 82-83
3. Bloom BA, Valentine BA, Gleed RD, et al.: Postanaesthetic recumbency in a Belgian filly with polysaccharide storage myopathy. Vet Rec 144:73-75, 1999
4. Jackson CA, Divers TJ: Nervous system, in Orsini JA, Divers TJ (eds): Manual of Equine Emergencies. Philadelphia, WB Saunders, 1998, pp 356-357
5. Valentine BA: Equine polysaccharide storage myopathy. Equine Vet Educ 15:254-262, 2003
6. MacLeay JM, Sorum SA, Valberg SJ, et al.: Epidemiologic analysis of factors influencing exertional rhabdomyolysis in Thoroughbreds. Am J Vet Res 60:1562-1569, 1999
7. Lentz LR, Valberg SJ, Herold LV, et al.: Myoplasmic calcium regulation in myotubes from horses with recurrent exertional rhabdomyolysis. Am J Vet Res 63:1724-1731, 2002
8. MacKenzie EC, Valberg SJ, Godden SM, et al.: Plasma and urine electrolyte and mineral concentrations in thoroughbred horses with recurrent exertional rhabdomyolysis after consumption of diets varying in cation-anion balance. Am J Vet Res 63:1053-1060, 2002
9. MacLeay JM, Valberg SJ, Pagan JD, et al.: Effect of diet on thoroughbred horses with recurrent exertional rhabdomyolysis performing a standardised exercise test. Equine Vet J Suppl 30:458-462, 1999
10. Edwards JE, Newtont JR, Ramzan PH, et al.: The efficacy of dantrolene sodium in controlling exertional rhabdomyolysis in the Thoroughbred racehorse. Equine Vet J 35:707-711, 2004
11. McKenzie EC, Valberg SJ, Godden SM, et al.: Effect of oral administration of dantrolene sodium on serum creatine kinase activity after exercise in horses with recurrent exertional rhabdomyolysis. Am J Vet Res 65:74-79, 2004
12. Koterba A, Carlson GP: Acid-base and electrolyte alterations in horses with exertional rhabdomyolysis. J Am Vet Med Assoc 180:303-306, 1982
13. Beech J: Chronic exertional rhabdomyolysis. Vet Clin North Am Equine Pract 13:145-168, 1997
14. Valberg SJ, Mickelson JR, Gallant EM, et al.: Exertional rhabdomyolysis in quarter horses and thoroughbreds: one syndrome, multiple aetiologies. Equine Vet J Suppl 30:533-538, 1999
15. Valentine BA: Polysaccharide storage myopathy in Draft and Draft-related horses and ponies. Equine Pract 21:16-21, 1999
16. Valberg SJ, Geyer C, Sorum SA, et al.: Familial basis of exertional rhabdomyolysis in Quarter horse related breeds. Am J Vet Res 57:286-290, 1996
17. Annandale EJ, Valberg SJ, Mickelson JR, Seaquist ER: Insulin sensitivity and skeletal muscle glucose transport in horses with equine polysaccharide storage myopathy. Neuromusc Disord 14:666-674, 2004
18. Firshman AM, Valberg SJ, Bender JB, Finno CJ: Epidemiologic characteristics and management of polysaccharide storage myopathy in quarter horses. Am J Vet Res 64:1319-1327, 2003
19. Valentine BA, Reynolds AJ, Ducharme NG, et al.: Dietary therapy of polysaccharide storage myopathy. Equine Pract 19:30-37, 1997

15.5 Monitoring horses with implants

Louise L. Southwood

Implants are used for surgical repair of various lesions in horses. Types of implants commonly used include plates, screws, pins, and wires for fracture repair; meshes for hernioplasty; and large synthetic nonabsorbable suture for laryngoplasty. The two most important complications associated with implant use are (1) repair breakdown and (2) infection. Patients should be monitored closely during hospitalisation for these complications. When an implant-associated infection is identified, a sample of fluid or tissue should always be aseptically collected for bacterial culture and sensitivity prior to treatment with empirical antimicrobial drugs.

Musculoskeletal implants

Failure of a fracture repair can occur catastrophically during recovery from general anaesthesia, in which case the horse usually becomes acutely non–weight-bearing lame in the affected limb and disruption of the repair may be diagnosed by observing or palpating the limb. Definitive diagnosis should always be obtained using radiography. Repair breakdowns can also occur gradually during hospitalisation. Horses will become lame in the affected limb with preferential weight-bearing on the supporting limb. Any worsening of lameness in the repaired limb warrants radiographic assessment. Several radiographic views should be taken. Radiographic signs that should be assessed are movement of fracture fragments, backing out of screws, and bending or breaking of screws, plates or pins in the case of a transfixation pin cast or external skeletal fixator (Figure 15.10, A and B).

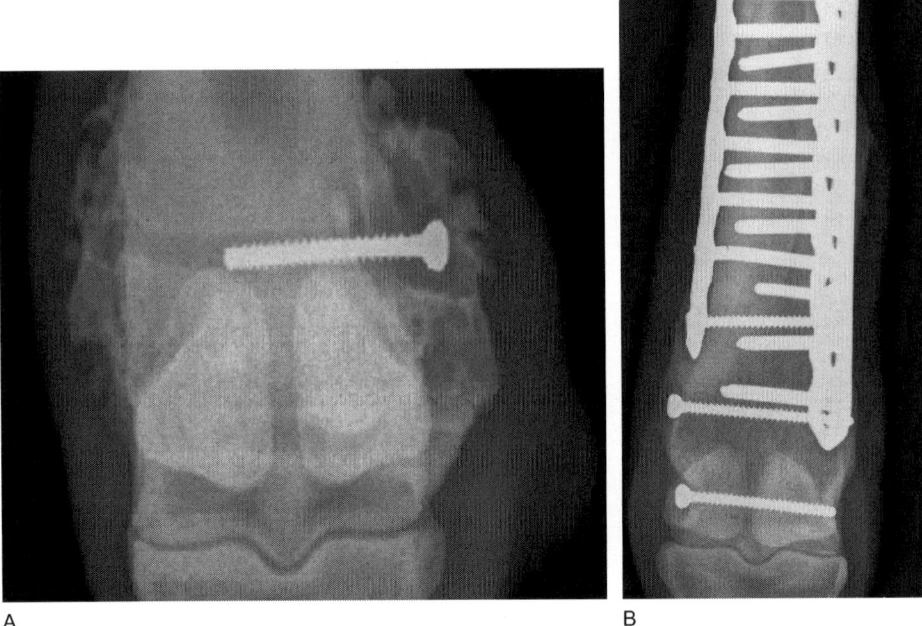

Figure 15.10A-B Radiography can be used to detect implant failure, for example screws backing out (15.10A) and breaking (15.10B). Figure 15.10A is a horse with chronic infection and periosteal proliferation and screw-associated bone lysis are radiographically apparent. Radiographic images courtesy of Drs. Midge Leitch, Janet Johnston (15.10A), and Dean Richardson (15.10B).

Implant associated infection

Implant-associated infection is unfortunately common in equine orthopaedic patients. Impaired fracture healing and osteomyelitis are the most common causes of treatment failure following long-bone fracture repair, with an occurrence rate of 30% to 40%.[1–4] Rubor, dulor, calor, tumour (redness, pain, heat and swelling) and drainage are signs consistent with infection. Signs of infection can occur from days to weeks after surgery. Redness may be observed in areas of white skin but is not often recognised in areas with pigmented skin. Horses should be monitored closely for an increase in lameness in the affected limb. Horse with an implant infection may raise and lower the limb while standing, lie down more frequently, or have a grade 4/5 or 5/5 lameness. In addition to lameness, there is usually pain on palpation of the affected limb. While an increase in heat compared to normal is associated with infection, this finding can be difficult to interpret because the affected limb is often clipped and bandaged or cast, both of which increase the skin temperature compared to that of surrounding areas. During bandage or cast changes, the limb may be more swollen than expected or the swelling may have increased compared to that at a previous bandage or cast change. Drainage from the surgical incision should raise concern regarding implant infection. Granulation tissue forms around the draining track. Orthopaedic implant infection should be suspected in horses demonstrating any of these signs and this should prompt further diagnostic tests and treatment.

Box 15.6. Sources of post-operative fever following surgical placement of orthopaedic implants

- Respiratory (pneumonia/pleuropneumonia)
- Gastrointestinal (enterocolitis, including salmonellosis or clostridiosis)
- Intravenous catheter-related (septic thombophlebitis)
- Viral infection
- Superficial (incisional) surgical site infection
- Deep (including implant-associated) surgical site infection

Fever

Horses should not have a fever postoperatively. Any signs of fever (rectal temperature >38.5° C [101.3° F]) warrants a thorough work-up (see Chapter 7.1). Sources of postoperative fever following surgical placement of orthopaedic implants are given in Box 15.6. Each possible fever source should be investigated and ruled out. Haematology and measurement of serum fibrinogen should be performed. Horses with infection will often have a leukocytosis, left shift (increase in nonsegmented neutrophils compared to normal) and hyperfibrinogenaemia. While these findings can also be associated with surgery and trauma, a left shift and persistent or severe leucocytosis and hyperfibrinogenaemia should raise concern of an infection... somewhere!

Radiography

Radiographic evaluation of the repair is easy, quick, economical and readily available. While radiography is the most commonly used diagnostic tool for diagnosing orthopaedic implant infection, it is important to remember that radiography is insensitive for early detection of bone lysis. A spherical lesion in trabecular bone needs to be greater than 15 mm in diameter and 30% to 50% of the calcium lost before it can be discerned radiographically.[5] Radiographic signs of osteomyelitis may not be visible for up to 14 days after the onset of disease[6]; changes consistent with osteomyelitis were visible in less than 5% of human patients initially, less than 30% at 1 week and 90% were positive at 3 to 4 weeks.[7] In a canine osteomyelitis model, radiography had a sensitivity of 62.5% and a specificity of 57.1% at 8 weeks after inoculation for diagnosing osteomyelitis.[8] Early radiographic signs of implant-associated orthopaedic infection and osteomyelitis are soft tissue swelling and loss of fascial planes, which is followed sequentially by periosteal thickening and elevation, osteopaenia, cortical destruction, sequestration, bone necrosis and involucrum-cloaca formation.[9] With chronicity, periosteal reaction, lysis and sclerosis are observed[9] (Figure 15.11, A and B).

Ultrasonography

Sonography can be useful for diagnosing osteomyelitis and implant-associated infection. Sonography is simple, rapid, noninvasive and inexpensive; however, skill and experience are necessary to obtain good-image quality and for interpretation of findings. Sonographic findings of fluid directly adjacent to the bone are consistent with osteomyelitis.[10] If there is soft tissue interposed between the fluid and the bone, then a diagnosis of osteomyelitis cannot be made and the patient is more likely to have an abscess or cellulitis.[10]

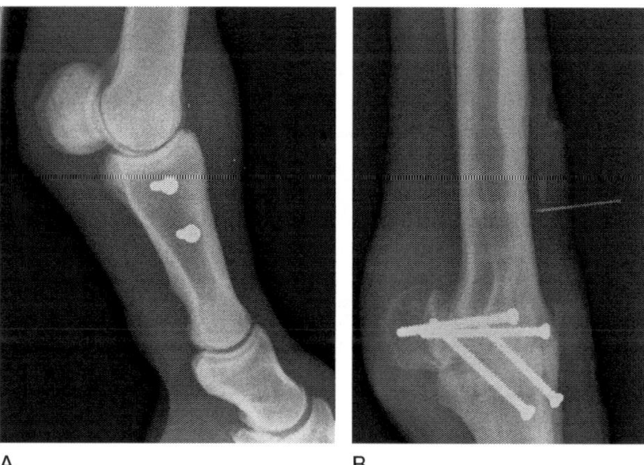

A B

Figures 15.11A-B Radiographic signs of early implant-associated infection include soft tissue swelling and loss of fascial planes (15.11A) and chronic implant-associated infection with periosteal proliferation and screw-associated bone lysis. Figure 15.11B is a fetlock arthrodesis and several implants have previously been removed. Radiographic images courtesy of Drs. Dean Richardson and Midge Leitch.

Other sonographic signs that are consistent with osteomyelitis include gas associated with an anaerobic infection, fluid-filled tracts, irregular bone surface and fragments or sequestra.[11] Sonographic signs consistent with osteomyelitis were detected prior to radiographic signs.[10,11] Sonographic changes were seen 1 to 2 days after the onset of clinical signs in human patients with acute primary osteomyelitis,[12] and sonography has a reported sensitivity of 83% for diagnosing osteomyelitis.[13] False-positive findings associated with soft tissue infection have been reported.[14] Sonography has not gained widespread use for diagnosis of implant-associated infection, most likely because the sonographic findings may be difficult to interpret in light of recent trauma and surgery and many experienced clinicians rely on clinical and radiographic findings.

Scintigraphy

Scintigraphy can be used to assess bone healing, vascular supply and osteomyelitis using technetium-labeled methylene diphosphonate (Tc-HDP), leukocytes, antigranulocyte antibodies or ciprofloxacin. Tc-HDP accumulates in areas of hyperaemia, as well as hydroxyapatite and immature collagen deposition.[15] In three horses with metacarpal or metatarsal fractures, Tc-HDP was used to evaluate vascularity and fracture healing. Horses with an increase in radionuclide uptake ratio healed the fracture, whereas one horse that did not have an increase in uptake developed an atrophic nonunion, with sequestration of the metacarpus and the horse was euthanised.[16] Tc-HDP can be used for identifying a site of infection or osteomyelitis in, for example, a case of fever of unknown origin; however, is not necessarily useful for diagnosing infection following surgical repair of a long-bone fracture because both fracture healing and infection will cause an increase in radionuclide uptake. Similarly, technetium-labeled leucocytes and antigranulocyte antibodies are not useful for differentiating infection from inflammation. The overall accuracy of labeled antigranulocyte antibodies was 72% with a sensitivity of 95% but a specificity of only 57% for diagnosing osteomyelitis.[17]

Technetium-labeled ciprofloxacin was developed specifically to differentiate infection from inflammation. Ciprofloxacin binds to bacterial DNA gyrase of both sensitive and resistant bacteria, as well as both resting and actively multiplying bacteria, and does not bind to dead bacteria. Ciprofloxacin reportedly penetrates abscesses, does not localise in the bone marrow as do labeled leukocytes and is independent of the patient's leukocyte count. Technetium-labeled ciprofloxacin is stable *in vivo*. Advantages of technetium-labeled ciprofloxacin compared to other scintigraphy methods for detecting infection include the theoretical high specificity for infection, blood handling is unnecessary, and the minimum time, technical skills and laboratory equipment required for preparation. When technetium-labeled ciprofloxacin was investigated experimentally for its ability to differentiate infected and noninfected fractures, there was no difference in radionuclide uptake ratio between the two groups at 4 and 8 weeks. There was a low specificity for diagnosing infected fractures, with a high percentage of false-positive diagnoses. Hyperaemia and oedema can cause an increase in the uptake of technetium-labeled ciprofloxacin. Technetium-labeled ciprofloxacin was no better than Tc-HDP for identifying infection.

Advanced imaging

While computerised tomography (CT) and magnetic resonance imaging (MRI) can be useful for diagnosing osteomyelitis, they are not useful for assessing implant-related infections. Metallic implants cause CT artifacts and stainless steel implants are contraindicated in MRI because of the strong magnetic field. Additionally, these diagnostic procedures are expensive, usually require general anaesthesia, and are not commonly available.

Laminitis

Horses with orthopaedic implants should also be monitored closely for laminitis because any worsening of lameness on the affected limb leads to an increase in weight-bearing on the contralateral limb and ultimately support-limb laminitis (see Chapter 15.2).

Mesh hernioplasty

A mesh is often used to repair large body wall hernias following trauma or a ventral midline celiotomy surgical site infection. Complications associated with mesh hernioplasty include hernia recurrence, persistent incisional drainage, adhesion between the hernia and abdominal viscera, peritonitis, implant infection and general anaesthesia complications.[17,18] Because these wounds were contaminated or infected, it is common for the mesh to become infected. Swelling (oedema or cellulitis) and drainage of purulent material from the site of mesh implantation are associated with infection (Figure 15.12). Horses may also

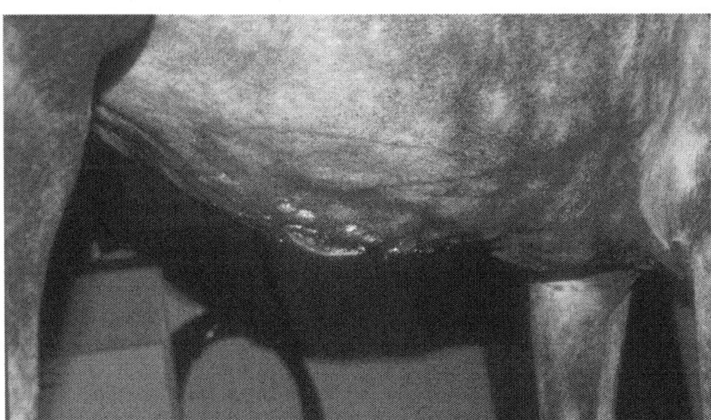

Figure 15.12 Drainage from a mesh hernioplasty site. Several areas of skin necrosis are apparent with drainage of purulent material from these sites. © Louise Southwood 2006.

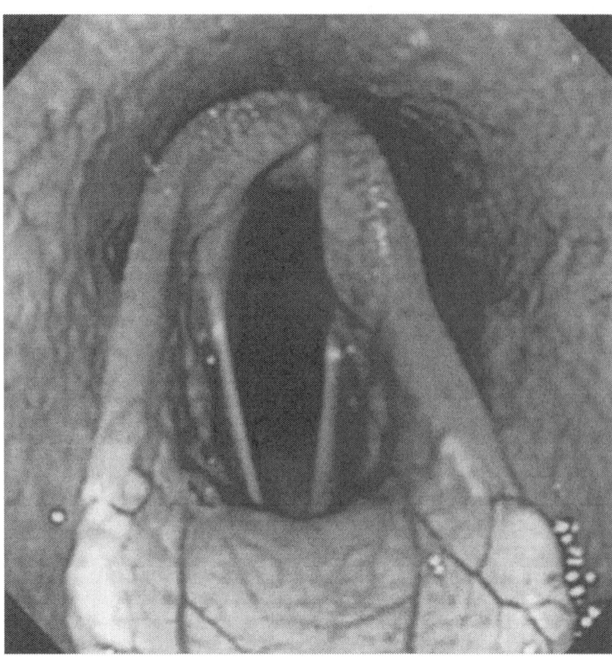

Figure 15.13 Endoscopy of the upper respiratory tract showing loss of abduction of the left arytenoid cartilage following laryngoplasty. Endoscopic image courtesy of Dr. Eric Parente, New Bolton Center, University of Pennsylvania. © Eric Parente 2006.

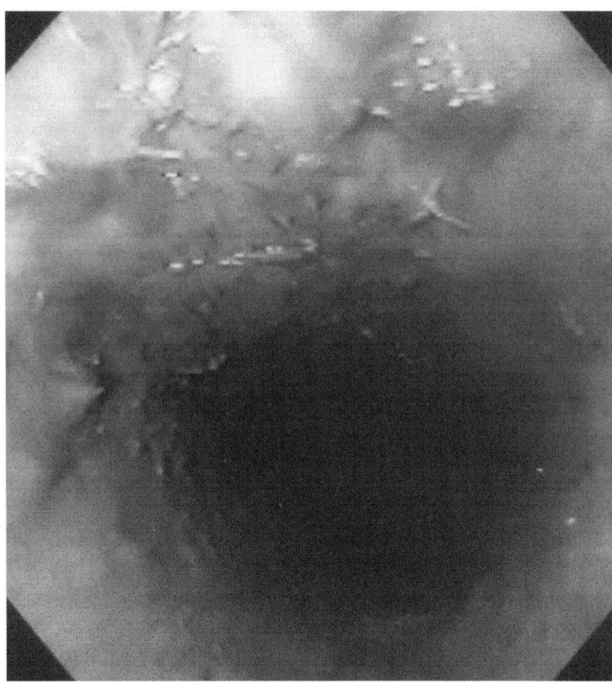

Figure 15.14 Endoscopy of the trachea in a horse following laryngoplasty. Aspirated feed material is seen in the tracheal lumen. Endoscopic image courtesy of Dr. Eric Parente, New Bolton Center, University of Pennsylvania. © Eric Parente 2006.

be painful to palpation. Often, these horses are treated with antimicrobial drugs for long time periods, and if drainage persists following discontinuing antimicrobial drugs, then the mesh can be removed once there is adequate fibrous tissue to close the body wall.

In a recent study evaluating mesh hernioplasty in 13 large horses,[19] all horses exhibited signs of abdominal pain during the initial 24 hours following mesh hernioplasty. All horses had seroma or haematoma formation at the surgical site. Sixty-two percent of horses had drainage from the surgical site and 23% of horses the obliquus internus abdominus (OIA) tore near the mesh-tissue interface. In 2 horses with OIA tearing, haematoma formation was extensive and required a blood transfusion in 1 horse, and in both horses skin necrosis occurred. The 3 horses with OIA tearing weighed more than 590 kg and 2 were midgestation mares. Other complications occurring in these horses were diarrhoea, laminitis and abdominal pain. Based on the findings of this study, large horses in particular should be monitored closely for swelling and drainage associated with the surgical site, anaemia associated with haemorrhage and haematoma formation, body wall tearing adjacent to the mesh hernioplasty, skin necrosis, abdominal pain, diarrhoea and laminitis. Sonographic examination can be used to identify and characterise fluid accumulation adjacent to the mesh hernioplasty and intestinal adhesions to the surgical site. Fluid accumulations can be identified and then drained with a sample collected for bacterial culture and sensitivity.

Laryngoplasty

Failure to maintain abduction is the most common complication following laryngoplasty (Figure 15.13). The incidence of failure ranges from 2% to 15%.[20–22] Loss of abduction is usually noted within the first month of surgery. Endoscopic reevaluation is recommended the day after surgery and at least 1 month postoperatively. Dysphagia with aspiration of gross feed material is the second most common complication, occurring in an estimated 5% to 10% of cases (Figure 15.14). Nasal discharge and coughing are clinical signs that should prompt another endoscopic evaluation. Many horses that aspirate in the immediate postoperative period will resolve spontaneously without further treatment within the first 2 weeks. If they do not, reoperation is recommended.

Implant infection is uncommon (0.5%–6.0%) following laryngoplasty.[20–22] Horses should be monitored for signs of swelling associated with the laryngoplasty surgical site. If marked swelling occurs, it is most often a seroma and drainage is recommended (Eric Parente, personal communication). Additional signs consistent with infection include fever, dysphagia and coughing. A fever should be investigated thoroughly for a source of infection other than the surgical site. If a surgical site infection occurs, it is not always associated with the implant and implant removal is not always indicated.

References

1. Auer JA, Watkins JP: Treatment of radial fractures in adult horses: an analysis of 15 clinical cases. Equine Vet J 19:103-110, 1987
2. Sanders-Shamis M, Bramlage LR, Gable AA: Radius fractures in the horse: a retrospective study of 47 cases. Equine Vet J 18:432-437, 1986
3. Crawford WH, Fretz PB: Long bone fractures in large animals. A retrospective study. Vet Surg 14:295-302, 1985
4. Hance SR, Bramlage LR, Schneider RD, Embertson RM: Retrospective study of 38 cases of femur fractures in horses less than one year of age. Equine Vet J 24:357-363, 1992
5. Letts RM, Afifi A, Sutherland JB: Technetium bone scanning as an aid in the diagnosis of atypical acute osteomyelitis in children. Surg Gynecol Obstet 140:899-902, 1975
6. Munoz P, Bouza E: Acute and chronic adult osteomyelitis and prosthesis-related infections. Bailliere's Clin Rheumatol 13:129-147, 1999
7. Wegener WA, Alavi A: Diagnostic imaging of musculoskeletal infection. Orthop Clin N Am 22:401-418, 1991
8. Braden TD, Tvedten HW, Mostosky UV, et al.: the sensitivity and specificity of radiology and histopathology in the diagnosis of posttraumatic osteomyelitis. Vet Comp Orthop Traum 3:98-103, 1989
9. Sammak B, Abd El Bagi A, Al Shahed M, et al.: Osteomyelitis: a review of currently used imaging techniques. Eur J Radiol 9:894-900, 1999
10. Nath AK, Sethu M: Use of ultrasound in osteomyelitis. Br J Radiol 65:649-652, 1992
11. Reef VB, Reimer JM, Reid CF: Ultrasonographic findings in horses with osteomyelitis. Proc Am Assoc Equine Pract 37:381-391, 1991
12. Sammak B, Abd El Bagi A, Al Shahed M, et al.: Osteomyelitis: a review of currently used imaging techniques. Eur Radiol 9:894-900, 1999
13. Abiri M, Kirpekar M, Ablow RC: Osteomyelitis: detection with US. Radiology 172:509-511, 1989
14. Abiri MM, DeAngelis GA, Kirpekar M, et al.: Ultrasound detection of osteomyelitis. Invest Radiol 27:111-113, 1992
15. Rosenthall L, Lisbona R, Hernandez M, et al.: 99mTc-PO4 and Ga-67 imaging following the insertion of orthopaedic devices. Radiology 133:717-721, 1979
16. Markel MD, Snyder JR, Hornof WJ, et al.: Nuclear scintigraphic evaluation of third metacarpal and metatarsal bone fractures in three horses. J Am Vet Med Assoc 191:75-77, 1987
17. Tulleners EP, Fretz PB: Prosthetic repair of large abdominal wall defects in horses and food animals. J Am Vet Med Assoc 182:258-262, 1983
18. van der Velden MA, Klein WR: A modified technique for implantation of polypropylene mesh for the repair of external abdominal hernias in horses: a review of 21 cases. Vet Quart 16:S108-S110, 1994
19. Elce YA, Kraus BM, Orsini JA: Mesh hernioplasty for repair of incisional hernias of the ventral body wall in large horses. Equine Vet Educ 17:252-256, 2005
20. Kraus BM, Parente EJ, Tulleners EP: Laryngoplasty with ventriculectomy or ventriculocordectomy in 104 draft horses. Vet Surg 32:530-538, 2003

21. Dixon P M, McGorum B C, Railton D I, et al.: Long-term survey of laryngoplasty and ventriculocordectomy in an older, mixed-breed population of 200 horses. Part 1: maintenance of surgical arytenoid abduction and complications of surgery. Equine Vet J 35:389-396, 2003
22. Hawkins J F, Tulleners E P, Ross M W, et al.: Laryngoplasty with or without ventriculectomy for treatment of left laryngeal hemiplegia in 230 racehorses. Vet Surg 26:484-491, 1997

15.6 Monitoring surgical incisions

Ehud Eliashar

In some procedures, surgical wound infection is considered a significant postoperative complication and an important cause of morbidity and even mortality.[1] Therefore, postoperatively, all surgical wounds have to be routinely monitored, mainly for signs of developing infection and/or dehiscence. The implications of wound infection are closely associated with the type and location of the procedure performed. For example, in orthopaedic procedures, because there is relatively little soft tissue overlying the bones and joints in the distal limb, excessive swelling or motion may lead to sutures cutting into the skin, and thus the surgical incision becomes an important pathway for bacteria to invade and colonise the superficial tissues and facilitate the progress of infection deeper.[2] The ventral aspect of the abdomen is another important location where infection of midline incisions following abdominal surgery occurs in approximately 7% to 37% of horses[3–5] and is closely associated with wound dehiscence and hernia formation[3]. It has been suggested that classifying the surgical wound as clean/clean-contaminated/contaminated/dirty and infected may allow the surgeon to anticipate if the wound is likely to become infected or not.[1] In the horse, however, this association varies greatly between soft tissue procedures where no such association exists and orthopaedic procedures where clean-contaminated surgeries are 24 times more likely to develop a postoperative surgical site infection compared to clean procedures.[6] However, some controversy exists with regards to the latter as contaminated and infected synovial structures resulting from traumatic wounds, were converted to a clean-contaminated state using arthroscopy/tenoscopy, and successfully treated and closed primarily with very low rate of surgical site infection.[7]

Routinely, whenever possible, surgical incisions should be protected by sterile dressing materials. If the incision is over a high motion area, immobilising the limb should be considered to minimise the tension created on the sutured skin. It is important that postoperatively every wound is inspected frequently, the horse is closely monitored for clinical signs associated with wound infection and all attempts are made to maintain a clean, dry seal of the surgical incision in order to avoid complications from infection. If infection is suspected, the horse should be assessed for clinical signs, and ultrasonographic evaluation of the surgical site should be considered (see Chapter 15.7). Cytologic examination of fluid obtained from a potential infected space or organ is valuable to determine if infection is present, and fluid obtained from incisional infection should be cultured in order to identify the correct antimicrobial therapy.[1]

Clinical signs of surgical site infection vary, but the earliest and most consistent sign of wound infection is low grade persistent elevation in body temperature or alternatively high temperature (39°–40° C) during the first 14 days post operatively.[1,2] Accumulation of fluid at the surgery site that can be palpated or imaged ultrasonographically is another early sign of infection and other local signs include swelling and increased heat around the incision, and the skin may appear reddened or pink and may start to thin out. The horse may respond with pain to palpation at the site, and horses that had an orthopaedic procedure may be lamer than expected. As a result of the local swelling, the sutures are subjected to increased tension and may cut into the skin, and there may be drainage through the incision or along the sutures with/without partial dehiscence. Incisions may drain clear serous or serosanguineous fluid without infection, but these horses are at a greater risk of developing one compared to those in which the incision remains dry and sealed.[2] Occasionally, only superficial infection is present with no involvement of the deeper tissues, and in these cases minimal interference is required (Figure 15.15). If, however, a pocket of fluid is identified, or the wound has partially dehisced and is draining, removal of some skin sutures at the most dependent part of the incision to improve drainage is recommended. If a synovial cavity is infected, either as a complication or as recurrence of condition, the horse should be subjected to

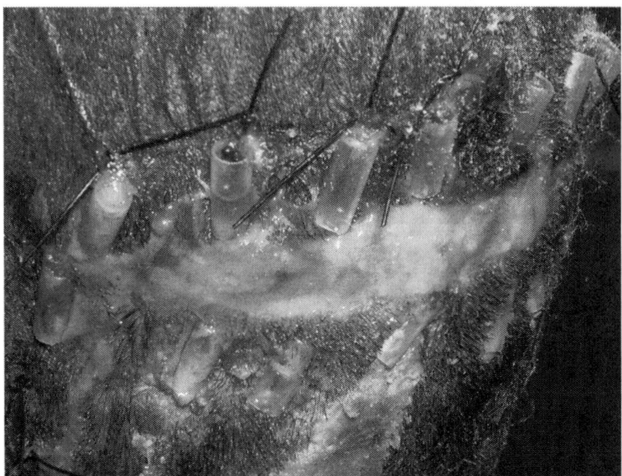

Figure 15.15 Appearance of a wound over the tarsal sheath which was closed primarily following tenoscopic lavage of the sheath. Note the superficial infection of the wound and the partial dehiscence despite using tension relieving suture pattern. The tarsal sheath was not infected and therefore only gentle cleaning of the wound was required. © Ehud Eliashar 2006.

arthroscopic lavage rather than the synovial cavity left open to drain. It is also important to note that postoperative oedema of celiotomy incisions is extremely common and is not necessarily indicative of infection.

In order to minimise interference with the early stages of the healing process, the first bandage change should ideally take place not earlier than 3 days from the procedure. A stent protecting a ventral midline incision should be removed 12 to 24 hours postoperatively, as delay in removal appears to be associated with increased risk of wound infection,[4] and similarly, a bandage/stent soaked with blood or other secretion should be removed or replaced. Routinely, the bandage should be changed every 3 to 5 days until the skin sutures are removed approximately 12 to 14 days postoperatively, at which stage aggregation of collagen macromolecules into fibrillar bundles has peaked, providing the wound with stability and tensile strength.[9]

Special attention is required for surgical incisions in which a drain has been placed, whereby the wound and the amount of fluid excreted through the drain have to be assessed daily. Drains should be removed as soon as possible, once the volume of fluid is significantly reduced and its consistency changed to serous, nonodiferous slightly turbid fluid. On average drains should be maintained for no more than 2 to 4 days postoperatively, as they may act as a potential source of ascending infection.[8] Surgical wounds protected by a cast are even more challenging to monitor, as visual assessment is impossible. Additional worrying signs may include inappropriate use of the limb in the cast, staining (strikethrough) and significantly increased heat of the cast over the wound. However, these signs may result from cast sore as well, and therefore decision making in these cases may be difficult because removal of the cast for the purpose of further wound assessment leads to lose of the support/protection of the cast.

References

1. Waguespack RW, Burba DJ, Moore RM: Surgical site infection and the use of antimicrobials, in Auer JA, Stick JA (eds): Equine Surgery, ed 3. Philadelphia, Saunders Elsevier, 2005, pp 70-87
2. Schneider RK: Synovial and osseous infections, in Auer JA, Stick JA (eds): Equine Surgery, ed 3. Philadelphia, Saunders Elsevier, 2005, pp 1121-1130
3. French NP, Smith J, Edwards GB, Proudman: Equine surgical colic: risk factors for postoperative complications. Equine Vet J 34:444-449, 2002.
4. Mair TS, Smith LJ: Survival and complication rates in 300 horses undergoing surgical treatment of colic. Part 2: Short-term complications. Equine Vet J 37:303-309, 2005
5. Phillips TJ, Walmsley JP: Retrospective analysis of the results of 151 exploratory laparotomies in horses with gastrointestinal disease. Equine Vet J 25:427-431, 1993
6. MacDonald DG, Morley PS, Bailey JV, Barber SM, Fretz PB: An examination of the occurrence of surgical wound infection following equine orthopaedic surgery (1981-1990). Equine Vet J 26:323-326, 1994
7. Wright IM, Smith MR, Humphrey DJ, Eaton-Evans TC, Hillyer MH: Endoscopic surgery in the treatment of contaminated and infected synovial cavities. Equine Vet J 35:613-619, 2003
8. Auer JA: Drains, bandages, and external coaptation, in Auer JA, Stick JA (eds): Equine Surgery, ed 3. Philadelphia, Saunders Elsevier, 2005, pp 202-218
9. Theoret CL: The pathophysiology of wound repair. Vet Clin North Am Equine Pract 21:1-13, 2005

15.7 Ultrasonography of surgical incisions

Ehud Eliashar

The extent of some postoperative complications associated with a surgical procedure is difficult to ascertain as the subdermal tissues are not visible. In these cases, ultrasonographic assessment of the surgical site offers the best and cheapest imaging modality of all soft tissue structures to the level of and including the surface of the bone in musculoskeletal conditions, and the internal organs in abdominal/thoracic procedures. Indications for performing an ultrasound scan include focal/general swelling of the surgical site which may/may not be painful to palpation, drainage of exudate or pus through the surgical site, partial or full dehiscence of the suture line and any clinical signs that may be indicative of surgical site infection such as peak in body temperature a few days postoperatively, when the cause cannot be identified elsewhere.

Equipment

Scanning directly over the surgical wound requires some preparation in order to minimise the risk of contamination. The horse should be restrained in stocks and sedated if required. Commonly, only a short time has elapsed from surgery; therefore, clipping around the site may not be required. However, if clipping is indicated, the incision should be gently covered with sterile K-Y Jelly beforehand, and clipping should be carried out carefully in order to avoid cutting the skin sutures. The surgical site should then be gently cleaned with sterile saline or diluted povidone-iodine solution. If the wound appears dry and clean, performing the scan under sterile conditions is recommended, and this can be easily achieved by using sterile gloves, placing the ultrasound probe within a sterile sleeve/rectal glove filled with coupling gel and applying sterile K-Y Jelly on the incision and the covered probe. Such measures are of less importance if the wound is obviously infected and/or draining; however, general cleanliness is still advisable.

A linear 7.5- to 10-MHz transducer with/without a standoff should be used to image the incision and immediate structures. Occasionally, when a celiotomy incision is being scanned, a lower-frequency sector transducer may be required to follow any draining tract towards the peritoneal cavity.

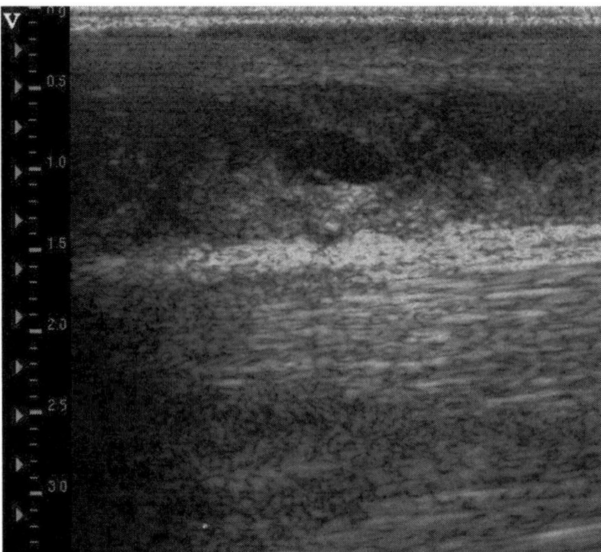

Figure 15.16 A longitudinal ultrasonographic image of the plantar aspect of a hind limb in a horse following neurectomy of the deep branch of the lateral plantar nerve. An echogenic capsule containing anechoic fluid, indicative of abscess, is present subcutaneously and plantar to the superficial digital flexor tendon (SDFT). © Ehud Eliashar 2006.

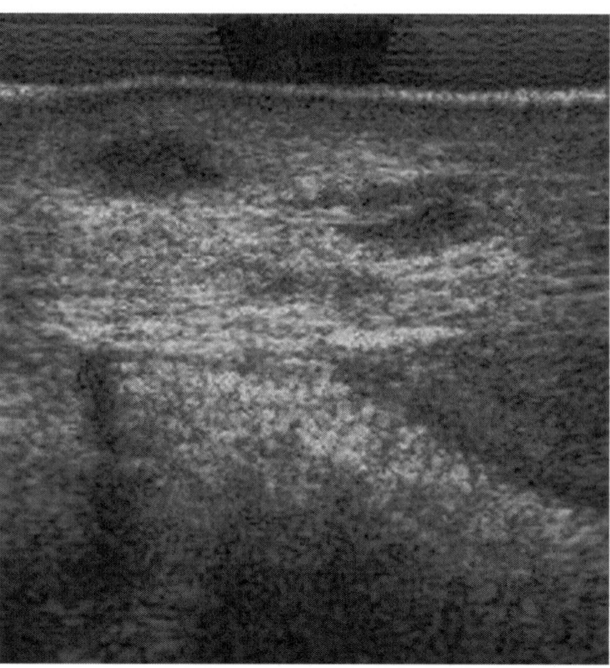

Figure 15.17 A longitudinal ultrasonographic image of a ventral midline incision in a horse following an abdominal surgery. Note two hyperechoic capsules surrounding hypoechoic material (fluid) and echogenic suture material contained within the one on the right, and appears to traverse towards the other, indicative of suture sinus formation. © Ehud Eliashar 2006.

Images obtained

Ultrasonography can demonstrate oedema, haematoma/seroma, abscessation, draining tracts, suture sinus formation and fluid accumulation around bones/implants. Suture material is commonly seen as short straight lines with homogeneous hyperechogenicity casting variable acoustic shadow.[1] Ultrasonographically, oedema appears like a hypoechoic area, extending 5 to 10 cm on either side of the incision. It is important to note that peri-incisional oedema is extremely common following abdominal ventral midline incisions. Pus/exudate draining incisions may reveal hypoechoic to anechoic tracts from the surface of the skin to the suture lines in the deeper layers, which are often surrounded by fluid forming suture sinus.[1] Multiple sutures may be involved, and if a tract is identified, it should be followed to its deepest extent, in order to identify any involvement of the deepest parts of the surgical site, such as the bone, peritoneum or peritoneal cavity. If an abscess has formed, it appears as a region of heterogeneous echogenicity surrounding hypoechoic fluid (Figure 15.16), and when suture material is involved, this abscess will contain a small focal hyperechoic area thought to represent the suture material[2] (Figure 15.17). In cases of orthopaedic infection, the ultrasound scan may demonstrate accumulation of hypoechoic fluid around bones/implants, and tendon sheaths may contain echogenic material thought to be clumps of fibrin.

Ultrasound image of a haematoma varies with its stage, the tissue into which the bleeding has occurred and the involvement of adjacent structures. The typical appearance is of anechoic fluid-filled structure containing fibrinous loculation, but recent haematoma may have a homogeneous echogenic appearance.[1] The haematoma may contain masses with variable echogenicity, associated with organising clots, while an organised haematoma may appear encapsulated by a thick echogenic capsule, and the contents remain echogenic and loculated. Seroma is indistinguishable from haematoma in most instances.

Ultrasonography can be used not only to identify the cause but also, in postoperative surgical site infection, it can be used for a guided sample collection with a needle for cytology, culture and sensitivity. In other cases, ultrasonography can identify pockets/abscesses that can be drained or sutures that can be removed[3] (Figure 15.17).

References

1. Reef VB: The use of diagnostic ultrasound in the horse. Ultrasound Q 9:1-33, 1991
2. Reef VB: Ultrasonographic evaluation of small parts, in Reef VB (ed): Equine Diagnostic Ultrasound, Philadelphia, WB Saunders, 1998, pp 480-547
3. Byars TD, Halley J: Uses of ultrasound in equine internal medicine. Vet Clin North Am Equine Pract 2:253-258, 1986

15.8 Management of surgical site infections

Louise L. Southwood

Recognition and acceptance compose the most critical part of managing surgical site infections (SSIs). Infection should be suspected in any postoperative patient that develops a fever, particularly if the first signs of fever occur longer than 48 hours after surgery. Leucocyte count and serum fibrinogen concentration should be measured in any case in which the horse develops a postoperative fever. The source of the fever should be localised. Common sources of a fever include deep and superficial SSI, respiratory tract infection, catheter site infection and enterocolitis.

Signs of swelling (oedema and cellulitis), heat, pain on palpation, redness and drainage are indications of a superficial SSI. A deep SSI can have similar signs but be more difficult to definitively diagnose. Sonographic examination of deeper structures can be used to diagnose infection. For example, abdominal sonographic examination can be used to identify an increase in peritoneal fluid volume and echogenicity compared to normal, which is suggestive of septic peritonitis, or a large volume of fluid within the colonic lumen, which may be an indication of colitis, and sonographic examination can be used to identify fluid accumulation adjacent to bone and implants in a case following internal fracture fixation.

When the infection source is localised, a sample should be obtained for culture and sensitivity testing. Sonographic examination can be used to identify fluid accumulation that can be collected for culture and sensitivity testing. Empiric antimicrobial drug therapy can then be started depending on the severity and consequences of the infection. If the infection is mild and not likely to be life-threatening, such as a laparotomy incisional infection, antimicrobial drugs therapy can be postponed until culture and sensitivity results are available. Implant-related infections often result in chronic drainage from the surgical site, and implant removal may be necessary if the infection becomes chronic and unresponsive to antimicrobial drugs.

Investigating and monitoring nosocomial infections

Culture and sensitivity testing is critical not only for individual case management but also for monitoring hospital SSI rate and antimicrobial drugs resistance patterns (see Chapter 3.3). The SSI rate should be monitored, and if it is higher than published values or than that previously recorded for the hospital, reasons for SSI should be investigated. Patient and surgeon skin preparation, operating room procedure, instrument and implant sterilisation and immediate postoperative management (wound dressing techniques, procedure for recovery from general anaesthesia) should be investigated in instances of a high SSI rate in a hospital population. For example, the author has experienced two instances of a high postlaparotomy SSI rate following abdominal surgery; the reason in the first instance was an inadequately cleaned and sterilised visceral retainer, and in the second instance the operating room nurses were not cleaning the ventral abdomen prior to commencing the sterile skin preparation. In both instances, the SSI rate had increased from approximately 15% to almost 100%.

Ideally, each hospital should have documentation of the most common bacteria isolated from the various SSIs as well as the antibiogram for the common bacteria isolated. Empirical antimicrobial drug selection can then be made based on the most likely bacteria and antimicrobial drug sensitivity. Antimicrobial drug resistance patterns can also be monitored. Human hospitals have numerous programs to control antimicrobial drug use and minimise resistance emergence.

Laparotomy wounds

Superficial SSI (defined as incisional drainage) rates following abdominal exploration are reported to range from 24% to 37%.[1–4] Some of the variability in SSI rates is attributed to different definitions of SSI and patient inclusion criteria for the study. Predisposing factors for SSI postlaparotomy include caecum/large colon obstruction, repeat laparotomy during the early healing period, duration of surgery greater than 2 hours, patients older than 1 year or more than 300 kg and near-far-far-near suture pattern.[1–4] Horses undergoing repeat laparotomy during the early healing period are reported to have had an SSI rate of 60 to 88%.[1,3,4] Incisional trauma was proposed to be a major contributing factor for SSI in horses with caecum/large colon obstruction and repeat laparotomy. Incisional trauma influences the ability of the host's local immunity to suppress contaminating bacteria. Multiple studies have indicated that clean-contaminated surgeries (enterotomy/enterectomy) are not predisposed to developing an SSI,[1,2,4] supporting the notion that trauma rather than contamination is a major contributing factor to SSI postlaparotomy.

Horses with an SSI postlaparotomy often have a fever, which is usually mild to moderate (38.5°–39.5° C [101.3°–103.1° F]) or rarely severe (>40° C [104° F]). While 62% of horses developed a fever following exploratory laparotomy, only 29% of febrile horses developed an SSI.[2] However, a positive association was found between fever and SSI.[2] An association was also found between a high number of non-segmented neutrophils (left shift) preoperatively and SSI.[2] Similarly, in human patients undergoing abdominal surgery, 38% developed a postoperative fever, but only 16% of the febrile patients had a bacterial infection; leucopaenia/leucocytosis and a fever identified after the second postoperative day were some of the factors associated with a bacterial infection.[5] Both of these studies support the recommendation that antimicrobial drugs should not be used routinely in any horse with a fever following a laparotomy. The use of antimicrobial drugs should be reserved for patients with an identified site of infection and ideally following bacterial culture and sensitivity testing.

Local signs of oedema or cellulitis, pain on palpation and drainage are seen in horses with a postlaparotomy SSI (Figure 15.18, A and B). In patients with extensive oedema, the use of an abdominal support bandage ("belly bandage") is recommended (Figure 15.19, A and B). The bandage can be applied for the minimal time necessary to reduce the oedema formation (for example, on for 6 hours and then

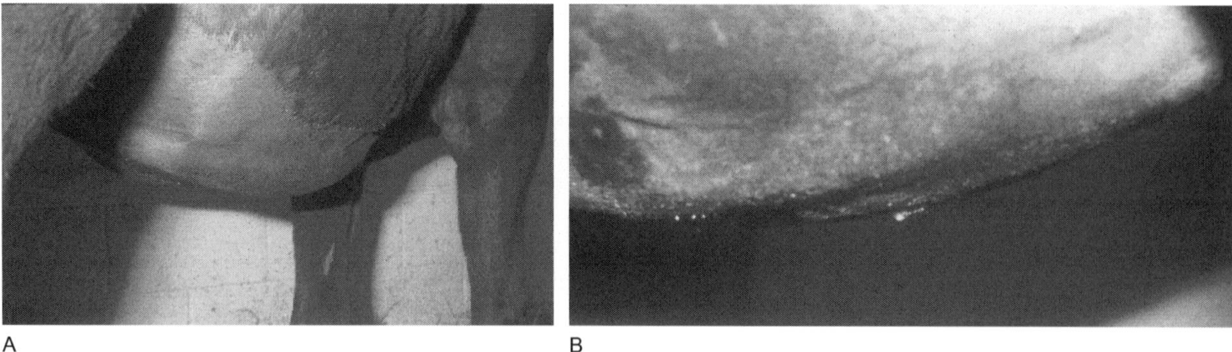

Figure 15.18A-B A post-laparotomy ventral midline incision with (15.18A) peri-incisional oedema and (15.18B) drainage. The amount of peri-incisional oedema can be minimized by using an abdominal support bandage ("belly bandage"; Figure 15.19A). When drainage from the surgical site is identified, a sample for bacterial culture and sensitivity testing should be aseptically collected. Staples or sutures adjacent to the affected area should be removed to facilitate drainage. The area should be cleaned several times daily. © Louise Southwood 2006.

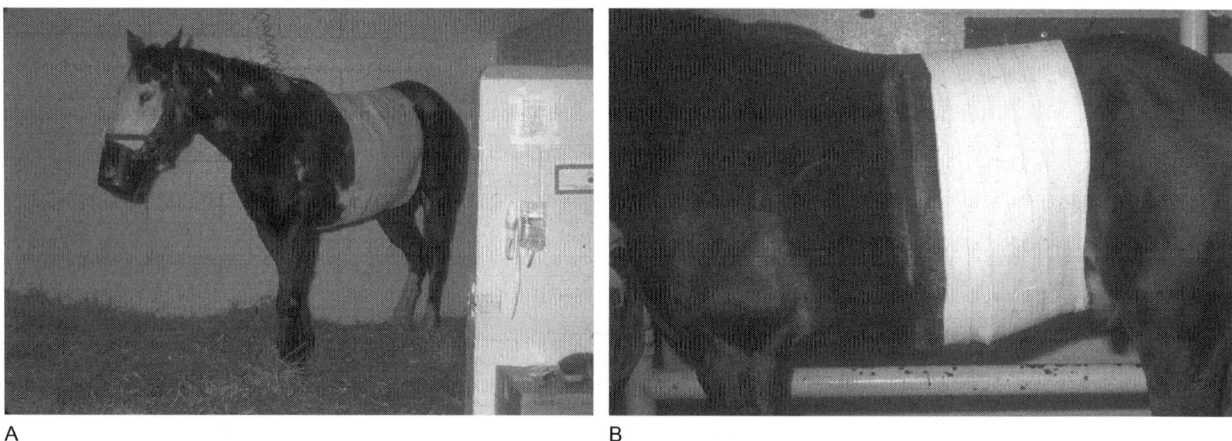

Figures 15.19A-B Abdominal support bandage ("belly bandage"). (15.19A) Commercially available, re-usable elastic bandage and (15.19B) disposable elastic adhesive bandage. The disposable elastic adhesive bandage is expensive and cannot be re-used, particularly in cases with incisional drainage. The authors usually place a sterile dressing under the abdominal support bandage adjacent to the wound to keep the wound clean and protected as well as to supply material to absorb any drainage from the incision. © Louise Southwood 2006.

off for 6 hours). Peri-incisional oedema also occurs in patients that do not have an SSI because of surgical trauma and the dependent location of the surgical site. If incisional drainage is present, the incision should be cleaned several times a day using either a chlorhexidine- or povidone iodine–based scrub and wiped thoroughly with sterile saline or alcohol if deep tissue is not exposed. Sterile gloves should be used when examining or cleaning the incision. Skin staples or sutures should be removed adjacent to the area of infection to facilitate wound drainage if staples or an interrupted suture pattern was used to appose the skin. If an abdominal support bandage is used, it should be changed frequently to avoid having copious amounts of purulent material adjacent to the incision for any length of time. Occasionally, the infection is severe and the skin and subcutaneous tissue layers of the incision will dehisce, exposing the linea alba and the sutures holding the abdominal wall together (Figure 15.20). These horses should obvi-

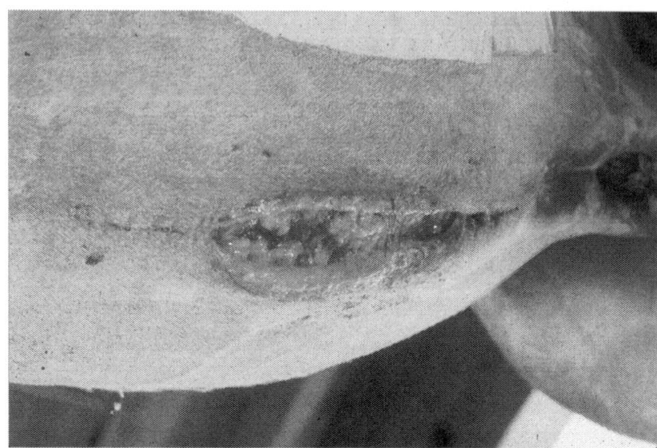

Figure 15.20 In severe cases of infected laparotomy wounds, the skin and subcutaneous tissue may dehisce and expose suture material apposing the body wall incision. © Louise Southwood 2006.

ously be confined to a stall with brief periods of hand walking.

Topical antimicrobial drugs can be used, including triple antibiotic ointment and amikacin in dimethylsulphoxide (DMSO). DMSO should not be applied to exposed subcutaneous tissue, muscle or fascia. Other topical treatments are usually not used by the author. A sample can be collected for bacterial culture and sensitivity testing by aseptically preparing the skin surrounding the incisional drainage site and then expressing a sample of the drainage fluid onto a culture swab or into a culture vial or small syringe. Sample collection should be performed aseptically. Aerobic and anaerobic bacterial culture should be performed.

Common bacterial isolates from laparotomy incisional infections in our hospital are *Escherichia coli*, *Enterobacter cloacae* and *Enterococcus faecium* and *faecalis* (Dr. Helen Aceto, personal communication). Hospital-acquired infections with enteric bacteria are frequently multidrug resistant and culture and sensitivity testing is necessary (Dr. Helen Aceto, personal communication). Interestingly, in the majority of cases, the bacteria cultured at the exploratory laparotomy (*Streptococcus* spp., *Staphylococcus* spp. and *E. coli*) were different to the bacteria cultured from an SSI postlaparotomy. However, there was an association between positive bacterial culture and subsequent incisional drainage.[2] It is possible that the contaminating bacteria are sensitive to routine antimicrobial drug prophylaxis, but the resistant bacteria proliferate and cause SSIs if in sufficient numbers at the completion of surgery. Alternatively, contamination can occur in the immediate postoperative period during recovery from general anaesthesia. Within 24 hours of a surgical procedure, the surgical site is believed to be sufficiently sealed and resistant to microorganism entry[6]; therefore, the immediate postoperative period is critical for infection prevention. Because of the high percentage of resistant organisms associated with SSI, bacterial culture and sensitivity testing is strongly recommended. Antimicrobial drug selection should be based on the results of these tests or the most likely antimicrobial drugs effective against the common infecting bacteria for the hospital. The latter requires diligent surveillance of hospital SSIs (see Chapter 3.3).

Horses should be confined to a stall for at least 4 weeks following complete healing of the skin wound to minimise the risk of evisceration and hernia formation. Stall confinement can be followed by 4 weeks in a stall and small run and then pasture turnout for 4 weeks prior to gradual return to exercise. Hand walking and grazing during periods of stall confinement are recommended.

Hernia formation is common following a postlaparotomy SSI, with a reported incidence of 9% to 16% following laparotomy.[1,2] There was a significant association between incisional drainage and hernia formation, with the odds of herniation being 62.5 times greater in horses with incisional drainage compared to horses that did not have incisional drainage. Hernioplasty is usually not performed until at least 3 to 4 months following SSI resolution. The necessity of hernioplasty depends on the hernia size and the horse use.

Occasionally, relaparotomy is necessary in horses with an SSI. In these cases, an approach can be made through a paramedian incision or through the infected incision. The approach selected depends on the anticipated lesion type and location and surgical procedures to be performed, as well as surgeon preference. If an approach is made through the infected incision and the body wall integrity is in question, the body wall incision can be apposed using monofilament stainless steel wire in an interrupted vertical mattress pattern supported with hard rubber tubing stents.[7]

Orthopaedic implants

Infection is one of the most devastating complications in horses and foals with orthopaedic implants. While "bone can heal in the face of infection if stability is provided," often the implants loosen and stability is lost and the horse or foal becomes severely lame, resulting in support-limb laminitis in adult horses and angular limb deformities in foals. Fracture healing is prolonged in patients that develop implant-associated osteomyelitis. Early recognition of infection associated with orthopaedic implants is essential for a favourable outcome (see Chapter 15.5).

Obtaining a sample of fluid, tissue, a deep culture using a swab or an implant (such as a screw) for bacterial culture and sensitivity testing is important because often infecting bacteria are resistant to commonly used antimicrobial drugs. Antimicrobial drug therapy is obviously critical for successful management of orthopaedic implant-related infections and can be delivered systemically and locally.

Local antimicrobial drug delivery methods have several advantages over systemic antimicrobial treatments, including high antimicrobial drug concentrations at the infection site and minimal systemic side effects. There are several methods of local antimicrobial drug delivery. Topical antimicrobial drugs, such as triple antibiotic ointment, can be used on any wound. Biodegradable and nonbiodegradable implants containing antimicrobial drugs can be used. Polymethylmethacrylate (PMMA) is a nonbiodegradable implant and is most commonly used for delivering antimicrobial drugs. Examples of biodegradable implants are collagen, hydroxyapatite, plaster of Paris, polyanhydrides, hyaluronan and polylactide-polyglycolide.[8] Antimicrobial drugs can be delivered to septic synovial structures using a constant rate infusion or an indwelling antimicrobial drug delivery system or via direct intrasynovial injection. Regional limb perfusion (RLP) is, however, becoming a very popular method for antimicrobial drug delivery for traumatic or infected surgical wounds, septic synovial structures and infected orthopaedic implants in the distal limb of horses. Regional limb perfusion is discussed later.

Implant removal is often necessary for infection resolution because a biofilm (glycocalyx) forms on the implant

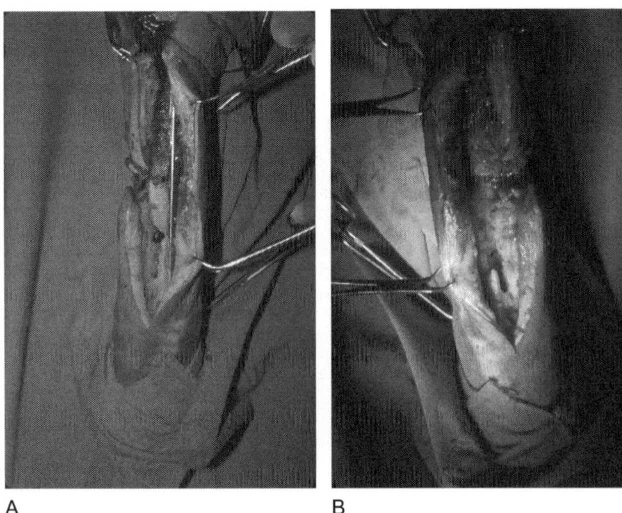

Figure 15.21A-B A neonatal foal that had an open displaced transverse mid-metatarsal fracture that was repaired using two dynamic compression plates and cortical screws. The foal developed a chronic draining tract associated with the implants and was persistently lame. A resistant Staphylococcus aureus was cultured from the wound. The infection was treated unsuccessfully with intraosseous regional limb perfusion using amikacin. After several months of medical treatment the foal was re-operated to remove and/or replace the implants (15.21A); however, the foal was euthanized because of the severity of the osteomyelitis and metatarsal necrosis (15.21B). © Louise Southwood 2006.

surface, making the bacteria inaccessible to antimicrobial drugs and the patient's immune system. Similarly, necrotic bone should be removed because it can also be a source of bacterial sequestration by a biofilm. The challenge becomes deciding when to take the horse back to surgery for implant removal and debridement. Concerns with reoperation are the expense to the client and risks associated with induction and recovery of general anaesthesia. The use of a pool recovery system can lower the risk associated with recovery from general anaesthesia and is recommended depending on availability. Indications for reoperation include implant-associated bone lysis, implant loosening, loss of stability at the fracture site and persistent severe lameness.

Reoperation involves lavage and debridement of the infected tissue and replacing loose screws or all implants (Figure 15.21, A and B). Alternatively, the fracture can be supported using an external fixator or a transfixation pin cast; however, the ability to do this depends on which bone is affected and the availability of normal bone through which pins can be placed. Placement of pins for external fixation through osteopenic or osteomyelitic bone can result in fracture through the pin holes or rapid pin loosening.

Support-limb laminitis is usually the reason adult horses with implant-associated infections are euthanised. Adult horses with osteomyelitis associated with implants can be placed in a sling in an attempt to minimise the load on the contralateral limb and to prevent laminitis. Analgesia is also important. Phenylbutazone is used most commonly. Additional methods of analgesia that are being used more often in equine patients include constant rate infusions of lidocaine, butorphanol, ketamine, and detomidine and fentanyl patches. If a hind limb is affected, an epidural catheter can be placed and epidural morphine administered.

Laryngeal implants

Eric Parente

Infection of laryngeal implants is uncommon. Diffuse swelling which obscures the normal definition of the caudal angle of the mandible, or incisional discharge may be an indication of seroma or infection. Needle aspiration or drainage via a needle is ill advised since it can potentially seed bacteria into an uninfected seroma. Removing several skin sutures to provide drainage, obtain a culture and manual expression of fluid twice daily is the most beneficial method of resolving fluid accumulation while minimising the risk promoting infection. Ascending infection is unlikely and flushing the surgical site or placement of a Penrose drain is also unnecessary and ill advised. Antimicrobial therapy based on culture results should be instituted as soon as possible.

It is also uncommon for the laryngoplasty sutures to require removal. When suture inadvertently penetrates the laryngeal mucosa and can be seen within the lumen, the suture should be removed. Use of an endoscope at the time of surgery should prevent this from occurring. Infection is often associated with abduction loss, but reoperation and suture replacement should not be considered unless there is no evidence of infection.

Like many surgeries, laryngoplasty infections are more common in cases of reoperation. The amount of fibrous tissue requiring transaction to access the laryngeal structures and haemorrhage associated with reoperation are factors that promote infection.

Regional limb perfusion

Louise Southwood

Regional limb perfusion with antimicrobial drugs can be used to treat septic arthritis, osteomyelitis, cellulitis and surgical or traumatic wound infections.[9] The principle of RLP is that by injecting the antimicrobial drug under pressure into a section of the vasculature or medullary cavity that is isolated from the systemic circulation, high intravascular pressures are created that force antimicrobials into the tissue down the pressure gradient created between the intravascular and extravascular spaces and through the gaps created between the endothelial cells and pericytes by the high pressure.[10] Using RLP, antimicrobial drugs reach poorly perfused tissues and the soft tissues acts as a depot for gradual antimicrobial drug release over time following RLP.[11] The antimicrobial drug concentrations achieved with RLP in the region of the limb isolated from the systemic circulation are several times higher than the minimal inhibitory concentration (MIC) of common equine pathogens for periods up to 20 to 36 hours and higher than concentrations achieved with systemic administration.[12] However, synovial fluid antimicrobial drug concentrations after RLP were not as high as the concentrations achieved with intra-articular injection.[13] contrary to what was initially thought, high concentrations of antimicrobial drugs are also achieved distal to the injection site.[14]

Regional limb perfusion can be performed using intravenous and intraosseous techniques. Intravenous RLP is simple to perform and results in higher concentrations of antimicrobial drug in the synovial fluid and soft tissues compared to intraosseous RLP.[15] Intravenous RLP is performed in the author's hospital. Either procedure can be performed with the horse standing or under general anaesthesia. There may be a difference in the antimicrobial drug distribution and concentration following RLP under general anaesthesia compared to standing sedation. The site for either intravenous or intraosseous perfusion is cleaned or clipped and aseptically prepared, respectively. The horse is sedated using butorphanol and xylazine or detomidine, or general anaesthesia is induced. A tourniquet is placed on the limb proximal to the site of RLP. In some cases, a tourniquet can be placed proximal and distal to the site of infection and RLP. Exsanguination (Esmarch bandage) and nonexsanguination (for example, rubber tubing) tourniquet techniques can be used (see Chapter 1.53). Elastic rubber tubing, elastic bandage (Esmarch bandage), pneumatic cuff and rolled gauze secured with an elastic bandage have been used as a tourniquet[9] (Figure 22, A and B). A pneumatic tourniquet will provide optimal vascular occlusion to prevent leakage while avoiding tissue damage,[9] and particular care should be taken with neonates to prevent osteonecrosis.[16] The effect of exsanguination on drug distribution is currently unknown; however, the perfusate volume should be lower in cases where exsanguination is not used to avoid excessive intravascular pressures as a result of the combined blood and perfusate volume.[17] Needle or catheter placement prior to exanguination is recommended if this technique is used.[9]

Ideally, antimicrobial drug selection should be based on culture and sensitivity testing or the most common pathogens associated with infection (see Chapter 6.3). Antimicrobial drugs that are most often used for RLP are amikacin and gentamicin. Amikacin was found to be most efficacious against Gram-positive and Gram-negative bacterial isolates from musculoskeletal infections.[18] RLP using ceftiofur has not been reported.[9] Enrofloxacin is reported to cause vascular damage and its use for RLP is not recommended.[19] Highly effective narrow-spectrum antimicrobial drugs, such as vancomycin, timentin and imipenem, have been used in cases with resistant microorganisms.[9] The use of concentration-dependent antimicrobial drugs, such as the aminoglycosides, for RLP may be ideal when RLP is

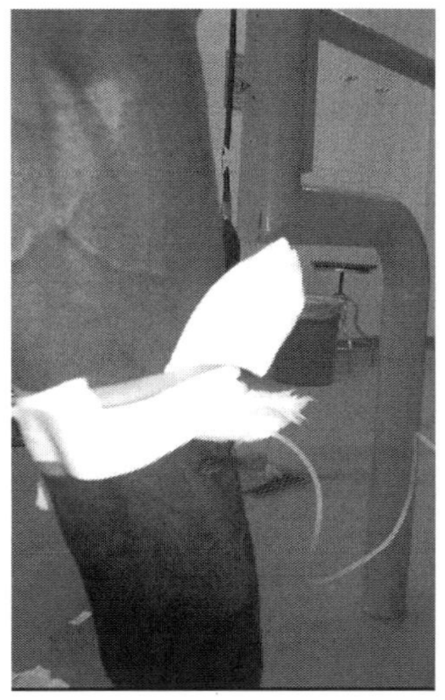

A

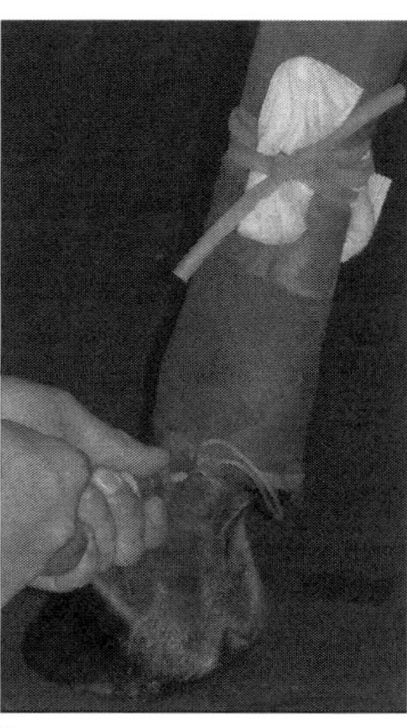

B

Figures 15.22A-B Intravenous regional limba perfusion using a small vein proximal to the carpus (15.22A) or the palmar digital vessels (15.22B). A tourniquet is applied using a rubber tubing (Penrose drain) and gauze over the vessel proximal to the injection site. Injection is performed using a 25-gauge 1-inch butterfly needle. Note that the gauze is placed over the cephalic vein (15.22A) or digital vessels in the groove between the suspensory ligament and flexor tendons (15.22B). © Louise Southwood 2006.

performed once a day or once every 2 to 3 days. However, because the soft tissues provide a depot for sustained antimicrobial release, time-dependent antimicrobial drugs, such as penicillins, could also be used.[20] The dose of antimicrobial used for RLP varies between reports and between clinicians. For example, gentamicin and amikacin have been used at one-third of the daily dose, gentamicin at 1 g/limb, and amikacin at 500 mg and 1 g/limb. Lower doses of aminoglycosides, 100 to 300 mg/limb, have also been used with high synovial fluid aminoglycoside concentrations achieved.[12] Potassium penicillin and ampicillin have been administered as one systemic dose (10×10^6 IU/limb). While dosing according to the weight of the limb would be ideal, currently this is impractical.[9] Monitoring peak and trough drug concentrations of aminoglycosides is important if systemic administration is used in conjunction with RLP to prevent toxicity with these drugs.

The antimicrobial drug is diluted in 20 to 60 ml of saline depending on the site of injection and infection (i.e., a smaller volume can be used for distal injection and infection sites) and the size of the patient (i.e., a smaller volume can be used in foals). The volume of saline is important because it is necessary to increase the intravascular pressure via a volume effect causing venous distension and diffusion of the antimicrobial drug into the tissues. However, too high of a volume can cause leakage through the vessels under the tourniquet. Higher antimicrobial concentrations were achieved with a 60-ml compared to a 30-ml perfusate volume.[15] Studies on the volume necessary for RLP are lacking, and often it is based on clinician preference. The perfusate is usually administered slowly by hand; however, an infusion pump can be used.[9] A high-pressure infusion pump is necessary for intraosseous RLP.[21] RLP is usually performed every 24 to 48 hours.

Intravenous regional limb perfusion

Intravenous RLP can be performed using any superficial vein, small or large.[9] Vessels that are often used include the saphenous and cephalic veins proximal to the tarsus and carpus, respectively, or the palmar/plantar metacarpal/metatarsal veins distally. Use of arteries is not recommended because of endothelial damage.[22] Figure 15.22, A and B, shows illustrations of intravenous RLP. While 18- or 20-gauge 1-inch (adults) or 22-gauge 1-inch (foals) butterfly needles or an intravenous over-the-needle catheter can be used,[9] smaller-diameter butterfly needles (25-gauge) are used in the author's hospital because they cause less endothelial damage, enabling RLP to be repeated daily for several days. Minimising endothelial damage is critical if multiple RLPs are to be performed. If a larger catheter or needle is used, repeated attempts at placement should be avoided because leakage of perfusate through the created holes in the vessel will occur.[9] Following sedation, the skin overlying the vessel is cleaned with alcohol, the tourniquet is applied and the butterfly needle is inserted into the selected vein.

Intraosseus regional limb perfusion

Intraosseous RLP can be performed in cases of severe cellulitis with no easily identified superficial vessel.[9] The antimicrobial drug is injected directly into the marrow cavity when the intraosseous technique is used. Intraosseous RLP is performed using a cannulated cortical screw with a Luer connection attached, which is placed into the medullary cavity of the metacarpal/metatarsal bone, tibia or radius following creation of a drill hole.[9] The distal end of an intravenous extension tubing or administration system can also be pushed into a drill hole.[9] Human intramedullary needles can be used as an alternative in foals.[23] Cyanoacrylate ester glue can be used to seal the interface between the tubing or needle to prevent leakage.[21] While high intraosseous pressures are created with intraosseous RLP, horses are not lame postperfusion, most likely because fluid can leak through the created hole in the bone.[9]

References

1. Phillips TJ, Walmsley JP: Retrospective analysis of the results of 151 exploratory laparotomies in horses with gastrointestinal disease. Equine Vet J 25:427-431, 1993
2. Ingle-Fehr JE, Baxter GM, Howard RD, et al.: Bacterial culturing of ventral median celiotomies for prediction of postoperative incisional complications in horses. Vet Surg 26:7-13, 1997
3. Kobluk CN, Ducharme NG, Lumsden JH, et al.: Factors affecting insional complication rates associated with colic surgery in horses: 78 cases (1983-1985). J Am Vet Med Assoc 195:639-642, 1989.
4. Wilson DA, Baker GJ, Boero MJ: Complications of celiotomy incisions in horses. Vet Surg 24:506-514, 1995
5. Mellors JW, Kelly JJ, Gusberg RJ, et al.: A simple index to estimate the likelihood of bacterial infection in patients developing fever after abdominal surgery. Am Surg 54:558-564, 1988
6. Altemeier WA, Culbertson WR, Hummel RP: Surgical considerations of endogenous infections—sources, types, methods of control. Surg Clin N Am 48:227-240, 1968
7. Stick JA: Abdominal hernias, in Auer JA, Stick JA, (eds): Equine Surgery, Philadelphia, WB Saunders, 2005, pp 491-499
8. Cruz AM, Rubio-Martinez L, Dowling T: New antimicrobials, systemic distribution, and local methods of antimicrobial delivery in horses. Vet Clin N Am Equine Pract 22: 297-322, 2006
9. Rubio-Martinez LM, Cruz AM: Antimicrobial regional limb perfusion in horses. J Am Vet Med Assoc 228:706-712, 2006
10. Langer K, Seidler C, Partsch H: Ultrastructural study of the dermal microvasculature in patients undergoing retrograde intravenous pressure infusions. Dermatology 192:103-109, 1996
11. Finsterbusch A, Weinberg H: Venous perfusion of the limb with antibiotics for osteomyelitis and other chronic infections. J Bone Joint Surg Am 54-A:1227-1234, 1972
12. Murphey ED, Santschi EM, Papich MG: Regional intravenous perfusion of the distal limb of horses with amikacin sulfate. J Vet Pharmacol Ther 22:68-71, 1999
13. Lloyd KC, Stover SM, Pascoe JR, et al.: Synovial fluid pH, cytologic characteristics and gentamicin concentration after intra-articular administration of the drug in an experimental model of infectious arthritis in horses. Am J Vet Res 51:1363-1369, 1990
14. Butt TD, Bailey JV, Dowling PM, et al.: Comparison of 2 techniques for regional antibiotic delivery to the equine forelimb: intraosseous perfusion vs. intravenous perfusion. Can Vet J 42:617-622, 2001
15. Scheuch BC, Van Hoogmoed LM, Wilson WD, et al.: Comparison of intraosseous or intravenous infusion for delivery of amikacin sulfate to the tibiotarsal joint of horses. Am J Vet Res 63:374-380, 2002
16. Bertone AL: Infectious arthritis, in Ross MW, Dyson SJ (eds): Diagnosis and Management of Lameness in the Horse. Philadelphia, WB Saunders, 2003, pp 598-605
17. Grice SC, Morell RC, Balestrieri FK, et al.: Intravenous regional anesthesia: evaluation and prevention of leakage under the tourniquet. Anesthesiology 65:316-320, 1986
18. Moore RM, Schneider RK, Kowalski J, et al.: Antimicrobial susceptibility of bacterial isolates from 233 horses with musculoskeletal infection during 1979-1989. Equine Vet J 24:450-456, 1992
19. Richardson DW: Local antimicrobial delivery in equine orthopedics. Proc Annu Symp Am Coll Vet Surg 74, 2003
20. Rubio-Martinez L, López-Sanromán J, Cruz AM, et al.: Evaluation of safety and drug pharmacokinetics of vancomycin after intravenous regional limb perfusion in horses. Am J Vet Res 66:2107-2113, 2005

21. Whitehair KJ, Blevins WE, Fessler JF, et al.: Regional perfusion of the equine carpus for antibiotic delivery. Vet Surg 21:279-285, 1992
22. Gottlob R: Endothelschäden nach intravasalen Injektionen und Infusionen. Verh Dtsch Ges Pathol 56:563-565, 1972
23. Hughes D, Beal MW: Emergency vascular access. Vet Clin N Am Small Anim Pract 30:491-507, 2000

15.9 External coaptation (splinting)

Jennifer O. Stephen

Techniques for equine fracture repair have progressed to the point where the limiting factor in the repair is often the condition of the soft tissue of the injured limb at the time of presentation. Without firm stabilisation, horses can rapidly traumatise the soft tissues to a point where orthopaedic repair is impossible or severely compromised. In this section, the use of splints and bandaging is discussed, as these are the materials commonly available to the practitioner in emergency situations. The use of casting material may also be beneficial but is often not available immediately. Correct use of casts is discussed in the following section (Chapter 15.10).

Acute management of orthopaedic injury

After a fracture or severe tendon injury has occurred, the first objective must be to prevent further damage to the limb. The horse must be calmed and brought under control and the limb stabilised before any other treatment or procedures are carried out.

The overall plan for emergency treatment of a horse with a limb fracture is given in Box 15.7. The objectives of first aid are to protect the horse and facilitate repair of the injury (see also Box 1.58).

The most important goal is to protect the skin and avoid an open fracture. Keeping the skin intact will halve the cost of treatment and double the likelihood of a good prognosis.[1] Equine skin is very thin and can be easily penetrated by sharp bone fragments, especially in the distal limb. If the skin has been penetrated, the wound should be covered with a water-soluble antibiotic ointment and a sterile dressing as soon as possible. Sedation should be used if necessary, starting with low dose and giving further doses as required. Xylazine (0.2–1.0 mg/kg IV) is probably the drug of choice for first aid procedures; it has good analgesic effect, short duration and minimal side effects.[1] Phenothiazine tranquilisers should be avoided due to their hypotensive effects.

An initial assessment of the degree of damage to the limb should be made. Some limbs may be too severely damaged for repair. Severe loss of bone or soft tissue indicates a poor prognosis. Fractures that are routinely treated with reasonable prognosis for return to soundness in the adult horse are listed in Box 15.8.

The prognosis for adult horses with complete fractures of long bones, especially if comminuted and or compound is still generally hopeless. There are some reports of successful treatment of shaft fractures of the radius,[2,3] tibia,[4] and cannon bones[5] in adult horses.

Box 15.9 lists fractures for which surgical repair may be attempted in the foal, in addition to those listed in Box 15.8.

If there is any doubt as to the possibility of repair, or as to the owner's wishes, then splinting should be applied immediately to give the best prognosis if surgical repair is attempted. Radiographs should be taken *after* proper stabilisation has been achieved; a good splint will facilitate better radiographs and priority has to be given to maximising the chances of repair.

Proper splinting protects bone ends and facilitates reconstruction. Splint application does not encourage the horse to walk on the affected limb; it encourages the horse to rest the limb until treatment may begin. An unsplinted horse with an unstable limb will make repeated attempts to stand on the limb and to place its limb in its normal position.

Box 15.8. Routinely treated fractures with a reasonable prognosis in adult horses

- Fractures of the olecranon
- Chip or slab fractures of the carpus
- Fractures of the lateral condyle of the third metacarpus or metatarsus
- Apical fractures of the proximal sesamoid bones
- Sagittal fractures of the first phalanx
- Pedal bone fractures

Box 15.7. Emergency steps for horses with limb fractures

1. Calm the patient and achieve restraint
2. Perform a cursory examination to determine if repair might be possible
3. Apply splints, bandages or cast
4. Arrange transportation to a suitable treatment facility

Box 15.9. Additional fractures for which surgical repair may be attempted in foals

- Humerus: reasonable prognosis with intra-medullary nailing and pinning
- Radius simple transverse fractures
- Cannon bone fractures
- Femoral fracture

Splinting the equine limb

Materials for splinting

When called to an emergency, veterinarians may not have commercial splints, or even sufficient bandage material, as large amounts are required to produce adequate stabilisation of the limb. PVC pipe, broomsticks, twitches, boards from hay pallets, towels and gaffer tape may all be successfully used to produce good coaptation if the correct principles are applied.

General principles when applying any splint include the following:

1. Protect the soft tissues and vasculature. Adequate padding should be used so that bandages may be applied firmly, yet protect the soft tissue circulation and not cause pressure points.
2. Never have a rigid splint end in the middle of a long bone; always use a splint of sufficient length (see below).
3. Ensure that splints are fixed tightly in place so they cannot slip. Avoid the use of elastic adhesive bandages (e.g., Elastoplast) to apply splints. Strong tape (e.g., duct tape*) is preferable.
4. The ends of items used as splints must be padded if there is a risk of them pressing on soft tissues above them.

The equine fore limb and hind limb may be divided into four biomechanically important regions (see Figure 1.173).

Region one

Distal to the distal quarter of the metacarpus (including fractures of the sesamoids and distal metacarpus). Align the dorsal cortices (see Figure 1.174); this is easier if an assistant raises the leg off the ground by holding the limb firmly above the carpus. Two layers of padding should be applied to the limb from foot to carpus and a board or gutter splint taped firmly to the dorsal surface of the limb. The splint should run from the toe to just below the carpus or tarsus. The toe must be firmly secured and the end of the splint next to the carpus well padded to avoid soft tissue trauma.[6] If the horse has a closed fracture and requires transportation, it is also helpful to put a layer of cast material on top of the splint.[1] If the sole injury to the limb is complete disruption of the suspensory apparatus, then a commercial Kimzey splint† may be used.

Region two

This involves structures between the mid-metacarpus and the distal radius. The aim is to fix the limb to the splint proximal and distal to the fracture. A Robert Jones dressing with many layers should be applied from foot to elbow (see Box 1.60). Splints are then taped on tightly with nonelastic tape to the bandage on the lateral and caudal surfaces from the ground to the elbow (see Figure 1.175). Plastic guttering material is useful for the caudal splint.

Region three

This involves fractures of the mid and proximal radius. The aim of the splint is to prevent abduction of the limb. A Robert Jones bandage (see below) should be applied from the foot to the elbow and a lateral splint which extends from the ground to the shoulder or hip should be taped tightly to the Robert Jones from the foot to the axilla (see Figure 1.176). Extra tape to hold the free end of the splint against the body helps to stabilise it.

Region four

This includes fractures of the ulna, humerus and scapula (proximal to stifle joint). With these fractures in the fore limb, the triceps is disabled and therefore fixing the carpus allows the horse easier control of the distal limb. Padding should be placed from the elbow to the fetlock and a splint taped on to the caudal aspect of the limb to extend the carpus.

Region five

Distal to the distal quarter of the metatarsus. In the hind limb, this splint may be applied as in the fore limb (region one).

Region six

Distal metatarsus to the tarsus. A slightly less extensive Robert Jones bandage should be placed to aid application of the splints, which is harder in the hind limb than in the fore limb. The splints are applied caudally and laterally from the tuber calcis to the ground.

Region seven

Tibia and tarsus. A Robert Jones should be applied from foot to stifle. A splint should be made to fit the limb on its craniolateral and craniocaudal surfaces from the ground to the level of the tuber coxae (see Figure 1.177). A 12-mm steel rod can be bent to do this and is stiff enough to support the limb. A splinting device with a steel walking bar frame and side supporting bars has also been used.[6]

Region eight

Proximal to the stifle joint. In the femur and pelvis, the large surrounding muscle mass provides splinting and little else can be done.

Robert Jones bandage

This method of bandaging was developed by Sir Robert Jones in the early 1900s to reduce bleeding, tissue oedema and joint stiffness after human knee surgery.[7] The bandage is a bulky compression dressing with multiple layers. It is

* Duct tape, Henkel Consumer Adhesives, Avon, OH, USA.
† Kimzey Metal Products, Woodland, CA, USA.

designed to limit swelling and oedema with uniform and controlled pressure to avoid adverse haemodynamic effects to the limb.[7] As well as providing first aid, the bandage may be used to provide support to the limb after removal of a cast or internal fixation device.[8]

Application of the bandage is described in Box 1.60. The bandage should prevent the horse from bending the carpus or hock. However, without splinting, a Robert Jones bandage will not be sufficient to completely immobilise the limb. If the bandage is being used to provide long-term support instead of first aid, then loose adhesive bandages should be used to "seal" the bandage to the skin or hoof top and bottom to prevent bedding or dirt wicking into the inner bandage layers. The bandage should be checked regularly and changed immediately if there is any sign that the bandage has slipped, as this can result in serious creasing and pressure in the inner layers. Dirty or wet bandages must also be changed immediately.

Treatment and transportation

After the limb is splinted antimicrobial drugs (see Chapter 6.3), anti-inflammatory drugs should be administered as necessary. The horse should be transported with the damaged limb to the rear of the box or trailer if possible. Horses should be restricted within the trailer as much as possible to give support, but the head should not be tied up so tight that it cannot be used to help balance. An attendant may be useful if this can be safely achieved and should be used when transporting foals with splints on.

References

1. Bramlage LR: Current concepts of emergency first aid treatment and transportation of equine fracture patients. Compend Cont Ed Pract Vet 5:S564-S574, 1983
2. Baxter GM: Repair of an open radial fracture in an adult horse. J Am Vet Med Assoc 199:364-367, 1991
3. Auer JA: Treatment of radial fractures in adult horses: an analysis of 15 clinical cases. Equine Vet J 19:103-110, 1987
4. Bramlage LR: Internal fixation of a tibial fracture in an adult horse. J Am Vet Med Assoc 180:1090, 1982
5. McClure SR: Complete fractures of the third metacarpal or metatarsal bone in horses: 25 cases (1980-1996). J Am Vet Med Assoc 213:847, 1998
6. Walmsley JP: First aid splinting for the equine fracture patient. Equine Vet Educ 5:61-63, 1993
7. Beroza GA: Splinting device for hindlimb fractures in horses. J Am Vet Med Assoc 186:1204-1206, 1985
8. Brodell JD: The Robert Jones bandage. J Bone Joint Surg 68:776-779, 1986

15.10 Application of casts

Ehud Eliashar

Applying a cast to a horse is indicated as the sole method of fracture fixation, support of a repaired fracture during recovery from general anaesthesia, and support of joints following luxation or significant damage of the collateral ligaments, severely strained or severed flexor tendons and suspensory apparatus, and wounds of the distal limb closed primarily under tension or left to heal by second intension.[1,2] Casts can be listed according to their location and length (Box 15.10).

Generally, it is advisable to apply the cast under general anaesthesia as this avoids dealing with the horse movements during the application and setting of the cast, which may weaken the cast and/or create pressure points.[1] General anaesthesia, however, is not required for hoof or sleeve casts, and in some horses adequate sedation may suffice for applying the other types as well.

Plaster of Paris is still considered a viable casting material because of its ease of use, good moulding capability and inexpensive price. However, its disadvantages when wet, its nonporous characteristics that do not allow for exchange of air and its inferior strength requiring an application of overall heavier cast to prevent breakage[1,3] make it less favourable. The most commonly used casting material in horses is resin-impregnated fibreglass or polyurethane, which in comparison to plaster of Paris is about 20 times stronger and 4 times lighter. A variety of synthetic materials are available on the market, but from a practical point of view there are no significant differences between them.[3] Furthermore, the ability of air exchange achieved by the porosity of synthetic material is thought to make the cast more comfortable and thus more suitable for a prolonged time.[4] Some clinicians, however, prefer to have the advantages of both the moulding capability of plaster of Paris and the durability of the synthetic materials by forming a combination cast, which is made by using plaster of Paris for the first few layers of the cast, followed by synthetic rolls.

Appropriately applied cast should terminate in the proximity of a joint to minimise the stress imposed on the bone

Box 15.10. Classification of casts according to their location and length

Name	Description
Hoof cast	covers the sole and hoof to just below the coronary band
Foot (distal limb) cast	includes the foot and extending to just below the metacarpo/metatarsophalangeal joint
Half limb cast	similar to the distal limb cast and extending to just below the carpus/tarsus
Full limb cast	covers the foot and extending as proximal as possible on the radius or tibia
Sleeve cast	similar to a full limb cast, but starting just above the metacarpo/metatarsophalangeal joint, thus not incorporating the pastern and foot

by the edge of the cast. The technique of applying the cast varies between clinicians, mainly with regards to the type and amount of padding, the size and number of cast rolls and limb positioning. The following description is the author's preferred method of applying a half limb cast. Preparing the limb includes thoroughly cleaning of the hoof and trimming if required and circumferentially clipping the part of the limb under the cast. Any wound/surgical incision is protected by a nonadherent pad covered by a thin layer of padding material. The limb is held in neutral position such as the phalanges and the third metacarpal bone are aligned in the same plane,[3] or in the hind limb, the metatarsophalangeal joint is held in slight (10°) extension. Orthopaedic felt, 5 to 7 cm wide, is applied to the limb at the expected proximal end of the cast, and a double layer of stockinet, about 10 cm longer than the expected length of the cast, is applied next. A second layer of thin padding is placed over the stockinet to complete the padding. Alternatively, if the cast is not applied over a wound or incision, the stockinet is applied first, followed by two thin layers of padding material. It is paramount that padding is applied to the whole area under the cast, including the coronary band.

The first layers of the cast are composed of two rolls of 7.5-cm (3-inch) casting material, which is easier to conform to the limb,[2] and an additional roll is used to cover the hoof and sole. The rolls should be applied firmly with just enough tension to lightly compress the padding, and each turn overlaps by half roll width. These are then followed by three wider rolls (12.5 cm, 5 inches), allowing the cast to reach a total thickness of 7 to 8 mm throughout its total length.[3] A wooden wedge is incorporated to the sole region of the cast in order to allow the horse to bear weight on the entire bottom of the cast rather than just the toe, and the cast is completed by applying a sturdy casting material such as Hexalite* to the bottom of the cast and this significantly reduces the risk of wearing. The top of the cast is sealed with elastic tape to prevent accumulation of shavings or other bedding material.

Recovery from anaesthesia is usually well tolerated with a half or distal limb cast; however, assisted recovery is recommended for horses with a full limb cast as it may be difficult and even dangerous because of the inability of the horse to flex the limb under the body.[2] As commonly the cast makes the limb longer, the contralateral limb can be kept shoed, or lengthened by securing a wooden block to the sole.

The cast should be checked for cracks or creases, excessive heat over a surgical site or areas prone for pressure sores, and signs of wear, mainly at the toe and discoloration. The elastic tape on top of the cast should be changed on a daily basis, and the skin checked for sores. By far the most important sign that something is wrong with the cast is refusal of the horse to use the limb. It is, however, important to remember that occasionally horses require a few days to adjust, especially to a full limb cast. Horses should be strictly stall rested as long as the limb is in the cast and only walked out a short distance daily to assess how well the cast is tolerated.

References

1. Murray RC, DeBowes RM: Casting techniques, in Nixon AJ (ed): Equine Fracture Repair. Philadelphia, WB Saunders, 1996, pp 104-113
2. Riggs CM: Indications for and application of limb casts in the mature horse. Equine Vet Educ 9:190-197, 1997
3. Auer JA: Drains, bandages, and external coaptation, in Auer JA, Stick JA (eds): Equine Surgery, ed 3. Philadelphia, Saunders Elsevier, 2005, pp 202-218
4. Stone WC: Drains, dressings, and external coaptation, in Auer JA, Stick JA (eds): Equine Surgery, ed 2. Philadelphia, Saunders Elsevier, 1999, pp 104-112

* Hexalite; Veterinary Specialty Products, Boca Raton, FL, USA.

16

Management of horses with problems of the integument

16.1 Wound management in hospitalised horses
16.2 Simple skin grafting techniques

16.1 Wound management in hospitalised horses

Louise L. Southwood

Wounds can be created surgically or caused traumatically. Surgical wounds associated with clean procedures should heal without complications. The surgical site infection rate for clean procedures is low (<5%; see Table 16.1). For example, reported infection rates for laryngoplasty were 3.3%[2]; for arthroscopy, 0.5%[3]; for cryptorchidectomy, 0.9%[4]; and for ovariectomy, 5%.[5] These wounds, however, should be kept clean, particularly during the immediate perioperative period, and monitored closely for signs of infection (heat, pain, swelling, redness and drainage). Sutures or staples should be removed 10 to 14 days following surgery. Prophylactic antimicrobial drugs should be unnecessary in most clean surgical procedures. Antimicrobial drug prophylaxis is indicated in clean procedures in which a surgical site infection would have devastating consequences and should be given as a single dose immediately before surgery.

Table 16.1. Categories of surgical wounds based on the National Research Council Operative Wound Classification

Category	Definition
Clean	Elective, primary closure, no drains, nontraumatic, no infection, no inflammation, aseptic technique maintained.
Clean-contaminated	Gastrointestinal, respiratory, urogenital tracts entered under controlled conditions and with expected amount of contamination; or minor break in aseptic technique.
Contaminated	Open, fresh traumatic wound; gross contamination from gastrointestinal tract; opening of urogenital or biliary tract with infected bile or urine; incisions in which noninfected purulent material is encountered; or major break in aseptic technique.
Dirty and infected	Traumatic wound with retained devitalised tissue and foreign bodies, faecal contamination, or delayed treatment or from a dirty source; perforated viscus encountered; or acute bacterial inflammation with purulent exudate encountered.

Modified from Trostle and Hartmann.[1]

Clean-contaminated and contaminated surgical procedures have a considerably higher infection rate compared to clean procedures. Reported surgical site infection rates for procedures that may be classified as clean-contaminated or contaminated were 10% to 37% for emergency exploratory celiotomy[6–8] and 52.6% for clean-contaminated orthopaedic procedures.[9] Antimicrobials are used in clean-contaminated and contaminated surgical procedures prophylactically to reduce the rate of surgical site infection. Numerous studies have demonstrated that a single preoperative dose is as effective as a multiple perioperative dose prophylactic antimicrobial regimen. Within 24 hours of a surgical procedure, the surgical site is believed to be sufficiently sealed and resistant to microorganism entry,[10] so antimicrobial use beyond this time should be unnecessary. For example, there was no difference in infection rates in human patients that received a single- versus a triple-dose cefuroxime undergoing elective abdominal surgery (gastric, biliary, pancreatic, jejunal, ileal or colorectal).[11] Antimicrobials should never be used in place of meticulous aseptic and atraumatic surgical technique. If signs of surgical site infection occur, wound drainage should be provided, the wound kept clean and a sample obtained for culture and antimicrobial sensitivity. Dirty and infected surgical wounds have a high infection rate, and antimicrobial use is therapeutic rather than prophylactic, and a course of antimicrobial drugs (at least 5–10 days) is probably indicated.

Traumatic wounds are classified as contaminated or dirty. Management of traumatic wounds has been reviewed in detail at several other texts.[12,13] The objective of this chapter is to discuss some of the important aspects of traumatic wound management as well as new research in this area.

A schematic outline of traumatic wound management is given in Figure 16.1. Controlling severe haemorrhage is

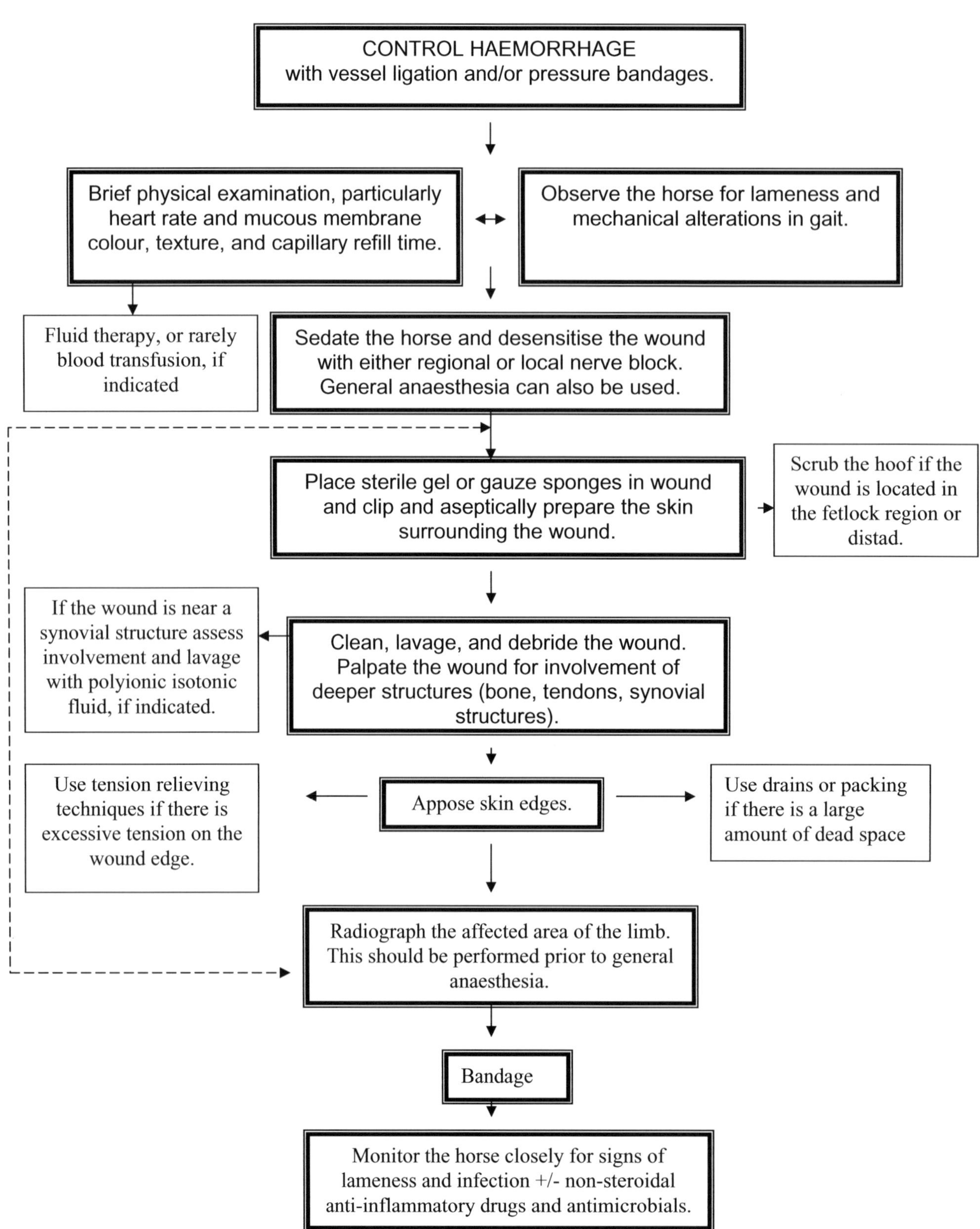

Figure 16.1 Schematic outline of traumatic wound management. ©Louise Southwood 2006.

the first and most important thing to do when treating a horse with a laceration. Wounds often have capillary haemorrhage, which is not life threatening. Haemorrhage from large vessels, however, can lead to life-threatening blood loss. Haemorrhage can be controlled by vessel ligation using 2-0 synthetic absorbable suture material or by applying a pressure bandage. Often, a pressure bandage will only control haemorrhage temporarily, and if the vessel cannot be ligated with the horse standing, general anaesthesia is indicated.

Initial assessment and treatment

A brief physical examination of the horse (heart and respiratory rates, mucous membrane colour, capillary refill time) should always be performed to assess the cardiovascular stability of the patient. If there are signs of hypovolaemic or haemorrhagic shock (tachycardia, pale and dry mucous membranes), intravenous fluid therapy (and, on very rare occasions, blood transfusion) is indicated.

It is important to pay close attention to the gait and assess the horse for lameness prior to sedation and local nerve block. The degree of lameness is quite variable between horses. If a horse is grade 4/5 or 5/5 lame (i.e., lame at a walk or non–weight-bearing lame, respectively), it is particularly important to rule out involvement of deeper structures, including a nondisplaced fracture of the underlying bone. Alterations in gait, such as elevation of the toe during weight-bearing indicating transection of the deep digital flexor tendon, should also be noted and addressed. The limb should be carefully palpated for areas of soft tissue swelling and effusion of synovial structures.

Sedation and regional or local nerve blocks are important for facilitating wound treatment because the horse is more likely to stand quietly and comfortably while the wound is examined and repaired. The horse can be sedated with xylazine (0.3–0.4 mg/kg IV) and butorphanol (0.01–0.02 mg/kg IV), or detomidine (0.01 mg/kg IV). A peripheral nerve (abaxial sesamoid or 4-point) or ring block should be performed proximal to the wound if possible. If this is not possible, local anaesthetic infiltration of the wound edge prior to suturing is usually performed. Infiltration of the wound from the wound edge rather than through the skin is less likely to be resented by the horse and does not appear to increase the infection rate.

Sterile lubricant* should be applied to the wound or the wound covered with sterile moist gauze to prevent hair adhering to the exposed tissue. Clip and aseptically prepare the skin surrounding the wound. It is important to clip and prepare a wide circumferential area around the wound (Figure 16.2, A–E). If adjacent hair and skin is soiled, it is likely to recontaminate the wound when bandaged. The skin and wound can be cleaned with a chlorhexidine gluconate†, chloroxylenol‡, or povidone-iodine§–based scrub. It is critical to scrub the wound gently and to remove all of the scrub from the wound because the detergent base is irritating to the tissue and may alter local defences and potentiate infection.[13] Alcohol should never be used near a wound because it will damage the exposed tissues. The entire hoof should also be scrubbed clean if the laceration is in the fetlock region or distal to the fetlock.

Wound lavage

The wound can be lavaged with sterile saline or saline containing 0.01% to 0.02% povidone-iodine solution (1–2 ml of 10% concentrate/1 L sterile saline) or 0.05% chlorhexidine diacetate solution (25 ml of 2% concentrate/1 L sterile saline). At these concentrations, these solutions were bactericidal and did not inhibit granulation tissue formation, wound contraction or epithelialisation.[14–16] Faster wound contraction was reported in wounds treated with chlorhexidine diacetate or povidone- iodine solutions compared with saline; however, the differences were only significant for chlorhexidine diacetate.[17] While the addition of antiseptic solutions to the lavage fluid may be of benefit, the addition of antimicrobials does not appear to offer any advantage except if indicated based on the results of bacterial culture and sensitivity testing.[13] Lavage fluid should be delivered with at least 7 pounds per square inch (psi) of pressure, which can be achieved with a spray bottle or by forcefully expressing lavage solution from a 35- to 60-ml syringe through an 18-gauge needle.[18] A pressure of 10 to 15 psi was shown to remove 80% of the soil infection-potentiating fractions from the wound and can be generated using a Water-Pik at an intermediate setting and a flow rate of 40 to 50 ml/min.[13] While ideally a wound should be rinsed and lavaged with sterile saline or other isotonic fluid, this is often not practical for extensive wounds (Figure 16.3, A and B). The use of a hose and tap water to clean these wounds is often more practical and clinically does not appear to adversely affect wound healing. Lavage should remove most of the gross contamination of the wound but should be discontinued before tissues appear water-logged.[13]

Exploration

Exploration of the wound, digitally using a sterile glove or using a sterile probe, should be performed to determine the extent of the wound, as well as the affected soft tissues, synovial structures, and bone. It then needs to be decided whether the wound is best treated with the horse under standing sedation or general anaesthesia.

* Priority Care 1; First Priority Incorporated, Elgin, IL, USA; K-Y Jelly, Johnson and Johnson, New Brunswick, NJ, USA.

† Betasept, 4% chlorhexidine gluconate; The Purdue Frederick Company, Stamford, CT, USA.

‡ TechniCare, 3% chloroxylenol USP; Care-Tech Laboratories Incorporated, O-T-C Pharmaceuticals, St. Louis, MO, USA.

§ Betadine Surgical Scrub, 7.5% povidone-iodine; Purdue Frederick Company, Stamford, CT, USA.

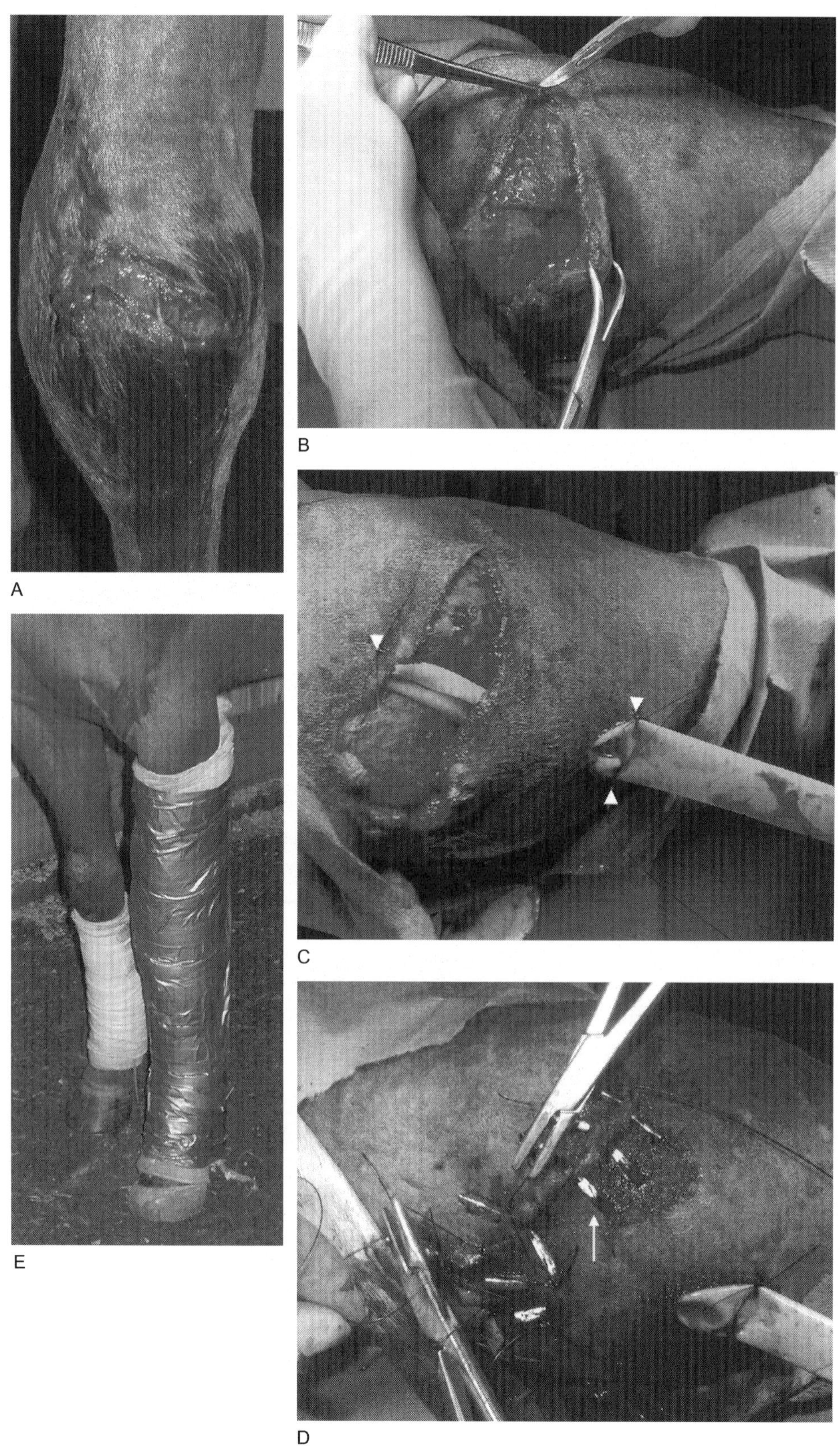
A
B
C
D
E

Debridement

The wound should be debrided prior to closure. Debridement can be accomplished by complete excisional or simple debridement.[13] While compete excisional debridement is most effective, simple debridement is most commonly used and involves systematic examination of the wound and removal of nonviable tissue and gross contamination (soil and hair) using sharp excision (Figure 16.2, B). Wounds involving several tissue planes with a lot of dead-space can be difficult to debride. In these cases, the skin wound can be extended to debride heavily contaminated "pockets" or a curette can be used gently to remove debris from the deeper tissues. Often, vessels that have stopped bleeding with digital pressure will begin bleeding again during cleaning and debridement and may require ligation. It is important to not transect vital structures during debridement.

Assessment of joint involvement

If involvement of a synovial structure is suspected based on wound exploration, the location of the wound and/or synovial effusion, the joint can be further assessed by aseptically inserting a sterile needle into the synovial structure at a site remote from the wound (see Chapter 15). Synovial fluid should be collected for analysis if possible. Values diagnostic for infection are total protein greater than 35 g/L (>3.5 g/dl), white cells greater than 30×10^9/L (>30,000/μl) and greater than 80% neutrophils. However, cell counts and protein concentrations less than this do not rule out contamination or infection. With the needle still inserted in the joint, the joint is distended with fluid to determine if the wound and the synovial structure communicate (i.e., fluid comes out of the wound). It is often beneficial to take the joint through a range of motion with the joint distended because fascial planes can obstruct fluid leakage through the wound. The wound should be dry and examined closely for fluid leakage because often only a few drops of fluid will appear in the wound. If deeper structures do not appear to be affected, begin treatment with broad-spectrum antimicrobial drugs if necessary and monitor the horse closely for signs of septic arthritis. If deeper structures are affected, prompt treatment is critical for a successful outcome.

Wound healing

Most lacerations in horses can be treated by clipping and aseptically preparing the surrounding skin, thoroughly lavaging and debriding the wound with primary, delayed-primary or secondary skin apposition. Primary closure is ideal and used for wounds that have mild to moderate tissue damage and can be adequately cleaned and debrided.[13] Delayed-primary closure is performed prior to granulation tissue formation (within 4–5 days) and is used for wounds with severe contamination and tissue damage.[13] Secondary closure is performed following formation of granulation tissue in wounds that are chronic, severely contaminated or infected.[13] Most equine wounds can be closed primarily if they are seen within 24 to 48 hours of injury and are thoroughly cleaned and debrided. When the wound is closed primarily, leaving 1 to 2 cm of the most distal or dependent aspect of the wound open can allow for drainage. In some instances, partial wound dehiscence may occur following primary closure and the wound will heal by second intention. Second intention healing is when the wound heals by contraction and epithelialisation and is used in cases with severe tissue damage, tissue loss, and contamination or infection. Additionally, second-intention healing may be used in cases in which economics are a concern and the procedure cannot be performed standing. Systemic antimicrobial and nonsteroidal anti-inflammatory drugs are also administered in most cases; however, they are probably only necessary preoperatively (i.e., immediately prior to wound debridement and repair) and may be unnecessary in many cases with relatively minor wounds.

Upper limb, body and head wounds

Most wounds on the upper limbs, body and head heal without complication; however, extensive lacerations may take several months to heal (Figures 16.3, A and B, and 16.4). These wounds can be cleaned, debrided and closed primarily (Figure 16.4) or allowed to heal by second

Figures 16.2A-E **(A)** A 10-cm wound to the dorsal aspect of the carpus. **(B)** Sterile gel was used to cover the wound and the skin surrounding the wound was clipped circumferentially for a distance of approximately 20 cm proximal and distal to the wound. The wound was gently scrubbed and thoroughly lavaged. The radiocarpal and middle carpal joints were assessed to determine if they communicated with the wound and they did not based on the absence of synovial effusion, normal synovial fluid, and there was no fluid exiting the wound when the joint was distended with sterile isotonic fluid. The wound was debrided using a sharp scalpel blade. **(C)** There was a relatively large area of dead space extending distal from the wound and a Penrose drain was placed. Note that the penrose drain did not exit through the proximal aspect of the wound (i.e., there is no ingress) and that a suture was placed blindly to keep the drain in place proximally (*white arrowhead*). The drain exited through a 2-cm stab incision at the most distal or most dependent aspect of the wound and was kept in place using two sutures (*white arrowheads*). It is important to use sutures of different colour to those used to close the wound to secure the drain in place or to have suture ends longer so that these sutures can be easily distinguished when the drain is removed 48 to 72 hours after surgery. **(D)** Tension-relieving sutures (quill technique) were placed using No. 2 (5 metric) nylon in a vertical mattress pattern. Rubber tubing using an extension set was used (*white arrow*). The skin edge was apposed with 2-0 (3 metric) nylon in a cruciate suture pattern. **(E)** A full limb bandage was applied and the limb splinted using polyvinylchloride and duct tape. The horse was also treated with nonsteroidal anti-inflammatory drugs for 3 to 4 days and broad-spectrum antimicrobials for 14 days. The wound healed without complication.

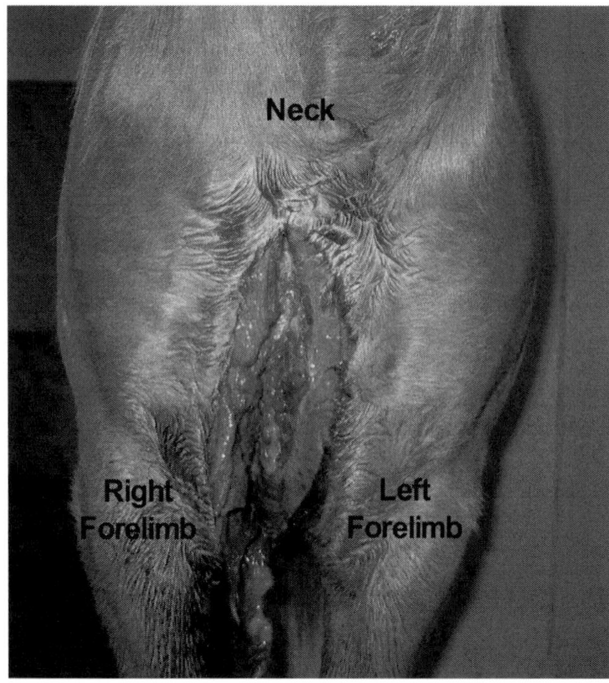

A

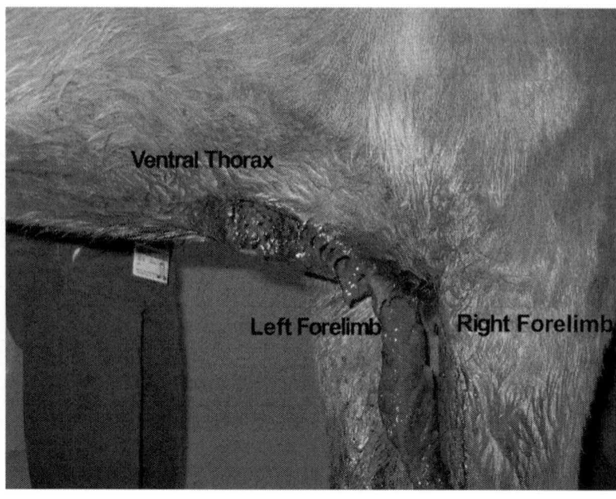

B

Figures 16.3A-B An extensive wound to the ventral thorax, (**A**) cranial-caudal and (**B**) lateral views. The laceration was approximately 70 cm long and extended from immediately dorsal to the manubrium sterni to 15 cm caudal to the point of the elbow. The laceration was approximately 35 cm in depth. A physical examination, haematology and serum biochemistry were performed to assess the horse's cardiovascular status, and it appeared that blood loss had not been excessive. The horse was able to walk normally. The wound was examined for involvement of deeper structures. The thorax was not penetrated and there was no haemorrhage from large vessels. The wound was cleaned and lavaged. An attempt was made to pack the wound, but this was unsuccessful because of the dependent location of the wound and the motion in the area. The wound was treated by daily cleaning with chloroxylenol scrub and hosing. Vaseline was placed on the skin distal to the wound to prevent serum scalding. The horse was treated with intravenous fluid therapy for 12 to 24 hours, nonsteroidal anti-inflammatory drugs for 4 to 5 days, and broad-spectrum antimicrobials for 4 weeks. Two months following the injury, the wound was healing well. ©Louise Southwood 2006.

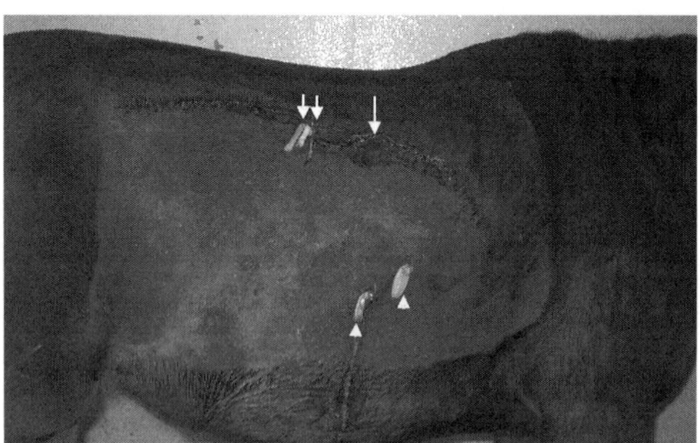

Figure 16.4 An extensive wound that involved the entire lateral aspect of the thorax and abdomen of a horse. The wound was treated by clipping and scrubbing the surrounding skin, lavaging and debriding the wound, and primary closure. Following lavage and debridement, the skin edges were desensitised using 2% lidocaine (lignocaine). The wound was apposed using #2 (5 metric) nylon in a vertical mattress and cruciate pattern. Because there was a lot of tension on the wound, a couple of vertical mattress sutures using umbilical tape were placed (double white arrow). There was a large amount of dead space and penrose drains were placed with the egress at the most dependent aspect of the wound (white arrow heads). The horse was also treated with nonsteroidal anti-inflammatory drugs and broad-spectrum antimicrobials. The wound healed well but there was an area at the skin edge that was non-viable and sloughed (white arrow). This area healed by second intention. ©Louise Southwood 2006.

intention (Figure 16.3, A and B). Drains should be placed in extensive wounds if there is a large amount of deadspace. Alternatively, these wounds can be packed with gauze. If packing is to be used, it should be made of material that does not fray and leave pieces of material in the wound. Packing should consist of one continuous piece of material, such as several rolls of gauze tied together, to ensure that there is no packing left in the wound following removal. The gauze packing can be soaked in dilute povidone-iodine solution; however, the advantage of this compared to sterile saline is unknown. Packing should be changed daily and wounds should only be packed during the debridement phase of healing (days 1–3 postinjury).

Recently, the use of vacuum-assisted closure for management of an extensive laceration in the cervical region of a horse was reported.[19] Vacuum-assisted closure involves applying a subatmospheric pressure (125 mm Hg) to the wound and is reported to cause an increase in blood flow and granulation tissue formation and a decrease in oedema and bacterial count in the wound.[19]

Some complications associated with upper limb and body wounds include septic synovitis, bone fracture, penetration of the thorax or abdomen, bone sequestration or osteomyelitis, and persistence of foreign material deep in the wound resulting in a chronic draining tract.

Small lacerations and puncture wounds of the distal limb

While extensive lacerations on the body usually heal without complications, very small lacerations or puncture wounds of the distal limb that are often ignored by owners can involve deeper structures and if not treated appropriately can lead to persistent severe lameness and support limb laminitis requiring euthanasia (Figures 16.5, A and B, 16.6 and 16.7). Lacerations of the distal limb often involve a synovial structure (joint or the digital sheath), tendon(s), ligament(s) and/or bone. In a recent report, 17% of heel bulb lacerations involved a synovial structure, with the distal interphalangeal (coffin) joint being affected most commonly.[20] It is important to attempt to identify if any of these structures are involved with the laceration or puncture wound. A thorough knowledge of anatomy is needed. A laceration affecting a synovial structure may result in a very favourable outcome for both survival and athletic performance if appropriately treated immediately postlaceration. The prognosis is excellent if the wound and affected synovial structure are treated within 6 to 8 hours of injury and if the amount of soft tissue and bone damage and gross contamination is not extensive. If treatment is delayed until signs of sepsis are recognised (i.e., severe lameness, synovial effusion, oedema, drainage and heat and pain on palpation), which can take up to 7 to 10 days, treatment is expensive and the prognosis decreases with increasing duration of time between injury and treatment. Treatment may be carried out in the field or at a referral hospital. Advantages of hospitalisation include access to inhalation anaesthesia, padded surgery table, and clean surgery room, technical assistance, lighting and surgical supplies. While many procedures can be performed standing, wound debridement and exploration, as well as joint lavage, is facilitated with the horse under general anaesthesia.

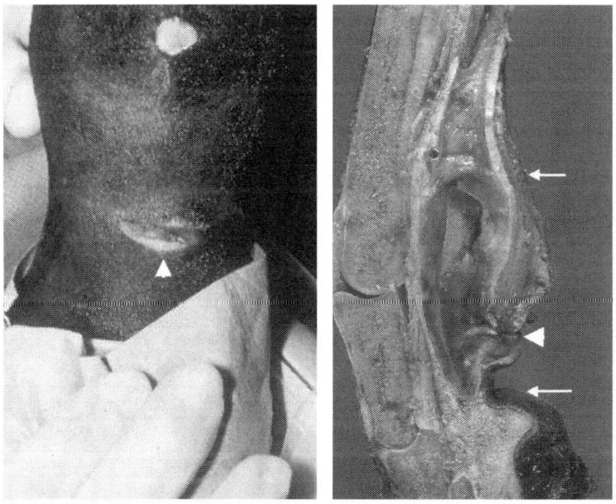

Figures 16.5A-B Small laceration to the palmar aspect of the pastern region (**A** and **B**, *white arrowhead*) that was not treated promptly. The laceration penetrated the digital sheath and because treatment was delayed septic tenosynovitis developed. Despite repeated synovial lavage as well as treatment with local and systemic antimicrobials and analgesia, the horse developed support–limb laminitis and was euthanised. At necropsy diagnosis of a septic digital sheath was confirmed (**B**, *white arrows*). ©Louise Southwood 2006.

Involvement of a synovial structure

If a synovial structure is involved, joint lavage on an emergency basis is indicated. The horse is sedated or anaesthetised and the skin aseptically prepared. Using sterile technique, a 14- to 18-gauge needle is inserted into the affected synovial structure. It is important to be familiar

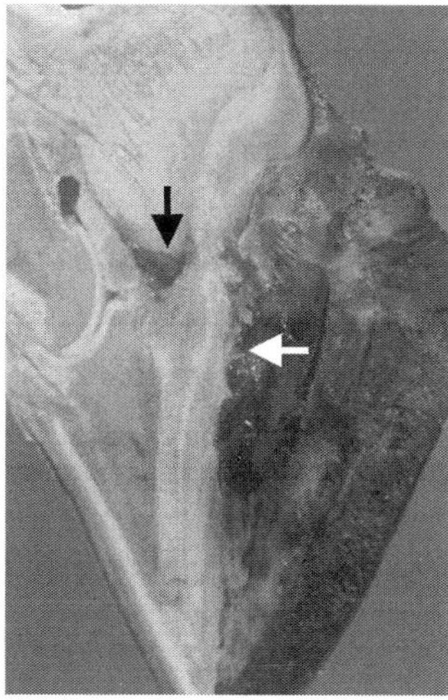

Figure 16.6 Septic navicular bursitis (*black arrow*) in a horse that sustained a penetrating wound to the middle third of the frog (*white arrow*). As was the case for the horse in Figure 16.5 **A**, treatment was delayed and the horse ultimately developed support-limb laminitis in the contralateral limb and was euthanised. ©Louise Southwood 2006.

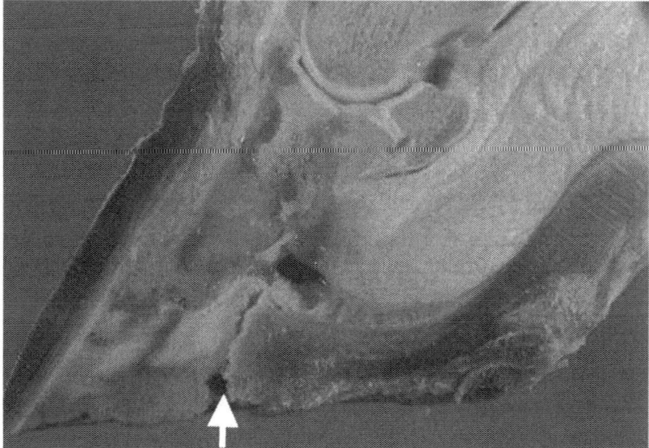

Figure 16.7 Septic osteitis of the third phalanx (coffin bone) as a result of a nail penetrating the sole of the hoof at the apex of the frog (*white arrow*). Note that most of the bone has been destroyed by infection and that septic arthritis of the distal interphalangeal (coffin) joint developed as a result of the infection extending through the articular surface of the third phalanx. ©Louise Southwood 2006.

with multiple injection sites for each joint (see Chapter 15). Needle insertion must be performed aseptically, preferably though an area with the least amount of swelling and cellulitis. Attempts at needle insertion and removal should be kept to a minimum to avoid lavage fluid leakage through the holes and subcutaneous accumulation of fluid during the procedure. The use of a smaller needle (16- to 18-gauge) and leaving poorly positioned needles in place may also reduce this complication. Synovial fluid should be collected for bacterial culture and sensitivity testing. The synovial structure is then lavaged with 3 to 6 L polyionic isotonic fluid. Holding the needle in place during synovial lavage, especially if using fluid pump, reduces the risk of the needle slipping out of the joint or sheath. If possible, multiple ingress/egress sites should be used to adequately flush the entire synovial structure. A fluid pump will greatly facilitate lavage. Wound debridement can be performed during synovial structure lavage to reduce general anaesthesia time. Dimethylsulphoxide (10% DMSO; 100 ml of the 90% solution/1 L sterile polyionic isotonic fluid) may be used in the lavage solution, although experimental and clinical evidence of its benefit are lacking. The use of a 1 to 2 L of triple antibiotic lavage solution (neomycin, bacitracin, polymixin B) may be of benefit. Lavage using solutions containing chlorhexidine diacetate or povidone-iodine is not recommended. Intra-articular antimicrobials (e.g., 2 ml amikacin or gentamicin) should be placed in the joint at the completion of the lavage. Regional limb perfusion can also be performed to increase the local concentration of antimicrobial drugs (see Chapters 1.53 and 15.8).

Wound closure

The wound may be closed primarily or allowed to heal by second intention. Primary closure is always recommended for acute lacerations (within 24 hours) and a laceration in which debridement is adequate. Primary closure can be accomplished using No. 2 (3 to 5 metric) synthetic absorbable monofilament suture material. Various suture patterns, including simple interrupted, cruciate or split-thickness vertical mattress, can be used to appose the skin edges[13] (see Chapter 1.56). There is usually a lot of tension on traumatic wounds because of swelling and skin edge retraction. Methods to relieve tension include using tension relieving suture patterns such as vertical mattress or near-far-far-near (Figure 16.2, D). Quill patterns provide additional support from buttons, rubber tubing or gauze preplaced under the suture before it is tied to reduce suture cut out. The use of quill patterns in wounds that will be covered with a pressure bandage can result in pressure necrosis of the skin under the supporting object; however, clinically this is less significant than the problem of wound dehiscence. Tension at the wound edge can also be relieved by meshing the flap of skin to be sutured with stab incisions (1–2 cm). Skin flap meshing also provides drainage in wounds with a large amount of deadspace. While the subcutaneous tissue should be closed in surgically created wounds, it is generally not closed in traumatic wounds. The presence of suture material can potentiate the development of infection and other techniques, such as drains, packing, skin meshing and pressure bandaging, can be used to prevent wound complications associated with deadspace.

Treatment after debridement, lavage and closure

The wound should be bandaged (see later and Chapter 1.51 for the limb and Chapter 1.54 for the head). Systemic parenteral antimicrobial drugs should be administered for 2 weeks. Low-dose nonsteroidal anti-inflammatory drugs (e.g., phenylbutazone [1–2 g/450-kg horse every 24 hours]) can be given for 3 to 4 days. Low doses of nonsteroidal anti-inflammatory drugs should be used so that early signs of mild lameness can be identified. Tetanus antitoxin should be given depending on the horse's vaccination status. Confine the horse to a clean, dry stall. Monitor the horse closely for 7 to 14 days. Signs of infection (lameness, heat, pain and swelling) often appear following wound healing and closure of the synovial structure. Intrasynovial antimicrobial drug administration, regional limb perfusion with antimicrobial drugs and lavage may be repeated at 24- to 72-hour intervals. If the joint or sheath becomes infected, more thorough lavage and debridement using arthroscopy is recommended.

Problems and more complicated wounds

Involvement of the tendons

If the superficial or deep digital flexor tendons or suspensory ligament is lacerated, the percentage of fibre damage should be assessed. Lacerations affecting less than 50% to 60% of a tendon/ligament should be splinted for 14 to 28 days to avoid further damage to the tendon. Lacerations affecting more than 60% of a tendon or ligament should either be sutured (locking loop or three-loop pulley) or cast for 4 to 6 weeks. The same principles apply to extensor tendon lacerations, but the horse will most likely return to normal function if splinted for 2 to 4 weeks with no suturing. The prognosis for horses with extensor lacerations was reported to be 87% (13 of 15) and 82% (47 of 57) for survival and 47% (7 of 15) and 44% (25 of 57) for return to their intended use.[21,22] The prognosis for horses with flexor tendon lacerations was less favourable, with 91% (20 of 22) and 65% (11 of 17) surviving and 18% (4 of 22) and 47% (8 of 17) of horses returning to their intended use.[21,22]

Bony involvement

Radiographs are important for evaluating the extent of damage following lacerations and puncture wounds and are particularly important for horses with blunt trauma and obvious bone involvement. If a horse is lamer than expected, radiographs should be taken initially, and if the horse is persistently lame, then radiographs should be repeated in 7 to 10 days to evaluate the presence of non-displaced fracture lines. Radiographs should always be taken prior to general anaesthesia in trauma cases because an unrecognised nondisplaced fracture will have devastating consequences during induction or recovery.

If bone is affected, curettage of the damaged and contaminated bone should be performed and any fragments removed. Degloving lacerations of the third metacarpus, for example, with extensive damage to the periosteum may result in sequestrum formation. If bone is exposed, it is important to attempt to cover the bone with as much skin as possible.

Sole of the hoof and frog puncture wounds

Puncture wounds to the sole of the hoof may result in septic pedal osteitis and septic navicular bursitis[23] (Figures 16.6 and 16.7). Radiographs should be taken prior to removal of the penetrating foreign body if possible or a retrograde contrast radiographic study performed to diagnose penetration of the navicular bursa. It can be difficult to locate the site of penetration if the object has been removed previously. Alternatively, a needle can be inserted into the navicular bursa from a remote site, a fluid sample collected if possible and the bursa distended to assess communication with the puncture wound. The site of penetration should be debrided and drainage established. The horse should be started on broad-spectrum antimicrobial drugs and a low dose of phenylbutazone. Traditionally, a street-nail procedure has been performed to manage septic navicular bursitis. The prognosis for survival with this procedure was guarded and the prognosis for return to athletic activity was grave.[23] Recently, endoscopic lavage of the navicular bursa following foreign body penetration has resulted in return of horses to performance, including racing, and is currently recommended for treatment of septic navicular bursitis.[24] Early treatment is essential for a favourable outcome. Therefore, even if navicular bursa penetration is suspected but not confirmed, endoscopic lavage is recommended.

Nonhealing wounds

Occasionally, wounds on the lower limb do not heal by second intention and skin grafting is necessary. The most commonly used skin grafting techniques are pinch and punch grafts. While these grafting techniques are practical and result in wound healing, the cosmetic and functional outcome is not as favourable as that achieved with primary closure. Grafting techniques are described in Chapter 16.2.

Prognosis

The prognosis for horses with a laceration or puncture wound depends on the structures affected, the duration of time between injury and treatment and the number and type of bacteria contaminating or infecting the wound. Early identification and appropriate treatment of lacerations, particularly those affecting deeper structures, are imperative for a favourable outcome.

Bandaging

A detailed description of bandaging has been provided in Chapters 1.51 and 1.54. Bandaging of wounds is important to reduce oedema, protect the wound from trauma and contamination, provide immobilisation of wound edges for healing, provide haemorrhage control and reduce serum accumulation in deadspace. Bandages should be changed every 1 to 3 days depending on the amount of wound drainage and the condition of the bandage. If a wound has been created surgically or repaired aseptically under general anaesthesia, it is recommended to leave the initial bandage change for 24 to 48 hours after surgery.

Surgical wounds

Bandaging of surgically created wounds is variable and depends on the procedure performed, the location of the wound, and the surgeon's preference. Following orthopaedic procedures, many surgeons bandage the limb until suture removal at 10 to 14 days and often a light bandage is placed for 24 hours following suture removal. Bandaging following abdominal surgery is usually used for the initial recovery period. Types of bandages used to protect an abdominal incision during recovery from general anaesthesia include stent bandages and iodine-impregnated drapes. It is critical to remove these bandages as soon as possible following recovery because blood and sweat accumulation can predispose to surgical site infection. An abdominal bandage can be created with gauze and elastic adhesive bandage material or by using commercially available elastic bandages. Abdominal bandages should be reserved for cases with extensive severe oedema postoperatively, a lot of deadspace, following a repeat celiotomy or in horses that spend a lot of time being recumbent. Generally, following recovery from general anaesthesia after abdominal surgery, the wound is left unbandaged. Bandaging is generally not performed following minimally invasive procedures such as laparoscopy.

Traumatic wounds

Bandaging of traumatic wounds is also dependent on clinician preference. Traumatic wounds that have been surgically repaired, particularly wounds on the distal limb and wounds where the skin was apposed under tension, should be bandaged. Wounds that are apposed with a lot of tension on the sutures, particularly those over a mobile joint, can be further stabilised using a splint or a cast[26] (Figure 16.2, E). Splints should be made of strong, light material, such as polyvinyl chloride plastic. Metal splints are heavy and wooden splints tend to break. Splints are applied using inelastic adhesive material to stabilise the joint adjacent to the wound (see Chapters 1.52 and 15.9). Wounds that are not infected and not associated with a deeper structure can be cast, which facilitates healing and lowers the cost of bandage material. Heel bulb lacerations heal well in a foot cast that incorporates the hoof and pastern regions.

Complications associated with the use of casts, such as cast sores and discomfort, should be taken into consideration. Routine use of full-limb casts for management of lacerations is not recommended because of the difficulty some horses have rising from recumbency and the risk of ligament injury and long-bone fracture proximal to the cast.

As an alternative to a routine cast, a bandage cast can be created by casting the limb over a bandage using fibreglass cast material, bi-valving the cast and then reapplying the cast as a conforming splint.[27] Conforming splints can also be made with fibreglass cast material by layering the cast material up and down the bandaged limb multiple times and allowing it to cure before applying it to the limb with inelastic adhesive material.

Wounds on the upper limb and body are also often closed with a lot of tension on the sutures. In many cases, these wounds cannot be bandaged with pressure bandages because of their location. The use of a stent bandage can provide tension relief in addition to wound protection and is recommended for these types of lacerations. Stent bandages can be made from rolled gauze sponges for small wounds through to rolled sterile surgery towels for large wounds and are kept in place using No. 2 (5 metric) non-absorbable suture material in an interrupted horizontal mattress pattern.

Bandaging of open wounds on the distal limb increases granulation tissue formation compared to unbandaged wounds[28]; therefore, distal limb wounds that have exuberant granulation tissue may heal best with stall confinement without bandaging. Wounds in which deadspace is extensive, for example, the wound in Figure 16.4, should be bandaged to reduce blood and serum accumulation within the deadspace. Dead space can also be addressed by packing, by drain placement or by placing stab incisions in the flap of skin over the deadspace.

The hoof should be incorporated in the bandage when the laceration is at the level of or distal to the fetlock region. The entire hoof should be covered with duct tape or other impermeable material to keep the area dry. Dressing types are discussed in Chapter 1.51, and more specific types of dressings and topical treatments are discussed later.

Drains

Drains are used in traumatic and surgical wounds when there is a large volume of deadspace that would delay wound healing and potentiate infection. Dead space results in accumulation of blood and serum, which inhibit healing by reducing the blood supply to the healing tissue, provide a medium for bacterial proliferation and inhibit bacterial killing by leucocytes. Drains facilitate the debridement phase of healing by providing a means of cellular debris removal; however, should never be used in place of meticulous surgical debridement. Drains should always be placed and maintained aseptically and should be removed ideally within 48 to 72 hours (following the debridement phase of healing) or as soon as possible after drainage is minimal (usually 2–4 days after surgery). If drainage persists or increases after an initial decrease, a foreign body response to the drain should be suspected and the drain removed. Patients are often treated with broad-spectrum antimicrobial drugs up to 24 hours after drain removal; however, this particular use of antimicrobial drugs may increase the risk of infection with a resistant pathogen. Wounds with drains should be bandaged to reduce the risk of ascending infection. Culture of the drain following removal is recommended.

Drains can be used in traumatic as well as surgical wounds. Active or negative-pressure suction drains, Figure 16.8, are most commonly used at sterile surgical sites with a large deep deadspace. Polyvinylchloride*† and Silastic‡ fenestrated drain tubes can be used in active drain systems. The drain is placed in the tissue plane that is expected to accumulate fluid and is attached to an extension set and 60-ml syringe (Figure 16.8) or a commercially available vacuum system§. The drain should be secured to the skin using a Chinese finger trap suture pattern (Figure 1.19). Examples of surgical wounds that may require a negative pressure suction drain include ventral stabilisation of vertebral instability ("wobbler syndrome") and femoral fracture repair. Because implants are used in these procedures, it is imperative that the drain is maintained aseptically. The connections between the different components of this drain system should never be separated. Aseptic management of these drains involves maintaining negative pressure to prevent ingress of air, fluid, and microbes, keeping the drain entry site clean and covered and using aseptic technique to empty the syringe.

Passive drains, such as Penrose drains*, are generally used for traumatic wounds. Penrose drains are manufactures from soft latex, which does not cause discomfort, and drainage is driven by gravity and surface tension. Intraluminal drainage is minimal and therefore fenestration is unnecessary and actually contraindicated because it decreases the surface tension and increases the risk of the drain breaking during removal. Appropriate latex Penrose drain placement is described in Figure 16.9. It is important to note that there is only an egress and not an ingress and egress hole. The egress hole for drain placement is located at the most distal or most dependent area of the deadspace. The drain should not be placed directly underneath the healing wound. If the deadspace is particularly large, multiple drains may be used (as in Figure 16.4).

Alternative methods for addressing deadspace and drainage have been discussed previously and include creating

* Polyvinylchloride multifenestrated drain; Zimmer Incorporated, Dover, OH, USA.

† Argyle Trocar Catheter; Sherwood Medical, St. Louis, MO, USA.

‡ Flat Silastic multifenestrated drain—Jackson-Pratt type drain; Zimmer Incorporated, Dover, OH, USA.

§ Snyder Hemovac-100 ml; Zimmer incorporated, Dover, OH, USA.

* Latex Penrose drains; Sherwood Medical, St. Louis, MO, USA.

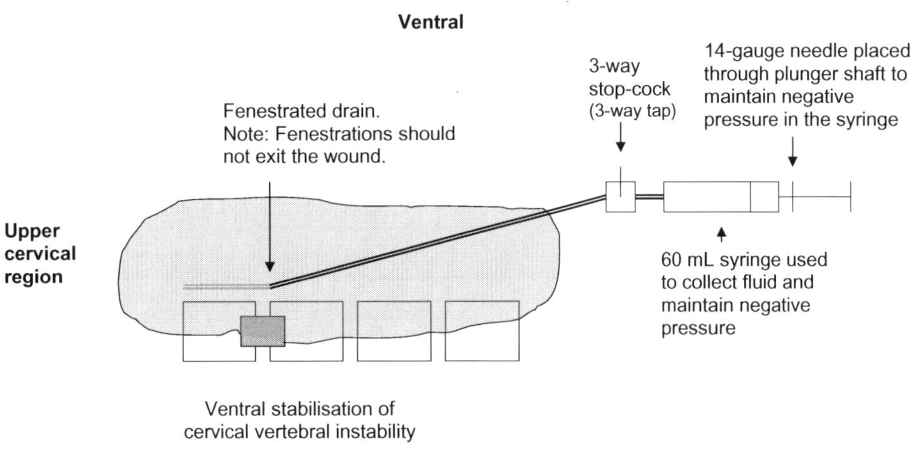

Figure 16.8 Principles of a negative pressure suction drain that can be used to drain deep wounds with a large dead space postoperatively. A fenestrated polyvinylchloride or silastic drain is used. The fenestrations should not exit the wound so that negative pressure is created. Negative pressure should be maintained at all times to prevent ingress of air, fluid, and bacteria. Periodically, the fluid should be removed from the syringe by turning the three-way stop-cock (three-way tap) off toward the patient and emptying the syringe through the three-way stop-cock. The system should never be disconnected. The amount of fluid should be recorded and when drainage is minimal, the drain should be removed, usually 2 to 4 days. The wound and drain should be aseptically bandaged. Horses are usually treated with antimicrobials for up to 24 hours following drain removal. ©Louise Southwood 2006.

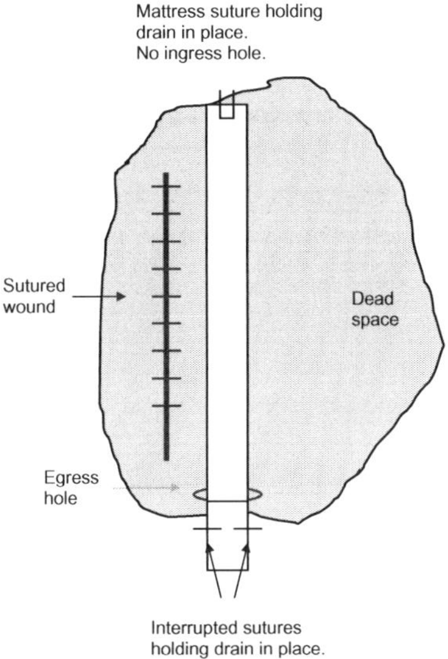

Figure 16.9 Schematic representation of correct placement of a latex Penrose drain in a traumatic wound. It is important to recognize that the drain is not placed directly underneath the wound because this can inhibit nutrient supply to the wound during the early phases of healing as well as inhibit neovascularisation. The drain exists through a stab incision through the most distal or most dependent aspect of the dead space (egress). Note that there is no hole for ingress. The drain is secured in place with a suture proximal and one or two sutures distal. These sutures should be easily distinguished from the sutures apposing the wound edge. The drain should generally be removed 48 to 72 hours following placement. ©Louise Southwood 2006.

several small stab incisions in the skin, leaving the most dependent part of the wound open to allow drainage through the wound, or packing the wound with gauze-soaked in dilute povidone-iodine solution. The deadspace can also be closed by tacking the subcutaneous tissue together. However, this increases the amount of foreign material (suture) in the wound. Drains can also be used in synovial structures and body cavities.[29]

Topical treatments and dressings

The goal of topical treatments is to enhance wound healing and lower the surgical site infection rate. The basic principles of wound dressing have been discussed in Chapters 1.51 and 1.54. In general, clean and clean-contaminated surgical wounds do not require specific topical treatment and should be treated with a nonadherent dressing. The use of occlusive and semiocclusive dressings to treat equine wounds prolongs wound healing and results in exuberant granulation tissue formation.[30] Topical treatments are commonly used on dirty and infected or open wounds and wounds that are not healing normally or develop exuberant granulation tissue. Burn injuries are a special category of wounds and have been discussed in a recent review.[31] Topical treatment should never replace surgical debridement and repair and meticulous wound management. Many commonly used topical treatments can inhibit wound healing[32] and care should be taken in deciding which patients should benefit from a topical treatment and which topical treatment to select. Studies investigating topical treatments are often experimental and involve *in vitro* studies investigating the effect of treatment on cells in culture or surgical creation of a standardised excisional wound on the metacarpus, metatarsus or body of the horse. The application of the findings from some experimental studies to traumatically created wounds is unknown. Most clinical studies, however, are not blinded and are limited by a lack of appropriate controls and treatment randomisation. The types of topical treatments that are often used to treat equine wounds include antiseptics and antimicrobials, topical treatments and dressings to enhance wound healing including biological dressings, and growth factors. The list of topical treatments that have been used in human and veterinary medicine is long; therefore, this section will focus on some of the more commonly used and more recently addressed treatments.

Topical antimicrobial and antiseptic treatments

Commonly used topical antiseptic and antimicrobial treatments include antibiotic ointments (Neosporin* [neomycin, bacitracin zinc, polymixin B sulphate], Polysporin† [bacitracin zinc, polymixin B sulphate], Furacin§ [nitrofurazone]), and Silvadene§ (silver sulphadiazine) and Betadine** (povidone-iodine) creams. In severely contaminated wounds, combined treatment with systemic and topical antimicrobials was more effective in preventing infection compared to placebo or either systemic or topical treatment alone; however, with mild contamination, systemic antimicrobial drugs alone were as effective as the combined antimicrobial treatment.[33] The antibacterial efficacy of topical treatments has been demonstrated in several studies. Topical treatment with bacitracin zinc and Neosporin decreased traumatic wound infection rates (5.5% and 4.5%, respectively) in patients seen at a military community hospital compared to Silvadene and petrolatum (12.1% and 17.6%, respectively).[34] The use of a topical antimicrobial gel containing cetrimide, bacitracin, and polymixin B sulphate reduced the infection rate in mild traumatic wounds in school children from 12.5% (control) to 1.6% (antimicrobial treated). There was no difference, however, in infection rates between wounds treated with povidone-iodine and the antimicrobial gel.[35] Whilst antimicrobial ointments may decrease infection rates, there is always concern that infection with an antimicrobial resistant pathogen will occur. Some authors suggest that antimicrobial ointments predispose to infection with resistant pathogens compared to antiseptic creams; however, there have been no studies to support or refute this concern.

Many topical antimicrobial and antiseptic treatments have been shown experimentally to negatively affect wound healing; however, the effect of these treatments on wound healing in clinical cases is essentially unknown. In an *in vitro* study, Neosporin was the only topical treatment that was not cytotoxic to fibroblasts and keratinocytes.[32] In an experimental study in pigs, Neosporin ointment increased the rate of reepithelialisation by 25%; Silvadene and its vehicle, by 28% and 21%, respectively; and Furacin decreased healing by 24%.[36] Povidone-iodine ointment did not affect the rate of healing.[36] In yet another study, treatment with silver sulphadiazine or povidone-iodine did not alter wound healing compared to untreated control wounds,[28] suggesting that the beneficial antimicrobial effect was not overshadowed by a negative effect on wound healing. Chlorhexidine diacetate (0.5%) reportedly delayed wound healing,[37] and 0.5% chlorhexidine diphosphanilate cream was more painful and more difficult to apply to burn injuries in human patients compared to silver sulphadiazine cream.[38] Therefore, the use of chlorhexidine-based ointments and creams is not recommended.

* Neosporin; Pfizer Incorporated, New York, NY, USA.
† Polysporin; Pfizer Incorporated, New York, NY, USA.
‡ Furacin; Schering-Plough Corporation, Kenilworth, NJ, USA.
§ Silvadene; Marion Laboratories, Kansas City, MO, USA.
** Betadine; Purdue Frederick Company, Stamford, CT, USA.

Growth factors and growth hormone

The application of topical granulocyte-macrophage colony-stimulating factor to acute and chronic granulating wounds infected with *Escherichia coli* in an experimental rat model resulted in enhanced wound healing and decreased bacterial counts compared to controls[39] and may ultimately be useful in treating infected wounds in horses. Growth factors have also been evaluated clinically and experimentally to enhance wound healing. Silver sulphadiazine cream containing epidermal growth factor (10 μg/ml) accelerated the rate of epidermal regeneration in skin graft donor sites[40] and stimulated healing in chronic wounds[41] compared to controls in human patients. The experimental studies investigating the use of growth factors to treat equine wounds have been less encouraging. There was no beneficial effect of intramuscular administration of recombinant equine growth hormone on healing of full-thickness skin wounds on equine limbs[42] or on full-thickness wounds in the pectoral region of horses.[43] Topical treatment with recombinant human transforming growth factor-β_1 (TGF-β, 50 and 500 ng/wound) had no beneficial effects on healing of excisional wounds on the metacarpus or metatarsus of horses.[44] The expression of TGF-β in equine wounds has been investigated and the results of these studies may lead to a focused approach to developing growth factor–based treatments to improve wound healing in horses. The expression of TGF-β_1 was upregulated following injury in cells associated with wound repair.[45] Bandaged wounds healing with exuberant granulation tissue had higher concentrations of fibrogenic TGF-β_1 and lower concentrations of antifibrotic TGF-β_3 compared to unbandaged wounds that did not develop exuberant granulation tissue formation.[46] Additionally, limb wounds healing with exuberant granulation tissue had more receptors for TGF-β_1 associated with an increase in cellularity compared to thoracic and nonbandaged limb wounds without exuberant granulation tissue.[47] Other growth factors that have shown benefit for healing of chronic wounds include platelet-derived growth factor and vascular endothelial growth factor.[48,49] The results of these studies suggest areas to target in the future to enhance wound healing and prevent exuberant granulation tissue formation.

Biological dressings

Biological dressings provide a favourable environment for wound healing and some biological dressings, such as platelets and small intestine submucosa, provide growth factors that may enhance wound healing. Biological dressings reduce wound pain and desiccation, enhance epithelialisation and neovascularisation, reduce exuberant granulation tissue formation and have antibacterial properties because of their preparation and storage with antiseptic and antibiotic-containing solutions.[50] Recently, a platelet gel dressing, produced by treating platelets with autologous thrombin, substantially improved healing in human patients with chronic skin wounds.[51] Small intestine submucosa was used to successfully treat equine wounds and resulted in less exuberant granulation tissue formation, less wound exudate, enhanced epithelialisation, faster wound healing and less cost compared to untreated wounds.[52] The small intestine submucosa was easy to handle and there were no adverse effects.[52] However, experimentally, compared to nonbiological dressings, split-thickness allogenic skin, allogenic peritoneum and xenogenic porcine small intestine submucosa had no benefits on healing in equine metacarpal or metatarsal wounds and allogenic peritoneum and xenogenic porcine small intestine submucosa were reportedly less practical to use because of the requirement for numerous dressing changes compared to split-thickness allogenic skin and the nonbiological dressing.[53] Equine amnion, on the other hand, decreased healing time, exuberant granulation tissue formation and the number of pathological bacteria compared to controls in experimentally created full-thickness metacarpal and metatarsal wounds in horses[54,55] and enhanced healing compared to biosynthetic hydrogel dressing and other nonbiological dressings in experimentally created full-thickness trunk wounds in dogs.[56] While these dressings have been evaluated experimentally, their widespread use in equine wound management has not occurred. Large prospective randomised clinical trials are needed to evaluate the usefulness of biological dressings for treating equine wounds.

Other topical wound dressings

There are a plethora of topical wound dressings and treatments that have been evaluated experimentally in laboratory animals and clinically in human and veterinary patients. Cyanoacrylate adhesive was used successfully to repair small (2 cm) experimental skin incisions in the scapular region of horses,[57] and cyanoacrylate spray was used successfully to protect wounds from dirt, debris and insects by providing a water-proof barrier, as well as stabilising wound edges by bridging normal to traumatised tissue facilitating granulation tissue formation and epithelialisation.[58] In the latter clinical report, the successful use of bovine collagen and various wound dressings were described.[58] Chitin (chitin-sponge, -cotton and -flake) was shown to result in good healing with no complications in 89% of veterinary patients with wounds from trauma, abscesses, surgical defects and herniorrhaphy; however, the study was not controlled.[59] Vedaprofen, a topical nonsteroidal anti-inflammatory drug, resulted in drier lesions with less oedema compared to controls in experimentally created wounds in the lumbar region of horses.[60] In the latter study, vedaprofen reduced epithelialisation compared to controls but did not affect wound healing overall.[60] Beta aminopropionitrile (β-APN) is an antifibrotic agent that resulted in more organised lesions compared to controls in an equine metacarpal wound model; however, wounds treated with β-APN had more exuberant granulation tissue formation.[61] Ketanserin, which is a 5-hydroxytryptamine antagonist, was more effective in preventing granulation tissue formation and resulted in successful healing in 2 to 5 times more equine clinical cases compared to topical wound treatments that were commonly used to prevent exuberant granulation tissue in horses such as malic, benzoic, and salicylic acid and ethacridin lactate solution.[62] Corticosteroids delay wound healing by stabilising lysosomal membranes and delaying the inflammatory phase of wound healing, and suppressing fibroplasia, ground substance formation, collagen formation, capillary proliferation and granulation tissue formation. Because of these effects, topical corticosteroids are commonly used to manage exuberant granulation tissue formation. Topical treatment with scarlet oil is often used to stimulate formation of granulation tissue in extensive wounds; however, it is irritating to the exposed tissue and may increase wound exudation.

Hydrogel dressings are reported to improve wound healing in human patients by creating a biocompatible environment, penetrating nonviable organic material and modifying it to become inhospitable to microbes, and facilitating autolytic debridement by increasing the water content of necrotic tissue and increasing collagenase production within the wound.[63] However, in an equine full-thickness open metacarpal wound model, one of these hydrogel dressings†† did not improve wound healing compared to dressing with saline-soaked gauze.[63] The lack of benefit observed with the hydrogel dressing in this model may have been because the wounds were created surgically and the debridement phase of healing was short and uncomplicated. Other similar products that are reported to facilitate wound debridement and epithelialisation are copolymer flakes‡‡ and dextranomer beads. The use of these products should never replace thorough surgical debridement of wounds. Based on clinical experience, treatment of wounds with meticulous surgical debridement results in improved and faster wound healing compared to treatment with any topical treatment or dressing.

Most recently, a commercially available resorbable naturally occurring extracellular matrix scaffold§§ anecdotally has been reported to enhance healing of extensive wounds by providing a biologically compatible scaffold for cell migration and neovascularlisation. Controlled studies evaluating this product have not been performed.

†† Solugel; Johnson and Johnson Medical, North Ryde, NSW, Australia.

‡‡ Copolymer Flakes; Avalon, Summit Hill Labs, Avalon, NJ, USA.

§§ Acell Vet; Acell Incorporated, Jessup, MD, USA.

Several available topical treatments can delay wound healing and should not be used. Examples of such topical treatments that can delay healing include gentian violet, hydrogen peroxide and acetic acid. Hydrogen peroxide (3%) is cytotoxic to fibroblasts, exceeding its bactericidal activity,[64] and may cause microvascular thrombosis adjacent to the wound margins.[13] Acetic acid solutions (0.25% or 0.5%) are reported to be active against *Pseudomonas* spp.; however, they retard epithelialisation and fibroblast migration, and the cytotoxicity is also thought to exceed its bactericidal effect.[13]

Conclusion

In conclusion, it is important to remember that many topical wound treatments may adversely affect wound healing and should never be used to replace optimal wound management. Most equine wounds will heal without any topical treatment if they are kept clean and the horse confined to a stall to prevent excessive movement at the wound edges. Early and appropriate treatment is critical for successful wound healing and a favourable outcome.

References

1. Trostle SS, Hartmann FA: Surgical infection, in Auer JA, Stick JA (eds): Equine Surgery, ed 2. Philadelphia, WB Saunders, 1999, pp 47-54
2. Spiers VC, Bourke JM, Anderson GA: Assessment of the efficacy of an abductor muscle prosthesis for treatment of laryngeal hemiplegia in the horse. Aust Vet J 60:294-298, 1983
3. McIlwraith CW, Yovich JV, Martin GS: Arthroscopic surgery for the treatment of osteochondral chip fractures in the equine carpus. J Am Vet Med Assoc 191:531-540, 1987
4. Wilson DG, Reinertson EL: A modified parainguinal approach for cryptorchidectomy in horses. Vet Surg 16:1-4, 1987
5. Meagher DM, Wheat JD, Hughes JP, et al.: Granulosa cell tumors in mares: a review of 78 cases. Proc Am Assoc Equine Pract 23:133-137, 1977
6. Kobluck CN, Ducharme NG, Lumsden JH, et al.: Factors affecting incisional complication rates associated with colic surgery in horses. J Am Vet Med Assoc 195:639-642, 1989
7. Honnas CM, Cohen ND: Risk factors for wound infection following celiotomy in horses. J Am Vet Med Assoc 210: 78-81, 1997
8. Wilson DA, Baker GJ, Boero MJ: Complications of celiotomy incisions in horses. Vet Surg 24:506-514, 1995
9. MacDonald DG, Morley PS, Baley JV, et al.: An examination of the occurrence of surgical wound infection following equine orthopedic surgery (1981-1990). Equine Vet J 26:323-326, 1994
10. 7. Altemeier WA, Culbertson WR, Hummel RP: Surgical considerations of endogenous infections—sources, types, methods of control. Surg Clin N Am 48:277-285, 1968
11. Aberg C, Thore M: Single versus triple dose antimicrobial prophylaxis in elective abdominal surgery and the impact on bacterial ecology. J Hosp Inf 18:149-154, 1991
12. Caron JP (ed): The integumentary system, in Auer JA, Stick JA (eds): Equine Surgery, ed 2. Philadelphia, WB Saunders, 1992, pp 121-188
13. Stashak TS: Equine Wound Management. Philadelphia, Lea & Febiger, 1991
14. Lozier S, Pope E, Berg J: Effects of four preparations of 0.05% chlorhexidine diacetate on wound healing in dogs. Vet Surg 21:107-112, 1992
15. Tvedten HW, Till GO: Effect of povidone, povidone-iodine, and iodine on locomotion (in vitro) of neutrophils from people, rats, dogs, and rabbits. Am J Vet Res 46:1797-1800, 1985
16. Lineaweaver W, Howard R, Soucy D, et al.: Topical antimicrobial toxicity. Arch Surg 120:267-270, 1985
17. Sanchez IR, Swaim SF, Nusbaum KE, et al.: Effects of chlorhexidine diacetate and povidone-iodine on wound healing in dogs. Vet Surg 17:291-295, 1988
18. Rodeheaver GT, Pettry D, Thacker JG, et al.: Wound cleaning by high pressure irrigation. Surg Gynecol Obstet 141:357-362, 1975
19. Gemeinhardt KD, Molnar JA: Vacuum-assisted closure for management of a traumatic neck wound in a horse. Equine Vet Educ 7:35-42, 2005
20. Janicek JC, Dabareiner RM, Honnas CM, Crabill MA: Heel bulb lacerations in horses: 101 cases (1988-1994). J Am Vet Med Assoc 226:418-423, 2005
21. Foland JW, Trotter GW, Stashak TS, et al.: Traumatic injuries involving tendons of the distal limbs in horses: a retrospective study of 55 cases. Equine Vet J 23:422-425, 1991
22. Gasthuys F, Brantegem L, van Vlaminck L, et al.: Retrospective study of tendon wounds of the distal limb segments in horses. Vlaams Diergeneeskundig Tijdschrift 67:172-180, 1998
23. Harreveld PD, van Gaughan EM, Biller DS: Diagnosis and treatment of septic navicular bursitis in horses. Equine Pract 22:10-13, 2000
24. Wright IM, Phillips TJ, Walmsley JP: Endoscopy of the navicular bursa: a new technique for the treatment of contaminated and septic bursae. Equine Vet J 31:5-11, 1999
25. Stashak TS: Principles of free skin grafting, in Stashak TS (ed): Equine Wound Management. Philadelphia, Lea & Febiger, 1991, pp 218-237
26. Booth TM, Knottenbelt DC: Distal limb casts in equine wound management. Equine Vet Educ 11:273-280, 1999
27. Hogan PM: How to make a bandage cast and indications for its use. Proc Am Assoc Equine Pract 46:150-152, 2000
28. Berry DB II, Sullins KE: Effects of topical application of antimicrobials and bandaging on healing and granulation tissue formation in wounds of the distal aspect of the limbs in horses. Am J Vet Res 64:88-92, 2003
29. Stone WC: Drains, dressings, and external coaptation, in Auer JA, Stick JA (eds): Equine Surgery. Philadelphia, WB Saunders, 1999, pp 104-113
30. Howard RD, Stashak TS, Baxter GM: Evaluation of occlusive dressings for management of full-thickness excisional wounds on the distal portion of the limbs of horses. Am J Vet Res 54:2150-2154, 1993
31. Hanson RR: Management of burn injuries in the horses: clinical management. Proc N Am Vet Conf 18:135-136, 2004

32. Cooper ML, Laxer JA, Hansbrough JF: The cytotoxic effects of commonly used topical antimicrobial agents on human fibroblasts and keratinocytes. J Traum Inj Inf Crit Care 31:775-782, 1991
33. Bergamini TM, Lamont PM, Cheadle WG, Polk HC Jr: Combined topical and systemic antibiotic prophylaxis in experimental wound infection. Am J Surg 147:753-756, 1984
34. Dire DJ, Coppola M, Dwyer DA, et al.: Prospective evaluation of topical antibiotics for preventing infections in uncomplicated soft-tissue wounds repaired in the ED. Acad Emerg Med 2:4-10, 1995
35. Langford JH, Artemi P, Benrimoj SI: Topical antimicrobial prophylaxis in minor wounds. Ann Pharm 31:559-563, 1997
36. Geronemus RG, Mertz PM, Eaglstein WH: Wound healing. The effects of topical antimicrobial agents. Arch Derm 115:1311-1314, 1979
37. Lee AH, Swaim SF, McGuire JA, Hughes KS: Effects of chlorhexidine diacetate, povidone iodine, and polyhydroxideine on wound healing in dogs. J Am Anim Hosp Assoc 24:77-84, 1988
38. Miller LM, Loder JS, Hansbrough JF, et al.: Patient tolerance study of topical chlorhexidine diphosphanilate: a new topical agent for burns. Burns 16:217-220, 1990
39. Robson M, Kucukcelebi A, Carp SS, et al.: Effects of granulocyte-macrophage colony-stimulating factor on wound contraction. Eur J Clin Micro Infect Dis 13:S41-S46, 1994
40. Brown GL, Nanney LB, Griffen J, et al.: Enhancement of wound healing by topical treatment with epidermal growth factor. N Engl J Med 321:76-79, 1989
41. Brown GL, Curtsinger L, Jurkiewicz MJ, et al.: Stimulation of healing of chronic wounds by epidermal growth factor. Plast Reconst Surg 88:189-194, 1991
42. Dart AJ, Cries L, Jeffcott LB, et al.: The effect of equine recombinant growth hormone on second intention wound healing in horses. Vet Surg 31:314-319, 2002
43. Smith LA, Thompson DL Jr, French DD, Leise BS: Effects of recombinant equine somatotropin on wound healing, carbohydrate and lipid metabolism, and endogenous somatotropin responses to secretagogues in geldings. J Anim Sci 77:1815-1822, 1999
44. Steel CM, Robertson ID, Thomas J, Yovich JV: Effect of topical rh-TGF-beta1 on second intention wound healing in horses. Aust Vet J 77:734-737, 1999
45. Theoret CL, Barber SM, Gordon JR: Temporal localization of immunoreactive transforming growth factor beta 1 in normal equine skin and full thickness dermal wounds. Vet Surg 31:274-280, 2002
46. Theoret CL, Barber SM, Moyana TN, Gordon JR: Preliminary observations on expression of transforming growth factor beta 1 and beta 3 in equine full-thickness skin wounds healing normally or with exuberant granulation tissue. Vet Surg 31:266-273, 2002
47. De Martin I, Theoret CL: Spatial and temporal expression of types I and II receptors for transforming growth factor beta in normal equine skin and dermal wounds. Vet Surg 33:70-76, 2004
48. Galiano RD, Tepper OM, Pelo CR, et al.: Topical vascular endothelial growth factor accelerates diabetic wound healing through increased angiogenesis and by mobilizing and recruiting bone marrow-derived cells. Am J Pathol 164:1935-1947, 2004
49. Higgins KR, Ashry HR: Wound dressings and topical agents. Clin Podiatr Med Surg 12:31-40, 1995
50. Caron JP: Management of superficial wounds, in Auer JA, Stick JA (eds): Equine Surgery. Philadelphia, WB Saunders, 1999, pp 129-140
51. Mazzucco L, Medici D, Serra M, et al. The use of autologous platelet gel to treat difficult-to-heal wounds: a pilot study. Transfusion 44:1013-1018, 2004
52. Dressel C, Furst A, Imhof A: Clinical use of small intestine submucosa in wound repair in 11 horses. Wiener Tierarztliche Monatsschrift 91:142-150, 2004
53. Gomez JH, Schumacher J, Lauten SD, et al.: Effects of 3 biologic dressings on healing of cutaneous wounds of the limbs of horses. Can J Vet Res 68:49-55, 2004
54. de Oliveira VA, de Alvarenga J: Equine amniotic membrane preserved in glycerin for repairing cutaneous wounds in equine limbs. Ciencia Rural 28:623-628, 1998.
55. Goodrich LR, Moll HD, Crisman MV, et al.: Comparison of equine amnion and a nonadherent wound dressing material for bandaging pinch-grafted wounds in ponies. Am J Vet Res 61:326-329, 2000
56. Ramsey DT, Pope ER, Wagner-Mann C, et al.: Effects of three occlusive dressing materials on healing of full-thickness skin wounds in dogs. Am J Vet Res 56:941-949, 1995
57. Magalhaes AC, Borges APB, da Silva JCP, et al.: Comparative study of methyl-2-cyanoacryate adhesive and nylon in wound repair of experimentally created wounds on equine skin. Rev Brasil Ciencia Vet 8:133-136, 2001
58. Bello TR: Practical treatment of body and open leg wounds of horses with bovine collagen, biosynthetic wound dressing and cyanoacrylate. J Equine Vet Sci 22:157-164, 2002
59. Okamoto Y, Minami S, Matsuhashi A, et al.: Application of polymeric N-acetyl-D-glucosamine (chitin) to veterinary practice. J Vet Med Sci 55:743-747, 1993
60. Hussni CA, Gianini CG, Alves ALG, et al.: Second intention skin wound healing in equines under vedaprofen treatment. Arch Vet Sci 9:87-92, 2004
61. Hussni CA, Wludarski ARL, Alves ALG, et al.: Evaluation of topical beta-aminopropionitrile on equine wound healing. Ars Vet 19:26-34, 2003
62. Engelen M, Besche B, Lefay MP, et al.: Effects of ketanserin on hypergranulation tissue formation, infection, and healing of equine lower limb wounds. Can Vet J 45:144-149, 2004
63. Dart AJ, Cries L, Jeffcott LB, et al.: Effects of 25% propylene glycol hydrogel (Solugel) on second intention wound healing in horses. Vet Surg 31:309-313, 2002
64. Lineweaver W: Topical antimicrobial toxicity. Arch Surg 120:267-270, 1985

16.2 Simple skin grafting techniques

Jennifer O. Stephen

The surgical techniques used for skin grafting range from very simple to very sophisticated. Choosing the correct technique and correct time for intervention is also a complex issue. This section is intended to give an overview of the basic techniques available to equine clinicians without specialist equipment. For a full discussion of skin grafting, surgical texts should be consulted.[1]

Preparing to graft

Recipient Site

Ideally, the recipient site should be a level healthy bed of tissue with good blood supply. Sites with infection, necrotic debris, sarcoid cells, foreign material, "proud flesh", exposed bone, tendon or fat are unlikely to support grafts. If there is excessive granulation tissue, it should be excised to 0.5 cm below skin level and a pressure bandage applied for 7 to 10 days.[2] Generally, granulation tissue that has proliferating epithelium at its margin is healthy enough to accept a skin graft.[1] As with the donor site, the recipient site should be aseptically prepared and then thoroughly rinsed with saline prior to grafting.

Donor site

The hair colour and direction of hair growth of the donor site should be matched to the recipient site as far as is possible. The donor site is clipped, aseptically prepared and then thoroughly rinsed with saline. Local anaesthetic is used to desensitise the area unless the graft is being taken under general anaesthesia.

Graft techniques

Punch grafts, pinch grafts and tunnel grafts are three simple techniques for skin grafting. The advantages and disadvantages of these techniques is given in Box 16.1.

Punch grafts

First, the recipient site is aseptically prepared and rinsed with saline. Next, a 5-mm skin biopsy punch is used to create holes in the granulation tissue (starting at most distal part of granulation tissue to prevent operative site being obscured by haemorrhage). After the holes are created, cotton-tipped swabs are embedded in them to reduce bleeding (Figure 16.10, A). Uncontrolled haemorrhage will literally "float" the grafts out of position. The recipient holes should be placed about 6 mm apart.[3]

The donor site is then surgically prepared and rinsed with saline. Small blemishes will be created by harvesting the grafts, which should be born in mind when selecting the site. Common donor sites include the ventrolateral abdomen, the perineum and the skin on the neck, which is covered by the mane.

A 7-mm skin biopsy punch is then used to take grafts from the donor site. It is unnecessary to close the wounds created; however, suturing or stapling the sites may give a better cosmetic result. Once harvested, all subcutaneous fascia and fat should be sharply excised from the graft. An alternative to harvesting multiple grafts directly from the horse is to take a large elliptical piece of skin (10 cm × 4 cm) from the cranial pectoral region. The skin harvested is then secured to a section of sterile cardboard and the punch biopsy samples are taken. This allows primary closure of the wound created and may be slightly more efficient.[3] Once harvested, all grafts should be kept sterile and moist until implanted.

The grafts are firmly pushed into each recipient hole. When all grafts have been placed, the area should be covered with a nonadherent dressing and bandaged. Grafts are susceptible to mechanical dislodgement in the first few days postoperatively so bandage changes should be kept to a minimum. While "island" grafts such as punch grafts are more resistant to movement than other forms of skin grafting, it is still important to keep the recipient site relatively immobile. If the wound is over a joint, a splint or cast may be necessary to achieve this.

After 10 days, it is expected to have lost about 25% to 40%[4] of the grafts. The grafts will appear as small grey islands in the granulation tissue (Figure 16.10, B). By 21 days, each graft will be surrounded by a red ring, which is a thin layer of epithelial cells; this spreads outwards until it coalesces with the other grafts at about 28 to 35 days

Box 16.1. Advantages and disadvantages of three different simple techniques for skin grafting

Punch grafts

Advantages
- Inexpensive
- Technically easy
- Can be performed without general anaesthesia

Disadvantages
- Blemishes caused at donor site
- Poor cosmetic result (divergent sparse hair cover produced)

Pinch grafts

Advantages
- General anaesthetic not necessary
- Easy technique, no specialist equipment required
- Relatively resistant to infection

Disadvantages
- Poor cosmetic end result: "cobblestone" appearance[5] and abnormal hair growth[6]
- Tendency for skin to crack and bleed with movement

Tunnel grafts

Advantages
- Overcome problem of graft displacement seen with other techniques
- Useful in areas of high motion, particularly recommended over the dorsal tarsal region[7]
- High success rate, both functional and cosmetic[8]

Disadvantages
- Requires two procedures, time consuming
- May require a general anaesthetic

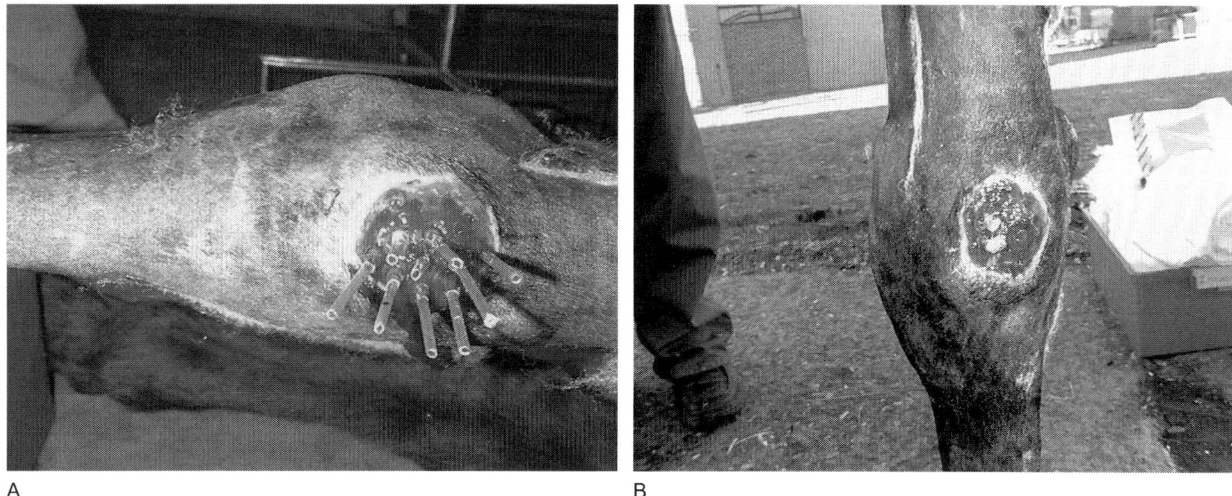

Figure 16.10A-B Punch graft of a nonhealing wound over the hock. (**A**) Cotton-tipped swabs placed in recipient sites for punch grafting. It is important to control haemorrhage or the grafts will be displaced. (**B**) The recipient site 10 days after the graft. ©Jennifer Stephen 2001.

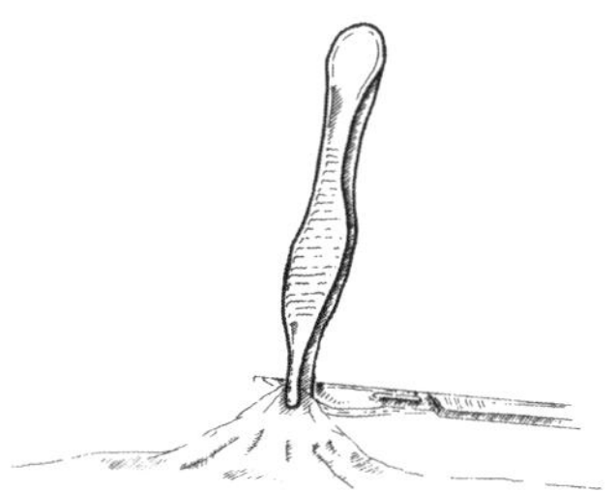

Figure 16.11 Pinch graft: Using forceps to tent the skin to harvest donor skin.

postgrafting. By 42 days, the surface will appear grey, as hair appears, and by 49 to 56 days, pigmentation of the skin should be seen, as well as contraction of the entire wound.[3]

Pinch grafts

The donor skin should be relatively thin and free from hair to obtain the most viable grafts.[5] The skin is elevated using a cutting needle or fine forceps to tent the skin (Figure 16.11). A split-thickness (as thin as possible) disc, 2 to 3 mm in diameter, is excised. Donor sites may be left open to heal or, if a full-thickness incision has been made, sutured.

Starting at the distal end of the wound, the recipient sites are made using a number 15 scalpel blade to create "pockets". The pockets should be 1 to 2 mm below the surface of the wound, 1 cm deep and open in an upwards direction (Figure 16.12). A density of one graft per centimetre squared should be aimed for.[5]

The pinch graft should be flattened out and inserted into the pocket epithelial side out. Grafts may be sealed into pocket using a bleb of tissue adhesive over the entry point or with manual pressure over site. The recipient site should be covered with a nonadherent dressing and bandaged.

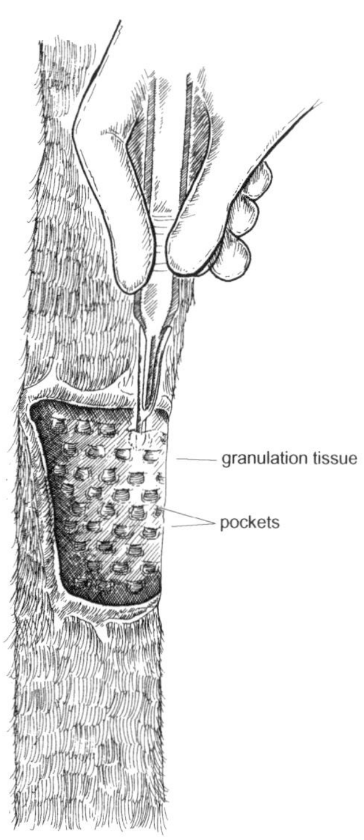

Figure 16.12 Pinch graft: Technique for preparing recipient sites. Starting at the distal end of the wound, the recipient sites are made using a number 15 scalpel blade to create "pockets". The pockets should be 1 to 2 mm below the surface of the wound, 1 cm deep and open in an upwards direction.

From 50% to 75% of the grafts may be expected to survive using this technique. Small dark specks should be seen on the wound surface around 12 to 14 days after grafting, with sloughing of the surface of the "pocket". The grafts should then double in size every week so that an epithelial covering is produced 3 to 4 weeks postgrafting.[5]

Tunnel grafts

The horse may require an anaesthetic depending on the size and location of wound to be grafted. Donor skin may be taken from the neck below the mane or the ventral flank or abdomen.[8] Prior to harvesting the graft, local anaesthetic or saline is injected into the subcuticular tissue to make a wheal or bleb 2- to 3-cm wide and slightly longer than the graft to be collected. Straight intestinal forceps are then applied along this line so that the skin is pinched and protrudes above the forceps. The graft should be long enough to bridge recipient site.[7] If a longer strip of skin is required, two intestinal forceps placed end to end may be used. The protruding skin is then sharply excised with a scalpel blade. The strip taken should be about 2 mm wide and can be split thickness[7] or full thickness.[8] If a full-thickness graft is taken, the subcutaneous tissue should be removed and the donor site closed primarily with sutures. Taking a full-thickness graft may be associated with less scarring at the donor site.[8] Alternatively, the grafts may be taken without forceps by simply making a series of parallel incisions 2 mm apart. Four or five strips may then be taken and the donor site is closed as single incision.

Originally, authors advocated attaching the grafts to tape for implantation.[7] The grafts were stuck to strips of sterile white adhesive tape, hair side down. One end of the tape was extended about 5 cm beyond the graft, for attachment to a needle. At the other end of the graft 1 cm of tape was folded over the graft to secure it. The grafts were then placed 5 to 6 mm below the granulation tissue, tape side up, by threading the tape across the wound with a large cutting needle (10 to 12 cm long). A modified version of this technique where tape is not applied to the grafts is also described.[8] In this technique, the grafts are implanted with 2-mm-diameter alligator forceps. The forceps are used to tunnel under granulation tissue to a depth of 5 to 10 mm. The graft is then grasped and pulled back under the wound surface (Figure 16.13). If the wound is wider than the forceps, the graft should be tunnelled to the extent of the forceps and brought out to the surface, then reinserted and advanced as before until the wound is traversed.

Whichever technique is used, the grafts should be placed parallel to each other at 2-cm intervals along the length of the wound.[8] The exposed ends of the graft should be sutured or glued at wound margin. When the grafting takes place on a limb, a tourniquet may be useful to decrease haemorrhage and improve visualisation of the strips during placement.[6]

About 60% to 80% of the grafts may be expected to take using this technique.[1] If placed sufficiently superficially, the granulation tissue over the grafts should slough 6 to 10 days after surgery; otherwise, the granulation tissue should be excised at around day 8 to expose the grafts. This procedure will require either heavy sedation or anaesthesia.[8] The sutures at the ends of the grafts are removed. The granulation tissue can then be excised either by passing a double piece of 0.3-mm wire through the tunnel and sawing through[7] or by passing a malleable metal probe and making a V-shaped incision over this[1] (Figure 16.14). The tape, if used, should have separated from the graft at this time and should be easily removed.[7]

Some authors recommend that bandages are changed daily from grafting and the wound gently cleaned until epithelialisation is complete.[6] Others recommend that the wound is kept bandaged with minimal bandage changes until the grafts are exposed and then the area is left uncovered.[7] It is important that granulation tissue between the grafts is kept trimmed down to the level of the grafts. Where excessive granulation is a problem, a water-soluble

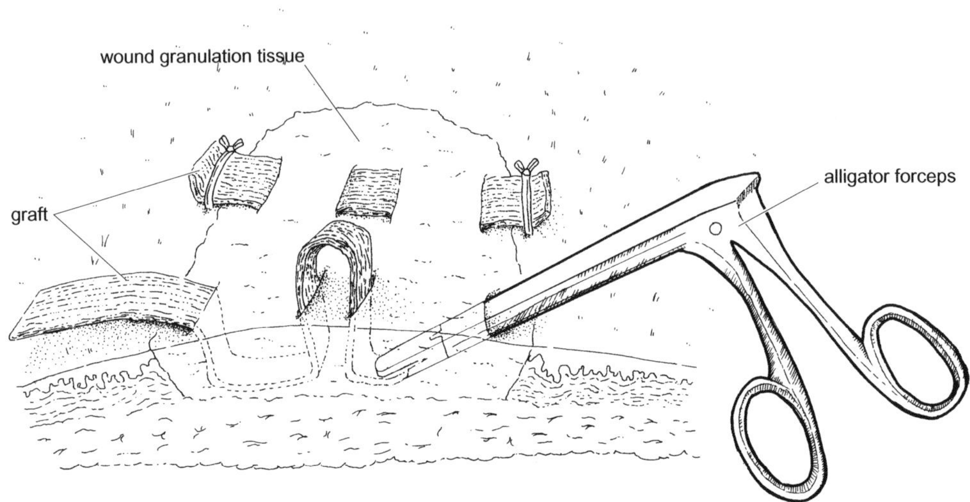

Figure 16.13 Tunnel graft: Technique for placing the graft. Alligator forceps are used to tunnel under granulation tissue to a depth of 5 to 10 mm. The graft is then grasped and pulled back under the wound surface. If the wound is wider than the forceps the graft should be tunnelled to the extent of the forceps and brought out to the surface, then reinserted and advanced as before until the wound is traversed.

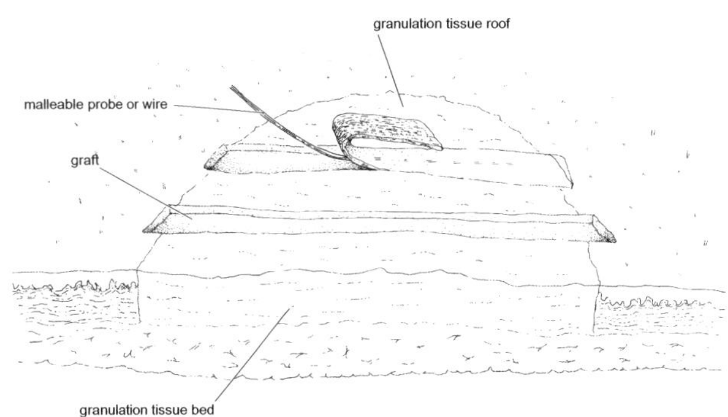

Figure 16.14 Tunnel graft: Technique for removing granulation tissue after the graft has taken. A malleable metal probe is passed under the granulation tissue, and a V-shaped incision is made over this.

antibacterial cortisone cream may be used in conjunction with daily debridement.[8] Epithelialisation may be complete in 12 weeks in successful cases.[7] The cosmetic appearance of the donor site should be good to excellent.[8]

References

1. Schumacher J: Skin grafting, in Auer JA, Stick JA (eds): Equine Surgery, ed 3. St. Louis, Elsevier, 2006, pp 269-287
2. Knottenbelt DC: Skin grafting, in Knottenbelt DC (ed): Equine Wound Management. St. Louis, Saunders, 2003, pp 79-86
3. Boyd CL: A skin punch technique for equine skin grafting. J Am Vet Med Assoc 158:82-88, 1971
4. Stashak TS: Skin grafting in horses. Vet Clin N Am 61:215-225, 1984
5. Mackay-Smith MP: A skin grafting technique in horses. J Am Vet Med Assoc 152:1633-1637, 1968
6. Bristol DG: Skin grafts and skin flaps in the horse. Vet Clin North Am Equine Pract 21:125-144, 2005
7. Bjork G: Tunnel grafting in the equine species. Proc Am Assoc Equine Pract 313-321, 1971
8. Lees MJ, Andrews GC, Bailey JV, et al: Tunnel grafting of equine wounds. Compend Contin Educ Pract Vet 11:962-968, 1989

17

Monitoring and treatment of eyes

Mary E. Utter

17.1 Ophthalmic examination
17.2 Management of horses with specific ophthalmic conditions
17.3 Management of ocular problems in the neonatal foal

17.1 Ophthalmic examination

For horses presented to the hospital with an ocular complaint, a timely and thorough examination is critical to appropriately direct their therapy. The history should provide information regarding the presenting complaint, duration of clinical signs and past and current treatment. It is not uncommon for a horse to arrive at hospital with someone who does not know what medications have been administered, and thus it is a good idea to try to obtain this information prior to arrival if possible or to instruct the shipper to bring eye medications along with the horse. Frequency of administration of topical medications is important in determining the appropriate course of therapy; for example, a horse that arrives with severe blepharospasm, a corneal ulcer and a miotic pupil that has had neither atropine nor flunixin carries a better prognosis for response to treatment than one that has already had two doses of topical atropine and systemic flunixin.

The eye examination should begin with visual inspection, prior to even laying hands on the horse, evaluating facial symmetry, lid position, and the presence of any ocular discharge, and globe integrity, symmetry and position. Determining whether there are any vision deficits and testing the menace response, dazzle reflex and pupillary light reflexes (direct and indirect) are best performed prior to sedation if possible. Following sedation and blocking lids (see Chapter 1.48), if necessary, a complete eye examination from anterior to posterior may ensue. To open the eyelids and view the eye, the index finger can be placed gently at the crease in the superior lid and used to carefully push the lid upwards toward the orbital rim but avoiding putting any pressure on the globe. Another technique for opening the lid is to gently grasp the crease in the superior lid between thumb and index finger, pull it slightly away from the globe to avoid putting pressure on it and lift the crease upward until the dorsal orbital rim is contacted. The superior lid can then be held firmly against the bony orbital rim, without putting any pressure on the globe. Repeated lid elevation should be avoided; once the lid has been grasped and secured against the orbital rim, allow an occasional blink but do not continuously grasp the lid and then let it go, as most horses are annoyed by prolonged lid elevation.

Depending on the presenting complaint, further diagnostics beyond an ophthalmic examination (e.g., culture, ocular ultrasonography, electroretinography) may be necessary and are discussed with the appropriate ocular disorder. Aside from patients that present to hospital for an ocular complaint, patients at risk of developing ophthalmological disorders during hospitalisation include, in particular, those that are recumbent due to illness (e.g., a neonatal foal that is on a bed, may be dehydrated, and is potentially not blinking enough), those undergoing general anaesthesia and anaesthetic recovery (who may sustain an ulcer from corneal desiccation while not blinking frequently enough under anaesthesia, or from trauma in recovery), those thrashing due to severe pain, as in colic, and those with inflammatory disease that may have multisystem manifestations (e.g., laminitis, sepsis). Patients with facial nerve paralysis will have desiccated corneas that develop severe and persistent ulcers if the cornea is not properly lubricated. Finally, sedated horses and those recently undergoing a lid block may not blink frequently enough to maintain the corneal surface and thus are also at risk for corneal ulceration.

17.2 Management of horses with specific ophthalmic conditions

Management of horses with corneal ulcers

One of the most common presenting complaints amongst horses hospitalised for ocular disease is corneal ulceration. Following examination of the ocular surface, prior to instilling topical anaesthesia or fluorescein stain, a corneal culture should be collected. It is not uncommon even for a cornea that has been treated with topical antibiotics to still be culture positive for a bacterial organism, typically one that is resistant to whatever has been used prior to treat the cornea. Therefore, it is still clinically worthwhile to collect a corneal culture from a horse that has received prior antibiotic treatment. To collect the culture, hold the eyelids open so as not to contaminate the swab with lid or conjunctival flora. The corneal lesion should be carefully swabbed making sure to contact the periphery of the ulcer, where infectious organisms can most reliably be found. It is important to either plate out the swab or to store the swab in a refrigerator on the day of sampling. After collecting a culture, fluorescein stain should be instilled to determine the location and extent of the ulcer. A cobalt blue filter is preferred to ensure the fluorescein is adequately seen. There is a cobalt blue light on the standard slit lamp biomicroscope, but direct and Pan-Optic ophthalmoscope heads can be obtained that have a cobalt blue light as well. In addition, a small sleeve can be purchased very inexpensively (about 1% of the cost of a slit lamp biomicroscope) for the transilluminator head that has a cobalt blue filter at the tip. In this manner, fluorescein uptake can clearly be evaluated.

Next, to perform corneal cytology, use a topical anaesthetic (e.g., 0.5% proparacaine or 1% tetracaine) to numb the cornea and conjunctiva. This can easily be applied by drawing up about 0.5 to 1.0 ml of the anaesthetic in a 3-ml syringe with a 25-gauge needle, breaking the needle off the hub by rocking the needle back and forth several times in the cap, and squirting the anaesthetic onto the ocular surface. To collect a corneal sample, use the blunt end of a scalpel blade (NOT the end used to cut tissue) as a spatula to gently scrape the corneal epithelium and superficial stroma until no further tissue is loosened. The heel of the hand should rest on the horse's face so only a small thumb and index finger movement ensues, and no undue pressure is put on the globe. This way, too, if the horse moves, the hand holding the blade will move with the horse, avoiding stabbing anyone in the eye. The sample obtained should be spread onto a glass slide, and stained with either Diff-Qwik or a Gram's stain. It is useful to collect three slides, one for each of the stains just mentioned and a third to save for any special stain that may be warranted (e.g., a Gomori methamine silver stain for suspected fungal keratitis). In preparing the Diff-Qwik–stained slide, there is no need to heat fix the slide as you should for a Gram stain. The slide should be inspected for the presence of bacterial rods or cocci, fungal hyphae, white blood cells including eosinophils, and corneal epithelial cells. It is not uncommon to see light brown translucent rod-shaped structures associated with epithelial cells; these represent melanin.

For severe corneal ulcers in globes at risk of rupture (Figures 17.1, 17.2 and 17.3), evaluation of the lens and posterior segment is often not possible due to corneal

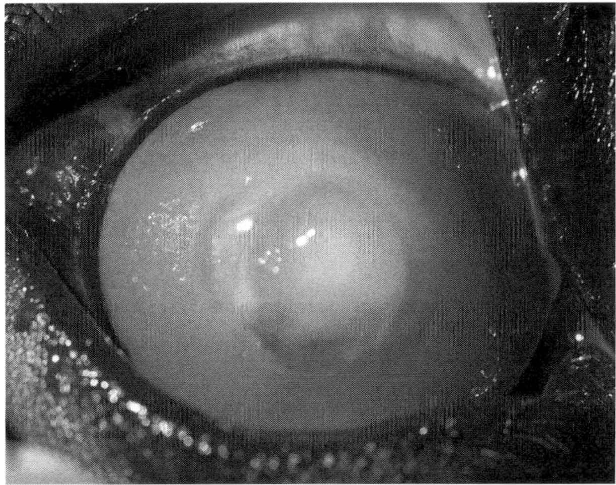

Figure 17.1 Right eye of an 8-year-old Percheron mare with a melting iris and focal iris prolapse. Diffuse corneal oedema precludes a view of intraocular structures. ©Mary Utter 2007.

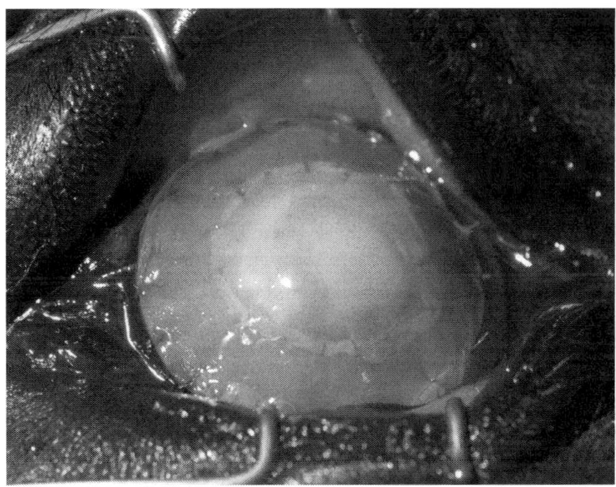

Figure 17.2 Surgical repair of the eye shown in Figure 17.1, with an amniotic membrane. ©Mary Utter 2007.

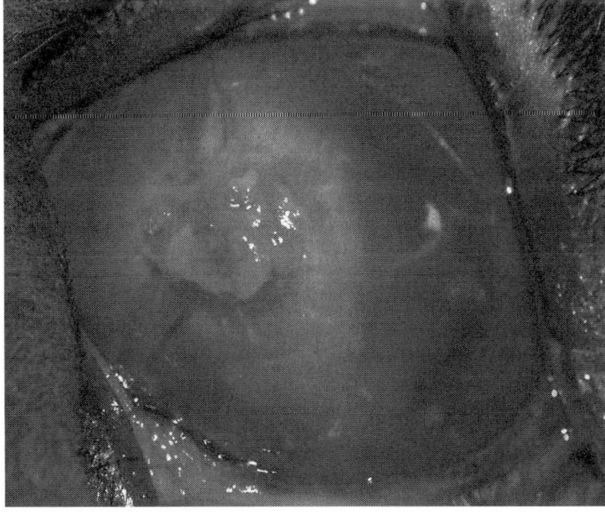

Figure 17.3 Postoperative photograph of the eye shown in Figure 17.1. The procedure resulted in a comfortable visual eye. ©Mary Utter 2007.

oedema, miosis and ocular pain. The contralateral eye should still receive a complete exam, but in some cases that can be deferred until after a subpalpebral lavage has been placed, if warranted, cytology results are examined, and therapy is under way. If there is any doubt that a patient will be easily treated with frequent topical medications without a subpalpebral lavage catheter (SPL), put one in. There are rarely complications with the SPL if it is properly placed and maintained (see Chapter 1.49), and it will be straightforward to ensure that medications are being delivered as intended.

For patients with an SPL, vigilant monitoring to ensure that the tubing remains patent and no complications have developed is critical. Each time medication is delivered through the SPL, fluid should be seen dripping from the palpebral fissure, indicating that medications pushed through the tubing are making it to the ocular surface, rather than running subcutaneously. The face below the inferior lid should be wiped dry after every medication to prevent development of dermatitis, and an ointment (like Vaseline or one containing vitamins A and D) may be used after cleaning to protect the skin from scalding. Butterfly sutures holding the tubing in place should be checked daily to ensure that they have not pulled through the skin, and they should replaced if they have. The injection port at the distal end of the tubing should be changed every several days, as one on an intravenous catheter would be. One of the more frustrating, although rare, complications associated with SPL placement is development of a lid abscess. Based on clinical impression, these occur in less than 5% of cases, and typically resolve in several days with systemic antibiotics and hotpacking the affected lid. In cases in which the lid abscess interferes with delivery of medication to the ocular surface, the SPL may need to be pulled, and another SPL placed in the lid without the abscess. Horses with SPL abscesses are often very painful, precluding examination of the eye itself until the lid swelling improves.

Therapy for horses with corneal ulcers can be organised into the "five A's" of ulcer therapy: antibiotics, antifungals, anticollagenases, atropine and anti-inflammatories.

Antibiotics

Drug selection should be based on cytology. After examining the horse, collecting diagnostic samples (culture and cytology) and placing the SPL if necessary, cytology should be examined prior to starting therapy. Frequency of administration should be quite often initially, but decreasing as clinical condition allows (e.g., every 1–2 hours for the first day, then every 4 hours for a few days, then only 3–4 times daily until the ulcer is healed). Antibiotic therapy should be continued until there is no more fluorescein uptake in the cornea, at which point the ulcer can be considered "healed", although it can take 4 to 6 weeks until the epithelium is firmly adhered to the basement membrane, and thus corneal oedema and the risk of deepithelialisation may persist for weeks.

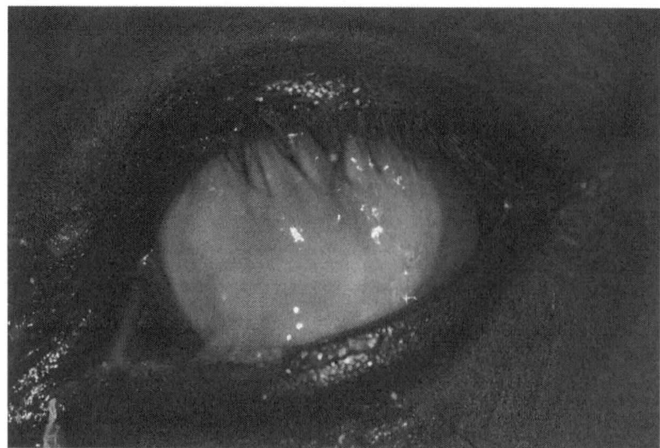

Figure 17.4 Keratitis due to *Pseudomonas* infection in a 2-year-old Thoroughbred filly. The filly had dirt kicked in her left eye during a race, and after rinsing of the eye, it appeared normal for 2 days following the race. Then, a large superficial ulcer developed, which progressed in 4 days to this appearance. The eyelids were held comfortably open, uncharacteristic for an ulcer of this severity. The filly had profuse mucopurulent ocular discharge. The conjunctiva was profoundly hyperaemic, and the cornea took up fluorescein stain everywhere but a 3-mm ring peripherally. The cornea was diffusely malacic. The eye was without a menace response but dazzle reflex and pupillary light reflex in the contralateral eye were positive. Ocular structures posterior to the cornea were not visible. ©Mary Utter 2007.

With the caveat that there are regional differences in susceptibility, and susceptibility patterns change over time, topical cefazolin,* is a good choice for severe Gram-positive corneal infections, and topical ciprofloxacin† remains a good choice for severe Gram-negative corneal infections (Figure 17.4). Topical antibiotics are epitheliotoxic (although varying in degree); thus once infection is controlled and frequency of topical antibiotic administration decreases, ulcers often heal faster. In an *in vitro* study using canine corneal epithelial cells, cefazolin and ciprofloxacin were the most epitheliotoxic, neomycin-polymyxin B-gramicidin‡ and gentamicin sulphate§ were intermediate, and chloramphenicol** and tobramycin had minimal epitheliotoxicity.[1] This should be taken into account when determining antibiotic choice and frequency of administration.

If bacterial cocci or rods are identified, therapy can be directed based on susceptibility patterns established by prior cases. In one study of 123 cases of ocular disease in

* Not currently available commercially as an ophthalmic solution. Intravenous preparations (e.g., Ancef; GlaxoSmithKline, Research Triangle Park, NC, USA) can be compounded at 55 to 60 mg/ml into ophthalmic solutions in some countries.

† Ciloxan; Alcon Inc, Fort Worth, TX, USA.

‡ Generic triple-antibiotic ophthalmic is available in many countries.

§ Generic gentamicin ophthalmic is available in many countries.

** Generic chloramphenicol ophthalmic is available in many countries.

horses, *Streptococcus* (44%), *Staphylococcus* (24%) and *Pseudomonas* (14%) spp. were the most common bacterial isolates, but susceptibility data from this study must be interpreted with caution due to its age.[2] Geographic variability may be seen in drug resistance across different bacterial species. In a retrospective study of 51 bacterial isolates from equine corneal ulcers over approximately 10 years in Tennessee, *Streptococcus equi* spp. *zooepidemicus* and *Pseudomonas aeruginosa* were the most frequently isolated organisms. No significant resistance was noted to aminoglycosides or fluoroquinolones among these organisms, but *S. equi* spp. *zooepidemicus* tended to be resistant to bacitracin.[3] Over an 8-year period in Missouri, 58% of the bacterial organisms isolated from 63 horses with corneal ulcers were Gram-positive (79% of these were *Staphylococcus* or *Streptococcus* spp.), and 42% were Gram-negative (most commonly *Pseudomonas* spp.). At the time of this study, 11 years ago, topical ticarcillin was the most effective against Gram-positive organisms, and topical ciprofloxacin§ was amongst those highly effective against Gram-negative organisms.[4] More recently, β-haemolytic *Streptococcus* spp. have been associated with aggressive keratomalacia, with the capability to digest conjunctival graft tissue.[5] Although newer ophthalmic fluoroquinolones, including ofloxacin (0.3%††), a second-generation fluoroquinolone, and gatifloxacin (0.3%‡‡) and moxifloxacin (0.5%§§), both fourth generation, are available, these should be reserved for resistant infections to prevent development of multidrug-resistant organisms.

Corneal ulcers are commonly treated with multiple topical medications. Combining selected ophthalmic therapeutic agents do not seem to alter their *in vitro* efficacy. In one study, atropine*** was added to gentamicin or tobramycin, and miconazole to gentamicin, in combination for as long as 6 hours prior to administration, with no apparent decrease in efficacy.[6] In another *in vitro* study in which tobramycin, cefazolin, natamycin and serum were administered as a drug combination, there was no loss of efficacy of the antimicrobials or of the antiproteinase activity of the serum.[7]

Antifungals

Although it is unclear why horses are prone to severe fungal keratitis over other domestic species, environment has been suggested as a contributing factor. That fungi are isolated more commonly from stabled than from pastured horses supports this notion.[8] The prognosis for retention of vision and of the eye in horses with fungal corneal ulcers is good with aggressive and appropriate therapy. In one study of 39 cases, 92% retained vision (100% following medical treatment without surgery and 84% following combined medical and surgical treatment) and only 5% lost the eye (none of those treated without surgery and 11% of those requiring surgery).[9] Early fungal keratitis may not show fluorescein uptake but, due to fungus-induced changes in the mucin layer of the tear film, may stain positive with rose Bengal.[10] Corneal fungal infections may rapidly progress to melting (Figure 17.5).

Antifungals that have been commonly used topically to treat fungal keratitis in the horse include fluconazole, itraconazole, ketoconazole, miconazole and voriconazole (azoles); and amphotericin-B, natamycin and nystatin (polyenes). Most antifungal compounds target either the formation or the function of ergosterol, an important component of the fungal cell membrane. Azoles are fungistatic agents that work by interfering with the synthesis and permeability of fungal cell membranes. The polyene antifungals act by binding to membrane sterols to produce a complex that alters membrane permeability, allowing contents of the fungus to leak out.

Choice of antifungal agent can be challenging, and fungal susceptibility results are often not available to guide therapy until the eye is either better or gone. In one study of fungal susceptibility, filamentous fungi had highest susceptibility to natamycin (97%), but *Fusarium* and *Aspergillus* were 100% susceptible to miconazole.[8] In an *in vitro* study of

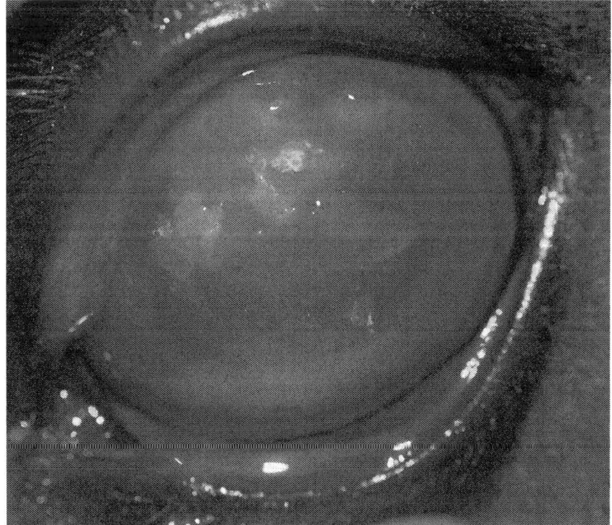

Figure 17.5 Keratitis due to a fungal infection in a 9-year-old Thoroughbred mare. Fungal hyphae were noted on cytology, and *Aspergillus flavus* was cultured from this cornea. This photograph was taken after excision of a large fungal plaque, performed under standing sedation. At the time of this photograph, the eye was very painful with profound epiphora. Menace response was absent but dazzle reflex and indirect pupillary light reflex were positive. The corneal ulcer involved over half the corneal surface area and was over 1/2 corneal depth at its periphery. Corneal vascularisation extended from the limbus to the ulcer margin dorsally and almost to the ulcer margin ventrally. There was hypopyon in the anterior chamber, and the pupil was fixed and miotic even on daily atropine. Structures posterior to the iris were not visible. ©Mary Utter 2007.

†† Ocuflox; Allergan Inc, Irvine, CA, USA.

‡‡ Zymar; Allergan Inc, Irvine, CA, USA.

§§ Vigamox; Alcon Inc, Fort Worth, TX, USA.

*** Isopto Atropine; Alcon Inc, Fort Worth, TX, USA.

antifungal suscepitiblity of fungi isolated from horses with keratomycosis in Florida, fungi were most susceptible to natamycin and miconazole equally, then to itraconazole, and then to ketoconazole, although no significant difference was found among drugs. Fungi were significantly less susceptible to fluconazole than to the other four drugs. An ointment containing 1% itraconazole with 30% dimethylsulphoxide developed at Cornell University is used commonly in the northeastern United States. In one study, this ointment resolved keratomycosis in 8 of 10 eyes, with a mean duration of treatment of about 1 month.[11] Itraconazole has been used orally but absorption following oral administration is variable, depending upon the formulation. In one study, an oral itraconazole solution had higher, more consistent absorption than orally administered capsules, and the oral solution attained plasma concentrations that were inhibitory against fungi that infect horses.[12]

Voriconazole is a new imidazole antifungal that has been increasingly used to treat fungal keratitis. This drug has been shown to effectively penetrate the cornea in clinically normal eyes and reach detectable concentrations in the aqueous humor and low plasma concentrations, after topical administration of a 1% solution. Voriconazole also penetrated noninflamed equine eyes after oral administration (at a 4 mg/kg/24 hr dose).[13] Natamycin* is the only antifungal that is commercially available for ophthalmic use; all others must be compounded. Silver sulphadiazine is a commercially available dermatological preparation that has been shown to have fungicidal activity against equine corneal fungal isolates.[14]

Antiproteases

Melting corneal ulcers can progress rapidly to perforation. Even with appropriate antimicrobial therapy and after infection has been cleared, corneal melting can proceed as a result of remaining corneal and tear film proteases. Combining appropriate antibiotic or antifungal therapy with topical protease inhibitors can speed corneal healing, because proteases play an important role in corneal stromal melting. Protease inhibitors used include EDTA, *N*-acetylcysteine, doxycycline and serum. These should be used as often as possible to halt aggressive corneal melting, hourly initially and then with the frequency decreasing as clinical signs improve.

Proteases are released by white cells, corneal epithelial cells and corneal fibroblasts as well as by microorganisms. There are four groups of proteases: serine, aspartic, thiol, and matrix metalloproteinases (MMPs). MMP-2 is produced by keratocytes and is involved in normal remodeling, whereas MMP-9 is produced by epithelial cells and polymorphonuclear cells following wounding. Neutrophil elastase (NE) is a serine protease involved in corneal melting. MMP inhibitors work by chelating zinc, which is an MMP cofactor, or calcium, an MMP stabilising ion. MMP inhibitors include doxycycline, EDTA and *N*-acetylcysteine.

Serum contains α_2-macroglobulin, a nonspecific antiprotease active against all four classes of proteases, and as such can be considered a broad-spectrum anticollagenase. To use topical serum, collect a sufficient quantity of whole blood to produce enough serum to last 5 to 7 days, and place in the appropriate number of red top tubes. (For example, if 0.2 ml serum is to be administered every 2 hours, about 2.5 ml is needed per day, and assuming serum comprises about half of the blood volume, 25 ml of whole blood should yield enough serum for 5 days.) The blood should be allowed to clot and then centrifuged. Serum may then be aseptically poured (if tiger-top tubes with a serum separator are used to collect blood) or aspirated through the rubber top (if red top tubes without a serum separator are used) into a separate sterile container. Fresh red top tubes work well to store the separated serum. Because the serum contains no preservatives or antimicrobials, care should be taken to store it in the refrigerator and replace it with fresh serum after 5 to 7 days, or sooner if any cloudiness is noted.

Atropine

Topical atropine is used in horses with corneal ulcers as a cycloplegic, to temporarily paralyse the iris sphincter muscle and thus relieve pain caused by ciliary spasm, and as a mydriatic, to dilate the pupils and thereby prevent adhesion formation between the iris and lens, as well as to open the drainage angle. The duration of mydriasis after administration of 1% atropine ophthalmic solution in the normal equine eye is greater than 14 days but is much shorter when uveitis is present. Mydriasis may last longer in Arabians and mares.[15] A side effect of topical atropine is decreased gastrointestinal motility, which can potentially lead to colic. Ensuring that hospitalised horses treated with ophthalmic atropine are getting sufficient exercise to maintain adequate gastrointestinal motility is critical. Such horses should be hand walked or turned out in a small paddock if their condition allows, and gut sounds and faecal output monitored closely. Atropinised horses do not necessarily need to wear a fly mask when outside or be protected from bright light because a pupil is dilated—they can squint if the ambient light is too bright. Getting exercise is more important than protecting a dilated eye from bright light.

Anti-inflammatories

Systemic nonsteroidal anti-inflammatories (NSAIDs) are an important part of the therapeutic regimen used to treat horses with corneal ulcers to relieve pain and reduce inflammation that can delay healing and potentiate scar formation. Side effects of systemic NSAID use can include kidney damage (particularly when horses are dehydrated),

* Natacyn (5% natamycin ophthalmic suspension); Alcon Inc, Fort Worth, TX, USA.

gastric ulceration and right dorsal colitis. Creatinine and total protein should be monitored regularly in hospitalised horses receiving chronic NSAID therapy. Use of topical NSAIDs (including diclofenac, flurbiprofen, indomethacin) should be avoided when an ulcer is present, due to the association between topical NSAID use and full-thickness corneal melts in people.[16]

The most commonly asked questions regarding medical therapy for horses hospitalised with corneal ulcers that require intensive treatment include choice of drug, frequency of treatment, frequency of ophthalmic evaluation and, finally, when to treat medically versus surgically and medically. In the absence of cytological findings to more specifically guide therapy, a good combination therapy for a melting ulcer would include serum every 1 to 2 hours; cefazolin and tobramycin each every 2 to 4 hours; natamycin and voriconazole every 4 to 6 hours; atropine 1 to 3 times daily and systemic flunixin (1 mg/kg twice daily). Surgical intervention should ensue when the ulcer progresses despite appropriate therapy, and the ulcer threatens the integrity of the globe.

Management of horses with corneal lacerations

Surgical repair is indicated if a corneal laceration extends deeply into, or full thickness through, the cornea. For corneal lacerations that do not extend deeply enough to threaten integrity of the globe, and thus surgical intervention is not warranted, excision of any corneal flaps that are likely to become necrotic and cause collateral damage is recommended. A typical scenario is a corneal laceration in which a flap has been undermined such that the dorsal border is attached but the ventral edge is hanging free, sometimes protruding between the closed lids. To excise such a flap, good sedation and topical anaesthesia are necessary to avoid movement during the procedure. The flap may be grasped with small ocular forceps (with 0.5- to 0.8-mm teeth) and cut free from the corneal base with tenotomy scissors by holding the scissors parallel to the corneal surface and sliding one blade of the scissors under the flap. In some cases, it is easier to isolate the hanging flap without using forceps, which may pull and cause pain and subsequent movement, rather simply elevating the flap with one blade of the scissors than excising by closing the blades, without any other movement.

Management of horses with iris prolapse

Iris prolapse is a surgical emergency (Figure 17.6). Absence of a menace response and dazzle reflex in the affected eye, along with an inability to view the pupil, is not uncommon in cases of iris prolapse. The indirect pupillary light reflex to the contralateral eye is important to the prognosis for return of vision. If this is present, repair rather than enucleation may be warranted. Other positive prognostic factors for return of vision and retention of the surgically repaired globe, identified in a retrospective study of 32 cases of iris prolapse, include traumatic rather ulcerative iris prolapse,

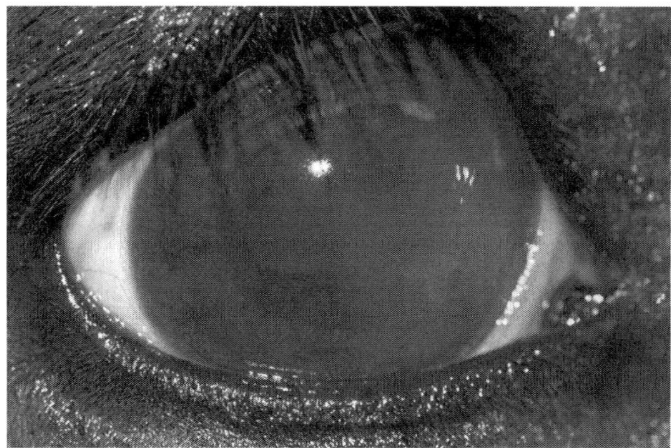

Figure 17.6 Right eye of a 12-year-old warmblood gelding who perforated his globe on a nail in his stall. There is a large full-thickness corneal laceration with iris prolapse through the laceration. Intraocular structures were not visible due to complete hyphaema. Surgical repair with a corneal transplant resulted in a quiet comfortable globe with a large corneal scar but good functional vision. ©Mary Utter 2007.

ulcerative keratitis of fewer than 15 days' duration, traumatic iris prolapse of less than 15 mm in length and traumatic iris prolapse that does not extend beyond the limbus. If there is keratomalacia or hyphaema, visual outcome is negatively affected. Retention of the globe following surgical repair was 80% for traumatic iris prolapse and 67% with ulcerative prolapse.[17] Surgical choices for repair include conjunctival grafting, full-thickness corneal transplantation (or penetrating keratoplasty) with or without adjunctive conjunctival grafting and the placement of other biomaterials like porcine small intestinal submucosa (SIS graft) or urinary bladder matrix (Acell graft). Following surgical repair, medical therapy should proceed as for a corneal ulcer.

Management of horses with a corneal stromal abscess

Corneal stromal abscesses are characterised clinically by a focal white to yellow corneal opacity, often deep within the stroma, that does not take up fluorescein stain and causes more pain that would be expected for the severity of the lesion. Other clinical signs often associated with a stromal abscess include blepharospasm, epiphora, conjunctival hyperaemia, corneal oedema and miosis. Stromal abscesses form when an infectious agent seeds the cornea through an epithelial defect (which may not be detected) and then the epithelial defect heals, leaving the agent inside the cornea. Stromal abscesses are often fungal in aetiology, with fungal hyphae found deep within the corneal stroma and even within Descemet's membrane. Typical medical therapy for a stromal abscess includes four of the five A's used to treat melting ulcers—antifungal, antimicrobial, atropine and anti-inflammatory—minus the antiprotease. In cases in which the abscess progresses even in the face of appropriate medical therapy, surgical intervention may be warranted. In a retrospective of 24 horses with a stromal abscess, surgical intervention was undertaken when corneal rupture was imminent, the iridocyclitis was intractable or there was minimal response to intensive medical therapy. The surgical procedure performed in most cases was a deep keratectomy. In this study, all except one horse had vision at discharge.[18]

Surgeries for corneal disease

Surgical choices for eyes with corneas that worsen in the face of appropriate medical therapy include conjunctival grafts (e.g., pedicle, bridge, advancement, island), corneal grafts (full thickness, posterior lamellar) and grafts using other biomaterials (amniotic membrane, SIS‡‡‡, Acell§§§) (Figure 17.2). Conjunctival grafts bring a blood supply to an otherwise avascular region of the cornea and thus may halt stromal lysis in cases of melting corneal ulcers, but conjunctiva does not provide a significant degree of structural support and thus is not useful to replace missing tissue as in cases of deep ulcers or descemetoceles, or iris prolapse. Conjunctiva is not appropriate, therefore, as the sole tissue graft in situations where tissue is missing. Conjunctival grafts do result in variable degrees of scarring over the affected area. The degree of scarring depends on numerous factors including thickness of the graft, degree of stromal degradation present at the time of surgery and ongoing postoperatively and age of the horse. Based on clinical impression, conjunctival grafts for melting ulcers tend to have better survival rates and remodel more quickly, leading to shorter duration of therapy and less significant scarring, in foals relative to adult horses. Corneal grafts are a good choice when tissue is missing and the structural integrity of the globe needs to be restored, as in deep ulcers, iris prolapse or corneal lacerations too large to allow primary closure. Frozen corneal grafts are typically transplanted after the nonviable epithelial and endothelial layers have been removed, resulting in transplantation of a layer that is effectively a plug of stroma. For this reason, these grafts are often best covered with an adjunctive layer (e.g., conjunctiva or amnion) if used to repair full-thickness defects, to prevent profound stromal swelling and to prevent potential graft dehiscence. For replacement of stroma when the globe remains intact, the frozen cornea does not necessarily need to be covered with another layer. In cases of profound keratomalacia involving a large proportion of the corneal surface area, in which there is little healthy tissue into which to suture conjunctiva or cornea, and in which a potentially blinding scar would result, use of preserved equine amnion may be a good option for tissue transplant. Results of a small number of equine amniotic membrane transplants suggest that amnion can be used successfully to preserve both globe structure and limited vision, as well as optimise cosmesis, in horses' eyes with corneal ulceration and severe keratomalacia.[19] Amnion has antifibrotic, antiangiogenic, antimicrobial and anti-inflammatory properties and appears to be tough enough to hold up to severe protease activity.

Placement of a temporary tarsorrhaphy (either partial or complete) is advised following corneal surgery to provide protection during anaesthetic recovery and in the postoperative period. To place a temporary tarsorrhaphy, nonabsorbable suture should be used in a horizontal mattress pattern with stents to prevent the suture pulling through the eyelid margin. Autoclaved rubber bands cut into segments are ideal to use as stents, because they are flat and are thus less likely to cause pressure necrosis of the underlying skin than are stents with a round surface, like intravenous tubing. Sutures may be removed individually to allow examination of the cornea at any point postoperatively.

Management of horses with nonulcerative keratitis

Horses may present to hospital for nonulcerative keratitis, typically characterised by corneal opacity that does not retain fluorescein but that can be associated with variable levels of discomfort, and may or may not be associated with additional ocular signs including blepharospasm, epiphora, conjunctival hyperaemia, aqueous flare and miosis (Figure 17.7). Nonulcerative keratitis may be classified based on depth within the cornea, including superficial stromal keratitis, which appears as a superficial stromal cellular infiltrate with diffuse vascularisation; midstromal

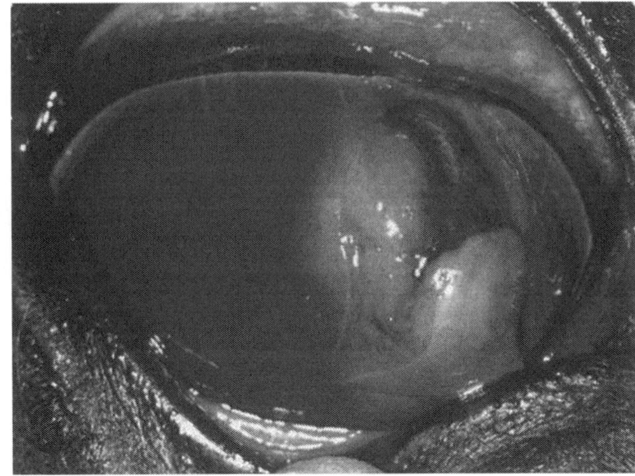

Figure 17.7 Nonulcerative keratitis in a 9-year-old Quarter Horse gelding. This horse had a 6-month history of corneal opacity that cleared and then recurred. There was no blepharospasm or ocular discharge. The corneal opacity involved the epithelium and superficial and middle stroma. There was superficial corneal vascularisation that extended from the medial limbus toward the centre of the opacity. Several large stromal bullae were noted in the centre of the opacity. No response was seen with systemic or topical treatment with a nonsteroidal anti-inflammatory but treatment with a topical steroid did increase corneal clarity and reduce corneal vascularisation. ©Mary Utter 2007.

‡‡‡Cook Medical Inc, Bloomington, IN, USA.
§§§Acell Inc, Jessup, MD, USA.

keratitis, which appears as midstromal cellular infiltrate with surrounding corneal oedema and vascularisation; and endothelial disease, which appears as endothelial cellular infiltrate with diffuse corneal oedema. Superficial keratitis may response to topical medical therapy, but surgical excision is warranted if the opacity persists or any discomfort develops. Topical cyclosporine is a good choice for midstromal keratitis, and endothelial disease is typically the least amenable to therapy.[20]

Management of horses with uveitis

Uveitis may be acute and associated with a traumatic event or chronic and recurrent as in equine recurrent uveitis (ERU). Post-traumatic uveitis in horses is often characterised by corneal vascularisation and oedema, with a moderate to severe anterior uveitis. In a series of cases of post traumatic keratouveitis, topical and systemic nonsteroidal drugs and atropine were used to control the anterior uveitis while allowing spontaneous corneal healing. Among these cases, eyes previously treated with local corticosteroids took significantly longer to resolve compared with eyes in which corticosteroids had not been administered, because locally administered corticosteroids inhibit healing of damaged corneal stroma and, by prolonging the keratitis, perpetuate the concurrent anterior uveitis.[21]

ERU is characterised in acute stages by blepharospasm, blepharitis, epiphora, corneal oedema, aqueous flare, miosis and vitreal haze and in chronic quiescent stages as iris hyperpigmentation, posterior synechia, cataract formation and retinal detachment (Figures 17.8 and 17.9). In severe cases, there may be lens luxation (Figure 17.10). ERU is a leading cause of blindness in horses and may develop as a sequela to systemic leptospirosis. In one study examining serum *Leptospira* titers in horses with and without uveitis, seropositive horses were 13.2 times more likely to have uveitis than were seronegative horses, and seropositive horses with uveitis were 4.4 times more likely to lose vision than were seronegative horses with uveitis. Thus, there is a strong positive relationship between uveitis and leptospiral seroreactivity in horses, and seropositive horses with uveitis are at increased risk of losing vision, compared with that in seronegative horses with uveitis. In that same study, of the horses with uveitis, 25% were Appaloosas, compared with only 4% of horses without uveitis. Sixty-eight percent of Appaloosas with uveitis developed blindness, compared with only 36% of non-Appaloosas with uveitis that lost vision in one or both eyes. Therefore, Appaloosas are at increased risk of developing uveitis and associated blindness compared with non-Appaloosas.[22]

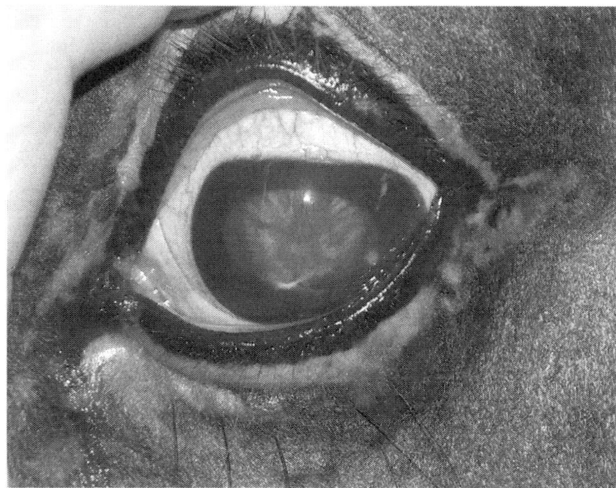

Figure 17.9 Left eye of a 12-year-old Appaloosa mare with chronic uveitis bilaterally. The cornea is ulcerated with superior neovascularisation. There is a mature cataract in the lens. ©Kevin Corley 2007.

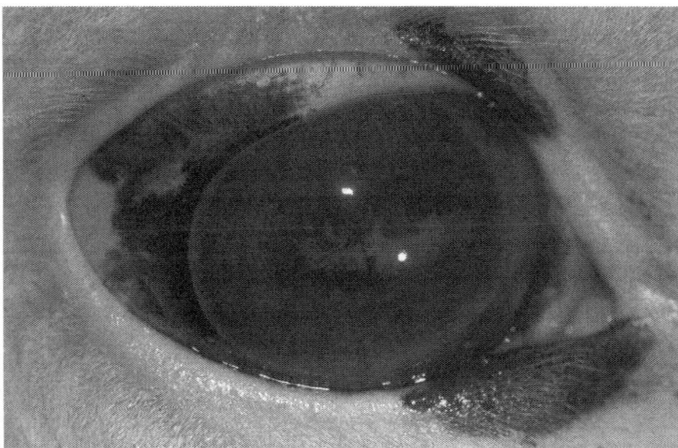

Figure 17.8 Right eye of a 6-year-old Paint mare with chronic uveitis bilaterally. This eye is currently in a quiescent phase but has posterior synechia (adhesions between the iris and anterior lens capsule), persistent miosis, iris hyperpigmentation and hypermature cataract. ©Mary Utter 2007.

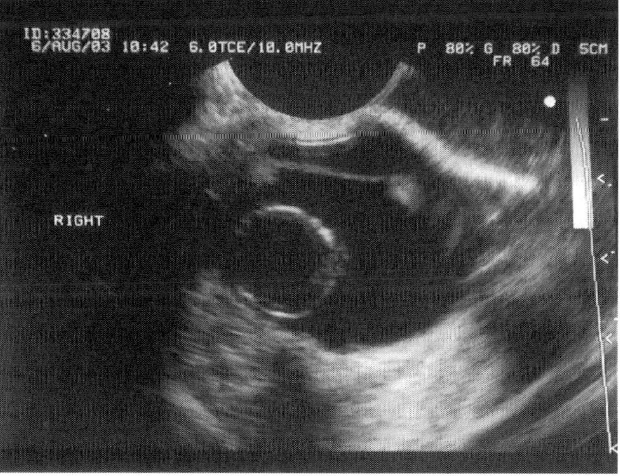

Figure 17.10 Transpalpebral ultrasound image of the right eye of the mare with chronic uveitis shown in Figure 17.7. The probe is held vertically against the closed eyelid, with dorsal to the right of the image. The lens lies ventrally in the posterior chamber of the eye (it has a hyperechoic circular border). ©Kevin Corley 2007.

Significantly more horses with uveitis than without uveitis have *Leptospira* spp. in their aqueous humor, although serological results do not typically correlate well with the presence of *Leptospira* DNA or organisms in the aqueous humor.[23]

Therapeutic choices for horses with ERU include systemic NSAIDs, systemic steroids, topical NSAIDs and steroids, typical cyclosporine and systemic antibiotics used against any infectious cause of uveitis as well as for their anti-inflammatory effect (e.g., doxycycline). Choices for surgical treatment of ERU include pars plana vitrectomy, intravitreal cyclosporine implant and suprachoroidal cyclosporine implant. Pars plana vitrectomy in horses has been successful in decreasing the frequency of episodes of ERU and of sequelae like cataracts or secondary glaucoma.[24] Intravitreal cyclosporine implants tend to be well tolerated with no long-term complications from the implants themselves; however, complications may occur from inadvertent implantation trauma or contamination during surgery.[25] Following intravitreal cyclosporine implantation, episodes of recurrent uveitis decreased in one study from 75 to 0.36 episode per year; only three horses developed episodes of recurrent uveitis after surgery; and 14 of 16 horses retained vision after 1 year.[26]

A second type of cyclosporine implant was developed that is less prone to perioperative complications due to its ease of surgical placement. The suprachoroidal implant is placed dorsolaterally underneath the conjunctiva and Tenon's capsule, not intraocularly, eliminating the need to enter the eye through a sclerotomy and puncture through the pars plana. Frequency of uveitic flareups decreased after implantation of the suprachoroidal cyclosporine implant, as well as after implantation of the intravitreal device.[27]

17.3 Management of ocular problems in the neonatal foal

Ocular problems observed in neonatal foals include subconjunctival haemorrhage associated with dystocia; entropion and ulcerative keratitis associated with recumbency, dehydration and generally poor systemic health; keratitis, hyphaema, uveitis and retinal disease associated with sepsis; and congenital cataract. For otherwise healthy foals that are born with ocular conditions secondary to dystocia, most commonly subconjunctival haemorrhage, these traumatic lesions will typically resolve without treatment. Recumbent foals should have their corneas lubricated every 4 to 6 hours. These foals may develop entropion and subsequent secondary corneal ulceration (caused by exposure from insufficient blinking or from direct eyelid-corneal contact). With adequate corneal lubrication and temporary correction of entropion, these ulcers typically resolve uneventfully. Entropion in foals will often resolve as their systemic health improves, and thus temporary correction is all that is required to prevent corneal ulceration. To place temporary tarsorrhaphy sutures, the foal should be adequately sedated (with level of sedation required depending upon the condition of the foal; 1 ml diazepam, 5 mg/ml, given intravenously, is a safe choice for most foals) and restrained (see Chapter 2.4). Usually, one assistant is sufficient to keep the head immobilised and prevent injury if the foal kicks; if it takes more than one person to restrain the foal, then sedation is probably not adequate. The inferior lower lid skin should be blocked with a local anaesthetic (e.g., 2% lidocaine). This is accomplished by inserting a 25-gauge needle up to the hub subcutaneously, parallel to and about 3 to 5 mm distal to the inferior lid margin at one end of the region to be blocked. The needle is then pointed toward the unblocked region, and a small amount of anaesthetic is injected. The needle is then removed and reinserted into the already blocked skin, in such a manner so as to "walk" the needle down the lid, with only the first injection being into an area that has not already been blocked. The line block will result in a curvilinear raised area parallel to the inferior lid margin. A second line block should be performed similarly, about 5 to 7 mm distal to the first line, to form a second curvilinear raised, blocked area. These two line blocks correspond to the entry and exit points of suture used to imbricate and evert the inferior lid. Simple interrupted suture of an absorbable material should be placed by taking a partial-thickness bite of skin through the first line block and a second partial-thickness bit through the second line block, both perpendicular to the lid margin, such that when the suture is tied, the lid is imbricated and everted. The degree of lid eversion is controlled by how tight the suture is tied. Three sutures are usually sufficient to adequately evert the lid and prevent lid-corneal contact. These sutures can easily be replaced if they are pulled out and can be removed as the condition corrects. Entropion has also been temporarily corrected by injecting procaine penicillin G in a curvilinear area parallel to the lid margin, as in the line block discussed above, but the degree and duration of eversion are more precisely controlled with sutures than with penicillin, so the tarsorrhaphy is recommended for hospitalised foals.

Septic foals may have concurrent uveitis that manifests as corneal oedema and vascularisation, aqueous flare and fibrin in the anterior chamber, and miosis. This often resolves without treatment as systemic health improves, but judicious use of topical steroids to control inflammation and topical atropine to prevent posterior synechia and provide relief from ciliary spasm may be warranted. Tissue plasminogen activator may be injected into the anterior chamber to dissolve fibrin and, in so doing, prevent permanent adhesion formation, if fibrin does not resolve without therapy.

Treatment for congenital cataracts is surgical extraction. Prior to undertaking cataract surgery in a foal, good systemic health and the absence of concurrent retinal disease must be clearly established. Ocular ultrasound can be used to rule out retinal detachment, and electroretinography used to rule out poor retinal function, either of which would preclude cataract surgery, as cataract extraction is unlikely to improve vision if there is a second cause of visual impairment beyond the cataract.

References

1. Hendrix DV, Ward DA, Barnhill MA: Effects of antibiotics on morphologic characteristics and migration of canine corneal epithelial cells in tissue culture. Am J Vet Res 62:1664-1669, 2001
2. McLaughlin SA, Brightman AH, Helper LC, Manning JP, Tomes JE: Pathogenic bacteria and fungi associated with extraocular disease in the horse. J Am Vet Med Assoc 182:241-242, 1983
3. Keller RL, Hendrix DV: Bacterial isolates and antimicrobial susceptibilities in equine bacterial ulcerative keratitis: 1993-2004. Equine Vet J 37:207-211, 2005
4. Moore CP, Collins BK, Fales WH: Antibacterial susceptibility patterns for microbial isolates associated with infectious keratitis in horses: 63 cases (1986-1994). J Am Vet Med Assoc 207:928-933, 1995
5. Brooks DE, Andrew SE, Biros DJ, et al.: Ulcerative keratitis caused by beta-hemolytic *Streptococcus equi* in 11 horses. Vet Ophthalmol 3:121-125, 2003
6. Hinkle KM, Gerding PA, Kakoma I, Schaeffer DJ: Evaluation of activity of selected ophthalmic antimicrobial agents in combination against common ocular microorganisms. Am J Vet Res 60:316-318, 1999
7. DE Brooks, Schuman CD, Barrie KP, Plummer CE, Kallberg ME: In vitro efficacy of an ophthalmic drug combination against common equine corneal pathogens. Proc ACVO 2006
8. Moore CP, Heller N, Majors LJ, Whitley RD, Burgess EC, Weber J: Prevalence of ocular microorganisms in hospitalized and stabled horses. Am J Vet Res 49:773-777, 1988
9. Andrew SE, Brooks DE, Smith PJ, Gelatt KN, Chmielewski NT, Whittaker CJ: Equine ulcerative keratomycosis: visual outcome and ocular survival in 39 cases (1987-1996). Equine Vet J 30:109-116, 1998
10. Brooks DE, Andrew SE, Denis H, et al.: Rose Bengal positive epithelial microerosions as a manifestation of equine keratomycosis. Vet Ophthalmol 3:83-86, 2000
11. Rebhun WC: Corneal stromal abscesses in the horse. J Am Vet Med Assoc 181:677-679, 1982
12. Davis JL, Salmon JH, Papich MG: Pharmacokinetics and tissue distribution of itraconazole after oral and intravenous administration to horses. Am J Vet Res 66:1694-1701, 2005
13. Clode AB, Davis JL, Salmon J, Michau TM, Gilger BC: Evaluation of concentration of voriconazole in aqueous humor after topical and oral administration in horses. Am J Vet Res 67:296-301, 2006
14. Betbeze CM, Wu CC, Krohne SG, Stiles J: In vitro fungistatic and fungicidal activities of silver sulfadiazine and natamycin on pathogenic fungi isolated from horses with keratomycosis. Am J Vet Res 67:1788-1793, 2006
15. Davis JL, Stewart T, Brazik E, Gilger BC: The effect of topical administration of atropine sulfate on the normal equine pupil: influence of age, breed and gender. Vet Ophthalmol 6:329-332, 2003
16. Guidera AC, Luchs JI, Udell IJ: Keratitis, ulceration, and perforation associated with topical nonsteroidal anti-inflammatory drugs. Ophthalmology 108:936-944, 2001
17. Chmielewski NT, Brooks DE, Smith PJ, Hendrix DV, Whittaker C, Gelatt KN: Visual outcome and ocular survival following iris prolapse in the horse: a review of 32 cases. Equine Vet J 29:31-39, 1997
18. Hendrix DV, Brooks DE, Smith PJ, et al.: Corneal stromal abscesses in the horse: a review of 24 cases. Equine Vet J 27:440-447, 1995
19. Lassaline ME, Brooks DE, Ollivier FJ, Komaromy AM, Kallberg ME, Gelatt KN: Equine amniotic membrane transplantation for corneal ulceration and keratomalacia in three horses. Vet Ophthalmol 8:311-317, 2005
20. Gilger BC, Michau TM, Salmon JH: Immune-mediated keratitis in horses: 19 cases (1998-2004). Vet Ophthalmol 8:233-239, 2005
21. Moore CP, Halenda RM, Grevan VL, Collins BK: Post traumatic keratouveitis in horses. Equine Vet J 30:366-372, 1998
22. Dwyer AE, Crockett RS, Kalsow CM: Association of leptospiral seroreactivity and breed with uveitis and blindness in horses: 372 cases (1986-1993). J Am Vet Med Assoc 207:1327-1331, 1995
23. Faber NA, Crawford M, LeFebvre RB, Buyukmihci NC, Madigan JE, Willits NH: Detection of *Leptospira* spp. in the aqueous humor of horses with naturally acquired recurrent uveitis. J Clin Microbiol 38:2731-2733, 2000
24. Fruhauf B, Ohnesorge B, Deegen E, Boeve M: Surgical management of equine recurrent uveitis with single port pars plana vitrectomy. Vet Ophthalmol 1:137-151, 1998
25. Gilger BC, Malok E, Stewart T, et al.: Long-term effect on the equine eye of an intravitreal device used for sustained release of cyclosporine A. Vet Ophthalmol 3:105-110, 2000
26. Gilger BC, Wilkie DA, Davidson MG, Allen JB: Use of an intravitreal sustained-release cyclosporine delivery device for treatment of equine recurrent uveitis. Am J Vet Res 62:1892-1896, 2001
27. Gilger BC, Salmon JH, Wilkie DA, et al.: A novel bioerodible deep scleral lamellar cyclosporine implant for uveitis. Invest Ophthalmol Vis Sci 47:2596-2605, 2006

18

Physiotherapy: indications and treatment techniques

Bairbre Sharkey and Patrick Herbots

Introduction

In 1983, Oliver and Lorenz[1] wrote "Physical rehabilitation is often as important as specific medical or surgical treatment in the outcome of a patient with neurological disease. However, physical therapy is often neglected in veterinary practice". Although physiotherapy is increasingly receiving recognition as an important adjunct to veterinary medicine, it remains underutilised in many equine patients. Expertly applied physiotherapy, in properly selected candidates, may shorten time to healing and improve both the range of movement of an affected joint or limb and the quality of the healed tissue. Early motion has been shown to be efficacious in hastening recovery and limiting the effects of disuse on bone, cartilage, periarticular soft tissue, ligaments, muscles and tendons.[2–4]

The advancement of equine surgical techniques, such as in the repair of orthopaedic injuries, and the concurrent pressure to achieve athletic outcomes has led to greater interest in postoperative care. Pharmaceutical treatments and surgical techniques are often already optimised, so in order to obtain better outcomes, veterinarians should consider complementary modalities such as physiotherapy. The extra costs involved by introducing physiotherapy are counterbalanced by the decreased number of hospitalisation days and the improvement in functional results, which are often remarkable.

It is important that every physiotherapy examination is preceded by a thorough examination by a veterinarian, including orthopaedic and neurological elements as necessary. Where relevant, the lesion must be thoroughly investigated with appropriate diagnostic imaging and documented. Positive communication between the veterinarian and the physiotherapist is essential.

The best result will be obtained when treatment and evaluation of the patient are carried out with full cooperation and communication between the owner, the trainer, the veterinarian, the physiotherapist and the farrier.

Frequently, physiotherapists can add an extra dimension to the diagnosis and analysis of subtle soft tissue injuries, which may not be apparent with imaging techniques.

Many different techniques can be used in physiotherapy, including mobilisations, manipulation, massage, stretching, electrical stimulation, therapeutic ultrasound, laser therapy, thermal therapy and design of controlled exercise programmes. These techniques are discussed in detail here.

This chapter aims to increase the knowledge of veterinarians to enable them to select patients that may benefit from physiotherapy and to understand the rationale behind the use of various treatment modalities. The focus will be on practical information, rather than on the theoretical background.

Qualifications

Veterinary physiotherapy is a fast emerging speciality whose profile has been highlighted by the use of animal physiotherapists both at Olympic and international equestrian competitions, by countries including Ireland, the United Kingdom, Australia and New Zealand. The credibility of veterinary physiotherapy has been greatly increased by the establishment of the Masters in Veterinary Physiotherapy programme at the Royal Veterinary College London, UK, the Masters in Animal Studies programme at the University of Queensland, Australia, and various postgraduate training programmes for people who have already completed a recognised degree qualification in physiotherapy. These postgraduate programmes involve training in the areas of animal anatomy, physiology, biomechanics and pathology. They aim to ensure that anyone specialising in this area has an in-depth understanding of the rationale behind the use of various forms of treatment and their relevance to equine pathologies. It should be noted that in different countries, different regulations exist as to whom can call themselves a "veterinary physiotherapist", "chartered physiotherapist" or an equivalent title. Many of these titles are not protected and can effectively be used by anyone. It is therefore important that the veterinarian understand the level of training and competence of any "physiotherapist" with whom they are working.

Indications for physiotherapy

Physiotherapists receive training in three main areas; neurology, respiratory and musculoskeletal physiotherapy. In veterinary medicine, physiotherapy is primarily an intervention used in the treatment of musculoskeletal conditions. However physiotherapy can function in many areas of veterinary medicine.[1–4]

Physiotherapy may be a useful tool when the following clinical signs and symptoms are present:

1. **Pain.** Pharmaceutical limitations may indicate a need for physiotherapy intervention. The underlying pathology will determine which treatment modality or combinations of modalities are most suitable. Some treatment options include manual therapy to release painful muscle spasm, laser or ultrasound to reduce inflammation and thus reduce pain, and transcutaneous electrical nerve stimulation (TENS) to provide symptomatic relief of pain.
2. **Muscle atrophy (localised neurogenic/disuse atrophy).** Physiotherapy may consist of a combination of electrical muscle stimulation and a specific rehabilitation exercise programme addressed at increasing both muscle strength and power and returning the limb or spine to normal function (Figure 18.1).
3. **Oedema.** The choice of treatment will depend on the cause and duration of the swelling. Immediate swelling (onset within 1–2 hours) may be due to bleeding in a joint; therefore, initial treatment will be aimed at reducing blood flow and metabolism in the area. Acute inflammation and oedema are treated with ice for the first 48 hours. Following this, modalities such as massage, alternate hot/cold, drainage/pressure bandaging and electrotherapy may be used.
4. **Inflammation.** Drugs alone may be insufficient to stop this cycle. Electrotherapy and thermal therapy can be a useful adjunct to reduce and prevent the development of chronic inflammation.
5. **Decreased range of motion.** Physiotherapy aims to restore normal range of motion through all joints (both spinal and peripheral), using a variety of techniques.

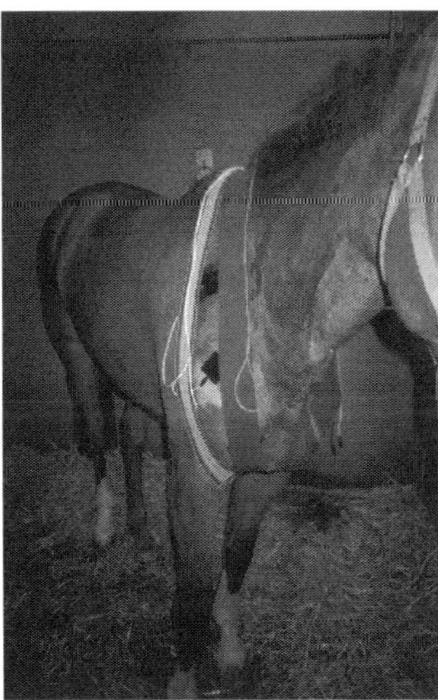

Figure 18.1 Muscle stimulation for the treatment of a suprascapular nerve injury. ©Patrick Herbots 2006.

An overview of some specific conditions that can benefit from physiotherapy intervention is given in Box 18.1.

Neurological conditions

Neurological physiotherapy is based on the principle of reestablishing neural pathways to restore normal movement. This may be achieved through the release of muscle spasm, decreasing pain and introduction of a rehabilitation programme. The rehabilitation programme aims to increase muscle strength, targeting either the whole body or specific muscle groups, and to improve proprioception. Techniques such as taping, long reining and pole work can give the horse an increased proprioceptive awareness and thus help improve gait pattern.

Facial nerve paralysis

A patient with facial nerve paralysis/palsy (Figure 18.2) can benefit greatly from specific stretching exercises to prevent

Box 18.1. Conditions that may benefit from physiotherapy intervention

Neurological
- Nerve injuries
- Facial nerve paralysis
- Brainstem/cranial nerve disease
- Spinal cord disease (dependent on differential diagnosis)
- Post neurological surgery

Musculoskeletal
- Dorsal spinous process impingement
- Sacroiliac and lumbosacral joint dysfunction
- Muscle imbalance or weakness
- Muscle rupture/tears or strains
- Myofascial pain syndrome
- Joint stiffness
- Post orthopaedic surgery

Other soft tissue
- Wounds nonhealing and acute
- Tendon and ligament injury

Respiratory
- Manual techniques to loosen secretions
- Positioning

General
- Immobility
- Saddle-fitting problems
- Performance problems
- Compensatory problems
- Care of the aged horse

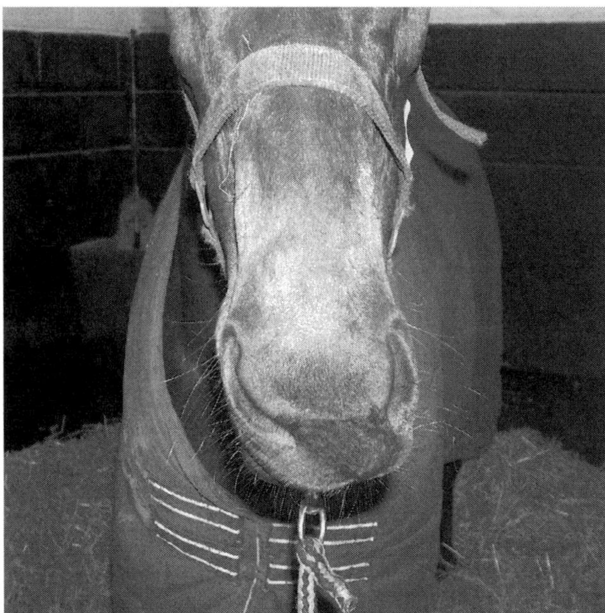

Figure 18.2 Facial palsy in a horse. ©Kevin Corley 2007.

adaptive shortening and active strengthening exercises (an example is lip tickling). Neuromuscular electrical stimulation similar to that used in Bell's palsy of humans can help to prevent or limit atrophy of the associated muscles. Certain taping techniques can help to encourage normal alignment and prevent unwanted lengthening of the weakened muscles. Taping involves the use of sports tape to keep those tissues that have become flaccid and lengthened in a normal position. It may be necessary to attach a straight bar rubber snaffle to the horse's head collar to keep the lips in normal alignment and prevent lengthening of these tissues due to the effects of gravity. This can be removed for feeding.

Other peripheral nerve injuries

More common peripheral nerve injuries include those that affect the radial nerve or the suprascapular nerve (Figure 18.1). Brachial plexus traction injuries also occur affecting a number of peripheral nerves. These can benefit from electrical stimulation, which aims to strengthen the affected myotomes and to restore the neuromuscular communication. This then counteracts any instability that may occur at the associated joints. Laser therapy has been shown to have a role in nerve regeneration. Specific stretching exercises try to prevent muscle shortening due to disuse. A suspended haynet (Figure 18.3) can stimulate proprioception of the affected limb.

Respiratory physiotherapy

Thoracic physical therapy for human patients has been associated with decreased duration of mechanical ventilation and reduced incidence of pulmonary infection. The baseline respiratory rate, heart rate and rhythm should be recorded prior to therapy and compared with those during

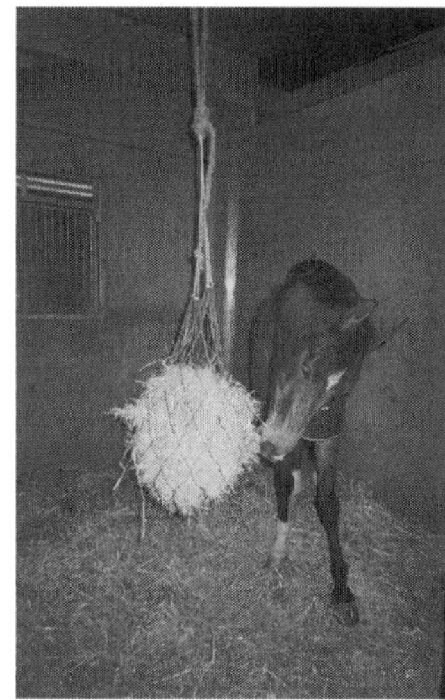

Figure 18.3 A haynet suspended in the centre of the horse's stable to encourage forelimb weight transference and increased proprioceptive input. ©Patrick Herbots 2006.

> **Box 18.2. Factors that contribute to respiratory dysfunction**
>
> - Increased venous admixture resulting in lowered oxygen partial pressure
> - Maldistribution of perfusion by hydrostatic forces (lower lung is overperfused whilst the upper lung is underperfused)
> - Hypoventilation of the lower lung caused by compression from the weight of the thoracic and abdominal viscera
> - Increased exposure to pathogens
> - Depressed immune function

treatment to assess the patient's tolerance of each procedure. The thorax should be auscultated to attempt to locate affected lung lobes, and to establish a baseline of lung sounds to help judge the effectiveness of therapy.[5,6] The factors that contribute to respiratory dysfunction are listed in Box 18.2.[7]

In situations of prolonged immobilisation and inflammatory processes, foals often encounter a productive respiratory distress with restricted functional capacity, due to mucus embedded in the lung structures and nasal discharge. To help evacuate the mucus, sterile saline nebulisation should be applied to humidify lung secretions. Immediately after nebulisation, the rehydrated, loosened secretions must be mobilised and cleared out of the lungs. Coupage or tapotage, tracheal manipulation to stimulate the cough reflex, postural drainage and mild exercise (to improve tidal ventilation) are methods of physiotherapy that can accomplish this. Most of these foals will also benefit from humidified intranasal oxygen therapy.

The creation of waves of air to loosen secretions in the lungs is called *percussion*. For manual percussion, the chest is struck with the hand held slightly cupped with fingers and thumb closed so that a cushion of air is trapped between the hand and the chest wall. Best results come from using both hands alternately in rapid sequence for several seconds, moving from ventral to dorsal lung fields and from the caudal to cranial lobes, to move secretions out of the tract. When done properly, this is a noisy procedure; however, it is not painful to the patient. Care must be taken to strike the chest wall without causing discomfort and bruising. Percussion may be contraindicated in patients with a bleeding disorder, fractured ribs or fragile bones. If the animal is ambulatory, a brief walk after coupage will aid in mobilisation of respiratory secretions.[8,9]

Vibration describes high-frequency compression of the chest wall. An electric hand vibrator or belt can be used to set up fine vibration that will also aid the drainage of secretions. During and between coupage treatments, a vibration belt may be kept around the thorax. A further benefit of continuous vibration is that lymphatic drainage may be stimulated, avoiding the deposit of mucus in the lungs.

To prevent cooling down of the body temperature, the animal should be covered with a blanket—eventually an infrared lamp or padded with hot packs—and should lay on insulated comfortable bedding.

Care should be taken to regularly reposition the animal from lateral to sternal position, to allow redistribution of blood flow and to influence gas exchanges in the lung tissues. Positioning of the foal on a slightly inclined surface can be beneficial to clear secretions by gravity. Every 3 to 4 hours, the foal can be hung in a sling, allowing it to stand and to help gravity evacuate fluids from the lungs and trachea. In order to ventilate adequately, the patient must be able to support its own weight while in the sling. A patient that hangs in the sling could easily asphyxiate. During this standing period, the therapist should mildly tapotage the complete surface of the thorax. Through rhythmic clapping on the wall of the thorax with cupped hands, mucus is released from the bronchi and brought into the trachea. Natural mucus removal works at a velocity of only some millimeters per hour, due to ciliary activity.

By stimulating the tracheal reflex, we can enhance active coughing, to obtain active removal of the secretions. The initial phase of the coughing is the most efficient because of the hyperpressure moment and also the highest velocity in air propulsion. Stimulation of the cough reflex by compressing the trachea will also expand the lungs maximally to help prevent atelectasis.

Contraindications for thoracic physical therapy are listed in Box 18.3.[5,7,10]

Musculoskeletal conditions

Spinal pain and stiffness

This can manifest itself in many ways. There may be an associated lameness or reduction in spinal range of movement, or it may present as a performance-related problem.[11]

Box 18.3. Contraindications to thoracic physical therapy

- Rib fractures
- Pneumothorax
- Low platelet count
- Subcutaneous emphysema
- Pain
- Unstable haemodynamics

It is important in the former case to exclude the possibility of distal limb lameness as the two conditions may coexist concurrently. Treatment may consist of manual therapy, trigger point release, electroneuromuscular stimulation, specific stretches and/or dry needling to address the muscle spasm and tightness often found with this condition. Laser therapy and acupuncture may be administered to help with management of the associated pain. When pain relief, muscle spasm and tightness have been managed, a specific exercise rehabilitation programme is introduced. Prognosis and follow-up treatment often depend on the presence or absence of an underlying spinal pathology (e.g., dorsal spinous process impingement [DSPI] or degenerative changes to the transverse and facet joints). It has been recommended that in horses that have been diagnosed with DSPI, initial treatment should include conservative treatment of physiotherapy and intra-articular injection, before surgical intervention is undertaken.[12] Due to regulations restricting the use of some medications close to competition, physiotherapy is at times the only option and can be very effective in managing the symptoms of this condition.

Sacroiliac dysfunction

These can be challenging cases, especially when associated with a malalignment of the tuber sacrale (Figure 18.4). It is essential that in these cases an ultrasound scan of the pelvis be performed by the referring veterinary surgeon to exclude the presence of an ilial wing fracture.[13] It is not uncommon for horses to present with a mild or no visible lameness following an ilial wing fracture. In these cases it is not advisable to treat the horse by releasing the associated muscle spasm as this may be splinting a deeper fracture, restricting movement at the joint and preventing further injury.

Physiotherapy is an essential adjunct to the management of sacroiliac dysfunction. Initially, muscle spasm or tightness is released by one of the methods listed in Table 18.1. Pain relief is also addressed at this time. Following symptomatic treatment, a specific rehabilitation programme can be developed. This aims to strengthen the musculature surrounding the injured joint in order to provide more strength and stability to that joint. It is well documented in human physiotherapy that joints with poor core stabilisation are more susceptible to sheering forces and increased physiological movement, which increases their susceptibility to injury.[14] These patients respond extremely well to a rehabilitation programme addressing the core stabilising muscles of the problematic joint. The equine rehabilitation programme will be dependent on a number of factors, including degree of lameness, which sacroiliac joint is affected, provoking factors and associated muscle atrophy.

Lumbosacral dysfunction

For those horses that present with bilateral pain on palpation and no asymmetry of the tuber sacrale, it is important not to forget the lumbosacral junction as a possible source of pain. At this level, a large intervertebral disc, diverging spinous processes and poorly developed interspinous ligament allow a significant amount of flexion and extension,[15] particularly during gallop and jumping activities.[16] This condition often responds well to physiotherapy and rest during the acute phase. Recurrent acute-on-chronic inflammatory conditions may require intra-articular injection. Intra-articular medication alone is often not sufficient to treat back pain, and a combination of medication and physiotherapy may yield far better results. Further research in this area will help to lead to best practice treatment programmes being established in the area of spinal pain and dysfunction.

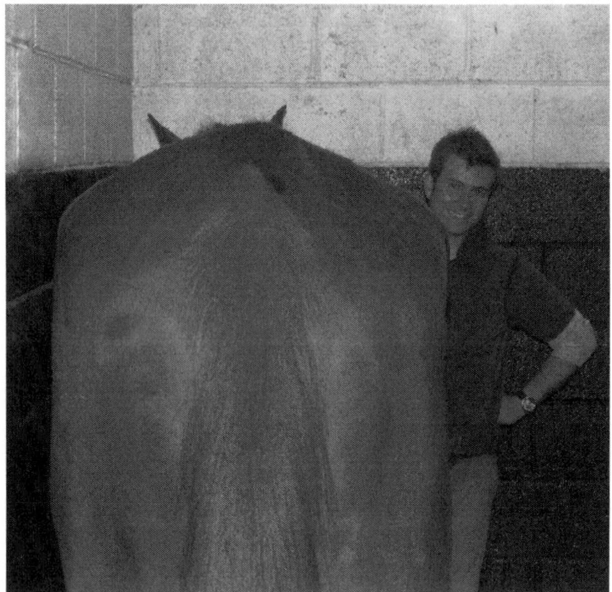

Figure 18.4 Asymmetry of the tuber sacrale, with wasting of the right gluteal muscles. ©Kevin Corley 2007.

Muscle rupture, tear or strain

In the treatment of these injuries, physiotherapy aims to prevent further injury, reduce inflammation and pain, promote healing and return the patient to normal function (Figure 18.5). Treatment modalities that may be used include laser, ultrasound, massage, electrical muscle stimulation, stretches and a rehabilitation programme. The severity of the injury will determine the choice of modalities and the short- and long-term goals.

Soft tissue injuries

Wounds, nonhealing and acute

Scientific research has suggested wound healing in animals can be accelerated by the use of various forms of electrotherapy.[17,18] The appropriate introduction of stretches and a rehabilitation programme may also assist in limiting scar tissue formation and earlier return to normal function.

Tendon and ligament injuries

Depending on the severity of the lesion, tendons and ligaments can benefit from a combination of ultrasound, laser

Table 18.1. An overview of the properties of some commonly used manual techniques in veterinary physiotherapy

Treatment	Indications for use	Physiological effects	Contraindications/precautions
Mobilisations/ manipulation	Joint stiffness Pain relief To increase range of movement	Increases in joint range of movement Pain modulation Stimulate joint lubrication	Ataxia Joint instability Neoplasia Non–weight-bearing lameness, refer to veterinary surgeon Severe splinting spasm as may indicate presence of a fracture
Massage	Pain relief Muscle stiffness/tightness	Increase blood flow Decrease pain via the pain gate mechanism Increase tissue length	As mobilisations Infection
Trigger point therapy/ myofascial release	Myofascial pain syndrome, causing movement dysfunction and pain	Biomechanical stretch releasing the actin and myosin contracture.	As mobilisations
Stretches	Increase range of movement Treatment and prevention of adaptive shortening/contractures	Lengthen the muscle tendon unit	As mobilisations Caution with recently repaired tissues

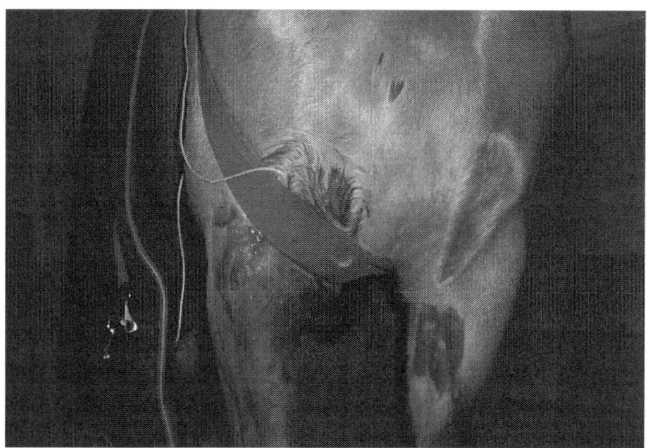

Figure 18.5 Treatment of a horse with traumatic injury to the pectoral muscles. ©Patrick Herbots 2006.

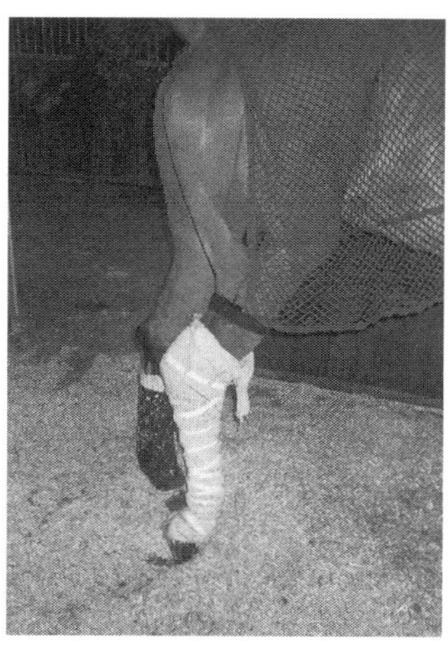

Figure 18.6 Rupture of the Achilles tendon in a horse. ©Patrick Herbots 2006.

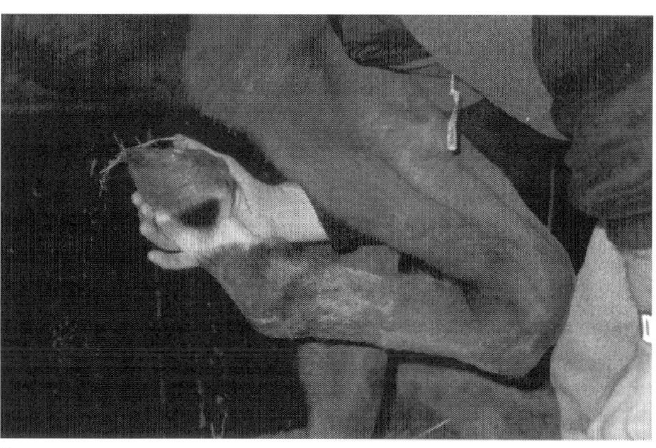

A

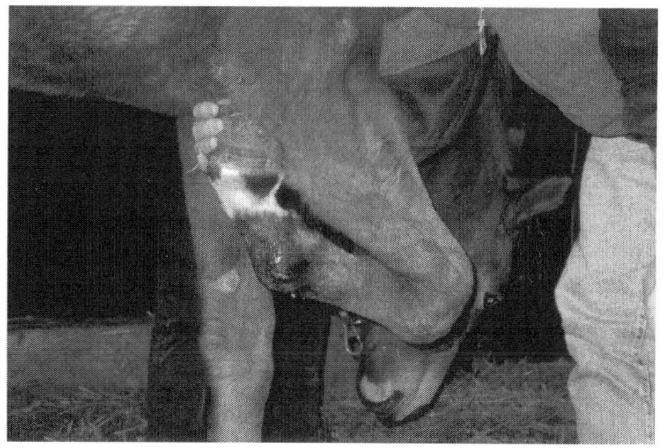

B

Figures 18.7 (A, B) Limited articular mobility in the fetlock. ©Patrick Herbots 2006.

and stretches and a rehabilitation programme (Figure 18.6). Treatment progress should be monitored with ultrasonography of the affected region by the referring veterinary surgeon.

General conditions

Postorthopaedic surgery

The physiotherapy treatment and rehabilitation programme will depend on the surgery performed. Treatment will aim to address any dysfunction to the musculoskeletal system and related structures. Postoperative outcomes following resection of the dorsal spinous process improve when physiotherapy is a component of postoperative rehabilitation.[4]

Immobilisation

Injury of the joint and surrounding tissues (Figure 18.7, A and B) and arthritis can lead to reduced joint mobility. It is important that all is done to prevent the detrimental effects of immobilisation to bone, muscle and tendon tissue (Box 18.4). Manual therapy, deep frictions, heat, electrical stimulation, ultrasound and stretches are often used to avoid pain and contractures or to increase circulation and joint mobility.

Saddle-fitting problems

Most horses with saddle-fitting problems present with spinal pain and stiffness. These clinical findings are treated and the horse is then referred to a qualified saddle fitter for assessment.

Performance problems

A detailed assessment needs to be carried out to determine the cause of the poor performance. In some instances, a joint veterinary and physiotherapy assessment is most appropriate as many sport horses, in particular, have a combination of mild lameness and back pain and stiffness. The symptoms may also be related to muscle imbalance, that is, differences in muscle development between sides, or muscle weakness.

Box 18.4. Pathological effects of immobilisation

- Decreased blood and lymphatic circulation
- Chemical and histological deterioration
- Decreased tissue elasticity
- Decreased sensation and proprioception
- Muscle atrophy and ligament strain
- Decreased mobility

Compensatory problems

These can cause as many problems as the primary dysfunction that initiated them. Usually, the primary problem is treated first. Then, the physiotherapist may be requested to treat the compensatory problems. Occasionally, however, the veterinarian may request that the compensatory problems are addressed in order to get a clearer picture of the primary problem. The benefits of this treatment will not last long but often will increase the severity of a lameness, temporarily making it easier to examine, until the compensatory components have developed again.

Care of the aged horse

A combination of stretches, joint mobilisations and massage techniques is used in the management programme tailored to the older horse. Aspects of this programme can be taught to the owner to enable the older horse to continue performing the activities it is required to do.

Treatment techniques

The treatment programme will be developed following a thorough and in-depth subjective and objective assessment. This will often involve close liaison between the physiotherapist and veterinary surgeon and other relevant members of the multidisciplinary team, such as the farrier, dentist and master saddler. Each treatment programme is specifically tailored to the individual patient's presenting signs and symptoms. Most treatment programmes will involve a combination of treatment techniques. The following section will explain the scientific basis and rationale behind the more frequently used treatment modalities (Box 18.5) and how they can be used in veterinary medicine to optimise outcomes.

Box 18.5. List of treatment techniques

Manual therapy
- Mobilisation/manipulation
- Massage
- Trigger point release/myofascial release technique
- Stretches

Electrotherapy
- Laser therapy
- Ultrasound
- Muscle stimulator
- TENS
- Magnetic field therapy

Thermal therapy
- Heat
- Cold

Exercise therapy
- Neuromuscular reeducation
- Proprioceptive rehabilitation

Hydrotherapy

Acupuncture/dry needling techniques

Facilities required for physiotherapy

Before starting examination or treatment, the environmental conditions should be considered for comfort and safety of both the physiotherapist and the horse. Physiotherapy requires spending time with and building up a rapport with the horse. It is therefore best to have the horse in a stable where it has had a chance to relax.

As physiotherapy includes the use of manual and electrical techniques, a clean, dry stable floor is a must. Machines that run on batteries are more practical and safer than those dependent on a main electricity supply. As horses are shod with metal shoes and stabled on floors that tend to be damp, it is a sensible idea when possible to carry out electrical treatment in stables with rubber matting as part of the flooring. Before starting to use physiotherapy devices and techniques, their indications and contraindications must be thoroughly understood. Proper training in physiotherapy, biomechanics and anatomy is essential.

Manual therapy

"Manual therapy (or manipulative therapy) refers to the practice of therapist applied passive or active assisted movement techniques for the management of pain and impairments in the articular, neural and muscular systems".[19] A list of frequently used manual treatment techniques, the indications for their use, their physiological effects and their contraindications or precautions to use are given in Table 18.1.

Mobilisations and manipulations

Mobilisations are therapist-applied passive movements, applied to peripheral or spinal joints, within the joint's physiological and accessory range of movement. *Manipulations* are large-amplitude accessory movements applied with a high-velocity thrust. These may include movements in various planes, including craniocaudal translation, flexion/extension, rotation and lateral glides. The availability of movement is dependent upon the anatomy of the joint involved.

They have been shown to be effective in the treatment of conditions of both spinal joints[20] and peripheral joints[21,22] in humans. In horses, using kinematic assessment of the range of motion of joints, it has been demonstrated that mobilisations and manipulation can increase range of motion of the equine spine.[23,24] This provides promise for further research and future treatment, as back pain in horses is associated with a reduction in spinal mobility.[25] Other studies have concentrated on the neurophysiological effects of mobilisation or manipulation.[21,26] It is thought that afferent neural input caused by this technique can have an analgesic effect at both a spinal cord level[27] and also involving higher centres of the central nervous system, via the descending inhibitory pathways.[26] Mobilisation and manipulation may be used in addition to stretches, exercise and electrotherapy.

Massage

Massage can involve a range of techniques applied at various tissue depths aimed at increasing tissue length and blood and lymph circulation and promoting relaxation. It is hypothesised that massage will lengthen tissue and reduce spasm through its mechanical effects, and reduce pain by increasing blood flow to the area and via the pain gate mechanism.[28] Massage is normally used in association with other techniques.

Trigger point therapy/myofascial release

A myofascial trigger point (MTrP) is defined as "a highly localised and hyperirritable spot in a palpable taut band of skeletal muscle fibres".[29,30] Trigger points are painful on palpation, prevent full muscle lengthening and thus shorten muscles, weaken the muscle without atrophy and can refer pain. The mechanisms that cause MTrPs are unknown but are thought to involve a dysfunction of the motor end plate.[31,32] Acute or chronic overload of a muscle, direct injury and overexertion of a muscle are thought to be some of the aetiological factors associated with trigger points.

The technique of MTrP release involves locating the trigger point of a muscle and applying a stretch to it via direct compression. This compression must be maintained until the clinician feels the release of the MTrP. Myofascial release involves massaging along the taut band of the trigger point outwards on both sides. These techniques are often used in conjunction with each other and other treatments such as electrotherapy, ice and stretch. In practice, MTrPs can be measured objectively using pressure algometry to measure any reduction in MTrP pain threshold levels and thus treatment effectiveness.[33] Pressure algometry also provides a quantitative and repeatable method for assessing the presence of musculoskeletal pain in horses.[34,35]

Stretches

Passive static stretches are the most applicable to veterinary physiotherapy. The therapist applies the stretch to the myofascial and neurological tissues. One of the main therapeutic uses of stretching is to lengthen the muscle tendon unit and thus achieve greater increase in range of movement at a particular joint or group of joints. An example of a stretch, which is useful as an assessment and treatment tool, is the sacral reflex stretch. The clinician may use their fingers or two pens, with equal force, and run them along the quarters from rump to hamstring. This will cause the horse to flex its spine. It should do so equally in a straight line. Should the quarters swing to one side, this may indicate a dysfunction on that side causing tightening or adaptive shortening of the paraspinal tissues of that side. This stretch can also be performed along one hindquarter (unilaterally) to stretch the spine laterally.

In lengthening the musculotendinous unit, stretching has a very important role to play in both the treatment and prevention of contractures and fibrosis. In equine veterinary medicine, one of the more common indications for stretching is in the treatment of foals with preexisting contractures and those with a non–weight-bearing lameness, which are at risk of developing contractures. It may also be necessary to introduce stretching programmes postoperatively, in certain surgeries, to prevent contractures and fibrosis (Figure 18.8). Baited and assisted stretches are also commonly used in dysfunction of the cervical spine. These can be performed in a way to maximise stretch of the upper, mid and lower cervical spine and involve bringing the horse's nose to the point of the shoulder, elbow and back towards the flank. A comparison is made between right and left.

Electrotherapy

Electrotherapy refers to the electrical modalities that can be used therapeutically in physiotherapy. The main electrotherapy machines used, their indications for use, physiological effects and contraindications or precautions are given in Table 18.2.

Low-level laser therapy

Low-level laser therapy is a form of electromagnetic radiation in the visible and near visible part of the spectrum. Laser light is absorbed by the chromophores in the cell

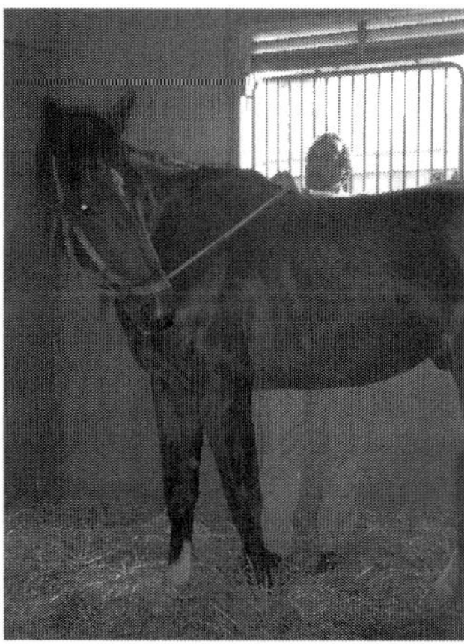

Figure 18.8 Static neck stretch in a horse. ©Patrick Herbots 2006.

Table 18.2. Electrical treatment modalities and their indications for use, physiological effects and contraindications or precautions

Treatment modality	Indications for use	Physiological effects	Contraindications/precautions
Laser	Wound healing Pain relief Inflammatory conditions Swelling/oedema Splints Tendon Injuries	Stimulate cell proliferation ↑ Fibroblast proliferation Stimulate collagen synthesis Vasodilation ↑ ATP production ↑ Metabolism of endogenous opiates	Infection Neoplasia Areas of haemorrhage Over pregnant uterus Eyes, gonads Altered skin sensitivity
Therapeutic ultrasound	Tissue healing Fracture healing, special unit Pain relief Oedema Ligament sprain Tendonitis Bursitis	↑ Metabolic activity ↑ Blood flow and vasodilation ↑ Cell membrane permeability ↑ Proliferation of fibroblasts ↑ Production of collagen and its extensibility ↑ Tensile strength of scar tissue	As for laser Particular caution over epiphyseal plates in growing animals Metal implants DVT
TENS	Pain relief	Pain modulation via segmental inhibition and descending pain suppression	As for laser and ultrasound No application over indwelling electronic stimulators
Neuromuscular electrical stimulation	Muscle atrophy; disuse and neurogenic Muscle tightness or contracture Prevention of post operative weakness Muscle spasm	Stimulate rhythmic muscle contraction Pain modulation as for TENS ↑ Blood flow and metabolism Promote nutrition Eliminate pain induced vasoconstriction by reversing muscle spasm ↓ Lactate levels ↑ O_2 uptake, CO_2 levels and local temperature	Caution over broken skin In the presence of decreased sensation When a strong muscle contraction could lead to joint or muscle damage In the presence of haemorrhages. Burns from heating of tissues or chemical buildup of waste products of contraction

mitochondria. This affects cell function and stimulates tissue-repair mechanisms.[36,37]

In Bjordal and Couppé's review,[38] different articles were checked for their aims and parameters used for treatment. It was reported that doses lower than 0.1 J/cm^2 did not produce significant results, while doses in excess of 4.5 J/cm^2, and power density higher than 10 mW/cm^2, produced an inhibitory effect on the fibroblasts' metabolism and collagen production. Therefore, the following treatment parameters are suggested[38]:

- Power density = Mean output/exposure area: 5 to 21 mW/cm^2
- Dose = Power density × Treatment time: 0.1 to 3 J/cm^2
- Treatment frequency: 3 to 5 times per week

In human medicine, laser therapy has been found to be effective in pain relief,[39,40] wound healing[41,42] and the treatment of chronic ligament and tendon injuries.[43]

However, studies in equine medicine have given conflicting results. One study reported significantly improved performance times,[44] whilst two others showed no significant effect on healing rates of wounds or tendons.[45,46] The literature on the effect of laser on wound healing is very controversial.[47,48] Authors are divided and the methods used and materials are different. Most of the controlled, scientific studies have focused on fresh wounds and do not report advantages in using laser therapy. Articles on the treatment of chronic wounds have reported more positive effects but tend to be based on anecdotal clinical cases. In the authors' experience, laser therapy has been beneficial in treating pain associated with sore shins and splints and in accelerating healing in chronic inflammatory conditions, particularly wound and tendon tissue. Further research is required to support the use of laser in equine veterinary medicine and to determine the most appropriate parameters for various acute and chronic conditions.

Ultrasound therapy

Ultrasound waves are high-frequency sound waves. Therapeutic ultrasonographic treatment can be thermal or athermal. The most commonly used therapeutic frequencies are 1 MHz and 3 MHz. The 1-MHz treatment penetrates deeper tissues (3–4 cm), and 3 MHz is used for more superficial tissues (2–4 cm). Greater pulse widths (e.g., 1:4) are used for acute injuries, and opinions vary regarding appropriate intensity settings.

Studies of the effect of therapeutic ultrasound on the healing of tendons show improvement in the degree of swelling, pain on palpation and lameness.[49–51] Treated tendons had a histological image closer to normal tissue and fewer peritendineous adhesions than nontreated tendons.[19,52,53] When applied to fresh fractured bone in humans, ultrasound has been shown to substantially accelerate the rate of repair with minimal risk of tissue damage.[54] In delayed and nonunion fractures, the ultrasound resulted in union in over 80% of cases. The synovial membrane and articular cartilage of animals treated with ultrasound (1 W/cm^2) showed accelerated healing.[55] Ultrasound accelerates not only the resolution of the inflammatory process but also the healing process in wound healing by increasing the rate of growth of replacement tissues at the site of injury.[49]

Electrical stimulation

Electrical neuromuscular stimulation is often used in one of two ways:

1. Stimulation of the sensory nerves for pain relief (TENS)
2. Stimulation of the motor nerves and muscle to produce a muscle contraction (neuromuscular stimulation)

In order to understand how both of these methods work, it is important to review the basic anatomy of peripheral nerves and how they function. Most peripheral nerves are made up of Aα, Aβ, Aδ and C fibres. These combine to give a mixture of motor and sensory afferent and efferent information to the spinal cord and the central nervous system (Table 18.3).

Electrical stimulation is a treatment that can be used in combination with medication or other physiotherapy techniques, such as massage, vibration, ultrasound, laser and rehabilitation exercises (Box 18.6).

Transcutaneous electrical nerve stimulation

TENS is a method of electrical stimulation that primarily aims to provide a degree of pain relief (symptomatic) by specifically exciting sensory nerves. A clear diagnosis must be given before TENS is used, as this treatment option may mask symptoms. There are primarily two types of TENS that are used: "conventional" and "burst, acupuncture-like". Rectangular, short-duration pulses (250 μsec) are used in both as the sensory nerves have relatively low thresholds and are therefore easy to excite.

The body uses nonmyelinated C-nerve fibres to transport pain stimuli at low speed to the brain.

To control pain sensation, we can manipulate two pathways:

Box 18.6. Goals for electrical muscle stimulation

- **Pain management**, through the principle of gate control or endorphin release
- **Eliminating pain-induced vasoconstriction**, by reversing muscle spasm
- **Increasing blood and lymphatic circulation**, due to muscle pumping effect
- **Turn down muscle atrophy**, reduce spasm or stimulate reinforcement
- **Effects on muscle enzyme**: After training muscles with electrical stimulation, it was stated that muscles fibres showed a better resistance to fatigue and lower lactate levels were measured.[45]
- **Rhythmic muscle contraction**: When the animal refuses to use this body part, this form of therapeutic exercise can help to restore movement in muscles and joints.
- **Wound healing**, due to increased blood/lymphatic circulation

Table 18.3. Characteristics of peripheral nerves

Fibre type	Function	Diameter and conduction velocity	Characteristics
Aα	Motor	13–22 μm 70–120 msec	Myelinated Respond to changes in the muscle spindle and Golgi tendon organ
Aβ	Sensory	5–15 μm 40–70 msec	Myelinated High discrimination touch
Aγ	Sensory	4–8 μm 15–40 msec	Thinly myelinated High threshold High discrimination touch Primarily involved in acute pain and the flexor withdrawal reflex
Aδ	Sensory	1–4 μm 5–15 msec	Thinly myelinated Respond to prickling pain, crude touch, cold Also motor to muscle spindles
C	Sensory	0.5–1 μm 0.5–2 msec	Unmyelinated Nociceptive—aching pain, tickle, cold and warmth Involved in chronic pain and muscle spasm.

- Segmental inhibition via the pain gate mechanism—Conventional, or
- Descending pain suppression via endogenous opioid release—Burst

Conventional TENS

Using "conventional" TENS (high frequency, low intensity, rectangular current), we can stimulate Aβ nerve vessels. This causes presynaptic inhibition of the Aδ and C fibres at that level of the dorsal horn in the spinal cord. The nociceptive pain transmission is blocked, the so-called "pain gate mechanism". So, the painful stimuli of the C-vessels to the brain will be overwhelmed. This can be compared to the situation where you rub your leg after somebody kicked it.

Pain alleviation from gate control stimulation has a rapid but short-lived effect and is indicated for acute or intense pain. Because conventional TENS does not produce muscle contraction in the equine, it is very difficult to judge the strength of sensation received by horse.

"Burst" TENS

The second pathway, "Burst" TENS, uses low-frequency (3 Hz), 250-μsec pulse widths and higher intensities. It is used to stimulate the Aδ fibres, which will activate the opioid mechanisms and provide pain relief by causing the release of endogenous endorphins in the spinal cord, which inhibits C-fibre–type pain. Clear muscle twitches are obtained. In humans, repeated muscle contractions for 15 minutes, at higher intensities, will lead to endorphin release. Pain alleviation due to endorphin release has a more longstanding effect and is indicated for the treatment of chronic pain and muscle atrophy.

Neuromuscular stimulation

Atrophied muscles decrease local circulation and predispose joint surfaces to structural changes. The associated pain hinders the animal from using the limb, thus promoting adhesions to occur. Neuromuscular stimulation artificially stimulates a muscle contraction by activation of the peripheral nerve to that muscle. A complementary effect of "burst TENS" stimulation is the benefit of the muscle contractions, which stimulate blood supply to the tissues, due to the muscle-pumping effect. This will clear the injured muscle from metabolic deposits and new nutricients will arrive. The arising muscle contraction will implicate more contracting muscle cells as intensity increases. This will lead to relaxation of the intrafusal muscle spindle and muscle relaxation. As a result of the endorphin release, most horses will go into a sleepy relaxation during treatment.

Where to place the electrodes: The current will remain relatively superficial if the electrodes are spaced closely together. If the electrodes are spaced farther apart, the current will flow through those tissues, providing the least resistance. To get the best contraction at the lowest intensity, one should look for the motor point of the muscle to place the electrodes. One can place gel on the skin surface above the target muscle, and by moving a small electrode at a set intensity, one can obtain better contractions at different zones. These zones, with the best muscle twitch at the lowest intensity, are defined as the *motor point*.[56–59]

By using sufficient conducting gel and wetting the coat, one can avoid hair clipping.

In humans, self-adhesive electrodes can be used. In animals, carbon-rubber electrodes are used with conducting gel. They are easier to apply and less expensive. The carbon electrodes can be cut to the appropriate size. In the authors' opinion, 7 × 7 cm electrodes are the most suitable. The larger the electrode, the greater is the intensity that is required to ensure the same result. One can keep the electrodes in place with tape, elastic bandages or surcingles to lead the wires. Electrodes can be placed over the lesion or following the dermatomes or covering the associated spinal nerve. Most of the research suggests treatment is beneficial when reinforced with a functional training programme.

Magnetic field therapy

Reviewing the literature on magnetic therapy also leads us to a very controversial range of interpretations. Articles conflict in describing effects on tendon healing,[60] non-union fractures[61,62] and stimulation of blood circulation.[63,64] There is no established mechanism of action to explain how either pulsating electromagnetic field or static magnetic field therapy could affect tissue. It is claimed that magnetic fields allow cells to stabilize following cellular damage, secondary to tissue disruption. One of the problems of evaluating effects described in different articles is the use of different parameters, such as Hertz (1 cycle per second) and Gauss (1 Volt per centimetre per second).

Thermal therapy

The effects of hot and cold therapy are listed in Table 18.4.

Cryotherapy

Cold therapy is an important form of therapy that is often forgotten in the initial stage of an injury. The application of a cold medium results in removal of heat from the tissue. Management of initial swelling and the deleterious effect it has on neuromuscular function are important in minimising recovery time from soft tissue injury.

There are a variety of modalities on the market for the application of cold to equine limbs.[52,53,65,66] Some are more effective than others at maintaining the limb at a prescribed temperature. The options range from cold hosing, the application of ice packs, cold whirlpool baths, cold spas, ice boots that are filled with ice and water, leg boots that contain ice packs and more expensive options such as the cryotherapy gun. Hyperbaric CO_2 used for acute pain can make limping disappear in the minutes following cryotherapy. Using this technique, frozen gas at −78° C (−108° F) is sprayed on the skin surface for 30 seconds.

Table 18.4. The effects of hot and cold therapy

Treatment modality	Indications for use	Physiological effects	Contraindications/precautions
Cold	Initial 24 to 48/72 hours following injury Pain relief Inflammatory conditions Swelling/oedema Laminitis Tendon injuries Lymphoedema	↓ Metabolism Vasoconstriction ↓ Haemorrhage ↓ Oedema ↓ The release of chemical mediators (pain) ↓ Afferent nerve conduction Inhibit histamine and neutrophil activation Inhibit collagenase activity	Altered skin sensation
Heat	For use in subacute/chronic phase of healing Effective precursor to stretching Promote tissue healing	↑ Metabolism ↑ Vasodilation and blood flow ↑ Oxygenation ↑ Cell permeability ↑ Tissue extensibility	Infection Neoplasia Areas of haemorrhage Altered skin sensitivity Burns

The skin temperature drops suddenly to 4° C (39° F), and cutaneous and subcutaneous pain receptors are deactivated. However, it is unclear how long the benefits last. Water immersion is the most effective cheaper form of cryotherapy; the desired ice-water temperature should be about 4° C. Cooling the equine foot has been shown to decrease soft tissue perfusion and reduce laminar-tissue temperatures within 30 minutes of treatment. Cooling the foot could decrease enzymatic reactions associated with laminitis,[67,68] and possibly other foot conditions where inflammation is excessive.

Heat therapy

The application of heat causes an elevation in tissue temperature, which subsequently produces vasodilatation and hypermetabolism. Therefore, heat therapy must be delayed until at least 48 hours after injury to avoid stimulation of the acute inflammation or haemorrhage. Heat therapy can be administered simply such as applying heat packs or hot towels or using electrotherapy such as thermal doses of ultrasound or electrical neuromuscular stimulation. Care must be taken to avoid burning. Single-leg whirlpools, with iodine concentrate added to the water, reduce the possibility of transmitting infections and aid in cleansing abraded skin. A thermometer to monitor water temperature is essential for the safety and effectiveness of hydrotherapy. The water temperature should be at a maximum of 40° C (104° F). It has been suggested that warming of the equine foot can increase local perfusion.[67] Therefore, application of heat to the foot could be an effective method of distributing/perfusing medication administered locally. Tissue extensibility can be improved as a result of local heating, and warming up is an excellent precursor to stretching. An increase in cutaneous blood flow will promote wound healing.

Exercise rehabilitation

Exercise affects the neuromuscular, orthopaedic, cardiovascular and metabolic systems; hence, all must be considered when formulating a rehabilitation programme.[69] An exercise programme should be progressive regarding duration and intensity of work. The purpose of a rehabilitation programme is to address injury and recovery of the musculoskeletal system, which may affect performance and function. Rehabilitation is often an essential part of the multimodal approach to the treatment of equine pathologies. Hence, it needs to be formulated following a detailed veterinary and physiotherapy assessment procedure involving diagnostic and prognostic evaluation.

Box 18.7. Elements of an exercise rehabilitation programme

- Strength training
- Proprioceptive training
- Increasing range of motion
- Stretching
- Gait reeducation

Exercise leads to improved conduction of nerve impulses and improved muscle activity.[70] Elements of the programme are given in Box 18.7. Strength training in the horse may involve strengthening of the global muscles of the body or may address a unilateral weakness or imbalance, by conducting exercise primarily in one direction. For example, should atrophy of the right gluteal muscle exist, it may be recommended that 70% of exercise is performed on the left rein. This is based on the hypothesis that the outside limb requires more force to propel the body forward and will have a longer stride length than the inside hind leg, when worked on a circle or in an arena. Intensity may be increased through the use of a variety of paces and degrees of collection. Poles and cavalletti at varying stride lengths can allow the physiotherapist to recruit specific muscle groups.

It has been suggested the use of distal leg weights can increase muscle activity and strength.[4] Wickler et al.[71] concluded that the application of leg weights to the distal limb significantly increased the range of motion of the stifle, tarsus and hind fetlock joint. General metabolic demands were significantly increased. Experimental surface electromyographic data were collected from the triceps brachii muscle, during treadmill exercise, with and without a 0.75-kg mass attached to both digits. The results showed significantly more activity in the long and lateral heads at canter.[72]

Proprioception can be addressed in a number of ways. This may include exercise on different surfaces, alternate stimuli to legs like chains and attachment of bells to the limbs, which can increase elevation. Denoix and Pailloux[4] suggest building a "sensory re-education path", where the horse encounters a number of terrains in sequence. Surfaces varying in depth and hardness (sand, asphalt, pebbles, water) are placed close to each other. Walking over the path creates a variety of plantar sensations and movements that enhance the rapidity of response and functioning of the neuroceptors.[4] At a later stage, walking up and down hills, reining back, circling, figures-of-eight and cavalletti can be added to the programme. Other techniques such as taping and long reining can also give the horse an increased proprioceptive awareness. Athletic taping of the fetlock has been shown to alter limb kinematics including reduced peak vertical forces.[73] The authors hypothesise that this is due to an increased proprioceptive awareness of the limb.

To encourage fore limb weight transference and increased proprioceptive input, a haynet suspended in the centre of the horse's stable is very useful (Figure 18.3). By grasping the haynet, this encourages the horse to move constantly; focusing on the hay, the horse will reprogramme its pathological movement pattern. The repeated incentive to move will improve the voluntary activation of the muscle group and reaction time of the associated nerves. Alternating weight-bearing will stimulate sensory information from the hoof to the brain.

Hydrotherapy

Hydrotherapy may refer to swimming horses or exercising them on a water treadmill.

Indications for swimming

Swimming provides a medium to high-intensity workout without subjecting the musculoskeletal system to high levels of concussive forces. This can allow earlier return to weight-bearing activity postinjury.

In a later stage of rehabilitation, swimming can be used to:

- Increase movement amplitude, with varying levels of weight-bearing. The degree of weight-bearing is directly proportional to the depth of the water, due to the buoyancy of the water. Warm water has less resistance to movement. The converse is also true.
- Restore muscle activity and strength. Research has shown swimming increases the aerobic capacity of muscle, based on histochemical analysis, when compared with land-based training in 2-year-old horses.[74]
- Provide cardiorespiratory training.
- Stimulate articular movement amplitude after healing of skeletal problems, including carpus injuries.[75]

In addition,

- Animals with poor balance on land may find it easier to stand in water due to the viscosity and surface tension of the water.
- Hydrostatic pressure is the pressure exerted by the water. It also is directly proportional to the depth of water. This can help to reduce pooling in the extremities in deep water and can assist in the reduction of oedema. It can affect lung volumes, and care needs to be taken with horses in respiratory distress.

Biomechanics of hydrotherapy

Horses normally swim in a trotting gait. The back of the horse will be held just under the surface of the water, the head will be raised and the nostrils shut except during inhalation. Large thrusts from the hindquarters produce significant lumbosacral flexion in an effort to push forwards through the water. Walking horses in water or underwater treadmills will encourage, at trot, a high degree of vertical displacement compared with overland locomotion. It has been reported that walking on the underwater treadmill recruits more electromyographic activity of extensor digitorum communis than does swimming or land-based exercise.[76] Flexor digitorum profundus, brachiocephalicus and triceps brachii caput longum were most active during swimming. This information can help the clinician decide which therapy is appropriate. For example, a horse with weakness and atrophy of the extensor tendons of the forelimb may benefit from a programme of exercise walking on the underwater treadmill.

Physiological effects of swimming

Swimming may improve respiratory muscle strength, as during inspiration the horse has to expand the chest wall against pressure of water. The respiratory strategy adopted by horses during swimming is entirely different than that on land. The respiratory rate during swimming exercise is much lower than that on land, where respiration rate is linked to stride frequency.

Water walking does not lead to high heart rates and can therefore be safely done with a horse that is at relatively low level of fitness. However, trotting in water requires considerable coordination and effort from the horse and can produce heart rates of up to approximately 170 beats per minute. Immersing horses in warm spring water to the level of the olecranon increases parasympathetic nervous activity and thus may provide a means of relaxation for horses.[77]

During swimming, a substantial amount of heat can be dissipated by conductive transfer to the surrounding pool water. It can be dangerous for a horse to swim in a pool where the water is at the same temperature as the horse's body temperature. In this situation, no conductive heat transfer can occur, and marked hyperthermia will be induced easily. The water is usually heated to between about 12° and 19° C.[71,78]

Safety rules

As a rule, patients with skin incisions that have been present less than 10 to 14 days should not be immersed and leg protection should always be worn. For most rehabilitation purposes, partial immersion is preferred above swimming. Care should be taken in horses with back problems. Remember that having horses swim exercises them in an unnatural fashion. It is generally agreed that different muscles are used for swimming and for running. A team of well-educated trainers is vital to detect early signs of fatigue such as hyperpnoea, anxious expression and dissention of superficial blood vessels. Horses that are fatigued after swimming show a peculiar gait impediment, evident even at walk.[79]

Contraindications

Stifle lameness is reported to be adversely affected by swimming. Also listed as being worse after swimming are shoulder or back lameness and joints that are nearly ankylosed.[79] The increased effort needed to overcome the extrathoracic hydrostatic effects of immersion may contribute to an increased incidence of pulmonary oedema in horses. This means that horses with signs of cardiac or respiratory distress should be excluded from swimming.

Acupuncture/dry needling

Acupuncture

Acupuncture is the application of needles to specific acupuncture points throughout the body for the management of many conditions. Traditional Chinese medicine views this as a method of balancing energy flow. Acupuncture analgesia is thought to be due to stimulation of the Aδ fibres by the needle, thus causing a descending inhibition of pain from the central nervous system resulting in both opioid and nonopioid analgesia.[80] There is limited support for the effectiveness of acupuncture in the management of pain. Randomised controlled trials investigating the use of acupuncture in veterinary medicine need to be conducted to support the existing anecdotal evidence.

Dry needling

Dry needling is a technique used to treat MTrPs (see earlier). The technique requires the clinician to palpate the taut band and localise the MTrP. A disposable stainless steel needle is then inserted into the MTrP. The needle is then partially withdrawn and reinserted, repeatedly until a local twitch response or "jump sign" is elicited. This is usually continued until no more twitches occur.

Many studies have reported significant pain relief following dry needling of MTrPs in human studies.[80–82] Janssens successfully treated 34 of 48 lame dogs with dry needling that had not responded to pharmaceutical treatment or acupuncture.[83] It is unclear precisely how this technique works. It has been suggested there are both mechanical and physiological effects of dry needling. The mechanical effect appears to apply a local stretch to the contracted sarcomeres, in addition to a stimulated contraction resulting in relaxation and normal alignment of the sarcomeres. The needle is also thought to produce greater activation of sensitised polymodal-type receptors at the MTrP, resulting in pain relief.[81,83] This is a relatively new and developing area of interest in veterinary medicine.

Conclusion

At present, limited research exists to evaluate the efficacy of physiotherapy treatments in equine veterinary medicine, and much of the rationale behind the treatment is based on evidence extrapolated from human studies and anecdotal evidence. However, with increasing support from veterinary surgeons, the advent of university-based postgraduate animal physiotherapy courses and scientific developments in measuring and analysing kinematic data, the potential exists to produce randomised controlled trials in the area of veterinary physiotherapy. This is essential in these times of evidence-based practice, to demonstrate the efficacy of veterinary physiotherapy.

Acknowledgments

Patrick Herbots would like to thank the following colleagues for the efforts they made to teach him how to touch and look at horses, so to be able to help and treat them: Jean-Pierre Pailloux, Marvin Cain, Dominique Giniaux, Prof. Pierre Lievens, Mary Bromiley and Pascal Evrard. He would also like to thank all the veterinary colleagues who take the time to refer, discuss and evaluate cases.

Bairbre Sharkey would like to thank all those who have helped and supported her to develop her clinical skills as an equine physiotherapist. She would especially like to thank the staff of Anglesey Lodge Equine Hospital—in particular, Ned Gowing, Marcus Swail and Marie Harty.

References

1. Oliver JE, Lorenz MD: Handbook of Veterinary Neurological Diagnosis, ed 2. Philadelphia, WB Saunders, 1983, p 130
2. Taylor R: Physical therapy in veterinary medicine. Proceedings of the World Small Animal Veterinary Association Congress, Vancouver, August 8-11, 2001
3. Bromiley M: Equine Injury and Therapy, ed 2. Ames, IA, Blackwell SP Professional Books, 1991, p 39

4. Denoix J-M, Pailloux J-P: Physical Therapy and Massage for the Horse, ed 2. North Pomfret, VT, Trafalgar Square, 1998, p 224
5. Manning AM: Physical therapy for critically ill veterinary patients. I. Chest physical therapy. Compend Cont Educ Pract Vet 19:675-689, 1997
6. Ciesla ND: Chest physical therapy for patients in the intensive care unit. Phys Ther 76:609-625, 1996
7. McConnico R: Supportive medical care of the recumbent horses. Compend Contin Educ Pract Vet 13:1287-1295, 1991
8. Sirois M: Principles and Practice of Veterinary Technology, ed 2. St. Louis, Mosby, 2004, p 744
9. McCurning DM: Clinical Textbook for Veterinary Technicians, ed 6. Philadelphia, WB Saunders, 2005, p 1280
10. Frownfelter DL: Percussion and vibration, in Frownfelter DL, Haugh C (eds): Chest Physical Therapy and Pulmonary Rehabilitation. St. Louis, Mosby, 1987, p 496
11. Jeffcott LB, Dalin G, Ekman S, et al.: Sacroiliac lesions as a cause of chronic poor performance in competitive horses. Equine Vet J 17:111-118, 1985
12. Walmsley JP, Pettersson H, Winberg F, et al.: Impingement of the dorsal spinous processes in two hundred and fifteen horses: case selection, surgical technique and results. Equine Vet J 34:23-28, 2002
13. Shepherd MC, Pilsworth RC: The use of ultrasound in the diagnosis of pelvic fractures. Equine Vet Educ 6:223-227, 1994
14. Hides JA, Richardson CA, Jull GA: Multifidus muscle recovery is not automatic after resolution of acute, first-episode low back pain. Spine 21:2763-2769, 1996
15. Haussler KK, Stover SM, Willits NH: Pathologic changes in the lumbosacral vertebrae and pelvis in Thoroughbred racehorses. Am J Vet Res 60:143-153, 1999
16. Johnston C, Holmt K, Faber M, et al.: Effect of conformational aspects on the movement of the equine back. Equine Vet J Suppl:314-318, 2002
17. Meagher J: Beating Muscle Injuries. Hamilton, MA Hamilton Horse Associates, 1985, pp 78-83
18. Ghamsari SM, Taguchi K, Abe N, et al.: Evaluation of low level laser therapy on primary healing of experimentally induced full thickness teat wounds in dairy cattle. Vet Surg 26:114-120, 1997
19. Goff L, Jull G: Manual therapy, in McGowan C, Goff L, Stubbs N (eds): Animal Physiotherapy: Assessment, Treatment and Rehabilitation of Animals. Oxford, Blackwell Publishing, 2007, pp 164-176
20. Bronfort G, Haas M, Evans RL, et al.: Efficacy of spinal manipulation and mobilization for low back pain and neck pain: a systematic review and best evidence synthesis. Spine J 4:335-356, 2004
21. Vicenzino B, Paungmali A, Buratowski S, et al.: Specific manipulative therapy treatment for chronic lateral epicondylalgia produces uniquely characteristic hypoalgesia. Manual Ther 6:205-212, 2001
22. Abbott JH, Patla CE, Jensen RH: The initial effects of an elbow mobilization with movement technique on grip strength in subjects with lateral epicondylalgia. Manual Ther 6:163-169, 2001
23. Faber MJ, van Weeren PR, Schepers M, et al.: Long-term follow-up of manipulative treatment in a horse with back problems. J Vet Med A Physiol Pathol Clin Med 50:241-245, 2003
24. Haussler KK, Hill AE, Puttlitz CM, et al.: Effects of vertebral mobilization and manipulation on kinematics of the thoracolumbar region. Am J Vet Res 68:508-516, 2007
25. Wennerstrand J, Johnston C, Roethlisberger-Holm K, et al.: Kinematic evaluation of the back in the sport horse with back pain. Equine Vet J 36:707-711, 2004
26. Wright A: Hypoalgesia post-manipulative therapy: a review of a potential neurophysiological mechanism. Manual Ther 1:11-16, 1995
27. Christian GF, Stanton GJ, Sissons D, et al.: Immunoreactive ACTH, beta-endorphin, and cortisol levels in plasma following spinal manipulative therapy. Spine 13:1411-1417, 1988
28. Wang HL, Keck JF: Foot and hand massage as an intervention for postoperative pain. Pain Manage Nurs 5:59-65, 2004
29. Simmons DG, Travell JG, Simons LS, Cummings BD: Travell and Simons' Myofascial Pain and Dysfunction: The Trigger Point Manual, ed 2. Baltimore, Williams & Wilkins, 1999, pp 1664
30. Dommerholt J: Dry needling in orthopaedic physical therapy practice. Orthop Pract 16:11-16, 2004
31. Cornwall J, Harris A, Mercer SR: The lumbar multifidus muscle and patterns of pain. Manual Ther 11:40-45, 2006
32. Gerwin RD, Dommerholt J, Shah JP: An expansion of Simons' integrated hypothesis of trigger point formation. Curr Pain Headache Rep 8:468-475, 2004
33. Fischer AA: Pressure algometry over normal muscles. Standard values, validity and reproducibility of pressure threshold. Pain 30:115-126, 1987
34. Haussler KK, Erb HN: Mechanical nociceptive thresholds in the axial skeleton of horses. Equine Vet J 38:70-75, 2006
35. Varcoe-Cocks K, Sagar KN, Jeffcott LB, et al.: Pressure algometry to quantify muscle pain in racehorses with suspected sacroiliac dysfunction. Equine Vet J 38:558-562, 2006
36. Baxter DG, McDonough SM: Principles of electrotherapy in veterinary physiotherapy, in McGowan C, Goff L, Stubbs N (eds): Animal Physiotherapy: Assessment, Treatment and Rehabilitation of Animals. Oxford, Blackwell Publishing, 2007, pp 177-186
37. Ramey DW, Basford JA: Laser therapy in horses. Compend Contin Educ Pract Vet 22:263-273, 2000
38. Bjordal JM, CouppéC: Low-level laser therapy for tendinopathy. Evidence of a dose-response pattern. Phys Ther Rev 6:91-99, 2001
39. Ekim A, Armagan O, Tascioglu F, et al.: Effect of low level laser therapy in rheumatoid arthritis patients with carpal tunnel syndrome. Swiss Med Wkly 137:347-352, 2007
40. Bjordal JM, Johnson MI, Lopes-Martins RA, et al.: Short-term efficacy of physical interventions in osteoarthritic knee pain. A systematic review and meta-analysis of randomised placebo-controlled trials. BMC Musculoskelet Disord 8:51, 2007
41. Hawkins D, Abrahamse H: Influence of broad-spectrum and infrared light in combination with laser irradiation on the proliferation of wounded skin fibroblasts. Photomed Laser Surg 25:159-169, 2007
42. Hawkins DH, Abrahamse H: The role of laser fluence in cell viability, proliferation, and membrane integrity of wounded

human skin fibroblasts following helium-neon laser irradiation. Lasers Surg Med 38:74-83, 2006
43. Yamada H, Kameya T, Abe N, et al.: Low level laser therapy in horses. Laser Ther 1:31-35, 1989
44. McKibbin LS, Paraschak DM: A study of the effects of lasering on chronic bowed tendons at Wheatley Hall Farm Limited, Canada, January, 1983. Lasers Surg Med 3:55-59, 1983
45. Petersen SL, Botes C, Olivier A, et al.: The effect of low level laser therapy (LLLT) on wound healing in horses. Equine Vet J 31:228-231, 1999
46. Marr CM, Love S, Boyd JS, et al.: Factors affecting the clinical outcome of injuries to the superficial digital flexor tendon in National Hunt and point-to-point racehorses. Vet Rec 132:476-479, 1993
47. Petersen SL, Botes C, Olivier A, et al.: The effect of low level laser therapy (LLLT) on wound healing in horses. Equine Vet J 31:228-231, 1999
48. Yamada H, Kameya T, Abe N, et al.: Low level laser therapy in horses. Laser Ther 1:31-35, 1989
49. Dyson M, Pond JB: The effect of pulsed ultrasound on tissue regeneration. Physiotherapy 56:136-142, 1970
50. Lievens P: Electrotherapy course. Brussel, University of Brussels, 1991
51. Saini NS, Roy KS, Bansal PS, et al.: A preliminary study on the effect of ultrasound therapy on the healing of surgically severed Achilles tendons in five dogs. J Vet Med A Physiol Pathol Clin Med 49:321-328, 2002
52. Kaneps AJ: Tissue temperature response to hot and cold therapy in the metacarpal region of a horse. Proc AAEP 46:208-213, 2000
53. Herbots P: Comparison between cooling modalities: cold packs, gel bandages and cooling gel. Unpublished thesis, 1995
54. Warden SJ, Wong WT, Bennell KL, et al.: Facilitation of fracture repair using low-intensity pulsed ultrasound. Vet Comp Orthop Traumatol 13, 158-164, 2000
55. Lang DC: Ultrasonic treatment of musculoskeletal conditions in the horse, dog and cat. Vet Rec 106:427-431, 1980
56. Herbots PG, Raemdonck D: Electrodiagnostics in horses. A comparative study on gluteal and longissimus muscle. Thesis, University of Ghent, 2000
57. Herbots PG, Vallaert M: S/D-curve in horses. Determining normal values for supra-spinatus and longissimus muscle. Thesis, University of Ghent, 1995
58. Denoix JM: Electrical muscle stimulation in the horse. Effects on morphometric and hematologic parameters. Pract Vet Equine 29:173-178, 1997
59. Fraser AC: The treatment of lameness in horses by Faradism: a report on one hundred cases. Vet Rec 73:94-100, 1961
60. Watkins JP, Auer JA: Healing of surgically created defects in the equine SDFT: effects of pulsing electromagnetic field therapy on collagen-type transformation and tissue morphologic reorganization. Am J Vet Res 46:2097-2103, 1985
61. Sanders-Shamis M: A preliminary investigation of the effect of selected electromagnetic field devices on healing of canon bone osteotomies in horses. Equine Vet J 21:201-205, 1989
62. Auer JA, Burch GE, Hall P: Review of pulsing electromagnetic field therapy and its possible application to horses. Equine Vet J 15:354-360, 1983
63. Kobluk CN, Johnston GR, Lauper L: A scintigraphic investigation of magnetic field therapy on the equine third metacarpus. J Comp Orthop Traumatol 7:9-13, 1994
64. Ramey DW: Magnetic and electromagnetic therapy in horses. Compend Contin Educ Pract Vet 21:553-560, 1999
65. Turner TA: Effects of topical therapeutic modalities on skin circulation in the horse. World Equine Vet Rev 5:12, 26-29, 2000
66. Ramey DW: Cold therapy in the horse. Equine Pract 21:19-21, 1999
67. Worster AA, Gaughan EM, Hoskinson JJ, et al.: Effects of external thermal manipulation on laminar temperature and perfusion scintigraphy of the equine digit. N Z Vet J 48:111-116, 2000
68. van Eps AW, Pollitt CC: Equine laminitis: cryotherapy reduces the severity of the acute lesion. Equine Vet J 36:255-260, 2004
69. Goff L, Stubbs N: Equine treatment and rehabilitation, in McGowan C, Goff L, Stubbs N (eds): Animal Physiotherapy: Assessment, Treatment and Rehabilitation of Animals. Oxford, Blackwell Publishing, 2007, pp 238-251
70. Tellington-Jones L, Bruns U: An Introduction to the Tellington-Jones Equine Awareness Method. New York, Breakthrough, 1988, p 177
71. Wickler SJ, Hoyt DF, Clayton HM, et al.: Energetic and kinematic consequences of weighting the distal limb. Equine Vet J 36:772-777, 2004
72. Marlin D, Nankervis K: Equine Exercise Physiology. Oxford, Blackwell Science, 2002, p 304
73. Ramon T, Prades M, Armengou L, et al.: Effects of athletic taping of the fetlock on distal limb mechanics. Equine Vet J 36:764-768, 2004
74. Misumi K, Sakamoto H, Shimizu R: Changes in skeletal muscle composition in response to swimming training for young horses. J Vet Med Sci 57:959-961, 1995
75. Auer J: Diseases of the carpus. Vet Clin North Am Large Anim Pract 2:81-99, 1980
76. Tokuriki M, Ohtsuki R, Kai M, et al.: EMG activity of the muscles of the neck and forelimbs during different forms of locomotion. Equine Vet J Suppl 30:231-234, 1999
77. Irwin DH, Howell DW: Some thoughts on swimming horses in a pool. J S Afr Vet Assoc 51:189-191, 1980
78. Kato T, Ohmura H, Hiraga A, et al.: Changes in heart rate variability in horses during immersion in warm springwater. Am J Vet Res 64:1482-1485, 2003
79. Swamstrom O, Lindy M: Therapeutic swimming. Proc Annu Conv Am Assoc Equine Pract 315-322, 1973
80. DiLorenzo L, Traballesi M, Morelli D, et al.: Hemiparetic shoulder pain syndrome treated with deep dry needling during early rehabilitation: a prospective, open-label, randomized investigation. J Musculoskelet Pain 12:367-376, 2004
81. Itoh K, Katsumi Y, Hirota S, et al.: Effects of trigger point acupuncture on chronic low back pain in elderly patients—a sham-controlled randomised trial. Acupunct Med 24:5-12, 2006
82. Itoh K, Katsumi Y, Kitakoji H: Trigger point acupuncture treatment of chronic low back pain in elderly patients—a blinded RCT. Acupunct Med 22:170-177, 2004
83. Janssens LA: Trigger points in 48 dogs with myofascial pain syndromes. Vet Surg 20:274-278, 1991

19

Appendix

19.1 Drug doses
19.2 Normal physiological values
19.3 Anticoagulants needed for various blood tests
19.4 Haematology
19.5 Biochemistry and electrolytes
19.6 Blood gas analysis
19.7 Peritoneal fluid analysis
19.8 Transtracheal and bronchoalveolar fluid analysis
19.9 Normal values for pleural fluid
19.10 Normal values for cerebrospinal fluid
19.11 Normal values for urine and urine production
19.12 Normal and abnormal values for joint fluid
19.13 Normal haemodynamics of adults and foals
19.14 Diagnosis of pituitary pars intermedia dysfunction (Cushing's disease)
19.15 The oral glucose tolerance test
19.16 Ageing horses by dentition

19.1 Drug doses

The following are approximate drug doses used in equine medicine. The inclusion of a drug or indication in this list does not imply recommendation by the authors. Many of the drugs have not been approved for use in horses. Drug doses change as new information is published, and clinicians should always use their own experience and judgement when using these doses (Tables 19.1 and 19.2).

19.2 Normal physiological values

Physical examination is discussed in Chapter 1.3 and the various organ system chapters. Some normal physiological values are given in Boxes 19.1 and 19.2.

19.3 Anticoagulants needed for various blood tests

Blood samples need to be collected in different anticoagulants for various different analyses. An outline of the appropriate anticoagulants for more commonly used tests is given in Box 19.3.

19.4 Haematology

Approximate normal values are given in Tables 19.3 and 19.4. If possible, normal values generated on the analyser to be used, from the local population of horses should be used in preference to these.

19.5 Biochemistry and electrolytes

Approximate normal values and ranges are given in Tables 19.5, 19.6, 19.7, 19.8 and 19.9. If possible, normal values generated on the analyser to be used, from the local population of horses should be used in preference to these. Interpretation of biochemistry results is outlined in Boxes 19.4 to 19.23.

19.6 Blood gas analysis

Normal values for arterial blood gas (adults and neonatal foals) and venous blood gas are given in Table 19.10.

19.7 Peritoneal fluid analysis

Normal values for peritoneal fluid are given in Table 19.11.[1–4] Interpretation of peritoneal fluid samples is discussed in Box 19.24.

References

1. Grindem CB, Fairley NM, Uhlinger CA, et al.: Peritoneal fluid values from healthy foals. Equine Vet J 22:359-361, 1990
2. Milne EM, Doxey DL, Gilmour JS: Analysis of peritoneal fluid as a diagnostic aid in grass sickness (equine dysautonomia). Vet Rec 127:162-165, 1990
3. Parry BW, Crisman MV: Serum and peritoneal fluid amylase and lipase reference values in horses. Equine Vet J 23:390-391, 1991
4. Mair T: Analysis of peritoneal fluid, in Mair T, Divers T, Ducharme N (eds): Manual of Equine Gastroenterology Philadelphia, WB Saunders, 2002, pp 16-20

Table 19.1. Approximate drug doses used in equine medicine

Drug	Dose	Route	Frequency	Notes	Reference
Acepromazine	0.02–0.06 mg/kg	IV		For standing sedation	Chapter 6.1
	0.03–0.1 mg/kg	IM		For standing sedation	Chapter 6.1
	0.01 mg/kg	IM	At surgery, and then q4–6h	Dose for use as prokinetic. Use only in well hydrated horses.	Chapter 11.2
Acetazolamide	2.2–4.4 mg/kg	PO	q12h	Dose for prophylaxis of hyperkalaemic periodic paralysis. May be insufficient dose to decrease ocular pressure.	Am J Vet Res 61:965, 2000
Acetylcysteine	200 ml of 4% solution (40 ml of 20% solution with 160 ml of water)	Enema	once	Used as a retention enema for treatment of meconium impaction in foals.	Equine Vet Educ 16:133, 2004
	10% topical solution	Ophthalmic	q1–4h	Treatment of melting corneal ulcers	CTEM5
ACTH (adrenocorticotrophic hormone)	100–250 μg	IM	q24h	Neonatal foals only. Approximate dose used to attempt to increase endogenous cortisol production in premature foals. Also suitable dose for testing adrenal function	J Vet Intern Med 21:314, 2007
Acyclovir	10 mg/kg	IV	q12h	For treatment of equine herpesvirus-1 (EHV-1)	J Vet Emerg Crit Care. 15:174, 2006
	Not recommended	PO		Bioavailability very poor. Valacyclovir is an oral alternative.	
Adequan (polysulphated glycosaminoglycans)	250 mg	Intra-articular	Once weekly		CTEM5
	1 mg/kg	IM	q24h	Once daily for 5 days	CTEM5
	0.1 ml of 5% IM product	Ophthalmic	q2h until cornea stable then q2–8h	Treatment of melting corneal ulcers	R Hepburn, personal communication
Adrenaline	0.01–0.02 mg/kg	IV	q3–5 minutes	Dose for CPR	Chapters 1.2 and 2.2
Albendazole	25 mg/kg	PO	q12h	For *Dictyocaulus arnfeldi*. 5-day course.	CTEM5
	50 mg/kg	PO	q24h	For *Strongylus vulgaris* larvae. 2-day course.	CTEM5
Albuterol	360–720 μg	Via MDI	As required	Short-acting, most useful in treatment of acute bronchoconstriction or intermittent therapy as needed in the management of chronic lower respiratory conditions	Chapter 10.2
Allopurinol	6 mg/kg	PO pNGT	Once	Neonatal foals: As a treatment for perinatal asphyxia syndrome	Irish Vet J 57:707, 2004
Altrenogest	0.044–0.088 mg/kg	PO	q24h	Maintenance of pregnancy in the first 8 weeks. Suppression of behavioural oestrous. To hasten oestrous in transitional mares (10–15 day course, then withdrawal in late transition).	Chapter 11.2
Amikacin	10 mg/kg	IV or IM	q24h	Adults	Chapter 6.3
	25 mg/kg	IV or IM	q24h	Foals	Chapter 6.3
	25–33% of systemic dose	Direct instillation via endoscope	q24h	Instil into affected bronchus. Dilute to 2–4 times the volume with saline	Chapter 10.2

Table 19.1. *Continued*

Drug	Dose	Route	Frequency	Notes	Reference
Aminocaproic acid (EACA)	20–40 mg/kg	IV	Can be repeated q6h as required	Dilute 1 : 9 in saline, deliver by slow infusion (30–60 minutes)	Chapter 8.2
Aminophylline	5–10 mg/kg	PO	q12h	Bronchodilator.	J Vet Pharmcol Ther 7:255, 2004
Aminoproparazine fumurate	0.5 mg/kg	IM IV	q12h	Smooth muscle relaxant	CTEM5
Ammonium chloride	20–520 mg/kg	PO	q24h	Used as an acidifier	CTEM5
Amoxicillin trihydrate	30 mg/kg	PO	q8h	Foals only	Chapter 6.3
Amphotericin B	0.5–0.9 mg/kg	IV	q24h	Empirical dose based on human dose, clinical cases and anecdotal positive clinical response. Dilute in 5% dextrose and give over 2–4 hours.	Chapter 6.3
Ampicillin sodium	20 mg/kg	IV or IM	q6–8h	Must be used when diluted, cannot be stored	Chapter 6.3
Ampicillin trihydrate	20 mg/kg	IM	q12h	Foals only; 20 mg/kg, q8h PO	Chapter 6.3
Arginine vasopressin	60 IU	IV	q6h	For diabetes insipidus	CTEM5
Ascorbic acid	30 mg/kg	In IV fluids	q12h		CTEM5
Aspirin	10–100 mg/kg 20 mg/kg	PO Per rectum	q12h		Can J Vet Res. 67:297, 2003
Atropine	0.005–0.01 mg/kg	IV		Ileus, mydriasis, supraventricular dysrhythmias	Chapter 9.2.1
Aurothioglucose	1 mg/kg	IM	Once weekly	Has been used for pemphigus foliaceous in the foal	JAVMA 180:400, 1982
Azathioprine	3 mg/kg	PO	q24h	Dose is safe, but bioavailability poor, therefore efficacy uncertain	Am J Vet Res 66:1578, 2005
Azithromycin	10 mg/kg	PO	q24–48h	Once a day for 5 days then q48h	Chapter 6.3
Bacampicillin	25 mg/kg	PO	q12h		Chapter 6.3
Beclomethasone	500–3750 μg/450-kg horse	MDI	q12–24h		Chapter 10.2
Benztropine mesylate	8 mg/horse	Slow IV		Given as a slow IV drip as a treatment for priaprism	JAVMA 199:1183, 1991
Bethanechol	0.025 mg/kg	SQ	q3–4h	Given after dose of 2.5 mg/500 kg SQ at 2 and 5 hours post surgery	Chapter 11.2
Bismuth subsalicylate	0.5–1 ml/kg	PO	q4–6h		CTEM5
Boldenone undecylenate	1.1 mg/kg	IV or IM	Every 3 weeks	Anabolic steroid. Detectable for greater than 6 weeks after administration	J Vet Pharm Ther 30:101, 2007
Botulinum antitoxin	200 ml/foal 500 ml/adult	IV or IM		Dose is for 100–150 U/ml concentration antitoxin	CTEM5
Botulinum toxin type B	1000 U	Into anal sphincter	once	May reduce dehiscence after repair of perineal lacerations. Causes reduction in anal tone from day 2 to day 84.	Am J Vet Res 65:26, 2004

Bretylium tosylate	3–5 mg/kg	IV	Total dose ≤10 mg/kg	Gastrointestinal side effects	Chapter 9.2.1
Bromocriptine mesylate				Very poor oral absorption. Causes local reactions if given subcutaneously. Not recommended.	
Buparvaquone	5 mg/kg	IV	q48h	Total of 4 doses. Treatment of piroplasmosis (*Babesia*)	Am J Vet Res 53:1396, 1992
Buprenorphine	0.004–0.010 mg/kg	IV			Chapter 6.1
Butorphanol	0.01–0.04 mg/kg 0.04–0.2 mg/kg	IV IM			Chapter 6.1 Chapter 6.1
Caffeine	10 mg/kg loading, then 2.5 mg/kg	PO or per rectum	As required (PRN)	For hypercapnia without hypoxaemia in neonatal foals. New evidence suggests a lack of efficacy.	Chapter 10.2
Calcium borogluconate 40%	0.1–0.5 ml/kg	IV		Over 2–3 hours. Treatment of hypocalcaemia	Chapter 6.5
Calcium gluconate 23%	0.2–1.0 ml/kg	IV		Over 2–3 hours. Treatment of hypocalcaemia	Chapter 6.5
Cambendazole	20 mg/kg	PO		For *Strongyloides westeri.*	CTEM5
Captan	3% solution	Topical			CTEM5
Carbamazepine	4 mg/kg	PO	See notes	Given q8h for 20 days, then q12–24h for 14 days. Treatment of headshaking.	Equine Vet J 32:308, 2000
Carprofen	0.5–1.1 mg/kg 0.7 mg/kg 0.7–1.3 mg/kg	IV IM PO	q24h q24h q24h		Chapter 6.2 Chapter 6.2 Chapter 6.2
Cefadroxil	20–40 mg/kg	PO	q8h	Foals only	Chapter 6.3
Cefazolin	20 mg/kg 20 mg/kg	IM IV	q8h q6–8h		Chapter 6.3 Chapter 6.3
Cefepime	11 mg/kg 2.2 mg/kg	IV IV	q8h q8h	Foals Adults	Chapter 6.3 Chapter 6.3
Cefoperazone	30 mg/kg	IV or IM	q6–8h		Chapter 6.3
Cefotaxime	40 mg/kg	IV	q6h		Chapter 6.3
Cefoxitin	20 mg/kg	IV or IM	q6h		Chapter 6.3
Cefpodoxime	10 mg/kg 20–30 mg/kg	PO IV	q8h q6h		Chapter 6.3 Chapter 6.3
Cefquinome	1–2 mg/kg 1–4 mg/kg	IV or IM IV or IM	q24h q6–12h	Adults Foals	
Ceftiofur	2.2–5 mg/kg 25–33% of systemic dose	IV or IM Direct instillation via endoscope	q12–24h q24h	 Instil into affected bronchus. Dilute to 2–4 times the volume with saline	Chapter 6.3 Chapter 10.2
Ceftriaxone	25 mg/kg	IV or IM	q12h		Chapter 6.3
Cephalexin	30 mg/kg	PO	q8h		Chapter 6.3
Cephalothin	20 mg/kg	IM	q8h		Chapter 6.3

Table 19.1. *Continued*

Drug	Dose	Route	Frequency	Notes	Reference
Cephapirin	20 mg/kg	IM	q8h		Chapter 6.3
	20–30 mg/kg	IV	q6h		Chapter 6.3
Cephradine	25 mg/kg	IV	q6h		Chapter 6.3
	25 mg/kg	PO	q6–8h	Foals only	Chapter 6.3
Charcoal (activated)	1–3 g/kg as slurry	PO		Repeat in 8h if necessary	CTEM5
Chloral hydrate	10–50 mg/kg	IV		Use a solution of less than 12%	Chapter 6.1
Chloramphenicol (palmitate or base)	50 mg/kg	PO	q6 or 12	Administer BID in foals less than 5 days of age then QID afterwards	Chapter 6.3
Chloramphenicol (sodium succinate)	25–50 mg/kg	IV	q6 or 12	Administer BID in foals less than 5 days of age then QID afterwards	Chapter 6.3
Cimetidine	6.6 mg/kg	IV	q6h		CTEM5
	16–20 mg/kg	PO	q8h	Oral absorption is very slow and variable in the horse.	Equine Vet J 22:48, 2000
Ciprofloxacin	5.5 mg/kg	IV	q12–24h	Should not be used in young growing horses: Risk of arthropathy	Chapter 6.3
Clarithromycin	7.5 mg/kg	PO	q12h		Chapter 6.3
Clenbuterol	0.8–3.2 μg/kg	PO	q12h		CTEM5
	0.8 μg/kg	IV	q12h		CTEM5
	200 μg	IM or slow IV		For uterine relaxation	CTEM5
Cloprostenol Na	250–500 μg/450-kg horse	IM		For parturition induction. Can repeat in 30–120 minutes.	CTEM5
Cromolyn Sodium	80–300 mg	Inhalation			CTEM5
Cyclophosphamide	200–300 mg/m^2	IV	q2–3 weeks		CTEM5
Cyproheptadine	0.25 mg/kg	PO	q12h	For treatment of pituitary pars intermedia dysfunction (Cushing's) and Headshaking	Equine Vet J 34:679, 2002
	0.5 mg/kg	PO	q24h	For treatment of pituitary pars intermedia dysfunction (Cushing's) and Headshaking	Equine Vet J 34:679, 2002
Cytosine arabipnoside	200–300 mg/m^2	IM or SQ	q1–2 weeks	For administration with cyclophosphamide	CTEM5
Dalteparin	50 U/kg	SQ	q24h		Chapter 8.2
Dantrolene	2–4 mg/kg	PO	q 2–7 days	For control of recurrent exertional rhabdomyolysis	Equine Vet J 35:707, 2003 Am J Vet Res 65:74, 2004
	10 mg/kg loading dose, then 2.5 mg/kg	PO	q2h	Treatment of acute rhabdomyolysis	CTEM5
	2–2.5 mg/kg	Slow IV		Dilute in saline. Treatment of acute rhabdomyolysis	CTEM5
Dembrexine	0.3–0.5 mg/kg	PO		Efficacy questioned	CTEM5
Demecarium bromide	0.25%	Ophthalmic	q12h	Treatment of glaucoma	CTEM5

Detomidine	0.004–0.02 mg/kg	IV		For standing sedation	Chapter 6.1
	0.02–0.05 mg/kg	IM		For standing sedation	Chapter 6.1
Dexamethasone	0.05–0.2 mg/kg	IV		Anti-inflammatory dose. Side effects: laminitis, immunosuppression.	Chapters 9.2.1 and 12
	0.02–0.2 mg/kg	PO			CTEM5
	100 mg/kg	IV	q24h	For 5 days to induce parturition	CTEM5
Diazepam	0.02–0.1 mg/kg	IV			Chapter 6.1
	0.1–0 2 mg/kg	IM			Chapter 6.1
	0.01–0.04 mg/kg	IV	As required	For control of seizures. Multiple doses may accumulate in the foal	Chapter 14.2
Difloxacin	7.5 mg/kg	PO	q24h	Should not be used in young growing horses: Risk of arthropathy	Chapter 6.3
Digoxin	0.0022 mg/kg	IV		Depression, anorexia, colic, dysrythmia. Monitor plasma levels.	Chapter 9.2.1
	0.011 mg/kg	PO	q12h	Depression, anorexia, colic, dysrythmia	Chapter 9.2.1
Dimercaprol	2.5–5 mg/kg	IM		Lead poisoning. Give 10% solution in oil q4h for 2 days, then q12h until recovery	CTEM5
Dimethylsulphoxide (DMSO)	0.5–1 g/kg as a 10% solution	IV	q12h	Control of cerebral oedema	Chapter 14.2
Dinoprost	10 mg/450-kg horse	IM			CTEM5
Dipyrone	5–22 mg/kg	IV or IM		As analgesic or antipyretic	CTEM5
Domperidone	1.1 mg/kg	PO	q24h	To treat poor milk production in postparturient mares. Also for Fescue toxicosis.	J Vet Intern Med 16:472, 2002
Doxepin hydrochloride	0.5–0.75 mg/kg	PO	q12h		CTEM5
Doxycycline	10 mg/kg	PO	q12h	Administer orally only. More effective in foals than in adults. IV doxycycline has severe cardiovascular side effects in horse including collapse and death	Chapter 6.3
EDTA	0.5% solution	Ophthalmic	q2–4h	For treatment of melting ulcers	CTEM5
Eltenac	0.5 mg/kg	IV	q24h		Am J Vet Res 59:1447, 1998
Enalapril	0.5 mg/kg	IV		Intravenous dose has short half-life. Bioavailability poor, and oral dose of 0.5 mg/kg not effective.	J Vet Intern Med 18:231, 2004
Enoxaparin	0.5 mg/kg	SQ	q24h		Chapter 8.2
Enrofloxacin	5.5 mg/kg	IV	q24h	Should not be used in young growing horses: Risk of arthropathy	Chapter 6.3
	7.5 mg/kg	PO	q24h	Should not be used in young growing horses: Risk of arthropathy	Chapter 6.3
Epinephrine	0.01–0.02 mg/kg	IV	q3–5 minutes	Dose for CPR	Chapters 1.2 and 2.2
Epsilon (ε)-aminocaproic acid (EACA)	20–40 mg/kg	IV	Can be repeated q6h as required	Dilute 1:9 in saline, deliver by slow infusion (30–60 minutes)	Chapter 8.2

Table 19.1. *Continued*

Drug	Dose	Route	Frequency	Notes	Reference
Erythromycin (lactobionate)	5 mg/kg	IV	q6h	Dilute and give by slow IV infusion. Dose for use as antimicrobial	Chapter 6.3
	2.2 mg/kg	IV	q6h	Dilute in 1 L of saline and give over 1 hour. Dose for use as prokinetic	Chapter 11.2
Erythromycin (phosphate, stearate, ethylsuccinate, estolate)	25 mg/kg	PO	q6–8h		Chapter 6.3
Estradiol	0.004–0.008 mg/kg	IM	q48h	For urinary incontinence	CTEM5
Estrone sulfate	0.04 mg/kg	IM	q24h		CTEM5
Ethamsylate	10–15 mg/kg	IV			Chapter 8.2
Etodolac	23 mg/kg	IV or PO	q12–24h	Bioavailability is approximately 77%. Only slightly selective for COX-2	J Vet Pharm Ther 30:43, 2007
Famotidine	4 mg/kg	PO	q8h	For treatment of gastric ulcers. Omeprazole and ranitidine may be more effective	J Vet Emerg Crit Care 11:141, 2001
	0.5 mg/kg	IV	q24h		J Vet Emerg Crit Care 11:141, 2001
Fenbendazole	5 mg/kg	PO			CTEM5
	10 mg/kg	PO		For treatment of *Parascaris equorum*	CTEM5
	50 mg/kg	PO		For treatment of *Strongyloides westeri*	CTEM5
Fenoprostalene	0.5 mg/450-kg horse	SQ			CTEM5
Fenoterol	2–4 μg/kg	MDI			CTEM5
Fentanyl	0.01–0.04 mg/kg	IV		Duration of action 15–30 minutes	Chapter 6.2
	0.22 mg/kg	IM		Duration of action 30–60 minutes	Chapter 6.2
	2 × 100 μg/hr patches/500-kg horse	Transdermal		Duration of action 48–72 hours	Chapter 6.2
Fleroxacin	5 mg/kg	IV or PO	q24h	Should not be used in young growing horses: Risk of arthropathy	Chapter 6.3
Florfenicol	20 mg/kg	IM or PO	q48h	Risk of colitis, mild diarrhoea seen in one study—change of faecal flora in another. Owners should be warned about risks of severe colitis with this drug.	Chapter 6.3
Fluconazole	14 mg/kg	PO	Loading dose		Chapter 6.3
	5 mg/kg	PO	q24h		Chapter 6.3
Flumazenil	0.5–2 mg	Slow IV		Benzodiazepine antagonist	CTEM5
Flumethasone	0.002–0.008 mg/kg	PO			CTEM5
Flunixin meglumine	0.25–1.1 mg/kg	IV	q12–24h		Chapters 6.2 and 11.2
	0.5 mg/kg	IV	q6h		Chapter 11.2
	1.1 mg/kg	IM	q24h		Chapter 6.2
Fluphenazine	25 mg/horse	IM		Duration of action 4–6 weeks. May cause muscle spasms and restlessness	Chapter 6.1

Fluprostenol	250–500 μg/horse	IM		Causes parturition in 1–36hs after dosage in mares after 320 days parturition. No effect before 320 days parturition.	Equine Vet J 16:264, 1984
Fluticasone	1000–2500 μg/450-kg horse	MDI	q12–24h		Chapter 10.2
Folic acid	40–75 mg	IM			CTEM5
Folinic acid	50–100 mg	IM			CTEM5
Follicle-stimulating hormone (FSH)	10–50 mg/450-kg horse	IV, IM or SQ			CTEM5
Furosemide (frusemide)	0.5–2 mg/kg	IV	q4–6h	For acute renal failure	Chapter 13
Gentamicin	6.6 mg/kg	IV or IM	q24h	Adults	Chapter 6.3
	12 mg/kg	IV or IM	q24h	Foals	Chapter 6.3
	25–33% of systemic dose	Direct instillation via endoscope	q24h	Instill into affected bronchus. Dilute to 2–4 times the volume with saline	Chapter 10.2
Glucagon	25–50 mg	IV			CTEM5
Glutamine	0 4 g/kg/day	PO		Divide into multiple feeds or doses.	Human dose
Glycopyrrolate	0 05–0.1 μg/kg	IV			Chapter 9.2.1
Glycosaminoglycans polysulphated (Adequan)	250 mg	Intra-articular	Once weekly		CTEM5
	1 mg/kg	IM	q24h	Once daily for 5 days	CTEM5
	0 1 ml of 5% IM product	Ophthalmic	q2h until cornea stable then q2–8h	Treatment of melting corneal ulcers	R Hepburn, personal communication
Gonadotrophin-releasing hormone	0 05 mg	SQ		120 and 30 minutes before breeding for poor libido	CTEM5
	0.04 mg	IM		6 hours before breeding to induce ovulation	CTEM5
Griseofulvin	10 g/450-kg horse	PO	q24h	After 2 weeks, reduce dose to 5 g/450 kg	CTEM5
Guaifenesin	25–100 mg/kg	IV		Induction of anaesthesia	Chapter 4
Heparin	40–60 IU	IV or SQ	q8–12h	Causes erythrocyte agglutination	Chapter 8.2
Hetastarch	2–10 ml/kg	IV		Maximum daily dose 10 ml/kg	Chapter 6.5
Hyaluronate Na	10–50 mg/joint	Intra-articular		See manufacturer's recommendation	CTEM5
	500 mg	IM	q4days	For 7 doses	CTEM5
Hyaluronic acid	20–50 mg	Intra-articular			CTEM5
	20–120 mg			Around inflamed tendon	CTEM5
Hydralazine	0.5 mg/kg	IV			CTEM5
Hydrochlorothiazide	0.7 mg/kg	PO	q12h		Res Vet Sci 59:95, 1995
Hydrocortisone sodium succinate	1–4 mg/kg	IV drip			CTEM5
Hydroxyethyl starch				See Hetastarch or Pentastarch	Chapter 6.5
Hydroxyzine	0.5–1 mg/kg	IM or PO			CTEM5

Table 19.1. *Continued*

Drug	Dose	Route	Frequency	Notes	Reference
Hyoscine	0.2 mg/kg	IV			Vet Rec 129:378, 1991
Hypertonic saline	2–4 ml/kg	IV		7–7.5% sodium chloride. Must be followed up by at least 5 times the volume of isotonic crystalloids	Chapter 6.5
Ibuprofen	25 mg/kg	PO	q8h	Foals: up to 6 days' duration of treatment	Am J Vet Res 60:1066, 1999
Imidocarb	2 mg/kg 4 mg/kg	PO PO	q24h q72h	For 2 doses. For treatment of *Babesia caballi* For 4 doses. For treatment of *Babesia equi*	Vet Parasit 138:147, 2006 Vet Parasit 138:147, 2006
Imipenem-cilastatin	10–15 mg/kg	IV or IM	q8–12h	Foals: for treatment of severe infections. Dilute IM prep in 1% lidocaine.	Human dose
Insulin (regular)	0.1–0.5 IU	SQ	q12h	Less reliable than constant rate infusion	Chapter 5
Insulin (protamine zinc)	0.1–0.3 IU/kg	SQ	q12h	Less reliable than constant rate infusion	Chapter 5
Interferon-alpha	50–90 U	PO	q24h	50-U dose for natural human interferon, 90 U for recombinant human interferon	Can Vet J 45:594, 2004
Ipratropium bromide	2–5 μg/kg (1200–2400 μg/horse)	MDI	q12h	Bronchodilator	Chapter 10.2
Isoflupredone acetate	10–14 mg	IM			CTEM5
Isoniazid	5–20 mg/kg	PO	q24h		CTEM5
Isoxsuprine	0.4–1.2 mg/kg	IM	q12h	Oral bioavailability is very poor	CTEM5
Itraconazole	5 mg/kg	PO	q24h		Chapter 6.3
Ivermectin	0.2 mg/kg	PO			CTEM5
Ketamine	1.7–2.2 mg/kg 0.2–0.80 mg/kg 1.0–2.0 mg/kg	IV IV IM		Induction of anaesthesia As an analgesic. Duration of action 15 minutes As an analgesic. Duration of action 30–60 minutes	Chapter 4 Chapter 6.2 Chapter 6.2
Ketoconazole	30 mg/kg (in 0.2N HCl)	Intragastric	q12h	Administer by nasogastric tube to prevent irritation by HCl	Chapter 6.3
Ketoprofen	2.2 mg/kg	IV or IM			Chapter 6.2
Lactulose	0.3 ml/kg	PO	q6–12h		Chapter 12.2
Levamisole	8–11 mg/kg	PO	q24h		CTEM5
Levothyroxine	10 mg	PO	q24h	Administer in 70 ml Karo syrup.	CTEM5
Lidocaine (lignocaine)	0.5–1 mg/kg	IV		Dose for ventricular tachycardia, acute onset. May cause CNS excitability.	Chapter 9.2.1
Lorazepam	0.1 mg/kg	IV	PRN	For control of seizures. Anticonvulsive effects longer lasting than diazepam in humans.	Human dose
Magnesium sulphate	1–2.5 g/450 kg/min 1 g/kg	IV pNGT	Total dose ≤25 gram q12–24h	 For treatment of large colon impactions. More frequent dosing may result in signs of toxicity.	Chapter 9.2.1 Chapter 11.2

Mannitol	0.25–2 g/kg as 20% solution	IV	q12–24h	For control of cerebral oedema	Chapter 14.2
Marbofloxacin	2 mg/kg	IV or PO	q24h	Should not be used in young growing horses: Risk of arthropathy	Chapter 6.3
Meclofenamic acid	2.2 mg/kg	PO	q12h		CTEM5
Medetomidine	0.004–0.01 mg/kg 0.01–0.02 mg/kg	IV IM		For standing sedation	Chapter 6.1 Chapter 6.1
Meloxicam	0.6 mg/kg	IV or IM			Chapter 6.2
Meperidine	0.4–2.0 mg/kg	IM		Intravenous administration can cause histamine release. Duration of action 90 minutes	Chapter 6.1
Mepyramine	1 mg/kg	IV, IM or SQ		Antihistamine	CTEM5
Methadone	0.12 mg/kg	IV		Duration of action approximately 60 minutes	Chapter 6.2
Methocarbamol	5–55 mg	Slow IV	q6h	High end of dose range for severe tetanus (controversial treatment)	CTEM5
Methylene Blue	8.8 mg/kg			As a 1% solution. Not effective for Red Maple toxicity	CTEM5
Methylprednisolone acetate	0.2–0.7 mg/kg	IM			CTEM5
Methylprednisolone sodium succinate	30 mg/kg	IV		For head trauma. Give within 8 hours of injury. Follow by 5.4 mg/kg/hr continuous infusion for 24–48 hours	Vet Clin N Am Equine Pract 20:199, 2004
Methylsulphomethane (MSM)	10 g/450-kg horse	PO	q12h		Am J Vet Res 53:1908, 1992
Metoclopramide	40–60 mg/450-kg horse	IV	q6h	Dilute in 1 L of saline and give over 1 hour. Not as effective as a constant rate infusion. Dose for use as prokinetic.	Chapter 11.2
Metronidazole	25 mg/kg 35 mg/kg 15 mg/kg loading dose, then 7.5 mg/kg 25–33% of systemic dose	PO Per rectum IV Direct instillation via endoscope	q12h q12h q6h q24h	Instil into affected bronchus. Dilute to 2–4 times the volume with saline	Chapter 6.3 Chapter 6.3 Chapter 10.2
Midazolam	0.02–0.1 mg/kg 0.1–0.2 mg/kg	IV IM			Chapter 6.1 Chapter 6.1
Misoprostol	1–4 µg/kg	PO	q24h		CTEM5
Morphine	0.02–0.2 mg/kg 0.2–0.6 mg/kg	IV IM		Can cause excitement in the absence of severe pain. Duration of action 30–90 minutes. Can cause excitement in the absence of severe pain. Duration of action 60–180 minutes.	Chapters 6.1 and 6.2 Chapters 6.1 and 6.2
MSM (methylsulphomethane)	10 g/450-kg horse	PO	q12h		Am J Vet Res 53:1908, 1992

Table 19.1. *Continued*

Drug	Dose	Route	Frequency	Notes	Reference
Naloxone	0.05 mg/kg	IV		Defaecation often follows the administration within approximately 15–20 minutes. Dose for use as prokinetic.	Chapter 11.2
Nandrolone decanoate	0.85 mg/kg	IM	q1week		
Neomycin	10–20 mg/kg	IM	q24h	Nephropathy at 10 mg/kg q12h after 4 days treatment.	Equine Vet J 17:30, 1985
	15 mg/kg	PO	q6h	Short course in combination with lactulose for treatment of hepatic encephalopathy	Chapter 12
Neostigmine	0.022–0.044 mg/kg	SQ or IV		If no clinical response (cramping/restlessness) dose may be increased by 2 mg to total of 10 mg per treatment	Chapter 11.2
Niclosamide	100 mg/kg			For treatment of tapeworms	CTEM5
Oestradiol	0.004–0.008 mg/kg	IM	q48h	For urinary incontinence	CTEM5
Oestrone sulfate	0.04 mg/kg	IM	q24h		CTEM5
Omeprazole	4 mg/kg	PO	q24h	For treatment of gastric ulcers	Equine Vet J Suppl 29:67, 1999
	1 mg/kg	PO	q24h	For prevention of gastric ulcers in horses in heavy work	JAVMA 230:1680, 2007
	0.5–1.5 mg/kg	IV	q24h		J Vet Intern Med 20:1202, 2006
Orbifloxacin	7.5 mg/kg	PO	q24h	Should not be used in young growing horses: Risk of arthropathy	Chapter 6.3
Oxacillin	25 mg/kg 25 mg/kg	IM IV	q8–12h q6h		Chapter 6.3 Chapter 6.3
Oxfendazole	10 mg/kg	PO			CTEM5
Oxibendazole	10–15 mg/kg 15 mg/kg	PO PO		 Dose for *Strongyloides westeri*	CTEM5 CTEM5
Oxymorphone	0.005–0.03 mg/kg 0.02–0.05 mg/kg	IV IM		Duration of action 45–60 minutes Duration of action 90–120 minutes	Chapter 6.2 Chapter 6.2
Oxytetracycline	5 mg/kg 44–70 mg/kg	IV IV	q12h Once only	Dilute and give by slow IV infusion Dose for tendon contracture in foals. Small risk of nephropathy, especially with repeated doses.	Chapter 6.3 CTEM5
Oxytocin	10–20 IU/450-kg horse 1–3 IU/450-kg horse 5–10 IU/450-kg horse 0.11–0.22 IU/kg	IV or IM IV or IM IV IV	 q15–20mins 	 For milk let-down To induce parturition For oesophageal obstruction. Controversy exists over the efficacy of this treatment	CTEM5 CTEM5 CTEM5 Equine Vet J32:151, 2000
Pancuronium	0.04–0.066 mg/kg	IV			CTEM5

Parvaquone	20 mg/kg	IM	once	Treatment of piroplasmosis (*Babesia equi*)	Am J Vet Res 48:1613, 1987
Penicillamine D	3–4 mg/kg	PO	q6h	For 10 days	CTEM5
Penicillin G (Na, K)	25000 IU/kg	IV	q6h		Chapter 6.3
Penicillin G (procaine)	25000 IU/kg	IM	q12h		Chapter 6.3
Pentastarch	2–15 ml/kg	IV		Maximum daily dose 15 ml/kg	Chapter 6.5
Pentazocine	0.99 mg/kg 2.2 mg/kg	IV IM			Chapter 6.2 Chapter 6.2
Pentobarbital	2–20 mg/kg	IV	q4h or as needed	For control of seizures. May cause excessive sedation and respiratory depression. Euthanasia solutions are usually not sterile.	Chapter 14.2
Pentoxifylline	10 mg/kg	PO	q12h	Plasma concentration decreases with repeated dosing. May need to increase dose with prolonged therapy	Am J Vet Res 67:1621, 2006
Pergolide	0.0017 mg/kg	PO	q24h	For treatment of pituitary pars intermedia dysfunction (Cushing's)	Equine Vet J 34:679, 2002
Perphenazine	0.375 mg/kg	PO	q12h	Excitability and hyperaesthesia have been reported after its administration	Chapter 6.1
Pethidine	0.4–2.0 mg/kg	IM		Intravenous administration can cause histamine release. Duration of action 90 minutes	Chapters 6.1 and 6.2
Phenobarbital	12 mg/kg loading dose, followed by 6.6 mg/kg	IV	q12h	For control of seizures. May cause excessive sedation and respiratory depression	Chapter 14.2
	11 mg/kg	PO	q24h	Clearance increases with prolonged treatment, and the dose may need to be increased. Ideally measure and maintain blood concentration of 20 µg/ml. Avoid ivermectin, chloramphenicol and tetracyclines in horses on treatment	Chapter 14.2
Phenoxybenzamine	0.7–1 mg/kg	Slow IV	q6–8h	Dilute in 500 ml saline. Has been used as a prokinetic agent.	CTEM5
Phenylbutazone	2.2–4.4 mg/kg 2.2–4.4 mg/kg	IV PO	q12h q12h	Irritant when used intramuscularly Do not exceed a total daily dosage of 8.8 mg/kg	Chapter 6.2 Chapter 6.2
Phenylephrine	4–10 mg/horse	Slow IV		Give over 15 minutes. For splenic contraction in horses with nephrosplenic entrapment.	Proc ACVS 1996
Phenytoin	1–2 mg/kg	PO	q8h	For maintenance control of seizures	Chapter 14.2
	20 mg/kg	PO	q12h	Treatment of ventricular tachycardia and ventricular premature depolarisations. Give for 3–4 doses then 10–15 mg/kg PO q12h. Sedation and drowsiness, excitability at high concentrations	Chapter 9.2.1
Physostigmine	0.1–0.6 mg/kg	IM or slow IV			CTEM5
Piperazine	88–110 mg/kg				CTEM5

Table 19.1. *Continued*

Drug	Dose	Route	Frequency	Notes	Reference
Pirbuterol	600 μg/450-kg horse	MDI	As required	Short-acting, most useful in treatment of acute bronchoconstriction or intermittent therapy as needed in the management of chronic lower respiratory conditions	Chapter 10.2
Pivampicillin	25 mg/kg	PO	q12h		Chapter 6.3
Plasma ("fresh frozen" or fresh equine plasma)	6–20 ml/kg approximate dose required	IV	Continue until bleeding stops	For emergency treatment of bleeding due to consumption of coagulation factors	Chapter 8.2
Polymixin B	1000–5000 IU/kg	IV	q8–12h	Dilute in 5% glucose or 5% dextrose. Higher dose effective 30 minutes after onset of endotoxaemia. Slight risk of nephropathy.	Chapter 11.2
Ponazuril	5 mg/kg	PO	q24h	For treatment of equine protozoal myeloencephalopathy. 28-day course recommended.	J Parasitol 92:637, 2006
Potassium chloride	0.1–0.2 g/kg	PO		For supplementation of potassium in hypokalaemia	Chapter 13
Potassium iodide	10–40 mg/kg	PO	q24h	May cause abortion in pregnant mares	Chapter 6.3
Pralidoxime chloride	20–50 mg/kg	Slow IV or IM		For organophosphate toxicity	CTEM5
Praziquantel	0.5–1.0 mg/kg	PO		Dose for tapeworms	CTEM5
Prednisolone	0.2–4.4 mg/kg	PO or IM	q12–24h		CTEM5
Primidone	1–2 g/foal	PO	q12–16h	Long-term or maintenance treatment of seizures	CTEM5
Procainamide	1 mg/kg/min	IV	Up to a total dose of 20 mg/kg	Causes GI disturbances as quinidine	Chapter 9.2.1
	22–35 mg/kg	PO	q8h		Chapter 9.2.1
Progesterone	300 mg	IM	q24h	To maintain pregnancy. Questionable efficacy beyond 8 weeks of gestation.	CTEM5
Promazine	0.25–1 mg/kg	IV		Acepromazine is preferred	CTEM5
Propafenone	0.5–1 mg/kg	IV		Gastrointestinal side effects, bronchoconstriction in horses with respiratory disease	Chapter 9.2.1
	2 mg/kg	PO	q8h	Gastrointestinal side effects, bronchoconstriction in horses with respiratory disease	Chapter 9.2.1
Propionibacterium acnes bacterin	4 ml/450 kg	IV		0.4 mg/ml preparation. Repeat administration 2 and 6 days after initial injection.	JAVMA 231:107, 2007
Propofol	1–3 mg/kg 1 mg/kg 0.15–0.3 mg/kg/min	IV IV IV	 PRN infusion	Anaesthetic induction of neonatal foals Maintenance of anaesthesia in foals Maintenance of anaesthesia in foals	Chapter 4 Chapter 4 Chapter 4
Propranalol	0.03 mg/kg	IV		Bronchoconstriction in horses with severe respiratory disease	Chapter 9.2.1
Psyllium mucilloid	1 g/kg	PO	q6–24h	Treatment of sand colic (controversial)	CTEM5
Pyrantel embonate	38 mg/kg	PO		Dose for tapeworms	CTEM5

Pyrimethamine	1 mg/kg	PO	q24h		Chapter 6.3
Quinidine gluconate	1 mg/kg	IV	Every 5–10 minutes	Up to a total dose of 12 mg/kg. Alternatively this 10–12 mg/kg may be given as infusion over 1–2 hours. May cause depression, GI signs.	Chapter 9.2.1
Quinidine sulphate	22 mg/kg	pNGT	q2h for up to 5 treatments then q6h	Treat until converted or toxic (plasma >5 μg/ml) May cause multiple side effects see Chapter 9.2.1.	Chapter 9.2.1
Ranitidine	6.6 mg/kg 1.5 mg/kg	PO IV	q8h q8h		CTEM5 CTEM5
Reserpine	1.0–2.0 mg/horse 1.0–2.5 mg/horse	IV IM	q48h q48h		Chapter 6.1 Chapter 6.1
Rifampin	5 mg/kg	PO	q12h		Chapter 6.3
Romifidine	0.05–0.12 mg/kg 0.1–0.2 mg/kg	IV IM		For standing sedation	Chapter 6.1 Chapter 6.1
Salbutamol	360–720 μg/450-kg horse	MDI	As required	Short-acting, most useful in treatment of acute bronchoconstriction or intermittent therapy as needed in the management of chronic lower respiratory conditions	Chapter 10.2
Selenium (Na Selenite)	5.5 mg/450-kg horse	IM			CTEM5
Sildenafil	0.5–2.5 mg/kg	PO	Up to q4h	Treatment of pulmonary hypertension in neonatal foals	Vet Clin N Am Equine Pract 21:457, 2005
Sodium bicarbonate	Up to 150 g/horse	PO	q8h	Management of horses with type I renal tubular acidosis	JAVMA 190:297, 1987
Sodium iodide (20% solution)	20–40 mg/kg	IV	q24h	May cause abortion in pregnant mares	Chapter 6.3
Sodium thiosulphate (20%)	0.22 ml/kg	Slow IV		Antidote for cyanide poisoning	CTEM5
Stanozolol	0.55 mg/kg	IM	Every 1–2 weeks	Anabolic steroid. Detectable for greater than 6 weeks after administration	J Vet Pharm Ther 30:101, 2007
Stilbestrol	30 mg/450-kg horse	IM			CTEM5
Sucralfate	1–4 g/foal	PO	q6–12h		CTEM5
Sulphadiazine	24 mg/kg	PO	q12–24h		Chapter 6.3
Terbutaline	0.02–0.06 mg/kg	IV or inhalation	q12h	This dose from CTEM5. However, oral bioavailability <1% and half-life after IV administration very short, meaning drug is highly unlikely to be useful	Am J Vet Res 61:761, 2000
Testosterone (aqueous)	0.1–0.2 mg/kg	SQ	q48h	For inadequate libido	CTEM5
Tetanus antitoxin	100 IU/kg	IM, SQ or IV	q3–5 days	For treatment of tetanus	CTEM5
Theophylline	5 mg/kg	PO	q12h		J Vet Pharm Ther 12:189, 1989
Thiabendazole	44 mg/kg	PO		Double this dose for *Parascaris equorum*	CTEM5
Thiamine HCl	0.5–5 mg/kg	IM			CTEM5

Table 19.1. *Continued*

Drug	Dose	Route	Frequency	Notes	Reference
Thiopental	6–10 mg/kg	IV		Induction of anaesthesia	Chapter 4
Thyroxine L	0.01 mg/kg	PO	q24h		CTEM5
Ticarcillin	50 mg/kg	IV	q6h		Chapter 6.3
Ticarcillin-clavulanic acid	50 mg/kg	IV	q6h		Chapter 6.3
Tinidazole	15 mg/kg	PO	q12h		Chapter 6.3
Tocopherol acetate	6000 IU/250–500 kg	PO	q24h		CTEM5
Tolazoline	0.5 mg/kg	IV			CTEM5
Tranexamic acid	5–25 mg/kg	IV, IM, SQ	q12h	Little published data regarding its use in horses	Chapter 8.2
Triamcinolone	0.02–0.1 mg/kg 1–3 mg/site	IM Intralesional		 Up to a total of 18 mg	CTEM5 CTEM5
Trichlormethiazide	200 mg/450-kg horse	PO			CTEM5
Trichlorphon	40 mg/kg	PO			CTEM5
Trimethroprim-sulphonamide	30 mg/kg (combined)	PO or IV	q12h	Give IV preparation slowly. Do not use IV preparation concurrently with detomidine, potentially fatal.	Chapter 6.3
Tripelennamine	1 mg/kg	IV or IM		H_1-receptor antagonist	CTEM5
Tulathromycin	2.5 mg/kg	IM	q1wk	Macrolide antibiotic. Efficacy against *R. equi* controversial	Vet J 174:418, 2007
Valacyclovir	40 mg/kg	PO	q8h	Anti–herpes virus drug	Antimicrob Agents Chemother 51:4308, 2007
Vancomycin	4.5–7.5 mg/kg	IV	q8h	Use only when organism resistant to all other antimicrobials. Dilute and administer over 1 hour	Chapter 6.3
Vedaprofen	2 mg/kg loading then 1 mg/kg	PO	q12h		Theriogenology 64:1867, 2005
Verapamil	2.2 mg/kg	SQ	q8h	Efficacy questionable	Vet Surg 22:496, 1993
Vicristine	0.01–0.025 mg/kg	IV	q7days		CTEM5
Vinegar	250 ml/450-kg horse	PO	q24h	For enterolith prevention	CTEM5
Vitamin C	30 mg/kg	IV infusion	q12h	Give in IV fluids	CTEM5
Vitamin K	0.5–2.5 mg/kg	IV, IM, SQ		Give for 3–5 days or until normalisation of PT value occurs	Chapter 8.2
Voriconazole	4 mg/kg	PO	q24h		Chapter 6.3
Xylazine	0.2–1.1 mg/kg 0.5–2.2 mg/kg	IV IM		For standing sedation	Chapter 6.1 Chapter 6.1
Yohimbine	0.075 mg/kg	IV		Give over 10 minutes. Dose for use as prokinetic.	Chapter 11.2

IV, intravenously; IM, intramuscularly; PO, by mouth; MDI, metered-dose inhaler; pNGT, by nasogastric tube; PRN, as needed; CTEM5, Robinson NE: Current Therapy in Equine Medicine, ed 5. Philadelphia, WB Saunders, 2003.

Table 19.2. Constant rate intravenous infusions

Drug	Loading dose	Loading dose administration time	Infusion rate	Comments	Reference
Butorphanol			13 μg/kg/hr	Dose for postoperative analgesia in colic patients	Chapter 11.2
	0.018 mg/kg		0.38 μg/kg/min	Analgesia	Chapter 6.1
Detomidine	0.006–0.015 mg/kg		0.1–0.6 μg/kg/min	For standing sedation	Chapter 6.1
Dobutamine			2–20 μg/kg/min	Foals. For support of cardiac output. May cause tachycardia and dysrhythmias, especially in under fluid-resuscitated animals.	Chapter 9.2.2
			0.25–5 μg/kg/min	Adults. For support of cardiac output. May cause tachycardia and dysrhythmias, especially in under fluid-resuscitated animals.	Chapter 9.2.2
Dopamine			3–25 μg/kg/min	For support of blood pressure and cardiac output. No evidence to support low-dose for acute renal failure. Norepinephrine/dobutamine combination preferred.	Chapter 9.2.2
Doxapram	0.5 mg/kg		0.03–0.08 mg/kg/min	For hypercapnia without hypoxaemia in neonatal foals. May induce tachycardia or increase oxygen consumption while increasing ventilatory drive, resulting in worsening of hypoxaemia.	Chapter 10.2
Epinephrine			0.1–2 μg/kg/min	For support of blood pressure. Patient must be monitored carefully during infusion.	Chapter 9.2.2
Fenoldopam			0.04 μg/kg/min	Possibly increases renal perfusion and might be beneficial in acute renal failure.	Chapter 13
Insulin (regular)			0.01–2.0 IU (units)/kg/hr	Start low and titrate upwards—see Tables 5.13 and 5.14.	Chapter 5
Ketamine	0.5–1 mg/kg		6.7–13.3 μg/kg/min	Dose for analgesia	Chapter 6.2
			10–50 μg/kg/min	Dose for control of seizures. Consider for seizures refractory to benzodiazepines.	Human dose
Lidocaine	1.3–3 mg/kg	15 minutes	0.03–0.05 mg/kg/min	Dose for ileus and analgesia. If discontinued for periods of greater than 45–60 minutes, bolus dose should be repeated. Do not use with IV cimetidine.	Chapters 6.2 and 11.2
	0.65 mg/kg	15 minutes	0.025 mg/kg/min	Dose for use in anaesthetised horses.	
			0.02–0.05 mg/kg/min	Dose for ventricular tachycardia, acute onset. May cause CNS excitability.	Chapter 9.2.1
Medetomidine	0.005 mg/kg		0.06 μg/kg/min		Chapter 6.1
Methylene Blue	2 mg/kg		0.25–1 mg/kg/hr	1% solution. Experimental human dose for increasing blood pressure in septic shock.	Crit Care Med 29:1860, 2001
Metoclopramide			0.04 mg/kg/hr	Dilute in 0.9% sodium chloride solution. May cause muscle spasms, motor restlessness and aggression.	Chapter 11.2
"MLK" infusion			2 ml/hr	Potent analgesic combination infusion. Add 20–60 mg morphine, 300 mg lidocaine and 60 mg ketamine per litre.	Am J Vet Res 64:1155, 2003
Morphine	0.3 mg/kg		0.05 mg/kg/hr	Must give α_2-agonist with loading dose to prevent excitement reaction. May cause decreased large intestinal motility and faecal production.	Chapter 11.2
Nitroprusside sodium			0.33 μg/kg/min	Starting rate. Monitor blood pressure very carefully. Dilute in 5% glucose or 5% dextrose and protect from light.	J Vet Intern Med 5:80, 1991
Norepinephrine			0.1–5 μg/kg/min	For support of blood pressure. Patient must be monitored carefully during infusion.	Chapter 9.2.2
Vasopressin			0.25 mU/kg/min	Starting rate. Can be increased to effect. May significantly reduce gastrointestinal perfusion, especially in under fluid resuscitated animals.	Chapter 9.2.2
Xylazine	1.0 mg/kg		12 μg/kg/min	For standing sedation	Chapter 6.1

Box 19.1. Normal physiological values for adult horse

Rectal temperature	37.5–38.5° C 99.5–101.5° F
Heart rate	30–40 bpm
Respiratory rate	8–16 bpm
Capillary refill time	1–2 seconds
Gut sounds	Mixing sounds: 2–4 times per minute Progressive sounds: every 2–4 minutes
Puberty (mare)	12–15 months
Reproductive cycle	19–35 days (average 21–22 days)
Puberty (stallion)	11–15 months
Testicle size (Thoroughbred)	8–12 cm long × 5 cm wide, total scrotal width 8 cm
Urine production	1.24 ml/kg/hr
Faecal production	20–28 g/kg/day (when fed 1.5 kg hard feed and ad libitum hay)

Box 19.2. Normal physiological values for neonatal foals

Gestation	341 days (315–365 days)
Rectal temperature	37.2–38.9° C 99.0–102.0° F
Heart rate	
• After delivery	40–80 bpm
• Attempting to stand	130–150 bpm
• First few days	70–100 bpm (greater if active)
Respiratory rate	
• First hour	60–80 bpm
• After first hour	20–40 bpm
Capillary refill time	<2 seconds
Righting reflex	Within 5 minutes of birth
Suckle reflex	Within 20 minutes of birth
Menace reflex	Negative
Time to stand	Average 57 minutes, range 15–165 minutes
Time to nurse	Average 111 minutes, range 35–420 minutes
First urination	Colts: 6 hours Fillies: 10.8 hours
Urine production	6.17 ml/kg/hr

Box 19.3. Anticoagulants for various blood tests

Haematology
EDTA—usually lavender, pink or purple lid or top

Platelet count
Usually done with haematology on EDTA sample
If query of clumping: Citrate—usually light blue top

Biochemistry and hormones (unless listed below)
Plain tube—usually red top
Clot activator and gel—usually red/black or gold top
Many biochemistry tests can be run on plasma
 Lithium heparin—usually green or orange top or lid

Glucose
Fluoride oxalate—usually grey top

Ammonia
Lithium heparin—usually green or orange top or lid. Must be run within 2 hours of taking

PT, aPTT and fibrinogen
Citrate—usually light blue top

Glutathionine peroxidase
Lithium heparin—usually green or orange top or lid

Blood lead
Lithium heparin—usually green or orange top or lid

ACTH
EDTA—usually lavender, purple top—separate plasma and freeze within 15 minutes

Table 19.3. Normal haematology values in adult horses

	Hot-blooded breeds	Cold-blooded breeds		Hot-blooded breeds	Cold-blooded breeds
Red blood cell ($\times 10^{12}$/L; $\times 10^{6}$/μl)	6.8–12.9	5.5–9.5	Lymphocytes (μl)	1,500–7,700	
Mean cell volume (fl)	37–58		Monocytes ($\times 10^{9}$/L; $\times 10^{3}$/μl)	0–1	
Mean cell haemoglobin (MCH) (pg)	12.3–19.9		Monocytes (/μl)	0–1,000	
Mean cell haemoglobin concentration (%)	31–36		Eosinophils ($\times 10^{9}$/L; $\times 10^{3}$/μl)	0–1	
Haemoglobin (g/dl)	11–19	8–14	Eosinophils (/μl)	0–1,000	
Packed cell volume (%)	32–53	24–44	Basophils ($\times 10^{9}$/L; $\times 10^{3}$/μl)	0–0.29	
Total leukocytes ($\times 10^{9}$/L; $\times 10^{3}$/μl)	5.4–14.3	6.0–12.0	Basophils (μl)	0–290	
Total leukocytes (/μl)	5,400–14,300	6,000–1,2000	Platelets ($\times 10^{9}$/L; $\times 10^{3}$/μl)	100–350	
Neutrophils ($\times 10^{9}$/L; $\times 10^{3}$/μl)	2.26–8.58		Fibrinogen (g/L)	1–4	
Neutrophils (/μl)	2,260–8,580		Fibrinogen (mg/dl)	100–400	
Lymphocytes ($\times 10^{9}$/L; $\times 10^{3}$/μl)	1.5–7.7				

Data from Kramer JW: Normal hematology of the horse, in Feldman BF, Zinkl JG, Jain NC (eds): Schalm's Veterinary Hematology, ed 5. Baltimore, Lippincott Williams and Wilkins, 2000, pp 1069–1074.

Table 19.4. Normal haematology values in foals, weanlings and yearlings

	One day	Seven days	One month	Four months	Twelve months
Red blood cell ($\times 10^{12}$/L; $\times 10^{6}$/μl)	8.2–11.0	7.4–10.6	7.9–11.1	8.9–12.7	7.7–10.9
Mean cell volume (fl)	36–46	35–44	33–40	31–37	35–44
Mean cell haemoglobin (MCH) (pg)	13.6 ± 1.2		11.8 ± 0.8		
Mean cell haemoglobin concentration (%)	32–40	35–40	34–40	34–40	34–40
Haemoglobin (g/dl)	12–16.6	10.7–15.8	10.9–15.3	11.6–17.2	11.0–15.4
Packed cell volume (%)	32–46	28–43	29–41	32–43	31–42
Total leukocytes ($\times 10^{9}$/L; $\times 10^{3}$/μl)	4.9–11.7	6.3–13.6	5.3–12.2	6.2–14.2	6.5–11.8
Neutrophils ($\times 10^{9}$/L; $\times 10^{3}$/μl)	3.36–9.57	4.35–10.55	2.76–9.27	3.01–7.48	2.66–5.90
Lymphocytes ($\times 10^{9}$/L; $\times 10^{3}$/μl)	0.67–2.12	1.43–2.28	1.73–4.85	2.8–7.32	2.01–6.53
Monocytes ($\times 10^{9}$/L; $\times 10^{3}$/μl)	0.07–0.39	0.03–0.54	0.05–0.63	0.08–0.66	0.04–0.44
Eosinophils ($\times 10^{9}$/L; $\times 10^{3}$/μl)	0–0.02	0–0.09	0–0.12	0–0.99	0–0.78
Basophils ($\times 10^{9}$/L; $\times 10^{3}$/μl)	0–0.03	0–0.18	0–0.08	0–0.07	0–0.09
Platelets ($\times 10^{9}$/L; $\times 10^{3}$/μl)	129–409	111–387	136–468	140–388	120–316
Fibrinogen (g/L)	1–4	1.5–4.5	2–7	2.5–8	2–5.5
Fibrinogen (mg/dl)	100–400	150–450	200–700	250–800	200–550
Serum amyloid A (mg/L)	0–36.6	0–29			

Data from Harvey JW: Normal hematological values, in Koterba AM, Drummond WH, Kosch PC (eds): Equine Clinical Neonatology. Philadelphia, Lea and Febiger, 1990, pp 561–570; Kramer JW: Normal hematology of the horse, in Feldman BF, Zinkl JG, Jain NC (eds): Schalm's Veterinary Hematology, ed 5. Baltimore, Lippincott Williams and Wilkins, 2000, pp 1069–1074; Stoneham SJ, Palmer L, Cash R, et al.: Measurement of serum amyloid A in the neonatal foal using a latex agglutination immunoturbidimetric assay: determination of the normal range, variation with age and response to disease. Equine Vet J 33:599–603, 2001; and Cohen ND, Chaffin MK, Vandenplas ML, et al.: Study of serum amyloid A concentrations as a means of achieving early diagnosis of *Rhodococcus equi* pneumonia. Equine Vet J 37:212–216, 2005.

Table 19.5. Normal biochemistry values in adult horses

	Adult horse		Adult horse
Albumin (g/L)	23–36	Creatine kinase (IU/L)	119–287
Albumin (g/dl)	2.3–3.6	γ-Glutamyl transferase (γGT) (IU/L)	8–22
Alkaline phosphatase (ALP) (IU/L)	86–285	Total globulin (g/L)	17–47
Aspartate aminotransferase (AST) (IU/L)	138–409	Total globulin (g/dl)	1.7–4.7
Total bilirubin (μmol/L)	9–39	Glucose (mmol/L)	4.9–6.2
Total bilirubin (μg/dl)	0.5–2.3	Glucose (mg/dl)	89–112
Conjugated bilirubin (μmol/L)	0–10	Total protein (g/L)	58–77
Conjugated bilirubin (mg/dl)	0–0.6	Total protein (g/dl)	5.8–7.7
Unconjugated bilirubin (μmol/L)	3–34	Iditol dehydrogenase (IDH)* (IU/L)	0–8
Unconjugated bilirubin (mg/dl)	0.2–2	Triglycerides (mmol/L)	<1.13
Cholesterol (mmol/L)	1.94–3.88	Triglycerides (mg/dl)	<100
Cholesterol (mg/dl)	75–150	Urea (mmol/L)	2–4.5
Creatinine (μmol/L)	80–177	Urea (mg/dl)	12–27
Creatinine (mg/dl)	0.9–2		

*Formerly referred to as sorbitol dehydrogenase (SDH).
Data from Carlson GP: Clinical chemistry tests, in Smith BP (ed): Large Animal Internal Medicine, ed 3. St. Louis, Mosby, 2002, pp 389–412; and Dunkel B, McKenzie HC: Severe hypertriglyceridaemia in clinically ill horses: diagnosis, treatment and outcome. Equine Vet J 35:590–595, 2003.

Table 19.6. Normal biochemistry values in foals, weanlings and yearlings

	One day	One week	One month	Four months	Twelve months
Alanine transaminase (ALT) (IU/L)	0–49	4–50	5–47	8–65	5–20
Albumin (g/L)	25–36	27–34	27–34	28–37	31–38
Albumin (g/dl)	2.5–3.6	2.7–3.4	2.7–3.4	2.8–3.7	3.1–3.8
Alkaline phosphatase (ALP) (IU/L)	861–2671	137–1169	210–866	124–222	
Aspartate aminotransferase (AST) (IU/L)	146–340	237–620	252–440	280–520	283–720
Total bilirubin (μmol/L)	22–77	13–51	19–29	5–17	7–24
Total bilirubin (mg/dl)	1.3–4.5	0.8–3.0	0.5–1.7	0.3–1.0	0.4–1.4
Conjugated bilirubin (μmol/L)	5–12	5–12	2–10	2–10	2–17
Conjugated bilirubin (mg/dl)	0.3–0.7	0.3–0.7	0.1–0.6	0.1–0.6	0.1–1.0
Unconjugated bilirubin (μmol/L)	17–65	9–39	7–21	3–7	3–10
Unconjugated bilirubin (mg/dl)	1.0–3.8	0.5–2.3	0.4–1.2	0.2–0.4	0.2–0.6
Cholesterol (mmol/L)	2.8–14.5	3.6–11.5	2.2–6.0	2.4–5.4	
Cholesterol (mg/dl)	110–562	139–445	83–233	91–207	—
Creatinine (μmol/L)	106–380	88–150	97–159	115–186	115–186
Creatinine (mg/dl)	1.2–4.3	1.0–1.7	1.1–1.8	1.3–2.1	1.3–2.1
Creatine kinase (IU/L)	40–909	52–143	81–585	60–266	
γ-Glutamyl transferase (γGT) (IU/L)	18–43	14–164	17–99	0–27	
Total globulin (g/L)	15–46	16–39	18–37	27–39	22–35
Total globulin (g/dl)	1.5–4.6	1.6–3.9	1.8–3.7	2.7–3.9	2.2–3.5
Glucose (mmol/L)	6.7–12.9	6.7–10.6	7.2–12.0	6.3–10.9	5.8–9.2
Glucose (mg/dl)	121–233	121–192	130–216	113–196	105–165
Total protein (g/L)	43–81	44–68	50–67	57–73	58–66
Total protein (g/dl)	4.3–8.1	4.4–6.8	5.0–6.7	5.7–7.3	5.8–6.6
Iditol dehydrogenase (IDH)* (IU/L)	0.6–4.6	0.8–8.2	1.2–5.9	1.5–4.4	—
Triglycerides (mmol/L)	0.34–2.2	0.34–2.7	0.5–1.75	0.16–1.67	—
Triglycerides (mg/dl)	30–193	30–239	45–155	14–148	—
Urea (mmol/L)	1.5–6.6	0.7–3.3	1–3.5	1.5–4.2	2.5–4
Urea (mg/dl)	9–40	4–20	6–21	9–25	15–24

*Formerly referred to as sorbitol dehydrogenase (SDH).
Data from Bauer JE, Harvey JW, Asquith RL, et al.: Clinical chemistry reference values for foals during the first year of life. Equine Vet J 16:361–363, 1984.

Box 19.4. Guide to interpretation of total protein concentrations

↓ Total protein

Possible interpretation
- Protein losing enteropathy
- Protein losing nephropathy
- NSAID toxicity
- Acute blood loss
- Excessive fluid therapy/water intake
- GI ulceration
- Strangulating GI obstruction
- Acute peritonitis
- Glomerulonephritis
- Rare causes: Blood-sucking parasite, intestinal lymphosarcoma, urinary blood loss, disseminated intravascular coagulopathy, immune-mediated thrombocytopaenia, congestive heart failure

Further action
- Check albumin and globulin
- Check urine for protein
- Check urine and faeces for blood
- Peritoneal tap

↑ Total protein

Possible interpretation
- Dehydration
- Increased globulin: inflammation, parasitism, multiple myeloma

Further action
- Check albumin and globulin
- Assess hydration status
- Identify potential cause of dehydration

Box 19.5. Guide to interpretation of albumin concentrations

↓ Albumin

Possible interpretation
- Colitis
- Parasitism
- Glomerulonephritis
- Pyelonephritis
- NSAID toxicity
- Chronic inflammatory disease
- Chronic liver disease
- Nephrotic syndrome
- Malnutrition/starvation
- Amyloidosis
- Tuberculosis
- Histoplasmosis

Further action
- Assess renal function
- Test for intestinal malabsorption
- Assess liver function
- Consider malnutrition

↑ Albumin

Possible interpretation
- Only occurs in severe dehydration

Box 19.6. Guide to interpretation of globulin concentrations

↓ Globulin

Possible interpretation
- Severe total protein loss
- Failure of passive transfer
- Combined immunodeficiency (Arabian foals)
- IgM deficiency

Further action
- Neonatal foals—measure IgG

↑ Globulin

Possible interpretation
- Common: intestinal parasitism, infection, abdominal or thoracic abscess, EIA, purpura haemorrhagica, dehydration
- Increased α-globulins: tissue injury or acute inflammation
- Increased β-globulins: intense immune response
- Increased γ-globulins: multiple myeloma or lymphoid neoplasm
- Polyclonal increase: chronic inflammatory disease, immune-mediated disease, lymphoid neoplasm.

Further action
- Rule out common causes
- Assess if monoclonal or polyclonal if necessary (serum protein electrophoresis)

Box 19.7. Guide to interpretation of fibrinogen concentrations

↓ Fibrinogen

Possible interpretation
- May decrease after major surgery
- Hepatic failure
- Disseminated intravascular coagulopathy

Further action
- Assess for liver disease
- Assess for disseminated intravascular coagulopathy

↑ Fibrinogen

Possible interpretation
- Indication of inflammation/infection
  - Pleuritis
  - Pneumonia
  - Osteomyelitis
  - Abscess
  - Septic arthritis
  - Thrombophlebitis
  - Vasculitis/cellulitis
  - Neoplasia
  - Cholelithiasis
  - GI inflammation
  - Salmonellosis

Further action
- Assess haematology
- Examine for source of infection/inflammation
- If haematology normal consider long standing abscess, abdominal/ thoracic ultrasound may be useful.

Box 19.8. Guide to interpretation of alkaline phosphatase (ALP) activity

↑ ALP activity

Possible interpretation
- Intrahepatic or extra-hepatic obstruction of biliary system
  - Acute liver failure
  - Chronic liver failure
  - Cholangiohepatitis
  - Cholelithiasis
  - Liver fluke
  - Pyrrolizidine alkaloid toxicity
- Increased activity of osteoblasts, therefore normal in young growing animals
- Pregnancy
- Can increase with steroid therapy

Further action
- Check other liver enzymes and bile acids
- Hepatic ultrasound/biopsy if other indicators of liver disease

Box 19.9. Guide to interpretation of aspartate aminotransferase (AST) activity

↑ AST activity

Possible interpretation
- AST has high activity in liver and muscle cells
- Muscle disease
- Rhabdomyolysis
- Polysaccharide storage myopathy
- *Streptococcus equi*–associated myopathy
- Nutritional myodegeneration
- Liver disease
- Acute liver failure
- Chronic liver failure
- Cholangiohepatitis
- Cholelithiasis
- Liver fluke

Further action
- Check creatine kinase and SDH (or γGT/bile acids if SDH not available)
- If CK is increased, investigate for muscle pathology
- If SDH/γGT/bile acids increased, investigate for liver damage
- AST has long half-life. increased AST with normal or declining CK/SDH indicates damage within 7–10 days that is no longer active. Increased AST with progressive increases in CK/SDH damage active

Box 19.10. Guide to interpretation of creatine kinase (CK) activity

↑ CK activity

Possible interpretation
- Exertional rhabdomyolysis
- Moderate increases (<10000 IU/L)
  - Transportation
  - General anaesthesia
  - Periodic hyperkalemia (check K^+ during episode)
  - Polysaccharide storage myopathy
  - Strenuous exercise
- Marked increase (>10000 IU/L)
  - Acute rhabdomyolysis
  - Nutritional muscular dystrophy (confirm with biopsy)

Further action
- If symptoms of muscle stiffness postexercise, perform exercise tolerance test: Baseline CK/AST, slow trot for 20 minutes, CK/AST 4 hours postexercise. CK/AST four times baseline value = recurrent equine rhabdomyolysis. Confirm with muscle biopsy
- Muscle biopsy (see Chapter 1.55)
- Potentially check isoenzymes:
  CKMM = skeletal muscle
  CKMB = cardiac muscle
  CKBB = brain

Box 19.11. Guide to interpretation of γ-glutamyltransferase (γGT) activity

↑ γ-GT activity

Possible interpretation
- Acute liver failure
- Chronic liver failure
- Pyrrolizidine alkaloid toxicity
- Aflatoxicosis
- Liver fluke
- Cholangiohepatitis
- Cholelithiasis
- Hyperlipemia
- Obstructive disease of the duodenum

Further action
- Hepatic ultrasonography/biopsy
- Gastroscopy/duodenoscopy

Note: High levels may be expected in nursing foals as a result of absorption maternal γGT in colostrum.
Burros, donkeys and asses have a different normal range to horses: 2–3 times higher than horses.

Box 19.12. Guide to interpretation of iditol dehydrogenase (IDH) (sorbitol dehydrogenase [SDH]) activity

↑ IDH activity

Possible interpretation
- Acute hepatic cellular damage
- Anoxia from shock, anaesthesia, acute anaemia may cause moderate increase.
- Half-life of IDH is short (few hours), continued increase indicates ongoing liver damage

Further action
- Hepatic ultrasonography/biopsy
- Repeat measurement if horse is acutely ill

Box 19.13. Guide to interpretation of bile acid concentration

↑ Bile acids

Possible interpretation
- Decreased liver function
- Brief marked increases are seen in some acute colic cases, especially with strangulating small intestinal lesions

Further action
- Hepatic ultrasonography/biopsy

Box 19.14. Guide to interpretation of bilirubin concentration

↑ Bilirubin concentration

Possible interpretation
- Foals
  - Neonatal isoerythrolysis
  - Rarely—internal bleed
- Adults
  - Anorexia or starvation
  - Haemolysis
  - Intrahepatic obstruction
  - Extrahepatic obstruction

Further action
- Determine proportion of unconjugated (indirect) and conjugated (direct) bilirubin
- Relative increase in unconjugated points to prehepatic (anorexia or haemolysis)
- Relative increase in conjugated points to post hepatic (biliary tree)
- These differences may be blurred or inconsistent in the horse

Box 19.15. Guide to interpretation of calcium concentrations

↓ Calcium concentration

Possible interpretation
- Hypoalbuminaemia (total calcium concentration)
- Cantharidin (blister beetle) toxicosis
- Lactation tetany
- Transport tetany
- Acute renal failure
- Decreased intake
- Gastrointestinal disease
- Excess sweating

Further action
- Measure ionised calcium if possible
- Check albumin
- Check creatinine

↑ Calcium concentration

Possible interpretation
- Excessive calcium intake/supplementation
- Chronic renal disease
- Hyper–vitaminosis D
- Maximal exercise.
- Plant toxicosis *(Cestrum diurnum, Solanum malacoxylon)*
- Hyperparathyroidism
- Neoplasms (gastric squamous cell carcinoma, lymphosarcoma)

Further action
- Check creatinine
- Check globulin

Box 19.16. Guide to interpretation of chloride concentrations

↓ Chloride concentration

Possible interpretation
- Gastrointestinal loss (diarrhoea/reflux)
- Blood loss
- Sequestration of fluid (peritonitis/ascites/ruptured bladder)
- Renal disease
- False hypochloraemia (hyperlipidaemia, hyperproteinaemia, hyperglycaemia)
- Psychogenic polydipsia
- Inappropriate ADH secretion
- Adrenal insufficiency

Further action
- Check sodium

↑ Chloride concentration

Possible interpretation
- Water deficit
- Burns
- Intrinsic renal disease
- Diuretics
- Diabetes insipidus
- Hypertonic saline administration
- Mineralocorticoid excess

Further action
- Check sodium
- If chloride increased without a proportional increase in sodium, consider hyperchloraemic metabolic acidosis, renal tubular acidosis or uncommonly compensation for respiratory alkalosis

Box 19.17. Guide to interpretation of creatinine concentrations

↑ Creatinine concentration

Possible interpretation
- Prerenal azotaemia
  - Reduced renal blood flow
  - Hypovolaemia
  - Heart failure
  - Dehydration
- Renal azotaemia
  - Acute/chronic renal failure
- Postrenal azotaemia
  - Renal calculi
  - Ureteral calculi
  - Urethral calculi
  - Ruptured bladder
- In neonatal foals in first 48 hours of life
  - Placental insufficiency

Further action
- Check urine specific gravity
  - If isotonic (1.008–10.12), suspect renal failure
  - If hypertonic (>1.020), suspect hypovolaemia or dehydration
- Urinalysis
- Response to fluids—if creatine stays high, likely renal failure
- Renal ultrasound
- Possible renal biopsy

Box 19.18. Guide to interpretation of glucose concentrations

↓ Glucose concentration

Possible interpretation
- Inappropriate sample (unless measured immediately, should be fluoride/oxalate tube [see Box 19.3])
- Starvation
- Malabsorption
- Septicaemia
- Adrenocortical insufficiency
- Liver failure
- Extreme exertion

Further action
- Assess haematology
- Assess liver function
- Oral glucose tolerance test

↑ Glucose concentration

Possible interpretation
- Transient
  - Postprandial
  - Pain/fear
  - CNS disease
  - Transport/stress
- Pituitary pars intermedia dysfunction
- Equine metabolic syndrome
- Hyperpituitarism
- Xylazine administration
- Glucocorticoid administration

Further action
- Repeat test if patient stressed/recently transported
- Test for pituitary pars intermedia dysfunction and other metabolic diseases if persistent

Box 19.19. Guide to interpretation of magnesium concentrations

↓ Magnesium concentration

Possible interpretation
- Intestinal disease
- Renal failure
- Excessive sweating
- Hypoaldosteronism
- Cantharidin toxicosis

Further action
- Assess renal function
- Electrocardiogram

↑ Magnesium concentration

Possible interpretation
- Renal failure
- Maximum exercise
- Iatrogenic (usually magnesium sulphate [Epsom salts] overdose)

Further action
- Assess renal function

Box 19.20. Guide to interpretation of phosphate concentrations

↓ Phosphate concentration

Possible interpretation
- Chronic renal failure
- Starvation
- Refeeding syndrome
- Hyperparathyroidism
- *Brassica* toxicity

Further action
- Assess renal function

↑ Phosphate concentration

Possible interpretation
- Foals have a higher normal range
- Acute renal failure
- Nutritional secondary hyperparathyroidism

Further action
- Assess renal function

Box 19.22. Guide to interpretation of sodium concentrations

↓ Sodium concentration

Possible interpretation
- Diarrhoea
- Excessive sweating
- Gastric reflux
- Pleural drainage
- Concurrent hyperkalaemia
  - Adrenal insufficiency
  - Uroperitoneum
- Fluid sequestration (peritonitis, ascites, ruptured bladder)
- Renal disease

Further action
- Assess renal function
- Assess potassium
- Assess chloride

↑ Sodium concentration

Possible interpretation
- Dehydration
- Salt poisoning

Further action
- Assess hydration status

Box 19.21. Guide to interpretation of potassium concentrations

↓ Potassium concentration

Possible interpretation
- Common after major surgery (mineralocorticoid and glucocorticoid release)
- High-flow sodium-containing fluids
- Anorexia
- GI losses
- Excessive sweating
- Urinary loss
- Alkalaemia

↑ Potassium concentration

Possible interpretation
- False hyperkalaemia (*in vitro* haemolysis, storage over 6 hours prior to plasma separation, markedly increased leukocyte count)
- Acidaemia
- Uroperitoneum
- Tissue necrosis
- Insulin deficiency
- Oliguria
- Adrenal insufficiency
- Hereditary periodic hyperkalaemia
- Maximal exercise

Further action
- Assess renal function

Box 19.23. Guide to interpretation of urea concentrations

↓ Urea concentration

Possible interpretation
- Liver failure
- Low-protein diet
- Anabolic steroid use
- Low in neonates

↑ Urea concentration

Possible interpretation
- Prerenal azotaemia
  - Reduced renal blood flow
  - Hypovolaemia
  - Heart failure
  - Dehydration
- Renal azotaemia
  - Acute/chronic renal failure
- Postrenal azotaemia
  - Renal calculi
  - Ureteral calculi
  - Urethral calculi
  - Ruptured bladder
- Protein catabolism

Further action
- Assess creatinine
- Check urine specific gravity
  - If isotonic (1.008–10.12), suspect renal failure
  - If hypertonic (>1.020), suspect hypovolaemia or dehydration
- Urinalysis

Table 19.7. Normal electrolyte concentrations in adult horses

	Adult horse
Sodium (mmol/L)	134.7–142
Potassium (mmol/L)	3.53–4.64
Chloride (mmol/L)	97.3–103.6
Ionised calcium (mmol/L)	1.45–1.73
Ionised calcium (mg/dl)	5.8–6.9
Total calcium (mmol/L)	2.8–3.4
Total calcium (mg/dl)	11.2–13.6
Ionised magnesium (mmol/L)	0.4–0.57
Ionised magnesium (mg/dl)	0.98–1.39
Total magnesium (mmol/L)	0.9–1.15
Total magnesium (mg/dl)	2.2–2.8
Phosphate (mmol/L)	1.0–1.8
Phosphate (mg/dl)	3.1–5.6

Data from Carlson GP: Clinical chemistry tests, in Smith BP (ed): Large Animal Internal Medicine, ed 3. St. Louis, Mosby, 2002, pp 389–412; and Corley KTT (unpublished data).

Table 19.9. Normal lactate concentrations in the adult horse and foal

		Lactate concentration (mmol/L)
Adult		0.2–0.7
Foal	0 hours	0.4–4.4
	24 hours	0.6–1.9
	48 hours	0.5–1.6

Data from Magdesian KG: Blood lactate levels in neonatal foals: normal values and temporal effects in the post-partum period [abstract]. J Vet Emerg Crit Care 13:174, 2003; and Corley KTT (unpublished data).

Table 19.8. Normal electrolyte concentrations in foals, weanlings and yearlings

	One day	One week	One month	Four months	Twelve months
Sodium (mmol/L)	141 ± 18	142 ± 12	145 ± 9	147 ± 12	146 ± 12
Potassium (mmol/L)	4.6 ± 1.0	4.8 ± 1.0	4.6 ± 0.8	4.8 ± 1.0	3.8 ± 1.6
Chloride (mmol/L)	102 ± 12	102 ± 8	103 ± 6	105 ± 11	104 ± 5
Total calcium (mmol/L)	2.9 ± 0.5	3.1 ± 0.3	3 ± 0.3	3.1 ± 0.4	3.2 ± 0.35
Total calcium (mg/dl)	11.7 ± 2.0	12.5 ± 1.2	12.2 ± 1.2	12.3 ± 1.6	12.7 ± 1.4
Total magnesium (mmol/L)	1.0 ± 0.75	0.8 ± 0.25	0.8 ± 0.4	1.0 ± 0.3	
Total magnesium (mg/dl)	2.4 ± 1.8	2.0 ± 0.6	2.0 ± 1.0	2.4 ± 0.7	
Phosphate (mmol/L)	1.8 ± 0.6	2.4 ± 0.65	2.3 ± 0.7	2.2 ± 0.6	1.95 ± 0.25
Phosphate (mg/dl)	5.6 ± 1.8	7.4 ± 2.0	7.1 ± 2.2	6.7 ± 1.8	6.0 ± 0.8

Values are given as mean ± SD. Data from Bauer JE, Harvey JW, Asquith RL, et al.: Clinical chemistry reference values for foals during the first year of life. Equine Vet J 16:361–363, 1984.

Table 19.10. Normal values for blood gases in adults horses and foals

	ADULT		FOAL in Lateral Recumbency (Arterial)	
	Arterial	Venous	2 Hours of age	7 Days of age
pH	7.364–7.444	7.33–7.41	7.362 ± 0.012	7.374 ± 0.014
Po_2 (mm Hg)	89–115	28.7–48.6	66.5 ± 2.3	86.9 ± 2.2
Po_2 (kPa)	11.86–15.33	3.83–6.48	8.66 ± 0.31	11.59 ± 0.29
Pco_2 (mm Hg)	37–49	46–64	47.7 ± 1.7	46.7 ± 1.1
Pco_2 (kPa)	4.93 ± 6.53	6.13–8.53	6.36 ± 0.23	6.23 ± 0.15
Base excess (mmol/L)		6.4–12.3	0.9 ± 1.0	1.4 ± 0.9
Bicarbonate (mmol/L)	23–30	31.6–37.7	25.0 ± 0.9	25.6 ± 0.8

Data from Aguilera-Tejero E, Estepa JC, Lopez I, et al.: Arterial blood gases and acid-base balance in healthy young and aged horses. Equine Vet J 30:352–354, 1998; Stewart JH, Rose RJ, Barko AM: Respiratory studies in foals from birth to seven days old. Equine Vet J 16:323–328, 1984; Corley KTT (unpublished data); and Soma LR, Uboh CE, Nann L: Prerace venous acid-base values in Standardbred horses. Equine Vet J 28:390–396, 1996.

Table 19.11. Normal and abnormal peritoneal fluid values in horses

	Adult	Foal	Medical colic	Surgical colic	Grass sickness
Colour	Clear, pale yellow	Clear, pale yellow	Slightly turbid, yellow	Clear to turbid. Yellow, red, brown, black	Clear to turbid ± floccules Deep yellow-orange
Protein (g/L)	<25	<25	6.2–20.6 (mean 10.6 ± 4.1)	14.6–82.3 (mean 30.2 ± 20.4)	Acute: 32 ± 14.1 Subacute: 22.4 ± 11.6
Protein (g/dl)	<2.5	<2.5	0.62–2.06 (mean 1.06 ± 0.41)	1.46–8.23 (mean 3.02 ± 2.04)	Acute: 3.2 ± 1.41 Subacute: 2.24 ± 1.16
Total nucleated cell count (×10^9/L)	<5.0–10	<1.5	1.1–9.4 (mean 3.1 ± 3.1)	1.4–11.0 (mean 4.0 ± 3.3)	Acute: 1.1–39.6 (mean 10.0 ± 10.6) Subacute: 1.1–39 (mean 11.4 ± 14.4)
Total nucleated cell count (cells/µl)	<5000	<1500	1100–9400	1400–11000	1100–39600
Neutrophils (%)	20–90				
Mononuclear cells (%)	5–60				
Lymphocytes (%)	0–35				
Eosinophils (%)	0–5				
Basophils (%)	0–1				
Total RBC count	Negligible				
Fibrinogen g/L	<0.1 (<10 mg/dl)				
Glucose	4.9–6.4 mmol/L (88–115 mg/dl)				
Urea nitrogen	3.9–8.2 mmol/L (11–23 mg/dl)	1.96 mmol/L (11.8mg/dl)			
Creatinine	161–237 µmol/L (1.8–2.7 mg/dl)				
Lactate	0.4–1.2 mmol/L (3.8–10.9 mg/dl)				
Total bilirubin	5–13 µmol/L (0.3–0.8 mg/dl)				
Alkaline phosphatase (IU/L)	19.3–129.2 (mean 59.3 ± 33.5)		2.0–179.5 (mean 76.3 ± 56)	209–1833 (mean 936.8 ± 697)	Acute: 8.0–531.5 (mean 175.4 ± 140) Subacute: 9.5–496 (mean 166.1 ± 166)
Specific gravity	<1.016		1.008–1.038	1.016–1.043	Acute: 1.015–1.041 Subacute: 1.01–1.032
Inorganic phosphate	0.9 ± 0.07 mg/dl (2.78 ± 0.21 mg/dl)				
Amylase	0–14 IU/L				
Lipase	0–36 IU/L				
γGT	0–6 IU/L				

Box 19.24. Guide to interpretation of peritoneal fluid

Colour abnormality

Action

- Measure total protein, RBC and WBC and make Gram smear

Interpretation

- Serosanguinous appearance indicates vascular injury
- Orange or brown red indicates necrosis, can be associated with duodentis/proximal jejunitis
- Red discolouration (if not iatrogenic) is a consistent indication of a surgical lesion.
- If sample brown-black bowel rupture should be suspected, especially if venous PCV very high

Increased total nucleated cell count

Interpretation

- Severe tissue inflammation or obstructive lesion
- Obstructive lesion to bowel: simple obstruction would expect counts in region of 3.0–8.0 $\times$ 10^9cells/L, strangulating obstruction >10 $\times$ 10^9cells/L
- Post abdominal surgery: counts may be as high as 400 $\times$ 10^9cells/L within 24 hours and remain elevated for at least 6 days. If concerned about post-operative case, measure serum and peritoneal glucose concentration difference of (>50 mg/dl) suggests septic peritonitis
- Post castration: open castration can induce nonseptic peritonitis with cell count 30 $\times$ 10^9 cells/L for 5 days should be normal 7 days postoperative

Increased total protein

Action

- Consider in view of colour of sample

Interpretation

- Red peritoneal fluid with total protein >20 g/L in horse with clinical signs of colic suggests surgical lesion may be present
- If sample is dark yellow/orange, consider grass sickness as differential. If possible, measure alkaline phosphatase activity. Grass sickness cases have lower activity (8.0–531.5 IU/L) compared to surgery cases (209–1833 IU/L)
- Colour normal, early inflammation

Increased red blood cell count

Action

- Take a PCV of peritoneal fluid and jugular blood samples.

Interpretation

- PCV peritoneal fluid = PCV jugular blood: suggests blood contamination of sample
- PCV peritoneal fluid > PCV jugular blood: suggests blood may be from puncture of spleen
- PCV peritoneal fluid < PCV jugular blood: peritoneal bleeding or strangulated infarctive lesion. Measure WBC. Increased RBC without increased WBC suggests vascular damage.

Increased urea

Action

- Take a PCV of peritoneal fluid and jugular blood samples

Interpretation

- If peritoneal creatinine is twice that of plasma creatinine confirms uroperitoneum

Intestinal content in sample

Action

- Make a smear and perform a Gram-stain

Interpretation

- Intracellular bacteria and toxic changes of neutrophils suggest rupture of bowel. If absent, sample may have been enterocentesis.

Low glucose content

Action

- Culture peritoneal fluid

Interpretation

- Low glucose is associated with infectious peritonitis

No peritoneal fluid obtained

Action

- Repeat tap distal to first attempt; use ultrasound to find good site.
- Check for dehydration. Measure PCV/total protein/lactate of serum if necessary.
- If need further information on medical/surgical colic decision, take serum.

Interpretation

- Serum phosphate >1.07 mmol/L (>3.3 mg/dL) is a predictor of major intestinal injury (sensitivity 60%, specificity 73%)

Table 19.12. Normal values for transtracheal aspirate and bronchoalveolar lavage cytology

Parameter	Transtracheal aspirate	Bronchoalveolar lavage[1–5]
% Neutrophils	<20,[6–8] <40[9,10]	<10
% Lymphocytes	5–10[6,7,9,10]	28–38
% Macrophages	24–35,[9,10] 44–65[6,7]	55–65
% Mast cells	<2[6,7,10,11]	<1
% Eosinophils	<4[7,9–11]	<2
% Epithelial cells	0–30[6,7,10]	<2

Table 19.13. Normal values for pleural fluid cytology

	Normal value
Volume	2–8ml
Colour	Reddish yellow
RBC	22–540 × 10^9/L
Nucleated cell count	<8000 cells/μl
Neutrophils	32–91% 450–10290/μl 0.5–10.3 × 10^9/L
Lymphocytes	0–22% 0–680/μl 0.07 × 10^9/L
Large mononuclear cells	5–66% 50–2620/μl 0.1–2.6 × 10^9/L
Eosinophils	0–9% 0–170/μl 0–0.2 × 10^9/L
Total protein	<25 g/L
Total protein	<2.5 g/dl

Total protein is best assessed after centrifugation.
Data from Wagner AE, Bennett DG: Analysis of equine thoracic fluid. Vet Clin Pathol 11:13, 1983; and Bain FT: Cytology of the respiratory tract. Vet Clin North Am Eq Pract 13:477–486, 1997.

19.8 Transtracheal and bronchoalveolar fluid analysis

Harold McKenzie

Normal values are given in Table 19.12.[1–11]

References

1. Clark CK, Lester GD, Vetro T, et al.: Bronchoalveolar lavage in horses: effect of exercise and repeated sampling on cytology. Aust Vet J 72:249-252, 1995
2. Fogarty U, Buckley T: Bronchoalveolar lavage findings in horses with exercise intolerance. Equine Vet J 23:434-437, 1991
3. Hare JE, Viel L, O'Byrne PM, et al.: Effect of sodium cromoglycate on light racehorses with elevated metachromatic cell numbers on bronchoalveolar lavage and reduced exercise tolerance. J Vet Pharmacol Ther 17:237-244, 1994
4. McKane SA, Canfield PJ, Rose RJ: Equine bronchoalveolar lavage cytology: survey of thoroughbred racehorses in training. Aust Vet J 70:401-404, 1993
5. McKenzie HC 3rd, Murray MJ: Concentrations of gentamicin in serum and bronchial lavage fluid after once-daily aerosol administration to horses for seven days. Am J Vet Res 65:173-178, 2004
6. Mair TS, Stokes CR, Bourne FJ: Cellular content of secretions obtained by lavage from different levels of the equine respiratory tract. Equine Vet J 19:458-462, 1987
7. Sweeney CR, Humber KA, Roby KA: Cytologic findings of tracheobronchial aspirates from 66 thoroughbred racehorses. Am J Vet Res 53:1172-1175, 1992
8. Malikides N, Hughes KJ, Hodgson DR, et al.: Comparison of tracheal aspirates and bronchoalveolar lavage in racehorses. 2. Evaluation of the diagnostic significance of neutrophil percentage. Aust Vet J 81:685-687, 2003
9. Derksen FJ, Brown CM, Sonea I, et al.: Comparison of transtracheal aspirate and bronchoalveolar lavage cytology in 50 horses with chronic lung disease. Equine Vet J 21:23-26, 1989
10. Larson VL, Busch RH: Equine tracheobronchial lavage: comparison of lavage cytologic and pulmonary histopathologic findings. Am J Vet Res 46:144-146, 1985
11. Hughes KJ, Malikides N, Hodgson DR, et al.: Comparison of tracheal aspirates and bronchoalveolar lavage in racehorses. 1. Evaluation of cytological stains and the percentage of mast cells and eosinophils. Aust Vet J 81:681-684, 2003

19.9 Normal values for pleural fluid

Normal values for pleural fluid are given in Table 19.13.

19.10 Normal values for cerebrospinal fluid

Martin Furr

Normal values for cerebrospinal fluid are given in Table 19.14.

References

1. Green E, Constantinescu G, Kroll R: Equine cerebrospinal fluid: analysis. Compend Contin Educ Pract Vet 15:288-301, 1993
2. Furr M, Bender H: Cerebrospinal fluid variables in clinically normal foals from birth to 42 days of age. Am J Vet Res 55:781-784, 1994

19.11 Normal values for urine and urine production

Normal values for urine and urine production are given in Table 19.15. A guide to possible interpretation of urinalysis is given in Box 19.25.

Table 19.14. Normal values for cerebrospinal fluid cytology and biochemistry

Parameter	Adult[1]		Neonates (<2 days of age)[2]
	AO site	LS site	AO
Total protein (g/L)	1–12	1–12	9.9–12
Total protein (mg/dl)	10–120	10–120	99–120
Nucleated cell count (/μl)	0–7	0–7	<5
Red blood cell count (/μl)	0–600	0–600	0–100
Glucose (mmol/L)	1.7–3.9 35–75% of plasma value	2.2–4.2 45–75% of plasma value	4.9–6.2
Glucose (mg/dl)	30–70 35–75% of plasma value	40–75 45–75% of plasma value	88–112
Creatine kinase (IU)	0–8	0–8	
Aspartate transaminase (SF units)	15–50	15–50	
Lactate dehydrogenase (IU)	0–8	0–8	
Sodium (mmol/L)	140–150	140–150	141–155
Potassium (mmol/L)	2.5–3.5	2.5–3.5	2.8–3.2
Chloride (mmol/L)	95–123	95–123	
Calcium (mmol/L)	0.63–1.5	0.63–1.5	
Calcium (mg/dl)	2.5–6.0	2.5–6.0	
Phosphorus (mmol/L)	0.16–0.48	0.16–0.48	
Phosphorus (mg/dl)	0.5–1.5	0.5–1.5	
Urea nitrogen (mmol/L)	0.83–3.32	0.83–3.32	
Urea nitrogen (mg/dl)	5–20	5–20	
Magnesium (mmol/L)			0.95–1.07
Magnesium (mg/dl)			2.3–2.6

Table 19.15. Normal values for urine and urine production

	Adult normal values	Foal normal values
Urine production	1.24 ml/kg/hr	6.17 ml/kg/hr
Urine pH	7.0–9.0	5.5–8.0
Urine specific gravity	1.028	1.004–1.008
Red blood cells	<5 per high-power field	<5 per high-power field
White blood cells	<5 per high-power field	<5 per high-power field
Creatinine clearance	1.2–2.38 ml/min/kg	1.78–2.17 ml/min/kg
Fractional excretion sodium	0.0002–0.87%	0.31 ± 1.8%
Fractional excretion potassium	1–75.1%	13.26 ± 4.49%
Fractional excretion chloride	0.012–3.47%	0.42 ± 0.32%
Fractional excretion phosphorus	0.023–5.53%	3.11 ± 3.81%
Fractional excretion calcium	0–6.723%	2.85–3.26%
Fractional excretion magnesium	20.8–43.1%	
γGT:creatinine ratio	<25 IU/g	8.2 ± 5.7 IU/g

Box 19.25. Guide to interpretation of urinalysis

Urinary casts

Possible interpretation
- Renal tubular disease

Further action
- Measure γGT/creatinine ratio
- Fractional excretion measurement
- Plasma creatinine, electrolytes

Increased epithelial cells

Possible interpretation
- Renal tubular inflammation
- Urinary tract inflammation
- Neoplasia

Further action
- Identify cell type, squamous, transitional or renal tubular. Identify if cells have normal morphology

Increased erythrocytes

Possible interpretation
- Neoplasia
- Cystic calculi
- Renal calculi
- Inflammation
- Acute tubular disease
- Coagulopathy
- Trauma during catheterisation

Increased leukocytes

Possible interpretation
- Inflammatory process of genitourinary tract

Increased glucose

Possible interpretation
- Stress
- α_2-Agonist administration
- Pituitary adenoma
- Diabetes mellitus

Further action
- Check plasma glucose

Intestinal protein

Possible interpretation
- Haemorrhage
- Inflammation
- Glomerulonephritis
- Amyloidosis
- False positive (urine dipstick in alkaline urine)

Further action
- Confirm true positive with acid-precipitation technique
- Examine urine for WBC/RBC, persistent strong reactions for protein with no haemorrhage or inflammation suggestive of glomerular disease

Occult blood (positive for haemoglobin)

Possible interpretation
- Haematuria
- Myoglobinuria
- Haemoglobinuria (haemolysis)

Further action
- Centrifuge sample, haematuria will clear when RBC sediment
- Take haematology, haemoglobinaemia associated with anaemia and discoloured plasma
- Myoglobinaemia does not discolour plasma

Increased pH

Possible interpretation
- Renal tubular acidosis (rare)

Decreased pH

Possible interpretation
- Metabolic acidosis
- Hypokalaemia
- Renal tubular acidosis

Decreased specific gravity

Possible interpretation
- Suckling neonate
- Psychogenic polydipsia
- Altered renal function
- Primary renal disease
- Chronic liver disease

Further action
- Measure plasma creatinine concentration
- Monitor in relation to hydration status
- Consistent isosthenuria (1.008–1.012) reflects loss of around 1/3 renal function

Greatly increased specific gravity (>1.050)

Possible interpretation
- Severe dehydration

Increased fractional excretion of electrolytes

Possible interpretation
- Increased $FeNa^+$
  - Renal disease
- Endotoxaemia
- Decreased FeK^+
  - Potassium deficit
- Increased $FePO_4^{2-}$
  - Hyperparathyroidism
  - Endotoxaemia

Further action
- Measure plasma creatinine concentration

Table 19.16. Normal synovial fluid cytology and values for common clinical conditions

	Normal	Osteoarthritis	Sepsis	Post arthrocentesis (24 hours)	Post medication gentamicin (24 hours)	Post lavage balanced electrolyte solution (24 hours)	Post lidocaine/ mepivacaine (24 hours)
Colour	Pale yellow, clear				Straw/yellow		
Viscosity	Viscus; if stretched between thumb and finger can make strand 2.5–5cm long.	Reduced viscosity	Reduced viscosity				
Total protein (g/L)	<20	8–35	>40	15–25	45–60	41–53	25–40
Total protein (g/dl)	<2	0.8–3.5	>4.0	1.5–2.5	4.5–6.0	4.1–5.3	2.5–4.0
Nucleated cell count ($\times 10^9$/L; $\times 10^3$/μl)	<0.5	≤1	>30 suggestive >100 pathognomic	1–4	4 ± 2.62	15–39	2–10
Nucleated cell count (cells/μl)	<500	≤ 1000	>30000 suggestive >100000 pathognomic	1000–4000	4400 ± 2615	15000–39000	2000–10000
Neutrophils (%)	<10	<15	>90	50	50	80	60
Mononuclear cells (%)	>90	>85	<10	50	50	20	40

19.12 Normal and abnormal values for joint fluid

Normal and abnormal values for joint fluid are given in Table 19.16.

References

1. Trotter GW: Clinical features and diagnosis of equine joint disease, in McIlwraith CW, Trotter GW (eds): Joint Disease in the Horse. Philadelphia, WB Saunders, 1996, pp 120-145
2. Caron JP: Osteoarthritis, in Ross MW, Dyson SJ (eds). Diagnosis and Management of Lameness in the Horse. Philadelphia, WB Saunders, 2003, pp 572-591
3. Kent Lloyd KC, Stover SM, Pascoe JR, et al.: Effect of gentamicin sulphate and sodium bicarbonate on the synovium of clinically normal equine antebrachiocarpal joints. Am J Vet Res 49:650, 1988
4. Bertone AL, McIlwraith CW, Powers BE, et al.: Effect of four antimicrobial lavage solutions on the tarsocrural joint of horses. Vet Surg 15:305-315, 1986
5. White KK, Hodgson DR, Hancock D, et al.: Changes in equine carpal joint synovial fluid in response to the injection of two local anaesthetic agents. Cornell Vet 79:25, 1989

19.13 Normal haemodynamics of adults and foals

The normal haemodynamics for adult horses are given in Table 19.17. The normal haemodynamics of foals are given in Table 19.18. Calculations for derived parameters and the normal values for 1-day-old neonatal foals are given in Table 19.19.

Table 19.17. Haemodynamics in the normal conscious horse and pony

Source	Cardiac output (L/min)	Cardiac index (ml/kg/min)	SVR (dynes·sec·cm^{-5})	Stroke volume (ml/min)
Horses				
Skarda (1996)[1]	40.6 ± 4.8	86 ± 9	217 ± 38	1126 ± 214
Hinchcliff (1991)[2]	33.6	70.9 ± 5.5		980
Muir (1976)[3]	32.5	73.8 ± 9.8		
Clark (1991)[4]	35.7–40.9	70 ± 10	202–217	
Muir (1992)[5]	≈33.5	70 ± 8	250 ± 15	
Garner (1977)[6]		83 ± 4.21	214 ± 25.25*	
Steffey (1987)[7]	32.32 ± 0.97	68.9 ± 3.1	333 ± 18*	889 ± 55
Hedenstierna (1987)[8]	40.2 ± 2.0			
Average	**36.2**	**74.7**	**223**	**998**
Ponies (154–313 kg)				
Geimer (1995)		71 (61–82)	525 (465–675)	

SVR, systemic vascular resistance.
*Calculated MAP ×80/CO (CVP not measured)—not included in average.

Table 19.18. Haemodynamics in the normal conscious neonatal foal

Age	Cardiac output (L/min)	Cardiac output (ml/kg/min)	SVR (dynes·sec·cm^{-})	Stroke volume (ml/min)
Thoroughbred foals[9]				
2 hours	7.1	155.3 ± 8.1	1027 (853–1201)	85.8
4 hours	8.98	197.8 ± 25.3	772 (653–891)	106.7
6 hours	8.24	181.5 ± 13.4	865 (759–971)	99.0
8 hours	7.9	173.9 ± 11.6	882 (808–956)	98.1
10 hours	8.5	188.1 ± 10.4	803 (718–888)	107.1
12 hours	8.0	180.5 ± 10.3	858 (788–928)	90.6
16 hours	8.24	181.5 ± 20.7	859 (736–982)	94.9
20 hours	8.9	195.5 ± 9.8	726 (672–780)	105.8
1 day	9.0	197.3 ± 12.0	708 (634–782)	107.1
2 days	9.86	204.1 ± 11.8	723 (673–773)	99.5
3 days	9.1	185.6 ± 14.3	814 (746–882)	100.7
4 days	11.3	222.8 ± 20.3	629 (583–675)	117.1
5 days	12.4	223.4 ± 20.3	623 (573–673)	117.1
6 days	12.25	214.5 ± 18.1	613 (540–686)	126.8
8 days	14.1	233.9 ± 16.3	543 (505–581)	130.6
10 days	13.0	205.8 ± 8.5	596 (551–641)	132.7
12 days	15.5	235.2 ± 35.1	520 (440–600)	143.4
14 days	15.7	222.1 ± 21.6	497 (410–584)	162.4
Quarter Horse/Thoroughbred cross foals[10]				
3–5 days	8.9–10.1	191 ± 31	818 ± 80	111 ± 10

Table 19.19. Calculations for derived haemodynamic parameters

Parameter	Calculation	Units	Normal values for 1-day-old foals
Cardiac index (CI)	$\frac{\text{Cardiac output (L/min)} \times 1000}{\text{Body weight (kg)}}$	ml/kg/min	197.3 ± 12.0
Stroke volume (SV)	$\frac{\text{Cardiac output (L/min)} \times 1000}{\text{Heart rate}}$	ml	107 ± 6.4
Stroke volume index (SVI)	$\frac{\text{Stroke volume}}{\text{Body weight (kg)}}$	ml/kg	2.35 ± 0.14
Systemic vascular resistance (SVR)	$\frac{(\text{MAP} - \text{CVP}) \times 80}{\text{Cardiac output}}$	dynes·sec·cm⁻	708 ± 74
Arterial oxygen content (Cao_2)	$1.34 \times [Hb] \times Sao_2 + 0.0031\ Pao_2$	ml/L	158 ± 13*
Venous oxygen content (Cvo_2)	$1.34 \times [Hb] \times Svo_2 + 0.0031\ Pvo_2$	ml/L	130 ± 13*
Global oxygen delivery (Do_2)	$\frac{CaO_2 \times \text{Cardiac index}}{1000}$	ml O_2/kg/min	31†
Global oxygen uptake (Vo_2)	$\frac{(CaO_2 - CvO_2) \times \text{Cardiac index}}{1000}$	ml O_2/kg/min	5.6†
Oxygen extraction ratio (O_2ER)	$\frac{(CaO_2 - CvO_2) \times 100}{CaO_2}$	%	18.0 ± 0.02*
Pulmonary vascular resistance (PVR)	$\frac{(\text{PAP} - \text{PAOP}) \times 80}{\text{Cardiac output}}$	dynes·sec·cm⁻	194 ± 37

MAP, mean arterial pressure; CVP, central venous pressure; [Hb], haemoglobin concentration (g/L); Sao_2, arterial haemoglobin saturation (%); Pao_2, arterial oxygen tension (mm Hg); Svo_2, venous oxygen saturation (%); Pvo_2, venous oxygen tension (mm Hg); PAP, mean pulmonary arterial pressure (mm Hg); PAOP, pulmonary arterial occlusion pressure (mm Hg). Normal values from Thomas et al. (1987),[9] except *data from five conscious, healthy 30–46-hour-old mixed-breed foals in lateral recumbency.

†Calculated from other data presented, intended as a guide only. From Corley KTT: Monitoring and treating haemodynamic disturbances in critically ill neonatal foals. Part I: haemodynamic monitoring. Equine Vet Educ 14:270–279, 2002. Used with permission.

References

1. Skarda RT, Muir WW: Analgesic, hemodynamic, and respiratory effects of caudal epidurally administered xylazine hydrochloride solution in mares. Am J Vet Res 57:193-200, 1996
2. Hinchcliff KW, McKeever KH, Muir WW: Hemodynamic effects of atropine, dobutamine, nitroprusside, phenylephrine, and propranolol in conscious horses. J Vet Int Med 5:80-86, 1991
3. Muir WW, Skarda RT, Milne DW: Estimation of cardiac output in the horse by thermodilution techniques. Am J Vet Res 37:697-700, 1976
4. Clark ES, Gantley B, Moore JN: Effects of slow infusion of a low dosage of endotoxin on systemic haemodynamics in conscious horses. Equine Vet J 23:18-21, 1991
5. Muir WW: Cardiovascular effects of dopexamine HCl in conscious and halothane-anaesthetised horses. Equine Vet J Suppl 11:24-29, 1992
6. Garner HE, Hahn AW, Salem C, et al.: Cardiac output, left ventricular ejection rate, plasma volume, and heart rate changes in equine laminitis-hypertension. Am J Vet Res 38:725-729, 1977
7. Steffey EP, Dunlop CI, Farver TB, et al.: Cardiovascular and respiratory measurements in awake and isoflurane-anesthetized horses. Am J Vet Res 48:7-12, 1987
8. Hedenstierna G, Nyman G, Kvart C, et al.: Ventilation-perfusion relationships in the standing horse: an inert gas elimination study. Equine Vet J 19:514-519, 1987
9. Thomas WP, Madigan JE, Backus KQ, et al.: Systemic and pulmonary haemodynamics in normal neonatal foals. J Reprod Fert Suppl 35:623-628, 1987
10. Lavoie JP, Madigan JE, Cullor JS, et al.: Haemodynamic, pathological, haematological and behavioural changes during endotoxin infusion in equine neonates. Equine Vet J 22:23-29, 1990

19.14 Diagnosis of pituitary pars intermedia dysfunction (Cushing's disease)

Jocelyn Habershon-Butcher

Pituitary pars intermedia dysfunction (PPID) is associated with an adenoma of the intermediate lobe of the pituitary gland, which causes abnormally high levels of several different hormones. These form the basis of the various tests for pituitary dysfunction. Clinical and laboratory signs are listed in Box 19.26.

Box 19.26. Clinical and laboratory signs and their prevalence in pituitary pars intermedia dysfunction

Clinical signs and percent of clinical cases affected
- Haircoat changes: 94%
- Weight loss: 88%
- Lethargy: 82%
- Laminitis: 82%
- PU/PD: 76%
- Hyperhydrosis: 59%
- Tachypnoea: 41%
- Tachycardia: 29%
- Skin/other infections: 24%
- Oral ulceration: 18%
- Bulging supraorbital fat pad: 12%
- Neurological signs: 6%

Laboratory signs and percent of clinical cases affected
- Leucocytosis: 12%
- Leucopenia: 6%
- Neutrophilia: 75%
- Lymphopenia: 25%
- Eosinopenia: 69%
- Eosinophilia: 12%
- Liver enzyme elevation: 6%
- Glucosuria: 77%
- Proteinuria: 10%
- Hyperglycaemia: 94%
- Increased basal cortisol levels: 53%

Basal tests

ACTH

Samples should be collected into a **plastic** EDTA blood tube, separated and frozen immediately and sent to a suitable laboratory on ice. This type of sample handling limits usefulness in the field.

Cortisol

Baseline cortisol levels are not that meaningful as there is a variation in levels throughout a 24-hour period. Urinary cortisol : creatinine ratio is also unreliable.

Insulin

Resting levels can be very high in some cases of PPID >250 to 1000 µIU/ml, but interpretation is difficult as insulin resistance is also associated with obesity, inflammatory conditions such as laminitis, infection, injury and pregnancy. The sample should be collected in a plain tube not within 2 hours of receiving a short feed. Insulin levels in grazed-only animals are reasonably stable.

Blood glucose

Collection should be made into a fluoride tube. Glucose levels vary throughout a 24-hour period, so results should be interpreted with caution. However, hyperglycaemia with normal or low insulin levels may be suggestive.

Dynamic tests

Low-dose dexamethasone suppression test

1. Collect baseline serum or heparinised blood sample.
2. Immediately inject 40 µg/kg dexamethasone intramuscularly.
3. At 18 to 24 hours later, collect a second serum or heparinised blood sample.
4. Submit both samples to laboratory for **cortisol** analysis.

Results interpretation

Normal horses show suppression of cortisol levels of at least 70% to 80% from the baseline value.

Combined dexamethasone suppression, TRH stimulation test

1. Collect baseline serum sample.
2. Inject 40 µg/kg dexamethasone intramuscularly.
3. At 3 hours later, collect a second serum sample.
4. Then inject 1.0 mg TRH intravenously.
5. Collect further serum samples at 30 minutes after TRH injection and at 24 hours after dexamethasone injection.
6. Submit all samples to the laboratory for **cortisol** analysis.

Results interpretation

PPID horses can have low or low-normal baseline cortisol levels, suppressed cortisol levels 3 hours after dexamethasone administration, a return to baseline cortisol level 30 minutes after TRH injection, or a return to baseline cortisol level 24 hours after dexamethasone administration.

The disadvantage of this test is time and cost.

Other tests

ACTH stimulation test, TRH stimulation test and combined ACTH/dexamethasone suppression test are no longer recommended for diagnosis of PPID.

Further reading

1. Chandler KJ, Dixon RM: Urinary cortisol:creatinine ratios in healthy horses and horses with hyperadrenocorticism and non-adrenal disease. Vet Rec 150:773-776, 2002
2. Dybdal NO, Hargreaves KM, Madigan JE, et al.: Diagnostic testing for pituitary pars intermedia dysfunction in horses. J Am Vet Med Assoc 204:627-632, 1994
3. Eiler H, Oliver JW, Andrews FM, et al.: Results of a combined dexamethasone suppression/thyrotropin-releasing hormone stimulation test in healthy horses and horses suspected to have a pars intermedia pituitary adenoma. J Am Vet Med Assoc 211:79-81, 1997
4. Hillyer MH, Taylor FGR, Mair TS, et al.: Diagnosis of hyperadrenocorticism in the horse. Equine Vet Educ 4:131-134, 1992
5. Love S: Equine Cushing's disease. Br Vet J 149:139-153, 1993
6. McGowan C: Diagnostic and management protocols for equine Cushing's syndrome. In Pract 25:586-592, 2003

19.15 The oral glucose tolerance test

Jocelyn Habershon-Butcher

The horse should be fasted for 12 to 16 hours prior to testing. The horse should not be sedated to perform the test as this can interfere with gastrointestinal transit time and falsely increase blood glucose levels. All blood samples are collected into a tube containing sodium fluoride anticoagulant.

Protocol

1. A baseline (0 minutes) blood sample is taken.
2. The horse is given 1 g/kg D-glucose powder as a 20% solution via a nasogastric tube.
3. Serial blood samples are then taken at 30, 60, 90, 120, 150, 180, 210, 240 (300, 360) minutes after glucose administration.

Interpretation of results

In a normal test, peak glucose concentrations will be seen at 90 to 120 minutes, and this peak should be greater than 85% above baseline glucose value. The glucose value should return back to baseline level within 4 hours.

Complete malabsorption is a peak glucose value at less than 15% above the baseline glucose value.

Partial malabsorption is a peak glucose value between 15% and 85% above the resting value.

Further reading

1. Roberts MC, Hill FWG: The oral glucose tolerance test in the horse. Equine Vet J 5:171-173, 1973
2. Mair TS, Hillyer MH, Taylor FGR, et al.: Small intestinal malabsorption in the horse: an assessment of the specificity of the oral glucose tolerance test. Equine Vet J 23:344-346, 1991

19.16 Ageing horses by dentition

Eruption of the incisor teeth gives a fairly reliable guide to the age of the horse up to 5 years old (Table 19.20).[1] The incisors come into wear approximately 6 to 9 months after eruption, and the wear gradually results in disappearance of the infundibulum (Box 19.27). Beyond 5 years of age, it becomes increasingly more difficult to age the horse accurately. The infundibulum is the "cup" present on the occlusal surface of the tooth, which is darker because it is covered in cement (Figure 19.1). As wear progresses, the secondary dentin within the pulp cavity (Figure 19.1) becomes visible, representing the "Dental Star" (Box 19.27). Hooks appear on the upper and lower corner incisors with wear. These are not a reliable guide to ageing, but generally do not appear before the age of 6.[1]

Galvayne's groove is a darkly stained groove on the outside (labial surface) of the upper corner incisor. It generally becomes visible at 10 years of age and reaches the occlusal surface at approximately 20 years of age.[1] The groove may be lost in very old horses. As the horse ages, the angle made between the upper and lower cheek teeth becomes more acute. With further ageing, this angle becomes straighter again, and the teeth become more triangular in appearance.

Table 19.20. Age for eruption of the incisor teeth

	Foal (deciduous teeth)	Permanent teeth
Central	0–7 days	2.5 years
Lateral	4–6 weeks	3.5 years
Corner	6–9 months	4.5 years

The permanent teeth come into wear 6–9 months after eruption.

Reference

1. Richardson J: Ageing horses: an illustrated guide. In Pract 19:486-489, 1997

Box 19.27. Changes with age to the incisors

Time of disappearance of the infundibulum
- Central incisor: 5–7 years
- Lateral incisor: 6–9 years
- Corner incisor: 7–10 years

Time of appearance of the dental star
- Central incisor: 6–7 years
- Lateral incisor: 7–9 years
- Corner incisor: 8–10 years

Time of appearance of Galvayne's groove
- Corner incisor: 10 years

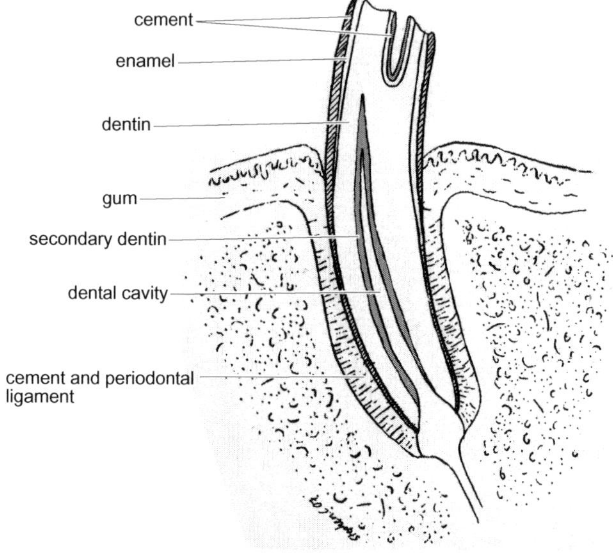

Figure 19.1

Index

A
AAAs. *See* Aromatic amino acids
Abaxial sesamoid nerve block, *98*
  for analgesia of pastern and foot, 97
  equipment for, 97 (box 1.56)
Abdomen
  auscultation of, 8
    gastrointestinal system exam and, 487–488
  extensive wound involving entire lateral aspect of, *614*
Abdominal compartment syndrome, 24
Abdominal drains
  inserting in standing horse, 19
  inserting under general anaesthesia, 19
  securing, 19–20
Abdominal size, of foal, monitoring, 305
Abdominal support bandages, 514
  laparotomy wounds and use of, 599, *600*
Abdominal surgery, longitudinal ultrasonographic image of ventral midline incision in horse after, *598*
Abdominal ultrasound, recording results of (form), *220–223*
Abdominal visceral pain
  acupuncture and, 328
  other causes of, 328
Abdominal wall, right and left, visceral projections on, *223*
Abdominocentesis, 16–18
  equipment for, 16, 16 (box 1.10)
  preparation, 16–17
  site for, 17
  teat cannula pushed through sterile gauze swab for, *17*
  technique for, 17–18
Abducens nerves, testing, 558
Abscesses
  within abdominal cavity, 490
  intra-abdominal, ultrasonography of, 497–498
Absorber function, determining, 231
ACE inhibitors. *See* Angiotensin-converting enzyme inhibitors
Acepromazine, 245
  approximate uses in equine medicine, 655*t*
  equine sedation and, 313*t*, 314
  foetal heart rate and, 319
  ileus treatment and, 502
  intraocular pressure and, 251
  musculoskeletal conditions and, 316
  neurological disease and, 317
Acetazolamide, approximate uses in equine medicine, 655*t*
Acetic acid, delay in wound healing and, 622
Acetylcysteine, approximate uses in equine medicine, 655*t*
Achilles tendon, rupture of, *643*
Acid-base balance, electrolytes, renal failure and, 546
Acid-base disturbances
  causes of, 380 (box 6.4)
  classification of, 381
Acidosis, 525
ACT. *See* Activated clotting time
ACTH test, anticoagulants for, 670 (box 19.3)
Actinobacillus spp., 337
  isolation of, from septic arthritis in foals, 580
Activated clotting time, 405
Active drains, peritoneal lavage and, 18
Active humidifiers, 475
Acupuncture, 644 (box 18.5), 651
  acute abdominal pain and use of, 328
Acute renal failure
  complications of, 543*t*
  incidence of, 533
  management priorities for patients with, 543 (box 13.5)
  symptomatic treatment for complications of, 543
  transabdominal ultrasonographic images
    of enlarged left kidney, *541*
    of enlarged right kidney, *541*
Acute seizures, treatment of, 565–566
ACV. *See* Assist-control ventilation
Acyclovir
  approximate uses in equine medicine, 655*t*
  EHV-1 myeloencephalopathy treatment and, 568
Adequan, approximate uses in equine medicine, 655*t*
Admixture bags
  PN, transfer lines with, 291
  PN, warning about transfer of solutions, 292
  PN formulation, 290
Adrenaline, approximate uses in equine medicine, 655*t*
Adrenocorticotrophic hormone, approximate uses in equine medicine, 655*t*
Adult horses
  critical care of, at equine hospital, 150
  normal biochemistry values in, 672*t*
  normal electrolyte concentrations in, 678*t*
  normal haematology values for, 671*t*
  normal haemodynamics for, 682, 685*t*
  normal physiological values for, 670 (box 19.1)
Adventitious sounds, 457, 458
AEF. *See* Assisted enteral feeding
Aerosol administration, of therapeutic substances for respiratory disorders, 466–468
  devices, 467–468
    metered dose and dry powder inhalers, 468
    nebulisers, 467–468
Aerosolised antimicrobials, 361–363
  administration of, 362–363
    devices, 362–363
    drug formulations for nebulisation, 363
  advantages with, 361
  aerosol theory, 362
  limitations with, 363
Aerosol theory, 362
AF. *See* Atrial fibrillation

Age, interpretation of peritoneal fluid and, 492
Aged horse, physiotherapy and care of, 644
Ageing horses by dentition, 688
Aggregometry, 406
Air bronchograms, 465, *465*
Air bubbles alarm, pumps and, 39
Air embolisms, 39
Air pumps, for insufflation of stomach, 21
Airway, Breathing, Circulation approach, in cardiopulmonary resuscitation, 122
Airway gases, 234–235
Airway narrowing, 457
Alanine aminotransferase, 521
Alaris IVAC P6000 syringe driver, *38*
Alaris Signature Gold dual-channel pump, *37*
Alarms, for pumps and syringe drivers, 39
Albendazole, approximate uses in equine medicine, 655*t*
Albumin, physiological functions of, 370
Albumin concentrations, guide to interpretation of, 673 (box 19.5)
Albuterol, 468
  approximate uses in equine medicine, 655*t*
  bronchoscopy technique and, 471
  cardiovascular and pulmonary support and use of, 243*t*
Albuterol Sulfate Solution for Inhalation, 64
Alfalfa hay, 266
  nutrient composition of, 265*t*
Alfentanil, equine sedation and use of, 315
Alkaline phosphatase (ALP) activity, guide to interpretation of, 674 (box 19.8)
Alkalosis, 525
Allopurinol, approximate uses in equine medicine, 655*t*
Alpha$_2$-adrenergic agonists
  colic pain and use of, 326
  constant rate infusions of, for standing chemical restraint and analgesia in horse, 327
  equine sedation and use of, 312, 313*t*
  pain management, adverse effects and use of, 325
ALT. *See* Alanine aminotransferase
Altrenogest
  approximate uses in equine medicine, 655*t*
  pregnant mares with colic and use of, 513
Alveolar pattern, lung tissue disease and, 465
Alveolar ventilation, deriving, 478
Alzheimer's disease, 568
Ambu bags, 5
Amikacin, 338, 344
  approximate uses in equine medicine, 655*t*
Amino acid mixtures/solutions, commercial, 272, 284
Amino acid supplementation
  future trends in, 271–272
    branched chain amino acids, 272
    glutamine, 271–272
Aminobenzyl penicillins, 343
Aminocaproic acid
  approximate uses in equine medicine, 656*t*
  hypocoagulable states in horses managed with, 411
Aminoglycoside antibiotics, renal insufficiency and, 533
Aminoglycosides, 342, 344–345
Aminophylline, approximate uses in equine medicine, 656*t*
Aminoproparazine fumarate, approximate uses in equine medicine, 656*t*
Amiodarone, 442
Ammonia test, anticoagulants for, 670 (box 19.3)
Ammonium chloride, approximate uses in equine medicine, 656*t*
Amniotic membrane, surgical repair of eye in Percheron mare and, *629*
Amoxicillin, 343
Amoxicillin trihydrate, approximate uses in equine medicine, 656*t*
Amphotericin B, 353
  fungal keratitis treatment and, 631
  spectrum of activity of, 353*t*
Ampicillin, 338, 343
Anaemia, severe, high heart rate and, 431
Anaesthesia, 226–254
  balanced, 243–244
  for colics, 249
  for foals, 246–248
  fractures and distal limb wounds that disrupt support structures and, 250–251
  gastrointestinal problems associated with, 485
  general, 226–246
  maintenance of, 240–242
  ocular, nasal, sinus and oral procedures and, 251–252
  postanaesthetic morbidity, 254
  for pregnant mares, 249–250
  pulley and rope system for assisted recovery of horses from, *156*
  regional, of eye, 91–93
  for some specific situations, 246–252
    colics, 249
    foals, 246, 248
    fractures and distal limb wounds that disrupt support structures, 250–251
    ocular, nasal, sinus and oral procedures, 251–252
    pregnant mares, 249–250
  standing surgery sedation and, 253–254
  total intravenous, 252–253
  triggers for initiating CPR during, 6 (box 1.3)
  for visceral pain, 328–329
Anaesthesia machines, for large animals, 228–231
Anaesthetic risk, 235–236
Anaesthetic stalls, at equine hospital, 154
Anaesthetised horse, cardiopulmonary resuscitation for, 5–7
Analgesia
  for colic patients, 326–327, 509
  for medical colic patients, 509
  regional, of limb, 96–100
  for surgical colic patients, 512
Analgesics, administration of, in caudal epidural space, 325*t*
Anal tone evaluation, 558
Anaphylactic reaction, transfusions and, 41
Ancillary neurological system tests, 559–561
  cerebrospinal fluid analysis, 559–561
    equine protozoal myeloencephalopathy, 561
    glucose, lactate, and enzyme concentration, 560–561
    red blood cells, 560
    white blood cells, 560
  cervical radiography, 559
Anderson sling, recovering horse and, 245
Angiotensin-converting enzyme inhibitors, 443
Anglesey Lodge Equine Hospital, The Curragh, Ireland
  arrangements for separating mares and foals during treatment of foal at, *151*
  Foal Intensive Care Programme
    daily sheet for ordering treatments for hospitalised neonatal foals, *210*
    neonatal foal admission form, *205*
    sheet for recording data on hospitalised neonatal foals, *209*
Anion acidosis, common causes of, in horses, 381 (box 6.6)
Anoplocephala perfoliata, caecal rupture and, 485
Anorexia, 263, 398
  electrolyte imbalances associated with, 266
  gastrointestinal problems and, 487
  protein requirements and, 270
  unconjugated hyperbilirubinaemia and, 522

Anthelmintic therapy
hepatic disease and, 527
hepatic disorders treated with, 527
Anthrax, nosocomial importance of, 186*t*
Antibacterial drugs, 337–342
aerosol administration of, 349–350
use of, in horses, 342–344
aminobenzyl penicillins, 343
antipseudomonal penicillins, 343
benzyl penicillin G, 342–345
β-Lactams, 342–344
cephalosporins, 343–344
Antibacterial therapy, hepatic diseases and, 527
Antibacterial treatment, nervous system and, 566
Antibiotic ointments, for wounds, 620
Antibiotics, corneal ulcers treated with, 630–631
Anticoagulants, for various blood tests, 654, 670 (box 19.3)
Anticonvulsant drugs, 565
long-term treatment with, 566
Antidysrhythmic drugs
classes of, 437
common use of, in horses, 437*t*
Antidysrhythmic therapy, 436–437
Antiendotoxic antibodies, 504–505
Antiendotoxic plasma, endotoxaemia treatment and, 504–505
Antifibrotic therapy, hepatic disorders treated with, 526–527
Antifungal drugs, 351–354
corneal ulcers treated with, 631–632
pharmacodynamics of, 352–353
spectrum of activity for, 353*t*
use of, in horses, 353–354
azoles, 353–354
polyenes, 353
systemic iodide therapy, 354
Antifungal susceptibility testing, 352
Antihaemorrhagic drugs
hypocoagulable states in horses managed with, 411
spontaneous bleeding episodes and, 413
Anti-inflammatory drugs
corneal ulcer treatment and, 632–633
neurological disorders and, 568
Anti-inflammatory therapy
hepatic disorders treated with, 527
liver disorders and, 527
Antimicrobial agents
aerosolised, 361–363
choosing, 337
enterocolitis associated with, 342
equine central nervous system infections and clinical choice of, 567–568
equine central nervous system or cerebrospinal fluid and, 567
intra-articular injections of, 350
for medical colic patients, 509
parenteral administration of, 361
pharmacokinetic-pharmacodynamic optimisation of doses, 341–342
regional perfusions of, 350–351
suggested choices of, for common bacterial pathogens of horses, 339t
suggested choices of, for selected bacterial infections of horses, 338*t*
for surgical colic patients, 511–512
Antimicrobial chemotherapy, role of, in treating equine infectious diseases, 337
Antimicrobial therapy, 337–354
aerosol administration of antibacterial agents, 349–350
antibacterial agents used in horses, 342–349
antibacterial drugs, 337–342
antifungal drugs, 351–354
local therapy for musculoskeletal infections, 350–351
pericardial fluid removal and, 428
value of in vitro susceptibility testing in predicting efficacy of, 340
Antiplatelet drugs
hypercoagulable states in horses managed with, 410
thrombocytopenia and administration of high doses of, 405 (box 8.5)
Antiproteases, corneal ulcer treatment and, 632
Antipseudomonal penicillins, 343
Antiseptic treatments, for wounds, 620
Antistaphylococcal isoxazolyl penicillins, 343
Antithrombin III, 406
Antithrombotic drugs, hypercoagulable states in horses managed with, 410
Antithrombotic therapy, spontaneous bleeding episodes and, 413
Antiviral drugs, neurological disorders and, 568
Anuria, 453
Aorta
two-dimensional, right parasternal short-axis echocardiogram of, *53*
two-dimensional left parasternal echocardiogram of, *54*
Aortic insufficiency, 425
severe, horse with, *425*
Aortic regurgitation, congestive heart failure and, 425
Aortic valves, 417
Aortoiliac thrombosis, 404
Appaloosas, polysaccharide storage myopathy in, 589
Aprons, lead, 167
Architects, hospital concept, siting and, 147–148
Archiving, of diagnostic image data, 175
Area under the serum concentration-time curve, 342
Arginine vasopressin, approximate uses in equine medicine, 656*t*
Argyle catheters, peritoneal lavage and, 18
Aromatic amino acids
failing liver and metabolisation of, 528
hepatic function and, 522
Arrow double-lumen catheters, 136
Arterial blood gas/arterial catheterisation
collection of, 139–141
dorsal metatarsal artery, 141
blood collection, 139–140
equipment for, 139 (box 2.12)
median artery, blood collection, 140
securing arterial catheter, 141
Arterial blood gas collection, 461–462
Arterial blood gas samples collection
arterial blood sampling from dorsal metatarsal artery, *43*
equipment needed for, 42, 42 (box 1.21)
procedure for, 42–43
Arterial blood gas tensions, strategies for improving, during ventilator treatment, 128 (box 2.8)
Arterial blood pressure measurement, 432–433, 452
direct, 45–46
indirect, 44–45
Arterial carbon dioxide tension, decreasing, during ventilator treatment, 128 (box 2.8)
Arterial catheterisation, 43–44
arterial catheter in transverse facial artery of horse after colic surgery, *44*
equipment needed for, 43, 44 (box 1.22), 139 (box 2.12)
procedure for, 43–44
transverse facial artery, palpating, *43*
Arterial catheters
in dorsal metatarsal artery, *46*
maintenance of, 44
securing, in foals, 141
Arterial hypercapnia, 473
Arterial oxygen tension, increasing, during ventilator treatment, 128 (box 2.8)
Arterial vasodilators, congestive heart failure treatment and, 443

Arthocentesis, 576
Arthritis, 643
Arthroscopy, reported infection rates for, 609
Arthroscopy patients, monitoring for septic arthritis, 574
Ascorbic acid, approximate uses in equine medicine, 656*t*
Aspartate aminotransferase
  acute rhabdomyolysis and increased serum activities of, 587
  biochemical monitoring of muscles and, 585–586
Aspartate aminotransferase activity, guide to interpretation of, 674 (box 19.9)
Aspartate transaminase, cerebrospinal fluid analysis and, 560
Aspartate transferase, cerebrospinal fluid analysis and, 561
Aspartic, 632
Aspergillus, miconazole and, 631
Aspiration catheter, for local lavage, 22
Aspiration pneumonia, avoiding, following improper nasogastric tube management in foal, 306
Aspirin, approximate uses in equine medicine, 656*t*
Assist-control ventilation, 476, 477
Assisted enteral feeding, 262, 275–276, 275 (box 5.11)
  complications associated with, 283–284
  suggested monitoring guidelines during, 283 (box 5.14)
AST. *See* Aspartate transaminase; Aspartate transferase
Astrocytes, 525
Asystole, irregular sinus rhythm progressing to, in horse, *5*
Atelectotrauma, 479, 480
Atlanto-occipital (AO) cerebrospinal fluid collection, 80–81
  after characteristic "pop" is felt, needle should not be advanced any further, *81*
  anatomy of site for collection of fluid, *81*
  equipment needed for, 81 (box 1.45)
  fluid collected via gravity flow, *81*
  procedure for, 80–81
Atracurium, intraocular surgery and, 252
Atrial fibrillation, 318, 440
  quinidine in treatment of, 438
  whole body potassium depletion and, 419
Atrium, left, two-dimensional left parasternal echocardiogram of, *54*
Atropine, 437*t*, 469
  approximate uses in equine medicine, 656*t*
  bradydysrhythmias and, 442
  cardiovascular and pulmonary support and use of, 243*t*
  corneal ulcer treatment and, 632
  gastrointestinal problems after surgery and, 485–486
  newborn foal, and contraindication of in resuscitation of, 124
AUC. *See* Area under the serum concentration-time curve
Aural lesions, bandaging, 112
Auricopalpebral nerves, anatomy of, *92*
Auriculopalpebral nerve block
  needle placed for, *92*
  performing, 92
  for placement of subpalpebral lavage catheter, 95
  regional anaesthesia of eye and use of, 91–92
Aurothioglucose, approximate uses in equine medicine, 656*t*
Auscultation
  abdominal, 487–488
  heart monitoring and, 417–419
    heart sounds, 418
    murmurs, 418–419
    rate, rhythm, and character of heart sounds, 418
a-wave, identification of, in complicated central venous pressure reading, *49*
Azathioprine, approximate uses in equine medicine, 656*t*
Azithromycin, 346
  approximate uses in equine medicine, 656*t*
Azoles, 353–354
  fungal keratitis treatment and, 631

B
B. Braun Medical Inc., 290, 308
Bacampicillin, approximate uses in equine medicine, 656*t*
Bacitracin zinc, 620
Backing test, 559
Bacteria
  minimal inhibitory concentration of, 339
  urine collection and, 536
Bacterial endocarditis
  severe, horse with, *425*
  treatment of, 444
Bacterial hepatitis, treating, 527
Bacterial infections
  in horses, 337–338
  in nervous system, 566
Bacterial pneumonia, treatment of, 471
Bacterial susceptibility, 338–339
Bacteriology, synovial fluid analysis and, 580
Bacteroides fragilis, 337, 338
BAL. *See* Bronchoalveolar lavage
Balanced anaesthesia, 243–244
Balanced electrolyte solutions, 372
BAL catheter, unguided technique, for bronchoalveolar lavage, 71
"Bandage bows," 574
  treating, 103
Bandage cast, creating, 618
Bandages
  abdominal support, 514
  changing, surgical incisions and, 597
  complications related to problems with, 574
  distal limb, 100, *102*, 105
  Esmarch, 108
  full limb, 105
    application of, *612*
  head, 110–112
  parts of, 103–104
  reusable, 105
  Robert Jones
    applying, 107 (box 1.60)
    for splinting equine limb, 606–607
  stent, 112
  uses for, 101
Bandaging of limb, 100–105
  avoiding problems and treating bandage "bows," 103
  commonly used materials for, 102 (box 1.57)
  monitoring and maintenance, 105
  procedure, 103–105
    distal limb bandages, 105
    full limb bandages, 105
    reusable bandages, 105
    splints, 105
Barbiturates, equine sedation and use of, 316
Barotrauma, 479
Base-apex ECG
  normal variations in P wave and T wave, *51*
  P, QRS, and T waves in, *50*
  placement of leads for recording of, *50*
Base-apex lead system, 49–50
Batch numbers, recording, for prescription-only medicines, 160
Baxter Flo-Gard GSP syringe driver, *38*
Baxter Flo-Gard 6301 dual-channel pump, *37*
Baxter Flo-Gard 6301 pump, fluid set pressed into fluid channel in, *38*
Baxter Healthcare, 290, 308
BCAA. *See* Branched chain amino acids
BCS. *See* Body condition score
BDZs. *See* Benzodiazepines
Becampicillin, 343

Beclomethasone, approximate uses in equine medicine, 656*t*
Beclomethasone dipropionate, inhaled corticosteroid therapy and, 470
Bedding, in stables at equine hospital, 150
Beet pulp, nutrient composition of, 265*t*
Behavioural modification, common equine sedatives used for, 313*t*
"Belly bandage," laparotomy wounds and use of, 599, *600*
Bench-top critical care analysers, 432
Benzodiazepines, 239
  adding constant rate infusions of, balanced anaesthesia and, 244
  equine sedation and use of, 313*t*
Benztropine mesylate, approximate uses in equine medicine, 656*t*
Benzyl penicillin G, 343–343
Bermudagrass hay, nutrient composition of, 265*t*
Beta aminopropionitrile, wound healing and, 621
Betadine, 620
β_2-adrenoreceptor agonists, clinical application with, 468–469
β_2-agonists, bronchodilators and types of, 468
β-lactams
  most significant factor in determining efficacy of, 342
  types of, used in horses, 342–344
Bethanechol, approximate uses in equine medicine, 656*t*
Bethanechol chloride, treatment of ileus and, 502
Bicarbonate-containing fluids, 372
Bilateral choanal atresia, 121
Bilateral fore limb and/or hind limb laminitis, 572
Bilateral jugular thrombophlebitis, 12
Bilateral pneumothorax
  in adult horse, caudo-dorsal thoracic radiograph showing, *73*, *74*
  in a horse, *466*
Bile acid concentration, guide to interpretation of, 675 (box 19.13)
Bilirubin, reagent strips and, 536
Bilirubin concentration, guide to interpretation of, 675 (box 19.14)
Bilirubinuria, 536
Biochemical monitoring, during PN therapy, 294
Biochemical profile
  evaluating, in hospitalised adult horse, 263, 265–267
    electrolyte imbalances, 266
    markers of glucose metabolism, 265
    markers of lipid metabolism, 265–266
    markers of protein metabolism, 265
    prolonged malnutrition and re-feeding syndrome, 266
    trace mineral and vitamin analysis, 266–267
  evaluating in hospitalised adult horse, 263, 265–267
    electrolyte imbalances, 266
    markers of glucose metabolism, 265
    markers of lipid metabolism, 265–266
    markers of protein metabolism, 265
    prolonged malnutrition and re-feeding syndrome, 266
    trace mineral and vitamin analysis, 266–267
Biochemistry
  electrolytes and, 654
  gastrointestinal system and, 490–491
Biochemistry tests
  anticoagulants for, 670 (box 19.3)
  neurological system and, 561
Biochemistry values, normal, in horses, 672*t*
Biocontainment, note on, 181
Biological dressings, wound management and use of, 620–621
Biopsies
  bone marrow, 89–91
  endometrial, 86–87, 542
  liver, 26–28, 524
  lung, 74–77
  muscle, 112–114
  rectal mucosal, 25–26
  renal, 88–89, 541
Biosecurity for equine hospitals, 180–186, 192
  concluding remarks about, 196–197
  education and awareness about, 196
  environmental surveillance and, 192
  hand hygiene and disinfection protocols, 194
  infectious/zoonotic diseases of hospitalised horse and, 196
  lessons from outbreaks, 182–183
  microbiological and other testing techniques, 192–194
    patient handling, 192–194
  need for, 182
  note on, 181
Biosecurity Officers, 183–184
Biosecurity programme, development and implementation of: focus on small to medium-sized clinics, 184 (box 3.7)
Biosensors, 185
Bismuth subsalicylate, approximate uses in equine medicine, 656*t*
Bite block, endotracheal intubation of adult horse and, 4
Bjordal, J. M., 646
Bladder
  endoscopy of, 86
  palpating, 10
  ultrasound of, 541
Bladder catheterisation, botulism and, 566
Blastomyces dermatidis, 352
Bleeding episodes in hospitalised horses, spontaneous, clinical approach and management of, 413
Bleeding form of disseminated intravascular coagulation, 402
  post-mortem of foal with, *402*
Blepharitis, 94
Blepharospasm, 633
Blister beetles (cantharidin)
  cantharidin toxicosis and, 534
  ingestion of, 420
Blocks
  in radiography rooms, in hospital, 168–169
  range of, used in equine radiography, *168*
Blood and blood component therapy, hypocoagulable states in horses managed with, 412
Blood and plasma transfusion
  administration of, 41
  design for homemade plasma collection device, *42*
  equipment needed for, 40, 40 (box 1.20)
  ideal donors for, 40 (box 1.19)
  parts of plasma collection kit, *41*
  procedure for, 40–41
  separation of plasma, 41
    by using homemade device, *41*
Blood gas collection and analysis, 461–463, 654
  arterial blood gas collection, 461–462
  venous blood gas collection, 462
Blood gases, normal values for, in adults and foals, 678*t*
Blood gas indices, 462
Blood gas machine, 234
Blood glucose levels, pituitary pars intermedia dysfunction and, 687
Blood lactate concentrations, haemodynamic therapy and, 453
Blood lead test, anticoagulants for, 670 (box 19.3)
Blood pressure machines, automated, 45, *45*
Blood pressure measurement, 432–433
  arterial, direct, 45–46
  arterial, indirect, 44–45
  indirect, in neonatal foal, 137–138
Blood samples
  collection of
    collection of blood and injection from jugular vein, 11–12
    collection of blood and injection into other veins, 12
    collection of blood for packed cell volume and total solids only, 12
    collection of blood from facial sinus, 12

Blood samples *(Continued)*
disinfection prior to venipuncture, 10–11
equipment needed for, 10, 10 (box 1.7)
Blood substitutes, 378
Blood tests, anticoagulants for, 654, 670 (box 19.3)
Blood transfusion, 376–377
Blood transfusion equation, 377
Body condition scores
adapting, to equine neonates, 298
assessing, for hospitalised adult horse, 262
guidelines for initiating diet therapy based on, 267 (box 5.7)
individual, description of, 263 (box 5.4)
patient evaluation and, 261
Body temperature, normal range of, in adult horse, 393
Body weight
assessing, for hospitalised adult horse, 262
equation for estimate of, using chest girth and body length, 261 (box 5.2)
of foals, monitoring, 302
in miniature horses, equation for using chest girth and body length, 262 (box 5.3)
Body wounds, 613–614
Boldenone undecylenate, approximate uses in equine medicine, 656*t*
Bone, common fungal pathogens in, 352*t*
Bone marrow
preparing smear of, for cytological evaluation, *91*
successful aspiration of, *91*
Bone marrow biopsy, 89–91
equipment needed for, 90 (box 1.53)
insertion of Jamshidi needle, *91*
longitudinal sections of sternae showing variation of anatomy, *90*
marking intersternebral space between two sternebrae to be aspirated, with marker pen, *90*
preparing smear of bone marrow for cytological evaluation, *91*
procedure for, 89–91
successful aspiration of bone marrow, *91*
ultrasonographic appearance of intersternal space between sternebrae A and B, *90*
use for, 89
Bony involvement, wounds and, 616–617
Book loss, at hospital libraries, 162
Borborygmi
assessment of, 8
abdominal auscultation and, 487–488
postoperative ileus and prolonged absence of, 510
Bottle-feeding, for foals, 301–302, *302*
Botulinum antitoxin, approximate uses in equine medicine, 656*t*
Botulinum toxin type B, approximate uses in equine medicine, 656*t*
Botulism, 566
Bowel prolapse, acute, steps to take in case of, through dehisced surgical wound, 514 (box 11.9)
Bradydysrhythmias, 442
Branched chain amino acids, 272
hepatic disease, diet and, 528
hepatic function and, 522
Breath control, mechanical ventilation and, 476
Breathing rate, CPR for neonatal foal and, 123
Bretylium, 437*t*
Bretylium tosylate
approximate uses in equine medicine, 657*t*
ventricular tachycardia treatment and, 439
Bromocriptine mesylate, approximate uses in equine medicine, 657*t*
Bronchial pattern, *465*
lung tissue disease and, 465
Bronchial tree, 471
Bronchoalveolar lavage, 70–71, 458, 460–461
equipment needed for, 70–71, 71 (box 1.39)
guided (endoscopic) technique, 71
primary utility of, 70
procedure for, 460
unguided (BAL catheter) technique, 71
uses for, 460
Bronchoalveolar lavage cytology
inflammatory, *460*
interpretation of, 460–461
normal, *460*
normal values for, 681*t*
Bronchodilators, 466, 468
Bronchoscopic examination, focal purulent drainage identified on, *460*
Bronchoscopic lavage, 471–472
bronchoscopy technique, 471–472
efficacy, 472
potential complications with, 472
Bronchoscopy
indications for, 471
sedation for, 318
technique for, 471–472
Bronchovesicular sounds, 457, 458
Broodmare
draining abdomen in, *20*
gravity-flow of fluids into abdomen via peritoneal drain into, *20*
Broth diffusion methods, 339
Bucket feeding, for foals, 301
"Bucking" the ventilator, 127
Bupivacaine, epidural analgesia and anaesthesia for visceral pain and, 328–329
Buprenorphine
approximate uses in equine medicine, 657*t*
equine sedation and use of, 313*t*, 315
Bursae, synoviocentesis of, 579
"Burst" TENS, 647, 648
Butorphanol, 238
approximate uses in equine medicine, 657*t*
bronchoscopy technique and, 471
constant rate infusions of, for analgesia after colic surgery, 327
equine sedation and use of, 313*t*, 314
head cases and use of, 317
for sedating neonatal foals, 320
somatic pain management and, 330
total intravenous anaesthesia and, 252
B vitamin supplementation, 274–275
hepatic insufficiency and, 528
in parenteral nutrition, 289

C
C. botulinum antiserum, 566
C. difficile, 342
Caecal impactions, after surgery or with hospitalisation, 485
Caecum
abnormalities of, 489
anatomy of, and site for percutaneous trocharisation, *25*
percutaneous trocharisation of, *25*
ultrasonography of, 496–497
Caesarean section delivery of foal, reasonable anaesthetic protocol for mares during, 250 (box 4.3)
Cafeteria feeding, of hospitalised adult horse, 267
Caffeine, approximate uses in equine medicine, 657*t*
Calcium
electrolyte assessment of cardiac disease and, 419
electrolyte imbalances and, 384
newborn foal, resuscitation of, and contraindication of, 124
total, formulas for correcting for measured albumin concentration, 384
Calcium borogluconate, approximate uses in equine medicine, 657*t*

Calcium concentrations, guide to interpretation of, 676 (box 19.15)
Calcium deficiency, clinical signs of, 266
Calcium disturbances, treatment of, 384–385
Calcium gluconate, cardiovascular and pulmonary support and use of, 243*t*
Calcium gluconate 23%, approximate uses in equine medicine, 657*t*
Calibrated scales, body weight measurement with, 262
Calorie-to-nitrogen ratio
  calculation of, 271 (box 5.9)
  ideal, for adult horses, 271
Cambendazole, approximate uses in equine medicine, 657*t*
Camera surveillance, on hospital grounds, 148
Canola oil, 279
Cantharidin toxicosis, renal insufficiency and, 534
Capillary refill time, 434
Capnography, 234
CAPS. *See* Central Admixture Pharmacy Services
Captan, approximate uses in equine medicine, 657*t*
Carbamazepine, approximate uses in equine medicine, 657*t*
Carbon dioxide, arterial and venous partial pressures of, 462
"Carboy" fluids, 371
Cardiac anatomy, function, and size, echocardiography and evaluation of, 52–55
Cardiac arrest, during general anaesthesia, 233
Cardiac conditions, equine sedation for, 318–319
Cardiac disease
  echocardiography and assessment of, 423–424
  rider safety and management of, 436
  specific indicators of, 420
Cardiac murmurs, grading of, 418 (ox 9.1)
Cardiac output, 55
  computer program calculating area under curve, to give volume of blood per unit time, *56*
  hydration status and determination of, 546
  measurement of, 55–58
    equipment needed for, 55, 56 (box 1.28)
    principle, 55
    procedure for, 55–57
    pulse contour analysis, 57–58
  monitoring of, 434
    lithium specific sensor for lithium dilution method, *56*
  optimising renal blood flow and, 543
  original LiDCO computer and sensor for calculation of, *56*
Cardiac performance, drugs aiding improvement of, 442–444
Cardiac rhythms
  disease processes related to, 421
  telemetric monitoring of, in horse during conversion of atrial fibrillation using quinidine sulphate, *421*
Cardiac stroke volume, 447
Cardiac troponins, 420
Cardiomyopathies, echocardiography and evaluation of, 426
Cardiopulmonary resuscitation
  in adult horse, 5–7
  during anaesthesia, 6 (box 1.4)
  for anaesthetised horse, 5–7
    procedure for, 6–7
    recognising need for, 5–6
  equipment needed for, 5, 5 (box 1.2), 122 (box 2.1)
    in dedicated box, *122*
  monitoring, 124
  for nonanaesthetised horse, 7
Cardiopulmonary resuscitation in neonatal foal, 122–124
  airway, 122–123
    mouth-to-nose resuscitation, 123
  breathing and, 123
  circulation and, 123
  defibrillation, 124
  drugs, 123–124
  equipment needed for, 122 (box 2.1)
  first 20 seconds, 122
  knowing when to stop, 124
  monitoring CPR, 124
  positive pressure ventilation and thoracic compressions in foal, *124*
Cardiovascular examination, form for recording results of, *212*
Cardiovascular monitors, 233–234
Cardiovascular shock, 431
Cardiovascular support
  for anaesthetised horses, 243*t*
  for pregnant mares, 250
Cardiovascular system, 417–453
  cardiac output monitoring of, 434
  derived haemodynamic parameters for, 435
  monitoring the heart, 417–428
  monitoring tissue perfusion, 430–433
  treating problems of heart, 436–444
  treatments aimed at improving tissue perfusion, 446–453
Carotid artery, 11
Carpal joints
  approaches to, for synoviocentesis, 578, *578*
  septic arthritis in, 573
Carprofen
  approximate uses in equine medicine, 657*t*
  endotoxaemia treatment, 506
  somatic pain management and, 330
Carpus
  analgesia of distal antebrachium and, 98, 100
  analgesia of limb distal to, 98
Cars, parking at equine hospital, 148–149, *149*
Caspofungin, spectrum of activity of, 353*t*
Cassette and cassette holders, in radiography room, at hospital, 167–168
Castration
  peritoneal fluid analysis and, 492
  total intravenous anaesthesia and, 252, 253
Casts
  application of, 607–608
  checking, 608
  classification of, according to their location and length, 607 (box 15.10)
  problems and complications related to, 574
  traumatic wounds and complications related to, 618
Cataract surgery, in foals, 636–637
Catheterisation
  arterial, 43–44
  of cephalic and lateral thoracic veins, 30–35
  epidural injection and, 81–84
  jugular, 28–30
  jugular vein, in neonatal foal, 133–137
  thrombophlebitis after, 394
  urinary, 84–85
Catheterisation of cephalic and lateral thoracic veins, equipment needed for, 31 (box 1.17)
Catheters
  for delivery of intravenous fluids, 369
  neonatal foals and care of, 137
  over-the-needle, placement of, for jugular catheterisation, 28–30
  over-the-wire, placement of, for jugular catheterisation, 30
  parenteral nutrition for hospitalised foals and placement of, 308
  subpalpebral, 630
  suitable, for jugular catheterisation, 28 (box 1.16)
Caudal epidural analgesia, 325
Caudal epidural space, analgesics administered in, 325*t*
Caudal maxillary sinus, as site for sinocentesis, 78
Caudo-dorsal radiograph, bilateral pneumothorax shown with, *73*, *74*
CCDs. *See* Charged-coupling devices

CCP. *See* Corpus cavernosum penis
CDC. *See* Centers for Disease Control and Prevention
Cefadroxil, approximate uses in equine medicine, 657*t*
Cefazolin, approximate uses in equine medicine, 657*t*
Cefepime, approximate uses in equine medicine, 657*t*
Cefoperazone, approximate uses in equine medicine, 657*t*
Cefotaxime, approximate uses in equine medicine, 657*t*
Cefoxitin, approximate uses in equine medicine, 657*t*
Cefpodoxime, approximate uses in equine medicine, 657*t*
Cefquinome, 344
  approximate uses in equine medicine, 657*t*
Ceftiaxone, approximate uses in equine medicine, 657*t*
Ceftiofur, 344
  aerosol administration of, 361
  approximate uses in equine medicine, 657*t*
Ceiling-mounted x-ray units, 166
Centers for Disease Control and Prevention, 180
Central Admixture Pharmacy Services, 290
Central venous pressure, 47, 434
  measurement of, 47–49, *48*
    electronic reading, 48–49
    equipment needed for, 47 (box 1.25)
    in horse with gastrointestinal disease, using manometer method, *48*
    manometer for, *48*
    manometer reading, 47
    procedure for, 47
  preload and, 546
Central venous pressure reading, complicated, identification of a-wave in, *49*
Central venous pressure trace, example of, taken during spontaneous breathing, *49*
Centrifugation, for separating plasma from cells, 378
CEPEF. *See* Confidential Enquiry into Perioperative Equine Fatalities
Cephalexin, approximate uses in equine medicine, 657*t*
Cephalic vein, 12
  catheter entry site, 31
  catheterisation of, 31–33
    catheter fed up wire and into vein up to the hub, *32*
    catheter hub sutured with cruciate stitch, 32, *33*
    dilator fed up the wire and pushed through skin into vein, *32*
    horse connected to fluids, parenteral nutrition and insulin through double-lumen cephalic catheter, *33*
    needle placed into vein, and wire fed into needle, *32*
    placing local anaesthetic over catheter entry site for cephalic catheter, *32*
  site of, *31*
Cephalosporins, 343–344
  equine central nervous system or cerebrospinal fluid and, 567
Cephalothin, approximate uses in equine medicine, 657*t*
Cephapirin, approximate uses in equine medicine, 658*t*
Cephradine, approximate uses in equine medicine, 658*t*
Cerebellar disease, signs of, 557–558
Cerebral oedema, treating, 569
Cerebrospinal fluid
  collection of, 79
  equine sedation and acquisition of, 317
  evaluation of, 559
Cerebrospinal fluid cytology and biochemistry, normal values for, 681, 682*t*
Cerebrospinal fluid taps, 252
Cervical examination, 541–542
Cervical radiographs, sagittal ratio measurements on, *559*
Cervix per rectum, ultrasonography of, 542
Cetiofur, intra-articular administration of, 350
Charcoal (activated), approximate uses in equine medicine, 658*t*
Charged-coupling devices, 167, 179
Chemical restraint and analgesia in horse, standing, constant rate infusions and, 327–328
CHF. *See* Congestive heart failure
"Chinese finger trap" suture
  around drain, *20*
  drains secured with, 618
  placement of, 19, *19*
  pleural drainage and, 473
Chitin, wound healing and, 621
Chloral hydrate
  approximate uses in equine medicine, 658*t*
  equine sedation and use of, 315–316
  gastrointestinal disorders and use of, 319
  gastrointestinal pain management and, 328
Chloramphenicol, 338, 348–349
  approximate uses in equine medicine, 658*t*
  equine central nervous system or cerebrospinal fluid and, 567
Chlorhexidine diacetate, 620
Chloride, electrolyte imbalances and, 384
Chloride concentrations, guide to interpretation of, 676 (box 19.16)
Chloride disturbances, treatment of, 384
Chlorpromazine, equine sedation and use of, 314
Choanal atresia, 121
Choke, 487
Cholangiohepatitis, 520
Choral hydrate, equine sedation and use of, 313*t*
Cimetidine, approximate uses in equine medicine, 658*t*
Ciprofloxacin, 345, 346
  approximate uses in equine medicine, 658*t*
Circulation, CPR for neonatal foal and, 123
Cisapride, 499
  treatment of ileus and, 501–502
CK. *See* Creatine kinase
Clarithromycin, 346, 347
  approximate uses in equine medicine, 658*t*
Clean-contaminated surgical procedures, infection rates for, 609
Clean-contaminated wounds, 609*t*
Cleaning and disinfection protocol, effective, broad application of, 195 (box 3.9)
Cleanliness/asepsis flow, central clinical area, at equine hospital, 154
Clean surgical wounds, 609*t*
Clenbuterol, approximate uses in equine medicine, 658*t*
Client education, at equine hospital, 161–162
Client information sheets, 225
Client waiting area, features and amenities for, at equine hospital, 152–153
Clindamycin, 342
Clinical and Laboratory Standards Institute, 339
Clinical area, main, at equine hospital, 153–154
Clinical condition, assessing, for hospitalised adult horse, 261–262
Clinical pathology panels, minimum recommended, 395 (box 7.2)
Clippers, ultrasonography and use of, 170
Cloprostenol Na, approximate uses in equine medicine, 658*t*
Clostridial enteritis
  biosecurity and, 182
  cross-sectional image of small intestine in 3-week-old foal with, *496*
  nosocomial importance of, 186*t*
Clostridium difficile, 277
  nosocomial diarrhoea and, 486
Clostridium perfringens type A, 342
Clostridium spp., 342
Closure time, 406
Clotrimazole, 353
CLSI. *See* Clinical and Laboratory Standards Institute
CMOS. *See* Complementary metal oxide semiconductor
CMV. *See* Controlled mandatory ventilation
CO. *See* Cardiac output

Coagulapathies, deficient activation of coagulation system and, 404
Coagulation activity, markers of, 406
Coagulation disorders
clinical approach and management of, in hospitalised horse, 413–414
therapy of, 409–413
Coagulation factors
coagulopathies due to consumption of, 405
disease conditions in which plasma transfusions recommended as replacement for, 412 (box 8.8)
measurement of, 406
Coagulation inhibitor activities, 406
Coagulation problems, main, clinical approach and management of, in hospitalised horses, 413–415
Coagulation system
dysfunctions of, in hospitalised horses, 401
laboratory tests for monitoring disorders in, 405–407
monitoring, 401–407
Coagulation testing profile, for diagnosing hypercoagulability and disseminated intravascular coagulation, 402–403
Coagulopathies
excessive activation of coagulation system and, 401
management of horses with, 409–415
treatments recommended in hospitalised horses with, 409 (box 8.6)
Coccidioides immitis, 352, 354
Coccygeal artery, indirect blood pressure cuff over, 137, *138*
Coffin bone, septic osteitis of, *615*
Coffin joint, approaches to, for synoviocentesis, *576*
Coils, equine magnetic resonance imaging and, 173
Cold therapy, effects of, 649*t*
"Colic checks," 510
Colic information sheet, post-operative, *211*
Colic patients
anaesthesia for, 249
anaesthetic risk and, 235
analgesia of, 326–327
collecting gastric reflux from foal with, *380*
feeding back, 512–515
nutritional management, 512–513
pregnant mare, 513–514
surgical wound management, 514–515
feeding changes and, 487
hepatopathy and, 520
lactate concentrations and hospital survival in, 432
medical, special considerations for, 507–509
analgesia, 509
antimicrobials, 509
fluid therapy, 508–509
monitoring, 507–508
thrombophlebitis and laminitis, 509
peritoneal and serum concentrations in horses with (U.S. units), 493*t*
peritoneal and serum phosphate concentrations in horses with (SI units), 493*t*
segregation of, 193
surgical, special considerations for, 509–512
immediate treatment after surgery, 509–510
monitoring fluid status, 511
monitoring intubation, 511
monitoring of, 510
Colic surgery
arterial catheter in transverse facial artery of horse after, *44*
LiDCO measurement of cardiac output in horse after, *57*
possible sources of fever in horses after, 510 (box 11.8)
Colitis
plasma used in horses with, 377
visceral pain and, 328
Collapse, rider injury and, 436
Colloidal oncotic pressure, 370
Colloidal osmotic pressure, formula for calculation of, 524–525
Colloid fluids, 375–376
dextrans, 376
gelatins, 376
hetastarch, 375
hydroxyethyl starches, 375
pentastarch, 375–376
Colloids, 371–372
Colon
large, abnormalities of, 489–490
ultrasonography of, 496–497
Colonic ammoniagenesis, reducing, 526
Colonic obstruction, risk factors for, 484
Colon impactions, large, stable confinement and, 484–485
"Comet tails," pleural, 463
Commercial compounding, of parenteral solutions, 290
Communication flow, in nurses' base at equine hospital, 153
Compendium of Veterinary Standard Precautions, 196
Compensated/subclinical form of disseminated intravascular coagulation, 401–402
Complementary metal oxide semiconductor, 167
Compounding parenteral solutions, 290–292
commercial compounding options, 290
in-house veterinary clinic compounding, 290–291
containers for total nutrient admixture parenteral nutrition formulations, 290–291
partial parenteral nutrition formulations, 290
instructions for, 291 (box 5.19)
preparation for, in laminar flow hood, *291*
preparing formulation, 291–292
supplements added to parenteral mixture, 292
Computed radiography system suppliers, 176 (box 3.3)
Computed tomography, 171–172, 178
Hounsfield units of various body tissues for, *171*
Computed tomography suppliers, 176 (box 3.3)
Computed tomography systems, horse-specific, suppliers, 176 (box 3.3)
Computerised radiography, 167
Computer tomography scanners, manufacturers of, 172
Confidential Enquiry into Perioperative Equine Fatalities, 235, 236
Confinement, complications related to, 574
Congestive heart failure, 318
atrial fibrillation and, 440
echocardiography and diagnosis of, 425
treatment of
arterial vasodilators, 443
digoxin, 442–443
dobutamine, 443
furosemide (frusemide), 443–444
milrinone, 443
Conidiobolus coronata, 351
Conjunctiva, anaesthesia of, 93
Conjunctival grafts, 634
Conjunctival hyperaemia, 633
Consent form, for University of Liverpool Equine Hospital, *201*
Consent forms, 200
Constant rate intravenous infusions, 669*t*
Constant rate of infusion, 244, 303
furosemide and, 443
lidocaine and, 501–502
pain management, adverse effects, and use of, 325
visceral pain management and, 327–328
Contaminated surgical procedures, infection rates for, 609
Contaminated surgical wounds, 609*t*
Contaminated traumatic wounds, 609
Continuous interlocking suture pattern, *119*
technique, advantages/disadvantages with, 119

Continuous positive airway pressure, 128, 476, 477
Controlled mandatory ventilation, 476, 477
"Conventional" TENS, 647, 648
COP. *See* Colloidal osmotic pressure
Cornea, anaesthesia of, 93
Corneal cultures, collecting, 629
Corneal cytology, performing, 629
Corneal disease, surgeries for, 634
Corneal grafts, 634
Corneal injuries, pain due to, 329
Corneal lacerations, management of horses with, 633
Corneal lesions, 94
Corneal melting, halting, 632
Corneal oedema, 633
Corneal stromal abscess, management of horses with, 633–634
Corneal ulcers, 329, 486
  anaesthesia and, 251
  management of horses with, 628–633
    antibiotics, 630–631
    antifungals, 631–632
    anti-inflammatories, 632–633
    antiproteases, 632
    atropine, 632
Cornell University, Ithacy, NY, arrangements for separating mares and foals during treatment of foal at, *151*
Corner suture pattern, technique, advantages with, 117
Corn oil, 279
Corpus cavernosum penis, lavage of, 548
Cortex, kidney, renal ultrasound and, 539
Corticosteroids, 466
  bradydysrhythmias and, 442
  decreased vasodilation and, 451–452
  inhaled, clinical application of, 470
  neurological disorders and, 568
  wound healing and, 621
Cortisol levels, pituitary pars intermedia dysfunction and, 687
Coupage, 640
  prior to suctioning airway, in neonatal foals, 128
Couppae, C., 646
Cow's milk, feeding of, to foals, 300
COX-1 inhibitors, 512
COX-2 inhibitors, 512
Coxofemoral (hip) joint, synoviocentesis of, 579
CPAP. *See* Continuous positive airway pressure
CPR. *See* Cardiopulmonary resuscitation
Crackles, 457
Cranial abscess, very large, with fluid line, on cranio-dorsal radiographic view of thorax, *466*
Cranial cervical radiograph, of fractured dens of C2, *560*
Cranial lobar bronchus, identifying, for respiratory endoscopy, 66
Cranial nerves, examining, 557–558
Cranial surgeries, anaesthesia and, 252
Creatine kinase
  acute rhabdomyolysis and increased serum activities of, 587
  biochemical monitoring of muscles and, 585
  cardiac isoenzyme of, 420
  cerebrospinal fluid analysis and, 560, 561
Creatine kinase activity, guide to interpretation of, 674 (box 19.10)
Creatinine, glomerular filtration rate and, 536
Creatinine concentrations
  guide to interpretation of, 676 (box 19.17)
  hypovolaemia and, 366
CRI. *See* Constant rate of infusion
Critical care nutrition, 261
Critical care stalls, at equine hospital, 150
Critical care ventilator, neonatal foals and use of, 125 (box 2.3)
Cromolyn sodium, approximate uses in equine medicine, 658*t*
CRT. *See* Capillary refill time
Cruciate stitch, catheter hub sutured with, in catheterisation of cephalic vein, 32, *33*
Cruciate suture pattern, *118*
  advantages/disadvantages with, 118
  placing over-the-wire catheter and, 136
  technique with, 117
Cryoprecipitate, 413
Cryotherapy, 648–649
Cryptorchidectomy, reported infection rates for, 609
Crystalloid fluids, 372–374
  balanced electrolyte solutions, 372
  glucose-containing solutions, 374
  hypertonic saline, 374
  normal saline, 372–373
  sodium bicarbonate, 373–374
Crystalloids, 370–371
Crystals, in equine urine, 536
CSF. *See* Cerebrospinal fluid
CT. *See* Computed tomography
cTn. *See* Cardiac troponins
Curschmann's spiral, 459, *459*, 461
Cushing's disease, diagnosis of, 686–687
Cushing's syndrome, laminitis and, 573
CVP. *See* Central venous pressure
Cyanoacrylate adhesive
  keeping Elastoplast/Elastikon in place with, *111*
  wound healing and, 621
Cyclophosphamide, approximate uses in equine medicine, 658*t*
Cyproheptadine, approximate uses in equine medicine, 658*t*
Cystic lavage, 547
Cystitis, 546–547
Cytology, synovial fluid analysis and, 579
Cytosine arabinoside, approximate uses in equine medicine, 658*t*

D
Daily record sheet, for hospitalised animals, University of Liverpool, *206*
Dalteparin, approximate uses in equine medicine, 658*t*
Danofloxacin, 345
Dantrolene, approximate uses in equine medicine, 658*t*
Dazzle reflex, 628
D-dimers, 406
Dead-horse removal vehicles, access for, at equine hospital, 158
Deadspace ventilation, 478
  equation for, 463 (box 10.2)
Debridement
  of wounds, 613
  wound treatment after, 616
Decompression, percutaneous trocharisation and, in standing horse, 24
Decubital ulceration, recumbency and, 563
Deep digital flexor, low four-point nerve block and, *98*
Deep fibular nerves, 100
Defibrillation, cardiopulmonary resuscitation of neonatal foal and, 124
Degree of rotation (angle T), radiographs evaluated for, 582, *582*
Dehydration, 379
  clinical signs of, 364–365, 365 (box 6.2)
  crystolloid fluids and treatment of, 370
  defined, 365
  laboratory signs for, 365, 366*t*
  urine specific gravity and, 366
Dembrexine, approximate uses in equine medicine, 658*t*
Demecarium bromide, approximate uses in equine medicine, 658*t*
Denoix, J-M, 650
Dental disease, computed tomography and evaluation of, 172
"Dental Star," 688, 688 (box 19.27)

Dentition, ageing horses by, 688
Dermatoses, nosocomial importance of, 186*t*
Descemetocoels, anaesthesia and, 251
Desflurane, 241
Detomidine, 246
  adding constant rate infusions of, balanced anaesthesia and, 244
  approximate uses in equine medicine, 658*t*
  bronchoscopy technique and, 471
  chemical restraint and use of, 327
  colic pain and use of, 326
  equine sedation and use of, 312, 313, 313*t*
  examination per rectum and use of, 9
  respiratory conditions and use of, 318
  somatic pain management and, 330
  total intravenous anaesthesia and, 252
Dexamethasone, 437*t*
  approximate uses in equine medicine, 659*t*
Dextrans, 376
Dextrose
  intravenous, administration of, for hospitalised adult horse, 267, 269
  in parenteral solutions, 287
Dextrose-supplemented fluid, for foals, 298
Diagnostic imaging
  archiving image data, 175
  central role of, 164–165
  computed tomography, 171–172
  equine magnetic resonance imaging, 172–175
  equine radiography, 165–166
    room dimensions and design, 165–166
  radiography equipment, 166–169
  scintigraphy, 169–170
  ultrasonography, 170
Diaphragmatic hernias, 490
  in foals, 246
Diarrhoea
  assisted enteral feeding and, 283
  daily cultures of faecal samples performed on horses with, 488
  fibre-free enteral diet and, 276
  fluid losses and, 364
  hepatopathy and, 520
  in hospitalised horses, 486
  human enteral formulations and, 278
  liquid enteral diet and, 283
  macrolides and derivatives and, 347
  oral or parenteral antimicrobial agents and, 342
Diastole, 418
Diastolic blood pressure, optimal accuracy of, 45
Diazepam
  acute seizure treatment and, 565
  approximate uses in equine medicine, 659*t*
  cardiac conditions and use of, 318
  equine sedation and use of, 313*t*, 315
  gastrointestinal pain management and, 328
  musculoskeletal conditions and, 317
  for sedating neonatal foals, 320
  total intravenous anaesthesia and, 252
DIC. *See* Disseminated intravascular coagulation
DICOM files, 175
Dictyocaulus arnfieldi, 458
Diet
  hepatic diseases and, 527–528
  preparation of, for enteral nutrition, 282
  recurrent exertional rhabdomyolysis and, 589
Diff-Quik stain, 458, 542
Difloxacin, 345
  approximate uses in equine medicine, 659*t*
Digital image systems, backup for, 175
Digitalis intoxication, hypokalaemia and, 419
Digital radiographic images, manipulating, on computer workstation, *160*
Digital sheath, synoviocentesis of, 579
Digoxin, 437*t*
  approximate uses in equine medicine, 659*t*
  congestive heart failure treatment and, 442–443
  supraventricular tachydysrhythmias and, 441
Dilution methods, principle behind, 55
Dimercaprol, approximate uses in equine medicine, 659*t*
Dimethylsulphoxide
  approximate uses in equine medicine, 659*t*
  laparotomy wounds and use of, 601
  neurological disorders and, 568–569
  solution of, urinary catheter disinfection and, 566
Dinoprost, approximate uses in equine medicine, 659*t*
Dipyrone, approximate uses in equine medicine, 659*t*
Dipyrone/hycosine, for colic pain, in United Kingdom, 326
Direct arterial blood pressure measurement, 45–46
  arterial catheter in dorsal metatarsal artery of anaesthetised horse, *46*
  equipment needed for, 46 (box 1.24)
  measurement, 46
  pressure transducer for direct monitoring of arterial pressure, *46*
  procedure for, 45
  setting up pressure transducer, 46
  zeroing pressure transducer, 46
Direct blood pressure monitoring, 234
Direct digital radiography, advantages/disadvantages with, 167
Direct digital radiography systems suppliers, 176 (box 3.3)
Dirty surgical wounds, 609*t*
Dirty traumatic wounds, 609
Discharge instructions, 225
Disinfection
  of critical care stalls at hospital, 150
  prior to venipuncture, 10–11
  protocols for, 194–195
Disk diffusions, 339
Disseminated intravascular coagulation, 401–403, 405
  clinical approach and management of hospitalised horses with, 414
  clinical considerations, 403
  clinical forms of, 401–402
    bleeding form of, 402
    compensated/subclinical form of, 401–402
    multiorgan failure form of, 402
  coagulation testing profile to diagnose hypercoagulability and, 402–403
  laboratory tests for diagnosis of, 403 (box 8.3)
  patients at risk for, 402
  primary diagnoses associated with increased risk of, 402 (box 8.1)
  results of specialised laboratory tests in diagnosis of, 403 (box 8.3)
  therapeutic protocol for, 410 (box 8.7)
  therapy for, 409–410
Distal interphalangeal (coffin joint), synoviocentesis of, 576
Distal leg weights, 649
Distal limb
  bandaging of, 100, 101, *102*
    granulation tissue formation and, 618
  magnetic resonance imaging of, 316
  puncture wounds of, 615
Distal limb bandages, 100, *102,* 105
  primary and secondary dressings for, *102*
Distal limb injuries
  anaesthesia for horses with, 250–251
  possible anaesthetic choices for horses with, 251 (box 4.4)
Distal limb oedema ("stocking up"), confinement and, 574
Distension colic, risk factors for, 484

DMSO. *See* Dimethylsulphoxide
Dobutamine, 447, 449
cardiovascular and pulmonary support and use of, 242, 243*t*
congestive heart failure treatment and, 443
guideline for diluting and preparation of, 449*t*
renal failure treatment and, 543–544
Documentation of care, 200
Domperidone
approximate uses in equine medicine, 659*t*
mare's milk production and, 300
Donkeys
gastric impaction in, 498
hyperlipaemia in, 399
Donors, for blood or plasma transfusions, 40 (box 1.19)
Donor site, skin grafts, 624
Doorway width, for radiography room, at hospital, 165
Dopamine
cardiovascular and pulmonary support and use of, 242, 243*t*
guideline for diluting and preparation of, 449*t*
renal failure treatment and, 543–544
tissue perfusion improvement and, 451
Doppler studies, 52, 423
Doppler technique, arterial blood pressure measurement with, 432
Dorothy Russell Havemeyer Foundation, Inc., 182
Dorsal aspect of carpus, 10-cm wound to, *612*
Dorsal hoof, percussion of, in early diagnosis of laminitis, *582*
Dorsal metatarsal artery
anatomical location of, *138*
arterial blood sampling from, *43*
arterial catheter in, *46*
catheterisation of, 141
foal restraint for collection of blood sample from, *140*
indirect blood pressure cuff over, 137
location of, and orientation of syringe for arterial blood collection, *140*
Dorsal metatarsal blood collection, from foal, 139, *140*
Dorsal recumbency
CT scanning of horse in, 172
foals placed in, on surgery table, 246
Dorsal spinous process impingement, 641
Dosemeters, 176
Dose rates, programmed, for pumps and drivers, 39
"Double circuit" design, 231
"Double clove-hitch pattern," 19
Double-lumen catheters, 136
in jugular vein of adult horse, *30*
parenteral nutrition treatment and use of, 293, *293*
Double-lumen guarded catheter, tracheal aspirate collection and, 458
Down horses, 562–563
Downstream occlusions, between bags and pumps, alarms and, 39
Doxapram, newborn foal, resuscitation of, and contraindication in use of, 124
Doxepin hydrochloride, approximate uses in equine medicine, 659*t*
Doxycycline, 347–348
approximate uses in equine medicine, 659*t*
CLSI breakpoint for susceptibility to, 341
DPIs. *See* Dry powder inhalers
DPJ. *See* Duodenitis-proximal jejunitis
Draft mares, retained foetal membranes and, 547
Drainage, for radiography room, at hospital, 165
Drains
"Chinese finger trap" suture around, *20*
in equine hospitals, 163–164
extensive wounds, and placement of, 614
surgical incisions and, 597
Drechslera spicifera, 351
Dress code, in operating theatre in hospital, 156
Dressings
biological, 620–621
for distal limb bandaging, *102*
hydrogel, 621
stretchy adhesive, catheterisation of lateral thoracic vein and use of, 35, *35*
wound management and, 619–622
Drinking, reluctance toward, by hospitalised horses, 398–399
Drip chamber, supplementary fluids added to, *36*
Drug doses, 654
approximate uses in equine medicine, 655–668*t*
Drug interactions, PN solution administration and, 293
Drugs, constant rate intravenous infusions of, 669*t*
Dry needling, 651
Dry powder inhalers, 467, 468
DSPI. *See* Dorsal spinous process impingement
Dual-channel pumps, *37*
operation of, 37–38
Duodenitis-proximal enteritis, 498
Duodenitis-proximal jejunitis, laminitis and, 573
Duodenoscopy, 23–24, 498–499
Duodenum
endoscopic view of major and minor papillae in, *24*
imaging of, 494–495
Duration, murmurs and, 418
Durham, A. E., 289
Dysmetria, 559
Dysphagia, 262, 563–564
botulism and, 566
laryngoplasty and, 595
neurological conditions leading to, 563 (box 14.3)
Dysrhythmias, 417, 420
antidysrhythmic therapy and, 436–437
echocardiography and assessment of, 423
electrocardiography procedures and risk of, 421

E
EACA. *See* Aminocaproic acid
Ear bandage, for horse after sarcoid removal, *112*
Early goal-directed therapy, 446
Ears, assessing, 7
ECGs. *See* Electrocardiograms
Echelon suture pattern, 116, *117*
Echinococus granulosus, 527
Echocardiograms
of foal with pericarditis, *427*
of heart, two-dimensional, right parasternal long-axis, *53*
large pericardial effusion and fibrin deposition on visceral pericardium in 2-year-old sport horse, *58*
predrainage and postdrainage, showing effect of fluid removal on the heart, *428*
Echocardiography, 52–55, 423–426
equipment needed for, 52 (box 1.27)
indications for, 423–424
myocarditis and cardiomyopathies, 426
pericardial disease and use of, 426
pericarditis and use of, 444
procedure for, 52–54
valvular lesions and, 424–426
Echogenicity, of abnormal kidney, 539–540
Ectoparasitis, nosocomial importance of, 186*t*
EDTA, approximate uses in equine medicine, 659*t*
Education, about hospital-acquired infections, 196
EEG. *See* Electroencephalography
EGDT. *See* Early goal-directed therapy

EHV-1. *See* Equine herpesvirus-1
EIA. *See* Equine infectious anaemia
EIPH. *See* Exercise-induced pulmonary haemorrhage
Elastic bandages, 104–105
  adhesive, for bandaging head wounds, 111
Elastoplast/Elastikon, 35, 104, 514
  keeping in place, cyanoacrylate adhesive and, *111*
Elective procedures, 236–244
Electrical defibrillation, use of, on neonatal foal, *124*
Electrical muscle stimulation, goals for, 647 (box 18.6)
Electrical stimulation, 638, 647
Electrical treatment modalities, indications, physiological effects and contraindications or precautions, 646*t*
Electrocardiogram leads, colour coding systems for, 50*t*
Electrocardiograms, 5
  radiotelemetry unit for recording of, *51*
Electrocardiographic recording, analysis of, 422–423
Electrocardiography, 49–51, 421–423
  ensuring electrical contact, 51
  equipment needed for, 49 (box 1.26)
  procedures for
    base-apex system, 49–50
    continuous and remote monitoring, 51
    other lead systems, 50
Electroencephalography, neurological system disease and use of, 561
Electrolyte abnormalities
  abnormalities of major electrolytes and their treatment, 381–386
    calcium, 384–385
    chloride, 384
    magnesium, 385
    phosphate, 385–386
    potassium, 382–384
    sodium, 382
  iatrogenic induction of, 386
  parenteral nutrition in foals and, 309
Electrolyte assessment of cardiac disease, potassium, magnesium, and calcium, 419
Electrolyte concentrations
  normal, in adult horses, 678*t*
  normal, in foals, weanlings, and yearlings, 678*t*
Electrolyte deficiencies, pareneral nutrition therapy and, 294–295
Electrolyte disturbances, gastrointestinal disease and, 491
Electrolyte imbalances
  anorexia, malnutrition, and gastrointestinal disease, 266
  correction of, 380–386
Electrolytes
  acid-base balance, renal failure and, 546
  biochemistry and, 654
  fractional excretion of, 537
Electronic infusion pumps, 37–38
  abbreviations used on, 38 (box 1.18)
  advanced operation of, 39
  alarms for, 39
  basic operation of, 37–38
Electronic medical records, 200
Electronic reading, in central venous pressure measurement, 48
Electrotherapy, 644 (box 18.5), 645–648
  "burst" transcutaneous electrical nerve stimulation, 648
  conventional transcutaneous electrical nerve stimulation, 648
  electrical stimulation, 647
  low-level laser therapy, 645–646
  magnetic field therapy, 648
  neuromuscular stimulation, 648
  transcutaneous electrical nerve stimulation, 647
  ultrasound therapy, 646–647
  wound healing and, 642
Eltenac
  approximate uses in equine medicine, 659*t*
  endotoxaemia treatment and, 506
  somatic pain management and, 330
Emergency admissions, infection threats to hospital and, 194
Emergency orthopaedic surgery cases, management of, 330
Emergency tracheotomy, 60–61
  after placement and potential complications, 61
  equipment needed for, 61 (box 1.30)
  indication for, 60
  procedure for, 60–61
EMND. *See* Equine motor neuron disease
EMRs. *See* Electronic medical records
Enalapril, approximate uses in equine medicine, 659*t*
Endocarditis, 425
Endogenous creatinine clearance
  description of, 537
  equation for, 537 (box 13.2)
Endometrial biopsy, 86–87, 542
  equipment needed for, 87 (box 1.50)
  procedures for, 86–87
    rectovaginal technique, 87
    vaginal technique, 87
Endometrial cytology, evaluating, 542–543
Endometritis, common fungal pathogens at, 352*t*
Endoscopes
  flexible, types of, 179
  second-hand, purchasing, 180
Endoscopic equipment, 179–180
  image recording equipment, 180
  light sources, 179–180
  purchasing a second-hand microscope, 180
  scope size, 180
Endoscopy
  of bladder and ureters
    equipment needed for, 86 (box 1.49)
    procedure for, 86
  of female genital tract, 542
  of the guttural pouch, 66–68
  of respiratory tract, 65–66
  of upper respiratory tract, *594*
  of urinary tract, 541
Endoscopy equipment and accessories, suppliers of, 180 (box 3.6)
Endotoxaemia
  clinical features of, 503 (box 11.6)
  disseminated intravascular coagulation and, 414
  ileus and, 499
  treatments for, 503–504, 504 (box 11.7)
Endotoxin, 371
Endotoxin binding, competitive inhibition of, 505
Endotracheal intubation
  in adult horse, 3–5
    equipment for, 4 (box 1.1)
  difficult intubations, 5
  equipment required for, 3
  procedure for, 4
Endotracheal tubes
  for cardiopulmonary resuscitation of neonatal foal, 122–123
  changing, mechanical ventilation and, 475
  checking for exudate accumulation, 479
  matching size of, to weight of foal, 120*t*
  matching size of, to weight of horse, 4*t*
End-tidal carbon dioxide (CO_2), monitoring cardiopulmonary resuscitation and, 124
Energy, hospitalised adult horse and, 269–270

Energy requirements
for adult horses using stall resting and maintenance energy equations, 270*t*
digestible, for horses in different physiological conditions, 270*t*
for neonatal foal, 298–299
Enilconazole, 353, 354
Enoxaparin, approximate uses in equine medicine, 659*t*
Enrofloxacin, 345, 346
approximate uses in equine medicine, 659*t*
Enteral diet ingredients, equine, estimated nutrient content of, 280*t*
Enteral diets
commercial, 278, 279*t*
feeds to avoid in, 280
protein in, 270
Enteral feeding bags, 133
Enteral fluid therapy, 367–368
composition, recipes and amounts to give, 368
delivery of nasogastric fluids, 367
free choice water, 367
intragastric fluid administration, 367
types of fluid for, 367–368
Enteral nutrition, 261, 262
for hospitalised foals, 300–301
Enteral nutritional therapy, indications for, in adult horse, 275 (box 5.11)
Enteral nutrition for hospitalised adult horses, 276–284
choice and use of indwelling nasogastric tubes, 280–281
oesophagostomy tube placement and contraindications, 281
diet formulations, 277–280
equine enteral diet recipes, 278–279
human formulations, 277–278
feeds to avoid in enteral diet, 280
fibre in enteral diets, 276–277
liquid diets, nutritional supplements in, 279–280
oil, 279
protein, 279
preparation and administration of, 282–283
diet preparation, 282
monitoring guidelines, 282–283
nutrition of, 282
return to voluntary feeding and, 284
Enteral nutrition formulation worksheet, 277 (box 5.12)
Enteral therapy
parenteral therapy *versus*, 275
for neonatal foals, 299–300
Enterobacter cloacae, isolates of, from laparotomy incisional infections, 601
Enterobacteriaceae, 338
antipseudomonal penicillins and, 343
cephalosporins and, 344
isolation of, from equine septic joints, 580
Enterobacter spp., 185, 337
Enterococcus, 185
Enterococcus faecium, isolates of, from laparotomy incisional infections, 601
Enterococcus spp., 338
Enterocolitis, antimicrobial agent-associated, 342
Environmental change, horses in hospital, gastrointestinal disorders and, 484
Environmental surveillance, infection control and, 192
Eosinophils, bronchoalveolar lavage cytology and presence of, 460
Ephedrine, cardiovascular and pulmonary support and use of, 243*t*
Epidural analgesia
for somatic pain, 331–332
for visceral pain, 328–329
Epidural injection and catheterisation, 81–84
anatomy of site for, *82*
epidural catheter in place, with filter and injection cap, *84*
equipment needed for, 82 (box 1.46)
hanging drop technique, *83*
Hustead epidural needle and Teflon catheter seated in coccygeal epidural space of horse, *83*
Hustead epidural needle used to tunnel 20-gauge 91.8 medical grade epidural catheter under skin, *84*
identification of appropriate intervetebral space for, *83*
indications, 81
injecting into epidural catheter, *84*
injecting into epidural space, via a needle, *84*
procedure for, 81–84
Epinephrine
approximate uses in equine medicine, 659*t*
guideline for diluting and preparation of, 449*t*
resuscitation of foal and, 123
tissue perfusion improvement and, 450–451
Epiphora, 633
Epistaxis, guttural pouch endoscopy and performing on patients with, 67–68
Epithelial cells, inflammation or neoplasia of renal tubules or urinary tract, 536
Epsilon-aminocaproic acid, approximate uses in equine medicine, 659*t*
EPSM. *See* Equine polysaccharide storage myopathy
Equi-analytical Laboratories, 253
Equine anaesthesia equipment, 229*t*
Equine colic admission form, Philip Leverhulme Equine Hospital, University of Liverpool, *203–204*
Equine feeds, common, estimated nutrient composition of, 265*t*
Equine Gastric Ulcer Council
grading system recommended by, 498
lesion grading system of, 494 (box 11.3)
Equine herpesvirus infection, nosocomial importance of, 187*t*
Equine herpesvirus myeloencephalitis, Florida outbreak of, 183
Equine herpesvirus-1, rectal impactions and, 566
Equine hospital feeding chart, 264 (box 5.5)
Equine hospitals
gates sited back from road, to allow lorries to pull of road when gates are shut, *148*
reasons for development of, 147
Equine infectious anaemia, 182, 560
nosocomial importance of, 187*t*
Equine influenza, 182
nosocomial importance of, 187*t*
Equine metabolic syndrome, 573
Equine motor neuron disease, 586
muscle biopsy and, 112
Equine neonate, healthy, enteral feeding for, 302
Equine polysaccharide storage myopathy
acute and long-term management of, 590
clinical signs of, 590
diagnosis of, 590
muscle biopsy and, 112
pathogenesis, 590
Equine protozoal myeloencephalopathy, 559
cerebrospinal fluid analysis and, 561
Equine recurrent uveitis, 635
Equine rhinovirus, 394
Equine Senior, 266
nutrient composition of, 265*t*
Equine Surgery (Stick), 281
Equine viral arteritis, 182
nosocomial importance of, 188*t*
Equipment storage, at equine hospital, 157–158
Equipment store, near stables, at equine hospital, 150
ERU. *See* Equine recurrent uveitis

Erythromycin, 346
approximate uses in equine medicine, 660*t*
treatment of ileus and, 501
ESBL. *See* Extended-spectrum ß-lactamase
Escherichia coli, 185, 337, 566
isolates of, from equine septic joints, 580
isolates of, from laparotomy incisional infections, 601
isolates of, from septic arthritis in foals, 580
Esmarch bandage
placement of, below hock for regional perfusion of distal limb, *109*
use of prior to application of tourniquet, 108
Estradiol, approximate uses in equine medicine, 660*t*
Estrone sulfate, approximate uses in equine medicine, 660*t*
E test, 339
Ethamsylate
approximate uses in equine medicine, 660*t*
hypocoagulable states in horses managed with, 411–412
Ether-a-go-go (ERG) potassium channel blocks, 502
Etodolac, approximate uses in equine medicine, 660*t*
Europe, example of parenteral nutrition formula used in, 307, 308 (box 5.25)
Euthanasia/Death in Hospital form, *202*
Euthanised horses, 162
EVA. *See* Equine viral arteritis
Evacuation of pneumothorax, 72–74
aspiration from thoracic catheter, *76*
caudo-dorsal thoracic radiograph showing bilateral pneumothorax in adult horse, *73*
equipment needed for, 74 (box 1.41)
insertion of thoracic trocar catheter for, *76*
intermittent, indwelling chest tube for, *76*
procedure for, 72, 74
site for, *75*
thoracic ultrasound at junction between dorsal surface of lung and air in pleural space, *75*
trocar removed from thoracic catheter, *76*
Examination rooms, specialised, at equine hospital, 158–159
Excess fluid administration, parenteral nutrition therapy and, 294
Exercise, maintenance of normal function of large intestine and, 485
Exercise-induced pulmonary haemorrhage, 412
bronchoalveolar lavage and, 461
Exercise rehabilitation, 649–650
elements of, 649 (box 18.7)
Exercise therapy, 644 (box 18.5)
Exertional myopathy, acepromazine and, 317
Extended-spectrum ß-lactamase, 182
Extensor tendon lacerations, prognosis for horses with, 616
External coaptation (splinting), 605–607
acute management of orthopaedic injury, 605
Robert Jones bandage, 606–607
splinting equine limb, 606
treatment and transportation, 607
Eyelids, anaesthesia of, 92–93
Eyes
examination of, 628
monitoring and treatment of, 628–637
regional anaesthesia of, 91–93

F
Facemasks
connecting to ultrasonic nebulisers, *467*
dry powder inhalers and, 468
nebulisers attached to, 467
Facial artery, palpating in adult horse, 431
Facial nerve paralysis, physiotherapy and, 639–640
Facial palsy, *640*
Facial sinus
collection of blood from, 12
location of, *12*
Facial symmetry, 558
Facility evaluation, biosecurity and, 195–196
Faecal balls, examination of, 488
Famotidine, approximate uses in equine medicine, 660*t*
Faraday cage, 170
Faraday shield, 174
Far-near-far suture pattern, *118*
disadvantage with, 119
technique, and advantage with, 118
Farrier at work, in dedicated hospital room, *160*
Farriery area, at equine hospital, 160, *160*
Fat-soluble vitamins, 274, 289
Feed chart, 253
Feeding back colic patients, 512–515
Feeding changes, colic patients and, 487
Feeding chart, equine hospital, 264 (box 5.5)
Feeding intolerance, enteral nutrition and, in neonatal foal, 306
Feeding mangers, at equine hospital, 150
Feeding schedule, hepatic insufficiency treatment and, 528
Feeding tubes, for foals, 303
Feet, gamma camera and obtaining images of, 170
Female foals
connection of urinary catheter to surgical drainage bag forming closed system in, *144*
equipment for urinary catheterisation of, 142 (box 2.13)
placement of urinary catheter in, *144*
urinary catheterisation of, 143–144, *144*
Female genital tract
investigating, 541–543
endometrial biopsy, 542
endoscopy of, 542
evaluating endometrial cytology, 542–543
ultrasonography of, 542
uterine lavage, 542
uterine swab, 542
Female horses, urinary catheterisation and, 85
Female urinary tract, scope size for endoscopy of, 180
Femoral fracture repair, 618–619
Femoropatellar joint, synoviocentesis of, 579
Femorotibial (stifle) joint, synoviocentesis of, 579
Fenbendazole, approximate uses in equine medicine, 660*t*
Fenoldopam mesylate, renal failure treatment and, 543–544
Fenoprostalene, approximate uses in equine medicine, 660*t*
Fenoterol, 468
approximate uses in equine medicine, 660*t*
Fentanyl
approximate uses in equine medicine, 660*t*
equine sedation and use of, 315
somatic pain management and, 330
Fetlock (fore limb)
analgesia of, 97
limited articular mobility in, *643*
Fetlock (hind limb), analgesia of, 98
Fetlock joints
septic arthritis in, 573
synoviocentesis and, 577, *577*
Fever
common causes of, in hospitalised horse, 393 (box 7.1)
implant surgery and, 592
remittent, 394
sustained, 394
unexplained, 393–395
investigation, 393–394
pathogenesis, 393

FgDP, 406
Fiberoptic endoscopes, 179
  collecting tracheal aspirate with use of guarded sampling catheter via, *458*
Fibre, in enteral diets, 276–277
Fibrin degradation products, 406
Fibrin deposits, post-mortem detection of, 406–407
Fibrin monomers, 406
Fibrinogen concentrations, 405
  guide to interpretation of, 674 (box 19.7)
Fibrinogen test, anticoagulants for, 670 (box 19.3)
Fibrinolytic activity, markers of, 406
Fibrinolytic drugs
  administration of, 405 (box 8.5)
  hypercoagulable states in horses managed with, 411
Fibrosis, 526–527
Fibular nerves, superficial and deep, 100
Fick method, cardiac output measurement and, 55
Field block, 97
Fight or flight response, equine sedation and, 318
Film badges, 176
  storage of, 169
Film/screen radiography, conventional, 166–167
Flax oil, 279
Flecainide, 442
Fleroxacin, 345
  approximate uses in equine medicine, 660*t*
Flexor tendon lacerations, prognosis for horses with, 616
Flood lighting, for yard at equine hospital, 152
Floors and flooring
  in equine hospitals, 162–163
  horses with neurological disorders and, 561–562
  ideal properties of, for hospitals, 163 (box 3.1)
  for main clinical area in hospitals, 154
  for MRI rooms, 174
  for operating theatres, 156
  for radiography rooms, 159, 165
  in rooms for performing nerve blocks, 160
Florfenicol, 349
  approximate uses in equine medicine, 660*t*
"Flow checks," 510
Flow cytometry, 406
Flowmeters, for large-animal anaesthesia machines, 229
Flow triggering, 476
Fluconazole, 353, 354
  approximate uses in equine medicine, 660*t*
  fungal keratitis treatment and, 631
  spectrum of activity for, 353*t*
Flucytosine, spectrum of activity for, 353*t*
Fluid administration sets, 36–37
  horse on continuous intravenous fluids, using infusion set with coil, *36*
Fluid bags, four, connecting to a giving set with two spikes, using transfer sets, 36, *36*
Fluid balance, monitoring in foals, 309
"Fluid challenge," 447, 453
Fluid control dials, 36
Fluid hangers
  intensive care patient and, *152*
  with swivel mechanism, *36*
Fluid overload, clinical signs of, 386
Fluid pumps, foal connected to, *37*
Fluid status, surgical colic patients and monitoring of, 511
Fluid therapy, 364–387
  acute renal failure and, 545–546
  approach to, in the horse, 364 (box 6.1)
  blood, blood components and blood substitutes, 376–378
  colloid fluids, 375–376
  correction of electrolyte imbalances, 380–386
  crystalloid fluids, 372–374
  enteral, 367–368
    composition, recipes and amounts to give, 368
    delivery of nasogastric fluids, 367
    free choice water, 367
    intragastric fluid administration, 367
    types of fluid for, 367–368
  hepatic disorders and, 524–525
  iatrogenic complications of, 386
    extravasation of fluids, 386
    fluid overload, 386
    hypothermia and energy loss, 386–387
    inatrogenic electrolyte abnormalities, 386
  improving tissue perfusion and use of, 446–447
    fluid challenge, 447
    uncontrolled haemorrhage and, 447
  intravenous, 368–372
    delivery systems, 369
    fluid types, 369–372
  matching fluid to needs, 379–380
    dehydration, 379
    maintenance, 380
    ongoing losses, 379–380
  for medical colic patients, 508–509
  during PN infusion, 294
  recognising need for, 364–366
  reversal of hypovolaemia, 378–379
  selecting route of administration for, 366
  treatment of ileus and, 499–500
Flumazenil, approximate uses in equine medicine, 660*t*
Flumethasone, approximate uses in equine medicine, 660*t*
Flunixin
  for colic pain, use of, in United States, 326
  endotoxaemia treatment, 505, 506
  somatic pain management and, 330
  subconjunctival, 329
Flunixin meglumine, 512
  approximate uses in equine medicine, 660*t*
Fluoroquinolones, 338, 342, 345–346
  equine central nervous system or cerebrospinal fluid and, 567
Fluoroscopy, 178
Fluphenazine, 316
  approximate uses in equine medicine, 660*t*
  equine sedation and use of, 313*t*, 314
Fluprostenol, approximate uses in equine medicine, 661*t*
Flushing catheter, percutaneous (transtracheal aspirate) and, 69–70
Fluticasone
  approximate uses in equine medicine, 661*t*
  inhaled corticosteroid therapy and, 470
Foal feeding tubes, 303
Foaling
  interpretation of peritoneal fluid and, 492
Foal milk replacers, 300
Foals. *See also* Neonatal foals
  ambulatory colt, closed urine collection system in, *144*
  anaesthesia for, 246–248
  anatomy of internal umbilical structures of, *145*
  arrangements for separating mares and, during treatment at hospitals, *151*
  bottle-feeding for, 301–302, *302*
  bucket or pan feeding for, 301
  cataract surgery in, 636–637
  catheter maintenance in, for intranasal oxygen administration, 62
  clinically ill, enteral feeding for, 303
    feeding protocol, 303–304
    volume to feed, 303
  with colic, collecting gastric reflux from, *380*

common indications for surgery in, 246
common microorganisms isolated from septic arthritis in, 580
connecting to fluid pump, *37*
connecting to ventilator, 126–127
correctly placed nasogastric feeding tube in, *133*
critically ill, rates of renal insufficiency and, 533
enteral feeding and monitoring of, 305–306
complications with, 306
external portion of catheter and tongue depressor affixed to face of, *63*
feeding, by providing milk in a bowl, *301*
feeding through indwelling nasogastric tube, *304*
fixing indwelling nasogastric feeding tube to, *131*
fluid rates for, 36
fracture repair in, 605 (box 15.9)
haemodialysis in, 544
healthy, average daily weight gain for, 298*t*
hospitalised, nutrition management of, 297–311
nutrient requirements for, 298–299
nutrition options: enteral nutrition, 300–306
nutrition options: parenteral nutrition, 306–309
patient evaluation and initiation of therapy, 297–298
selecting form of supplemental nutrition, 299–300
hospitalised neonatal, enteral feeding chart for, 305 (box 5.23)
hospitalised neonatal, weekly feeding plan for, 304 (box 5.22)
incorrectly placed nasogastric feeding tubes in, *133*
inhalant anaesthesia induction of, *247*
jugular thrombophlebitis in site of previous indwelling intravenous catheter in, *396*
measuring length of nasogastric feeding tube to place in, *131*
nasal intubation of, *247*
nebulisation of, with fitted, valved facemask, *64*
neonatal, guidelines for infusing regular insulin in (non-SI units), 310–311*t*
neonatal, guidelines for infusing regular insulin in (SI units), 310*t*
neonatal, matching size of endotracheal tube to weight of, 120*t*
neonatal, sedating, 320
neonates and older, anaesthetic choices for, 247*t*
normal biochemistry values in, 671*t*
normal electrolyte concentrations in, 678*t*
normal haemodynamics in, 682, 685*t*
normal haemotology values for, 671*t*
normal haustrated left ventral colon imaged transabdominally in, *497*
normal physiological values for, 670 (box 19.2)
opisthotonus in, with severe hyponatraemia, *558*
parenteral nutrition in, *306*
complications, 309
formulations, 306–308
infusion protocol, 308
monitoring, 308–309
parenteral nutrition worksheet for, 307 (box 5.24)
with pericadial effusion causing tamponade, *426*
pericardial effusion from foal with septic pericarditis, *420*
petechial haemorrhages in, with severe pneumonia, *404*
post-mortem of, with bleeding form of disseminated intravascular coagulation, *402*
readout from pulse contour analysis cardiac output determination in, *57*
reasonable anaesthetic protocol for mares during controlled vaginal or caesarean section delivery of, 250 (box 4.3)
recovering from general anaesthesia, 248
small and large intestine adhered to large abdominal *Rhodococcus equi* abscess in, *497*
small intestinal intussusception in, *496*
starting on nutrition, 133
with Tyzzer's disease, 527
of varying ages, volume of milk per day, 302*t*
ventilator adjusted to, 127–128
Foal unit, at equine hospital, 150
Foal-ventilator interactions, description of, in synchronised intermittent mandatory ventilation with pressure support (SIMV-PS) mode, 126 (box 2.5)
Focal iris prolapse, in Percheron mare, *629*
Focal pulmonary abscessation, detection of, on ultrasonographic examination, *464*
Foetal membranes, retained, 547
Foley catheter
filling balloon of, after being passed into bladder in male foal, *143*
placement of, into bladder of gelding, *85*
urinary catheterisation of male foal and, 143
Folic acid, approximate uses in equine medicine, 661*t*
Folinic acid, approximate uses in equine medicine, 661*t*
Follicle-stimulating hormone, approximate uses in equine medicine, 661*t*
Foot, analgesia of, 97
Foot cast, 607 (box 15.10)
Foot-related problems, equine magnetic resonance imaging and, 173
Forage analysis, 253
Forearm of horse, cross section of, *99*
Fore limb laminitis, 572
Fore limbs
biomechanically important regions of, for splinting, *106*
caudal aspect of, anatomy of, *100*
splinting applied to, 106–107
Formaldehyde, hypocoagulable states in horses managed with, 412
Formoterol, 468
Founder
defined, 572
lateral radiography of horse with, *582*
monitoring for, in hospitalised horses, 581
patients at risk of, 572–573
Founder distance (D), radiographs evaluated for, 582
Fractional excretion of electrolytes
equation for calculation of, 537 (box 13.3)
use for, 537
Fractional excretions, urinary, 590, 591
Fractional shortening, calculating, 52
Fractured limbs, objectives in first aid for, 106 (box 1.58)
Fracture patients
handling, at equine hospital, 150
install rail for tying up, *152*
Fractures
anaesthesia for horses with, 250–251
emergency steps for horses with, 605 (box 15.7)
possible anaesthetic choices for horses with, 251 (box 4.4)
routine treatment of, with reasonable prognosis in horses, 605 (box 15.8)
surgical repair of, in foals, 605 (box 15.9)
Free choice water, 367
French Argyle chest tube, large-bore, pericardiocentesis and use of, 59
Fresh (frozen) plasma
hypercoagulable states in horses managed with, 411
hypocoagulable states in horses managed with, 412
Friesian mares, retained foetal membranes and, 547
Frog puncture wounds, 617
Frontal block
for placement of subpalpebral lavage catheter, 95
in regional anaesthesia of eye, 93
Frontal nerve, regional anaesthesia of eye and block to, 93, *93*
Frontal sinus, as site for sinocentesis, 78
Frusemide, 366
FS. *See* Fractional shortening
FSH. *See* Follicle-stimulating hormone
Full-limb bandages, 105
application of, *612*
Full-limb casts, 607 (box 15.10)

Fungal infections
  keratitis due to, in 9-year-old Thoroughbred mare, *631*
  systemic therapy of, 352
Fungal pathogens, most common, at selected sites in horses, 352*t*
Furacin, 620
Furosemide (frusemide)
  approximate uses in equine medicine, 661*t*
  congestive heart failure treatment and, 443–444
Fusarium, miconazole and, 631

G
Gabapentin, pain management and, 332
Gag, opening mouth of horse with, prior to intubation, 4, *4*
"Gag" reflex, 558
Gait analysis, 558–559
  grading system for, 559 (box 14.2)
  wound management of hospitalised horse and, 611
Galvayne's groove, 688, 688 (box 19.27)
Gamma cameras, 169–170
  ceiling mounted rectangular, *170*
Gamma scintigraphy, 159
Gamma scintigraphy camera, using, *159*
Gantry-mounted radiographic tube head, using, *159*
Garden spray-pump, adapted, for insufflation of stomach, *21*
Gas distension, relieving, with percutaneous trocharisation, 24–25
Gastric mucosa, grading of, 498
Gastric reflux, collecting from foal with colic, *380*
Gastric squamous cell carcinoma, diagnosing, 498
Gastric ulceration, 486–487
Gastrointestinal disease
  electrolyte imbalances associated with, 266
  shedding of *Salmonella* in adult horses with, 486
Gastrointestinal disorders
  equine sedation and, 319
  management of horses with, 499–515
  patients at risk of developing, during hospitalisation, 484–487
    anaesthesia, 485
    atropine, 485–486
    caecal impactions, 485
    change of environment, 484
    diarrhoea, 486
    gastric ulceration, 486–487
    nonsteroidal anti-inflammatory drug toxicity, 485
    oesophageal obstruction (choke), 487
    postoperative ileus, 484
    stable confinement and large colon impactions, 484–485
Gastrointestinal infections, simplified guidelines for surveillance of, 181*t*
Gastrointestinal pain
  alpha$_2$-adrenergic agonist and, 328
  long-term modulation of, 327
Gastrointestinal perfusion, vasopressin, terlipressin and, 450
Gastrointestinal protein loss, fever associated with, 394
Gastrointestinal sounds, propulsive, commonly used drugs that decrease or abolish, 488 (box 11.2)
Gastrointestinal system
  abnormal findings in, 489–490
    caecum, 489
    large colon, 489–490
    late gestational mares, 490
    miscellaneous abnormalities, 490
    small colon, 490
    stomach and small intestine, 489
  haemotology, biochemistry and, 490–491
  monitoring, 484–499
  ultrasonography of, 494–498
Gastroscopy, 21–24, 498–499
  equipment for, 21–22, 21 (box 1.12)
  patient preparation, 22
  procedure for, 22–23
  scope size for, 180
Gates, car and lorry parking at hospital and, 148, *148*
Gatifloxacin, 346
Gauze packing, extensive wounds, and placement of, 614
Gelatins, 376
Gelding, Foley catheter placed into bladder of, *85*
Gemifloxacin, 346
General anaesthesia, 226–246
  anaesthetic risk, 235–236
  balanced anaesthesia, 243–244
  elective procedures, 236–239
    preanasthetic evaluation, 236–237
    premedication, 237–239
  equipment, 228–235
    large-animal anaesthesia machines, 228–231
    large-animal anaesthesia ventilator, 231–233
    pulse oximetry, capnography and airway gases, 234–235
    surgical table: positioning and padding, 228
  facilities for, 226–228
    induction area, 226–228
    recovery room, 228
    storage, 228
  gastrointestinal motility and, 485
  hypoventilation and hypotension, 242–243
  hypoxaemia, 244
  induction, 239
  intubation, 239–240
  maintenance of anaesthesia, 240–242
  monitoring equipment, 233–234
    blood gas, 234
    cardiovascular monitors, 233–234
    direct blood pressure monitoring, 234
  personnel, 235
  postoperative pain management, 245–246
  recovery, 244–245
    physical restraint and assisted recoveries, 245
Generators, in equine hospitals, 164
Genital disorders, 534
Gentamicin, 337, 338, 344
  aerosol administration of, 361
  intra-articular therapy and, 350
  percutaneous trocharisation and use of, 25
Gentian violet, delay in wound healing and, 622
George D. Widener Hospital for Large Animals (University of Pennsylvania), 182, 183, 185, 192
Gestational mares, late, gastrointestinal abnormalities and, 490
GFR. *See* Glomerular filtration rate
Giemsa techniques, cytology slides stained with, 458
Giving sets, from fluid pumps, 36
GKX. *See* Guaifenesin/ketamine/xylazine
GLDH. *See* Glutamate dehydrogenase
Global oxygen delivery, 435
Global oxygen uptake, 435
Globe perforation, in 12-year-old warmblood gelding, *634*
Globulin concentrations, guide to interpretation of, 673 (box 19.6)
Glomerular filtration rate, measurement of, 536–537
Gloves
  correctly stored, *166*
  prolonging life of, 167
Glucagon, approximate doses used in equine medicine, 661*t*
Glucocorticoids
  herpes simplex encephalitis and, 568
  laminitis and, 573
Glucose
  intravenous administration of, for hospitalised adult horse, 267, 269

in parenteral solutions, 287
reagent strips and, 535
Glucose concentrations
cerebrospinal fluid analysis and, 560–561
guide to interpretation of, 676 (box 19.18)
Glucose-containing solutions, 374
Glucose metabolism, markers of, in hospitalised horse, 265
Glucose-supplemented fluid, for foals, 298
Glucose test, anticoagulants for, 670 (box 19.3)
Glucosuria, 535
parenteral nutrition therapy and, 295
Glutamate dehydrogenase, 521
Glutamine, 271–272
approximate doses used in equine medicine, 661*t*
Glutathionine peroxidase test, anticoagulants for, 670 (box 19.3)
Gluteal muscle, site for surgical biopsy of, *113*
Glycopyrrolate, 437*t*
approximate doses used in equine medicine, 661*t*
bradydysrhythmias and, 442
cardiovascular and pulmonary support and use of, 243*t*
Glycosaminoglycans polysulphated, approximate doses used in equine medicine, 661*t*
Goat's milk, feeding of, to foals, 300
Gonadotrophin-releasing hormone, approximate doses used in equine medicine, 661*t*
Grafting. *See* Skin grafting
Gram-negative bacteria, 337
Gram negative microorganisms, suggested choices of antimicrobial agents for common bacterial pathogens of horses and, 339t
Gram-positive aerobic bacterial isolates, in vitro antimicrobial susceptibility of, from horses, 340*t*
Gram-positive microorganisms, 337
suggested choices of antimicrobial agents for common bacterial pathogens of horses and, 339t
Grass sickness, peritoneal fluid and, 493
Gravity flow system, enteral feeding for clinically ill foals and, 303
Grids, computerised radiography and use of, 168
Griseofulvin, approximate doses used in equine medicine, 661*t*
Growing horses
digestible energy requirements for, 270*t*
protein requirements for, 271*t*
Growth factors, wound management and, 620
Growth hormone, wound management and, 620
Guaifenesin, 239
approximate doses used in equine medicine, 661*t*
balanced anaesthesia and adding constant rate of infusions of, 244
total intravenous anaesthesia and, 252
Guaifenesin/ketamine/xylazine, total intravenous anaesthesia and use of, 252, 253
Guided (endoscopic) technique, for bronchoalveolar lavage, 71
Guttural pouch, anatomy of, *68*
Guttural pouch endoscopy, 66–68
biopsy forceps used to open salpingopharyngeal fold allowing entry of endoscope into guttural pouch, *67*
endoscopic view of normal guttural pouch, *68*
equipment needed for, 67 (box 1.37)
guttural pouch openings, *67*
procedure for, 67–68
purpose of, 66
Guttural pouch mycosis, common fungal pathogens at, 352*t*

H
Haematology, anticoagulants for, 670 (box 19.3)
Haematology tests, neurological system and, 561
Haematuria, 535
Haemodialysis, 544
Haemodynamic parameters, derived, calculations for, 686*t*
Haemodynamics
in normal conscious horse and pony, 685*t*
in normal conscious neonatal foal, 685*t*
Haemodynamic variables, 435
Haemoglobin, decreased vasodilation and, 452
Haemoglobin-based oxygen-carrying solutions, 452
Haemoglobinuria, 535
Haemolysis, unconjugated hyperbilirubinaemia and, 522
Haemophilia A, 405
Haemorrhages
uncontrolled, 379
exception to aggressive fluid therapy for hypovolaemia and, 447
wound management and control of, 611
Haemosiderin, 528
Haemostasis
markers not routinely available to study in depth, 406–407
aggregometry, 406
coagulation inhibitor activities, 406
flow cytometry, 406
markers of coagulation activity, 406
markers of fibrinolytic activity, 406
measurement of coagulation factors, 406
post-mortem detection of fibrin deposits, 406–407
thromboelastography and perfusion studies, 407
Haemostatic defect
coagulopathies due to, 404
hepatopathies, 404–405
thrombocytopenia, 404
vasculitis, 404
vitamin K deficiency, 404
Haemotology, 654
gastrointestinal system and, 490–491
Haemotology values, normal, in adult horses, 671*t*
HAIs. *See* Hospital-acquired infections
Half limb cast, 607 (box 15.10)
Hallebeek, J. M., 273
Halogen light sources, endoscopic equipment, 179
Halothane, 241
maintenance of anaesthesia and use of, 240
summary of subjective differences in clinical signs of anaesthesia in adult horses under isoflurane, sevoflurane and, 241*t*
Handheld analysers, for lactate measurement, 432, *432*
Handheld cassette holders, 168
Hand hygiene, critical importance of, 194–195
Hartmann's solution, 372
Haynet, suspension of, to encourage forelimb weight transference and increased proprioceptive input, *640*, 650
HBOC. *See* Haemoglobin-based oxygen-carrying solutions
HE. *See* Hepatic encephalopathy
Head bandaging, 110–112, *111*
commonly used materials for, 110 (box 1.62)
indications for, 110
procedure for, 110–112
soft helmet used to protect horse's head during recovery from general anaesthesia, *110*
Head cases, equine sedation and, 317
Heads of horses
adjustable stand for, 169
CT scanner for scanning of, *172*
examination of, 558
Head-to-toe approach, in physical examination, 7–8
Head wounds, 613–614
Heart
auscultation of, 8
predrainage and postdrainage echocardiograms, showing effect of fluid removal on, *428*
two-dimensional, right parasternal long-axis echocardiograms of, *53*

Heart monitoring, 417–428
auscultation, 417–419
heart sounds, 418
murmurs, 418–419
rate, rhythm, and character of heart sounds, 418
echocardiography, 423–426
indications for, 423–424
myocarditis and cardiomyopathies, 426
pericardial disease, 426
valvular lesions, 424–426
electrocardiography, 421–423
analysis of electrocardiographic recording, 422–423
electrolyte assessment: potassium, magnesium, and calcium, 419
laboratory investigations, 419–420
pericarditis, 426–428
clinical signs of, 426
evaluation of the fluid, 426–428
physical examination, 417
plasma biochemistry, 419–420
specific indicators of cardiac disease, 420
Heart problem treatments, 436–444
Heart rate
electrocardiographic recording and calculation of, 422
pulse contour analysis and, 57
Heart sounds, rate, rhythm, and character of, 418
Heating panels, intensive care patient and, *152*
Heat-moisture exchange filters, 126, 475
attachment of, to expiratory arm of ventilator circuit, *127*
Heat therapy, 649
effects of, 649*t*
Heavy metals, renal insufficiency and, 534
Heimlich valve, for thoracic drainage, *20*
Heparin
approximate doses used in equine medicine, 661*t*
hypercoagulable states in horses managed with, 410
thrombocytopenia and administration of high doses of, 405 (box 8.5)
Hepatic conditions, equine sedation and, 319–320
Hepatic diseases, specific diets for, 527–528
Hepatic disorders
management of horses with, 524–528
hepatic encephalopathy, 525–526
specific fluid therapy considerations, 524–525
patients at risk of developing, during hospitalisation, 520
specific therapies for, 526
Hepatic encephalopathy, 524, 525–526
clinical signs associated with, in horses, 525 (box 12.2)
head-pressing by horse with, *562*
treatment of, 526
Hepatic fibroplasia, 523, 526–527
Hepatic function, serum biochemical evaluation of, 522–523
Hepatic insufficiency, 522
Hepatic lipidosis, 266, 520
treatment for, 525
Hepatic stellate cells, 527
Hepatic system, monitoring and treating, 520–523
Hepatisation, consolidation of lung parenchyma with, *464*
Hepatopathies, 404
Hepatotoxicity, 520–521
Herbal remedies, hepatotoxins and, 528
Herbal substances, 253
Hernia formation, postlaporotomy infection and, 601
Herpesvirus myeloencephalitis, 182
Hetastarch, 375
approximate doses used in equine medicine, 661*t*
Hexalite, 608
Hickman block, 169
High four-point nerve block, 99
analgesia of limb distal to carpus and hock, 98
High-risk patients, biosecurity and, 185
Hind limbs
biomechanically important regions of, for splinting, *106*
laminitis in, 572
splinting applied to, 107
tibial and fibular (peroneal) block for, 100
Histoplasma capsulatum, 352
HMEs. *See* Heat-moisture exchange filters
Hock, analgesia of limb distal to, 98
Hock region, primary dressing applied to, 105
Hoists and hoisting
bar on hook and chin of hoist used to lift horses while putting less stress on back and legs, *227*
equine radiography and, 165
in induction area, 226
in operating theatre, 156
Holter monitors, use of, 421, 422
Holter recordings, ECG, 51
Hoof cast, 607 (box 15.10)
Hoof debridement, total intravenous anaesthesia and, 252, 253
Hoof testers, application of, for detection of laminitis, 581, *581*
Hoof wall thickness (WT), radiographs evaluated for, 582
Hooves, physical examination of, 575
Horizontal mattress suture pattern, *117*
with quills, *117*
technique, advantages/disadvantages with, 117
Hormonal secretion, in mares, sedative drugs and, 320
Hormone tests, anticoagulants for, 670 (box 19.3)
Horse handling, magnetic resonance imaging and, 174–175
Horses
antibacterial agents used in, 342–344
bacterial infections in, 337–338
intubation, getting past larynx of, *4*
opening mouth of, with gag, prior to intubation, *4*
Horse-specific scintigraphy systems suppliers, 176 (box 3.3)
Hospital, use of word, for describing clinic, 147
Hospital-acquired infections
deaths related to, 180–181
hand hygiene, disinfection protocols and, 194–195
increase in incidence of, 180
medical and economic consequences related to, in veterinary settings, 182
patient surveillance and, 185
Hospital design and organisation, 147–197
biosecurity for equine hospitals
concluding remarks about, 196–197
development and implementation of programme for: small to medium-sized clinics, 184 (box 3.7)
education and awareness, 196
facility evaluation, 195–196
hand hygiene and disinfection protocols, 194–195
infection control programme: overview, 183–184
infectious/zoonotic diseases of hospitalised horse, 196
microbiological and other testing techniques, 192
monitoring and surveillance, 185, 192
patient handling, 192–194
protecting the patient and the hospital, 180–185
steps in cleaning and disinfection, 195 (box 3.9)
why we need it; lessons from outbreaks, 182–183
buildings, 149–162
stabling and yard, 149–150, 152
designing and building equine hospital, 147–164
car and lorry parking, 148–149
concept and site, 147–148
diagnostic imaging, 164–180
endoscopic equipment, 179–180
facilities and equipment for, 164–174
radiation safety, 175–179

hospital building, 152–162
anaesthetic stalls and surgical facilities, 154–158
nurses' base and main clinical area, 153–154
reception and client waiting area, 152–153
vehicular access, 158
hospital design and organisation
farriery area, 160
laboratory, 160–161
library, 162
office and staff facilities, 161
pharmacy, 160
radiography rooms, 159–160
rooms for performing nerve blocks, 160
seminar and meeting rooms, 161–162
specialised examination rooms, 158–159
miscellaneous items, 162–164
drains, 163–164
flooring, 162–163
generators, 164
killing area and facilities for a post-mortem examination, 162
stocks, 163
treadmills, 164
Hospital Feeding Chart, 264 (Box 5.5), 267, 284
Hospital forms, 200–225
consent forms, 200
discharge instructions and client information sheets, 225
monitoring and treatment sheets, 225
progress notes, 225
record keeping, 200
samples of, *201–224*
specialist examination forms, 225
Hospitalisation
caecal impactions and, 485
diarrhoea and, 486
examination per rectum in, 488
gastric ulceration and, 486–487
horses at risk of developing neurological systems disorders during, 557
oesophageal obstruction (choke) and, 487
patients at risk of developing hepatic disorders during, 520
patients at risk of developing musculoskeletal disorders during, 572
patients at risk of developing respiratory disorders during, 457
patients at risk of developing urogenital disorders during, 533–534
Hospitalised horse
common problems encountered in, 393–400
hyperlipaemia, 399–400
inappetence, 397–398
thrombophlebitis, 395–397
unexplained fever, 393–395
unwillingness to drink, 398–399
Hounsfield units, of various body tissues for computed tomography, *171*
Housing, for horses with neurological disorders, 561
HR. *See* Heart rate
HSCs. *See* Hepatic stellate cells
Human formulations, enteral diet, 277–278
Human liquid enteral products, 278*t*
Humidified oxygen, delivery of, 63
Humidifiers
connecting inspiratory arm of ventilator circuit to, *126*
mechanical ventilation and, 475
Humoradial (elbow) joint, synoviocentesis of, 579
Husbandry, for horses with neurological disorders, 561
Hyaluronate Na, approximate doses used in equine medicine, 661*t*
Hyaluronic acid, approximate doses used in equine medicine, 661*t*
Hydralazine, approximate doses used in equine medicine, 661*t*
Hydration status, monitoring, in hospitalised foal, 305–306
Hydrochlorothiazide, approximate doses used in equine medicine, 661*t*
Hydrocortisone, 452
Hydrocortisone sodium succinate, approximate doses used in equine medicine, 661*t*
Hydrogel dressings, wound healing and, 621
Hydrogen peroxide, delay in wound healing and, 622
Hydromorphone, equine sedation and use of, 314
Hydronephrosis, 540
Hydrostatic pressure, 370
Hydrotherapy, 644 (box 18.5), 650–651
biomechanics of, 650
contraindications for, 651
indications for, 650
physiological effects of, 650–651
safety rules for, 651
Hydroxyethyl starch, 375
approximate doses used in equine medicine, 661*t*
Hydroxyzine, approximate doses used in equine medicine, 661*t*
Hyoscine, approximate doses used in equine medicine, 662*t*
Hyperammonaemia, in horses with hepatic encephalopathy, 526
Hypercalcaemia, 384, 546
fluids of choice for, 383*t*
treatment of, 385
Hypercapnia, ventilatory support and, 473
Hyperchloraemia
fluids of choice for, 383*t*
treatment of, 384
Hyperchloraemic acidosis, common causes of, in horses, 381 (box 6.6)
Hypercoagulable states, 401
treatments in horses with, 409 (box 8.6)
Hypercoagulation, 409–410
"Hyperdynamic shock," 431
Hyperechogenicity, 539
Hyperechoic material, abscessation of tip of the lung and, *464*
Hyperfibrinogenaemia, 394
Hyperglobulinaemia, 394, 522
Hyperglycaemia, 431
parenteral nutrition infusion in hospitalised foals and, 309
parenteral nutrition therapy and, 295
Hyperimmune plasma, 41
Hyperkalaemia, 546
fluids of choice for, 383*t*
treatment options for, 383–384
Hyperlipaemia, 265
enteral feeding via large bore nasogastric tube in pony with, *280*
in hospitalised horses, 399–400
clinical signs and diagnosis, 399
differences between horses, ponies and donkeys, 399–400
pathophysiology of hyperlipaemia and hyperlipidaemia, 399
treatment of, 400
inappetence in hospitalised horses and, 397
pathophysiology of, 399
risk factors for, in hospitalised equines, 520 (box 12.1)
Hyperlipidaemia
inappetence in hospitalised horses and, 397
pathophysiology of, 399
Hypermagnesaemia, 419
fluids of choice for, 383*t*
Hypermetria, 559
Hypernatraemia, fluids of choice for, 383*t*
Hypernatraemic alkalosis, common causes of, 382 (box 6.7)
Hypersthenuria, 535 (box 13.1)
Hyperthermia, 393
Hypertonic saline, 374
approximate doses used in equine medicine, 662*t*
Hypertriglyceridaemia
dietary lipids used for horses with, 273
malnutrition and, 266

Hypertriglyceridaemia *(Continued)*
parenteral nutrition infusion in hospitalised foals and, 309
parenteral nutrition therapy and, 295
Hypnosis, quieting horse with, 318
Hypnotics
equine sedation and use of, 313*t*
gastrointestinal pain management and, 328
for standing sedation, 312–314
Hypocalcaemia, 419, 546
clinical signs of, 41, 384
fluids of choice for, 383*t*
treatment of, 384–385
Hypochloraemia
fluids of choice for, 383*t*
pH and, 535
treatment of, 384
Hypochloraemic alkalosis, common causes of, 382 (box 6.7)
Hypocoagulable states, 404
treatments in horses with, 409 (box 8.6)
Hypocoagulation therapy, 411–413
Hypoechogenicity, 540
Hypoechoic renal cyst, transabdominal ultrasonographic image of, in left kidney, *540*
Hypoglossal nerve, tongue tone and, 558
Hypoglycaemia, 523
Hypokalaemia, 266, 419, 525
pH and, 535
polyuric renal failure and, 546
Hypomagnesaemia, 419
fluids of choice for, 383*t*
treatment of, 385
Hypometria, 558
Hyponatraemia
fluids of choice for, 383*t*
severe, opisthotonus in foal with, *558*
Hyponatraemic acidosis, common causes of, in horses, 381 (box 6.6)
Hypophosphataemia
clinical signs of, 385
fluids of choice for, 383*t*
Hypoproteinaemic alkalosis, common causes of, 382 (box 6.7)
Hyposthenuria, 535 (box 13.1)
Hypotension
algorithm for treatment of, in neonatal foals, *448*
maintenance of inhalant anaesthesia and, 242–243
Hypothermia, fluid therapy, energy loss and, 386–387
Hypoventilation
equine anaesthesia and, 231
hypercapnia and, 473
local and central causes of, 380 (box 6.4)
maintenance of inhalant anaesthesia and, 242–243
Hypovolaemia
addressing before anaesthesia and surgery, 249
clinical signs of, 364–365, 365 (box 6.2)
creatinine concentration and, 366
decreased urine output and, 431, 453
defined, 365
fluid therapy and reversal of, 378–379, 387
intravenous fluid therapy and, 368–378
intravenous fluid types and, 369–370
laboratory signs of, in the horse, 365, 365*t*
neonatal foals and, 365
packed cell volume, total solids and, 365–366
"shock doses" of fluids for reversal of, in both adult horses and foals, 372 (box 6.3)
Hypovolaemic shock, high heart rate and, 431
Hypoxaemia, 244
equine anaesthesia and, 231
pregnant mares and, 250
treatment of, 473–474
underlying causes of, in horses, 462 (box 10.1)
Hypozincaemia, 528

I
Iatrogenic complications of fluid therapy, 386–387
extravasation of fluids, 386
fluid overload, 386
hypothermia and energy loss, 386–387
iatrogenic electrolyte abnormalities, 386
Ibuprofen
approximate doses used in equine medicine, 662*t*
endotoxaemia treatment and, 506
ICPR. *See* International Commission on Radiological Protection
ICPs. *See* Infection control programmes
ICS. *See* Intercostal space
Iditol dehydrogenase activity
guide to interpretation of, 675 (box 19.12)
Iditol dehydrogenase (IDH), 521
Ileum, abnormalities of, 489
Ileus
pathophysiology of, 499
treatment of, 499–503
acepromazine and yohimbine, 502
bethanechol chloride, 502
choice of prokinetic drug, 502–503
cisapride, 501–502
decompression of stomach and fluid therapy, 499–500
erythromycin, 501
lidocaine (lignocaine), 500–501
metoclopramide, 501
naloxone, 502
neostigmine, 502
nonsteroidal anti-inflammatory drugs, 500
prokinetic drugs, 500
Image data, archiving, 175
Image recording equipment, for recording endoscopy images, 180
Imaging equipment suppliers, 176 (box 3.3)
Imidazole, 353
Imidocarb, approximate doses used in equine medicine, 662*t*
Imipenem-cilastatin, approximate doses used in equine medicine, 662*t*
Immobilisation, 643
pathological effects of, 644 (box 18.4)
Implant-associated infection, 592
laryngoplasty and, 595
radiographic signs of, *593*
Implants
monitoring horses with, 591–595
advanced imaging, 594
fever, 592
implant-associated infection, 592, 595
laminitis, 594
musculoskeletal implants, 591
radiography, 593
scintigraphy, 593–594
ultrasonography, 593
Inappetence
in hospitalised horse, 397–398
investigation of, 397–398
treatment of, 398
Incisor teeth, age for eruption of, 688, 688*t*
Indicator dilution methods, cardiac output measurement and, 55
Indirect arterial blood pressure measurement, 44–45
equipment for, 45, 45 (box 1.23)
procedure for, 45
Indirect arterial pressure monitor, *45*

Indirect blood pressure measurement in neonatal foal, 137–138
  cuff placement, 137
    coccygeal artery, 137
    dorsal metatarsal artery, 137
  equipment needed for, 137 (box 2.11)
  taking measurement, 137–138
  troubleshooting
    for failing to get a measurement, 138
    for inconsistent measurements, 138
Induction, 239
  equine inhalant-based anaesthetic drug choices, 237*t*
  of horses with unstable limbs, 250–251
Induction anaesthetic choices, for equine neonates and older foals, 247*t*
Induction area, general anaesthesia and, 226–228
Induction space, creation of, by a partition hinged on back wall and secured by a rope over the horse's head, *227*
Indwelling chest tube, for intermittent evacuation of pneumothorax, *76*
Indwelling nasogastric tubes, passage of, 16
Infection control programmes, 181
  overview of, 183–184
Infections
  avoiding, operating theatre in hospital and, 155
  implant-associated, 592
  laryngeal implants and, 602
  laryngoplasty and, 595
  nosocomial, investigating and monitoring, 599
  parenteral nutrition therapy and, 295
  surgical site, 596–597
  surgical site, management of, 598–602
Infectious diseases
  fever and, 394
  hospitalised horses and, 196
Infectious organisms, continued evolution of, 183
Inflammation, physiotherapy and, 639
Inflammatory bronchoalveolar lavage cytology, *460*
Inflatable floor, recovering horse and, 245
Information flow, nurses' base at equine hospital and, 153
Infratrochlear nerve, regional anaesthesia of eye and block to, 93, *93*
Infundibulum, 688
  time of disappearance of, 688 (box 19.27)
Infusion set with coil, horse on continuous intravenous fluids with use of, *36*
Inguinal hernias, 534
Inhalant anaesthesia induction, foals and, *247*
Inhalant-based anaesthetic drug choices, equine, 237*t*
Inhalation drug delivery systems, therapeutic aerosols and, 362
Inhaled bronchodilators
  clinical application of, 468–470
    β_2-adrenoreceptor agonists, 468–469
    inhaled corticosteroids, 470
    parasympatholytics, 469
Inhaled corticosteroids, application of, 470
Inherited haemostatic disorders, in young animals, 405
Inotropes, 447–449
  dobutamine, 447, 449
  guideline for diluting and preparation of, 449*t*
  isoproterenol, 449
  practical use of, 453
Insufflation of stomach, adapted garden spray-pump for, *21*
Insulin levels, pituitary pars intermedia dysfunction and, 687
Insulin (protamine zinc), approximate doses used in equine medicine, 662*t*
Insulin (regular)
  approximate doses used in equine medicine, 662*t*
  guidelines for infusion of, in neonatal foals (non-SI units), 310–311*t*
  guidelines for infusion of, in neonatal foals (SI units), 310*t*
Integument problems
  management of horses with, 609–627
  simple skin grafting techniques, 623–627
  wound management in hospitalised horses, 609–622
Intensity, of murmur, 418
Intensive care patient, fluids administered to, *152*
Intensive care sheet, *207*
Intercostal space, 52, 417
Interferon-alpha, approximate doses used in equine medicine, 662*t*
International Commission on Radiological Protection, 175
Internet
  access to, in equine hospital, 162
  MRI system supported and monitored for performance via, 174
Interstitial pattern
  diffuse, with patchy areas of alveolar density, *465*
  lung tissue disease and, 465
  pulmonary disease and, 465
Intertarsal joint, approaching for synoviocentesis, 578–579
Intestinal ammoniagenesis, reducing, 526
Intestinal disease, liver and, 520
Intestines, wall thickness and diameter of sections of, as measured by ultrasound, 495*t*
Intra-articular injections, of antimicrobial agents, 350
Intragastric fluid administration, of enteral fluid therapy, 367
Intragastric fluids, indwelling narrow nasogastric tube placed in polo pony for constant delivery of, *368*
Intramuscular administration, pain management, adverse effects, and use of, 325
Intramuscular injections, 13–15
  close up of hand holding needle, *15*
  complications with, 14
  equipment for, 13, 13 (box 1.8)
  "needle-shy" horses, 14–15
  site of, into pectoral muscles, *13*
  sites for, in horse, 13, *13*
  technique, 13–14
Intramuscular opioids, postoperative analgesia and use of, 252
Intranasal oxygen administration, 62–63, 470–471
  bilateral nasal oxygen administration in foal with severely compromised oxygenation, *63*
  catheter sutured to external nares in adult horse, *63*
  equipment needed for, 62 (box 1.31)
  external portion of catheter and tongue depressor affixed to foal's face, *63*
  nasal oxygen catheter taped to tongue depressor, *63*
  oxygen tank, flowmeter and humidifier, *62*
  piped oxygen outlet, flowmeter, and humidifier, *62*
  procedure for, 62–63
Intraosseous (IO) regional limb perfusion, 351, 604
Intravenous bolus, pain management and use of, 325
Intravenous catheters, 28
  infusion of parenteral formulations and, 293
Intravenous dextrose, administration of, 267
Intravenous fluids, infusion set with coil and administration of, *36*
Intravenous fluid therapy, 368–378
  delivery systems for, 369
  fluid types, 369–372
    dehydration and, 370
    general principles: colloids, 371–372
    general principles: crystalloids, 370–371
    general principles: oncotic pressure, 370
    hypovolaemia and, 369–370
    maintenance and, 370
Intravenous injection, equipment for collection of, 10 (box 1.7)
Intravenous regional limb perfusion, *603*, 604
Intubations, 239–240
  of adult horse, 3–5

Intubations, *(Continued)*
with horse in lateral recumbency, 239, *240*
with horse in sternal recumbency, 239, *240*
of neonatal foal, 120–122
checking that tube is correctly placed, 120–121
difficult, strategies for, 121–122
nasatracheal intubation, 120
orotracheal intubation, 120
In vitro antimicrobial susceptibility
of gram-negative aerobic bacterial isolates from horse, 340*t*
of selected gram-positive aerobic bacterial isolates from horse, 340*t*
In vitro susceptibility tests, 339
interpretive standards for, with selected antimicrobial agents used in horses, 341*t*
Iodides, spectrum of activity for, 353*t*
Iodide therapy, systemic, 354
Iodine-impregnated drapes, for surgical wounds, 617
Ionophore toxicosis, 420
Ipratropium bromide, approximate doses used in equine medicine, 662*t*
Iris problems, in Percheron mare, *629*
Iris prolapse, management of horses with, 633
Iron, liver disease in horses and, 528
Irregular sinus rhythm, progression of, to asystole in a horse, *5*
Ischaemia-reperfusion injury, 371
Isoflupredone acetate, approximate doses used in equine medicine, 662*t*
Isoflurane, 241
summary of subjective differences in clinical signs of anaesthesia in adult horses under halothane, sevoflurane and, 241*t*
Isolating equine patients, practical tips for, at small to medium-sized clinics, 193 (box 2.8)
Isolation and barrier flow chart, *191*
Isolation facilities, at equine hospital, 150
Isolation of horses, with diarrhoea, 486
Isolec, 372
Isoniazid, approximate doses used in equine medicine, 662*t*
Isoproterenol, 449
Isosthenuria, 535, 535 (box 13.1)
Isotonic sodium chloride, 372
Isoxsuprine, approximate doses used in equine medicine, 662*t*
Itraconazole, 353, 354
approximate doses used in equine medicine, 662*t*
fungal keratitis treatment and, 631, 632
spectrum of activity for, 353*t*
Ivermectin, approximate doses used in equine medicine, 662*t*

J
Jacob's chuck, sinocentesis and use of, 78
Jamshidi needle, bone marrow biopsy and use of, 90, 91, *91*
JD Medical LAV2000 large-animal ventilator, 232
Jejunum
distended loop of small intestine adjacent to spleen in horse after resection and anastomosis of, *495*
imaging, 495
Jet nebulisers, 362, 467
Joint fluid
cytological evaluation of, 576
normal and abnormal values for, 682, 684*t*
Joint involvement, wound management and assessment of, 613
Joint lavage, total intravenous anaesthesia and, 252
Joints
common fungal pathogens at, 352*t*
monitoring in neonatal foals, 575
Jones, Sir Robert, 606
Jugular catheterisation, 28–30
equipment needed for, 28 (box 1.16)
placement of over-the-needle catheter, 28–30
placement of over-the-wire catheter, 30
Jugular catheter placement, parenteral nutrition for hospitalised foals and, 308
Jugular thrombophlebitis, 401, 403–404
clinical considerations, 403–404
in horse with colitis, secondary to presumed endotaxaemia, *403*
in site of previous indwelling intravenous catheter in a foal, *396*
Jugular vein
collection of blood and injection from, 11–12
pre- and postdrainage, in foal with pericardial effusion causing tamponade, *426*
Jugular vein catheterisation, 133–137
in neonatal foal
catheter care, 137
catheter placement, 134–137
for over-the-needle catheter, 136–137
for over-the-wire catheter, 134–136
catheter types used in, 133
equipment needed for catheter placement, 134 (box 2.10)
preparation, 134
restraint, 133
Jugular venous filling and distension, assessing, 417
J-wire assembly, over-the-wire catheter and, 135, *135*

K
Kanamycin, 344
Keep vein open mode, on electronic infusion pumps, 38, 38 (box 1.18)
Keptoprofen, endotoxaemia treatment and, 505, 506
Keratitis
common fungal pathogens at, 352*t*
due to fungal infection, in 9-year-old Thoroughbred, *631*
due to *Pseudomonas* infection, in 2-year-old Thoroughbred filly, *630*
nonulcerative
management of horses with, 634–635
in 9-year-old Quarter Horse gelding, *633*
Ketamine, 239, 565
approximate doses used in equine medicine, 662*t*
balanced anaesthesia and adding constant rate infusions of, 244
intracranial pressure and, 251
pain management, adverse effects, and use of, 325
total intravenous anaesthesia and, 252
Ketanserin, wound healing and, 621
Ketoconazole, 353
approximate doses used in equine medicine, 662*t*
fungal keratitis treatment and, 631, 632
spectrum of activity of, 353*t*
Ketones, reagent strips and, 535–536
Ketonuria, 535
Ketoprofen
approximate doses used in equine medicine, 662*t*
colic pain and use of, 326
somatic pain management and, 330
Ketorolac, endotoxaemia treatment and, 506
Kidneys
biopsy of, 88–89
image acquisition for, 538
normal, 538–539
normal left, transabdominal ultrasonographic image of, in a weanling, *539*
normal right, transabdominal ultrasonographic image of, *539*
right, transabdominal ultrasonographic image of, from horse with chronic renal failure, *540*
right, transabdominal ultrasonographic image of, from 19-year-old "Teaser" with chronic renal failure, *539*
Kidney size, 540
Killing area, at equine hospital, 162
Kirby Bauer test, 339
Klebsiella, 185

Klebsiella spp., 337
  isolate of, from septic arthritis in foals, 580
Knots, suture, 114

L
Laboratory, at equine hospital, 153, 160–161
Laboratory tests for monitoring of coagulation system disorders, 405–407
  closure time, 406
  clotting time, 405
  fibrin degradation products/D-dimers, 406
  fibrinogen concentration, 405
  mean platelet component, 405
  platelet count, 405
  template bleeding time, 406
Lacerations, of distal limb, 615
Lacerations with impending global collapse, anaesthesia and, 251
Lacrimal nerve, regional anaesthesia of eye and block to, 93, *93*
Lactate, handheld analyser for measurement of, *432*
Lactate concentration, fluid therapy and, 366
Lactate concentrations, normal, in adult horse and foal, 678*t*
Lactate dehydrogenase, 521
  acute rhabdomyolysis and increased serum activities of, 587
  biochemical monitoring of muscles and, 585, 586
  cardiac isoenzymes of, 420
  cerebrospinal fluid analysis and, 560, 561
Lactated Ringer's solution, 372
Lactating mares
  digestible energy requirements for, 270*t*
  protein requirements for, 271*t*
Lactic acidosis, 380
  common causes of, in horses, 381 (box 6.6)
Lactulose, approximate doses used in equine medicine, 662*t*
Lame horses, managing, at equine hospital, 150
λ-glutamyltransferase activity, guide to interpretation of, 675 (box 19.11)
Lameness
  complete, workup form for recording results of, *216–217*
  laminitis and identification of, 581
  monitoring in hospitalised horse, 574–575
  wound management of hospitalised horse and, 611
Laminitic foot, supporting, 584–585
"Laminitic trigger factors," 583
Laminitis, 332, 581–584
  defined, 572
  detection and treatment of, 581–584
  grading system for horses with, 581, 582 (box 15.4)
  medical colic patients and, 509
  orthopaedic implant monitoring and, 594
  patients at risk of, 572–573
  percussion of dorsal hoof used in early diagnosis of, *582*
  predictors of outcome, 583
  predisposition to, 573
  radiography and, 582–583
  specific lesions associated with, 573 (box 15.1)
  support-limb, treatment of, 583–584
  treatment and prevention of, 583
LA neurologic examination, *218–219*
Laparotomy wounds
  investigating and monitoring, 599–601
  severe cases of, skin and subcutaneous tissue dehiscing due to, *600*, 600–601
Laporotomy incisions, postoperative infections of, 394
Large-animal anaesthesia circle system, with vaporiser(s) outside of circle, *230*
Large-animal anaesthesia equipment, sources for, 230 (box 4.1)
Large-animal anaesthesia machines, 228–231
Large-animal anaesthesia ventilator, 231–233
Large-animal circle system, 228, 229*t*
Large-animal ventilators
  electronic, control variable choices on, 233*t*
  with microprocessor control and ascending bellows, *232*
  with microprocessor controls, *233*
Large-bore CT scanners, 172
Large-bore nasogastric tube, enteral feeding via, in pony with hyperlipaemia, *280*
Large colon, abnormalities of, 489–490
Large-gauge catheters, jugular catheterisation and, 28
Laryngeal functional grading systems, 66 (box 1.36)
Laryngeal implants, infection of, 602
Laryngoplasty, 595
  endoscopy of trachea after, *594*
  endoscopy of upper respiratory tract after, *594*
  reported infection rates for, 609
Laser therapy, 638
  low-level, 645–646
Laser treatment, indications for use, physiological effects, and contraindications or precautions, 646*t*
Lateral recumbency
  CT scanning of horse in, 172
  intubation done with horse in, 239, *240*
  positioning during, under total intravenous anaesthesia, *253*
  restraining foal in, 130, *130*, 139
Lateral splint bone, high four-point nerve block and, *99*
Lateral thoracic vein
  catheterisation of, 33–35
    catheter covered with sterile gauze swab wrapped with stretchy adhesive dressing, *35*
    catheter fed onto wire, *35*
    catheter hub secured to skin with cruiciate suture, *35*
    catheter needle in vein, dripping blood, *34*
    dilator fed onto wire, and then pushed into vein, *34*
    long extension set attached to mane to allow fluid therapy, *35*
    raised, ultrasound of, *34*
    raising lateral thoracic vein, and placing anaesthetic bleb over it, *34*
    site for, *33*
    wire advanced into needle, taking care not to displace needle, *34*
    wire removed once catheter seated into vein, *35*
Lavage catheter, subpalpebral, placement of, 93–96
Lawsonia intracellularis infection, 495–496
  markedly thickened loop of small intestine in 8-month-old foal with confirmation of, *496*
Laying down a foal, 129
LDH. *See* Lactate dehydrogenase
Lead aprons, 167
  storage of, 166
Lead gowns, 179
  correctly stored, *166*
  x-ray rooms and, 177
Lead (Pb) protective clothing, 167
  scintigraphy and wearing of, 169
Lead syringe shields, 169
Leahurst Hospital, University of Liverpool, form for recording results of complete lameness workup at, *216–217*
Left frontal sinus, *78*
Left ventral colon, normal haustrated, imaged transabdominally in 3-month-old foal, *497*
Left ventricle, two-dimensional, right parasternal short-axis echocardiogram of, *53*
Left ventricular (LV) pressure, effect of ventricular premature beats on, *424*
Left ventricular volume overload, horse with, *425*
Legs, fixing splint to, 106 (box 1.59)
Leptospirosis, 533
Lesser curvature, endoscopic view of, 23, *23*

Leucocytes, inflammation in urogenital tract and increased numbers of, 536
Leuconostoc mesenteroides, 376
Leukocytosis, 490, 491
Leukopaenia, 491
Levamisole, approximate doses used in equine medicine, 662*t*
Levothyroxine, approximate doses used in equine medicine, 662*t*
Libraries, at equine hospital, 162
LiDCO computer, original, and sensor for calculation of cardiac output, *56*
LiDCO measurement, of cardiac output in horse after colic surgery, *57*
Lidocaine (lignocaine), 437*t*
 approximate doses used in equine medicine, 662*t*
 balanced anaesthesia and adding constant rate infusions of, 244
 CRI, as analgesic, for thermal stimulus applied to withers of normal horses, 331–332
 ileus treatment and, 500–501
 ventricular tachycardia treatment and, 438
 visceral pain management and, 328
Lifelong learning, libraries at equine hospital and, 162
Ligament injuries, physiotherapy and, 642–643
Lighting
 in MRI rooms, 174
 in operating theatres, 156
 in x-ray rooms, 177
Light sources, for endoscopic equipment, 179–180
Limb arteries, thrombosis of, 404
Limb bandage, full, for wound healing, wound protection, and wound edge immobilisation, *103*
Limb leads, electrocardiogram, placement of, 50
Limb placement test, 558
Limbs
 bandaging of, 100–105
 regional analgesia for, 96–100
 splints applied to, 106–107
Lincomycin, 342
Line block, 97
Linoleic, 272
Lipid metabolism
 markers of, in hospitalised horse, 265–266
 obese equine patients and derangements in, 261
Lipids
 adding last, in compounding of parenteral nutrition solution, 292
 contraindications for supplementation with, 273
 dietary, use of for horses with hypertriglyceridaemia, 273
 future trends in supplementation with, 273
 for hospitalised adult horse, 272–273
 for neonatal foals, 299
 in parenteral solutions, 287–289
Lipid-soluble vitamins, 289
Lipophilic drugs, 338
Liquid enteral diets
 commercial and pelleted equine feeds suitable for use in, 279*t*
 infusion protocol for, 282 (box 5.13)
 nutrition supplements in, 279
Lithium dilution, conversion of, to a voltage, displayed on the screen, *56*
Lithium dilution (LIDCO) method, 55
Lithium specific sensor, for lithium dilution method of cardiac output monitoring, *56*
Liver
 biochemical monitoring of, 521–523
  liver derived serum enzyme concentrations, 521
  serum biochemical evaluation of hepatic function, 522–523
 biopsy of, 524
 intestinal disease and, 520
 monitoring and treating, 520–523
 normal, transabdominal ultrasonographic image of, *523*
 sources of enzymes commonly measured for assessment of, 521*t*
 ultrasonography of, 523–524
Liver biopsy, 26–28
 equipment needed for, 27 (box 1.15)
 indications for, 26
 preferred site for, *27*
 technique, 27–28
Liver biopsy specimens, scores attributable to specific histopathologic findings in, 524*t*
Liver derived serum enzyme concentrations, 521
Liver function, dynamic testing of, 523
Loading ramps, at equine hospital, *149*
Local anaesthetics
 epidural analgesia and anaesthesia for visceral pain and, 329
 pain management, adverse effects and use of, 325
Locking loop suture, tendon involvement in wounds and, 616
Long-acting β_2-agonists, 468, 469
Long-chain triglycerides, 273
Loop diuretics, renal failure treatment and, 544
Lorazepam, approximate doses used in equine medicine, 662*t*
Lorenz, M. D., 638
Lorries
 gates sited back from road at hospital, to allow lorries to pull off road when gates are shut, *148*
 muck removal and, 148
 parking for, at equine hospital, 148–149
Low-dose dexamethasone suppression test, pituitary pars intermedia dysfunction and, 687
Low-four-point nerve block, *98*
 for analgesia of fetlock (fore limb), 97
 equipment for, 97 (box 1.56)
Low-level laser therapy, 645–646
Low-molecular-weight heparins, 506
 hypercoagulable states in horses managed with, 410
Low-six-point nerve block
 analgesia of fetlock (hind limb) and, 98
 equipment for, 97 (box 1.56)
Lumbosacral dysfunction, physiotherapy and, 642
Lumbosacral (LS) space, 79
Lumbosacral spinal fluid collection, 79–80
 anatomy of site for collection of fluid from lumbosacral space, *79*
 equipment needed for, 79 (box 1.44)
 plunger of syringe gently withdrawn to allow fluid to flow into syringe, *80*
 procedure for, 79–80
Lung biopsy, 74, 76–77
 careful removal of sample from open biopsy instrument using 25-gauge needles, *77*
 equipment needed for, 76 (box 1.42)
 indication for, 74
 insertion of automated lung biopsy device, *77*
 insertion of manual lung biopsy device, *77*
 percutaneous, most frequent complications with, 77
 procedure for, 74, 77
 sedation for, 318
Lung biopsy devices
 automated, insertion of, *77*
 manual, insertion of, *77*
Lung collapse, pneumothorax and, 465
Lung parenchyma, consolidation of, with hepatisation, *464*
Lungs
 common fungal pathogens in, 352*t*
 ultrasonography of, 463–464
Lung tissue disease, increased tissue density and, 465

M
MAC. *See* Minimum alveolar concentration
Macrolides, 338
  derivatives and, 346–347
Macromineral requirements, for adult horses at physiologic state of maintenance, 274 (box 5.10)
Macrominerals, in parenteral solutions, 289
Magnesium
  electrolyte assessment of cardiac disease and, 419
  electrolyte disturbances and, 385
Magnesium concentrations, guide to interpretation of, 677 (box 19.19)
Magnesium disturbances, treatment of, 385
Magnesium sulphate, 437*t*
  approximate doses used in equine medicine, 662*t*
  ventricular tachycardia treatment and, 439
Magnetic field therapy, 648
Magnetic resonance imaging, equine, 172–175
  building MRI facility, 173
  of distal limb, 316
  horse handling, 174–175
  operator, 175
  scanner, 173–174
  underlying technical principle of, 173
Magnetic resonance imaging suppliers, 176 (box 3.3)
Magnet strength, equine magnetic resonance imaging and, 173
Maintenance, equine inhalant-based anaesthetic drug choices, 237*t*
Maintenance anaesthetic choices, for equine neonates and older foals, 247*t*
Male foals
  equipment for urinary catheterisation of, 142 (box 2.13)
  filling balloon of Foley catheter, after it has been passed into bladder in, *143*
  urinary catheterisation of, 142–143, *143*
Male genital tract, examination of, 543
Male horses, urinary catheterisation of, 84–85
Malnutrition
  electrolyte imbalances associated with, 266
  hypertriglyceridaemia and, 266
  prolonged, 266
Manganese accumulation, hepatic insufficiency and, 528
Manipulations, 642*t*, 644–645
Mannitol, approximate doses used in equine medicine, 663*t*
Manometer
  central venous pressure measurement in horse with gastrointestinal disease and, *48*
  for measurement of central venous pressure, *48*
Manometer reading, in central venous pressure measurement, 47, *48*
Manual therapy, 644–645, 644 (box 18.5)
  massage, 645
  mobilisations and manipulations, 644–645
  stretches, 645
  trigger point therapy/myofascial release, 645
MAP. *See* Mean arterial pressure
Marbofloxacin, 345
  approximate doses used in equine medicine, 663*t*
Mare-foal bond, maintaining, while administering fluid to foal, 37
Mares
  acute laminitis in, 573
  arrangements for separating foals and, during treatment at hospitals, *151*
  with colic, measurement of foetal heart rate in, at 8 months of gestation, 513
  pregnant
    anaesthesia for, 249–250
    with colic, monitoring of, 513–514
    digestible energy requirements for, 270*t*
    protein requirements for, 271*t*
  thoroughbred, oesophagostomy tube in, *281*
  ventral abdominal ultrasound of, *18*
Mare's milk, for critically ill foals, 300
Massage, 638, 642*t*, 645
Matrix metalloproteinases, 527, 632
Maxillary sinus, *78*
MCT. *See* Medium-chain triglycerides
MDIs. *See* Metered-dose inhalers
Mean arterial pressure, pulse contour analysis and, 57
Mean platelet component, 405
Mechanical ventilation, 473–480
  attachment of nasotracheal tube to elastic tape bandage placed around muzzle to prevent displacement during, *475*
  complications with, 479–480
  decision to ventilate, 474
  indications for, 474
  initiation of, 474–475
  large-animal anaesthesia machine designed for use with, *230*
  modes of, 475–477
  monitoring, 478–479
  objective of, 232
  recruitment manoeuvres, 477–478
  ventilatory support, 473–474
  weaning, 479
Mechanical ventilation in neonatal foal, 125–129
  adjusting ventilator to foal, 127–128
  connecting foal to ventilator, 126–127
  connecting inspiratory arm of ventilator circuit to active humidifier, *126*
  equipment needed for, 125 (box 2.3)
  improving arterial blood gas tensions and, 128 (box 2.8)
  indications for, 125
  initial setting for, example of, 126 (box 2.4)
  maintenance for, 128
  preparation for, 125–126
  standing foal with assistance, whilst being ventilated with reverse-ratio pressure-controlled ventilation, *127*
  strategies for improving ventilator-patient synchrony, 127 (box 2.7)
  underlying disease conditions and, 125 (box 2.2)
  weaning, 128
Meclofenamic acid, endotoxaemia treatment, 506
Medetomidine
  approximate doses used in equine medicine, 663*t*
  balanced anaesthesia and adding constant rate infusions of, 244
  equine sedation and use of, 312, 313*t*
  visceral pain management and, 327
Medial cutaneous antebrachial nerve block, 100, *101*
  equipment for, 97 (box 1.56)
Medial splint bone, high four-point nerve block and, *99*
Median artery
  anatomical location of, *141*
  blood collection from foal, 140
Median nerve block, 100
  equipment for, 97 (box 1.56)
Medical colic patients
  analgesia for, 509
  antimicrobials for, 509
  determination of surgical colic *versus*, 492–493
  fluid therapy for, 508–509
  laminitis and, 509
  monitoring of, 507–508
  thrombophlebitis and, 509
Medium-chain triglycerides, 273
Medofenamic acid, approximate doses used in equine medicine, 663*t*
Medulla, kidney, renal ultrasound and, 539
Medullary rim sign, 539–540
Meeting rooms, at equine hospital, 161–162

Meloxicam
approximate doses used in equine medicine, 663*t*
endotoxaemia treatment, 506
somatic pain management and, 330
Melting iris, in Percheron mare, *629*
Menace response, 557–558, 628
Meperidine, approximate doses used in equine medicine, 663*t*
Mepyramine, approximate doses used in equine medicine, 663*t*
Mesh hernioplasty, 594–595
drainage from site of, *594*
Metabolic acidosis, 373, 380
common causes of, in horses, 381 (box 6.6)
Metabolic disturbances, specific, fluids of choice for, 383*t*
Metacarpophalangeal joint (fetlock joint), approaches to, for synoviocentesis, 577, *577*
Metapopulations, infectious organisms and, 183
Metatarsal IV, synoviocentesis and palpating head of, *578*, 579
Metered-dose inhalers, 467, 468
respiratory disease treatment and use of, 466–470
aerosol administration, 466–467
clinical application of inhaled bronchodilators, 468–470
devices, 467–468
single nostril delivery device for, *467*
valved facemask for delivery of aerosolised medications, with spacer for delivering drugs by, *467*
Methadone
approximate doses used in equine medicine, 663*t*
equine sedation and use of, 314
somatic pain management and, 330
Methicillin-resistant *Staphylococcus aureus*
biosecurity and, 182, 185
emergence of, in some equine veterinary hospitals, 343
Methocarbomal, approximate doses used in equine medicine, 663*t*
Methylene Blue, approximate doses used in equine medicine, 663*t*
Methylprednisolone acetate, approximate doses used in equine medicine, 663*t*
Methylprednisolone sodium succinate, approximate doses used in equine medicine, 663*t*
Methylsulphomethane, approximate doses used in equine medicine, 663*t*
Metoclopramide, treatment of ileus and, 501
Metodopramide, approximate doses used in equine medicine, 663*t*
Metronidazole, 337, 342, 348
approximate doses used in equine medicine, 663*t*
equine central nervous system or cerebrospinal fluid and, 567
MIC. *See* Minimal inhibitory concentration
Miconazole
fungal keratitis treatment and, 631
intranasal, 354
spectrum of activity of, 353*t*
Microbiological testing techniques, 192
Microscope room, at equine hospital, 161
Midazolam
approximate doses used in equine medicine, 663*t*
equine sedation and use of, 313*t*, 315
gastrointestinal pain management and, 328
musculoskeletal conditions and, 317
for sedating neonatal foals, 320
total intravenous anaesthesia and, 252
Mid cervical radiograph, of fractures of C3 and C4, *560*
Middle gluteal site, for muscle biopsy, 112
Milk
for ill neonatal foals, 300–301
nutrient content of, 301*t*
volume of, per day for foals of varying ages, 302*t*
Milk replacers, 300
nutrient content of, 301*t*
Milrinone, congestive heart failure treatment and, 443
Mineralised calculi, chronic renal disease and, 539–540
Mineral requirements
for hospitalised adult horse, 274–275
for neonatal foals, 299
Minerals, in parenteral solutions, 289
Mineral supplements, adding to PN mixture, 292
Miniature horses
equation for estimate of body weight in, using chest girth and body length, 262 (box 5.3)
hyperlipaemia in, 399
Minimal inhibitory concentration, 339
Minimum alveolar concentration, 240
Misoprostol, approximate doses used in equine medicine, 663*t*
Mitral regurgitation, congestive heart failure and, 425
Mitral valve lesions, 426
Mitral valves, 417
M-mode, 423
of left ventricle, *54*
M-mode techniques, with echocardiography, 52
MMPs. *See* Matrix metalloproteinases
Mobile operating table, 157
Mobile x-ray units, 166
Mobilisations, 642*t*, 644–645
MODS. *See* Multiple organ dysfunction syndrome
MOFS. *See* Multiorgan failure syndrome
Monitoring, radiation safety and, 176
Monitoring and treatment sheets, 225
Monitoring equipment, anaesthesia, 233–234
blood gas, 234
cardiovascular monitors, 233–234
direct blood pressure monitoring, 234
Monocyte tissue factor, hepatic insufficiency and, 522
Morbidity, postanaesthetic, 254
Morphine
approximate doses used in equine medicine, 663*t*
balanced anaesthesia and adding constant rate infusions of, 244
equine sedation and use of, 313*t*, 314, 315
gastrointestinal disorders and use of, 319
intra-articular, postoperative analgesia and, 246
Mortality rate
for postoperative ileus, 499
rushing stressed horses to surgery and, 251
Motilin receptors, 501
Mouth-to-nose resuscitation, for neonatal foal, 123, *123*
Moving beam, allowing use of both theatres and three anaesthetic boxes, 156, *156*
Moxifloxacin, 346
MPC. *See* Mean platelet component
MRI. *See* Magnetic resonance imaging
MRSA. *See* Methicillin-resistant *Staphylococcus aureus*
MTIV. *See* Metatarsal IV
MtrP. *See* Myofascial trigger point
Muck pit
screening, 152, *152*
siting, at equine hospital, 148–149, 150
Mucous membranes, color changes in, cardiovascular system and, 431
Mucus
in equine urine, 536
tracheal aspirate cytology and, 459, *459*
Multidrug-resistant bacterial infections, nosocomial importance of, 188*t*
Multiorgan failure form of disseminated intravascular coagulation, 402
Multiorgan failure syndrome, 402, 410
Multiparameter monitors, some sources of, 234 (box 4.2)
Multiple organ dysfunction syndrome, laminitis and, 572
Murmurs, 417, 418–419
echocardiography and assessment of, 423
grading of, 418 (ox 9.1)

Muscle associated enzymes, increases seen with mild, moderate and severe injury and, 585*t*
Muscle atrophy, physiotherapy and, 639
Muscle biopsies, 112–114
equipment for, 113 (box 1.63)
needle biopsy, 113
site of, 112
surgical biopsy, 113–114
Muscle rupture, tear, or strain, physiotherapy and, 642
Muscles
biochemical monitoring of, 585–586
aspartate aminotransferase, 585–586
assessing significance of result, 586
creatine kinase, 585
lactate dehydrogenase, 586
troponin I, 586
biological monitoring of, 585–586
Muscular weakness, testing for, 558
Musculoskeletal conditions
physiotherapy intervention and, 639 (box 18.1)
sedation and, 316–317
Musculoskeletal implants, 591
Musculoskeletal infections
local therapy for, 350–351
intra-articular therapy, 350
intravenous and introsseous regional limb perfusion, 350–351
Musculoskeletal problems in hospitalised horses, 572–608
biochemical monitoring of the muscles, 585–586
cast application, 607–608
external coaptation, 605–607
laminitis, 581–585
laryngeael implants, 602
management of rhabdomyolysis and myopathy, 587–591
monitoring, 572–580
horses with implants, 591–595
surgical incisions, 596–597
regional limb perfusion, 602–604
surgical site infections management, 598–602
ultrasonography of surgical incisions, 597–598
Musculoskeletal system, monitoring, 572–580
M.V.I. Adult, 292
Mydriasis, 317, 632
Myocarditis, 420
echocardiography and evaluation of, 426
horse with, and development of third-degree atri-ventricular block, *422*
Myofascial release, 642*t*, 645
Myofascial trigger point, defined, 645
Myoglobinuria, 535
Myopathies
management of, 587–591
patients at risk for, 574

N
N-acetylprocainamide, 438
Naloxone
approximate doses used in equine medicine, 664*t*
treatment of ileus and, 502
Nandrolone decanoate, approximate doses used in equine medicine, 664*t*
NAPA. *See* *N*-acetylprocainamide
"Nappy" systems, for urine and/or faecal collection, 534
Nasal catheter, positioning, for intranasal oxygen administration, 62–63
Nasal intubation, of foal, *247*
Nasal oxygen catheter, taping of, to tongue depressor, *63*
Nasal procedures, anaesthesia and, 252
Nasogastric fluids
enteral fluid therapy and delivery of, 367
recipes for, 367*t*
Nasogastric intubation
equipment for, 15, 15 (box 1.9)
passage of indwelling nasogastric feeding tube, 16
procedure for, 15–16
surgical colic patients and monitoring of, 511
Nasogastric tubes
enteral feeding for clinically ill foal and, 303–304
large-bore, enteral feeding via, in pony with hyperlipaemia, *280*
passing, in a horse, i15
uses for, 15
Nasogastric tubes, indwelling
checking placement of tube, 132
choice and use of, in enteral feeding, 280–283
correctly placed tube in foal, *133*
equipment needed for, 130, 131 (box 2.9)
feeding foal through, *304*
fixing feeding tube to foal, *131*
fixing to foal, 132
incorrectly placed tube in foal, *133*
measuring length of tube, to place in foal, *131*
placement of, 130–132
in neonatal foal, 130–133
in polo pony for constant delivery of intragastric fluids, *368*
testing and using the tube, 132–133
Nasotracheal and orotracheal intubation
in neonatal foal, 120–122
checking that tube is correctly placed, 120–121
equipment required for, 120
nasotracheal intubation, 120, *121*
orotracheal intubation, 120, *121*
strategies for difficult intubations, 121–122
Nasotracheal intubation, 3
for mechanical ventilation, 474
of neonatal foal, 120
preparation for mechanical ventilation and, 125–126
Nasotracheal tube, attachment of, to elastic tape bandage placed around muzzle to prevent displacement during mechanical ventilation, *475*
Natamycin, fungal keratitis treatment and, 631
National Research Council Nutrient Requirements of Horses (sixth revised edition), 270
National Research Council Operative Classification, categories of surgical wounds based on, 609*t*
Naylor diet, 278
Near-far far-near suture pattern, *612*, 616
Nebulisation, 63–64
aerosol administration and, 362
defined, 63
drug formulations for, 363
equipment needed for, 64 (box 1.32)
of foal, with fitted, valved facemask, *64*
procedure for, 64
respiratory disorders and, 466–470
Nebulisers, 467–468
pneumatic *vs.* ultrasonic, 64
using, 362
Neck
intramuscular injections in, 13, 14
passive and active flexion of, 559
Neck injuries, equine sedation and, 317
Needle biopsy, for muscle biopsy, 112–113
Needle hub technique, 12
"Needle-shy" horses, intramuscular injections and, 14
NEFAs. *See* Nonesterified fatty acids
Negative pressure ventilation, 474

Neomycin, 344, 620
  approximate doses used in equine medicine, 664*t*
Neonatal foal admission form, Anglesey Lodge Equine Hospital Foal Intensive Care Programme, *205*
Neonatal foals. *See also* Foals
  algorithm for treatment of hypotension in, *448*
  cardiopulmonary resuscitation of, 122–124
  causes of seizures in, 564 (box 14.4)
  collection of arterial blood gas/arterial catheterisation of, 139–141
  daily sheet for ordering treatments for, *210*
  dilute urine in, 366
  hypothermia in, 386
  hypovolaemia and, 365
  implant infection in, *602*
  indirect blood pressure measurement in, 137–139
  jugular vein catheterisation and, 133–137
  lactate concentrations and hospital survival in, 432
  maintenance formula fluids for, 370
  management of ocular problems in, 636–637
  mechanical ventilation of, 125–129
  monitoring joints in, 575
  nasotracheal and orotracheal intubation of, 120–122
  normal haemodynamics in, 685*t*
  placement of urinary catheter in, 141–144
  placing indwelling nasogastric tube in, 130–133
  plasma used in, 377
  restraint of, 129–130
  sedating, 320
  septic arthritis signs in, monitoring of, 573
  sequelae of septicaemia and, 337
  sheet for recording data on, *209*
  traditional approach to anaesthesia for, 246
  ultrasonography of the umbilicus, 144–146
  use of saline and risks for, 374
Neosporin, 620
Neostigmine
  approximate doses used in equine medicine, 664*t*
  treatment of ileus and, 502
Nephrotoxins, avoiding administration of, 543
Nerve blocks
  general procedure for placing, 96–97
  rooms for performing of, at hospital, 160
  types of, 97
  wound treatment and, 611
Nervous system
  clinical examination of, 557–559
    cranial nerves, 557–558
    gait analysis, 558–559
    limb placement and panniculus tests, 558
    tail and anal tone evaluation, 558
Neurological disease
  complications and sedation for horses with, 318
  equine sedation and, 317–318
Neurological disorders, management of horses with, 561–569
Neurological examination, form for recording results of, *218–219*
Neurological physiotherapy, 639–640
  facial nerve paralysis, 639–640
  peripheral nerve injuries, 640
Neurological sequelae, hospitalised horses and conditions related to, 557 (box 14.1)
Neurological system, monitoring, 557–561
Neuromuscular electrical stimulation, 646*t*, 648
Neutrophil elastase, 632
Neutrophils
  bronchoalveolar lavage cytology and presence of, 460
  degenerative, tracheal aspirate cytology and, 459, *459*
  inflammatory bronchoalveolar lavage cytology with increased numbers of, 460
Newborn foals
  creatinine concentrations in, 366
  preparing for cardiopulmonary resuscitation, 122
Niclosamide, approximate doses used in equine medicine, 664*t*
Nitrofurazone, 620
Nitroimidazoles, 348
Nonadherent dressings, 104
Nonanaesthetised horse, cardiopulmonary resuscitation for, 7
Nonesterified fatty acids, 265
Nonhealing wounds, 617
Nonpurposive movements in down horses, 563
Nonseptic inflammatory tracheal aspirate cytology, with increased mucus and increased number of neutrophils, *459*
Nonseptic lymphoplasmacytic hepatitis, 527
Nonsteroidal anti-inflammatory drugs
  avoiding administration of, in animals with acute renal failure, 543
  caecal perforation and, 485
  corneal ulcer treatment and, 632–633
  endotoxaemia treatment and, 505–506
  hepatotoxicity and, 521
  laminitis and use of, 332
  neurological disorders and, 568
  pain management, adverse effects and use of, 325
  pathophysiology of ileus and, 500
  renal insufficiency and, 533
  somatic pain management and, 330
  toxicity and right dorsal colitis related to, 485
Nonstructural carbohydrates, 273, 277
Nonulcerative keratitis
  management of horses with, 634–635
  in 9-year-old Quarter Horse gelding, *633*
Norepinephrine
  cardiovascular and pulmonary support and use of, 243*t*
  guideline for diluting and preparation of, 449*t*
  renal insufficiency and, 533
  tissue perfusion improvement and, 449–450
Norfloxacin, 345
Normal saline, 372–373
Normosol-R, 372
Nose twitch, examination per rectum and use of, 9
Nosocomial importance, equine contagious and zoonotic diseases of, 186–190*t*
Nosocomial infections
  investigating and monitoring, 599
  simplified guidelines for surveillance of, 181*t*
NSAIDs. *See* Nonsteroidal anti-inflammatory drugs
Nuclear medicine
  procedure, 178–179
  regulations, 178
Nurse mares, orphan foals and, 300
Nurses' base, at equine hospital, 153
Nursing mares, sedation and, 319
Nutrient Requirements Council, 253
Nutrient requirements for hospitalised adult horse, 269–275
  carbohydrates, 273–274
  energy, 269–270
  lipids, 272–273
    contraindications for supplementation with, 273
    future trends in supplementation with, 273
  minerals and vitamins, 274–275
  protein, 270–272
    contraindications for supplementation with, 271
    future trends in amino acid supplementation, 271–272
  water, 269

Nutrient requirements for hospitalised foals, 298–299
energy, 298–299
lipids, 299
minerals and vitamins, 299
protein, 299
Nutrient Requirements of Horses, 270
Nutrition, foal started on, 133
Nutrition administration, for enteral nutrition, 282
Nutritional history, reviewing, for hospitalised adult horse, 262–263
Nutritional management of hospitalised horse
adult horse, 261–295
assessing body weight and body condition, 262
biochemical profile evaluation, 263, 265–267
clinical evaluation of, 261–262
indications for enteral or parenteral nutritional therapy in, 275 (box 5.11)
initiating treatment with therapeutic nutrition, 267, 269
nutrient requirements, 269–275
nutritional history review, 262–263
nutrition options: enteral nutrition, 276–284
nutrition options: parenteral nutrition, 284, 287–295
patient evaluation, 261–267
return to voluntary feeding, 284, 295
selecting form of supplemental nutrition, 275–276
colic patient, 512–513
foal, 297–311
guidelines for, *268*
Nutritional requirements
for hospitalised adult horse, 269–275
carbohydrates, 273–274
energy, 269–270
lipids, 272–273
minerals and vitamins, 274–275
protein, 270–272
water, 269
Nutrition options for hospitalised adult horse
enteral nutrition, 276–284
administration of, 282
choice and use of indwelling nasogastric tubes, 280–281
complications associated with assisted enteral feeding, 283–284
diet preparation, 282
enteral diet formulations, 277–280
fibre in enteral diets, 276–278
monitoring guidelines, 282–283
return to voluntary feeding, 284
parenteral nutrition, 284–295
administration of, 292–295
formulating, 290–292
formulating parenteral solution, 284
ingredients in parenteral solution, 284, 287–290
return to voluntary feeding, 295
Nutrition support, early, acute renal failure and, 545
Nutrition therapy, goal of, in hospitalised equine, 261 (box 5.1), 264 (box 5.6)
Nystatin, 353
Nystatin (polyenes), fungal keratitis treatment and, 631

O
Oat hay, 266
nutrient composition of, 265*t*
Obel, N., 581
Obese equine patients, 261
Obligate intracellular pathogens, suggested choices of antimicrobial agents for common bacterial pathogens of horses and, 339t
Oblique internus abdominus, 595
Occlusive dressings, 104
Occult blood, reagent strips and, 535
Ocular examination, of horse with painful eye, 91
Ocular pain, 329–330
Ocular procedures, anaesthesia and, 251–252
Oculocardiac reflex, 252
Oculomotor nerve, testing, 558
Oedema, physiotherapy and, 639
Oesophageal obstruction (choke), 487
Oesophagostomy tube placement and contraindications, for hospitalised adult horse, 281
Oesophagus, endoscopic view of, *22*
Oestradiol, approximate doses used in equine medicine, 664*t*
Offices, at equine hospital, 161
OIA. *See* Oblique internus abdominus
Oil, in liquid enteral diets, 279
Oleander toxicity, uniform ventricular tachycardia in horse with, *420*
Oleander toxicosis, 420
Oliguria, 453
Oliver, J. E., 638
Omega-3 fatty acids, endotoxaemia and, 507
Omeprazole, approximate doses used in equine medicine, 664*t*
Omolene 100, nutrient composition of, 265*t*
Oncotic pressure, 370
Onestrone sulfate, approximate doses used in equine medicine, 664*t*
Operating room, 226
at equine hospital, 155
Operating table
in equine hospital, 157
horse positioned on, for spinal process resection, *158*
Ophthalmic examination, 628
Opioids
as analgesics, 245, 509
equine sedation and use of, 313*t*, 314–315
head cases and use of, 317
pain management, adverse effects and use of, 325
Opisthotonus, in foal with severe hyponatraemia, *558*
Oral cavity, common fungal pathogens at, 352*t*
Oral fluids, 368
recipes for, 367*t*
Oral glucose tolerance test, protocol and interpretation of, 688
Oral procedures, anaesthesia and, 251–252
Orbifloxacin, 345
approximate doses used in equine medicine, 664*t*
Orchardgrass hay, nutrient composition of, 265*t*
Orotracheal intubation, in neonatal foal, 120, *121*
Orphan foal, healthy, enteral feeding for, 302
Orthopaedic felt, 608
Orthopaedic implants
infection and, 601–602
sources of post-operative fever following surgical placement of, 592 (box 15.6)
Orthopaedic injury, acute management of, 605
Osmolarity, of parenteral solution, 289–290
Osmolyte HN, 275, 277, 278
Osmotic diuretics, renal failure treatment and, 543–544
Osteomyelitis, 575
Ovarian pain, 328, 329
Ovariectomy, reported infection rates for, 609
Ovaries, ultrasonography of, 542
Over-the-needle catheters
arterial catheterisation and use of, 43, 44
jugular catheterisation and placement of, 28–30
flattening catheter towards neck and advancing 5 to 10 cm, *29*
jugular catheter with extension set, *30*
pushing catheter through skin over jugular vein, *29*
sliding catheter off stylet and into vein, *29*
for jugular vein catheterisation in foals, 133
placing, in neonatal foal, 136–137

Over-the-wire catheters
jugular catheterisation and placement of, 30
double-lumen catheter in jugular vein of adult horse, *30*
for jugular vein catheterisation in foals, 133
lateral thoracic vein catheterised with, 33
placing, for jugular vein catheterisation in foals, 134–136
catheter sutured to skin, *136*
catheter threaded onto wire, *136*
needle placed into jugular vein, *135*
needle removed from vein and slid off end of wire, *135*
Oxacillin, approximate doses used in equine medicine, 664*t*
Oxfendazole, approximate doses used in equine medicine, 664*t*
Oxibendazole, approximate doses used in equine medicine, 664*t*
"Oxspring" block, 168, *168*, 169
Oxygen, arterial and venous partial pressures of, 462
Oxygen administration, intranasal, 62–63
Oxygen extraction ratio, 435
Oxygen flows, for induction in foals, 246
Oxygen tank, *62*
Oxygen therapy, 470–471
intranasal oxygen administration, 470–471
Oxymorphone
approximate doses used in equine medicine, 664*t*
equine sedation and use of, 314
Oxytetracycline, 347
approximate doses used in equine medicine, 664*t*
Oxytocin, approximate doses used in equine medicine, 664*t*

P
Pacemaker implantation, bradydysrhythmias and, 442
Packed cell volume
collection of blood for, 12
evaluation of, in foals, 301
gastrointestinal disease and monitoring of fluid status, 491
hypovolaemia and, 365–366
measuring, 283
PACs. *See* Picture archiving and communication systems
Padded anaesthetic rooms, at equine hospital, 154
Padded head covers, 562
Padded walls, horses with neurological disorders and, 561, *562*
Padding, primary dressings and, 104
PAF. *See* Platelet-activating factor
Paging system, for reception area in hospital, 153
PAH. *See* Para-aminohippuric acid
PAI. *See* Plasminogen activator inhibitor
Pailloux, J-P., 650
Pain, physiotherapy and, 639
Pain management in hospitalised horse, 324–332
considerations for, 324–326
objective of, 324–325
ocular pain, 329–330
postoperative, 245–246
secondary hyperalgesia or "wind up," 331–332
somatic pain, 330–331
systemic analgesics used in horse, 324*t*
visceral pain, 326–329
Palmar-digital nerve block, 96
Palmar nerves, analgesia of fetlock (fore limb) and, 97
Palpation
examination per rectum and, 9–10
physical examination and, 7
Pancuronium, approximate doses used in equine medicine, 664*t*
Pan feeding, for foals, 301
Panniculus tests, 558
Pao_2, hypoxaemia and, 244
PAP complexes. *See* Plasmin-[alpha] 2-antiplasm complexes
Para-aminohippuric acid, clearance of, as measure of renal blood flow, 538
Paradoxical aciduria, 535
Paradoxical bronchoconstriction, 468–469
Paralytic ileus, 484
Paranasal sinus disease, sinocentesis for, 77–78
Paraphimosis, 534, 548
Parasympatholytics, 469
Parenteral formulations, minerals added to, 274
Parenteral nutrition, 261, 262
carbohydrates and, 273–274
commercial mixtures, 285*t*
double- and triple-lumen catheters recommended for use during treatment with, 293, *293*
double-lumen catheters and administration of, 369
examples of vitamin and mineral supplements suitable for, 289 (box 5.18)
for horses with sustained ileus, 503
indications for, in adult horse, 275 (box 5.11)
ingredients in, 288*t*
jugular catheterisation and administration of, 28
suggested monitoring guidelines during, 283 (box 5.14)
treatment with, for hospitalised adult horse, 275 (box 5.11)
Parenteral nutrition for hospitalised adult horse, 276, 284–295
administration of parenteral solution, 292–295
instructions for, 293
intravenous catheters, 293
patient monitoring, 294
complications associated with PN therapy, 294–295
electrolyte deficiencies, 294–295
excess fluid administration, 294
hyperglycaemia, 295
hypertriglyceridaemia, 295
infections, 295
formulation of, 290–292
compounding parenteral solution, 290–291
preparing, 291–292
supplements added to mixture, 292
ingredients
dextrose and glucose, 287
fluid requirements, 290
lipids, 287–289
minerals and vitamins, 289
osmolarity, 289–290
protein, 284
return to voluntary feeding, 295
Parenteral nutrition for hospitalised foal, *306*, 306–309
complications with, 309
formulations for, 306–308
infusion protocol with, 308
monitoring of, 308–309
Parenteral nutrition formula, example of, used in Europe, 307, 308 (box 5.25)
Parenteral nutrition infusion, instructions for, 294 (box 5.21)
Parenteral nutrition solutions
compounding, instructions for, 291 (box 5.19)
drugs incompatible with, 292 (box 5.20)
preparing for compounding, in laminar flow hood, *291*
Parenteral nutrition therapy
complications associated with, 294–295
electrolyte deficiencies, 294–295
excess fluid administration, 294
hyperglycaemia, 295
hypertriglyceridaemia, 295
infections, 295
Parenteral nutrition worksheet for foals, 307 (box 5.24)
Parenteral therapy
enteral therapy *versus*, 275
for neonatal foals, 299–300
Partial parenteral nutrition, 273, 284

Partial parenteral nutrition formulations, in-house veterinary clinic, compounding of, 290
Partial parenteral nutrition worksheet, 285–286 (box 5.15)
Parvaquone, approximate doses used in equine medicine, 665*t*
PAs. *See* Pyrrolizidine alkaloids
Passive drains, peritoneal lavage and, 18
Passive humidifiers, 475
Passive static stretches, 645
Pastern, analgesia of, 97
Pastern joint, synoviocentesis approaches for, 577, *577*
Pastern region, small laceration to palmar aspect of, *615*
Pasteurella spp., 337, 338
Patient handling, biosecurity and, 192–194
Patient observation, from nurses' base at hospital, 153
Patient surveillance, infection control and, 185, 192
Patient-ventilator synchrony, mechanical ventilation of neonatal foal and, 127, 127 (box 2.7)
PCV. *See* Packed cell volume
Peak inspiratory pressure, 478
Pectoral muscles
  intramuscular injections in, 13, 14, *14*
  site of intramuscuar injection into, *13*
  treatment of horse with traumatic injury to, *643*
Pediculosis, nosocomial importance of, 187*t*
PEEP. *See* Positive end-expiratory pressure
Pelleted diets, preparation of, 282
Pelleted feeds, commercial, 278
Pelvic visceral pain management, 329
Penicillamine D, approximate doses used in equine medicine, 665*t*
Penicillin, 337, 338
  equine central nervous system or cerebrospinal fluid and, 566
  excretion of, 342
Penicillin G (Na, K), approximate doses used in equine medicine, 665*t*
Penicillin G (procaine), approximate doses used in equine medicine, 665*t*
Penis
  examining, 543
  of foal, holding for insertion of urinary catheter, 143, *143*
Penrose drain
  latex, correct placement of in traumatic wound, *619*
  placement of, *612*
Pentastarch, 375–376
  approximate doses used in equine medicine, 665*t*
Pentazocine
  approximate doses used in equine medicine, 665*t*
  equine sedation and use of, 315
Pentobarbital
  approximate doses used in equine medicine, 665*t*
  equine sedation and use of, 313*t*, 316
Pentoxifylline
  approximate doses used in equine medicine, 665*t*
  endotoxaemia treatment, 505
Percheron mare, iris problems, surgical repair and postoperative photograph of eye in, *629*
Percussion, 640–641
  prior to suctioning airway, in neonatal foal, 128
Percutaneous (transtracheal aspirate), 69–70
Percutaneous trocharisation, 24–25
  anatomy of caecum and site for, *25*
  of the caecum, *25*
  defined, 24
  equipment needed for, 23 (box 1.13), 24
  indications for, 24
  performing technique, 24–25
Performance problems, assessing, 643
Perfusion studies, 407
Pergolide, approximate doses used in equine medicine, 665*t*
Perianal skin reactions, evaluating, 558–559
Pericardial disease, 426
  determining aetiology of, 58
Pericardial effusion
  20F Argyle chest tube inserted in fifth ICS for drainage of, *60*
  in 2-year-old sport horse, echocardiogram showing, *58*
Pericardial sac
  catheter in, draining pericardial fluid, *60*
  fluid draining from chest tube placed in, *60*
Pericardial tamponade, 318
Pericardiocentesis, 58–60, 426, 444
  equipment needed for, 59 (box 1.29)
  indication for, 58
  procedure for, 58–60
  usual site for, *59*
  weanling foal with telemetric ECG set up for monitoring cardiac rhythm during, *59*
Pericarditis, 426–428
  clinical signs of, 426
  echocardiograms of foal with, *427*
  evaluation of the fluid, 426–428
    drainage, 427–428
  treatment of, 444
Perineural analgesia of limb
  analgesia of fetlock (fore limb), 97
  analgesia of fetlock (hind limb), 98
  analgesia of limb distal to carpus and hock, 98
  analgesia of pastern and foot, 97
Peripheral catheter placement, parenteral nutrition for hospitalised foals and, 308
Peripheral nerves, characteristics of, 647*t*
Peripheral perfusion, assessing, 417
Perirenal oedema, 541
Peristaltic pump, turning on, prior to taking cardiac output measurement, 57
Peritoneal dialysis, 544–545
Peritoneal drain, gravity-flow of fluids into abdomen via, in broodmare, *20*
Peritoneal fluid
  analysis of, 654
  guide to interpretation of, 680*t*
  interpretation of, 492–493
    determination of medical *versus* surgical colic, 492–493
    effect of age, surgery and foaling, 492
    grass sickness, 493
    septic peritonitis, 493
    total nucleated cell count, 493
  spectrophotometric assessment of, 493
  ultrasound of, 17, *17*
Peritoneal fluid values, normal and abnormal in horses, 679*t*
Peritoneal lavage, 18–21
  equipment needed for, 18, 18 (box 1.11)
  inserting abdominal drain under general anaesthesia, 19
  inserting drain in the standing horse, 19
  performing the lavage, 20
  possible complications, 21
  purpose of, 18
  securing drain, 19–20
Peritoneal phosphate concentrations
  in horses with colic (SI units), 493*t*
  in horses with colic (U.S. units), 493*t*
Peritonitis, 337
Peroneal nerve block, *101*
Perphenazine
  approximate doses used in equine medicine, 665*t*
  equine sedation and use of, 313*t*, 314
Personnel
  hospital team in anaesthesia, 235
  Salmonella and segregation of, 194

Petechial haemorrhages
clinical approach and management of hospitalised patient with, 414–415
in oral mucous membranes of 2-month-old foal presenting with severe pneumonia, *404*
Pethidine (meperidine)
approximate doses used in equine medicine, 665*t*
equine sedation and use of, 313*t*, 314, 315
PFGE. *See* Pulsed-field gel electrophoresis
PG. *See* Prostaglandins
pH, of adult horse urine, reagent strips and, 535
Pharmacies
commercial compounding, 290
at equine hospital, 160
Pharynx, common fungal pathogens in, 352*t*
Phenobarbital
acute seizure treatment and, 565
approximate doses used in equine medicine, 665*t*
equine sedation and use of, 313*t*, 316
neurological disease and use of, 318
Phenothiazines
equine sedation and use of, 313*t*, 314
genital disorders and, 534
hormonal secretion in mares and, 320
Phenoxybenzamine, approximate doses used in equine medicine, 665*t*
Phenylbutazone
approximate doses used in equine medicine, 665*t*
caecal rupture and, 485
endotoxaemia treatment and, 505, 506
somatic pain management and, 330
Phenylephrine
approximate doses used in equine medicine, 665*t*
cardiovascular and pulmonary support and use of, 242, 243*t*
intranasal spray, 245
Phenytoin, 437*t*
approximate doses used in equine medicine, 665*t*
supraventricular tachydysrhythmias and, 442
ventricular tachycardia treatment and, 439
Philip Leverhulme Equine Hospital, University of Liverpool, equine colic admission form, *203–204*
Phlebitis, 396
Phlebotomy
hepatic disorders and, 527
liver injury and, 527
Phosphate, electrolyte disturbances and, 385
Phosphate concentrations, guide to interpretation of, 677 (box 19.20)
Phosphate disturbances, treatment of, 385–386
Physical examination
of adult horse, 7–8
equipment needed for, 7–8, 7 (box 1.5)
findings from, 236
head-to-toe approach, 7–8
heart monitoring and, 417
of hospitalised adult horse, 261
monitoring of lameness and, 575
per rectum, 8–10
tissue perfusion and, 430–431
wound management of hospitalised horse and, 611
Physical rehabilitation, importance of, 638
Physical restraint and assistance, in recovering horse, 245
Physiological shunt fraction equation, 463 (box 10.2)
Physiological values, normal, 654, 670 (box 19.1)
Physiotherapy
conditions that may benefit from, 639 (box 18.1)
indications and treatment techniques
acupuncture, 651
electrotherapy, 645–649
exercise rehabilitation, 649–650
facilities required for, 644
hydrotherapy, 650–651
indications for, 639–640
manual therapy, 644–645
massage, 645
mobilisations and manipulations, 644–645
stretches, 645
trigger point therapy/myofascial release, 645
musculoskeletal conditions, 641–643
postorthopaedic surgery, 643–644
qualifications for, 638
respiratory, 640–641
thermal therapy, 648–649
cryotherapy, 648–649
heat therapy, 649
treatment techniques, 644–645
list of treatment techniques, 644 (box 18.5)
properties of commonly used manual techniques in, 642*t*
Physostigmine, approximate doses used in equine medicine, 665*t*
Picture archiving and communication systems, 175
Pigmenturia, 533
Pinch grafts
advantages and disadvantages with, 624 (box 16.1)
procedure for, 625
recipient site prepared for, *625*
PIP. *See* Peak inspiratory pressure
Piped anaesthetic gas, use of, in equine hospital, 156–157
Piped oxygen outlet, flowmeter, and humidifier, *62*
Piperacillin, 343
Piperazine, approximate doses used in equine medicine, 665*t*
Pipothiazine, equine sedation and use of, 314
Pirbuterol, 468
approximate doses used in equine medicine, 666*t*
Pituitary pars intermedia dysfunction (Cushing's disease), 573
basal tests, 686–687
blood glucose levels, 687
clinical and laboratory signs and their prevalence in, 687 (box 19.26)
combined dexamethasone suppression, TRH stimulation test, 687
cortisol levels, 687
diagnosis of, 686–687
dynamic tests, 687
insulin levels, 687
low-dose dexamethasone suppression test, 687
Pivampicillin, 343
approximate doses used in equine medicine, 666*t*
Placenta
common fungal pathogens in, 352*t*
retained, 547
Plantar digital nerve, abaxial sesamoid nerve block and, *98*
Plasma, 377–378
approximate doses used in equine medicine, 666*t*
separation of, 41
Plasma biochemistry, cardiac disease and, 419–420
Plasma collection device, homemade, design for, *42*
Plasma collection kit, parts of, *41*
Plasma fibrinogen, hepatic function and, 522
Plasma-lyte 148, 372
Plasmapheresis, 378
Plasma total solids, hypovolaemia and, 365–366
Plasma transfusions, as replacement for coagulation factors, disease conditions and, 412 (box 8.8)
Plasmin-[alpha] 2-antiplasm complexes, 406
Plasminogen, 406
Plasminogen activator inhibitor, 406
Plaster of Paris, as casting material, 607

Plate holders
ceiling-mounted x-ray units and, *165*, 166
range of, with 360° swivel handle, *168*
in x-ray rooms, 177–178
Platelet-activating factor, endotoxaemia and, 506–507
Platelet count, 405
Platelet count test, anticoagulants for, 670 (box 19.3)
Platelet-derived growth factor, wound healing and, 620
Platelet gel dressing, wound healing and, 621
Platelets and platelet-rich plasma, hypocoagulable states in horses managed with, 412–413
Pleural drainage, 472–473
Pleural effusion
"fluid line" caused by, on thoracic radiograph, *465*
in right ventral thorax, with consolidation of tip of the lung, *463*
Pleural fluid collection, 461
interpretation of cytology and, 461
procedure for, 461
Pleural fluid cytology, normal values for, 681*t*
Pleural friction rubs, 457
Pleurocentesis, 71–72
equipment needed for, 72 (box 1.40)
indication for, 71
potential complications with, 72
procedure for, 71–72
selecting site for, 461
site for placing thoracic drain for removal of pleural effusion, *73*
with use of teat cannula and three-way stopcock, *73*
Pleuropneumonia, 458
causes of, 337
pleural fluid and, 463, *463*
PMI, murmurs and, 419
PMMA. *See* Polymethylmethacrylate
PN. *See* Parenteral nutrition
Pneumatic nebulisers, 64
Pneumatic tourniquet, complications with, 109
Pneumonia, ventilator-associated, 479
Pneumothorax
bilateral, in a horse, *466*
evacuation of, 72–74
suggestion of, 72
unilateral, in a horse, *466*
Point block, 97
Polydipsia, liver failure and, 522
Polyenes, 353
Polyionic fluids, classes of, 372
Polymerised bovine haemoglobin, 378
Polymethylmethacrylate, antimicrobial drugs delivery and, 601
Polymixin B
approximate doses used in equine medicine, 666*t*
endotoxaemia treatment and, 504
Polymixin B sulfate, 620
Polysaccharide storage myopathy, 586, 589–590
acute management of, 590
diagnosis of, 590
long-term management of, 590
muscle biopsy and, 112
pathogenesis, 589–590
Polysporin, 620
Polyurethane, as casting material, 607
Polyuria, 453
liver failure and, 522
Polyvinylchloride fenestrated drain tubes, 618
Ponazuril, approximate doses used in equine medicine, 666*t*
Ponies, hyperlipaemia in, 399
Pool systems, recovering horse and, 245
Positive end-expiratory pressure, 126 (box 2.5), 475, 477, 478, 479
Positive pressure ventilation, 474
use of, in neonatal foal, *124*
Postanaesthetic morbidity, 254
Postanaesthetic myopathy, renal insufficiency and, 533
Post-mortem examination facility, at equine hospital, 162
Post-operative colic information sheet, *211*
Postoperative ileus, 484, 499
Postoperative pain, 330
management of, 245–246
Postorthopaedic surgery, physiotherapy treatment and, 643
Postrenal factors, correcting, 543
Postrenal failure, 533
Posttraumatic chronic pain syndromes, 332
Potassium
electrolyte assessment of cardiac disease and, 419
electrolyte imbalances and, 382–383
Potassium chloride, approximate doses used in equine medicine, 666*t*
Potassium concentrations, guide to interpretation of, 677 (box 19.21)
Potassium imbalances, treatment of, 383–384
Potassium iodide, approximate doses used in equine medicine, 666*t*
Potentiated sulphonamides, equine central nervous system or cerebrospinal fluid and, 567
PPID. *See* Pituitary pars intermedia dysfunction
PPN. *See* Partial parenteral nutrition
PPV. *See* Positive pressure ventilation
Pralidoxime chloride, approximate doses used in equine medicine, 666*t*
Praziquantel, approximate doses used in equine medicine, 666*t*
Preanaesthetic evaluation, 236–237
Preanaesthetic physical examination findings, anaesthetic concerns related to, in horses scheduled for elective anaesthesia, 238*t*
Preanaesthetic preparation, 239*t*
Precordial thrill, 417
Prednisolone, approximate doses used in equine medicine, 666*t*
Preepidural morphine, in horse with septic tarsal sheath, *331*
Pregnant mares
anaesthesia for, 249–250
with colic, monitoring of, 513–514
digestible energy requirements for, 270*t*
protein requirements for, 271*t*
sedation and, 319
Prekallikrein deficiency, 405
Premedication, 237–239
equine inhalant-based anaesthetic drug choices, 237*t*
Premedication anaesthetic choices, for equine neonates and older foals, 247*t*
Prerenal factors, correcting, 543
Prescriptions, recording batch numbers for, 160
Pressors
cautious use of, 447
guideline for diluting and preparation of, 449*t*
practical use of, 453
Pressure cuff, noninvasive blood pressure monitoring via, 432
Pressure cycled ventilators, 232
Pressure sores, minimising, 563
Pressure support, 128
Pressure support ventilation, 476, 477
Pressure transducer
for direct monitoring of arterial pressure, *46*
setting up, for direct arterial blood pressure monitoring, 46
zeroing, for direct arterial blood pressure monitoring, 46
Pressure triggering, 476
Priapism, 534, 548
Primary dressing
application of, to hock region, 105
bandages and, 103, *103*
for head bandaging, *111*
Primary hyperlipaemia, 399

Primary infusion
for pumps and drivers, 39
Primary wound closure, 616
Primidone, approximate doses used in equine medicine, 666*t*
Procainamide, 437*t*
approximate doses used in equine medicine, 666*t*
supraventricular tachydysrhythmias and, 442
ventricular ectopic depolarisations and use of, 440
ventricular tachycardia treatment and, 438
Procaine, 343
Profuse bleeding after surgery, clinical approach and management of hospitalised patient and, 415
Progesterone, approximate doses used in equine medicine, 666*t*
Progress notes, 225
Proinflammatory cytokines, 263
Prokinetic drugs
choice of, 502–503
examples of those used in horses, 500 (box 11.4)
possible choices for, based on condition or site of lesion, 503 (box 11.5)
Promazine
approximate doses used in equine medicine, 666*t*
equine sedation and use of, 314
ProNurse, 300
Propafenone, 437*t*
approximate doses used in equine medicine, 666*t*
supraventricular tachydysrhythmias and, 442
ventricular ectopic depolarisations and use of, 440
ventricular tachycardia treatment and, 438–439
Propionate, inhaled corticosteroid therapy and, 470
Propionibacterium acnes, approximate doses used in equine medicine, 666*t*
Propionylpromazine, equine sedation and use of, 314
Propofol
anaesthesia of foals and, 248
approximate doses used in equine medicine, 666*t*
Propranolol, 437*t*
approximate doses used in equine medicine, 666*t*
supraventricular tachydysrhythmias and, 442
ventricular tachycardia treatment and, 439
Proprioception, addressing, 650
Proprioceptive loss, clinical signs associated with, 558
Prostaglandins, 512
pain management and, 332
Protective clothing
radiation safety and, 176
safe handling of radiopharmaceuticals and, 179
Protein
for hospitalised adult horse, 270–272
contraindications for supplementation with, 271
in liquid enteral diets, 279
low intakes of, hepatic insufficiency and, 528
in parenteral solutions, 284
reagent strips and, 535
Protein C, 406
Protein metabolism, markers of, in hospitalised horse, 265
Protein requirements
for horses in different physiologic conditions, 271*t*
for neonatal foals, 299
Proteinuria, 535
Proximal interphalangeal joint (pastern joint), approaches to, for synoviocentesis, 577, *577*
PS. *See* Pressure support
Pseudallescheria boydii, 351
intranasal miconazole and, 354
Pseudomonas infection, keratitis due to, in 2-year-old Thoroughbred filly, *630*
Pseudomonas spp., 338
isolation of, from septic arthritis in foals, 580
PSSM. *See* Polysaccharide storage myopathy
PSV. *See* Pressure support ventilation
Psyllium mucilloid, approximate doses used in equine medicine, 666*t*
PT, anticoagulants for, 670 (box 19.3)
Ptosis, observing, 7
Pulley and rope system, for assisted recovery of horses from anaesthesia, *156*
Pulmonary artery, two-dimensional left parasternal echocardiogram of, *55*
Pulmonary disease, severe, arterial blood gases and, 420
Pulmonary function, mechanical ventilation and monitoring of, 478
Pulmonary mechanics, 462–463
Pulmonary support, for anaesthetised horses, 243*t*
Pulmonary thromboembolism, after orthopaedic surgery, 404
Pulmonic valves, 417
Pulse character, 417
PulseCO, calibration of to LiDCO, 57
Pulse contour analysis, cardiac output measurement and, 57–58
Pulse contour analysis cardiac output determination, readout from, in a foal, *57*
Pulsed-field gel electrophoresis, 192*n*
Pulse oximetry, 234
arterial haemoglobin oxygenation saturation monitored with, 432
Pulse oximetry probes, reflectance probe on gingival mucous membrane and finger probe on tongue, *234*
Pumps
electronic infusion, 37–38
fluid, 36–37
Punch grafts
advantages and disadvantages with, 624 (box 16.1)
of nonhealing wound over hock, *625*
procedure for, 624–625
Puncture wounds
of distal limb, 615
to sole of hoof, 617
Pupillary light reflex, 628
Pupils, evaluating, 558
Purse-string suture, placing, at base of drain, before continuing to "Chinese finger trap" suture, *19*
PVC (polyvinlychloride) drains, peritoneal lavage and, 18
P wave
analysis of electrocardiographic recording and, 422
normal variations in, in base-apex ECG, *51*
Pyelonephritis, 547
Pylorus
endoscope passage and viewing of, 23
endoscopic view of, *23*
Pyrantel embonate, approximate doses used in equine medicine, 666*t*
Pyrimethamine, approximate doses used in equine medicine, 667*t*
Pyrrolizidine alkaloids, 523
Pyrrolizidine alkaloid toxicity, 524
Pythium insidiosum, 351, 352
Pythium spp., 354

Q
QRST-complexes, uniform ventricular tachycardia and, *423*
QRS wave
analysis of electrocardiographic recording and, 422
in base-apex ECG, *50*
Quality, murmurs and, 418
Quarter Horses, polysaccharide storage myopathy in, 589
Quidding, 262
Quills, horizontal mattress suture pattern with, *117*
Quill suture patterns, 616

Quinidine, 421
ventricular tachycardia treatment and, 438
Quinidine gluconate, 437*t*
approximate doses used in equine medicine, 667*t*
supraventricular dysrhythmias and, 440
Quinidine-induced dysrhythmias, treatment of, 441*t*
Quinidine sulphate, 437*t*
approximate doses used in equine medicine, 667*t*
ventricular ectopic depolarisations and use of, 440

R
R. equi infections in foals, macrolides and derivatives and, 347
Rabies, nosocomial importance of, 188*t*
Racks and hangers, for radiography room, at hospital, 166, *166*
Radiation exposure, minimising, 175–176
Radiation hazard, minimising, basic principles for, 176 (box 3.4)
Radiation levels, monitoring, in imaging rooms, 176
Radiation safety, 175–179
computed tomography, 178
fluoroscopy, 178
ionising radiation and, 175
nuclear medicine, 178–179
procedure for, 178–179
regulations for, 178
principles of minimising radiation exposure, 175–177
monitoring and safety testing, 176
regulatory requirements, 175–176
training, 176–177
radiography, 177–178
equipment for, 177
outside designated room, 177
procedure for, 177–177
room requirements
x-ray machine features and, 177
Radioactivity, units of, 176*t*
Radiofrequency signals, equine magnetic resonance imaging and, 174
Radiographs, lacerations, puncture wounds and use of, 616–617
Radiography, 177–178
computerised, 167
conventional film/screen, 166–167
direct digital, 167
equipment, 177
implant evaluation with, 593
implant failure detected with, *592*
laminitis and use of, 582–583
outside designated room, 177
procedure for, 177–178
room requirements for, 177
Radiography equipment, 166–169
blocks, 168–169
cassette and cassette holders, 167–168
ceiling-mounted x-ray units, 166
computerised radiography, 167
conventional film/screen radiography, 166–167
direct digital radiography, 167
miscellaneous, 169
mobile x-ray units, 166
protective lead clothing, 167
Radiography of respiratory tract, 464–465
interpretation of, 465
procedure for, 464
Radiography room
designing, for equine hospital, 165–166
at equine hospital, 159–160
Radiography suite, equine, with ceiling-mounted x-ray machine and plate holder, *165*
Radiography suppliers, 176 (box 3.3)
Radiopharmaceuticals, 178
equipment for safe handling of, 179
Radiotelemetry, 51, 421
Radiotelemetry unit, for recording ECGs, *51*
"Railroad tracks" pattern, lung tissue disease and, 465
Range of motion, decreased, physiotherapy and, 639
Ranitidine, approximate doses used in equine medicine, 667*t*
RAO. *See* Recurrent airway obstruction
Rapid volume expanders, hypovolaemia treated with, 369
Rattles, 457
RCVS. *See* Royal College of Veterinary Surgeons
Reagent strips, urine samples and, 535
Rebreathing examination, 8, 457–458
Reception area, in equine hospital, 152–153, *153*
Recipes
enteral fluid therapy, 368
equine enteral diet, 278–279
Recipient site, for skin grafts, 624
Record keeping, hospital forms and, 200
Recovery
controlling in volatile and large animals, 244
equine inhalant-based anaesthetic drug choices, 237*t*
horse in sternal recumbency during, *246*
Recovery anaesthetic choices, for equine neonates and older foals, 247*t*
Recovery room
in equine hospital, 155
general anaesthesia and, 228
Recruitment manoeuvres, mechanical ventilation and, 477
Rectal examination, 488
Rectal impactions, 566
Rectal mucosal biopsy, 25–26
equipment needed for, 25, 26 (box 1.14)
holding uterine biopsy instrument for introduction into rectum, *26*
rectal mucosa pinched and placed in jaws of biopsy instrument, *26*
technique for, 25–26
value of, 25
Rectal sleeves, examination per rectum and use of, 9
Rectal tears, minimizing, 9
Rectangular block, *168*
Rectovaginal technique, for endometrial biopsy, 87
Rectum
examination per, 8–10
description of, 9–10
equipment needed for, 8, 8 (box 1.6)
preparation for, 8–9
structures palpable on, *10*
Recumbency, complications of, 563
Recurrent airway obstruction, 457, 459
parasympatholytics and, 469
Recurrent exertional rhabdomyolysis, 588–589
acute management of, 589
clinical signs of, 589
diagnosis of, 589
dietary management and, 589
exercise regimen and, 589
long-term management of, 589
Red blood cells
cerebrospinal fluid analysis and, 560
haematuria and, 536
Re-feeding syndrome, 266
Regional anaesthesia of the eye
anaesthesia of cornea and conjunctiva, 93
approximate areas of desensitisation with block to frontal, infratrochlear, lacrimal and zygomatic nerves, front and side view, *93*
auriculopalpebral nerve block used for, 91–92

Regional anaesthesia of the eye *(Continued)*
  blocks of ophthalmic branches of trigeminal nerve, 92–93
  equipment needed for, 92 (box 1.54)
Regional analgesia of limb, 96–100
  general procedure for placing nerve block, 96–97
  indications for, 96
  perineural analgesia of limb, 97–98, 100
    analgesia of distal antebrachium and carpus, 98, 100
    analgesia of fetlock (fore limb), 97
    analgesia of fetlock (hind limb), 98
    analgesia of limb distal to carpus and hock, 98
    analgesia of pastern and foot, 97
    equipment for, 97 (box 1.56)
    hind limb: tibial and fibular (peroneal) block, 100
  types of nerve block, 97
Regional limb perfusion, 108–109, 601, 602–604
  equipment for application of, 109 (box 1.61)
  Esmarch bandage placed below hock for, *109*
  intraosseus, 604
  intravenous, *603*, 604
Regional perfusions, of antimicrobial agents, 350–351
Regulatory requirements, radiation safety and, 175–176
Relaporotomy, 601
Relaxation, equine magnetic resonance imaging and, 173
Renal biopsies, 88–89, 541
  equipment needed for, 89 (box 1.52)
  indications for, 88
  procedure for, 88–89
Renal blood flow
  measurement of, 538
  optimising cardiac output and, 543
Renal calculi, 540
Renal enlargement, 540
Renal failure
  small kidneys and, 540
  specific treatment of, 543–546
    avoiding administration of nephrotoxins, 543
    correcting underlying conditions, prerenal and/or postrenal factors, 543
    dobutamine, 543–544
    dopamine, 544
    early nutritional support, 545
    electrolytes and acid-base balance, 546
    fenoldopam mesylate, 544
    fluid therapy considerations, 545–546
    loop diuretics, 544
    optimising cardiac output and renal blood flow, 543
    osmotic diuretics, 544
    other options, 544–545
    potential therapies for future, 544
    treating acute complications, 543
Renal function assessment, 536–538
  fractional excretion of electrolytes, 537
  measurement of glomerular filtration rate, 536–537
  measurement of renal blood flow, 538
  urinary enzyme activity, 537–538
Renal insufficiency
  disease states and increased risk of, 533
  drugs increasing risk of, 533–534
  incidence of, 533
  toxic causes of, 534
Renal oedema, 540
Renal papillary necrosis, 539
Renal ultrasound, 538–541
  abnormal kidney, 539–541
    echogenicity, 539–540
    other abnormalities, 541
    size, 540
  image acquisition, 538
  normal kidney, 538–539
Reoperation, orthopaedic implants and, 602
RER. *See* Recurrent exertional rhabdomyolysis; Resting energy requirement
Reserpine
  approximate doses used in equine medicine, 667*t*
  equine sedation and use of, 313*t*, 316
  musculoskeletal conditions and, 316, 317
Resin-impregnated fibreglass, as casting material, 607
Respiratory acidosis, common causes of, in horses, 380 (box 6.4)
Respiratory alkalosis, common causes of, in horses, 381 (box 6.5)
Respiratory conditions
  equine sedation and, 318
  physiotherapy intervention and, 640–641
Respiratory disorders
  management of horses with, 466–480
    bronchoscopic lavage, 471–472
    mechanical ventilation, 473–480
    metered-dose inhalers and nebulisation, 466–470
    oxygen therapy, 470–471
    pleural drainage, 472–473
  patients at risk of developing, during hospitalisation, 457
Respiratory dysfunction, factors contributing to, 640 (box 18.2)
Respiratory endoscopy, 65–66
  equipment needed for, 65 (box 1.33)
  general procedure for, 65–66
  laryngeal functional grading systems, 66 (box 1.36)
  scoring system for tracheal mucus, 66 (box 1.34)
Respiratory function testing, 462–463
  arterial and venous partial pressures of oxygen and carbon dioxide, 462
  blood gas analysis, 462
  blood gas indices, 462
  pulmonary mechanics, 462–463
Respiratory infections
  lower, causes of in adult horse, 337
  simplified guidelines for surveillance of, 181*t*
Respiratory physiotherapy, 640–641
Respiratory rate, normal, in adult horse, 457
Respiratory system
  monitoring, 457–465
    auscultation and rebreathing examination, 457–461
    blood gas collection and analysis, 461–463
    radiography of respiratory tract, 464–465
    ultrasonography of the lungs, 463–464
Respiratory system clinical examination sheet, *213–215*
Respiratory tract, radiography of, 464–465
Respiratory tree, collection of samples from, 458–459
Resterilised intravenous fluid delivery set, indwelling nasogastric tube connected to, *368*
Resting energy requirement
  for foal, 298
  for hospitalised horse, 269
Restraint of neonatal foal, 129–130
  in lateral recumbency, 130
  laying down a foal, 129
  recalcitrant and standing, *129*
  restraint of standing foal, 129
  in sternal recumbency, 130
Retained foetal membranes, 547
Reusable bandages, 105
Reverse-ratio pressure-controlled ventilation, foal ventilated with, *127*
Reynold's number, 418

Rhabdomyolysis
acute
diagnosis of
biochemistry, 587
history, 587
urinalysis, 587
management of, 587–588
clinical signs, 587
monitoring horses with, 588
chronic, 588–591
electrolyte depletion and, 590–591
detection of, 590
dietary analysis, 590
urinary fractional excretions, 591
management of, 587–591
patients at risk of, 574
recurrent exertional
acute management of, 589
clinical signs of, 589
diagnosis of, 589
dietary management, 589
drug therapy for, 589
exercise regimen for, 589
long-term management of, 589
pathogenesis, 588–589
renal insufficiency and, 533
Rhizobium spp., 505
Rhodobacter spheroides, 505
Rhodococcus equi, loop of markedly thickened small intestine in 3-month-old foal with, *496*
Rhodococcus equi abscess, small and large intestine adhered to, in 6-month-old foal, *497*
Rhodococcus equi infection
bilateral nasal oxygen administered to foal with, *63*
nosocomial importance of, 189*t*
Rice bran, nutrient composition of, 265*t*
Rifampicin, equine central nervous system or cerebrospinal fluid and, 567
Rifampin, 338, 349, 396
approximate doses used in equine medicine, 667*t*
Rifamycins, 349
Right dorsal colon, normal, in adult horse, *497*
Ring block, 97
Risk assessment, muck pit management and, 152
RLP. *See* Regional limb perfusion
RM. *See* Recruitment manoeuvres
Robert Jones bandage, 106 (box 1.59)
applying, 107 (box 1.60)
for splinting equine limb, 606–607
Roll cotton, for limb bandaging, 104
Romifidine, 245
approximate doses used in equine medicine, 667*t*
equine sedation and use of, 312, 313, 313*t*
respiratory conditions and use of, 318
total intravenous anaesthesia and, 252
Roof height, in equine hospital, 157
Ropivacaine, epidural analgesia and anaesthesia for visceral pain and, 329
Rossdale and Partners Hospital, Newmarket, UK
architectural plan for ground floor level of, *155*
arrangements for separating mares and foals during treatment of foal at, *151*
Ross Laboratories, osmolyte solutions produced by, 278, 278*t*
Rostral maxillary sinus, as site for sinocentesis, 78
Rotavirus infection, nosocomial importance of, 189*t*
Royal College of Veterinary Surgeons, 147
Royal Liverpool Children's Hospital (Alder Hey) Enquiry, 200
Royal Veterinary College, London
arrangements for separating mares and foals during treatment of foal at, *151*
Masters in Veterinary Physiotherapy programme at, 638
RR interval
analysis of electrocardiographic recording and, 422
uniform ventricular tachycardia and, *423*

S
SAA. *See* Serum amyloid A
Sacral reflex stretch, 645
Sacrocaudalis dorsalis medialis (tail head muscle), surgical biopsy from, 112
Sacroiliac problems, physiotherapy and, 641–642
Saddle-fitting problems, assessing, 643
Safety testing, radiation safety and, 176
Sagittal ratio measurements, on cervical radiographs, *559*
Salbutamol, 468, 469
approximate doses used in equine medicine, 667*t*
Salbuterol, 244
Saline
hypertonic, 374
normal, 372–373
Salmeterol, 468
Salmonella
environmental samples for detection of, and culturing using WHO/ISO technique, 192*n*
routine surveillance focused on, 185
shedding
animals with increased rates of, 194
risk factors associated with, amongst hospitalised horses, 486 (box 11.1)
Salmonella spp., 277, 337
critical care stall disinfection and, 150
isolation of, from septic arthritis in foals, 580
small colon impaction and, 486
Salmonellosis
biosecurity and, 182
nosocomial importance of, 189*t*
Salpingopharyngeal fold, opening, biopsy forceps used to allow entry of endoscopy into guttural pouch, *67*
Sand colic, 487
Sandhoff's disease, 568
Sarcoid removal, horse's ear bandaged after, *112*
Scanner, equine magnetic resonance imaging and, 173–174
Scapulohumeral (shoulder) joint, synoviocentesis of, 579
Scintigraphic examination
room for, 170
time required for, 169
Scintigraphy, 169–170
implant evaluation with, 593–594
sedation and, 179
software, 179
suppliers, 176 (box 3.3)
Scone Veterinary Hospital, Scone, NSW, Australia, arrangements for separating mares and foals during treatment of foal at, *151*
Scope size, for gastroscopy and endoscopy, 180
Scrotum, examining, 543
Scrub up and surgical trolley laying-up room, at equine hospital, 157
Secondary dressing, bandages and, 103, *103*
Secondary hyperalgesia, 331–332
Secondary infusion, for pumps and drivers, 39
Security
hospital grounds, 148
reception area, in hospital, 153

Sedation
preanaesthetic, 237–238
standing, 312–320
Sedatives, for standing sedation, 312–314
Sediment examination, after urine collection, 536
Seizures, 564–566
acute, treatment of, 565–566
causes of, in neonatal foal, 564 (box 14.4)
causes of, in older foal and adult horse, 564 (box 14.5)
fundamental objectives in treatment of, 564–565
long-term treatment for, 566
padded head covers used for horses with, 562
treatment goals for, in horses, 565*t*
Seldinger catheters, 43, 44
Selenium (Na Selenite), approximate doses used in equine medicine, 667*t*
Semimembranosis, surgical biopsy and, 112, 113
Seminar rooms
digital projector in, at hospital, 162, *162*
at equine hospital, 161–162
Semiocclusive nonadherent dressings, 104
Semitendinosis, surgical biopsy and, 112, 113
Sepsis
common metabolic effect of, 265
treatments for, 503–504
Septicaemia
bacterial, morbidity and mortality related to, 337
sources of bacteria in, 573 (box 15.2)
Septic arthritis, patients at risk of, 573–574
Septic cholangiohepatitis, 498, 524
Septic navicular bursitis, *615*
Septic osteitis, of coffin bone, *615*
Septic patients, corticosteroids and, 451, 452
Septic pericarditis
horses with, 427
pericardial effusion from foal with, *420*
Septic peritonitis, 493
Septic shock, high heart rate and, 431
Septic tarsal sheath, preepidural and 12-hour postepidural morphine in horse with, *331*
Septic thromboembolism, 396
Septic tracheal aspirate cytology, degenerate neutrophils and mucus in, *459*
Serine, 632
Serratia spp., possible outbreaks of infections caused by, 182
Serum amyloid A, 394
Serum biochemical evaluation, of hepatic function, 522–523
Serum biochemistry profile, 263
Serum phosphate concentrations
in horses with colic (SI units), 493*t*
in horses with colic (U.S. units), 493*t*
Serum urea nitrogen, 265
Sevoflurane, 241
maintenance of anaesthesia and use of, 240
summary of subjective differences in clinical signs of anaesthesia in adult horses under halothane, isoflurane and, 241*t*
S_4 heart sound, 418
Shape, murmurs and, 418–419
"Shock Dose" method, reversal of hypovolaemia and, 378
Short-acting β_2-agonists, 468, 469
"Sigh" manoeuvre, 478
Signage
about delivery protocol, at equine hospital, 149, *149*
for reception area in hospital, 153
for x-ray rooms, 177
Silastic fenestrated drain tubes, 618
Sildenafil, approximate doses used in equine medicine, 667*t*
Silicone abdominal drains, peritoneal lavage and, 18
Silvadene, 620
Silver sulfadiazine, 632
Simple continuous suture pattern, *116*
technique, advantages/disadvantages with, 116
Simple interrupted suture pattern, *115*
advantages/disadvantages with, 116
technique for, 115–116
SIMV. *See* Synchronised intermittent mandatory ventilation
SIMV-PS. *See* Synchronised intermittent mandatory ventilation with pressure support
Sinks, ultrasonography and use of, 170
Sinocentesis, 77–78
equipment needed for, 78 (box 1.43)
left frontal sinus, *78*
maxillary sinus, *78*
sites for, 78
technique, 78
Sinuses
facial, location of, *12*
left frontal, *78*
maxillary, *78*
Sinus procedures, anaesthesia and, 251–252
SIRS. *See* Systemic inflammatory response syndrome
Siting, for equine hospital, 147–148
Skin, common fungal pathogens at, 352*t*
Skin closure, suture materials and suture patterns for, 114–119
Skin flap meshing, 616
"Skin-flick" response, panniculus reflex and, 558
Skin grafts, 623–627
advantages and disadvantages with different techniques for, 624 (box 16.1)
pinch grafts, 624 (box 16.1), 625, *625*
preparing to graft, 624
recipient site and donor site, 624
punch grafts, 624–625, 624 (box 16.1), *625*
tunnel grafts, 624 (box 16.1), 626–627, *627*
Skin staples, *119*
technique, advantages/disadvantages with, 119
Skin ulcers, recumbency and development of, 563
Sleeve cast, 607 (box 15.10)
Slings
for horses with neurological disease, 562
priapism and use of, 548
Small colon, abnormalities of, 490
Small intestinal volvulus, multiple loops of moderately distended, amotile small intestine in horse with ileus 1 day after surgery for, *495*
Small intestine
abnormal findings in, 489
distended loop of, adjacent to spleen in horse after resection and anastomosis of jejunum, *495*
ultrasonography of, 494–495
Sodium, electrolyte imbalances and, 382
Sodium bicarbonate, 373–374
approximate doses used in equine medicine, 667*t*
Sodium concentrations, guide to interpretation of, 677 (box 19.22)
Sodium disturbances, treatment of, 382
Sodium iodide (20% solution), approximate doses used in equine medicine, 667*t*
Sodium thiosulphate, approximate doses used in equine medicine, 667*t*
Soft helmet, for protecting horse's head during recovery from general anaesthesia, *110*
Soft tissue injuries
physiotherapy intervention and, 639 (box 18.1)
tendon and ligament injuries, 642–643
wounds, nonhealing and acute, 642

Sole of hoof, puncture wounds to, 617
Somatic pain, 330–332
  epidural analgesia for, 331–332
S_1 heart sound, 418
Soy oil, 279
Spacer devices, use of, with metered-dose inhalers, *467*, 468
Spasticity, 559
Specialist examination forms, 225
Specific gravity, urine, 535
Spermatic cord, examining, 543
Speticaemia, simplified guidelines for surveillance of, 181*t*
Spinal fluid collection, lumbosacral, 79–80
Spinal pain and stiffness, physiotherapy and, 641
Spirochetes, suggested choices of antimicrobial agents for common bacterial pathogens in horses and, 339t
SPL catheter, 630
Splint application, 106–107
  equipment needed for, 106, 106 (box 1.59)
  for fore limb: region 1, 106, *107*
  for fore limb: region 2, 106, *108*
  for fore limb: region 3, 107, *108*
  for fore limb: region 4, 107
  for hind limb: region 5, 107
  for hind limb: region 6, 107
  for hind limb: region 7, 107, *109*
  for hind limb: region 8, 107
Splinting, 605–607
  of equine limb
    biomechanically important regions for, 606
    materials for, 606
    Robert Jones bandage, 606–607
    treatment and transportation, 607
Splints, 105
  general principles for application of, 606
  for traumatic wounds, 617
SPL system. *See* Subpalpebral lavage system
Spontaneous period duration
  improving ventilator-patient synchrony and, 127 (box 2.7)
  synchronised intermittent mandatory ventilation with pressure support mode and, 126 (box 2.5)
Spontaneous ventilation, large-animal anaesthesia machine designed for use with, *230*
Sporothrix schenckii, 351
Square knot, 114, *114*
SSIs. *See* Surgical site infections
Stable confinement, large colon impactions and, 484–485
Stable environment, for horses with neurological disorders, 562
Stabling facilities, at equine hospital, 149–150, 152
Staff facilities, at equine hospital, 161
Staff training, radiation safety and, 177–178, 178 (box 3.5)
Stall confinement, equine sedation and, 316
Stallion catheters, enteral feeding of critically ill foal and, 303
Stalls, at equine hospital, 149–150, 152
Standing chemical restraint, common equine sedatives used for, 313*t*
Standing sedation, 312–320
  anaesthesia and, 253–254
  clinical applications, 316–320
    cardiac conditions, 318–319
    conditions of head and neck, 317
    gastrointestinal disorders, 319
    hepatic and urogenital conditions, 319–320
    musculoskeletal conditions, 316–317
    neurological diseases, 317–318
    respiratory conditions, 318
  neonatal foals, 320
  opioids, 314–315
  other sedatives, tranquilisers and hypnotics, 315–316
  phenothiazines, 314
  tranquilisers, sedatives and hypnotics, 312–314
Stanozolol, approximate doses used in equine medicine, 667*t*
Staphylococcosis, nosocomial importance of, 190*t*
Staphylococcus aureus, 185, 566
  biosecurity and, 182
Staphylococcus zooepidemicus, 337
Staples, skin, 119
Static neck stretch, *645*
Steinmann pin, sinocentesis and use of, 78
Stent bandages
  for head wounds, 112
  for surgical wounds, 617
  for traumatic wounds, 618
Stents, vertical mattress suture pattern with, *117*
Sterile gel, for wound coverage, *612*
Sternal recumbency
  horse in, during recovery, *246*
  intubation done with horse in, 239, *240*
  restraint of foal in, 130
Stethoscope, physical examination of adult horse and, 7
S_3 heart sound, 418
Stick, John, 281
Stilbestrol, approximate doses used in equine medicine, 667*t*
Stockinets, 608
  for bandaging of head, 110
"Stocking up"
  confinement and, 574
  reduction of, 101
Stocks
  CSF collection and restraint of horses in, 79
  in equine hospitals, 163
  for radiography room, at hospital, 165
  ultrasonography and use of, 170
Stomach
  abnormal findings in, 489
  anatomy of, and path along which gastroscope should be passed for imaging purposes, *22*
  decompression of, and treatment of ileus, 499–500
  endoscopic view of lesser curvature, cardia, and pyloric antrum of, *23*
  enlarged, transabdominal ultrasound image of, in 4-month-old foal with duodenal stricture, *495*
  ultrasonography of, 494
Stopcock, three-way, in pressure transducer, 46
Storage, general anaesthesia and, 228
Storage area, for radiography room, at hospital, 166, *166*
Strangles, nosocomial importance of, 190*t*
Strangulated small intestine, ultrasonography of, 495
Streptococcus bovis, 277
Streptococcus equi, outbreaks of strangles caused by, 182
Streptococcus equi equi, 394
  emergency tracheotomy and, 60
Streptococcus equi subspecies *equi*, 337
Streptococcus zooepidemicus, 566
Streptomycin, 344
Stretches, 638, 642*t*, 645
Stroke volume, 435
  pulse contour analysis and calculation of, from arterial waveform, 57
Structural carbohydrates, 273
S_2 heart sound, 418
Subchondral bone disease, computed tomography and evaluation of, 172
Subcutaneous emphysema, 458
Subcutaneous tissues/cellulitis, common fungal pathogens at, 352*t*
Subcuticular suture pattern
  suture extended, *115*
  technique, advantages, 115

Subcuticular suture pattern *(Continued)*
  tying final knot, *115*
  tying first knot, *115*
Subpalpebral lavage catheter, 630
  placement of, 93–96
    equipment needed for, 93, 95 (box 1.55)
    indications for, 93
    in lower eyelid, *94*
    parts of commercial subpalpebral lavage catheter kit, *94*
    passing trochar through upper eyelid, *96*
    procedure for, 95–96
    site for, 93–95
    in upper eyelid, *94*
Subpalpebral lavage system, 93
Suckling reflex
  bucket or pan feeding for foals and, 301
  enteral feeding for clinically ill foals and, 304
  placement of indwelling nasogastric tube in foal and, 132
Sucralfate, approximate doses used in equine medicine, 667*t*
Suction pumps, for evacuating gastric fluid, 22
Sudden death, rider injury and, 436
Sulphadiazine, 348
  approximate doses used in equine medicine, 667*t*
SUN. *See* Serum urea nitrogen
Superficial and deep fibular nerves (peroneal) block, equipment for, 97 (box 1.56)
Superficial digital flexor, low four-point nerve block and, *98*
Superficial fibular nerves, 100
Supplemental nutrition
  categories of foals and, 298
  selecting form of, for hospitalised adult horse, 275–276
    assisted enteral feeding, 275–276
    enteral *versus* parenteral therapy, 275
    parenteral nutrition, 276
Supplemental nutrition for hospitalised foals, selecting form of: enteral *versus* parenteral therapy, 299–300
Suppliers, of imaging equipment, 176 (box 3.3)
Support-limb laminitis
  lesions predisposing horses to, 572
  treatment of, 583–584
Supraorbital block
  for placement of subpalpebral lavage catheter, 95
  in regional anaesthesia of eye, 93
Supraorbital nerves, anatomy of, *92*
Suprascapular nerve injury, muscle stimulation for treatment of, *639*
Supraventricular premature depolarisation, 424
Supraventricular premature depolarisations, 440
Supraventricular tachycardias, 40
Supraventricular tachydysrhythmias, 440–442
Surgeon's knot, 114, *114*
Surgery
  common indications for, in equine neonates, 246
  gastrointestinal problems associated with, 485
  interpretation of peritoneal fluid and, 492
  postoperative ileus and, 484
Surgery report form, *224*
Surgery table
  designed as part of induction/recovery floor, *227*
  fastening to wall beneath the wall/door of the induction/recovery stall in a transitional room between induction/recovery and the OR, *227*
Surgical biopsy
  for muscle biopsy, 113–114
  from *sacrocaudalis dorsalis medialis* muscle, *113*
  site for, of gluteal muscle, *113*
Surgical colic patients
  determination of medical colic *versus*, 492–493
  immediate treatment of, after surgery, 509–510
  monitoring, 510–511
    of fluid status, 511
    of nasogastric intubation, 511
Surgical facilities, at equine hospital, 154–158
Surgical gloves, examination per rectum and use of, 9
Surgical incisions
  monitoring, 596–597
  ultrasonography of, 597–598
Surgical instruments, storage of, at equine hospital, 158
Surgically-induced profuse bleeding, coagulopathies due to, 405
Surgical site infections
  clinical signs of, *596*
  management of, 598–604
    investigating and monitoring nosocomial infections, 599
    laparotomy wounds, 599–601
    orthopaedic implants, 601–602
  simplified guidelines for surveillance of, 181*t*
Surgical tables, positioning and padding of, 228
Surgical wound management, in colic patients, 514–515
Surgical wounds, 609
  bandaging of, 617
  categories of, based on National Research Council Operative Classification, 609*t*
  drains used in, 618–619
Surveillance
  environmental, infection control and, 192
  patient, infection control and, 185, 192
Suscepitibility testing, bacteria and, 338
Susceptibility tests
  antifungal, 352
  interpretation of, and correlation with clinical outocmes, 339–341
  in vitro, 339
Suspensory ligament, low four-point nerve block and, *98*
Suture materials, for skin closure, 114
Suture patterns, 115–119
  continuous interlocking, technique, advantages/disadvantages with, 119
  corner suture, technique and advantages with, 117
  cruciate
    disadvantage with, 119
    technique for, 117
  horizontal mattress, technique, advantages/disadvantages with, 117
  placement of over-the-needle catheter in jugular catheterisation and, 29
  simple continuous, technique, advantages/disadvantages with, 116
  simple interrupted
    advantages with, 116
    technique for, 115–116
  skin staples, technique, advantages/disadvantages with, 119
  subcuticular, technique and advantages with, 115
  vertical mattress, technique, advantages/disadvantages with, 116
Suture placement, for skin closure, 114
Suxibuzone, endotoxaemia treatment and, 506
SV. *See* Stroke volume
SVPDs. *See* Supraventricular premature depolarisations
SVR. *See* Systemic vascular resistance
SVTs. *See* Supraventricular tachycardias
Swallowing
  abnormalities in, 563–564
  evaluating, 558
Swallowing reflex, placement of indwelling nasogastric tube in foal and, 132
Swamp fever, nosocomial importance of, 187*t*
Sway test, 558
Swimming
  contraindications for, 651

indications for, 650
physiological effects of, 650–651
safety rules for, 651
Synchronised intermittent mandatory ventilation, 476, 477
Synchronised intermittent mandatory ventilation with pressure support, ventilation in foal and, 126
Syncope, rider injury and, 436
Synovial fluid analysis, 579–580
bacteriology, 580
cytology, 579
Synovial fluid cytology, normal, and values for common clinical conditions, 684*t*
Synovial structure, wound management and involvement of, 615–616
Synoviocentesis ("joint tap"), 575, 576
of bursae, 579
carpal joints and approaches to, 578, *578*
coffin joint approached for, *576*
of coxofemoral (hip) joint, 579
of digital sheath, 579
of distal interphalangeal (coffin joint), 576
equipment for, 576 (box 15.3)
of femoropatellar joint, 579
of femorotibial (stifle) joint, 579
fetlock joint and approaches to, for, 577, *577*
of humoradial (elbow) joint, 579
pastern joint and approaches to, for, 577, *577*
of scapulohumeral (shoulder) joint, 579
tarsal joints and approaches to, *578*, 578–579
Syringe drivers, *38–39*
advanced operation of, 39
advantages with, 38
alarms for, 39
designs for, 38
operation of, 39
Systemic analgesics, use of, 324*t*
Systemic blood pressure, anaesthesia and, monitoring in foal, 248
Systemic inflammatory response syndrome, 432, 435
laminitis and, 572
renal insufficiency and, 533
treatments for, 503–504
Systemic vascular resistance, 435
pulse contour analysis and, 57
vasoactive therapy and, 447
Systole, 418
Systolic blood pressure, optimal accuracy of, 45

T
Tachypnoea, common causes of, 381 (box 6.5)
Tail evaluation, 558
Tail head muscle, surgical biopsy of, 113
"Tail-pull" test, 558, 559
Talampicillin, 343
Tamm-Horsfall glycoprotein, urinary casts and, 536
Tapotage, 640
Tarsal bandage, application of, to control moisture and provide wound edge immobilisation of tarsal wound, *104*
Tarsal joints, approaches to, for synoviocentesis, *578*, 578–579
Tarsal wound, tarsal bandage applied to control moisture and provide wound edge immobilisation of, *104*
Tarsometatarsal joints, approaching for synoviocentesis, *578*, 578–579
Tarsorrhaphy, temporary, placement of, 634
TAT complexes, 406
Tc. *See* Technetium
Tc-DTPA. *See* Technetium-diethyletneaminopentacetic acid
Tc-HDP. *See* Technetium-labeled methylene diphosphonate
TDM. *See* Therapeutic drug monitoring
Teat cannula
for abdominocentesis, 17, *17*
pleurocentesis and, *73*
Technetium, 169, 178, 179
Technetium-diethyletneaminopentacetic acid, glomerular filtration rate measurement and, 536
Technetium-labeled methylene diphosphonate, scintigraphy to monitor implants and, 593
Telemetric electrocardiograms, 51
Telemetric electrocardiography, 421
Telemetry, pericardiocentesis and, 58
Telephone system, for reception area in hospital, 153
Temperature, pulse rate, respiratory rate values, monitoring during PN therapy, 294
Temperature control, in MRI rooms, 174
Temperature therapy, effects of, 649*t*
Template bleeding time, 406
Tendon injuries, physiotherapy and, 642–643
TENS. *See* Transcutaneous electrical nerve stimulation
Tension relieving suture patterns, 616
Tension-relieving sutures (quill technique), in wound management, *612*
Terbutaline, approximate doses used in equine medicine, 667*t*
Terlipressin, tissue perfusion improvement and, 450
Tesarowski, D., 468
Testicles, examining, 543
Testosterone (aqueous), approximate doses used in equine medicine, 667*t*
Tetanus antitoxin, approximate doses used in equine medicine, 667*t*
Tetracyclines, 338, 347–348
TG. *See* Triglycerides
Theophylline, approximate doses used in equine medicine, 667*t*
Therapeutic diets, 261
metabolic profile and, 263
protein in, 271
Therapeutic drug monitoring, aminoglycosides and, 345
Therapeutic nutrition
initiating, in hospitalised adult horse, 267, 269
cafeteria feeding, 267
intravenous dextrose, 267, 269
Therapeutic ultrasound, 638
indications for use, physiological effects, and contraindications or precautions, 646*t*
Thermal therapy, 638, 644 (box 18.5), 648–649
cryotherapy, 648–649
heat therapy, 649
Thiabendazole, approximate doses used in equine medicine, 667*t*
Thiamine deficiency, in hospitalised adult horse, 266
Thiamine HCl, approximate doses used in equine medicine, 667*t*
Thiol, 632
Thiopental, 239
approximate doses used in equine medicine, 668*t*
total intravenous anaesthesia and use of, 253
Thoracic catheter
aspiration from, *76*
trocar removed from, *76*
Thoracic compressions
ideal rate for, in adult horse, 6–7
in neonatal foal, *124*
number per minute, for neonatal foal, 123
stopping, in neonatal foal, 124
Thoracic drains, peritoneal lavage and, 18
Thoracic physical therapy, contraindications to, 641 (box 18.3)
Thoracic radiography, 464
Thoracic trocar catheter, insertion of, for evacuation of pneumothorax, *76*
Thoracic trochars, for percutaneous puncture, 19
Thoracic ultrasonography, indications for, 463

Thoracic ultrasound, at junction between dorsal surface of lung and air in pleural space, *75*
Thoracic visceral pain, 329
Thoracocentesis, sedation for, 318
Thorax
  auscultation of, 8
  extensive wound involving entire lateral aspect of, *614*
Thoroscopy, sedation for, 318
Thoroughbred horses, recurrent exertional rhabdomyolysis in, 588–589
Thoroughbred mare, oesophagostomy tube in, *281*
Three-loop pulley, tendon involvement in wounds and, 616
Three-way stopcock, pleurocentesis with use of, *73*
Thrombin time, 405
Thrombocytopenia, 404
  iatrogenic causes of, 405 (box 8.5)
Thromboelastography, 407
Thrombophlebitis
  after catheterisation, 394
  catheter care and monitoring neonatal foals for, 137
  catheterisation of cephalic and lateral thoracic veins and risk of, 30
  factors reported to be associated with, 403 (box 8.4)
  in hospitalised equine patients, 395–397
    diagnosis of, 396
    prevention of, 397
    treatment of, 396–397
  jugular, in site of previous indwelling intravenous catheter in a foal, *396*
  medical colic patients and, 509
  parenteral formulas, catheterisation of both jugular veins and risk of, 293
  patients at risk of, 574
Thrombosed medial plantar artery, ultrasonographic image of, *574*
Thrombosis, 401
  of limb arteries, 404
Thromboxanes, 512
Thyroid shields, 167
  correctly stored, *166*
Thyroxine L, approximate doses used in equine medicine, 668*t*
Tibial and fibular (peroneal) block, 100
Tibial nerve, 100
Tibial nerve block, *101*
  equipment for, 97 (box 1.56)
Tibiotarsal joints, approaching for synoviocentesis, *578*, 578–579
Ticarcillin, 343
  approximate doses used in equine medicine, 668*t*
Ticarcillin-clavulanic acid, approximate doses used in equine medicine, 668*t*
Tidal volume, 478
Time triggering, 476
Timing, murmurs and, 418
Timothy hay, nutrient composition of, 265*t*
TIMPs. *See* Tissue inhibitors of metalloproteinases
Tinidazole, 348
  approximate doses used in equine medicine, 668*t*
Tissue inhibitors of metalloproteinases, 527
Tissue perfusion
  monitoring, 430–433
    arterial blood pressure, 432–433
    lactate, 432
    physical examination, 430–431
    pulse oximetry, 433
    urine output, 431–432
  treatments aimed at improving, 446–447, 449–451
    early aggressive fluid resuscitation, 446–447
    inotropes, 447, 449
    vasoactive therapy, 447
    vasopressorrs, 449–451
TIVA. *See* Total intravenous anaesthesia
TNCC. *See* Total nucleated cell count
Tocopherol acetate, approximate doses used in equine medicine, 668*t*
Tolazoline, approximate doses used in equine medicine, 668*t*
Tongue depressors
  nasal oxygen catheter taped to, *63*
  placing indwelling nasogastric tube in foal and, 131, *131*, 132
Tongue tone, 558
Topical antimicrobial treatments, for wounds, 620
Topical medications, for corneal ulcers, 631
Topical treatments and dressings
  types of, used for treatment of equine wounds, 619
  wound management and, 619–622
Total intravenous anaesthesia, 235, 252–253
  positioning during lateral recumbency and, *253*
Total nucleated cell count, 493
Total nutrient admixture parenteral nutrition formulations, 284
  containers for, 290–291
Total nutrient admixture parenteral nutrition worksheet, 286 (box 5.16)
Total parenteral nutrition, 284
Total parenteral nutrition worksheet example, 287 (box 5.17)
Total protein concentrations, guide to interpretation of, 673 (box 19.4)
Total solids, hypovolaemia and, 365–366
Tourniquet
  application of, 107–108
  complications with application of, 109
  equipment for application of, 109 (box 1.61)
  successful perfusions and placement of, 351
t-PA, 406
TPN. *See* Total parenteral nutrition
TPR values. *See* Temperature, pulse rate, respiratory rate values
Trace mineral analysis, in hospitalised adult horse, 266–267
Trace mineral supplementation, 274
  in parenteral nutrition, 289
Trachea
  endoscopy of, in horse following laryngoplasty, *594*
  identifying, 60
    for respiratory endoscopy, 65
Tracheal aspirate, 458
  interpretation of tracheal aspirate cytology, 458–459
Tracheal aspirate cytology, normal, *459*
Tracheal aspiration, 68–70
  aspiration of instilled fluid from trachea via aspiration catheter, *70*
  equipment needed for, 69 (box 1.38)
  insertion of introducer needle through skin and tracheal wall, *70*
  methods for, 68
  percutaneous technique (transtracheal aspirate), 69–70
  polypropelene catheter slowly advanced and withdrawn during, *70*
  stylet introduced in mid-cervical region, just above strap muscles, *69*
  transendoscopic technique, 68–69
Tracheal mucus, scoring system for, 66 (box 1.34)
Tracheal rings, *61*
Tracheotomy
  emergency, 60–61
  site for and incisions for, *61*
Training, radiation safety and, 176–177
Tranexamic acid
  approximate doses used in equine medicine, 668*t*
  hypocoagulable states in horses managed with, 411
Tranquilisers, for standing sedation, 312–314
Transabdominal ultrasonographic images
  of enlarged left kidney showing acute renal failure, *541*
  of enlarged right kidney showing acute renal failure, *541*
  of hypoechoic renal cyst in left kidney, *540*
  of normal left kidney in a weanling, *539*
  of normal right kidney, *539*

of right kidney from horse with chronic renal failure, *540*
of right kidney from 19-year-old "Teaser" with chronic renal failure, *539*
Transabdominal ultrasonography, liver biopsy guided by, 523
Transabdominal ultrasound, percutaneous trocharisation and use of, 25
Transcutaneous electrical nerve stimulation, 647–648
"burst," 647, 648
conventional, 647, 648
indications for use, physiological effects, and contraindications or precautions, 646*t*
Transducers, ultrasound, 170
types and frequencies recommended for common applications in horses, 171 (box 3.2)
Transendoscopic technique, for tracheal aspiration, 68–69
Transfusion reactions, 41, 376
Transfusions, blood and plasma, 40–42
Transpalpebral ultrasound image, of right eye of mare with chronic uveitis, *635*
Transpleural pressure, 462
Transtracheal aspirate, 458
Transtracheal fluid analysis, normal values for transtracheal aspirate, 681*t*
Transvenous cardioversion, 442
Transverse facial artery, palpating, *43*
Traumatic wound management, schematic outline for, *610*
Traumatic wounds, 609
bandaging of, 617–618
correct placement of latex Penrose drain in, *619*
drains used in, 618–619
Treadmills, in equine hospitals, 164
Treatment ordering form, for hospitalised patients, *208*
Trendelenburg position, 157
Triamcinolone, approximate doses used in equine medicine, 668*t*
Triazoles, 353
Trichlormethiazide, approximate doses used in equine medicine, 668*t*
Trichlorphon, approximate doses used in equine medicine, 668*t*
Tricuspid valve, 418
Trigeminal nerve, blocks of ophthalmic branches of, 92–93
Trigger point therapy, 642*t*, 645
Triglycerides, 265
Trimethoprim, 338
Trimethroprim-sulphonamide (TMS) combination, 348
approximate doses used in equine medicine, 668*t*
Tripelennamine, approximate doses used in equine medicine, 668*t*
Triple-lumen catheters, parenteral nutrition treatment and use of, 293, *293*
Triple-lumen guarded catheter, tracheal aspirate collection and, 458
Trochar, passage of, through upper eyelid, *96*
Trochlear nerve, testing, 558
Troponin I, biochemical monitoring of muscles and, 585, 586
Trotting, access to soft surface for, at equine hospital, 152
TT. *See* Thrombin time
Tuber coxae, needle biopsy and, 113
Tuber sacrale, asymmetry of, *642*
Tulathromycin, approximate doses used in equine medicine, 668*t*
Tunnel block, *168*, 168–169
Tunnel grafts
advantages and disadvantages with, 624 (box 16.1)
granulation tissue removed after graft has taken, *627*
procedure for, 626–627
technique for placement of, *626*
T wave
in base-apex ECG, *50*
normal variations in, in base-apex ECG, *51*
12-hour postepidural morphine, in horse with septic tarsal sheath, *331*
20F Argyle chest tube, insertion of, in fifth ICS, to drain pericardial effusion, *60*
24-hour ambulatory (Holter) monitors, 51
Two-lead arthroscopic irrigation set, lavage performed with, 20
TX. *See* Thromboxanes
Tying up (rhabdomyolysis), patients at risk of, 574
Tyzzer's disease, 527

U
U.K. National Health Service guidelines, consent forms, 200
Ulnar nerve block
for analgesia of distal antebrachium and carpus, 98, 100
equipment for, 97 (box 1.56)
Ultrasonic nebulisers, 64, 362, 467
facemask connected to, *467*
Ultrasonograms
of bladder apex and left umbilical artery, *146*
of infected umbilical artery, *146*
of infected umbilical vein, *146*
of internal umbilical vein, *146*
of internal umbilicus, *146*
Ultrasonographic images
longitudinal, of plantar aspect of hind limb in horse following neurectomy of deep branch of lateral plantar nerve, *598*
longitudinal, of ventral midline incision in horse after abdominal surgery, *598*
of thrombosed medial plantar artery, *574*
Ultrasonography, 170, 597–598
determining site for abdominocentesis and, 17
of female genital tract, 542
implant evaluation with, 593
of liver, 523–524
of scrotum and testicles, 543
of surgical incisions, 597–598
equipment, 597
images obtained, 598
Ultrasonography of gastrointestinal system, 494–498
abscesses, 497–498
caecum and colon, 496–497
small intestine, 494–496
stomach, 494
Ultrasonography of lungs, 463–464
interpretation of, 463–464
procedure for, 463
Ultrasonography of umbilicus, 144–146
equipment needed for, 144–145, 145 (box 2.14)
indication for, 144
ultrasonographic examination, 145–146
Ultrasonography suppliers, 176 (box 3.3)
Ultrasound
of bladder, 541
of peritoneal fluid, *17*
renal, 538–541
wall thickness and diameter of sections of intestines, as measured by, 495*t*
Ultrasound guidance, liver biopsy with, 27
Ultrasound machines, imaging umbilical structures of foal with, 144
Ultrasound therapy, 646–647
Umbilical arteries
diameter of, 146
infected, ultrasonogram of, *146*
right and left, 145
ultrasonogram of left artery, *146*
Umbilical structures, of foal, anatomy of, *145*
Umbilical stump, 145, 146
Umbilicus, ultrasonography of, 144–146
Unguided (BAL catheter) technique, for bronchoalveolar lavage, 71
Unilateral pneumothorax, in a horse, *466*
University of Liverpool Equine Hospital, consent form for, *201*

University of Queensland, Australia, Masters in Animal Studies programme at, 638
Unwillingness to drink, by hospitalised horse, 398–399
Upper-airway obstructions, tracheotomies performed for, 60–61
Upper limb wounds, 613–614
Upper respiratory tract, endoscopy of, showing loss of abduction of left arytenoid cartilage following laryngoplasty, *594*
Upstream occlusion, between bags and pumps, alarms and, 39
Urachus, 145, *146*
Urea concentrations, guide to interpretation of, 677 (box 19.23)
Ureteritis, 547
Ureters, endoscopy of, 86
Urethral catheterisation, urinary tract infections and, 534
Urinalysis, 534–536
  acute rhabdomyolysis and, 587
  general appearance, 534
  guide to interpretation of, 683 (box 19.25)
  reagent strips, 535
    bilirubin, 536
    glucose, 535
    ketones, 535
    occult blood, 535
    pH, 535
    protein, 535
  sediment examination, 536
    bacteria, 536
    casts, 536
    crystals, 536
    epithelial cells, 536
    leucocytes, 536
    mucus, 536
    red blood cells, 536
  specific gravity, 535
  urine output, 534–535
Urinary casts, 536
Urinary catheterisation, 84–85
  ascending infection and, 432
  of female
    equipment needed for, 85 (box 1.48)
    procedure for, 85
  of male
    equipment needed for, 85 (box 1.47)
    procedure for, 84–85
Urinary catheter placement in foal, 141–144
  checking and connecting catheter, 144
  equipment for, 142 (box 2.13)
  female foal, 143–144
  functions served by, 141
  male foal, 142–143
Urinary enzyme activity, 537–538
Urinary fractional excretions, chronic rhabdomyolysis and, 590, 591
Urinary GGT: creatinine ratio, 538
  equation for calculation of, 538 (box 13.4)
Urinary tract, endoscopy of, 541
Urinary tract infections, 534, 546–547
  cystitis, 546–547
  pyelonephritis and ureteritis, 547
  simplified guidelines for surveillance of, 181*t*
Urine, radioactive, avoiding spread of, 179
Urine and urine production, normal values for, 682, 683*t*
Urine collection, 534
Urine collection bags, commercially available, 535
Urine concentration, description of, 535 (box 13.1)
Urine glucose, monitoring, in hospitalised foal, 309
Urine output, end-organ perfusion and, 431, 453
Urine specific gravity, 535
  dehydration and, 366
Urogenital conditions, equine sedation and, 319–320
Urogenital system
  monitoring, 533–543
  treating, 543–548
Urolithiasis, 534, 547
Uroliths, 488
Uterine biopsy instrument, holding for introduction into rectum, *26*
Uterine horns, ultrasonography of, 542
Uterine lavage, 87–88, 542, 547
  equipment needed for, 88 (box 1.51)
  fluid poured into uterus via stomach tube and funnel, *88*
  procedure for, 87–88
    obtaining cellular material, 87
    for uterine cleansing, 88
Uterine pain, 328, 329
Uterine swab, 542
  lost, 548
Uterine torsion, 490
UTIs. *See* Urinary tract infections
Uveitis
  bilateral, right eye of 6-year-old Paint mare with, *635*
  chronic, in left eye of 12-year-old Appaloosa mare, *635*
  chronic, transpalpebral ultrasound image of right eye of mare with, *635*
  management of horses with, 635–636

V
Vacutainer, collection of blood and injection from jugular vein and, 11, *12*
Vacuum-assisted closure, for management of extensive laceration in cervical region of horse, 614
Vaginal delivery of foal, reasonable anaesthetic protocol for mares during, 250 (box 4.3)
Vaginal examination, 541–542
Vaginal technique, for endometrial biopsy, 87
Valacyclovir, approximate doses used in equine medicine, 668*t*
Valved facemask
  for delivery of aerosolised medications, with spacer for delivering drugs by metered-dose inhaler, *467*
  nebulisation and use of, 64
  nebulisation of foal with, *64*
Valvular lesions, 424–426
Vancomycin, approximate doses used in equine medicine, 668*t*
Vancomycin-resistant *Enterococcus*, 185
VAP. *See* Ventilator-associated pneumonia
Vaporiser cleaning, 231
Vaporiser settings, for induction in foals, 246
Vascular catheter infections, simplified guidelines for surveillance of, 181*t*
Vascular endothelial growth factor, wound healing and, 620
Vasculitis, 404
Vasoactive therapy, 447
Vasopressin
  guideline for diluting and preparation of, 449*t*
  tissue perfusion improvement and, 450
Vasopressors, 449–451
  choice of, 451
  dopamine, 451
  epinephrine, 450–451
  guideline for diluting and preparation of, 449*t*
  norepinephrine, 449–450
  vasopressin and terlipressin, 450
V-block, *168*
Vedaprofen
  approximate doses used in equine medicine, 668*t*
  endotoxaemia treatment and, 506
  wound healing and, 621

Vehicular access, at equine hospital, 158
Veins
  collection of blood and injection into other, 12
Venipuncture
  disinfection prior to, 10–11
  minimisation of, in critically ill horses and prevention of thrombophlebitis, 397
Venous blood gas analysis, 419–420
Venous blood gas collection, 462
Ventilation-perfusion mismatching, 478
  respiratory function testing and, 462
Ventilator-associated pneumonia, 479
Ventilators
  adjustment of, to foal, 127–128
  foals connected to, 126–127
Ventilatory support, goals of, 473
Ventral abdominal ultrasound, of a mare, *18*
Ventral thorax, extensive wound to, *614*
Ventricle, left, M-mode of, *54*
Ventricular ectopic depolarisations, 439–440
Ventricular ectopy, in postsurgical colic horse, *421*
Ventricular fibrillation
  use of, on neonatal foal, *124*
  ventricular rhythm progressing to, in a horse, *5*
Ventricular premature beats, effect of, on left ventricular (LV) pressure, *424*
Ventricular premature depolarisations, 436–437
Ventricular rhythm, progression of, to ventricular fibrillation in horse, *5*
Ventricular septal defect, adult Standardbred horse with, *424*
Ventricular tachycardia, 436
  base-apex electrocardiograms from horse exhibiting different types of, *436*
  defined, 437
  treatment of, 438–439
    bretylium tosylate, 439
    general guidelines for, 439
    lidocaine (lignocaine), 438
    magnesium sulphate, 439
    phenytoin, 439
    procainamide, 438
    propafenone, 438–439
    propranolol, 439
    quinidine, 438
  uniform, *423*
    in horse with oleander toxicity, *420*
Verapamil, approximate doses used in equine medicine, 668*t*
Vertical mattress suture pattern, *116*, 616
  with stents, *117*
  technique, advantages/disadvantages with, 116
Vesicular stomatitis, nosocomial importance of, 190*t*
Veterinary Clinics of North America: Equine Practice, 182
Veterinary hospital, protection of phrase and RCVS practice standards, 147
Veterinary personnel, preventing zoonotic disease in, 196
Veterinary-specific PACS suppliers, 176 (box 3.3)
Vibration, of chest wall, 641
Vicristine, approximate doses used in equine medicine, 668*t*
Video endoscopes, 179
Viel, L., 468
Viewing window, for radiography room, at hospital, 165
VILI, types of, 479
Vinegar, approximate doses used in equine medicine, 668*t*
Visceral pain, 326–329
  abdominal, other causes for, 328
  acupuncture for, 328
  analgesia of colic patient, 326–327
  constant rate infusions, 327–328
  eqpidural analgesia and anaesthesia for, 328–329
  thoracic, 329
Vision, assessing, 557–558
Visitors car park, at equine hospital, 148, *149*
Vital HN, 277, 278*t*
Vitamin A, 274
Vitamin analysis, in hospitalised adult horse, 266–267
Vitamin C, approximate doses used in equine medicine, 668*t*
Vitamin D, 274
  deficiency of, hepatic insufficiency and, 528
Vitamin D intoxication, renal insufficiency and, 534
Vitamin E, 274
  hepatic insufficiency and supplementation with, 528
Vitamin K
  approximate doses used in equine medicine, 668*t*
  deficiency of, 404
    liver failure and, 528
  hypocoagulable states in horses managed with, 413
Vitamin K antagonists, hypercoagulable states in horses managed with, 411
Vitamin requirements, for neonatal foals, 299
Vitamins
  hepatic disease and dietary supplementation with, 528
  for hospitalised adult horse, 274–275
  in parenteral solutions, 289
Vitamin supplements, adding to PN mixture, 292
Vita Mix Blender Super 5000, 282
Volume controlled ventilation, 475–476
Volume to be infused button, on electronic infusion pumps, 37, 38, 38 (box 1.18)
Voluntary feeding
  enteral nutrition in hospitalised horse and return to, 284
  parenteral nutrition in hospitalised adult horse and return to, 295
Volutrauma, 479, 480
von Willebrand factor, hepatic insufficiency and, 522
von Willebrand's disease, 405
Voriconazole, 353
  approximate doses used in equine medicine, 668*t*
  fungal keratitis treatment and, 631, 632
  spectrum of activity for, 353*t*
VPDs. *See* Ventricular premature depolarisations
VRE. *See* Vancomycin-resistant *Enterococcus*
"V-shaped" flap or wound
  closing, *118*
  converting to "Y-shaped" deficit, *118*
VT. *See* Ventricular tachycardia

W
Water, for hospitalised adult horse, 269
Waterbeds, for recumbent foals, 563
"Water buffet," 399
Weaning
  from mechanical ventilation, 479
  neonatal foals from mechanical ventilation, 128
Weanlings
  normal biochemistry values for, 671*t*
  normal electrolyte concentrations for, 678*t*
  normal haemotology values for, 671*t*
Webcam connection, between nurses' base and foal or adult critical care, and isolation stalls, 153
Webcams, for hospital grounds, 148
Weight average molecular weight, 371
Weight loss, hepatic failure and, 527
Western blot testing, 559
West Nile virus encephalitis, 560
  corticosteroids and, 568

Wet-to-dry adherent dressings, 104
Wheat bran, nutrient composition of, 265*t*
Wheezes, 457
White blood cells, cerebrospinal fluid analysis and, 560
WHO. *See* World Health Organization
Whole blood transfusion, 376–377
  hypocoagulable states in horses managed with, 412
WHONET software, 185
Wickler, S. J., 649
Windows
  for operating theatre in hospital, 155
  for x-ray rooms, 177
"Wind up," 331–332
"Wobbler syndrome," 618
World Health Organization, 181
Wound cleaning, tarsal sheath and, *596*
Wound closure
  primary or healing by second intention, 616
  treatment after, 616
Wound dressings, 104
Wound exploration, 611
Wound healing, electrotherapy and, 642
Wound-induced profuse bleeding, coagulopathies due to, 405
Wound infection, monitoring surgical incisions and, *596*
Wound lavage, 611
  treatment after, 616
Wound management in hospitalised horses, 609–622
  bandaging, 617–618
    of surgical wounds, 617
    of traumatic wounds, 617–618
  clipping and aseptic preparation of skin, 611, *612*
  drains, 618–619
  initial assessment and treatment, 611, 613–616
    debridement, 613
    exploration, 611
    involvement of synovial structure, 615–616
    joint involvement and, 613
    small lacerations and puncture wounds of distal limb, 615
    upper limb, body and head wounds, 613–614
    wound healing, 613
    wound lavage, 611
  problems and complications, 616–617
    bony involvement, 616–617
    nonhealing wounds, 617
    prognosis, 617
    sole of hoof and frog puncture wounds, 617
    tendon involvement, 616
  topical treatments and dressings, 619–622
    beta aminopropionitrile, 621
    biological dressings, 620–621
    chitin, 621
    cyanoacrylate adhesive, 621
    growth factors and growth hormone, 620
    hydrogel dressings, 621
    topical antimicrobial and antiseptic treatments, 620
    vedaprofen, 621
  wound closure, 616
    treatment after debridement, lavage and closure, 616
Wounds, limb bandaging and healing of, 101, *103*

X
Xanthochromia, 560
Xenon light sources, for endoscopic equipment, 179
X-ray machine, maximum output of, 177
X-ray rooms, requirements for, 177
X-ray system, at equine hospital, 165
X-ray units
  ceiling-mounted, at equine hospital, 166
  mobile, at equine hospital, 166
Xylazine, 238, 245, 565
  approximate doses used in equine medicine, 668*t*
  colic pain and use of, 326
  equine sedation and use of, 312, 313, 313*t*
  examination per rectum and use of, 9
  foetal heart rate and, 319
  hormonal secretion in mares and, 320
  intraocular pressure and, 251
  neurological disease and use of, 317
  total intravenous anaesthesia and, 252

Y
Yearlings
  normal biochemistry values for, 671*t*
  normal electrolyte concentrations for, 678*t*
  normal haemotology values for, 671*t*
Yohimbine
  approximate doses used in equine medicine, 668*t*
  treatment of ileus and, 502
Yohimbine hydrochloride, 502
Y-piece extension set, for fluid administration, 36
y-port, for parenteral administration, checking for potential drug interactions and, 293
"Y-shaped" deficit, converting "V-shaped flap or wound to, *118*

Z
Zinc oxide tape "butterfly," catheter sutured to skin of foal and, 136, *136*
Zinc supplementation, liver disease and, 528
Zone of inhibition, 339
Zoonotic diseases, in hospitalised horses, 196

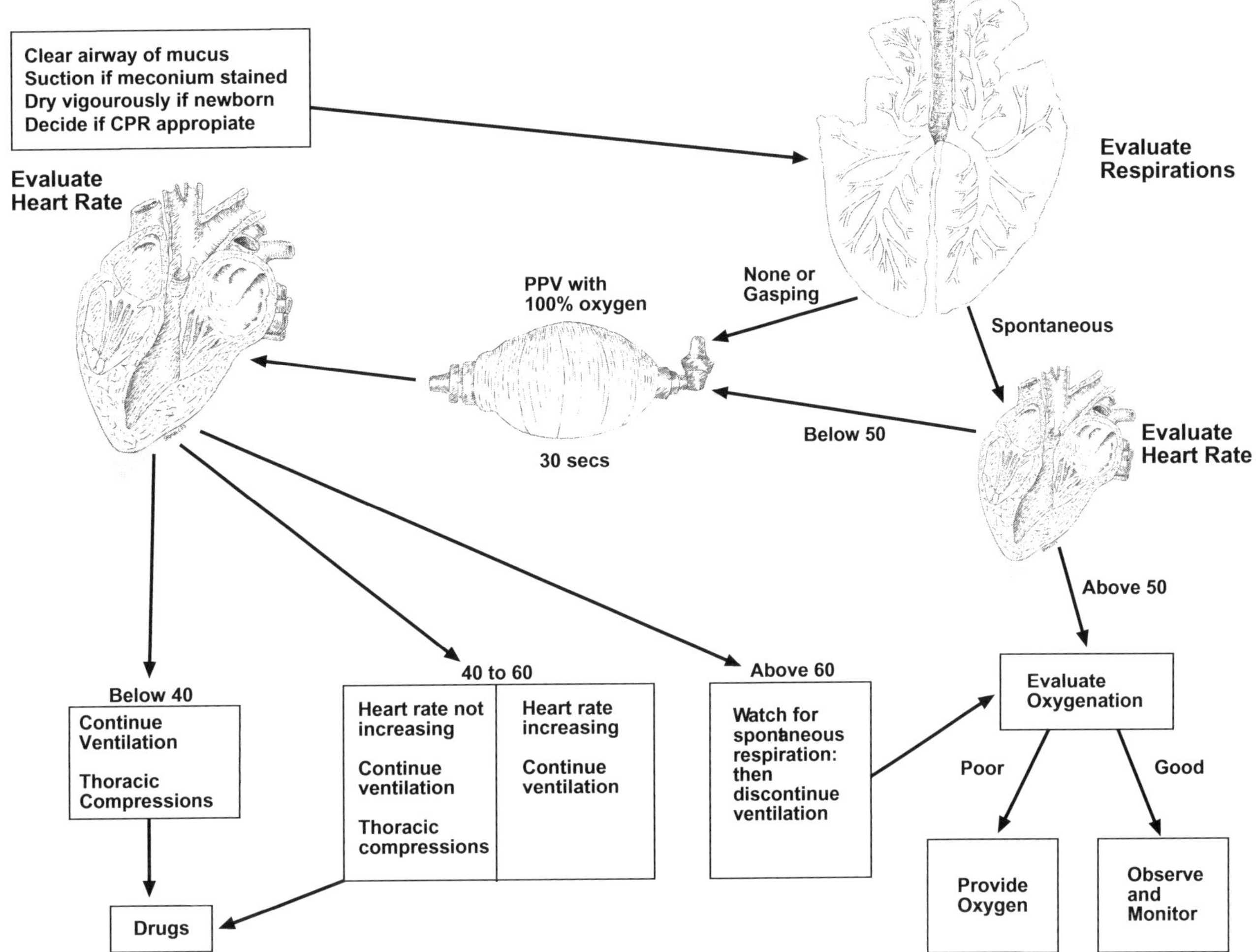

Flowchart for cardiopulmonary resuscitation (CPR) in the newborn foal (see Chapter 2.2).

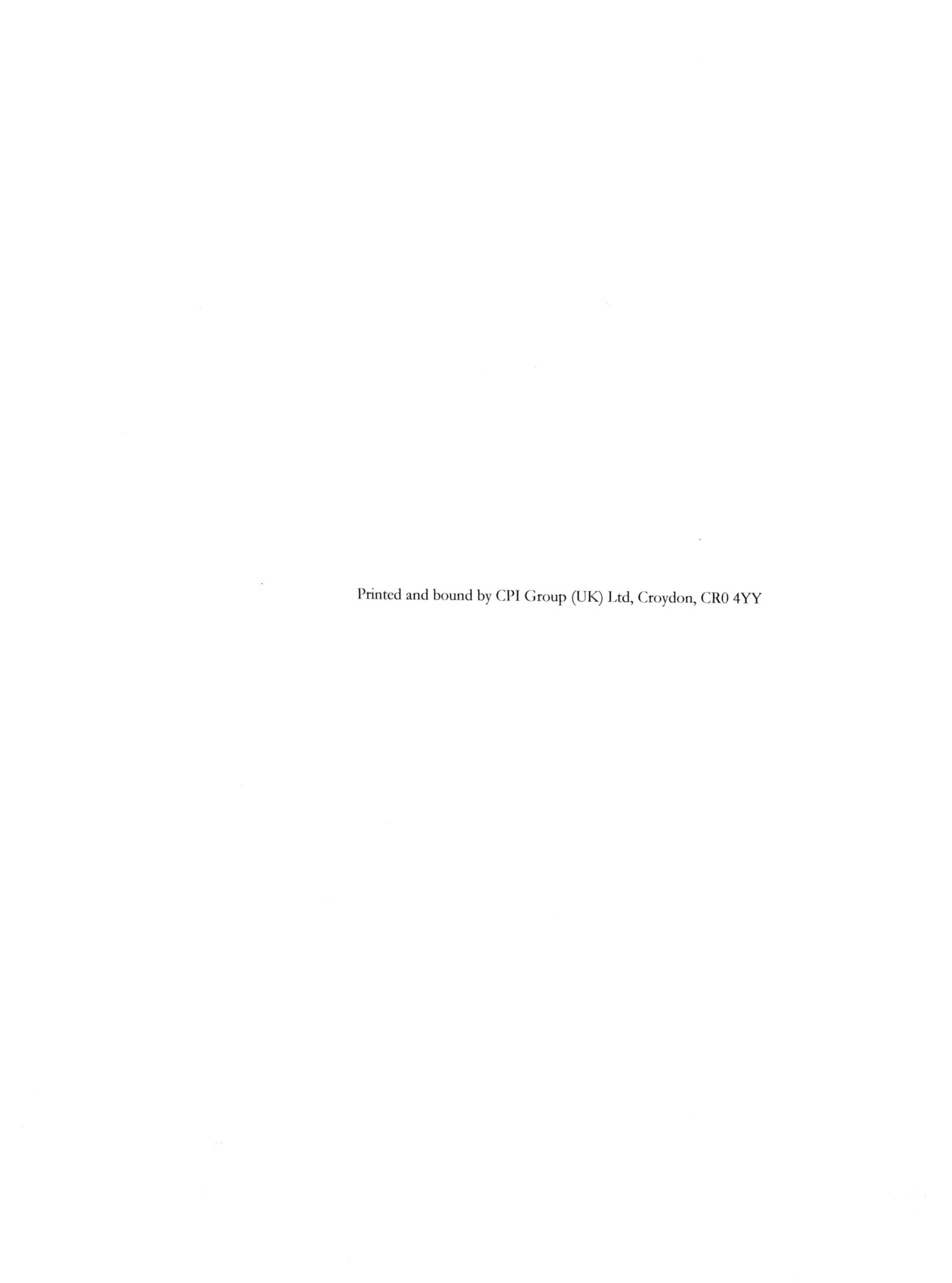

Printed and bound by CPI Group (UK) Ltd, Croydon, CR0 4YY